SECOND EDITION

CRUSH STEP 1

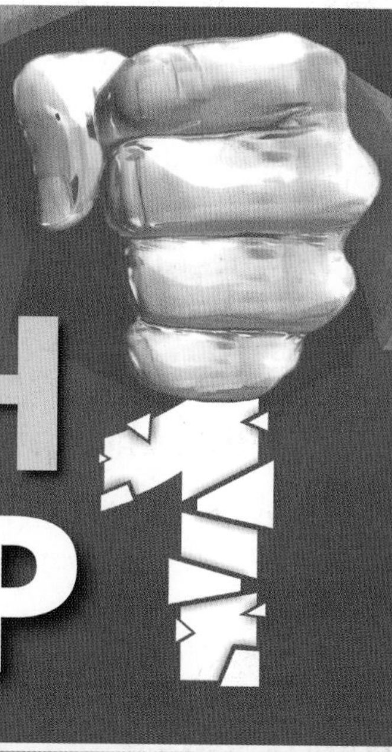

The Ultimate USMLE Step 1 Review

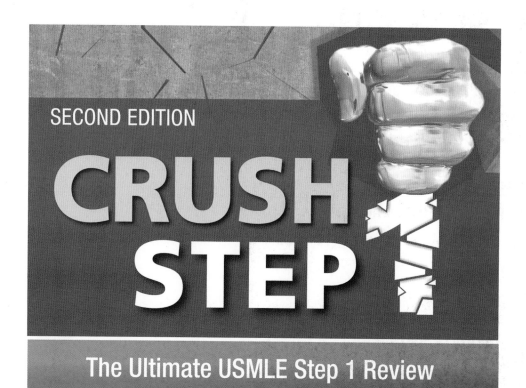

SECOND EDITION

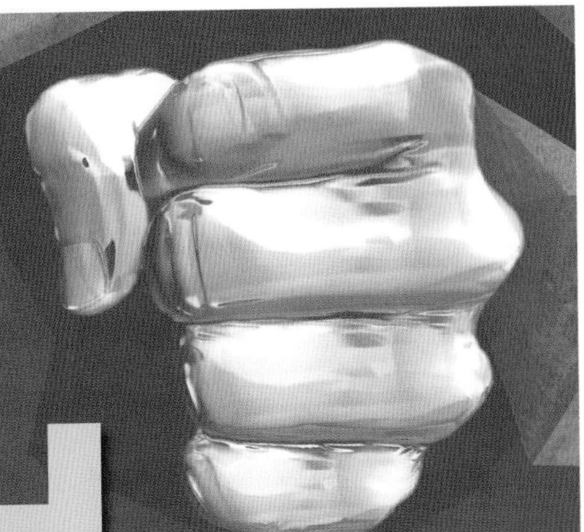

CRUSH STEP 1

The Ultimate USMLE Step 1 Review

Theodore X. O'Connell, MD
Program Director, Family Medicine Residency Program
Kaiser Permanente Napa-Solano, California
Assistant Clinical Professor, Department of Family and Community Medicine
University of California, San Francisco School of Medicine
San Francisco, California

Ryan A. Pedigo, MD
Director, Undergraduate Medical Education, Department of Emergency Medicine
Harbor-UCLA Medical Center
Assistant Professor of Emergency Medicine
David Geffen School of Medicine at UCLA, Los Angeles, California

Thomas E. Blair, MD
Resident Physician, Emergency Medicine
Harbor-UCLA Medical Center, Los Angeles, California

ELSEVIER

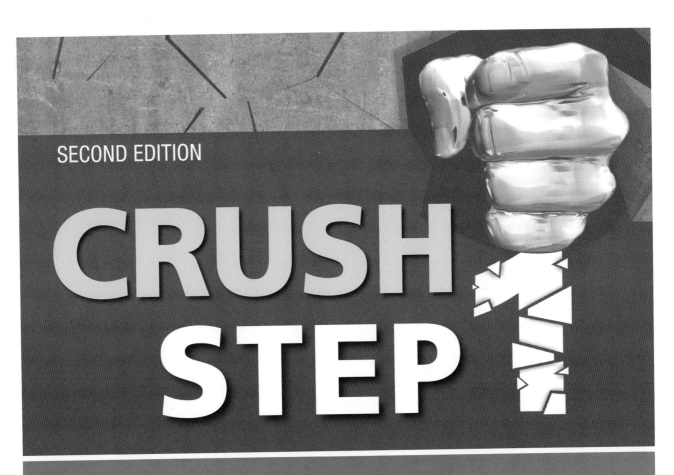

ELSEVIER

1600 John F. Kennedy Blvd.
Ste 1800
Philadelphia, PA 19103-2899

CRUSH STEP 1: THE ULTIMATE USMLE STEP 1 REVIEW, 2nd ed ISBN: 978-0-323-48163-2

Library of Congress Cataloging-in-Publication Data
Names: O'Connell, Theodore X., author. | Pedigo, Ryan A., author. | Blair, Thomas E. (Edward), 1984- author.
Title: Crush step 1 : the ultimate USMLE step 1 review guide / Theodore X. O'Connell, Ryan A. Pedigo, Thomas E. Blair.
Description: Second edition. | Philadelphia, PA : Elsevier, 2017. | Includes bibliographical references and index.
Identifiers: LCCN 2017026444 | ISBN 9780323481632 (pbk. : alk. paper)
Subjects: | MESH: Clinical Medicine | Examination Questions
Classification: LCC RC58 | NLM WB 18.2 | DDC 616.0076--dc23 LC record available at https://lccn.loc.gov/2017026444

Content Strategist: James Merritt
Content Development Specialist: Angie Breckon
Publishing Services Manager: Patricia Tannian
Project Manager: Ted Rodgers
Design Direction: Renee Duenow

Printed in China

Last digit is the print number: 9 8 7 6 5 4 3 2

FACULTY REVIEW BOARD

Nichole Bosson, MD, MPH, FAEMS
Assistant Medical Director
Los Angeles County EMS Agency
Adjunct Faculty
Department of Emergency Medicine
Harbor-UCLA Medical Center
Assistant Professor of Clinical Medicine
David Geffen School of Medicine at UCLA
Los Angeles, California

Samuel O. Clarke, MD, MAS, FACEP
Assistant Professor
Department of Emergency Medicine
UC Davis Health System
Sacramento, California

STUDENT REVIEW BOARD

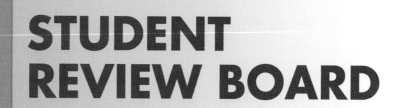

CONTRIBUTORS

Will Babbitt, MD
Attending Pediatrician
Kaiser Permanente
Daly City, California

John H. Baird, MD
Fellow Physician
Divisions of Hematology and Medical Oncology
Stanford University
Stanford, California

Brenton Bauer, MD
Fellow Physician
Division of Cardiology
Ronald Reagan UCLA Medical Center
Los Angeles, California

Thomas E. Blair, MD
Resident Physician
Emergency Medicine
Harbor-UCLA Medical Center
Los Angeles, California

Manuel Celedon, MD
VA Greater Los Angeles Healthcare System
Health Sciences Assistant Clinical Professor of Emergency Medicine
David Geffen School of Medicine at UCLA
Los Angeles, California

Edwin Li
Resident Physician
Department of Pediatrics
Stanford University
Stanford, California

Masood Memarzadeh, MD
Resident Physician
Department of Anesthesia and Perioperative Care
University of California
San Francisco, California

Theodore X. O'Connell, MD
Program Director, Family Medicine Residency Program
Kaiser Permanente Napa-Solano, California
Assistant Clinical Professor, Department of Family and Community Medicine
University of California, San Francisco School of Medicine
San Francisco, California

Gwen Owens, MD/PhD Candidate
David Geffen School of Medicine at UCLA
California Institute of Technology
Los Angeles, California

Ryan A. Pedigo, MD
Director, Undergraduate Medical Education, Department of Emergency Medicine
Harbor-UCLA Medical Center
Assistant Professor of Emergency Medicine
David Geffen School of Medicine at UCLA
Los Angeles, California

Tiffany Pedigo, MD
Fellow Physician
Division of Critical Care Medicine
Children's Hospital Los Angeles
Los Angeles, California

Tina Roosta Storage, MD
Fellow Physician
Division of Digestive Diseases
Ronald Reagan UCLA Medical Center
Los Angeles, California

Lauren Sanchez, MD
Fellow Physician
Division of Pediatric Allergy, Immunology, and Bone Marrow Transplantation
University of California, San Francisco
San Francisco, California

Manpreet Singh, MD
Faculty, Department of Emergency Medicine, Harbor-UCLA Medical Center
Assistant Professor of Emergency Medicine
David Geffen School of Medicine at UCLA
Los Angeles, California

Natalie Villa
Resident Physician
Division of Dermatology
UCLA Medical Center
Los Angeles, California

Andrew Yu, MD
Resident Physician
Department of Neurology
Brigham and Women's Hospital
Boston, Massachusetts

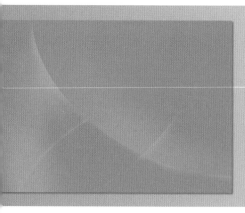

INTRODUCTION

The first edition of *Crush Step 1* was conceptualized, designed, and created by medical students, then edited by experts in their field, with the goal of being the best resource on the market for truly understanding the material that is tested on the USMLE Step 1. Our research showed that students were frustrated because review books were either too in-depth for the purposes of the test or too focused on memorization rather than understanding. We asked students like you before and after the test what they wish they would have had during their own preparation, and we sought to provide that for future students. This book has always been driven by what those preparing for the USMLE Step 1 want, and this concept has not changed as we took your feedback into account for this edition. The response to the first edition has been overwhelming, and we are truly privileged to be able to bring you a second edition of this text and take into account all of your feedback and requests.

When students understand the concepts of how anatomy, physiology, pathology, and pharmacology interact with one another, medicine becomes less about memorization and more about truly learning how the body works – and doesn't work! The second edition builds on the careful analysis and planning that went into creating the first edition, adding improved explanations and new information important for the USMLE Step 1 based on your feedback.

We sincerely hope you enjoy *Crush Step 1*. Continued feedback is always important to us. This is your book, and we want to make sure everything is clear, precise, and up to date and serves your needs. Although we have a rigorous editing process, it is possible that errors occur within the text. Please help us with our goal to make this text the best resource available for medical students by submitting any comments, suggestions, or corrections to our Facebook group https://www.facebook.com/CrushStep1/ where you can post, message the authors, and see the most up-to-date errata. If you do not use Facebook, you can also e-mail us at CrushStepOne@gmail.com.

Thanks again, and best of luck to you on your journey toward becoming an outstanding physician.

Sincerely,
The Crush Step 1 Team

CONTENTS

1 BIOSTATISTICS

Thomas E. Blair

MEAN, MEDIAN, AND MODE

- **Sample value set:** 1, 1, 2, 4, 5, 7, 7, 25, where $n = 8$
- **Mean:** The average of a sample. It is calculated by adding all values, then dividing by the number of values (n). In the sample set just given, $(1 + 1 + 2 + 4 + 5 + 7 + 7 + 25)/8 = 6.5$. The mean is sensitive to extreme values.
- **Median:** The middle value of a sample. It is equivalent to the 50th percentile such that half the sample values are above and half are below. It is identified by arranging the values in ascending order, then finding the middle-most number. If n is odd, the median is the $[(n + 1)/2]$th largest observation. If n is even, the median is the average of the $(n/2)$th and the $(n/2 + 1)$th largest observations. In this example, there is an even number of values, so the median is the average of the two middle-most numbers; that is, for 1, 1, 2, 4, 5, 7, 7, 25, the median = $(4 + 5)/2 = 4.5$. An advantage of the median is that it is not sensitive to extreme values. You may notice that in this sample the mean is greater than the median. This indicates that the distribution has a positive skew (see later discussion).
- **Mode:** The most frequently occurring value in a sample. In this example, both 1 and 7 are modes because they both appear twice. Therefore this data set can be said to be bimodal.
- **Standard deviation (SD):** A measure of the spread and variability of a data set, calculated as the square root of the variance. It represents the average deviation from the mean. The closer the values remain to the mean, the smaller the SD (Fig. 1.1). The concept, not the mathematics, may be tested on Step 1.
  - *Example:* Normal body temperature will have a small SD because an individual's anterior and posterior hypothalamus maintains temperature homeostasis within a very limited range. Blood sugars, on the other hand, will have a larger SD because glycemic loads change throughout the day.

> Mean: average value
> Median: middle value
> Mode: most frequent value

> Standard deviation represents the average deviation from the mean.

DEFINITIONS

- **Incidence:** The number of **new** cases of a disease in a population over a specific period (longitudinal).
- **Prevalence:** The total number of people in a population affected by a condition at one point (cross-sectional).
- **Duration** relates incidence to prevalence.
  - *Example:* Upper respiratory infections (URIs) have a high annual incidence, occurring often during winter months, but a comparatively low prevalence, because most URIs resolve quickly. Diabetes has a relatively low incidence but high prevalence, because a patient who has diabetes generally has it for life.
- **Normal distribution:** Also known as a Gaussian distribution or bell-shaped curve. A probability function in which values are symmetrically distributed around a central value, and the **mean, median, and mode are equal.** In a normal distribution, 1 SD accounts for 68% of all values, 2 SDs account for 95% of all values, and 3 SDs account for 99.7% of all values—the **68-95-99 rule** (Fig. 1.2). The area under the curve is 1 (100%).

> In a normal distribution, mean = median = mode.

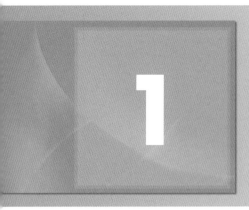

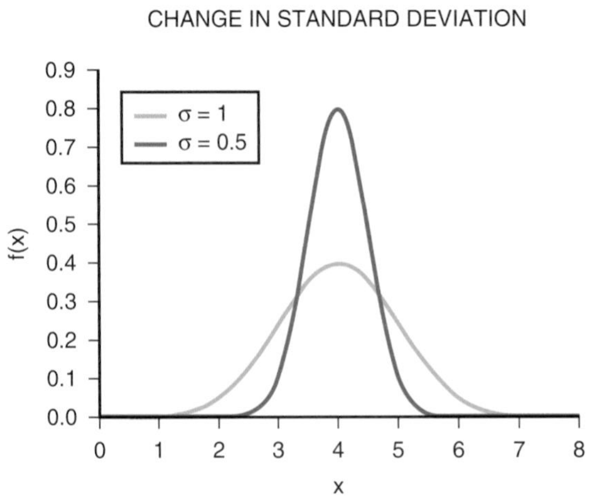

Fig. 1.1 Data sets with the same mean but different standard deviations. The wider curve has a larger standard deviation than the taller curve.

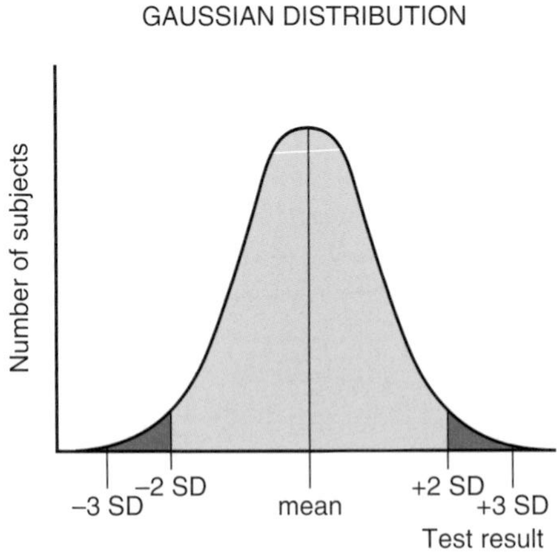

Fig. 1.2 In a normal distribution, 1 standard deviation (SD) accounts for 68% of all values, 2 SDs account for 95% of all values, and 3 SDs account for 99% of all values. *(From Marshall WJ, Bangert SK.* Clinical Chemistry. *6th ed. Philadelphia: Elsevier; 2008.)*

- *Example:* The intelligence quotient (IQ) test is constructed to follow a normal distribution with a mean of 100 and SD of 15. That means that 95% of the population (2 SDs) will have an IQ between 70 and 130. Of clinical import, intellectual disability is defined as an IQ of < 70.

- **Bimodal distribution:** A distribution with two modes.
  - *Example:* The incidence of Crohn's disease displays a bimodal distribution with the first peak between 15 and 30 years of age and the second peak between 60 and 80 years of age.
- **Negative skew:** An asymmetric distribution in which a tail on the left indicates that **mean < median < mode.** The tail is due to outliers on the left side of the curve.
  - *Example:* A graphic representation of age at death would show a negative skew, with most people clustered at the right end of the distribution and relatively few dying at a younger age (Fig. 1.3A).
- **Positive skew:** An asymmetric distribution in which a tail on the right side indicates that **mean > median > mode.** The tail is due to outliers on the right side of the curve.
  - *Example:* A graphic representation of age at initiation of smoking would display positive skew. Most people would be clustered around their late teens, but a small number of middle-aged and older adults, who initiated smoking later in life, create a positive tail (Fig. 1.3B).

Negative skew: tail on left

Positive skew: tail on right

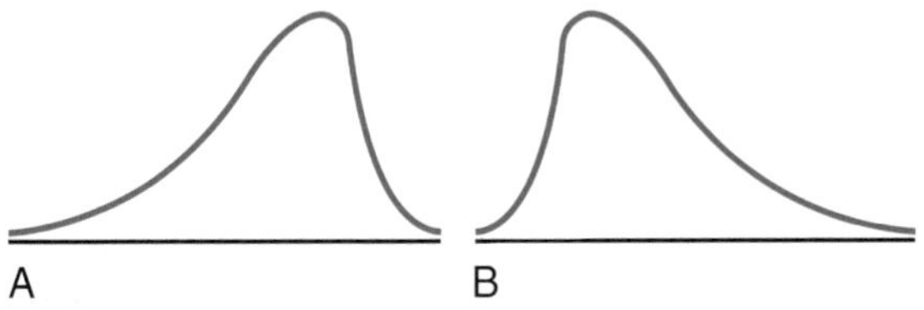

Fig. 1.3 A, Negative skew. **B,** Positive skew. *(From Jekel JF, Katz DL, Wild JG, Elmore DMG.* Epidemiology, Biostatistics, and Preventive Medicine. *3rd ed. Philadelphia: Elsevier; 2007.)*

Statistics for Diagnostic Tests

- **True positive (TP):** Disease is present and diagnostic test is positive (a correct result).
- **True negative (TN):** Disease is absent and diagnostic test is negative (a correct result).
- **False positive (FP):** Disease is absent and diagnostic test is positive (an incorrect result).
- **False negative (FN):** Disease is present and diagnostic test is negative (an incorrect result).
- **2 × 2 Table:** Consider drawing a 2 × 2 table whenever faced with a biostatistics question. To consistently put the table in the right order, try using the mnemonic "truth over test results"; that is, the truth is more important than the test. Intuitively, "yes" precedes "no" on both axes (Table 1.1).

Table 1.1 Example of a 2 × 2 Test Result for Calculating Biostatistics

		THE "TRUTH"	
		YES	**NO**
TEST RESULTS	**Yes**	**A** True +	**B** False +
	No	**C** False –	**D** True –

SN-N-OUT: For a test that is **S**e**N**sitive, a **N**egative result rules **OUT** the disease

- **Prevalence:** This is defined as (total number of people with disease)/(total number of people studied) or, from the 2 × 2 table, (TP + FN)/(TP + TN + FP + FN). Note that prevalence varies by population. For example, Chagas disease has a higher prevalence in South America than it does in the United States.
- **Sensitivity:** Given the disease is present, the probability that the test will be positive. In other words, ask yourself, "Of all the people who actually have this disease, how many will be detected as positive by this test?" It is defined as TP/(TP + FN) or TP/(total number of people with disease). Sensitive tests are useful for screening because there are few false negatives; nearly everyone who has the disease is detected as positive. Therefore, if you test negative with this test, it essentially rules out the disease. Consider the mnemonic **SN-N-OUT**—for a test that is **S**e**N**sitive, a **N**egative result rules **OUT** the disease. Keep in mind that the equation for sensitivity says nothing about false positives. You may have detected everyone with the disease as positive (high sensitivity), but you may have also told many who do not have the disease that they tested positive (FPs); see example 2.
  - *Example 1:* An HIV test with 98% sensitivity means that, when a disease is present, it will be detected 98% of the time.
  - *Example 2:* Consider a test that was positive 100% of the time regardless of the presence or absence of disease. It would technically have 100% sensitivity because it would be positive in all the patients with disease (but would be clinically useless because it would be positive in all the patients without disease too). Therefore sensitivity is not the whole picture when it comes to test characteristics; specificity is also important.

SP-P-IN: For a test that is **SP**ecific, a **P**ositive result rules **IN** the disease

- **Specificity:** Given the disease is absent, the probability that the test will be negative. In other words, ask yourself the question, "Of all the people who do not have this disease, how many will be correctly identified as negative by this test?" It is defined as TN/(TN + FP) or TN/(total number of people without disease). Tests with high specificity are useful to confirm a diagnosis because there are few false positives. Because a highly specific test can identify correctly most patients who do not have the disease, if you see a positive result, it likely rules in the disease. Consider the mnemonic **SP-P-IN**—for a test that is **SP**ecific, a **P**ositive result rules **IN** the disease.
  - *Example:* An HIV test with 98% specificity means that, when a disease is absent, the test will be negative 98% of the time.

In general, there is a tradeoff between sensitivity and specificity. For example, changing the cutoff value for an "elevated" serum lipase level will change the test's ability to detect a sick population with acute pancreatitis. Raising the cutoff value will increase the specificity (fewer false positives) but will also decrease the sensitivity (more false negatives) (Fig. 1.4). As another example, if the random blood sugar

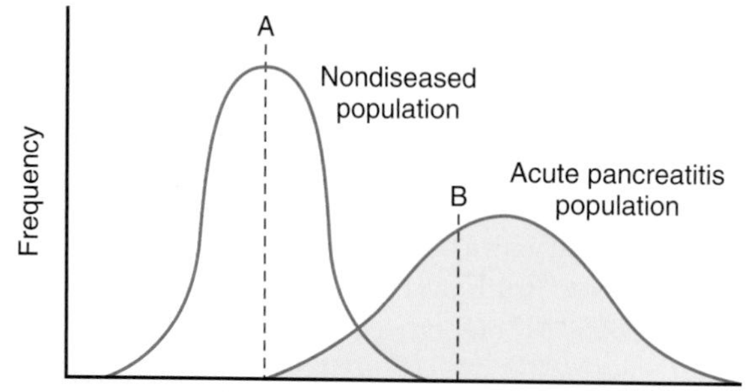

Fig. 1.4 Increasing the diagnostic cutoff (moving it to the right) will make the test more specific but less sensitive. In this example, if the cutoff point is at A, then the test will be 100% sensitive because all patients with acute pancreatitis will be detected. At cutoff A, however, the test is very nonspecific because many healthy people will be incorrectly classified as having acute pancreatitis. If the cutoff point is moved to B, the test will be 100% specific because all positive tests will be true positives. At cutoff point B, however, the test is not sensitive (many cases of acute pancreatitis will be missed). *(From Jekel JF, Katz DL, Wild JG, Elmore DMG.* Epidemiology, Biostatistics, and Preventive Medicine. *3rd ed. Philadelphia: Elsevier; 2007.)*

Table 1.2 Example of a 2 × 2 Table for Calculating Risk or Odds

		OUTCOME	
		YES	**NO**
Exposure	**Yes**	**A**	**B**
	No	**C**	**D**

cutoff for the diagnosis of diabetes were moved from 200 mg/dL to 400 mg/dL, then the test would be very specific because anyone with a blood sugar greater than 400 mg/dL very likely has diabetes (very few false positives). However, it would be very insensitive because people with diabetes with random blood sugar readings of 300 mg/dL would have false negatives.

Positive Predictive Value (PPV). Given the test is positive, the probability that the disease is present. PPV = TP/(TP + FP) or TP/(total number of positive tests). For example, if a computed tomography (CT) scan has 98% positive predictive value for appendicitis, then a patient with a positive CT scan will truly have appendicitis 98% of the time.

Increasing the diagnostic cutoff will make a test more specific but less sensitive.

Negative Predictive Value (NPV). Given the test is negative, the probability that the disease is absent. NPV = TN/(TN + FN) or TN/(total number of negative tests). For example, if an HIV test has 98% NPV, then given a negative test, the patient will truly be HIV negative 98% of the time.

- Once the result of a diagnostic test is known, PPV and NPV are extremely useful to clinicians. For example, if a diagnostic test for a pulmonary embolism (PE) is positive, PPV answers the clinician's question: "Given this positive result, what is the actual probability my patient has a PE?" Unfortunately for the clinician, PPV and NPV vary depending on the prevalence of the disease in a population. They must be used with caution if your patient population is not identical to the one studied. Sensitivity (and specificity), on the other hand, will not be affected because the ratio of TP/(total number of people with disease) will not change for a given test, but the ratio of TP/(total number of positive tests) will vary because an area with higher prevalence will have a higher number of positive tests.

Sens = TP/(TP + FN)
Spec = TN/(TN + FP)
PPV = TP/(TP + FP)
NPV = TN/(TN + FN)

Calculations of Risk Measures

2 × 2 Table. You can also draw a 2 × 2 table whenever faced with calculating risk or odds. To remember how to set up the table, think "outcome over exposure" (i.e., the outcome is more important than the exposure). Intuitively, "yes" precedes "no" on both axes. Note that the exposure can be "good," such as a beneficial treatment, or "bad," such as a carcinogen or harmful medication. A 2 × 2 table for exposure can be set up similar to a 2 × 2 table for diagnostic tests, where the exposure can refer to a known characteristic, an observed exposure, or an assigned treatment (Table 1.2).

The incidence (or prevalence in the setting of cross-sectional studies) is calculated for each group from the 2 × 2 table. The probability (p) that the event will occur in the exposed group is given by **risk in exposed = a/(a + b),** and in the unexposed (control) group it is given by **risk in unexposed = c/(c + d).**

- *Example:* One hundred patients are treated with a statin and five suffer a myocardial infarction (MI). What is the incidence of MI in the group treated with ("exposed to") a statin?
  - *Solution:* a/(a + b) = 5/100 = 0.05 = 5%.
- **Risk Difference (RD):** The difference between the two groups. RD = risk in exposed – risk in unexposed, or vice versa. There are several ways to express the risk difference.
- **Absolute risk reduction (ARR):** The reduction in incidence associated with a treatment. ARR = risk in control group – risk in treatment group.
  - *Example:* In one study, 5% of patients on a statin suffered an MI, whereas 9% of those on placebo suffered an MI. What is the ARR of statins?
    - *Solution:* ARR = 9% – 5% = 4%. The use of statins in this population is associated with a 4% decrease in the number of MIs.
- **Attributable risk:** The increase in disease incidence associated with an exposure. Attributable risk = risk in exposed – risk in unexposed.
  - *Example:* In one study, 9% of patients exposed to asbestos developed bronchogenic carcinoma, and 2% of those without exposure developed bronchogenic carcinoma. What is the attributable risk of asbestos?
    - *Solution:* Attributable risk = 9% – 2% = 7%; that is, asbestos exposure increased the incidence of bronchogenic carcinomas by 7%.
- **Number needed to treat (NNT):** The number of patients required to receive an intervention before an adverse outcome is prevented (e.g., death, MI). **NNT = 1/ARR.** The opposite concept is **number needed to harm (NNH),** used for interventions or exposures that may be detrimental (e.g., radiation exposure). **NNH = 1/attributable risk.**
  - *Example:* In one study, the ARR of statin therapy is calculated at 4%. What is the NNT?
    - *Solution:* NNT = 1/.04 = 25. Twenty-five patients would need to be treated with statins to prevent one MI.
- **Relative risk (RR, risk ratio):** The ratio of incidence in the two groups. **RR = risk in exposed/risk in unexposed.** For a negative outcome, a ratio greater than 1 indicates a harmful treatment/exposure and a ratio less than 1 indicates a beneficial treatment/exposure, whereas a ratio of 1 is a null effect.
  - *Example:* In one study, 50% of diabetic patients developed heart disease, compared with 10% of a control population. What is the relative risk of diabetic patients developing heart disease?
    - *Solution:* RR = 0.5/0.1 = 5. Diabetic patients are 5 times more likely to develop heart disease than nondiabetic patients.
- **Relative risk reduction (RRR):** The percentage of diseases prevented by a treatment. **RRR = (risk in unexposed – risk in exposed)/risk in unexposed = ARR/baseline risk.** For harmful exposure, the equivalent concept is excess relative risk = (risk in exposed – risk in unexposed)/risk in unexposed.
  - *Example:* Five percent of patients on a statin suffered an MI, whereas 9% of those on placebo suffered an MI. What is the RRR of being on a statin?
    - *Solution:* RRR = (0.09 – 0.05)/0.09 = 0.44 = 44%. That is to say, in the statin group, the risk of MIs was reduced by 44% relative to those in the control group.
- **Odds:** The ratio of the probability of the outcome to the probability of not having the outcome. **Odds = $p/(1 - p)$.**
- **Odds ratio:** A comparison of event rates between exposed and unexposed groups, calculated using odds instead of probabilities. It is the **odds of an event in the exposed group divided by the odds of the event in an unexposed group.** In a 2 × 2 table, it is calculated by OR = (a/b)/(c/d) = ad/bc, thus cross-multiplication of the values in the 2 × 2 table. Odds ratios are somewhat unintuitive; however, one can simplify understanding by considering that OR > 1 implies increased likelihood of an event in the exposed group, OR < 1 implies decreased likelihood of an event in the exposed group, and OR = 1 implies no difference between the exposed group and the control group. **ORs are used instead of risk ratios in case-control studies** because the risk ratio cannot be calculated from the study data as a result of purposeful oversampling of cases in the study design. The **OR will approximate the relative risk if the outcome is rare.**

Risk in exposed = a/(a + b)

Risk in unexposed = c/(c + d)

ARR = control group risk – treatment group risk

Attributable risk = risk in exposed – risk in unexposed

NNT = 1/ARR

RR = Risk in exposed/risk in unexposed

RRR = ARR/risk in unexposed

Odds ratio = ad/bc

- *Example:* Investigators conduct a case-control study to evaluate the risk for lymphoma as a result of radiation exposure from medical imaging. One hundred people are selected with lymphoma, and 100 people without lymphoma are selected as controls. Five patients with lymphoma had prior radiation exposure, whereas only two patients without lymphoma had prior radiation exposure. Calculate the odds ratio.
  - *Solution:* First refer to the 2 × 2 table in Table 1.3. OR = (a/b)/(c/d) = ad/cb = 2.6. The odds of having lymphoma in those with radiation exposure is 2.6 times those of patients who never had significant radiation exposure.

TABLE 1.3 Example of a 2 × 2 Table for Odds Ratio

		OUTCOME	
		YES	**NO**
Exposure	**Yes**	**A** = 5	**B** = 2
	No	**C** = 95	**D** = 98

STATISTICAL TESTS AND SIGNIFICANCE

Reliability is a measure of the consistency of a test—that is, the likelihood that, on repetition, it will deliver the same results in the same situation. Reliability decreases as random error increases in a test. **Validity** is the ability of a test to measure what it is intended to measure. Reliability does not necessarily imply validity. For example, a test may reliably measure serum concentrations of vitamin D; however, this does not inherently mean it is a valid predictor of a disease such as osteoporosis.

Accuracy: ability to obtain "true results"

Precision: ability to replicate results

Interrater reliability reflects to what degree test results will vary depending on who is administering the test. For example, body temperature has good interrater reliability when a thermometer is used but poor interrater reliability when simple touch is used.

Accuracy: Analogous to validity and a measure of a test's ability to obtain "true" results (Fig. 1.5B).

Precision: Analogous to reliability and a measure of a test's ability to replicate results (Fig. 1.5C).

Categorical Data: Data with a fixed number of nominal categories, or data that have been grouped as such (e.g., race, gender, or living/dead).

Continuous Data: Data that can take any value within a range (e.g., height or weight).

Categorical data: nominal categories

Continuous data: can take any value within a range

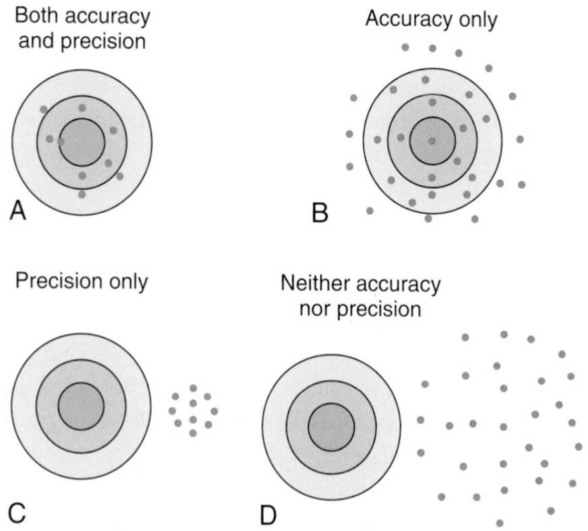

FIG. 1.5 Precision versus accuracy. (*From Jekel JF, Katz DL, Wild JG, Elmore DMG.* Epidemiology, Biostatistics, and Preventive Medicine. *3rd ed. Philadelphia: Elsevier; 2007.*)

Statistical Tests for Data Analysis

See Table 1.4 for a summary of statistical tests.

Two-Sample t-Test: Compares the means (continuous data) of two groups and determines whether there is a difference between the means based on a predetermined level of significance (α). For example, is there a significant difference in the average systolic blood pressure (continuous data) between men and women (categorical data)? As the name implies, only two groups can be compared in a two-sample t-test.

ANOVA (ANalysis Of VAriance): Serves a similar function to a t-test but can compare more than two groups. For example, is there a significant difference in the average systolic blood pressure (continuous data) of Asian Americans, European Americans, and African Americans (categorical data)?

Chi-Square Test: Compares proportions between groups of categorical data. There is no limit to the number of variables being compared. For example, is use of antibiotic x, y, or z (categorical) associated with a difference in survival from sepsis (categorical)?

Correlation Coefficient (*r*): The degree to which two continuous variables change together in a linear fashion. The correlation coefficient ranges from −1 to 1. A coefficient of 1 implies a perfect correlation, 0 implies no correlation, and −1 implies a perfect inverse correlation. For example, there is a positive correlation between height and forced expiratory volume (FEV), which increases as height increases. The square of the correlation coefficient is the coefficient of determination (R^2), which takes on a value between 0 and 1, and is a measure of how much the change in the dependent (y) variable is determined by the change in the independent (x) variable.

TABLE 1.4 Summary of Statistical Tests

NAME	NUMBER OF GROUPS	TYPE OF DATA	COMMENT
Two-sample t-test	2	Continuous	Compares 2 means
ANOVA	3 +	Continuous	Compares 3 + means
Chi-square test	2 +	Categorical	Compares 2 + groups
Correlation coefficient	2	Continuous	Measures covariance

ANOVA, Analysis of variance.

Causality

Although tempting, it is important to never assume that an association implies causation (i.e., "a" causes "b"). This simplification is often not the case because of the following:

- **Inverse causation:** "b" could actually be causing "a." One might conclude that immunosuppression predisposes people to lentivirus infection; however, the lentivirus (HIV) is actually the cause of the immunosuppression (AIDS).
- **Confounding:** A third variable "c" could be affecting both measured variables "a" and "b." For example, gingivitis may not cause diabetes, but lack of access to health care may predispose someone to both conditions.
- **Other sources of bias** (see later).

Correlation does not imply causation.

Hypothesis Testing

Null Hypothesis (H_0): The hypothesis of no association between two variables; for example, "a given treatment has no effect" or "two groups have identical risks despite different exposures." When constructing an experimental design, one attempts to statistically accept or reject the null hypothesis. The null hypothesis is paired with the **alternative hypothesis (H_a),** which takes the opposite assertion. For example, in a study comparing metronidazole to placebo for the treatment of giardiasis, the null hypothesis asserts that there would be no increased rate of resolution, whereas the alternative would assert that metronidazole hastens recovery (it does).

Alpha (Type 1) Error: Rejecting the null hypothesis when it is true, creating a "false alarm," or false positive. Mnemonic: Think **A** for **a**larm and type **1** because A is the **1**st letter of the alphabet. For example, a study finds the use of vitamin D improves recovery from a URI when, in fact, it does not. Alpha is sometimes called the level of significance because it is the predetermined level below which the differences are considered unlikely to be due to chance alone and the null hypothesis is rejected. Usually, the alpha is set at 0.05.

Beta (Type 2) Error: Failing to reject the null hypothesis when it is false, creating a "missed detection," or false negative. For example, a study finds that there is no significant decrease in mortality for patients who regularly exercise, when, in fact, there is.

Power: The ability of a test to reject the null hypothesis when it is false. Otherwise stated, the probability of avoiding type 2 error. Power = 1 − beta. Power is increased with increased difference between groups (i.e., effect size) and increased sample size.

P-Value: The probability of obtaining a test statistic (such as t-test or chi-square test statistic) as extreme or more extreme by chance alone if the null hypothesis is true and there is no bias. A P-value of less than 0.05 is usually said to be statistically significant.

Confidence Interval: A range of values around the point estimate such that, with repetition, the true value will be contained with a specified probability of 1 − α. Most often, the 95% confidence interval is reported, corresponding to an alpha level of 0.05. Increasing the sample size will narrow the confidence interval. A test in which the 95% confidence interval contains the "true" value is considered **accurate.** A test with a narrow confidence interval is considered **precise.**

If the 95% confidence interval does not contain the **null result, then there is a statistically significant difference in the groups.** The null result depends on the test. Rather than memorizing these results, think about which results would imply a difference and which would not. For ratios (RR, OR), the null value will be 1, whereas for differences (ARR), the null value will be 0.

> Alpha error: false alarm (false positive)
> Beta error: missed detection (false negative)

> Increasing sample size will narrow the confidence interval.

Clinical Study Design

- **Experimental study:** The investigator controls the exposure assignment. An example is randomized control trials.
- **Observational study:** The investigator observes the subjects without intervention. Cross-sectional, case-control, and cohort studies are observational studies.
  - **Cross-sectional study:** Subjects are enrolled without regard to exposure and disease status, which are then evaluated simultaneously—most often in the form of a survey. A cross-sectional study designed to determine the number of people with disease at a given time is a prevalence study.
    - *Example:* How many people in the United States have AIDS?
    - *Example:* How many people who have hyperlipidemia also currently have coronary artery disease?
  - **Case-control study:** Subjects are enrolled based on disease status, one group with disease (cases) and one group without (controls), and then exposure is assessed in the two groups. Case-control studies are retrospective studies where disease status is known before exposure assessment.
    - *Example:* Select subjects with and without mesothelioma and then ascertain the proportion of each group previously exposed to asbestos.
  - **Cohort study:** Subjects are enrolled based on exposure status, one cohort with the exposure and one without (controls), and followed over time for the disease of interest. Subjects must be free of the disease at enrollment. The study may be prospective (disease status is not known at the time of enrollment) or retrospective (chart review). The incidence in each group can be calculated. Relative risks are calculated for effect measure estimation.
    - *Example:* Does having elevated cholesterol increase your chances of having a myocardial infarction?
      - Prospective design: Patients with and without high cholesterol are enrolled and followed over time to see if they develop heart disease.
      - Retrospective design: Patients with and without high cholesterol are identified from 10-year-old hospital records. Their charts are then reviewed through the present date to determine whether they developed heart disease.
- **Randomized control trial (RCT):** Subjects without the outcome of interest are enrolled and then randomly assigned by the investigator to either the exposed or unexposed group. The groups are followed prospectively for the outcomes of interest. The advantage of randomization is that it makes the groups similar in characteristics other than the exposure of interest. Additionally, participants and/or researchers may be blinded to (kept unaware of) the treatment arm. If both are blinded, this is referred to as a "double-blinded" trial. Randomization makes systematic error (bias) random. It can fail to sufficiently control bias if the sample size is small or if there is differential loss to follow-up (selection bias). Clinical drug trials are the main example of RCTs. Randomized studies cannot

> Case-control studies select participants already diagnosed with the disease of interest.

> Use odds ratios in case-control studies.

> Cohort studies identify participants who have an exposure and follow them over time.

ethically be used to assess interventions thought to be harmful. For example, you cannot randomly assign someone to start smoking.
- *Example:* Are patients randomly assigned to receive statins less likely to have an MI than those receiving a placebo?

- **Crossover study:** A type of prospective study, usually an RCT but possibly a cohort study, in which each patient begins in either the control or treatment group and then crosses over to the other group. In this way, every patient serves as his or her own control.
  - *Example:* Patients are randomly assigned either placebo or a tricyclic antidepressant to treat their fibromyalgia. After a period receiving one treatment, the groups switch to see if the placebo group improves on the medication.
- **Meta-analysis:** A study that pools the results of several similar studies to increase statistical power by increasing the overall study size. If individual studies are of high quality, a meta-analysis can produce the most convincing level of evidence. However, a meta-analysis cannot compensate for poor research—"garbage in equals garbage out."

CLINICAL TRIALS

- **Phase I:** The first stage of testing in human subjects. A small group of **healthy** volunteers is given a medication to determine **safety, pharmacodynamics, and pharmacokinetics** of the medication.
- **Phase II:** In this stage, a slightly larger group of patients with the target condition is given the drug to determine **efficacy, optimal dosing, and side effects.** Many drugs fail in phase II because they are determined not to work as planned.
- **Phase III:** Large randomized controlled trials to determine efficacy of a drug compared with placebo or a "gold standard." Phase III trials must prove both **safety** and **efficacy** of a drug for it to be approved by the U.S. Food and Drug Administration (FDA).

Bias

Bias can turn a good experiment bad and comes in many flavors that you will have to recognize in Step 1. The best way to avoid bias is a well-designed, randomized, double-blind, controlled trial. However, these trials may be unethical, impractical, or even impossible to perform in some cases.

- **Confounding**: Another variable, related to both exposure and outcome, is unevenly distributed between groups and distorts the association of interest.
  - *Example:* A study finds that drinking coffee is associated with lung cancer because the study fails to recognize that coffee drinkers are also more likely to be smokers.
    - *Solution:* Matching is one solution, which distributes confounders evenly between groups.
- **Selection bias**: Groups are not similar at baseline because of nonrandom assignment.
- **Sampling bias (ascertainment bias):** A sample is selected that does not accurately represent the population it is intended to. These studies may have **internal validity** (accurate within the study) but lack **external validity** (results are not generalizable to the population as a whole).
  - *Example:* A study of an economically diverse population inadvertently overselects members of the lowest socioeconomic class by offering a small financial compensation for the study.
  - *Example:* A study to examine heart disease does not have any patients older than 65 years. The study may have **internal validity** but lacks **external validity** and cannot be extrapolated to the general population (in which most patients with heart disease would be older than 65 years).
    - *Solution:* Random sampling.
- **Susceptibility bias:** Patients who are sicker are selected for a more invasive treatment.
  - *Example:* Sicker patients get selected for surgical management over medical management of heart disease. Studies then show medical management to be associated with better outcomes simply because patients were healthier at baseline.
    - *Solution:* Randomization.
- **Attrition bias:** If **loss to follow-up** is unequal between the intervention and control groups, it can make an intervention seem more effective than it is.
  - *Example:* A new acne medication may work for some patients, but it causes unwanted side effects. Patients taking the medication who do not experience improvement in their acne drop out of the

> Confounding occurs when a variable related to exposure and outcome is unevenly distributed between groups.

> Sampling bias: The sample population does not represent the intended study population.

> Susceptibility bias: Sicker patients receive more invasive treatments.

trial at a higher rate than those without improvement taking placebo. In this case the medication appears more effective at resolving acne than it is because more unimproved patients dropped out of the treatment group.
    - *Solution:* Gather as much data as possible about dropouts.

- **Measurement bias (Hawthorne effect):** People change their behaviors when in a study.
  - *Example:* Participants in a medication trial to treat hypertension are more likely to adopt a healthy lifestyle if they know they are being studied. The decrease in blood pressure that occurs because of these lifestyle changes is attributed to the medication.
    - *Solution:* Include a placebo group.
- **Recall bias:** Patients' recall of an exposure may be affected by their knowledge of their current disorder.
  - *Example:* A nonsmoker with lung cancer reports significant exposure to secondhand smoke as a child. On the other hand, a healthy nonsmoker with the same degree of exposure forgot all about his uncle who smoked indoors.
    - *Solution:* Search for confirmatory or objective sources of information or conduct a prospective study.
- **Lead-time bias:** Detecting a disease earlier may be misinterpreted as improving survival.
  - *Example:* A 75-year-old patient with prostate cancer survives only 5 years after he presents with back pain. If a screening prostate-specific antigen (PSA) test had been done in the same patient at 60 years of age, it would have provided the diagnosis and the patient would have lived for 20 years after disease detection. However, he would not have an increased life span. It would be a mistake, therefore, to conclude the screening test improved survival.
    - *Solution:* Scrutinize any screening study for lead-time bias and ask, "Is this actually improving survival or only detection?" Adjust survival rates according to severity of disease (e.g., survival from stage T1, N0, M0 prostate cancer, rather than survival from date of detection).
- **Late-look bias:** Information is gathered too late to make useful conclusions because subjects with severe disease may be incapable of responding or deceased.
  - *Example:* A survey of patients with pancreatic cancer reveals only minimal symptoms because those with severe disease are too sick to respond or may be deceased.
    - *Solution:* Stratify by severity.
- **Procedure bias:** Subjects are treated differently depending on their arm of the study.
  - *Example:* Patients assigned to a surgical intervention arm of a study are followed more closely than those assigned to no intervention.
    - *Solution:* Perform a double-blind study.
- **Experimenter expectancy (Pygmalion effect):** The hopes of the experimenter influence the outcome of the study.
  - *Example:* A physician hoping to treat fibromyalgia conveys to a patient in the treatment arm his expectations that the medication will work.
    - *Solution:* Perform a double-blind study.

> Attrition bias: Loss to follow-up is unequal between study groups.

> Measurement bias: People change their behaviors when they are being studied.

> Recall bias: Recall of an exposure is influenced by knowledge of their current disorder.

> Lead-time bias: Early detection is mistaken for improved outcomes.

> Late-look bias: Information is gathered too late to make useful conclusions.

> Procedure bias: Different arms of the study are treated unequally.

> Experimenter expectancy: Hopes of the experimenter influence the study.

MEDICAL ETHICS

- **Basic principles:**
  - **Autonomy:** Principle that all patients have the right to make their own informed medical decisions for their own reasons. Competent patients have a nearly limitless ability to exercise autonomy even if it means their own death or if it conflicts with their physician's personal ethical principles.
  - **Nonmaleficence (do no harm):** Physicians should weigh the relative risks and benefits of an intervention, acknowledging that most treatments have inherent risk and that it may be better to do nothing at all.
  - **Beneficence:** Physicians have a duty to do what is best for their patients.
  - **Justice:** All people should be treated similarly regardless of age, race, or ability to pay. Medical resources should be allocated fairly.

- **Informed consent:** Requires a discussion with the patient that includes the procedural information from the **BRAIN** mnemonic: **B**enefits, **R**isks, **A**lternatives, **I**ndications for the procedure, and **N**ature of the procedure. Consent must be free from coercion. It may be oral or written and can be revoked at any time.
- **Exceptions to informed consent:** Follow the mnemonic WIPE.
  - **W**aiver: Patient legally expresses a desire not to know.
  - **I**ncompetence: A legal determination made by judge that a person is unable to manage his or her affairs because of mental limitations such as intellectual disability. Additionally, a physician can determine lack of decision-making capacity, for example, in a patient experiencing acute delirium. Note that, unlike competence, which is legally determined by a judge, decision-making capacity may change depending on the complexity of the decision. For example, a delirious and septic patient may be able to comprehend the decision to take an antiemetic and refuse the medication but may not be able to understand the complexities of consenting to or refusing a central venous catheter.
  - Therapeutic **P**rivilege: Disclosure is withheld because it could seriously harm the patient, for example, causing the patient to commit suicide, not just to refuse treatment.
  - **E**mergency/implied consent: Patient with an emergent condition is unable to provide consent—for example, an unconscious victim of a motor vehicle crash.
- **Futility:** A patient cannot demand unnecessary treatment from a physician. A physician may refuse to provide further intervention on the grounds of futility if the treatment has already failed, the treatment will not achieve the patient's goals, or there is no physiologic reason the treatment will work.
- **Advance directives:** If a patient is incapable of making medical decisions or determining goals of care, the focus should shift to what the patient would want if he or she could communicate. These may simply be inferences from statements the patient made earlier or may be formalized as a **living will**—a document that explains what care a patient wants or does not want in certain situations. **Durable power of attorney** is more flexible and allows a surrogate selected by the patient to make decisions that reflect the patient's wishes.
- **Minors and medicine:** Children younger than 18 years cannot refuse treatment or give informed consent except in select circumstances.
- **Parental consent for minors**: The need for parental consent should nearly always be respected. Consent only needs to be obtained from one parent of a minor. In some situations, parental consent needs to be circumvented.
  - In life- or limb-threatening emergencies, treatment should not be delayed despite parental objection.
  - In urgent situations, legal options can be pursued to make the child a ward of the court (e.g., parents cannot refuse lifesaving therapy for a minor with cancer).

> Minors do not require parental consent for reproductive health management, substance abuse treatment, or treatment immediately saving of life or limb.

- **Exceptions to the need for parental consent:**
  - Emancipated minors: married, serving in the military, financially independent, or parents to children.
  - Reproductive health: sexually transmitted diseases (STIs), birth control, prenatal care.
  - Substance abuse treatment.
- **Confidentiality:** Physicians cannot disseminate information about their patients without consent. This principle applies to speaking with families, friends, the court, or other doctors who are "just curious"; however, any communications for the purpose of patient care are acceptable (e.g., consultants). Exceptions to confidentiality are rare but are focused on preventing harm. They include the following:
  - **Tarasoff decision:** Physician–patient confidentiality **must** legally be breeched if the patient has threatened to harm another person. The health care provider should try to detain the patient, contact the police, and **warn the potential victim.**
  - **Child abuse/elder abuse**
  - **Dangerous driving:** Patients must be reported to the Department of Motor Vehicles if they experience a seizure or otherwise present a danger.
  - **Reportable diseases:** Many diseases must be reported to local authorities (and to the patient's partner in the case of STDs). Examples include the following:
    - Most STIs (HIV, gonorrhea, chlamydia, syphilis); bioterrorism agents (anthrax, smallpox); hepatitis A, B, and C; animal-/arthropod-borne disease (rabies, Lyme disease, tularemia); diseases preventable with vaccination (measles/mumps/rubella/varicella).

- **Waiver:** The patient may waive confidentiality so discussions can be held with family members or disclosures made to the insurance company.

❍ **Detainment:** Patients deemed to be a danger to self (suicidal) or a danger to others (homicidal), or to have grave disability (unable to care for self), can be detained against their will for a defined period depending on state laws. These patients retain all other rights, however, and may still refuse treatment if they have capacity to do so. Only a judge may take away other rights or detain a patient for longer.

❍ **Principles for ethics on the** United States Medical Licensing Examination (**USMLE**)**:**

- Even if it does not make sense to you, a patient has the right to forgo treatment unless the patient is deemed legally incompetent or lacks the capacity to make the decision.
- Assume that a patient has capacity to make medical decisions unless there is strong evidence otherwise. Examples include after a suicide attempt or if the patient is acutely psychotic or delirious. The burden of evidence falls on you to prove that the patient lacks capacity, not the other way around.
- If a patient is refusing a treatment plan you think is best, always ask why and explore the patient's reasoning.
- If a patient is angry, ask why and try to express empathy in regard to the patient's concerns. If the patient is angry with another physician, avoid condemning the other physician.
- Avoid escalating the problem if possible. Communication tactics are favored over legal tactics.
- If a patient makes sexual advances, establish boundaries and use a chaperone if needed. Focus on closed-ended questioning. Never establish a romantic relationship with a patient.
- State laws vary in regard to physician-assisted death. In most states, physicians cannot legally, actively assist a patient in dying. It is legal, however, to allow a patient to die by withholding life-sustaining care (according to the patient's wishes). Medications can be given to reduce pain that coincidentally shorten life.
- The amount of information a child is given about his or her disease is at the parents' discretion.
- Maternal autonomy legally supersedes fetal health in the first trimester (after that point, state laws vary and therefore are highly unlikely to be tested). A pregnant female patient can accept and refuse care regardless of risk to the fetus, and she can seek an abortion for medical or non-medical reasons.
- *Substituted judgment* means judging **what the patient would want (not what the decision maker wants).** In all instances, the patient's interests and wishes should be the basis of decision making. The feelings of family members should be respected but should not affect care at the expense of patient autonomy.
- A physician should not be allowed to practice medicine in a way that puts patients at risk. Whether sick with a contagious disease (e.g., tuberculosis), psychologically unsound, or practicing subpar medicine, the issue should be addressed either directly or with a supervisor.
- If a physician makes a medical error he should admit to it, apologize, and do everything possible to limit the complications from that error. The physician should not blame others or cover it up.
- A patient with medical capacity is allowed to refuse care or leave the hospital "against medical advice." The physician should discuss the risks of forgoing treatment and should offer available alternatives when possible. For example, a patient with pneumonia may benefit from intravenous (IV) antibiotics but refuses hospital admission. He could still be given a prescription for oral antibiotics and an appointment for follow-up.
- Avoid unnecessary treatments even if a patient requests them (but try to understand why the patient is requesting them).
- Do not accept referral fees or "kickbacks" from medical manufacturers or pharmaceutical companies.

> Patients who are suicidal, homicidal, or obviously unable to care for themselves can be temporarily detained.

> A competent patient can refuse even lifesaving treatment.

> Parents decide how much information to tell their children about their disease.

> Consent only needs to be obtained from one parent of a minor.

Preventative Medicine and Health Care

❍ **Primary prevention:** Preventing a disease process from ever occurring (e.g., vaccinations, sunscreen use).

❍ **Secondary prevention:** Recognizing disease early and preventing disease progression (e.g., mammography and colonoscopy for cancer screening).

- **Tertiary prevention:** Preventing disease sequelae and reducing disability from illness (e.g., diuretics for the treatment of congestive heart failure, hemoglobin A1c [HbA1c] monitoring for diabetic patients).
- **Health maintenance organization (HMO):** A type of managed care organization with integration of payment and delivery of health care, in which a group of providers contract with the insurance agency to provide complete care for a patient in exchange for a referral base. All care is coordinated by a primary care provider (PCP), who refers the patient to specialists as necessary. Kaiser Permanente is an example of an HMO.
- **Preferred provider organization (PPO):** A type of insurance in which the insurer develops a network of physicians to provide care to their clients at a reduced rate. In exchange, physicians receive access to a population of potential patients. In contrast to an HMO, patients may seek care from any PPO provider, including specialists, without a PCP referral.
- **Medicare:** Federal health insurance plan for those 65 years and older and people with certain disabilities. All qualifying citizens receive Part A but must opt in for Parts B and D.
  - Part A: In-patient care.
  - Part B: Outpatient care.
  - Part D: Prescription drug coverage.

Medicare: insurance for those older than 65 years.

Medicaid: insurance for the impoverished.

- **Medicaid:** Joint state and federal program that provides health insurance to impoverished citizens and permanent residents. Qualifications and benefits depend on the state.
- **Physician reimbursement:**
  - Fee-for-service: Each procedure is reimbursed to the physician. *Pitfall:* A financial incentive exists for physicians to overtreat patients.
  - Capitation: A physician is paid a fixed amount for each patient, usually on a monthly basis, regardless of time spent or treatment rendered. *Pitfall:* Physicians may select for healthier patients or be less likely to order tests.
  - Salary: Hospitals or HMOs pay a fixed salary to the physician regardless of procedures performed, tests ordered, or number of patients cared for. *Pitfall:* Physicians may have less productivity.
- **Malpractice:** A physician is at risk for a civil suit if the situation fits the **4 Ds:** If the physician has a **duty** to the patient, is **derelict** in the patient's care, and **directly** causes **damage** to the patient.
  - **Good Samaritan Law:** Limits the liability of physicians who help patients in an emergency when the physician is not receiving compensation for the patient's care.

Malpractice: dereliction of a physician's duty that directly causes damage.

REVIEW QUESTIONS

(1) During a hospitalization, a patient's serum K^+ value follows a normal distribution with a mean of 140 and an SD of 2.5. During his stay, what percentage of his K^+ values will be greater than 145?

(2) A new test for tuberculosis finds that 195 out of 200 people with tuberculosis test positive. A total of 35 people out of 150 without the disease also tested positive. Before calculation, decide whether this test is sensitive or specific. Next, draw a 2 × 2 table and calculate the sensitivity, specificity, PPV, and NPV.

(3) Investigators conduct a randomized control trial to study the benefits of a new asthma medication. Of 200 people on the medication, only 10 had asthma attacks. A total of 30 people out of 200 in the control group developed an asthma attack. Construct a 2 × 2 table and calculate the incidence in the exposed and unexposed, ARR, NNT, RR, and RRR for this medication.

(4) A case-control study is designed to study risk factors for developing Buerger's disease (thromboangiitis obliterans). Ten people are selected with Buerger's disease, and 10 subjects are selected as controls. Nine patients who developed Buerger's disease were heavy smokers, and two people without Buerger's disease smoked. Construct a 2 × 2 table and calculate the odds ratio. Using these data, can we calculate the prevalence of Buerger's disease? Why should we calculate odds ratio and not relative risk?

(5) You want to determine whether people are more likely to be alive 1 week after MI if they are older than 65 or younger than 65 years. Which statistical test should you use?

(6) Which test would you use to compare the age of menopause among whites, African Americans, and Asians?

(7) A 15-year-old girl presents to her physician with a 5-cm laceration extending through the dermis. When her mother leaves the room, she confides in you that she has been sexually active and would like to start an oral contraceptive. On further discussion, she describes vaginal discharge and on examination has cervical motion tenderness. Which of these concerns can be addressed without parental consent?

(8) A patient's wife knows that her husband has a diagnosis of terminal pancreatic cancer. She asks the physician not to inform her husband because it will upset him greatly. What should the physician do?

(9) A Jehovah's Witness has severe postpartum hemorrhage. Without a blood transfusion, she will likely die, but she refuses it on religious grounds. What should be done?

(10) A schizophrenic man on clozapine requires a bone marrow biopsy for evaluation of agranulocytosis thought to be caused by his antipsychotic medication. His positive and negative symptoms are well controlled. Can the schizophrenic patient legally consent to (or refuse) this procedure?

2 BIOCHEMISTRY

Gwen Owens

PROTEIN STRUCTURE AND FUNCTION

Amino Acid Structure

Amino acids are the building blocks of proteins. Amino acids are composed of an α-amino group ($-NH_3^+$) and an α-carboxyl group (–COOH), with different characteristic side chains. Twenty amino acids are naturally incorporated into polypeptides (Fig. 2.1). Nine of these amino acids are "essential," cannot be synthesized by humans, and must be obtained in the diet. These essential amino acids include **phenylalanine, valine, threonine, tryptophan, isoleucine, methionine, histidine, leucine,** and **lysine.** In children, an additional three amino acids are essential: arginine, tyrosine, and cysteine. In adults, the remaining 11 amino acids can be synthesized.

The nature of the amino acid side chain is critical to how proteins interact with their environment. Acidic, basic, and uncharged polar side chains tend to be found on the exterior of soluble proteins and on the interior of proteins found within membranes. Conversely, amino acids with nonpolar side chains are located in the interior of proteins that exist in aqueous environments and on the exterior of proteins in lipid environments (e.g., membranes).

Homocystinuria is elevated homocysteine and early-onset vascular disease.

- **Alanine** is an important substrate for gluconeogenesis.
- **Isoleucine, valine,** and **leucine** are branched-chain amino acids that are increased in maple syrup urine disease.
- **Methionine** is a precursor of homocysteine, a product associated with atherosclerosis. Increased levels of homocysteine are seen in patients with classic homocystinuria, with a deficiency in cystathionine β-synthase. These patients have early-onset vascular disease.
- **Phenylalanine** accumulates in phenylketonuria (PKU). **Tryptophan** is a precursor of serotonin, niacin, and melatonin. **Arginine** and **histidine** stimulate growth hormone and insulin. Arginine is a precursor of **nitric oxide**.
- **Glutamine** is the most common amino acid and is an important nitrogen donor in the synthesis of purines and pyrimidines.
- **Cysteine** forms disulfide bonds and is sensitive to oxidation state.
- **Proline** is different from other amino acids because its side chain forms a **five-membered ring.** Proline is often found in collagen and its unique side chain is used to interrupt α-helices in globular proteins.

Tryptophan is a precursor of serotonin, niacin, and melatonin.

The pK_a (-log of the acid dissociation constant, K_a) is a measure of the strength of an acid in solution. The pK_a of amino acid side chains gives insight into the pH characteristics of proteins and stability. Histidine is unique in that its side group, imidazole, has a pK_a of 6. This means that histidine has a positive charge at pH 7; and at physiologic pH, small shifts in pH change the charge on histidine, and the side group acts as a buffer. Aspartic acid and glutamic acid (acidic amino acids) have a negative charge at pH 7; albumin is a strong binding protein for positively charged molecules in part because of its high content of these acidic amino acids.

The isoelectric point (pI) is the pH value at which an amino acid, or any other molecule, has a net zero electrical charge. Amino acids are zwitterions, with positive and negative charges. When pH is greater than pI, the net charge on the molecule is negative. When pH is less than pI, the net charge on the molecule is positive. At physiologic pH, lysine, arginine, and histidine have a positive charge,

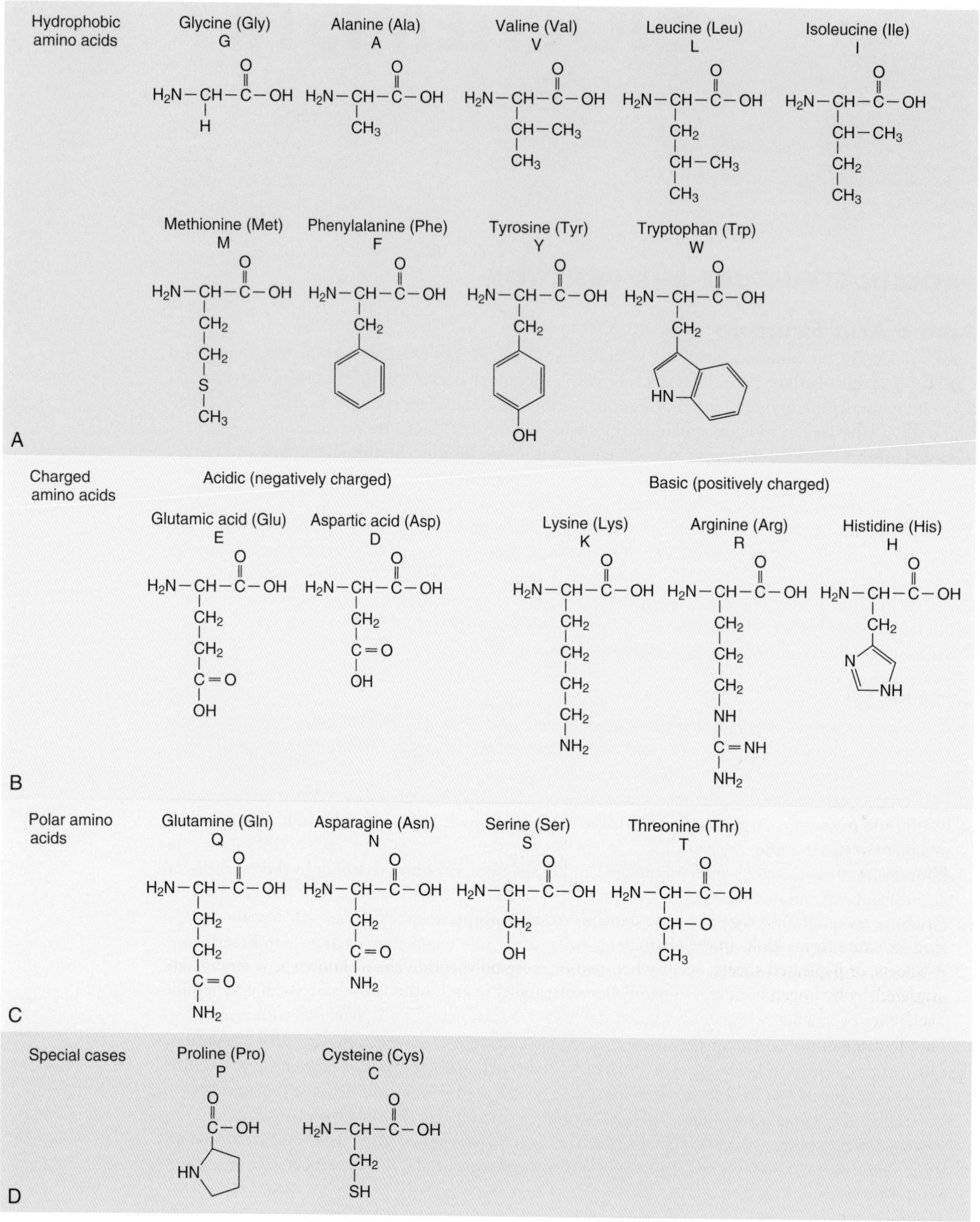

FIG. 2.1 The 20 naturally occurring amino acids.

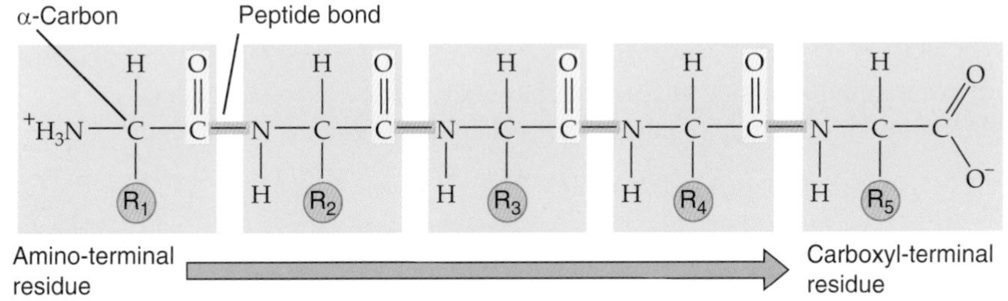

FIG. 2.2 Protein primary structure. By convention, the amino-terminal (N-terminal) residue is depicted at the far left of the protein sequence, and the carboxyl-terminal (C-terminal) residue is at the far right. (*From Boron WF, Boulpaep EL.* Medical Physiology. *2nd ed. Philadelphia: Elsevier; 2008.*)

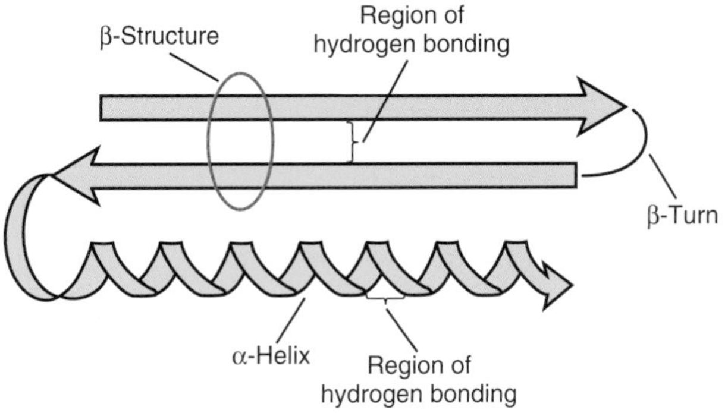

FIG. 2.3 Protein secondary structure components. (*From Pelley JW.* Elsevier's Integrated Biochemistry. *Philadelphia: Elsevier; 2007.*)

whereas aspartate and glutamate have a negative charge. Proteins can be separated based on their pI using **isoelectric focusing** on a polyacrylamide gel, which separates proteins using a pH gradient. This is the first step in two-dimensional gel electrophoresis.

Protein Structure

The *primary* structure of a protein is the linear sequence of amino acids (Fig. 2.2). Peptide bonds are formed between the α-carboxyl group and the α-amino group, creating a covalent amide linkage.

The *secondary* structure of proteins involves the arrangements of the amino acids located near each other in the amino acid sequence (Fig. 2.3). Important secondary structure components include α-helices and β-sheets.

- α-Helices are the most common kind of polypeptide helix. Extensive hydrogen bonding occurs between the peptide bonding of carbonyl oxygen and amide hydrogen. **Each α-helical turn contains 3.6 amino acids.** Therefore amino acids that are spaced 3 to 4 amino acids apart in the primary structure are quite close together in an α-helix. Proline disrupts α-helices because its five-membered ring structure forms kinks in the chain.
- β-Sheets, or β-pleated sheets, occur when two or more polypeptide chains known as β-strands are arranged, by hydrogen bonding, in parallel or antiparallel to each other. Bonds between polypeptide backbones of separate polypeptide chains are known as interchain bonds. Globular proteins tend to have β-sheets with a right-handed curl or twist, which form their core. Silk is a packed β-sheet.
- Proteins that bind to DNA also have important secondary structure motifs. For example, the DNA-binding zinc finger motif is found in many transcription factors.

The *tertiary* structure of proteins includes the three-dimensional shape of the folded protein chain. Several different kinds of interactions stabilize tertiary structures.

- Disulfide bonds are covalent links formed from the sulfhydryl group (–SH) of two cysteine residues. Disulfide bonds are important in proteins that are secreted from cells, such as immunoglobulins.
- Ionic interactions include negatively charged side groups interacting with positively charged groups.
- Hydrophobic interactions force amino acids with nonpolar side chains into the interior of polypeptide molecules, where they are able to associate with other hydrophobic residues. Amino acids with polar

side chains tend to be located on the surface of a protein and contact the polar solvent to be most energetically favorable.

- Hydrogen bonds can form between amino acid side chains that have oxygen- or nitrogen-bound hydrogen, such as serine and threonine. This can help to improve the solubility of proteins in aqueous environments.

The *quaternary* structure is the arrangement of polypeptide subunits in a protein structure that has more than one polypeptide chain. These subunits are usually held together by noncovalent interactions.

Proteins fold in a very short time (milliseconds to microseconds), whereas the translation of protein from messenger RNA (mRNA) progresses at a much slower rate (5 to 20 amino acids per second). Chaperone proteins such as the **heat shock proteins** are critical in keeping some proteins properly folded. Proteins can be denatured by heat, solvents, strong acids or bases, and detergents. Some proteins can also misfold, and deposition of these misfolded proteins is associated with several diseases.

- **Amyloidoses** are diseases in which an altered protein accumulates. In some amyloidoses, insoluble, fibrillar proteins aggregate in a form that resembles β-sheets. In Alzheimer disease, plaques form that contain amyloid β (Aβ), which is hypothesized to be neurotoxic. These Aβ peptides aggregate, forming amyloid in brain tissue and in blood vessels. Alzheimer disease is also defined by an accumulation of hypophosphorylated tau (τ) proteins known as neurofibrillary tangles.

> Amyloidosis is the accumulation and deposition of an abnormal protein in soft tissues and organs.

- **Prion diseases** are caused by the **prion protein (PrP),** an infectious protein that causes normal protein to change structure and form insoluble aggregates of fibrils. Prion diseases include transmissible spongiform encephalopathies (TSEs) such as Creutzfeldt-Jakob disease in humans, scrapie in sheep, and bovine spongiform encephalopathy (BSE) in cattle (mad-cow disease). It has been shown that **many α-helices present in noninfectious PrP are replaced by β-sheets in the infectious form**; this makes the protein highly resistant to proteolytic degradation.
- **Heinz bodies** are formed when red blood cells undergo oxidative stress, whereby hemoglobin is denatured to form aggregates on the membrane of red blood cells (RBCs). This occurs in conditions such as glucose-6-phosphate dehydrogenase (G6PD) deficiency, thalassemias, and exposure to oxidative compounds.

> Heinz bodies are formed when RBCs undergo oxidative stress (e.g., G6PD deficiency).

OXYGEN-BINDING PROTEINS: HEMOGLOBIN AND MYOGLOBIN

Hemoglobin A, the most common hemoglobin in adults, is composed of two α-globin subunits and two β-globin subunits ($\alpha_2\beta_2$). Each globin protein subunit is composed of an α- or β-protein chain plus a heme group. Heme, in turn, is composed of an Fe^{2+} held in a protoporphyrin IX ring. Hemoglobin has two primary forms. **Hemoglobin that is desaturated with oxygen is deoxyhemoglobin (T, tense form), which has a low oxygen affinity** and a lower degree of freedom. **Hemoglobin that is saturated with oxygen is oxyhemoglobin (R, relaxed form), which has a high oxygen affinity and a higher degree of freedom.**

> Normal hemoglobin is $\alpha_2\beta_2$. Fetal hemoglobin is $\alpha_2\gamma_2$. Sickle cell disease (SCD) is $\alpha_2\beta^s{}_2$

A single hemoglobin molecule can bind up to **four** oxygen molecules. The four globin subunits work **cooperatively** in hemoglobin, in which the binding of oxygen to one subunit of the tetramer increases the affinity of the other subunits for oxygen. The first oxygen binds with low affinity, but this leads to a transition from T to R form. The second through fourth oxygen molecules bind with increasing affinity, which leads to a **sigmoidal oxygen-binding (or oxygen-saturation) curve for hemoglobin** (Fig. 2.4).

> The O_2-binding curve shifts right with increase in CO_2, acidosis (low pH), increase in 2,3-BPG, exercise, and temperature.

Deoxyhemoglobin (T form) preferentially binds hydrogen ion (H^+), 2,3-bisphosphoglycerate (2,3-BPG), and CO_2. This leads to stabilization of the T state, decreased affinity for oxygen, and a rightward shift in the oxygen saturation curve. Exercise and an increase in temperature can also cause a rightward shift. Conversely, **a leftward shift in the oxygen saturation curve occurs in the presence of a decrease in CO_2, alkalosis (high pH, low hydrogen ion concentration), and decrease in 2,3-BPG.**

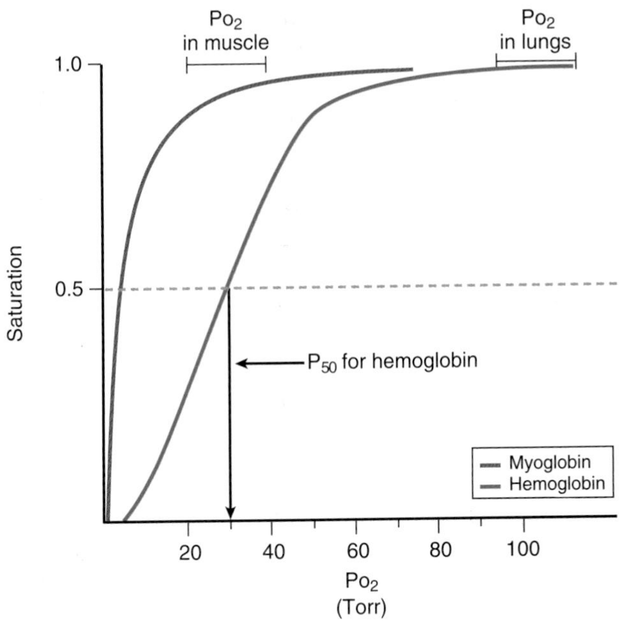

FIG. 2.4 Comparison of oxygen-binding curves for hemoglobin and myoglobin. The P_{50} is the Po_2 at half saturation. Having a lower P_{50} means having a greater affinity for oxygen. (*From Pelley JW. Elsevier's Integrated Biochemistry. Philadelphia: Elsevier; 2007.*)

Myoglobin is a single polypeptide chain with a single heme group. Myoglobin is present in heart and skeletal muscle and acts as an oxygen carrier and location for storage of oxygen. Myoglobin can only bind to one oxygen molecule; therefore the binding curve is hyperbolic rather than sigmoidal because the binding of O_2 is not cooperative (see Fig. 2.4).

Carbon monoxide (CO) binds to hemoglobin to form carboxyhemoglobin, which has a high affinity for CO and displaces O_2. This leads to stabilization of the R state, a leftward shift of the oxygen saturation curve, and an oxygen saturation curve for hemoglobin that resembles the curve for myoglobin.

Fig. 2.4 compares the oxygen-binding curves for hemoglobin and myoglobin. Myoglobin has a lower P_{50} than hemoglobin, meaning that it has a greater affinity for oxygen. This ensures that oxygen is bound to myoglobin in all cases except hypoxia.

Hemoglobinopathies (Fig. 2.5) are a group of genetic disorders caused by abnormal hemoglobin structure or insufficient synthesis of normal hemoglobin.

- **Sickle cell disease** (HbS disease) is a homozygous recessive genetic disorder that results from production of hemoglobin with an altered amino acid sequence, caused by a single point mutation in the β-globin gene. The mutation is a **glutamate-to-valine mutation at position 6 in the β-globin chain.** During electrophoresis at a basic pH, HbS migrates more slowly toward the anode (positive electrode) than does HbA, as a result of the absence of the negatively charged glutamate residues in the two β-globin chains, which makes HbS less negative. The mutant β-globin chain is designated β^S, and the resulting hemoglobin, $\alpha_2\beta_2{}^S$, is HbS. The α-globin chains are normal. This amino acid substitution forms a protrusion on the β-globin that polymerizes deoxygenated HbS into fibers. The resulting sickled erythrocytes occlude blood flow in the capillaries, causing mircoinfarcts leading to tissue anoxia and severe pain. An infant does not begin to show symptoms of the disease until sufficient HbF has been replaced by HbS so that sickling can occur. Sickling is increased by anything that increases the proportion of HbS in the deoxygenated state, such as decreased O_2 tension, increased Pco_2, decreased pH, dehydration, and increased concentration of 2,3-BPG in erythrocytes. **Hydroxyurea** is used to treat sickle cell disease because it increases circulating levels of HbF, which decreases RBC sickling. Sickle cell disease is tested for at birth to allow **prophylactic antibiotic therapy** to begin soon after because these children are at risk for sepsis.
- **Hemoglobin C disease** (HbC disease) results from production of hemoglobin with an altered amino acid sequence as a result of a glutamate-to-lysine substitution **at position 6 in the β-globin gene.** The substitution of a positively charged amino acid for a negatively charged amino acid causes HbC to move more slowly toward an anode than HbA or HbS does. Homozygous patients have a mild, chronic hemolytic anemia.

CO poisoning causes stabilization of the R state, a leftward shift in O_2 saturation curve, and a saturation curve for hemoglobin that resembles the curve for myoglobin.

Myoglobin has a lower P_{50} than hemoglobin; therefore it has a greater affinity for O_2. Thus O_2 is bound to myoglobin in all cases except hypoxia.

HbC disease is caused by an altered β-globin gene. It causes a mild hemolytic anemia.

HbSC disease is more severe than HbC disease but is generally milder than sickle cell disease.

Pattern	Type of anemia	Interpretation and discussion
A_2 S F A; 2% (A2), 1% (F), 97% (A)	None	Normal Hb electrophoresis
A_2 S F A; 2% (A2), 1% (F), 97% (A)	Microcytic	α-Thal trait. Note that the proportion of the Hb types remains the same; however, the patient has a microcytic anemia.
A_2 S F A; 5% (A2), 2% (F), 93% (A)	Microcytic	β-Thal minor. Note that HbA is decreased, because β-globin chain synthesis is decreased. There is a corresponding increase in HbA2 and HbF.
A_2 S F A; 10% (A2), 90% (F)	Microcytic	β-Thal major. Note that there is no synthesis of HbA.
A_2 S F A; 2% (A2), 45% (S), 1% (F), 52% (A)	No anemia	Sickle cell trait. Note that there is not enough HbS to cause spontaneous sickling in the peripheral blood.
A_2 S F A; 2% (A2), 90% (S), 8% (F)	Normocytic	Sickle cell disease. Note that there is no HbA. There is enough HbS to cause spontaneous sickling.

FIG. 2.5 Hemoglobinopathies. Hb, hemoglobin. (*From Goljan EF, Sloka KI. Rapid Review Laboratory Testing in Clinical Medicine. Philadelphia: Elsevier; 2007.*)

- **Hemoglobin SC** disease occurs when some β-globin genes have the sickle cell mutation, whereas others have the mutation found in HbC disease. These patients are compound heterozygotes because both of their β-globin genes are abnormal but are different from each other. Affected individuals have fewer vasoocclusive events than those with sickle cell disease, but their course is more serious than those with HbC disease.
- Thalassemias are caused by decreased production of normal hemoglobin as a result of defective synthesis of either the α- or the β-globin chain. In β-thalassemia, synthesis of β-globin chains is decreased or absent, but the α-globin chain synthesis is normal. Other forms of hemoglobin may be present in elevated amounts, including HbF ($\alpha_2\gamma_2$) in β-thalassemia and hemoglobin Bart (γ_4) in α-thalassemia. Because there are only two copies of the β-globin gene, individuals have either β-thalassemia trait (minor) or β-thalassemia major (Cooley anemia). Because β-globin is not expressed until late in gestation, symptoms of β-thalassemia appear only after birth. α-Thalassemias

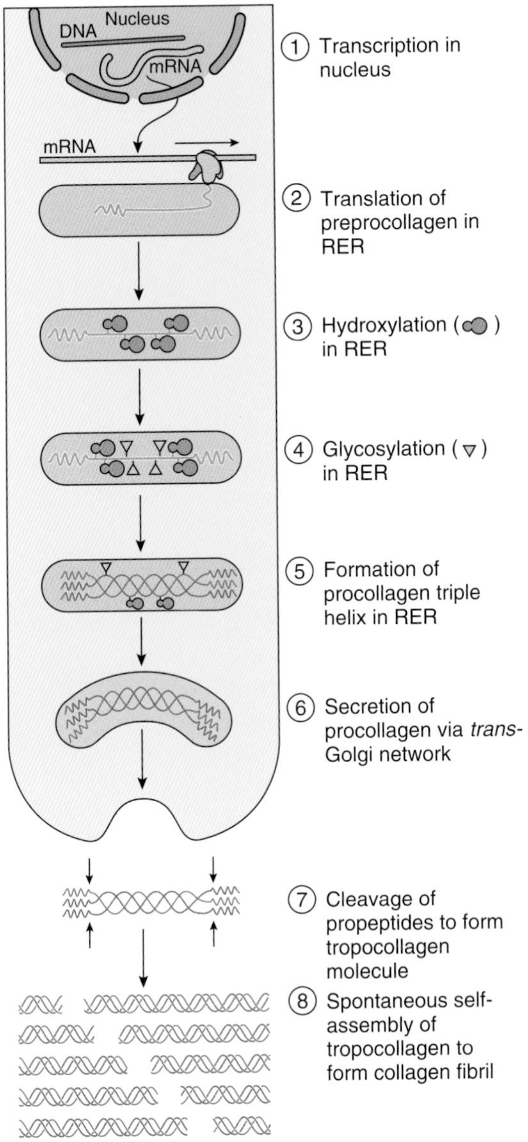

Fig. 2.6 Collagen synthesis and assembly. RER, rough endoplasmic reticulum. (*From Gartner LP, Hiatt JL: Color Textbook of Histology. 3rd ed. Philadelphia: Saunders; 2007:77.*)

occur when α-globin chains are decreased or absent. There are four copies of the α-globin gene, so there are several possible levels of deficiency. If one copy of the α-globin is absent or defective, the person is a silent carrier. Two defective genes lead to α-thalassemia trait. Three defective genes lead to hemoglobin H (HbH) disease. If all four α-globin genes are defective, hydrops fetalis and fetal death result because α-globin chains are required for the synthesis of HbF.

Fibrous Proteins

Collagen is the most abundant protein in humans and is found primarily in connective tissue and muscle. **Collagen is composed of a triple helix of three α-chains held together by hydrogen bonds.** There are more than 20 types of collagen; collagen I is the most common. Collagen has a large amount of **proline** and **glycine.** Proline helps in the formation of the α-chain, and **glycine is found in every third amino acid.** The sequence is –Gly–X–Y–, where X is often proline and Y is often hydroxyproline or hydroxylysine.

The biosynthesis of collagen (Fig. 2.6) occurs as follows:

1. It begins with mRNA transcription in the nucleus of a fibroblast or related cell.
2. mRNA is translated into **preprocollagen** on the **rough endoplasmic reticulum** (RER), and these peptide chains are directed into the lumen of the RER and become **pro-α-chains.**
3. Proline and lysine residues are next **hydroxylated by prolyl hydroxylase and lysyl hydroxylase.**
4. Some hydroxylysine residues are glycosylated with glucose and galactose.

5. Pro-α-chains form procollagen, which has a central triple helix with N- and C-terminal propeptide extensions; these prevent premature assembly of collagen within the endoplasmic reticulum.
6. Procollagen is transported to the Golgi apparatus, where it is released into the extracellular space.
7. After release of procollagen, peptidases remove the terminal propeptides, forming tropocollagen.
8. Tropocollagen then spontaneously assembles into collagen fibrils. **The collagen fibers are cross-linked by lysyl oxidase, which oxidatively deaminates lysyl and hydroxylysyl residues in collagen,** forming covalent cross-linked, mature collagen fibers.

- The hydroxylation reaction requires both oxygen and the reducing agent **vitamin C** (ascorbic acid) for the hydroxylating enzymes prolyl hydroxylase and lysyl hydroxylase to function. **Vitamin C deficiency leads to a lack of prolyl and lysyl hydroxylation,** making collagen fibers unable to be cross-linked, which decreases the tensile strength of the assembled collagen fiber. This is called **scurvy.** Because of the weak collagen structure, patients often have bruises, corkscrew hairs, and perifollicular hemorrhage caused by capillary fragility. Copper is also a cofactor for lysyl oxidase.

Vitamin C deficiency causes scurvy because collagen fibers cannot be cross-linked.

- **Ehlers-Danlos syndrome (EDS)** is a connective tissue disorder caused by defects in collagen synthesis. EDS arises from lysyl hydroxylase deficiency, procollagen peptidase deficiency, or mutations in collagen amino acid sequences, most importantly collagen type III. Skin hyperextensibility and joint hypermobility are seen in patients with EDS.
- **Osteogenesis imperfecta** (OI), also known as "brittle bone disease," is a genetic disorder caused by defects in connective tissue, usually type I collagen, such as decreased production of collagen α-chains, leading to bones that are prone to bending and fracture. OI is an autosomal dominant disorder but arises sporadically in one-third of cases. Type I OI is the most common form of OI and is known as osteogenesis imperfecta tarda. **Patients with type I OI have bones that fracture easily, early hearing loss, and a blue-gray tint to the sclera** caused by thinned scleral tissue. The blue tint of the sclera is secondary to defective type I collagen, which allows visualization of underlying choroidal veins.

Osteogenesis imperfecta is from a defect of type 1 collagen causing brittle bones and blue sclera.

Elastin is a connective tissue protein composed of elastin and glycoprotein microfibrils that are found primarily in the lungs, arterial walls, and elastic ligaments. Elastin is synthesized from tropoelastin, a precursor protein. After secretion from the cell, tropoelastin deposits onto fibrillin. **Mutations in fibrillin cause Marfan syndrome.** Marfan syndrome is noted by increased height, joint laxity, ectopia lentis (lens displacement) and cardiac abnormalities including aortic dilation and mitral valve prolapse. In the alveoli, elastin is broken down by elastase from activated neutrophils. **α_1-Antitrypsin, an enzyme produced in the liver, usually blocks elastase and protects the lungs.** However, genetic defects in **α_1-Antitrypsin** can lead to pulmonary emphysema at a young age because of increased breakdown of lung connective tissue.

Enzymes

Enzymes are protein catalysts. They have active sites, which permit substrate binding. Stabilization of the transition state leads to decreased activation energy, leading to increased rates of substrate to product (reaction rate) but no change in reaction equilibrium. Enzymes are described mathematically using Michaelis-Menton kinetics (Fig. 2.7):

A higher K_m means a lower affinity of the substrate for the enzyme.

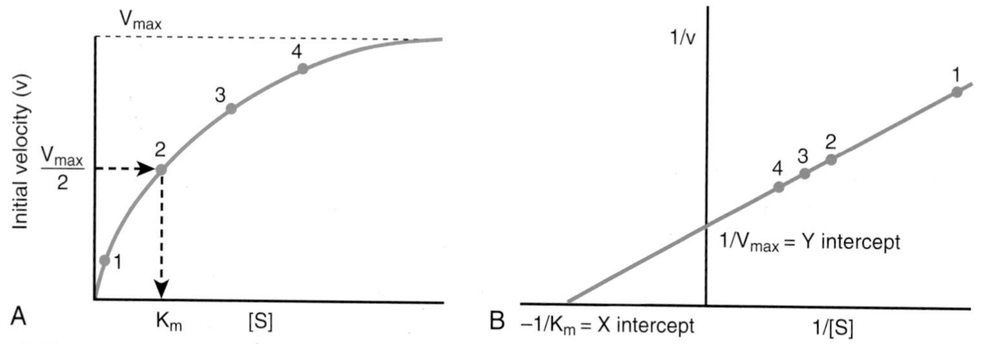

FIG. 2.7 Michaelis-Menton enzyme kinetics. **A,** Substrate concentration [S] versus initial velocity (V) for a reaction with Michaelis-Menton kinetics with a constant enzyme concentration. **B,** Lineweaver-Burk double reciprocal plot. K_m and V_{max} are determined from the intersection of the resulting straight line with the horizontal and vertical axes, respectively. (*From Pelley JW, Goljan EF.* Rapid Review Biochemistry. *3rd ed. Philadelphia: Elsevier; 2010.*)

K_m is the substrate concentration at which the reaction rate is $\frac{1}{2}V_{max}$, v is the velocity of the reaction, and [S] is the substrate concentration. A higher K_m means a lower affinity of the substrate for the enzyme.

- When [S] > > than K_m, the rate of the reaction is independent of [S]. This is known as zero-order kinetics.
- When [S] = K_m, then the initial velocity (v) = $V_{max}/2$
- When [S] < K_m, the reaction rate is proportional to [S]. This is first-order kinetics.
- V_{max} is the maximal reaction velocity. This occurs when the enzyme is saturated with substrate.
- A Lineweaver-Burk plot is a double reciprocal plot of $1/v$ versus 1/[S]. This produces a straight line. **The Y-intercept is $1/V_{max}$, and the X-intercept is $-1/K_m$.**

Enzyme kinetics are affected by inhibitors, which may be classified in several ways (Fig. 2.8).

- **Competitive inhibitors: K_m is increased, V_{max} is unchanged** (there is always competition between two lines so that they cross on graph; solute concentration changes, but velocity remains the same). Plots intersect on the vertical axis (V_{max} is the same). Competitive inhibitors include methanol and ethylene glycol (antifreeze), which compete with ethanol for binding to alcohol dehydrogenase. Giving a patient ethanol reduces methanol toxicity by competing for the enzyme active site, thereby slowing the build-up of toxic metabolites. For competitive inhibitors, high substrate concentration can reverse competitive inhibition because the enzyme is saturated with substrate.
- **Noncompetitive inhibitors: K_m is unchanged, V_{max} is decreased.** Plots intersect on the horizontal axis (K_m is the same). Noncompetitive inhibitors bind at a site distant from the active site and form unreactive complexes with the enzyme. Increased substrate amount does not change the level of inhibition. Physostigmine, a cholinesterase inhibitor, is a noncompetitive inhibitor.
- A third kind of enzyme inhibitor is an **irreversible inhibitor, which permanently inactivates enzymes.** Examples include heavy metals, aspirin (an irreversible inhibitor of cyclooxygenase), fluorouracil, and organophosphates. The effect of irreversible inhibitors is only overcome by synthesis of new enzymes.

Competitive inhibitors: K_m is increased, V_{max} is unchanged.

Enzymes may be useful in serum as diagnostic markers (Table 2.1).

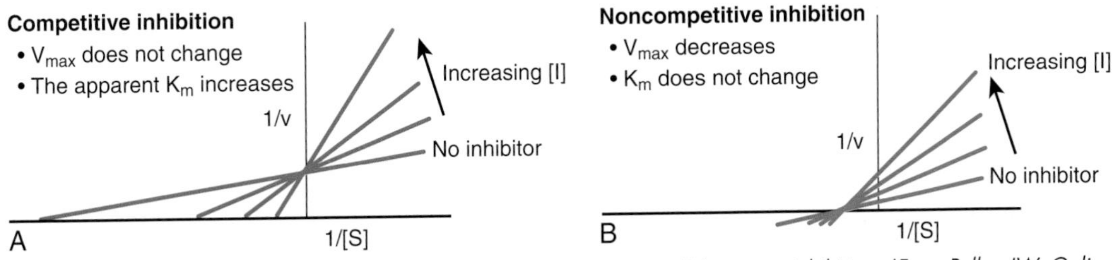

Fig. 2.8 Lineweaver-Burk plots of competitive (**A**) and noncompetitive (**B**) enzyme inhibition. (*From Pelley JW, Goljan EF. Rapid Review Biochemistry. 3rd ed. Philadelphia: Elsevier; 2010.*)

Table 2.1 Serum Enzyme Markers Used for Diagnosis

SERUM ENZYME	DIAGNOSTIC USE
Alanine aminotransferase (ALT)	Viral hepatitis (ALT > AST)
Aspartate aminotransferase (AST)	Alcoholic hepatitis (AST > ALT)
Alkaline phosphatase	Osteoblastic bone disease Obstructive liver disease
Amylase	Acute pancreatitis Mumps (parotitis)
Creatine kinase (CK)	Myocardial infarction (CK-MB) Duchenne muscular dystrophy (CK-MM)
γ-Glutamyltransferase (GGT)	Obstructive liver disease, increased in alcoholic patients
Lactate dehydrogenase (LDH, type I)	Myocardial infarction
Lipase	Acute pancreatitis (more specific than amylase)

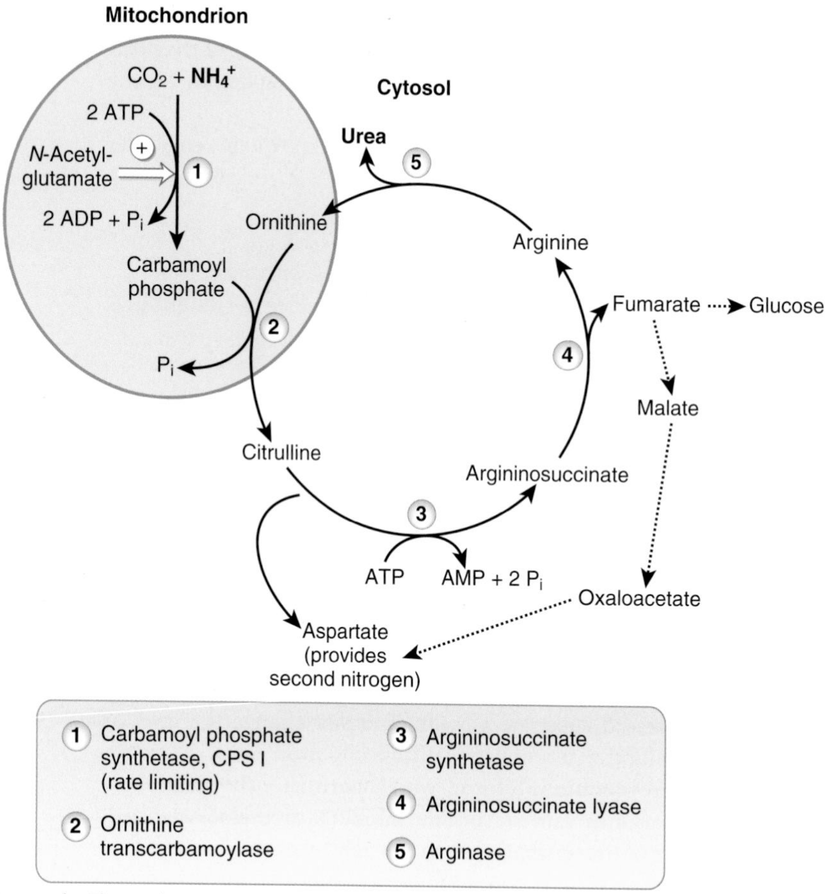

FIG. 2.9 Urea cycle. This pathway occurs in the liver and disposes of toxic ammonia (NH_3). ADP, adenosine diphosphate; AMP, adenosine monophosphate; ATP, adenosine triphosphate. (*From Pelley JW, Goljan EF.* Rapid Review Biochemistry. *3rd ed. Philadelphia: Elsevier; 2010.*)

NITROGEN METABOLISM

Heme synthesis, the urea cycle, and gluconeogenesis reactions occur in both the mitochondria and the cytosol.

Disposal of Amino Acid Nitrogen

Free amino acids are produced by degradation of dietary protein, synthesis of nonessential amino acids, and degradation of body protein. Nitrogen is removed from amino acids because amino acids cannot directly take part in energy metabolism. Amino groups are removed from amino acids by two sequential reactions:

- **Transaminases**, such as alanine aminotransferase (ALT) and aspartate aminotransferase (AST), transfer amino groups to α-ketoglutarate, producing an α-keto acid and glutamate. The α-keto acid can enter the citric acid cycle. Aminotransferases require pyridoxal phosphate for function (a derivative of vitamin B_6). Transaminases are intracellular enzymes found primarily in hepatic tissue; thus elevated serum levels of transaminases can be diagnostic of liver damage.
- Next, **glutamate dehydrogenase oxidatively deaminates glutamate** to α-ketoglutarate and free ammonia (NH_3). The NH_3 can be stored and transported to the liver as glutamine or as alanine (as part of the glucose-alanine cycle).

Aspartate and ammonia then enter the **urea cycle**, the body's primary method for disposing of amino groups from amino acids. The nitrogen of aspartate, CO_2, and NH_3 are incorporated into urea.

The urea cycle (Fig. 2.9) is a five-step metabolic pathway that takes place within the liver. It removes nitrogen waste from the amino groups of amino acids that occurs during protein turnover. The rate-limiting step for the urea cycle is **carbamoyl phosphate synthetase I**, which is activated by

Table 2.2 Inborn Errors of Urea Cycle Metabolism

DISORDER	DEFICIENCY	GENETICS	CLINICAL FEATURES
Carbamoyl synthetase deficiency	Carbamoyl phosphate synthetase (1)	AR	Hyperammonemia
Ornithine transcarbamylase deficiency	Ornithine transcarbamylase (2)	XD	Hyperammonemia
Citrullinemia	Argininosuccinate synthetase (3)	AR	Variable
Argininosuccinic aciduria	Argininosuccinate lyase (4)	AR	Hyperammonemia
Hyperargininemia	Arginase (5)	AR	Hyperammonemia

AR, Autosomal recessive; XD, X-linked dominant.

N-**acetylglutamate**, which is synthesized from acetyl coenzyme A (CoA). Two molecules of NH_3 and one of CO_2 are converted into urea. Urea is then transported in the blood to the kidneys for excretion in urine. Urea levels in patients with kidney failure are elevated. Urease produced by bacteria in the gut creates a significant amount of ammonia, which can lead to hyperammonemia. **Neomycin and rifaximin** orally administered can reduce the number of urease-producing bacteria and are used in the treatment of hepatic encephalopathy.

Hyperammonemia causes tremors, blurry vision, and cerebral edema.

Hyperammonemia occurs when there are genetic defects of the urea cycle, or liver disease. Ammonia has a toxic effect on the central nervous system (CNS), causing tremors, cerebral edema, and blurring of vision. Urea cycle disorders (Table 2.2) are rare and, with the exception of X-linked ornithine transcarbamylase deficiency (which is the most common hereditary hyperammonemia), are inherited as autosomal recessive traits. Deficiencies of enzymes in the urea cycle cause intolerance to protein from the accumulation of ammonia in the body (hyperammonemia). These increased ammonia levels are toxic to the CNS and can lead to coma and death. These hereditary hyperammonemia disorders include those listed in Table 2.2.

Urea cycle disorders can be treated with dietary protein elimination and amino acid–binding compounds.

In each of these disorders, urea is unable to be synthesized, which leads to hyperammonemia during the first weeks after birth. **Mental retardation** is common. Treatment of these disorders includes protein limitation in the diet and administration of compounds that bind covalently to amino acids so that they can then be excreted in the urine. For example, **phenylbutyrate**, a prodrug that is metabolized to phenylacetate, combines with glutamine to form phenylacetylglutamine, which can be excreted in the urine. This assists in clearance of nitrogen from the blood.

Amino Acid Synthesis and Degradation

Although essential amino acids must be obtained from the diet, nonessential amino acids can be synthesized by several different pathways.

- **Aspartate, alanine,** and **glutamate** are synthesized from **transamination of α-keto acids.** Aspartate is derived from oxaloacetate, glutamate from α-ketoglutarate, and alanine from pyruvate.
- **Glutamine** and **asparagine** are synthesized by **amidation.** Glutamine synthetase forms glutamine from glutamate. This reaction also helps to reduce ammonia levels. Asparagine synthetase forms asparagine from aspartate.
- **Serine** is synthesized from the glycolysis intermediate 3-phosphoglycerate. **Glycine,** in turn, can be synthesized from serine.
- **Proline** is synthesized from glutamate.
- **Arginine** is synthesized from citrulline, an intermediate in the urea cycle.
- Two amino acids can be synthesized from essential amino acids. **Cysteine** is synthesized from homocysteine and serine; homocysteine is derived from methionine. **Tyrosine** is synthesized from phenylalanine by **phenylalanine hydroxylase.** This reaction requires tetrahydrobiopterin (BH_4). Because tyrosine and cysteine are formed from essential amino acids, tyrosine and cysteine are only nonessential in the presence of adequate dietary intake of methionine and phenylalanine.
- When amino acids are catabolized, the α-amino group is removed and enters the urea cycle for excretion (see previous section, "Disposal of Amino Acid Nitrogen"), while the carbon skeleton

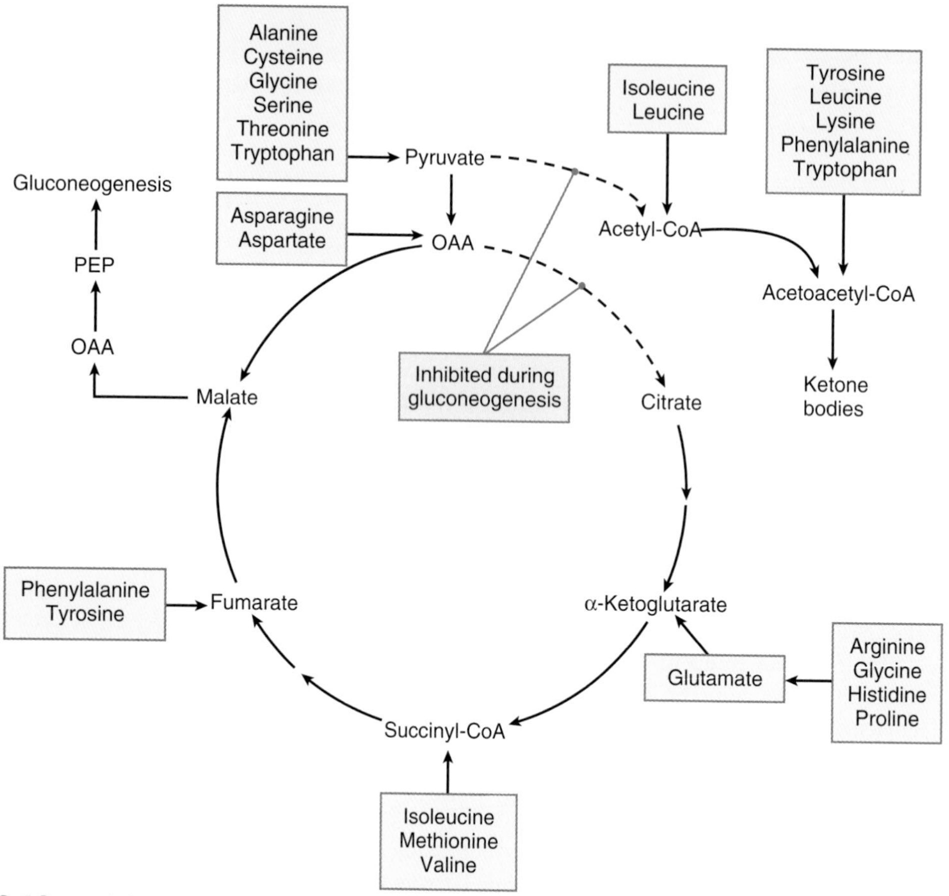

Fig. 2.10 Metabolic intermediates from amino acid degradation. CoA, coenzyme A; OAA, oxaloacetic acid; PEP, phosphoenolpyruvate. (*From Pelley JW.* Elsevier's Integrated Biochemistry. *Philadelphia: Elsevier; 2007.*)

is metabolized. Amino acids are classified as glucogenic, ketogenic, or both based on which intermediates are produced during catabolism.

- **Glucogenic amino acids** yield pyruvate or one of the intermediates of the tricarboxylic acid (TCA) cycle (oxaloacetate, α-ketoglutarate, succinyl CoA, or fumarate) when they are catabolized. This yields lipids and energy in addition to glucose. Most amino acids are exclusively glucogenic.
- **Ketogenic amino acids** yield acetoacetate or one of its precursors, such as acetyl CoA or acetoacetyl CoA, providing lipids and energy. **Leucine and lysine, the two exclusively ketogenic amino acids**, cannot therefore produce glucose or glycogen in the liver or glycogen in muscle.
- Four amino acids are both glucogenic and ketogenic. These include isoleucine, phenylalanine, tryptophan, and tyrosine.

Fig. 2.10 depicts the location at which each amino acid is integrated into the TCA cycle.

Several important disorders arise in patients with deficiencies in the enzymes of amino acid synthesis and degradation pathways, including maple syrup urine disease, albinism, and PKU (Fig. 2.11).

- **PKU** is a common disease of amino acid metabolism that can be effectively treated through changes in diet. **PKU is caused by a deficiency of phenylalanine hydroxylase.** Patients are characterized by a deficiency of tyrosine and elevated phenylalanine. High levels of phenylalanine lead to elevated levels of phenylalanine metabolites such as phenyllactate, phenylacetate, and phenylpyruvate, which give the **body and urine a characteristic "musty" or "mousey" odor.** Clinically, patients with PKU have mental retardation, seizures, tremor, microcephaly, and failure to thrive. Symptoms of mental retardation start by 1 year of age. The first step in the pigment melanin formation is hydroxylation of tyrosine by tyrosinase, which is competitively inhibited by the high levels of phenylalanine in PKU. Because of this, patients with PKU also often have hypopigmentation ("fair hair, blue eyes, light skin color"). Early screening and diagnosis are critical because PKU can be treated by diet. However,

Phenylketonuria is a deficiency of phenylalanine hydroxylase, causing a musty body and urine odor and mental retardation if not treated early with low phenylalanine diet.

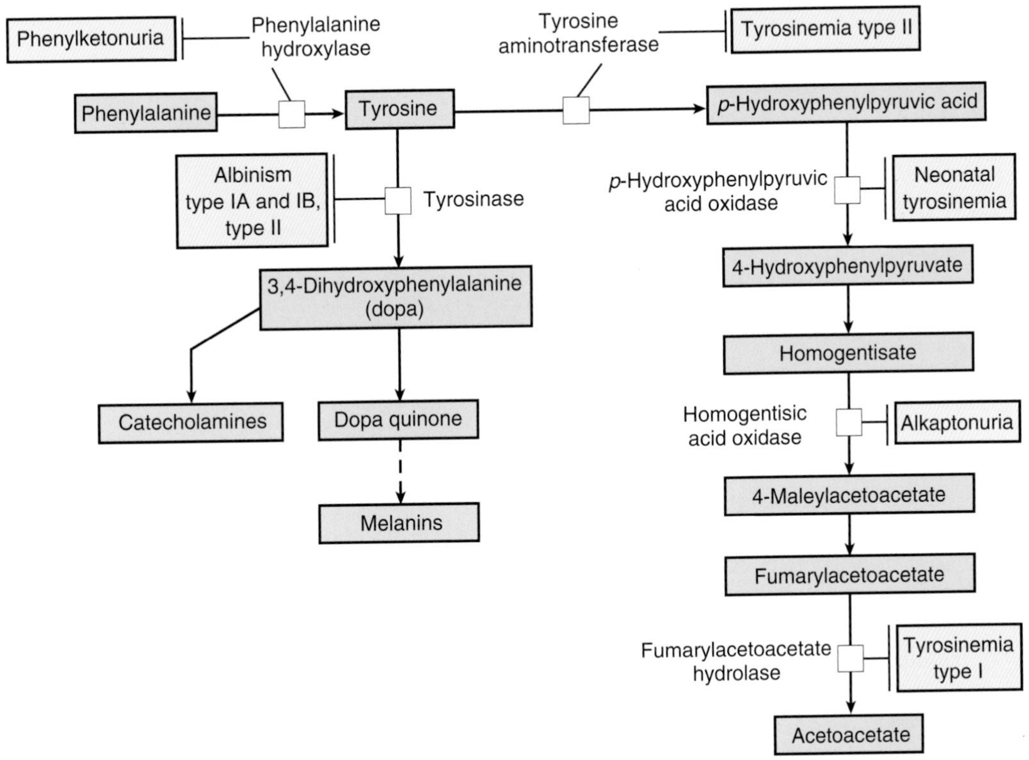

FIG. 2.11 Disorders of amino acid metabolism. *(From Adkison LR, Brown MD.* Elsevier's Integrated Genetics. *Philadelphia: Elsevier; 2007.)*

newborns with PKU may have normal phenylalanine levels at birth owing to maternal transfer; therefore screening tests are typically done at least 1 to 2 days after birth.

- **Albinism** is a group of conditions in which there is **a deficiency in melanin production caused by a defect in tyrosine metabolism**, causing decreased pigmentation of eyes, hair, and skin. The most severe kind of albinism is called complete albinism and is caused by a complete lack of tyrosinase activity.
- Alkaptonuria is a disorder caused by the deficiency of homogentisic acid oxidase, an enzyme in the pathway that degrades tyrosine. This leads to accumulation of homogentisic acid, causing homogentisic aciduria, in which the patient's urine has an elevated level of homogentisic acid. When allowed to stand, the homogentisic acid in the urine is oxidized to a dark pigment. Patients with Alkaptonuria also exhibit arthritis of large joints and black pigmentation of cartilage and collagen. Treatment includes diets low in phenylalanine and tyrosine. Although this is not a life-threatening disorder, arthritis may be severe.

> Alkaptonuria is a deficiency of homogentisic acid oxidase causing arthritis, dark pigmented cartilage, and urine that turns dark when left standing.

- **Maple syrup urine disease** is an autosomal recessive disorder in which there is a deficiency of **branched-chain α-keto acid dehydrogenase.** The inability to oxidatively decarboxylate the branched-chain amino acids **leucine, valine,** and **isoleucine** leads to the buildup of α-ketoisocaproic acid, α-ketoisovaleric acid, and α-keto-β-methyl-valeric acid, respectively. This leads to a buildup of branched-chain α-keto acids in the urine, causing a sweet odor. They also accumulate in the blood, leading to toxic effects on the brain. Typically, symptoms present within a few days of birth and include vomiting, severe metabolic acidosis, and a maple syrup odor to the urine. Treatment is with formula with reduced levels of leucine, valine, and isoleucine. However, branched-chain amino acids are important in growth, so low levels are present in the formula.
- **Homocystinuria** is a group of autosomal recessive disorders caused by abnormal homocysteine metabolism. Patients have high levels of homocysteine and methionine in the urine but a low level of cysteine. One important enzyme involved in homocysteine metabolism, cystathionine β-synthase, is mutated in a common form of homocystinuria. Without cystathionine β-synthetase to convert homocysteine to cystathionine, patients have **ectopia lentis, osteoporosis, and mental retardation, in addition to early vascular disease.** Some patients can improve with treatment with pyridoxine

Table 2.3 Inborn Errors of Amino Acid Metabolism

DISORDER	DEFICIENCY	GENETICS	CLINICAL FEATURES
Phenylketonuria	Phenylalanine hydroxylase	AR	Mental retardation, epilepsy, fair skin, body/urine has a "mousey" odor
Alkaptonuria	Homogentisic acid oxidase	AR	Homogentisic aciduria (dark urine), arthritis, darkly pigmented collagenous tissues
Oculocutaneous albinism	Tyrosinase	AR	Hypopigmentation, vision defects, photophobia, increased skin cancer risk
Homocystinuria	Cystathionine β-synthase	AR	Mental retardation, ectopia lentis (dislocation of lens), thrombosis, skeletal abnormalities
Maple syrup urine disease	Branched-chain β-ketoacid decarboxylase	AR	Mental retardation, metabolic acidosis, urine has a maple syrup odor

AR, Autosomal recessive.

(vitamin B_6), a coenzyme of cystathionine β-synthetase. Treatment of homocystinuria also includes reduced intake of methionine and administration of vitamin supplements.

Other disorders can also arise from genetic mutations in enzymes important in the amino acid metabolism pathways. These include tyrosinemia type I, methylmalonyl CoA mutase deficiency, histidinemia, and cystathioninuria.

A summary of several important hereditary disorders is included in Table 2.3.

Amino Acid Derivatives

In addition to their role in proteins, amino acids are the precursors of many nitrogen-containing molecules such as pyrimidines, purines, heme, neurotransmitters (glycine and glutamate), and other small molecules.

Fig. 2.12 depicts the synthetic pathway of the catecholamines dopamine, norepinephrine, and epinephrine from tyrosine. This synthetic pathway occurs primarily in the CNS, peripheral ganglia, and the adrenal medulla. First, tyrosine is hydroxylated by tyrosine hydroxylase into dopa, a reaction that requires tetrahydrobiopterin (BH_4). Second, dopa is decarboxylated, forming dopamine. Dopamine levels are reduced in Parkinson disease; one treatment for Parkinson disease is L-dopa, the precursor to dopamine. Norepinephrine is formed by hydroxylation of dopamine, and epinephrine is then formed by methylation.

The degradation of catecholamines is shown in Fig. 2.13. **Two enzymes are critical in catecholamine degradation: monoamine oxidase (MAO) and catechol-*O*-methyltransferase (COMT).** Homovanillic acid and vanillylmandelic acid are excreted in the urine. The catecholamine breakdown pathway is important in two different clinical scenarios.

- MAO inhibitors (MAOIs) are a class of medications used to treat depression. MAOIs can inhibit the breakdown of amines in the diet, which can cause hypertensive crisis if an individual taking an MAOI also consumes foods containing the sympathomimetic tyramine, such as cheese.
- Neuroendocrine tumors of the adrenal medulla are known as pheochromocytomas. The tumorous chromaffin cells secrete large amounts of catecholamines, leading to elevated heart rate, elevated blood pressure, and sweating. Diagnosis of pheochromocytoma includes measuring plasma for catecholamines and metanephrines or urine for vanillylmandelic acid (VMA). Neuroblastomas may also produce elevated levels of catecholamines and are tested for in a similar manner.

Consuming tyramine while taking MAOIs can lead to hypertensive emergencies.

Measuring urine VMA and plasma catecholamines/metanephrines can detect pheochromo cytoma and neuroblastomas.

The synthesis and breakdown of serotonin, also called 5-hydroxytryptamine (5-HT), is important in the balance of serotonin in the body (Fig. 2.14). Tryptophan is hydroxylated to form 5-HTP, which is then decarboxylated to form serotonin. Serotonin is degraded by MAO to 5-hydroxyindole acetic acid (5-HIAA). The presence of high levels of 5-HIAA in the urine is diagnostic of cancers that produce large amounts of serotonin (e.g., carcinoid tumors).

Several other important nitrogen-containing molecules synthesized from amino acids.

- Melanin, a pigment, is synthesized from tyrosine in melanocytes.
- Nitrogen oxide (NO), a neurotransmitter, plays a role in macrophage function and relaxes vascular smooth muscle, causing vasodilation. **NO is synthesized from arginine by NO synthase.**

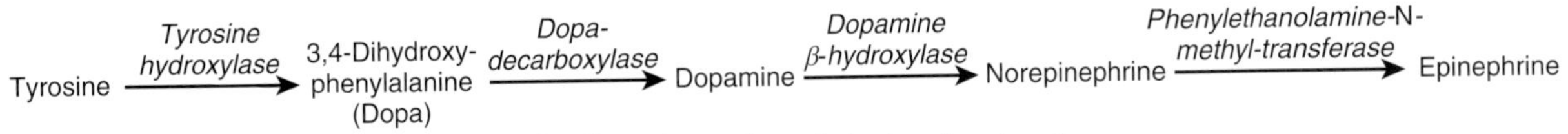

FIG. 2.12 Synthesis of catecholamines from tyrosine.

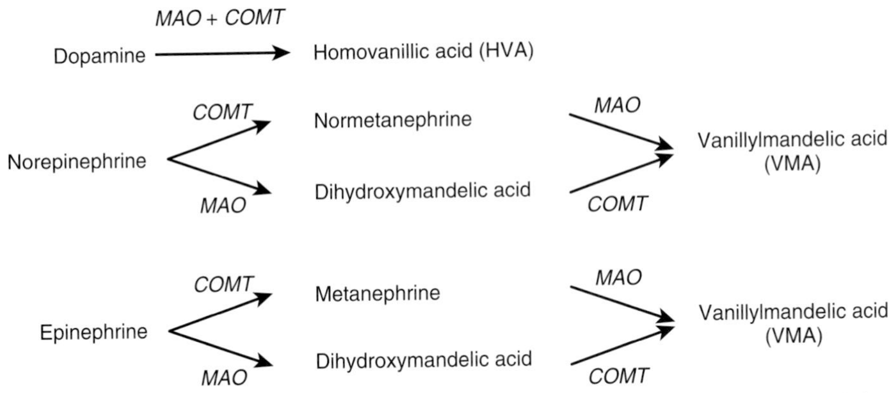

FIG. 2.13 Degradation of catecholamines with major degradation products. COMT, catechol-O-methyltransferase; MAO, monoamine oxidase.

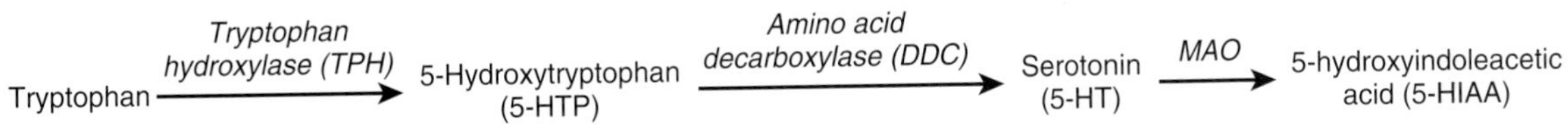

FIG. 2.14 Serotonin synthesis and degradation.

Heme Synthesis and Metabolism

Heme is composed of the tetrapyrrole ring, protoporphyrin IX, with one coordinating ferrous (Fe^{2+}) iron ion in the center. Heme is found not only in hemoglobin and myoglobin but also in cytochromes, catalase, and many other proteins. Heme is synthesized (Fig. 2.15) primarily in the liver (especially cytochrome P-450) and the bone marrow. **The first reaction and the last three reactions occur in the mitochondria, whereas the rest of the reactions occur in the cytosol.** Because reactions occur in the mitochondria, mature RBCs cannot synthesize heme because of their lack of mitochondria. The steps in heme synthesis include the following:

> The first step in heme synthesis is the rate-limiting step. It involves the enzyme ALA synthase.

- First, δ-aminolevulinic acid (ALA) is formed from glycine and succinyl CoA, in a reaction catalyzed by **ALA synthase** and requiring pyridoxal phosphate as a coenzyme. **This is the rate-limiting step of heme synthesis.** Hepatic ALA synthase is inhibited by hemin, a heme molecule with oxidized Fe^{2+} to Fe^{3+} that forms when porphyrin production is higher than its corresponding protein production. However, erythropoietic heme synthesis is instead controlled by erythropoietin and iron levels.
- When drugs that are metabolized by the cytochrome P-450 system are metabolized, there is increased production of cytochrome P-450 enzymes and a decrease in the heme concentration in the liver. This causes upregulation of ALA synthase production and activity.
- In the second step of heme synthesis, porphobilinogen is produced by **ALA dehydrase, an enzyme that is inhibited by lead. Another enzyme, ferrochelatase, is also inhibited by lead.** Thus anemia and elevation in ALA commonly seen in lead poisoning.

Porphyrias are disorders of heme synthesis (Table 2.4) leading to accumulation of heme precursors. (The term *porphyria* means "purple pigment," referring to the purple color of the urine of some patients.) There are two kinds of porphyria: deficiencies in liver heme synthesis, called *hepatic porphyrias;* and deficiencies in bone marrow heme synthesis, called *erythropoietic porphyrias.* In some of these porphyrias, there is photosensitivity caused by accumulation of tetrapyrrole intermediates, which form superoxide free radicals that destroy cellular components upon exposure to ultraviolet light.

> Porphyria cutanea tarda is photosensitivity and red urine caused by uroporphyrinogen decarboxylase deficiency.

- **Porphyria cutanea tarda** is the most common porphyria. It is caused by deficiency in uroporphyrinogen decarboxylase. Photosensitivity is caused by porphyrin accumulation. Urine has a characteristic red-brown color.

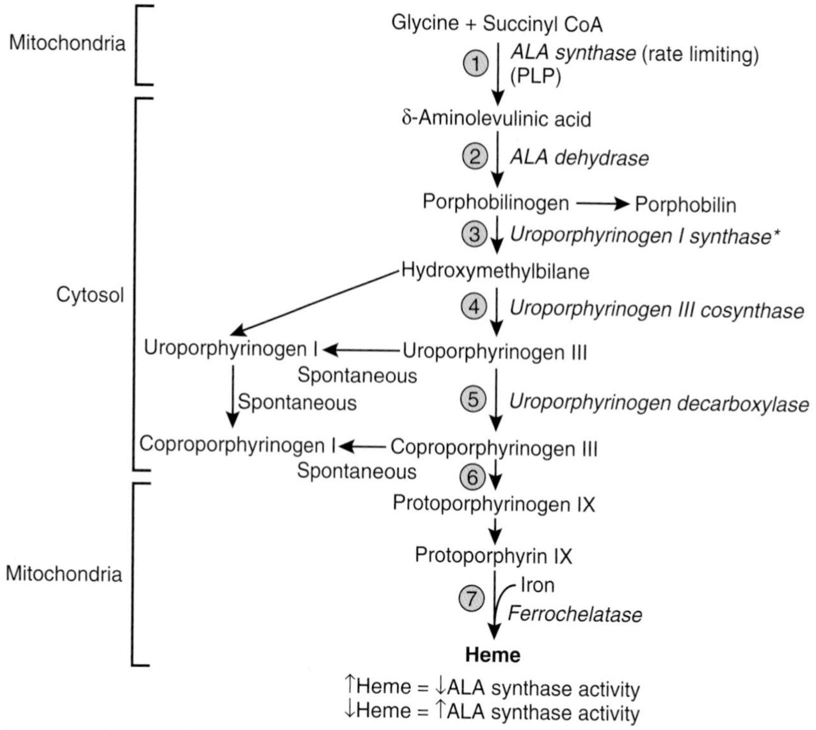

Fig. 2.15 Heme synthesis pathway. ALA, δ-aminolevulinic acid. (*From Pelley JW, Goljan EF.* Rapid Review Biochemistry. *2nd ed. St. Louis: Mosby; 2007, Fig. 8.7.*)

Table 2.4 Inborn Errors of Porphyrin Metabolism

DISORDER	DEFICIENCY	GENETICS	HEPATIC/ ERYTHROPOIETIC	CLINICAL FEATURES
Acute intermittent porphyria (AIP)	Uroporphyrinogen I synthetase	AD	Hepatic	Acute; CNS effects, abdominal pain
Congenital erythropoietic porphyria	Uroporphyrinogen III synthase	AR	Erythropoietic	Hemolytic anemia, photosensitivity
Porphyria cutanea tarda	Uroporphyrinogen decarboxylase	Acquired, AD (20%)	Both (primarily hepatic)	Photosensitivity, red/ brown urine
Hereditary coproporphyria	Coproporphyrinogen oxidase	AD	Hepatic	CNS effects, abdominal pain, photosensitivity
Porphyria variegate	Protoporphyrinogen oxidase	AD	Hepatic	CNS effects, abdominal pain, photosensitivity
Erythropoietic protoporphyria	Ferrochelatase	AD	Erythropoietic	Photosensitivity, liver disease

AD, Autosomal dominant; AR, autosomal recessive; CNS, central nervous system.

- Hepatic porphyrias (acute intermittent porphyria, hereditary coproporphyria, and porphyria variegate) cause acute abdominal pain, psychiatric symptoms, and cardiovascular problems. Drugs that induce cytochrome P-450 synthesis can precipitate attacks of hepatic porphyria because increased cytochrome P-450 synthesis reduces heme, increasing ALA synthase synthesis and thus increasing the accumulation of heme precursors.
- Erythropoietic porphyrias (congenital erythropoietic porphyria and erythropoietic protoporphyria) present with photosensitivity, blisters, and urine that changes to a red-brown color.

Heme degradation occurs in the spleen by macrophages and in the liver by hepatocytes. Within macrophages, hemoglobin and cytochromes are digested into heme, which is converted into biliverdin, a green pigment, by heme oxygenase. Biliverdin is reduced, forming bilirubin, a yellow pigment. Because bilirubin is relatively insoluble in plasma, bilirubin is bound to albumin for transport in the blood to the liver. Upon arrival in hepatocytes in the liver, bilirubin becomes bilirubin glucuronide (conjugated bilirubin) using the enzyme bilirubin glucuronyltransferase, an enzyme that is deficient in patients with Crigler-Najjar and Gilbert syndromes. The conjugated bilirubin is secreted into bile and transported to the intestine, where it is oxidized into stercobilin and excreted (brown pigment in feces), converted into urobilin and excreted in urine (yellow pigment in urine), or enters the entero-hepatic urobilinogen cycle.

NUCLEIC ACID STRUCTURE AND FUNCTION

Nucleic Acid Structure

Nucleic acids include DNA (deoxyribonucleic acid) and RNA (ribonucleic acid). Nucleic acids are assembled from nucleotides, which are composed of a 5-carbon sugar, a nitrogenous base, and one to three phosphate groups. The sugar can be ribose (RNA) or deoxyribose (DNA). The nitrogen-containing base may be a purine (adenine or guanine) or a pyrimidine (cytosine, thymidine, or uracil). Thymine is specific for DNA, whereas uracil is specific for RNA. DNA has several structural forms; the B form is active DNA, whereas the Z form is inactive.

Purine Metabolism

Purine nucleotides are synthesized *de novo* from several compounds, including CO_2, glycine, glutamine, aspartate, and N^{10}-formyl tetrahydrofolate. The synthesis of purines is an 11-step process (Fig. 2.16A) The first step is synthesis of PRPP (5-phosphoribosyl-1-pyrophosphate) from adenosine triphosphate (ATP) and ribose-5-phosphate, a reaction catalyzed by PRPP synthetase. The second step is the regulated step of purine synthesis, using the enzyme **glutamine phosphoribosyl pyrophosphate aminotransferase**. The next nine steps lead to the synthesis of IMP (inosine 5′-monophosphate). Two of these steps require N^{10}-formyl tetrahydrofolate. Several drugs target the purine synthesis pathway by inhibiting the formation of tetrahydrofolate (THF). Inhibition of purine synthesis leads to a lack of DNA synthesis, resulting in inhibition of cell growth and division (Fig. 2.16B).

Adenosine deaminase deficiency (severe combined immunodeficiency [SCID]), gout, and Lesch-Nyhan syndrome all arise from defects in purine salvage or purine degradation pathways.

The next steps in purine synthesis involve formation of adenosine monophosphate (AMP) or guanosine monophosphate (GMP) from IMP. **Mycophenolic acid**, an immunosuppressive drug used to prevent organ transplant rejection, **is an inhibitor of IMP dehydrogenase, the first reaction to convert IMP to GMP**. This reduces the proliferation of T and B cells, which are dependent on the *de novo* pathway of purine synthesis, resulting in mycophenolic acid's immunosuppressive effects. The final step in production of purines is synthesis of nucleoside diphosphates from nucleoside monophosphates using nucleoside monophosphate kinases.

Mycophenolic acid is an immunosuppressive drug. It inhibits IMP dehydrogenase thus reducing IMP→GMP conversion. This reduces T and B cell proliferation.

- **Sulfonamides are analogs of paraaminobenzoic acid (PABA) and competitively inhibit the synthesis of folic acid by bacteria.** This inhibits the synthesis of THF, which slows the purine synthesis pathway in microorganisms, leading to antibacterial effects. Humans do not synthesize folic acid, but instead obtain it from the diet, so sulfonamides affect only bacterial purine synthesis.
- **Methotrexate and trimethoprim inhibit dihydrofolate reductase.** The inhibition of dihydrofolate reductase inhibits growth of cancer cells (in the case of methotrexate) and bacterial growth (for trimethoprim, a specific inhibitor of *bacterial* dihydrofolate reductase) because these drugs inhibit synthesis of THF and slow the purine synthesis pathway. However, methotrexate has toxicity for all dividing cells, including cells in the bone marrow, skin, immune system, and gastrointestinal tract, leading to numerous drug side effects.

Methotrexate and trimethoprim inhibit dihydrofolate reductase.

Another pathway to obtain purines is the **purine salvage pathway**, in which purines from the diet or cellular breakdown can be recycled. Hypoxanthine and guanine are converted to IMP and GMP, respectively, by the enzyme hypoxanthine guanine phosphoribosyltransferase (HGPRT). **Lesch-Nyhan syndrome is an X-linked recessive disorder in which there is a deficiency of HGPRT.** These patients are unable to salvage guanine or hypoxanthine using the purine salvage pathway; this leads to increased PRPP and an increase in *de novo* purine synthesis. This then leads to increased purine turnover and hyperuricemia. Patients with Lesch-Nyhan syndrome present at an early age with neurologic features such as self-mutilation, spasticity, and cognitive defects. Orange uric acid crystals can be found in their diapers. Although there is no cure, treatment with allopurinol can decrease the hyperuricemia, but it does not alter the neurologic symptoms.

Lesch-Nyhan syndrome is an X-linked deficiency of HGPRT causing elevated PRPP, self-mutilation, cognitive defects, and uric acid crystals in their urine.

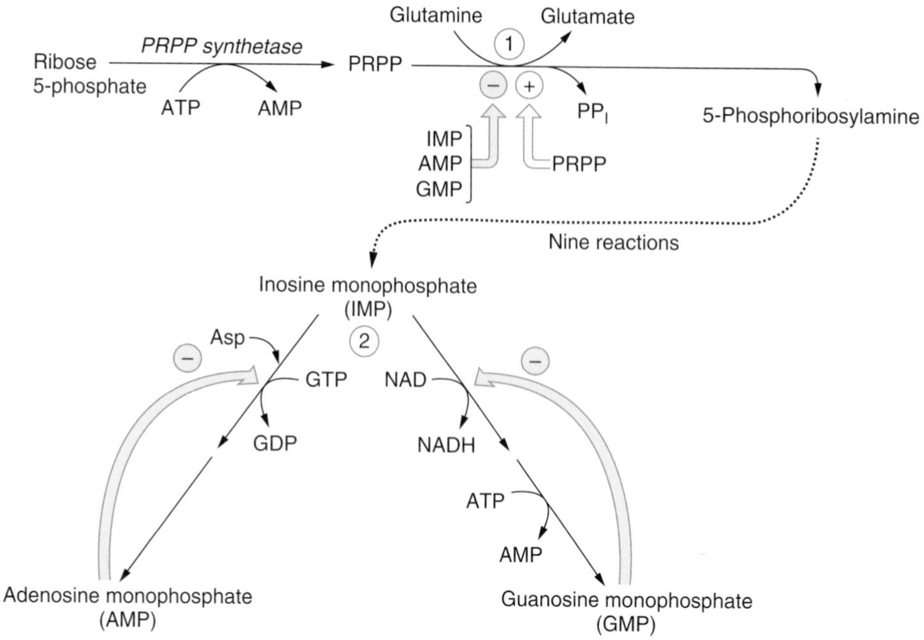

A

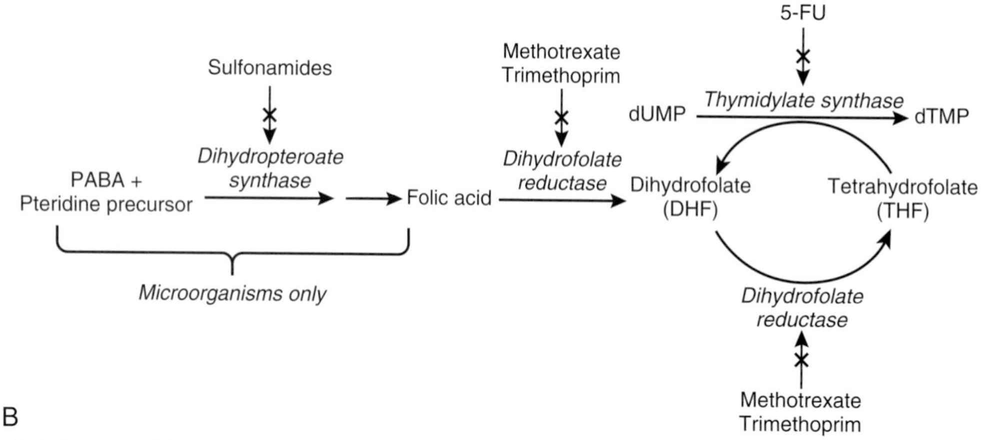

B

FIG. 2.16 A, Simplification of the purine synthesis pathway. **B,** Folate synthesis and inhibitors. 5-FU, 5-fluorouracil; dTMP, thymidine-5′-phosphate; dUMP, deoxyuridine monophosphate; PABA, paraaminobenzoic acid. (**A,** *from Pelley JW, Goljan EF.* Rapid Review Biochemistry. *3rd ed. Philadelphia: Elsevier; 2010.*)

Purines are degraded into uric acid, which is excreted in the urine. **Xanthine oxidase converts hypoxanthine to xanthine, and then converts xanthine to uric acid.** Two diseases are closely associated with degradation of purines.

❍ **Gout occurs when there are high levels of uric acid in the blood (hyperuricemia),** because of either overproduction or underexcretion of uric acid. Monosodium urate crystals deposit in the joints, leading to inflammatory arthritis. Most patients with gout underexcrete uric acid. These patients are treated with uricosuric drugs, such as probenecid or sulfinpyrazone, which help to increase the amount of uric acid that is excreted. Patients with gout that overproduce uric acid are treated with **allopurinol, an inhibitor of xanthine oxidase.** This leads to an increase in hypoxanthine and xanthine, which are more soluble than uric acid and do not form crystal deposits. For both kinds of patients, acute gout attacks are treated with antiinflammatory drugs, including nonsteroidal antiinflammatory drugs (NSAIDs) and colchicine. Colchicine stops the polymerization of microtubules, which inhibits migration of neutrophils into the inflamed area.

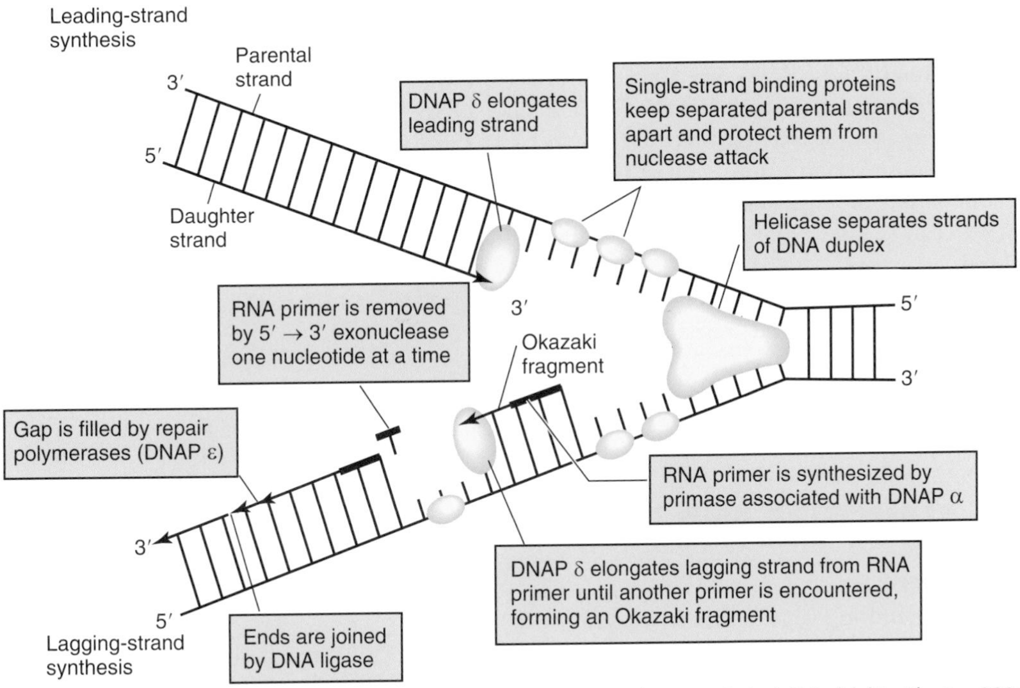
Leading-strand synthesis
Parental strand
3′
5′
Daughter strand
DNAP δ elongates leading strand
Single-strand binding proteins keep separated parental strands apart and protect them from nuclease attack
Helicase separates strands of DNA duplex
RNA primer is removed by 5′ → 3′ exonuclease one nucleotide at a time
3′
Okazaki fragment
5′
3′
Gap is filled by repair polymerases (DNAP ε)
RNA primer is synthesized by primase associated with DNAP α
3′
DNAP δ elongates lagging strand from RNA primer until another primer is encountered, forming an Okazaki fragment
5′
Lagging-strand synthesis
Ends are joined by DNA ligase

Fig. 2.17 DNA replication. (*From Pelley JW, Goljan EF.* Rapid Review Biochemistry. *3rd ed. Philadelphia: Elsevier; 2010.*)

- **Adenosine deaminase (ADA) deficiency** can lead to a form of SCID. The accumulation of adenosine inhibits ribonuclease reductase, preventing production of DNA and thereby the proliferation of lymphocytes. Patients with the most severe form have deficiencies in T cells, B cells, and NK cells.

Pyrimidine Synthesis

The first step in pyrimidine synthesis is the formation of carbamoyl phosphate (CAP) by carbamoyl phosphate synthetase II. This is the regulated step of pyrimidine synthesis. After several more steps, uridine 5′-monophosphate (UMP) is synthesized. UMP can then be converted into the pyrimidines thymidine monophosphate (TMP, also known as thymidylate), uridine triphosphate (UTP), and cytidine triphosphate (CTP). **Deficiency of UMP synthase** (which is a bifunctional enzyme composed of both orotidine phosphate decarboxylase and orotate phosphoribosyltransferase) **causes orotic aciduria.** Patients have severe anemia, poor growth, and orotate excreted in the urine. Treatment involves feeding synthetic uridine to supply the pyrimidine nucleotides that are needed for DNA and RNA synthesis.

DNA Replication

DNA replication begins at the replication fork, where helicases help to separate the strands of DNA (Fig. 2.17). Topoisomerases act to remove supercoiled structures that are formed by this process. Several anticancer agents, such as etoposide, inhibit topoisomerase II. Primase adds an RNA primer for DNA synthesis. DNA polymerases (DNAP) synthesize DNA in the 5′ → 3′ direction. Two daughter strands are formed: one leading strand, synthesized continuously in the 5′ → 3′ direction toward the replication fork; and one lagging strand, synthesized discontinuously in the 5′ →3′ direction away from the replication fork using short DNA fragments called Okazaki fragments.

DNA Repair

DNA may need repair because of environmental damage, such as ultraviolet (UV) light or chemicals; mistakes in DNA synthesis; or spontaneous loss of bases. Cells have three principal mechanisms to counteract single-stranded DNA damage.

- In **DNA mismatch repair (MMR),** mismatches in daughter DNA strands compared with the parent DNA are removed by an exonuclease and correctly filled in by a DNA polymerase. **Hereditary nonpolyposis colorectal cancer (HNPCC) is caused by defects in mismatch repair, most commonly in the *MSH2* gene,** and leads to an increased risk for colon and other types of cancer.

Hereditary nonpolyposis colorectal cancer is caused by a defect in mismatch repair and increases the risk for colon cancer.

- **Nucleotide excision repair (NER)** is used to correct errors created by UV radiation damage. UV light can cause DNA damage by covalent joining of two thymines that are next to each other, creating a **thymine dimer.** In NER, UV-specific endonucleases cut one side of the double helix, and then DNA polymerases synthesize a new DNA strand. DNA polymerase has an exonuclease activity, which excises the damaged strand from 5′ to 3′. Finally, DNA ligase joins the ends together. **Xeroderma pigmentosum is an autosomal recessive disorder that results from defective nucleotide excision repair caused by a mutant UV-specific endonuclease.** This leads to high rates of skin cancer after exposure to UV light, including melanoma, squamous cell carcinoma, and basal cell carcinoma.
- In **base excision repair (BER)**, altered bases are recognized by DNA glycosylases and cleaved from the DNA backbone, and several other enzymes assist in repair of the site.

Other diseases such as ataxia-telangiectasia, Fanconi syndrome, and Bloom syndrome are also associated with defects in DNA repair.

CARBOHYDRATE STRUCTURE AND METABOLISM

Carbohydrate Structure

Glucose oxidation provides much of the energy needed by cells in the fed state.

- **Monosaccharides** are classified as either **aldoses** (aldehydes) or **ketoses** (ketones). Although most sugars can exist as either D or L form optical isomers, most human sugars are D form. The general formula for monosaccharides is $(CH_2O)_x$, with the number of carbons being key. Triose sugars have 3 carbons; tetrose have 4 carbons; pentose/furanose have 5 carbons (ribose, fructose, deoxyribose); hexose have 6 carbons (glucose, galactose, fructose).
- Monosaccharides can link together through condensation reactions to form disaccharides and oligosaccharides. The bond linking sugars is called a **glycosidic bond**, which can be either α or β.
  - Maltose = glucose + glucose
  - Lactose = glucose + galactose
  - Sucrose = glucose + fructose
- Polysaccharides can be linear, such as amylose, or branched, such as glycogen. Starch is the primary glucose storage molecule in plants. Starch can be broken down by humans using amylase. Starch has two components: amylose (linear, α-1,4 linkages) and amylopectin (branched, α-1,4 linkages and α-1,6 linkages). Glycogen is the main way that animals store glucose. The linkages are α-glycosidic (branched, α-1,4 and α-1,6). Each glycogen has one reducing end and many nonreducing ends. Glycogen is produced by the liver and muscle from excess glucose.
- Cellulose **is an insoluble fiber** because it has **β-1,4 linkages** and humans only have enzymes that cleave α-glycosidic bonds, such as those contained in starch.

Sorbitol, a derivative of glucose, is osmotically active and causes formation of cataracts (lens damage), peripheral neuropathy (Schwann cell), and retinopathy (pericytes); these are associated with DM. This occurs through aldose reductase.

TCA steps: In the fasted state, citrate is the starting substrate for making oxaloacetate-citrate, isocitrate, ketoglutarate, succinyl CoA, fumarate, malate, and oxaloacetate.

Glycolysis

Glycolysis involves the oxidation of glucose and occurs in the **cytosol of all cells**. Glycolysis can be either aerobic or anaerobic.

- In aerobic glycolysis (with oxygen), glucose is oxidized to pyruvate. The pyruvate and NADH created in aerobic glycolysis can be used by the citric acid cycle and the mitochondrial electron transport system to generate 36 to 38 ATP molecules by oxidative phosphorylation.

In anaerobic glycolysis (without oxygen), glucose is oxidized to lactate. Lactate dehydrogenase converts pyruvate to lactate, forming 2 ATP molecules per glucose molecule and reoxidizing NADH to NAD^+. Anaerobic glycolysis occurs in anoxic tissues, red blood cells, and skeletal muscle during intense exercise.

There are nine steps in glycolysis. Three regulated enzymes catalyze irreversible reactions in glycolysis: hexokinase, phosphofructokinase, and pyruvate kinase (PK). The first step in glycolysis (Step 1, Fig. 2.18) is phosphorylation of glucose into glucose-6-phosphate by either hexokinase or glucokinase.

Phosphorylation of glucose into glucose-6-phosphate traps glucose inside cells.

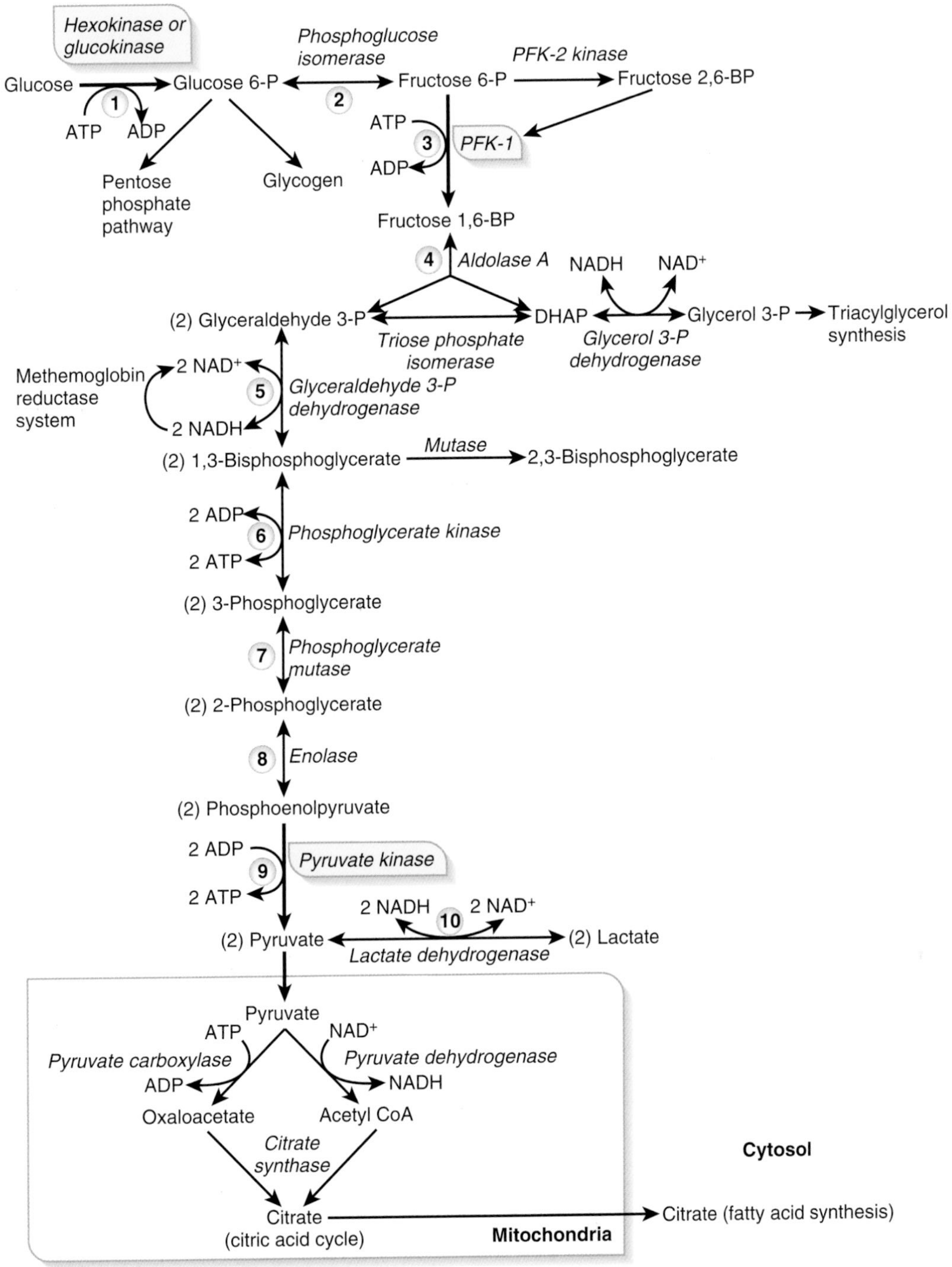

FIG. 2.18 Glycolysis pathway. ADP, adenosine diphosphate; ATP, adenosine triphosphate; CoA, coenzyme A; DHAP, dihydroxyacetone phosphate; PFK, phosphofructokinase. (*From Pelley JW, Goljan EF.* Rapid Review Biochemistry. *3rd ed. Philadelphia: Elsevier; 2010.*)

Phosphorylation traps glucose inside cells because phosphate is negatively charged and charged compounds cannot easily cross cell membranes, and there is no specific transporter for glucose-6-phosphate.

- Hexokinase is found in the cytosol of most tissues. Hexokinase has a low K_m (high affinity for glucose), ensuring that hexokinase is saturated at normal blood glucose concentrations. Hexokinase is not specific for glucose and can catalyze the phosphorylation of many different hexoses. Hexokinase is also inhibited by glucose-6-phosphate, which prevents too much glycolysis occurring and cells accumulating too much glucose.

- Glucokinase is present in the liver and beta cells of the pancreas. In contrast to hexokinase, glucokinase has a high K_m (low affinity for glucose), meaning that glucokinase is not saturated at normal blood glucose concentrations, but instead is able to act as a glucose sensor for the liver and beta cells to maintain glucose homeostasis. Glucokinase is highly specific for glucose. Glucokinase is inhibited by fructose-6-phosphate, which prevents glucose from being phosphorylated faster than it is metabolized.

The rate-limiting step of glycolysis is the phosphorylation of fructose-6-phosphate by phosphofructokinase-1 (PFK-1) (Step 3, see Fig. 2.18). Fructose 2,6-bisphosphate strongly activates PFK-1. Fructose 2,6-bisphosphate is created by phosphofructokinase-2 (PFK-2), a bifunctional enzyme that can either produce fructose 2,6-bisphosphate using kinase activity or produce fructose-6-phosphate using phosphatase activity. After a meal, insulin levels increase and glucagon levels decrease; this causes an increase in fructose 2,6-bisphosphate, activating PFK-1 and increasing the rate of glycolysis when glucose is plentiful. In contrast, in the fasting state, there is a decrease in fructose 2,6-bisphosphate, leading to a decrease in the rate of glycolysis.

The rate-limiting step of glycolysis is the phosphorylation of fructose-6-phosphate by PFK-1.

The final irreversible reaction of glycolysis is formation of pyruvate from phosphoenolpyruvate, which is catalyzed by pyruvate kinase (Step 9, see Fig. 2.18). **A mutation in pyruvate kinase causes hemolytic anemia.** When pyruvate kinase is mutated, the ATP generated by anaerobic glycolysis necessary for red blood cell function is not made, causing red blood cells to die prematurely and resulting in hemolytic anemia.

The final irreversible reaction of glycolysis is formation of pyruvate from phosphoenolpyruvate, which is catalyzed by pyruvate kinase.

Gluconeogenesis

Gluconeogenesis, the process by which glucose is synthesized, **occurs primarily in the liver and kidneys.** The carbon sources for the synthesis of glucose is from small precursors, including pyruvate, lactate, glycerol, and glucogenic amino acids. The glucose released from gluconeogenesis is released into the bloodstream. Gluconeogenesis is composed of the reversible reactions of glycolysis as well as several reactions specific to gluconeogenesis that bypass the irreversible reactions of glycolysis: (1) conversion of pyruvate to phosphoenolpyruvate (PEP), which bypasses pyruvate kinase; (2) conversion of fructose 1,6-bisphosphate to fructose-6-phosphate, which bypasses phosphofructokinase; and (3) conversion of glucose-6-phosphate to glucose, which bypasses hexokinase.

To convert pyruvate to PEP, pyruvate is first carboxylated to oxaloacetate by **pyruvate carboxylase.** In a second reaction, oxaloacetate is converted to PEP by **PEP-carboxykinase** (PEP-CK).

- Fructose 1,6-bisphosphate is converted to fructose-6-phosphate by **fructose-1,6-bisphosphatase.** Fructose 1,6-bisphosphatase is inhibited by fructose-2,6-bisphosphate, a molecule that activates PFK-1 in glycolysis. This ensures that both pathways are not active at the same time.
- Glucose-6-phosphate is converted to glucose by **glucose-6-phosphatase.** This enzyme is also essential for the last steps of glycogenolysis, and a deficiency of glucose-6-phosphatase leads to type 1a glycogen storage disease (Von Gierke disease). There is hypoglycemia in this disorder because the patients are unable to produce glucose by glycogenolysis or gluconeogenesis.

Von Gierke disease is a glycogen storage disease from glucose-6-phosphatase deficiency. Hypoglycemia occurs because of an inability to perform glycogenolysis or gluconeogenesis.

Glycogen Synthesis and Degradation

Glycogen, a polysaccharide, is the way that the body stores glucose in a form that can be rapidly mobilized to maintain glucose homeostasis and to serve as fuel for muscles. Glycogen is stored primarily in liver and muscle tissue, but small amounts are present in most cells.

Glycogenesis is the production of glycogen and occurs in the cytosol. The substrate for glycogenesis is uridine diphosphate (UDP) glucose. **Glycogen synthase** adds to the nonreducing ends of chains in $\alpha(1\rightarrow4)$ linkages. Branches with $\alpha(1\rightarrow6)$ linkages are created by a branching enzyme, amylo-$\alpha(1\rightarrow4)\rightarrow(1\rightarrow6)$-transglucosidase. Glycogenesis is stimulated by insulin and inhibited by glucagon and epinephrine.

Glycogenolysis is the breakdown of glycogen and also occurs in the cytosol. First, glycogen phosphorylase cleaves $\alpha(1\rightarrow4)$ glycosidic bonds between individual glucosyl residues' nonreducing ends, forming glucose-1-phosphate. Next, glucose-1-phosphate is converted to glucose-6-phosphate by phosphoglucomutase. Glucose-6-phosphatase can then convert the glucose-6-phosphate into glucose. The debranching enzyme releases free glucose from $\alpha(1 \rightarrow 6)$ bonds at the branch points. Glucagon stimulates glycogenolysis, while insulin inhibits glycogenolysis.

Table 2.5 Glycogen Storage Diseases

GLYCOGEN STORAGE DISEASE	DEFICIENCY	GLYCOGEN IN AFFECTED CELLS	GENETICS	CLINICAL FEATURES
Von Gierke (type I)	Glucose-6-phosphatase	Increased amount, but normal structure	AR	Hepatomegaly, hypoglycemia
Pompe (type II)	α-1,4-Glucosidase	Increased amount, but normal structure	AR	Cardiac and respiratory failure, early death
Cori (type III)	Debranching enzyme	Increased amount, short branches	AR	Similar to Von Gierke, but milder symptoms
Anderson (type IV)	Branching enzyme	Increased amount, long branches	AR	Liver cirrhosis, early death
McArdle (type V)	Phosphorylase	Small increase in amount, but normal structure	AR	Muscle cramps with exercise
Hers (type VI)	Phosphorylase	Increased amount	AR	Similar to Von Gierke, but milder symptoms

AR, Autosomal recessive.

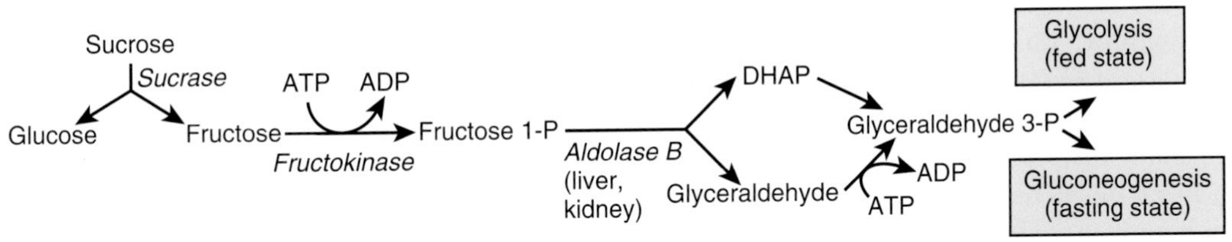

Fig. 2.19 Breakdown of sucrose. ADP, adenosine diphosphate; ATP, adenosine triphosphate; DHAP, dihydroxyacetone phosphate. (*From Pelley JW, Goljan EF.* Rapid Review Biochemistry. *3rd ed. Philadelphia: Elsevier; 2010.*)

Glycogen Storage Diseases

Several inherited deficiencies of glycogen metabolism lead to glycogen storage diseases (Table 2.5).

Metabolism of Sugars

Lactase metabolizes lactose to glucose and galactose. Galactokinase converts galactose to galactose-1-phosphate. In several reactions, galactose-1-phosphate becomes glucose-1-phosphate. **Lactase deficiency** leads to milk intolerance and causes bloating and diarrhea after ingestion of lactose-containing products. **Galactokinase deficiency causes a mild galactosemia,** leading to galactitol accumulation and cataracts formation. **Galactose-1-phosphate uridyl transferase deficiency causes severe galactosemia,** resulting in failure to thrive, mental retardation, liver dysfunction, cataracts, and susceptibility to infection.

Sucrase converts sucrose to glucose and fructose (Fig. 2.19). Note that hexokinase can convert fructose to fructose-6-phosphate by phosphorylation in the liver and kidney. **Fructokinase deficiency leads to essential fructosuria,** which is a benign disorder. However, **fructose-1-phosphate aldolase deficiency leads to hereditary fructose intolerance.** This causes severe hypoglycemia after ingesting fructose or sucrose.

Fructokinase deficiency leads to essential fructosuria, a benign disorder. Fructose 1-phosphate aldolase deficiency leads to hereditary fructose intolerance: hypoglycemia after ingesting fructose/sucrose.

Pentose Phosphate Pathway

The pentose phosphate pathway can be used either for glycolysis or for oxidation of glucose. The oxidative processes, which are irreversible, generate NADPH needed for pathways such as the synthesis of fatty acids and cholesterol. The nonoxidative processes, which are reversible, rearrange sugars so that they can enter glycolytic pathways. Additionally, ribose-5-phosphate can be formed by the pentose phosphate pathways and used for synthesis of nucleotides. G6PD is an enzyme of the pentose phosphate pathway that provides a key regulatory role. **Patients with G6PD deficiency, an X-linked recessive disorder, are unable to effectively produce NADPH through the pentose phosphate pathway.** This prevents cells from maintaining reduced glutathione, which results in increased oxidative stress on cells, particularly erythrocytes, leading to **hemolytic anemia.** Some patients with G6PD deficiency only develop anemia when they experience oxidative stress, such as by taking oxidant drugs (sulfamethoxazole, primaquine), eating fava beans, or infection.

TCA Cycle

The tricarboxylic acid (TCA) cycle (Fig. 2.20), also known as the citric acid cycle or the Krebs cycle, occurs in the mitochondria. Red blood cells do not have mitochondria. The pyruvate produced from glycolysis becomes acetyl coenzyme A (acetyl CoA) through the enzyme pyruvate dehydrogenase. Fatty acids can also yield acetyl CoA by beta oxidation. The TCA cycle begins when oxaloacetate condenses with acetyl CoA to form citrate. For one pass through the TCA cycle, oxaloacetate is regenerated, two moles of CO_2 are released, 1 guanosine triphosphate (GTP) is produced, and 11 molecules of ATP are produced by oxidative phosphorylation.

Glycolysis occurs in the cytosol. The TCA cycle occurs in the mitochondria.

Electron Transport and Oxidative Phosphorylation

The chemiosmotic hypothesis describes the coupling of the electron transport chain to the synthesis of ATP through flow of electrons. As electrons are pumped through the complexes of the electron transport system, hydrogen ions are pumped into the intermembrane space of mitochondria. This forms a **proton-motive force** from a pH and electrical potential gradient across the mitochondrial membrane. Hydrogen ions passing through ATP synthase down their concentration gradient drive the formation of ATP through ATP synthase.

Cyanide blocks the electron transport chain preventing the cell from forming ATP.

Uncoupling agents carry hydrogen ions across the inner mitochondrial membrane without transport through ATP synthase. This uncouples flow of electrons and ATP synthesis. This leads to energy dissipated as heat instead of synthesis of ATP. Uncoupling proteins play an important role in animals that hibernate, where stored energy generates heat. In newborn mammals, brown fat has thermogenin, which is an uncoupling protein. This allows energy to dissipate as heat. However, in humans, uncoupling agents such as 2,4-dinitrophenol (taken in the past for weight reduction) are poisonous.

Several compounds inhibit flow of electrons through the electron transport chain, including cyanide, carbon monoxide, hydrogen sulfide, and amobarbital.

LIPID STRUCTURE AND METABOLISM

Lipid Structure

Fatty acids are the building blocks of lipids (Fig. 2.21). Fatty acids are oxidized in the fasting state to provide energy to cells. Two fatty acids must be supplied in the diet: linoleic and α-linolenic acid. Fatty acids are made up of an unbranched hydrocarbon chain with a terminal carboxyl group. Most fatty acids have an even number of carbon atoms and 16 to 20 total carbons.

Essential fatty acids are linoleic and α-linolenic acid.

- Short-chain fatty acids have 2 to 4 carbons, and medium-chain fatty acids have 6 to 10 carbons. They can be directly absorbed in the small intestine. They can also diffuse into the mitochondrial matrix and be oxidized directly.
- Long-chain fatty acids have 12 or more carbons. They are in triacylglycerols (fat). To move from the cytosol into the mitochondria, they require the carnitine shuttle.

Unsaturated fatty acids have at least one double bond, most commonly *cis* (rather than *trans*) configuration. *Trans* fatty acids are formed during the production of hydrogenated vegetable oils and have been associated with an increase in atherosclerosis.

Triacylglycerols are formed by esterification of fatty acids with glycerol. These have 9 kcal/g and are stored in adipose tissues.

Steroids are a kind of lipid with a four-membered ring structure and a hydroxyl or keto group on the third carbon. There are five major groups of steroids:

- Cholesterol (27 carbons): the most abundant steroid in humans, important in cellular membrane fluidity, precursor of steroid hormones, skin-derived vitamin D, and bile acids
- Bile acids (24 carbons): includes cholic acid
- Progesterone and adrenocortical steroids (21 C)
- Androgens (19 carbons)
- Estrogens (18 carbons): derived from aromatization of androgens

Cholesterol aids in membrane fluidity and is a precursor of steroid hormones and bile acids.

Cholesterol synthesis is regulated by 3-hydroxy 3-methylglutaryl (HMG) CoA reductase, and a key intermediate in cholesterol synthesis is HMG CoA. Statins are HMG-CoA reductase inhibitors.

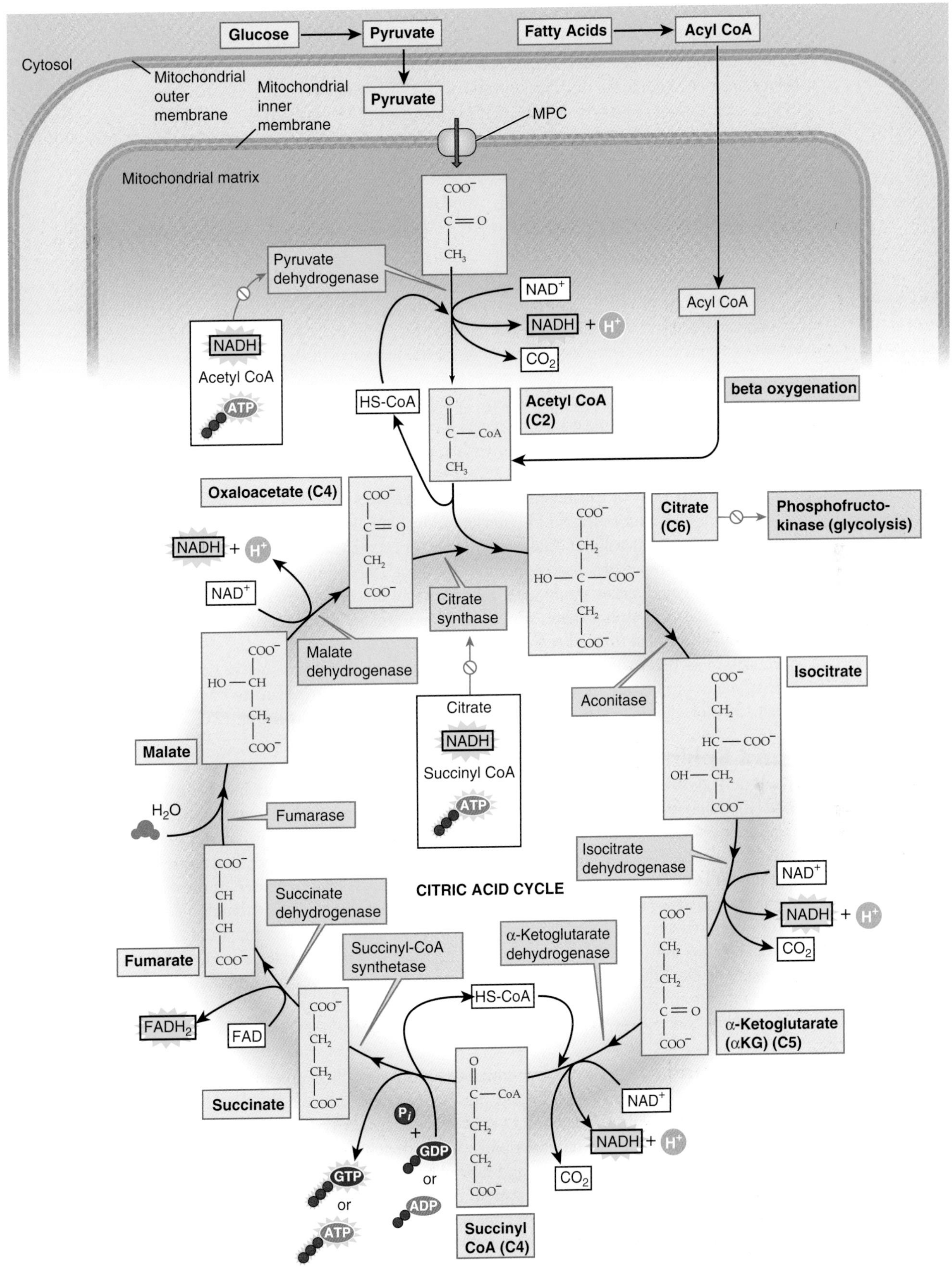

Fig. 2.20 Tricarboxylic acid cycle. ADP, adenosine diphosphate; ATP, adenosine triphosphate; CoA, coenzyme A; GDP, guanosine diphosphate; GTP, guanosine triphosphate; MPC, mitochondrial pyruvate carrier. (*From Boron WF, Boulpaep EL.* Medical Physiology. *2nd ed. Philadelphia: Elsevier; 2008.*)

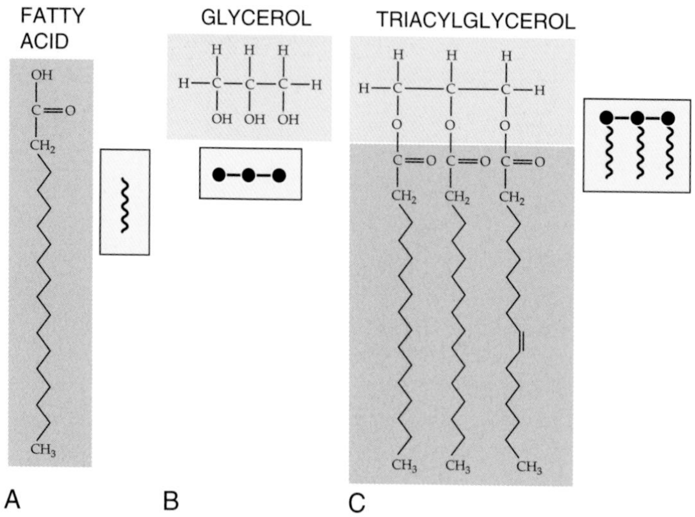

FIG. 2.21 Structure of **(A)** fatty acids, **(B)** 2-monoacylglycerol, and **(C)** triacylglycerol. (*From Boron WF, Boulpaep EL. Medical Physiology. 2nd ed. Philadelphia: Elsevier; 2008.*)

Phospholipids are a major component of cell membranes and are created from phosphatidic acid (diacylglycerol + phosphate group on C3). Phospholipids are cleaved by phospholipases. Phospholipase A1 and A2 remove fatty acyl groups. Phospholipase A2 in cell membranes is activated by cytosolic Ca^{2+}, which causes damage to cell membranes when tissues undergo hypoxia. Phospholipase A2 is inactivated by corticosteroids, reducing the release of arachidonic acid. Phospholipase C frees its component compounds, diacylglycerol and inositol triphosphate, which are important in intracellular signaling. Phospholipase D makes phosphatidic acid from phospholipids.

Lung surfactant is important in decreasing the surface tension in alveoli. It is particularly rich in phosphatidylcholines. Insufficient production of lung surfactant by premature infants leads to respiratory distress syndrome, which is characterized by poor gas exchange and partial lung collapse.

Sphingolipids and Sphingolipid Storage Diseases

Sphingolipids are derived from ceramide, a molecule that is formed by coupling a fatty acid and sphingosine (sphingosine + fatty acids = ceramide). Sphingolipids are essential components of membranes throughout the body and are particularly abundant in nervous tissue, especially in the white matter of the CNS. Lysosomal enzymes degrade sphingolipids to sphingosine using several hydrolytic reactions. Sphingolipidoses are a group of hereditary lysosomal enzyme deficiency diseases in which one of these hydrolytic enzymes in the degradative pathway is deficient (Table 2.6). Deficiencies of sphingolipid-degrading enzymes in lysosomes (lysosomes contain hydrolytic enzymes) lead to the accumulation of the substrate in lysosomes and thus to lysosomal storage diseases. In most of these diseases, neurologic deterioration and early death occur. Also note that Fabry disease is X-linked recessive rather than autosomal recessive.

> Fabry disease is X-linked recessive, whereas other sphingolipidoses are autosomal recessive.

Eicosanoids

Eicosanoids (icosanoids) are important short-range (autocrine/paracrine) signaling molecules that are formed by oxidation of 20-carbon essential fatty acids by phospholipase A2, including eicosapentaenoic acid (an omega-3 fatty acid) and arachidonic acid (an omega-6 fatty acid, synthesized from the essential fatty acid linoleic acid). There are four subtypes of eicosanoids: leukotrienes (LTs) and three types of prostanoids—prostaglandins (PG), prostacyclins (PGI), and thromboxanes (TX).

LTs are noncyclic. They are synthesized by hydroxylation of arachidonic acid by lipoxygenase. Leukotriene B_4 (LTB_4) is an important chemotactic agent for neutrophils, and also increases neutrophil adhesion. LTC_4, LTD_4, and LTE_4 are known as *slow-reacting substance of anaphylaxis* and increase bronchoconstriction, vasoconstriction, and vascular permeability. LT inhibitors are used for treatment of asthma and include zileuton, an inhibitor of lipoxygenase, and zafirlukast and montelukast, which are leukotriene receptor antagonists.

> PGE_2 is used to prepare the cervix for induction of labor.

Table 2.6 Genetic Disorders of Sphingolipid Degradation

SPHINGOLIPIDOSES	DEFICIENCY	ACCUMULATED MATERIAL	GENETICS	CLINICAL FEATURES
Tay-Sachs disease	Hexosaminidase A	GM_2 gangliosides	AR	Developmental regression, muscle weakness, blindness, cherry-red macular spot, deafness, no hepatosplenomegaly, death
Gaucher disease	β-Glucosidase	Glucocerebrosides	AR	Joint and limb pain, hepatosplenomegaly, macrophages appearing like "crinkled paper"
Niemann-Pick disease	Sphingomyelinase	Sphingomyelin	AR	Failure to thrive, hepatosplenomegaly, cherry-red spot, developmental regression, macrophages appear "bubbly"
Fabry disease	α-Galactosidase	Ceramide trihexosides	XR	Cataracts, kidney and heart failure, paresthesia
Krabbe disease	β-Galactosidase	Galactocerebrosides	AR	Progressive psychomotor retardation, "globoid bodies" in brain white matter, death
Metachromatic leukodystrophy	Arylsulfatase A	Sulfatides	AR	Mental retardation, peripheral neuropathy

AR, Autosomal recessive; XR, X-linked recessive.

PGs are created when cyclooxygenase acts on arachidonic acid. Prostaglandin H_2 (PGH_2) is the first stable prostaglandin produced in this pathway. PGs produce inflammation, inhibit or stimulate muscle contraction, and promote vasodilation or vasoconstriction depending on the vascular bed. PGE_2 interacts with several different prostaglandin receptors, which are G-protein-coupled receptors, and leads to vasodilation, inflammation, and an increase in gastric mucus secretion. PGE_2 is known as dinoprostone and is used in labor to prepare the cervix for induction of labor, but has also been demonstrated to sustain fetal ductus arteriosus patency. $PGF_{2\alpha}$ stimulates uterine contractions and also increases vasoconstriction. Analogs of $PGF_{2\alpha}$ include dinoprost, latanoprost, bimatoprost, and travoprost. They are used in medicine to induce labor and as abortifacients. Aspirin is an irreversible cyclooxygenase inhibitor.

Prostacyclin (PGI_2) is an effective vasodilator and bronchodilator and inhibits platelet activation. Synthetic prostacyclin analogs, such as iloprost and cisaprost, are used as vasodilators in severe Raynaud disease and pulmonary hypertension. As a drug, PGI_2 is known as epoprostenol. PGI_2 is produced in endothelial cells from PGH_2. Prostacyclin is in cardiovascular homeostasis with thromboxane A_2 (TXA_2).

TXA_2 promotes contraction of arterioles and aggregation of platelets.

TXA_2 is produced in platelets from PGH_2 by thromboxane synthase. TXA_2 promotes contraction of arterioles and aggregation of platelets. Dipyramidole inhibits thromboxane synthase. Aspirin and other NSAIDs acetylate and inhibit cyclooxygenase, leading to reduced synthesis of prostaglandins (antiinflammatory effect) and reduced synthesis of TXA_2 (antithrombotic effect caused by reduced platelet activation).

By inhibiting phospholipase A_2, corticosteroids inhibit the production of all the eicosanoids.

Fatty Acid Oxidation and Synthesis

Fatty acids are oxidized to CO_2 and H_2O in the mitochondrial matrix. Long-chain fatty acids must be shuttled into the mitochondrial matrix by the **carnitine transport system** because they cannot cross the mitochondrial inner membrane alone. Medium-chain fatty acids are able to pass directly through the mitochondrial membrane. The oxidation of fatty acids occurs by the **β-oxidation system of the mitochondria**, where each cycle produces 17 ATP molecules using the electron transport system and citric acid cycle.

Fatty acids are synthesized from acetyl CoA and malonyl CoA by fatty acid synthase (Fig. 2.22). Seven reaction cycles yield palmitate and fatty acid synthase. Palmitate acts as the precursor to other

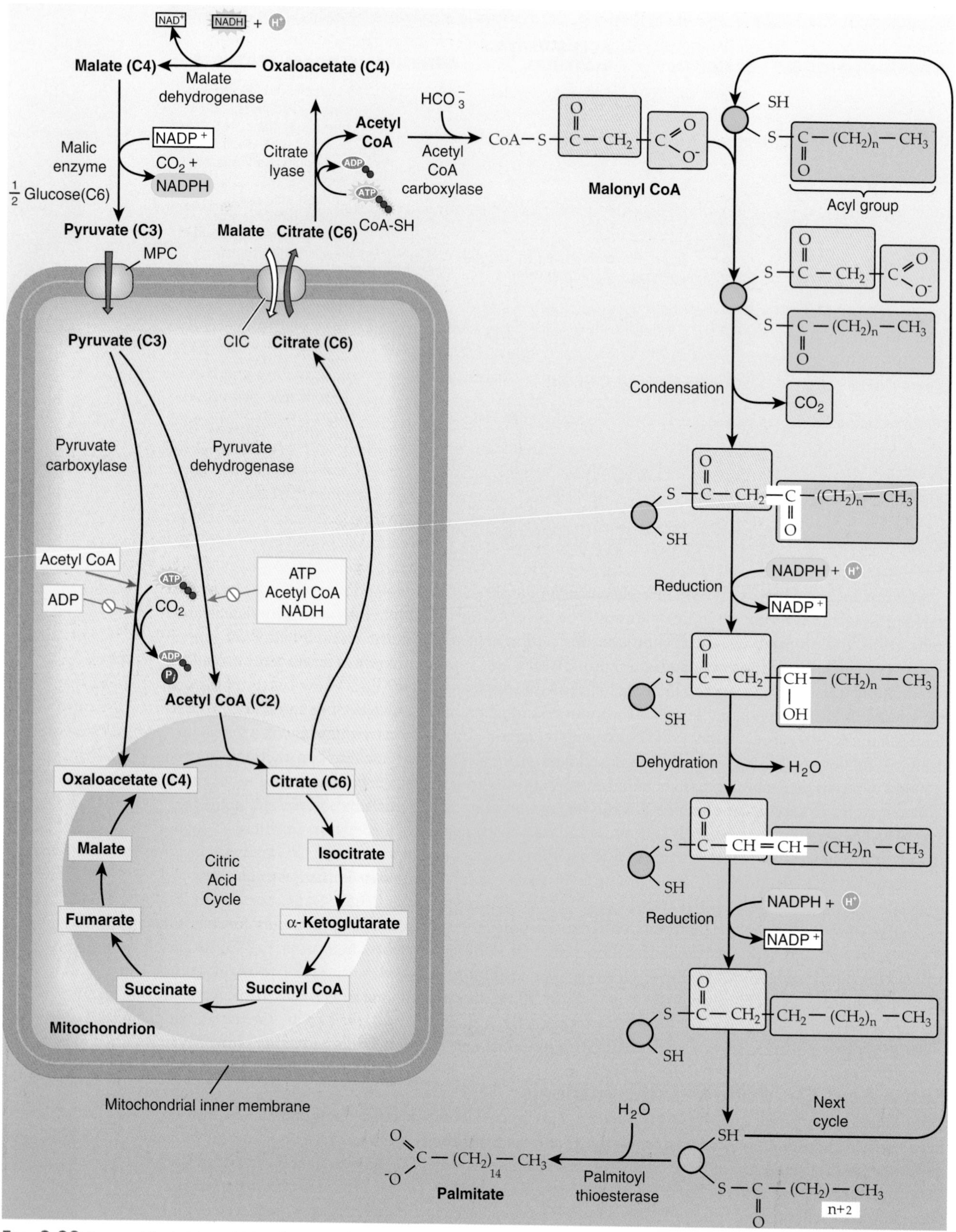

FIG. 2.22 Fatty acid synthesis. ADP, adenosine diphosphate; ATP, adenosine triphosphate; CIC, citrate carrier; CoA, coenzyme A; MPC, mitochondrial pyruvate carrier. (*From Boron WF, Boulpaep EL.* Medical Physiology. *2nd ed. Philadelphia: Elsevier; 2008.*)

fatty acids. Longer fatty acids are synthesized by chain-lengthening systems, and unsaturated fatty acids are synthesized by a desaturating system. However, the desaturating enzymes are only able to desaturate double bonds greater than 10 carbons from the C terminus. Therefore linoleic acid and linolenic acid are essential fatty acids.

INTEGRATION OF METABOLISM

Vitamins

Vitamins are classified as water soluble, excreted in the urine and rarely reach toxic levels, or fat soluble, functioning as hormones, cofactors, and antioxidants (Fig. 2.23). Because fat-soluble vitamins are transported in chylomicrons and stored in the liver and adipose tissue, toxicity can occur.

The water-soluble vitamins **include thiamine, riboflavin, niacin, pyridoxine, folic acid, vitamin B_{12}, and vitamin C.**

- **Thiamine (vitamin B_1)** is a water-soluble vitamin that acts as a coenzyme in the decarboxylation of pyruvate and α-ketoglutarate for the enzymes transketolase, pyruvate dehydrogenase, and α-ketoglutarate dehydrogenase. These pathways are important in cellular energy metabolism and production of ATP and are particularly important in the nervous system. Because of its role as a cofactor for transketolase, thiamine deficiency can be diagnosed by either low transketolase activity levels or increased erythrocyte transketolase activity on addition of thiamine. Two disorders are caused by thiamine deficiency.
- **Beriberi** is a disorder classically caused by malnutrition as a result of a diet consisting primarily of polished rice, which is thiamine deficient. Beriberi can occur in two forms: dry and wet.
- **Wernicke-Korsakoff syndrome** is seen primarily in chronic alcoholic patients and is due to dietary deficiency or reduced absorption of thiamine. Wernicke-Korsakoff syndrome is associated with atrophy of the mammillary bodies. Wernicke encephalopathy results from severe, acute deficiency of thiamine, whereas untreated Wernicke encephalopathy and chronic thiamine deficiency lead to Korsakoff syndrome (also known as Korsakoff psychosis), coma, and possibly death. Wernicke encephalopathy is characterized by ataxia, ophthalmoplegia, and confusion. Korsakoff syndrome is characterized by anterograde and retrograde amnesia, confabulation, and hallucinations. Glucose administration to malnourished patients should be preceded by thiamine treatment to avoid the risk for precipitating Wernicke encephalopathy. This is because glucose metabolism involves the action of pyruvate dehydrogenase, an enzyme that requires thiamine.
  - Dry beriberi affects the peripheral nervous system, causing wasting, difficulty walking, and paralysis.
  - Wet beriberi affects cardiac tissue, leading to congestive heart failure with marked edema.
- Riboflavin (vitamin B_2) is active as the central component of flavin mononucleotide (FMN) and flavin adenine dinucleotide (FAD), cofactors required for many key steps in energy metabolism. Riboflavin is rarely deficient alone but may accompany other vitamin deficiencies. Symptoms of riboflavin deficiency, known as ariboflavinosis, include dermatitis, glossitis, and fissures at the corner of the mouth (cheilosis).
- Niacin (vitamin B_3, nicotinic acid) is active as nicotinamide adenine dinucleotide (NAD^+) and nicotinamide adenine dinucleotide phosphate ($NADP^+$). **A severe deficiency in niacin causes the disease pellagra, which is characterized by dermatitis, diarrhea, and dementia (the three Ds). If untreated, it can lead to death (the fourth D).** Niacin can increase the levels of high-density lipoprotein (HDL) cholesterol but is not frequently used because of the side effect of flushing.
- Pyridoxine (vitamin B_6, pyridoxamine) is a cofactor in the metabolism of amino acids, heme, and neurotransmitters. Isoniazid (first-line treatment for tuberculosis) interferes with the action of pyridoxine, so supplementation may be necessary to prevent complications of isoniazid treatment such as peripheral neuropathy.
- Biotin (vitamin B_7) is a cofactor for carboxylase enzymes. Deficiency is rare and may be caused by eating raw egg whites, which bind biotin. Deficiency is noted by dermatitis, glossitis, as well as other nonspecific changes.

Wernicke encephalopathy includes ataxia, ophthalmoplegia, and confusion caused by thiamine deficiency and mammillary body dysfunction.

Niacin deficiency (pellagra) causes dermatitis, diarrhea, and dementia.

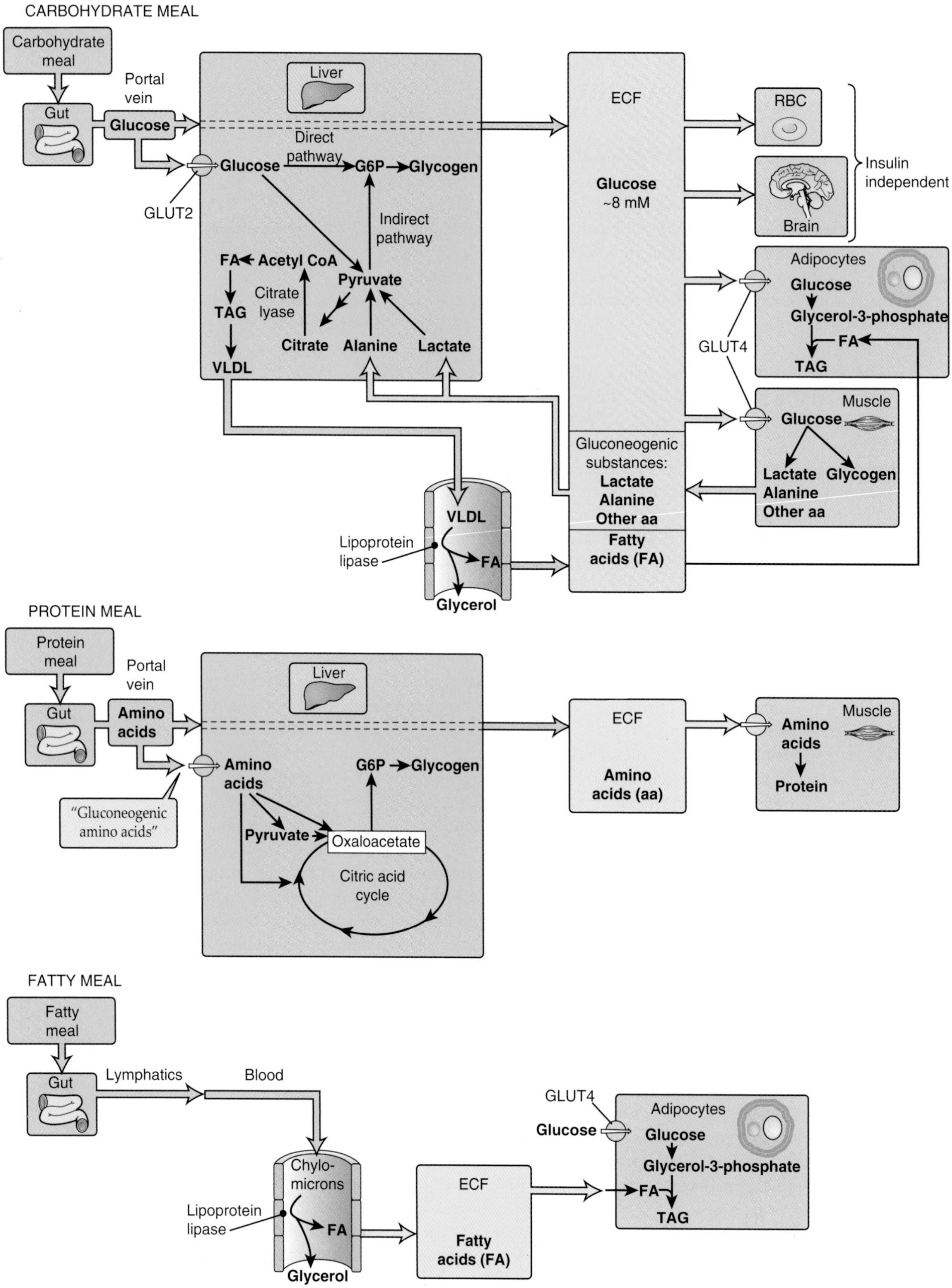

Fig. 2.23 Energy utilization and storage following meals. aa, amino acid; CoA, coenzyme A; ECF, extracellular fluid; RBC, red blood cell; TAG, triacyglycerol; VLDL, very-low-density lipoprotein. (*From Boron WF, Boulpaep EL.* Medical Physiology. *2nd ed. Philadelphia: Elsevier; 2008.*)

- Folic acid (vitamin B_9) is essential to the synthesis and repair of nucleic acids as its derivative tetrahydrofolate. Deficiency is caused by malnutrition (especially among alcoholic people) or increased utilization during pregnancy. Folic acid deficiency leads to macrocytic anemia, hypersegmented neutrophils, and in pregnancy, fetal neural tube defects (spina bifida occulta, meningocele, meningomyelocele). All women should take folic acid before conception and during pregnancy. Medications such as phenytoin, methotrexate, 5-fluorouracil, sulfonamides, and trimethoprim also cause folate deficiency and should be avoided in pregnancy.
- Vitamin B_{12} (cobalamin) is important in DNA and fatty acid synthesis. Like folic acid, deficiency leads to macrocytic anemia and hypersegmented neutrophils. Additionally neurologic deficits occur such as peripheral neuropathy and dementia (cobalamin deficiency is one of the few reversible causes of dementia). Cobalamin is absorbed in the terminal ileum when bound to intrinsic factor (produced by gastric parietal cells). In pernicious anemia, autoimmune destruction of gastric parietal cells causes vitamin B_{12} deficiency. Other causes of deficiency include surgical resection of the stomach/ileum, inflammation of the ileum (Crohn disease), the "fish tapeworm" *Diphyllobothrium latum,* or a vegan diet (because cobalamin is found only in animal products).
- Vitamin C (ascorbic acid), as discussed earlier, is a cofactor necessary for the cross-linking of collagen fibers. Deficiency leads to **scurvy.** Additionally, vitamin C reduces Fe^{3+} (from dietary plants) to Fe^{2+} (the absorbable form). Vitamin C deficiency can therefore cause iron deficiency anemia, and is commonly supplemented with iron for iron deficiency anemia for better absorption. Vitamin C is found in vegetables and fruits.

Treating tuberculosis with isoniazid may require B_6 supplementation to prevent peripheral neuropathy.

Folate and cobalamin deficiency cause macrocytic anemia and hypersegmented neutrophils.

The four fat-soluble vitamins are A, D, E, and K.

- Vitamin A (retinal, β-carotene) is present within the retina's rods and cones in the form of retinal. Retinal responds to light by changing shape. It is the first step in a cellular cascade that converts electromagnetic energy (light) into vision. Vitamin A, in its retinoic acid form, has an entirely different function as a growth factor. It plays an important role in developing the anterior-posterior axis during embryogenesis by interacting with *Hox* genes (which is why isotretinoin [Accutane] is teratogenic). Vitamin A also plays a role in the differentiation of cells (which is why it can be used to treat acne vulgaris and promyelocytic leukemia). Deficiency, usually caused by malnutrition, causes night blindness. Toxicity causes neurologic symptoms (headache, blurry vision, confusion). Vitamin A is a yellow pigment and contained in many yellow foods such as butter, vegetables, and egg yolks. Excessive consumption of β-carotene, a vitamin A precursor, will turn skin yellow similarly to jaundice– preferentially affecting the hands and soles but sparing the eyes (without scleral icterus, unlike jaundice).
- Vitamin D, when in its active form [1,25(OH)-vitamin D, calcitriol], **increases intestinal absorption and renal reabsorption of calcium and phosphate.** It also stimulates bone remodeling. The net effect of vitamin D is increasing serum calcium and phosphate levels through the kidneys, gut, and bone. **Vitamin D** is obtained in the diet or synthesized in the skin through **sunlight.** This inactive vitamin D then goes to the liver and kidney to become activated as calcitriol. Vitamin D deficiency can be caused by low dietary intake or low sunlight exposure. Renal dysfunction can also lead to a lack of activated calcitriol. Deficiency results in defective bone mineralization. This presents as osteomalacia in adults and rickets in children.
- Vitamin E is an antioxidant that protects cell membranes from free radical damage. Deficiency is rare but can lead to a hemolytic anemia caused by RBC membrane fragility.
- Vitamin K is a cofactor for an enzyme that carboxylates glutamate residues. This is required for the proper synthesis of clotting factors II, VII, IX, X. It is also important for anticoagulant protein C and protein S. Vitamin K is found in leafy green vegetables and is also synthesized by intestinal flora. It must be activated, however, by the hepatic enzyme epoxide reductase. Warfarin, an anticoagulant, functions by inhibiting epoxide reductase and thus inhibiting the formation of clotting factors. Vitamin K deficiency is most commonly characterized by excessive bleeding. It is most commonly seen in people taking warfarin or in cirrhotic patients who lack functional hepatic epoxide reductase. Neonates are supplemented with vitamin K to prevent hemorrhagic disease of the newborn because milk is low in vitamin K and they have no intestinal flora at birth. Patients on broad-spectrum antibiotics reduce their intestinal flora and may also be deficient.

Vitamin K is essential for clotting factors II, VII, IX, X, protein C, and protein S. It must be activated by epoxide reductase.

Warfarin inhibits epoxide reductase.

Trace Elements

Iodine is an important component of thyroid hormone. It is naturally found in seafood. Table salt is now fortified with iodine to prevent deficiency. Clinically, iodine deficiency causes hypothyroidism and goiters.

Zinc is second only to iron as the most abundant metal found in the human body. It plays an important role in many enzymes, particularly as zinc finger motifs in proteins that bind to DNA and collagenases that aid in wound remodeling. It also plays a role in spermatogenesis and is found in high concentrations in the prostate and in semen. Deficiency leads to poor wound healing, hypogonadism, and anosmia.

Copper is a cofactor in many enzymes. Notably, these enzymes are involved in the electron transport chain, iron absorption and transport, neurotransmitter synthesis, and collagen cross-linking (lysyl oxidase). Deficiency is rare but leads to iron deficiency anemia and poor wound healing. **Wilson disease** is an autosomal recessive disorder characterized by excessive total body copper. It is caused by a mutation in Wilson disease protein, an ATPase responsible for transporting copper and forming ceruloplasmin (the transport protein for copper). The inability to excrete copper leads to an increase in free serum copper. **Total serum copper may be high, low, or normal, given the relative lack of ceruloplasmin to transport copper.** Copper accumulates in the liver, causing **cirrhosis,** and in the basal ganglia, causing **parkinsonism**. Excess copper in the cornea is visible as **Kayser-Fleischer rings**. Diagnosis is based on a decrease in serum ceruloplasmin, an elevation in urinary copper, and copper deposits on liver biopsy.

Fluoride is important in the mineralization of teeth. Adequate consumption prevents dental caries. Excessive fluoride intake can stain teeth white. Fluoride is added to the drinking water in most U.S. communities.

GENETICS

Patterns of Inheritance

Pedigree Analysis

Being able to read a pedigree is critically important to understanding genetic disorders. First, the traditional symbols in pedigrees must be covered (Fig. 2.24). Females are depicted as circles, whereas males are shown as squares. If the sex is unknown, it is typically a diamond (such as in the case of an early fetus). Affected individuals have shaded circles (females) or squares (males), whereas unaffected individuals have unshaded shapes. Sometimes carriers are denoted with half-shaded shapes or dots, but often they are left blank as well. Reading a pedigree will allow you to deduce whether a condition is likely to be **autosomal dominant, autosomal recessive, X-linked dominant**, or **X-linked recessive**, or have **mitochondrial inheritance.** This distinction is important to understanding the risk for disease in future offspring.

Pedigree analysis helps deduce the mode of transmission of a genetic disease.

Basic Mendelian Inheritance

Genes are found on autosomes and on sex chromosomes. Each individual has two copies of each gene for all autosomes. For sex chromosomes, males only have one X chromosome (because they are XY) and therefore only possess one copy of any gene that lies on the X chromosome. Females are XX, and although they technically have two copies of each gene, because of a process called lyonization (X-inactivation), only one of the X chromosomes is active (in fact, if, because of a genetic defect, a female has more than two X chromosomes, all but one will be inactivated).

There are variations in the genes people have, called alleles. The alleles that an individual has define the individual's **genotype**. The expression of those alleles defines someone's **phenotype**. Dominant alleles are typically denoted by capital letters (e.g., H), whereas recessive alleles are denoted by lowercase letters (e.g., h). Someone with both alleles as dominant alleles (HH) would be called **homozygous dominant**, a person with one dominant and one recessive allele (Hh) would be called **heterozygous**, and a person with two recessive alleles (hh) would be called **homozygous recessive**. A condition that only requires one defective gene to cause the condition (display the phenotype) is called dominant (if the genes are on autosomes, it is called autosomal dominant; if the genes are on the X chromosome, it is called X-linked dominant). A condition that requires two defective genes to display the condition is referred to as recessive.

Genotype is what alleles people have. Phenotype is the expression of those alleles.

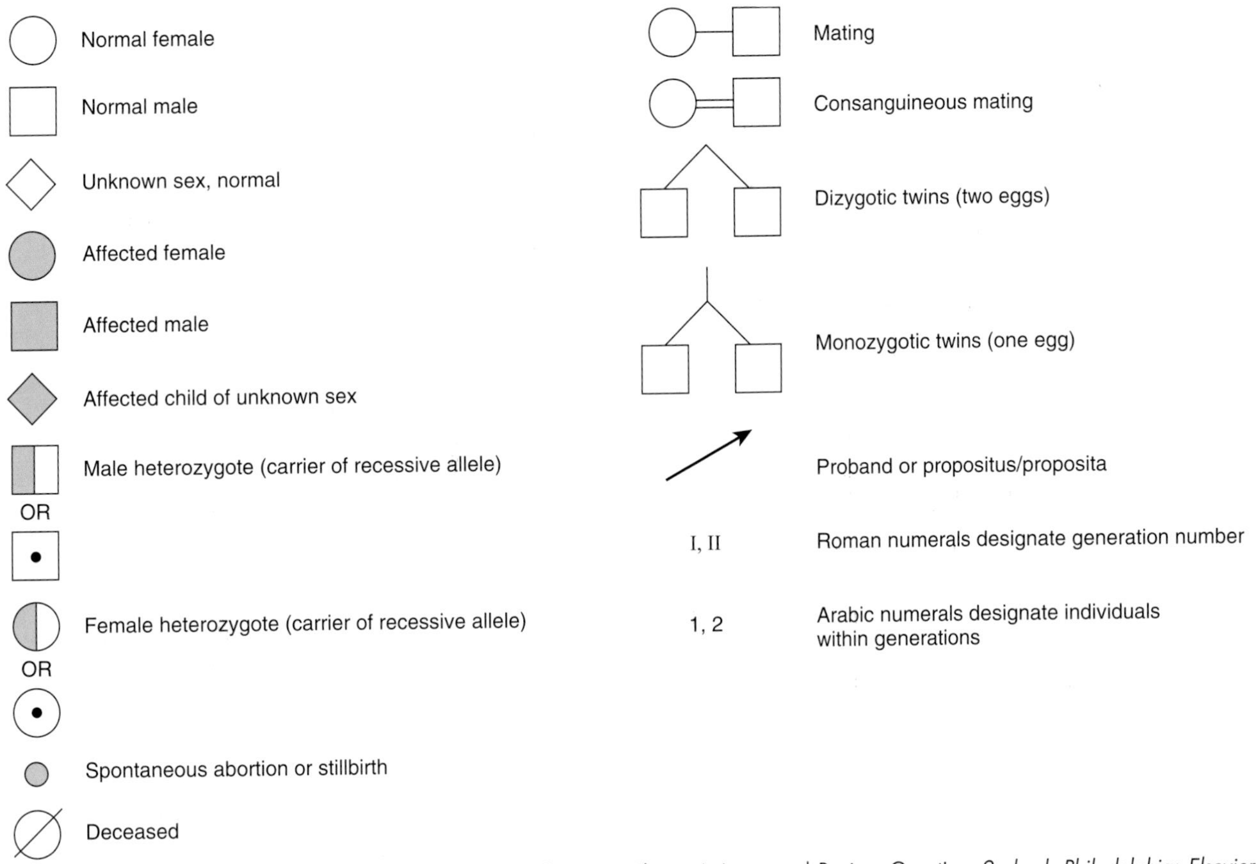

FIG. 2.24 Common symbols used in pedigrees. (*From Adkison LR.* Elsevier's Integrated Review Genetics. *2nd ed. Philadelphia: Elsevier; 2011.*)

Parents will give one of each of their chromosomes (with their alleles) to their children; therefore one allele for each gene will come from the father, one from the mother. To show which combinations of alleles in a child are possible, **Punnett squares** are drawn (Fig. 2.25). Punnett deduced the probability of the offspring getting certain combinations of alleles. In a Punnett square, the alleles of each parent are drawn at the end of a 2 × 2 table. Then, in each cell of the 2 × 2 table, write in the corresponding allele for each parent to see what combinations of alleles can occur.

Punnett squares deduce the probability of what genotypes the offspring of two individuals will be.

In Fig. 2.25A, it can be seen that when one parent is homozygous dominant (HH) and the other is homozygous recessive (hh), one parent will always give an H, and the other will always give an h, leading to only Hh (heterozygous) offspring. In Fig. 2.25B, it can be seen that both parents are heterozygotes. This leads to a diverse combination in which 25% off the offspring will be homozygous dominant (HH) if both parents give an H and 25% of the offspring will be homozygous recessive (hh) if both parents give an h. The other 50% of the time, the offspring will be heterozygous (Hh) when one parent gives an H and the other gives an h (or vice versa). Practice drawing Punnett squares to familiarize yourself with the concept.

Autosomal Dominant

Autosomal dominant means that for two alleles (which again are alternative forms of the same gene), only one must be present for the disease to manifest itself. For instance, **Marfan syndrome** is autosomal dominant caused by a mutation in fibrillin. Fibrillin is on chromosome 15 (an autosome, as it is not a sex chromosome); each individual has two copies of the gene that codes for fibrillin. Since Marfan syndrome is autosomal dominant, only one gene must be abnormal for an individual to have Marfan syndrome. Fig. 2.26 depicts what the pedigree for an autosomal dominant condition for Marfan syndrome might look like.

Autosomal dominant means that only one mutated allele is needed to express the disease.

To further familiarize yourself with Punnett squares and with pedigrees, refer again to Fig. 2.26. It can be seen that the father has Marfan syndrome (shaded square) and the mother does not (blank circle). If a

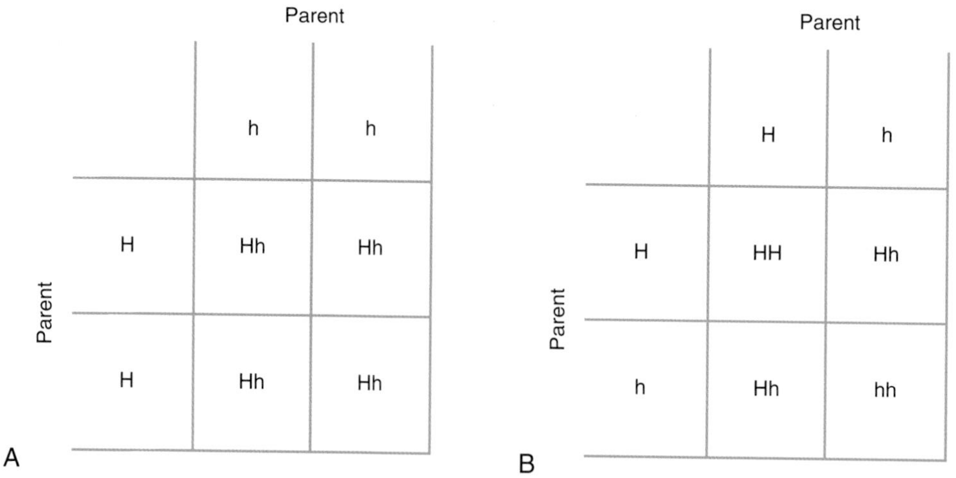

FIG. 2.25 Punnett squares demonstrating (**A**) the output when one parent who is homozygous dominant and one parent who is homozygous recessive (all offspring are heterozygotes), and (**B**) the output when both parents are heterozygotes (25% of offspring are homozygous dominant, 50% are heterozygous, and 25% are homozygous recessive). (*From Jorde LB, Carey JC, Bamshad MJ. Medical Genetics. 4th ed. Philadelphia: Elsevier; 2009.*)

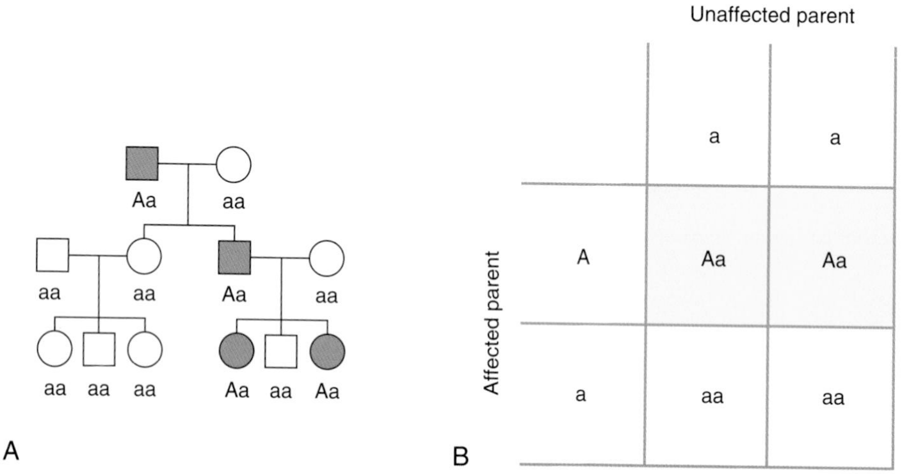

FIG. 2.26 **A,** Pedigree depicting an autosomal dominant condition. Note that all the affected individuals are shaded; they possess only one "A" (are all heterozygous by genotype) but display the features of the disease (phenotype). Therefore because only one allele had to be present for the disease to manifest, this is autosomal dominant. **B,** Punnett square showing one affected parent and one affected parent: half of their children will be affected. (*From Jorde LB, Carey JC, Bamshad MJ. Medical Genetics. 4th ed. Philadelphia: Elsevier; 2009.*)

Punnett square were to be drawn between the two (see Fig. 2.26B), it would be seen that there is a 50% chance of a child having Marfan syndrome. In this case one of the two children (50%) did have Marfan syndrome. The unaffected daughter (aa) went on to have children with an unaffected man, and therefore none of the children could possibly have Marfan syndrome. The affected son had children with an unaffected woman and subsequently still had a 50% risk for having children with Marfan syndrome.

Because only one allele must be present to display the disease, and having the allele causes expression of the disease, this brings a few "rules" for autosomal dominant inheritance. Note that **if a *de novo* (new) mutation occurred in one of the genes, these rules do not apply** (e.g., if one of the father's sperm had a new mutation for the fibrillin gene and subsequently caused a child with Marfan syndrome).

- The affected offspring **must** have had one affected parent (unlike recessive).
- Unaffected individuals cannot have children with the disease (unlike recessive).
- Males and females have an equal likelihood of getting and passing on the disease (unlike X-linked).
- As a general rule, patients with autosomal dominant conditions live to reproductive age. Otherwise, these conditions would be rapidly eliminated from the population (no carrier state). Consider Huntington disease, autosomal dominant polycystic kidney disease, and Marfan syndrome as examples.

Rules of autosomal dominant transmission: must have an affected parent; unaffected individuals cannot have children with disease (cannot be a carrier); males and females are equally affected.

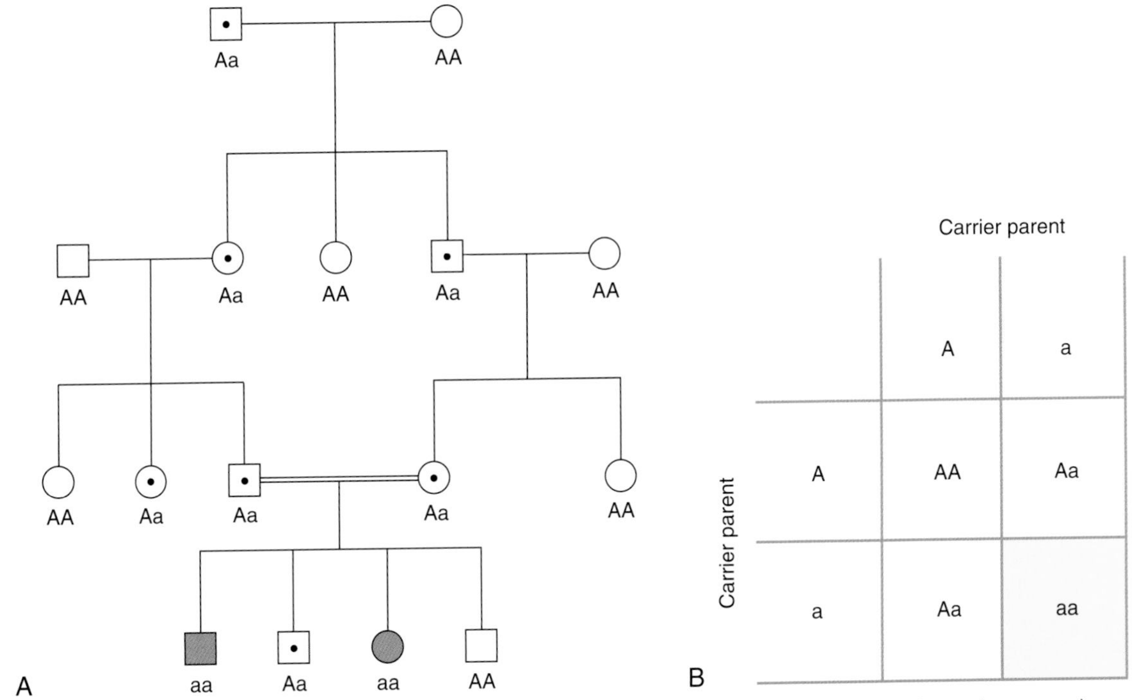

FIG. 2.27 Autosomal recessive disease. **A,** Pedigree showing affected children (*shaded*) at the bottom. The dots in this case indicate carriers. The two carriers who produced the affected children are both heterozygotes. The likelihood of them both being heterozygotes was increased because of consanguinity; both individuals were close relatives. **B,** Punnett square showing two heterozygotes with a one in four chance of having an affected child. (*From Jorde LB, Carey JC, Bamshad MJ. Medical Genetics. 4th ed. Philadelphia: Elsevier; 2009.*)

Autosomal Recessive

Autosomal recessive diseases are those in which **two** mutated alleles must be present for the disease to manifest itself (Fig. 2.27). Therefore, if a child has an autosomal recessive disease but neither parent displays the disease, the parents must have both been heterozygotes (Hh). Refer to Fig. 2.25B, which shows that when both parents are heterozygotes, they have a 25% chance of producing a homozygous recessive offspring (hh). An example of an autosomal recessive disease is **cystic fibrosis** (see Fig. 2.27 for details; see also Chapter 17). In cystic fibrosis, there is an abnormal chloride channel (called the cystic fibrosis transmembrane conductance regulator, or CFTR); loss of function of this channel leads to thickened mucus production in the lungs (predisposing to infections) and thickened pancreatic secretions (leading to pancreatitis and type 1 diabetes mellitus). **Having one functional *CFTR* gene allows for normal function.** Therefore because both genes must have mutant alleles, cystic fibrosis is homozygous recessive.

Autosomal recessive means that both mutant alleles are needed to express disease; therefore it can have carriers.

There are also "rules" for autosomal recessive inheritance.

- Suspect autosomal recessive inheritance when a child has a genetic disease but has two unaffected parents (who then must be heterozygotes themselves).
- If both parents are heterozygotes (carriers), only 25% of their children will be affected, on average.
- As with autosomal dominant inheritance, males and females are equally likely to be affected (unlike X-linked).
- Consanguinity (mating with close relatives) increases the likelihood of recessive diseases to manifest because the likelihood of close relatives being heterozygotes for a disease is higher than the likelihood of two unrelated individuals both being heterozygotes for a particular disease.

Rules of autosomal recessive transmission: highly suspicious if two unaffected parents (carriers) have affected offspring; increased frequency with consanguinity.

X-Linked Recessive

Males are XY and females are XX, so the likelihood of expression of disease differs in X-linked diseases (unlike autosomal diseases, which do not favor one sex or the other because males and females have the same autosomal chromosomes). Because males only have one X chromosome, an X-linked recessive disease will cause the male to have the phenotype of the disease with just one mutant allele.

X-linked recessive disease means that males exhibit the disease almost exclusively (because they only have one X chromosome).

Females, on the other hand, have two X chromosomes, and therefore having a single mutant allele will not necessarily cause disease (because they have another X chromosome with a functional allele). This is complicated somewhat by X-inactivation (lyonization), whereby the female cells inactivate one of the two X chromosomes in each cell. Therefore in females with one abnormal allele on an X chromosome, about 50% of the body's cells will have inactivated the chromosome with the abnormal allele, but 50% will have inactivated the other. Usually, this does not lead to significant disease.

The classic X-linked recessive disease is **hemophilia** (both hemophilia A and hemophilia B are X-linked recessive). Hemophilia A causes a deficiency in factor VIII, and hemophilia B causes a deficiency in factor IX; both of these deficiencies in clotting factors lead to deep tissue bleeding, joint bleeding, and other bleeding-related symptoms. Another common X-linked disease is **Duchenne muscular dystrophy** and its milder subtype, **Becker muscular dystrophy**. Both of these cause skeletal muscle degeneration, eventually leading to paralysis and death (with Duchenne muscular dystrophy almost always causing inability to walk by age 12 years; Becker muscular dystrophy patients may be able to ambulate for significantly longer).

In Fig. 2.28A, it is clear that only males are affected. This is a striking feature of X-linked recessive diseases. In Fig. 2.28B, the mating between a normal XY father and a carrier XX mother is shown (X_1 is the normal allele, X_2 is the abnormal allele). Because the female offspring are XX, one X must be from the father, and one must be from the mother. In this case in which the mother is the carrier, 50% of the daughters then will also be carriers. **Male offspring must receive the Y from the father** because the mother cannot provide a Y chromosome. Therefore an interesting finding in X-linked recessive disease

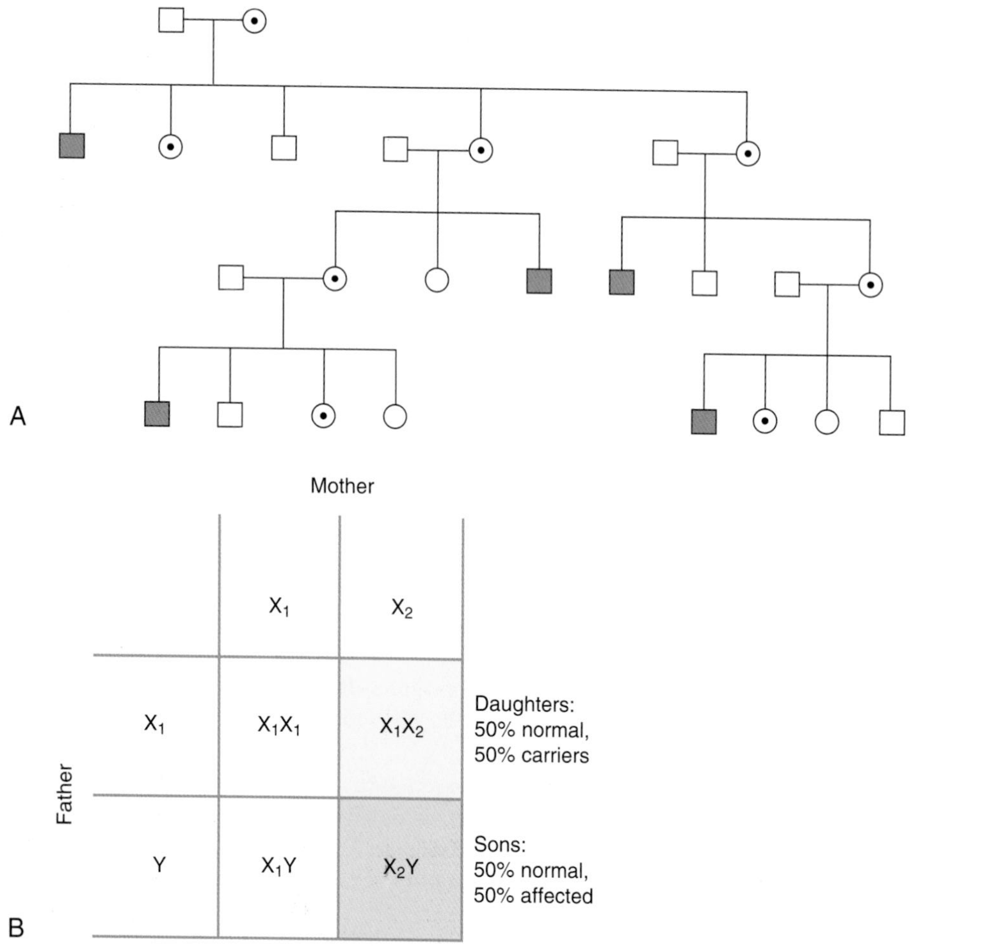

Fig. 2.28 X-linked recessive disease. **A,** Pedigree showing that only males are affected; there are numerous female carriers. **B,** Punnett square showing mating between an unaffected male (XY) and a carrier female (XX). X_1 is the normal allele, X_2 is the abnormal allele. (*From Jorde LB, Carey JC, Bamshad MJ.* Medical Genetics. *4th ed. Philadelphia: Elsevier; 2009.*)

is that **a male with the disease cannot give the disease to his son** (because by definition the male offspring X chromosome must have come from the mother and not the father).

Rules of X-linked recessive: no male to male transmission; affected males always make carrier daughters.

Knowing what we know now about X-linked recessive inheritance, we can form the "rules":

- Affected males cannot give the disease to their sons (because they have to give their Y chromosome to make a son); the only way that a son of an affected father can have the disease is if the mother is an asymptomatic carrier.
- Affected males will always give their X chromosome (with their mutated allele) to their daughters (because if they gave their Y chromosome, it would be a son). Therefore all daughters of affected males are carriers.
- Heterozygous women (**X*X**) will give their mutant allele away half the time. Therefore 50% of the daughters will be carriers, 50% of the sons will have the disease.

X-Linked Dominant

This is incredibly rare. Because it is dominant, there cannot be any carriers. However, the defining feature that separates X-linked dominant conditions from autosomal dominant conditions is that **affected males cannot transmit the disease to other males.** This is because if a male is affected, he is affected because he has an abnormal allele on his X chromosome. However, to have male offspring, he has to give his Y chromosome. Suspect X-linked dominant only if the transmission appears dominant but there are numerous affected males who have normal male offspring and affected female offspring. Fragile X syndrome and Rett syndrome are examples of X-linked dominant conditions.

Mitochondrial Inheritance

Mitochondrial inheritance is easy to detect if you remember to think of this as a possible mode of transmission. All mitochondria in your entire body initially came from your mother's egg. The sperm do not provide mitochondria. Therefore with mitochondrial diseases, **affected females will have 100% of their offspring affected**, but **affected males will have 0% of their offspring affected** (Fig. 2.29). Affected males do not give their mitochondria to their children, so it is impossible for males to transmit the condition to their offspring. Important conditions that are inherited through mitochondria are Leber hereditary optic neuropathy, mitochondrial encephalomyopathy with lactic acidosis and strokelike episodes (MELAS), and myoclonic epilepsy and ragged red fibers (MERRF).

Mitochondria are **only** transmitted to offspring by the mother. Therefore all offspring of affected females will have the disease; no offspring of affected males will have the disease.

CHROMOSOMAL ABNORMALITIES

Nondisjunction

Meiosis is the type of cell division that occurs to produce gametes (sperm and eggs). It is incredibly complex and therefore is prone to error. One type of error that can occur is **nondisjunction.** There are

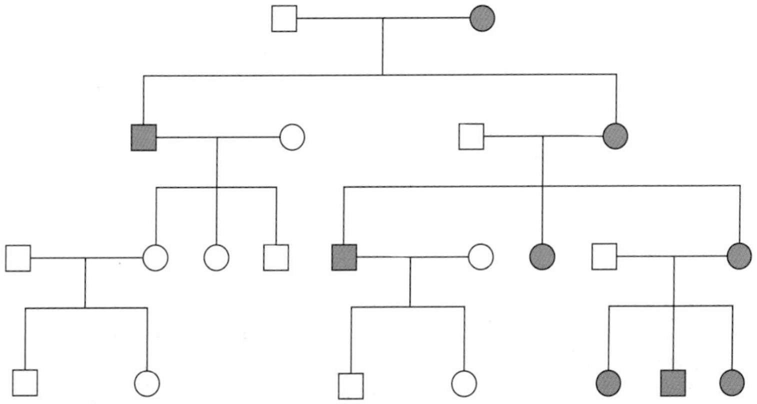

FIG. 2.29 Mitochondrial inheritance. It can be seen that affected females pass their mitochondrial disease onto 100% of their offspring. However, males do not contribute mitochondria to their offspring (because it is only present in the egg), so none of the affected males will have affected offspring. (*From Jorde LB, Carey JC, Bamshad MJ.* Medical Genetics. *4th ed. Philadelphia: Elsevier; 2009.*)

two opportunities for nondisjunction during meiosis: during the first round of meiosis (meiosis I), or during the second round of meiosis (meiosis II). Fig. 2.30 depicts a simplified illustration of this complex concept with only one pair of chromosomes. In the top image, nondisjunction has occurred during meiosis I. This means that a pair of homologous chromosomes has failed to separate. Imagine for the sake of discussion that this pair of homologous chromosomes was a pair of chromosome 21 and that this was meiosis for a female. This would lead to four eggs: Two eggs would have an additional 21st chromosome and would produce a child with trisomy 21 (Down syndrome) if fertilized by a normal sperm. The other two eggs would not have a 21st chromosome and would produce a child with monosomy 21 if fertilized by a normal sperm.

Monosomy means having only one copy of a given chromosome (e.g., Turner syndrome, Xo). Trisomy means having an extra copy of a given chromosome (e.g., Down syndrome [21], Patau syndrome [13], Edwards syndrome [18]).

Essentially all cases of monosomy are lethal in utero and lead to spontaneous abortion, except for Turner syndrome (monosomy X). Most **autosomal** trisomy cases are also lethal in utero, with the exception of trisomy 21 (Down syndrome), trisomy 13 (Patau syndrome), and trisomy 18 (Edwards syndrome). To remember which is which, think trisomy **18** for **Edwards** syndrome—at age **18** you can participate in the **elections**. These will be briefly discussed later; there are also abnormalities of increased numbers of sex chromosomes, which are typically not lethal.

Nondisjunction can also occur during meiosis II. Because the first division has occurred appropriately, the outcome is different. The first division produced two cells. Nondisjunction in meiosis II would only affect one of the two cells, so the unaffected cell would be expected to divide normally.

Nondisjunction in meiosis I leads to four abnormal gametes; nondisjunction in meiosis II leads to two abnormal gametes.

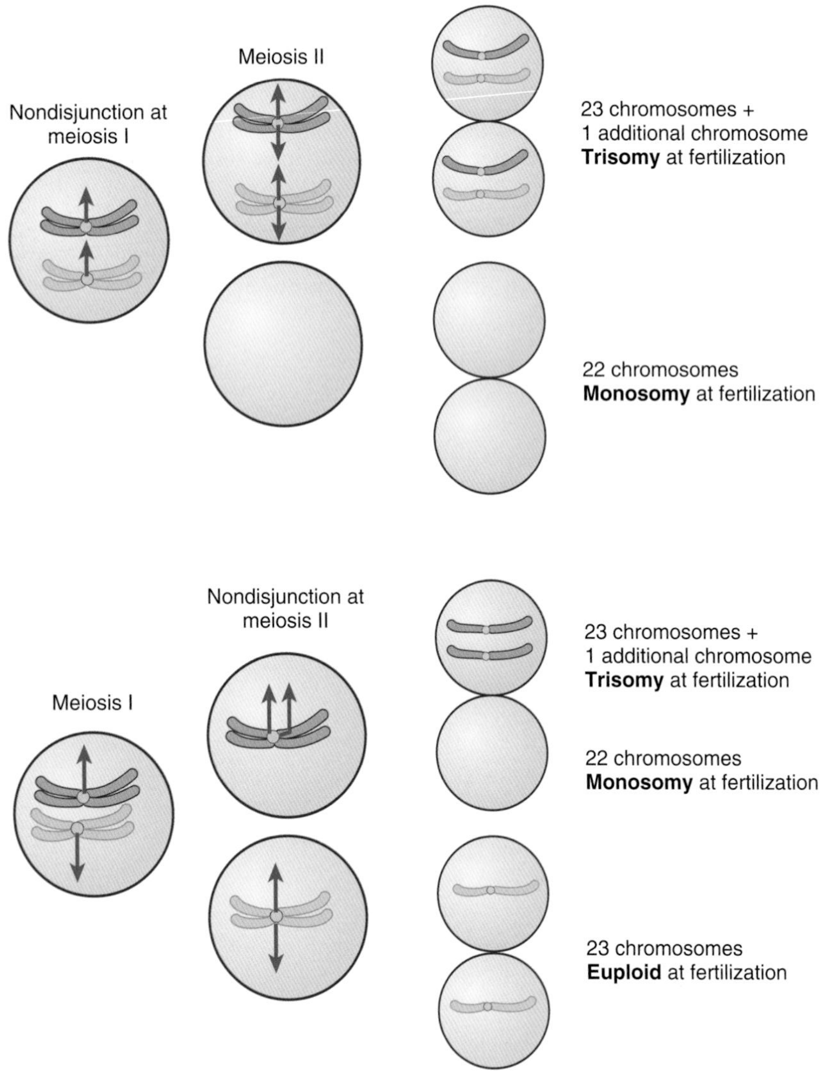

FIG. 2.30 Examples of nondisjunction in meiosis I (*top*) and meiosis II (*bottom*). (*From Adkison LR.* Elsevier's Integrated Review Genetics. *2nd ed. Philadelphia: Elsevier; 2011.*)

Therefore of the four gametes, two would be normal. The other gamete, which had nondisjunction in meiosis II, would produce two abnormal gametes: one with an extra chromosome (e.g., chromosome 21 causing trisomy 21), and one with a missing chromosome (e.g., causing monosomy of that chromosome).

In summary, nondisjunction in meiosis I leads to four abnormal gametes—two with an extra chromosome, two with a missing chromosome. Nondisjunction in meiosis II leads to only two abnormal gametes because the other normal gametocyte produced during meiosis I will divide normally. This leads to one gamete with an additional chromosome, one with a missing chromosome, and two normal gametes.

Autosomal Trisomies

As stated previously, there are only three autosomal trisomies that are not lethal in utero: Down syndrome (trisomy 21), Patau syndrome (trisomy 13), and Edwards syndrome (trisomy 18).

Down syndrome is also associated with congenital heart disease, acute lymphoblastic leukemia, and Alzheimer disease.

Down syndrome is the most common trisomy and also the only trisomy that allows for survival into adulthood. This is typically associated with **cognitive delays** and a set of distinguishing physical characteristics, including a **single palmar crease, protruding tongue, hypertelorism** (increased interorbital distance), and **epicanthic skin folds** on the inner corner of the eyes. Patients with Down syndrome are at increased risk for **acute lymphoblastic leukemia, Alzheimer disease, and congenital heart disease** (specifically endocardial cushion defects). Note that in addition to nondisjunction, patients with Down syndrome can also have an extra 21st chromosome if one of the 21st chromosomes attaches abnormally to another chromosome. This is called **translocation** and either can be asymptomatic in the mother (e.g., mother has two 21st chromosomes, but one of them is attached to another chromosome, leading to the potential for trisomy 21 in the offspring) or can occur during rearrangement in meiosis. The most common is a robertsonian translocation between chromosomes 14 and 21.

With Patau and Edwards syndromes, almost all affected babies die by 1 year of age. **P**atau syndrome includes cleft **p**alate and **p**olydactyly.

Both **Patau** and **Edwards** (Fig. 2.31) syndromes are associated with extremely high mortality by 1 year of age. They both have much in common: the risk for congenital heart defects is high, both have severe cognitive impairment, and they include numerous congenital defects. The features that set them apart are that patients with **trisomy 13** (Patau syndrome) have cleft lip and palate and polydactyly, and patients with **trisomy 18** (Edwards syndrome) have clenched hands with overlapping fingers and rocker-bottom feet.

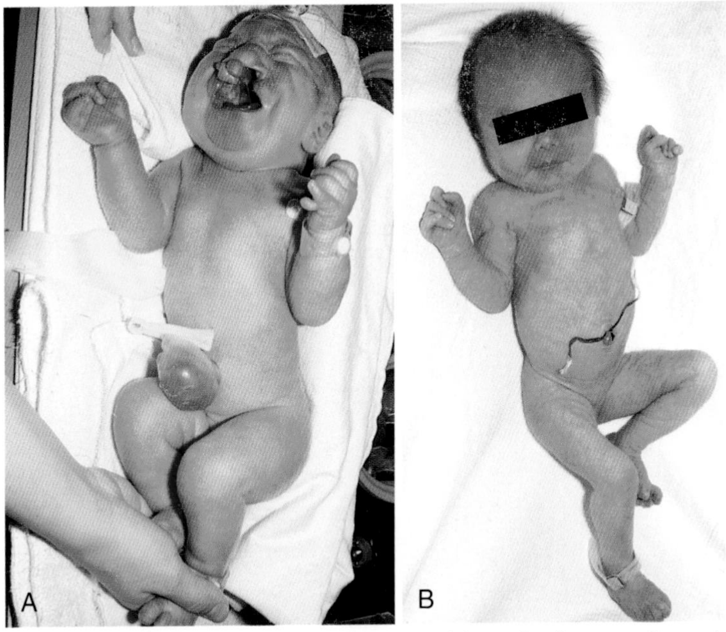

FIG. 2.31 **A,** Trisomy 13 (Patau syndrome) with characteristic cleft lip and palate as well as polydactyly. This baby also has an omphalocele. **B,** Trisomy 18 (Edwards syndrome) with characteristic clenched fists with overlapping fingers. (*From Adkison LR.* Elsevier's Integrated Review Genetics. *2nd ed. Philadelphia: Elsevier; 2011.*)

Sex Chromosome Aneuploidy

Turner syndrome (45,Xo) features include short stature, ovarian dysgenesis causing sterility and sexual infantilism, shieldlike chest, coarctation of the aorta, and bicuspid aortic valve.

Klinefelter syndrome (47,XXY) features include male gender, tall stature, small testes, and sterility.

It has been discussed how, through nondisjunction (or translocation), an extra (or one fewer) autosomal chromosome can occur. However, the same process can also occur in sex chromosomes. This leads to a few specific conditions, the most important of which are **Klinefelter syndrome** and **Turner syndrome**.

Klinefelter syndrome occurs when the individual is 47,XXY (extra X chromosome) Patients with Klinefelter syndrome are phenotypically male but have an inactivated X chromosome in each of their cells, just as females would. This can be seen microscopically as a Barr body (the remnant of the inactivated chromosome). Those with Klinefelter syndrome typically are **tall**, have long arms and legs, and have **small testes**. They are typically sterile.

Turner syndrome is a condition in which instead of being 46,XX (normal female), the patients are 45,Xo. This means they only have a single X chromosome. They typically are **short** and have **ovarian dysgenesis** ("streak" gonads, which are nonfunctional, causing sterility and lack of estrogen and sexual infantilism). They have a characteristic physical appearance that includes a broad **shieldlike** chest, lymphedema of the hands and feet, and a **webbed neck** (Fig. 2.32). They are also at risk for **coarctation of the aorta** and a **bicuspid aortic valve**.

Trinucleotide Repeat Disorders

Trinucleotide repeat disorders are several well-known neurogenetic diseases that result in dementias, ataxias, muscular atrophies, and mental retardation. Diseases within this classification include Huntington disease, Fragile X syndrome, Friedreich ataxia, and spinobulbar muscular atrophy. They are characterized by expansions of a certain three nucleotide repeating sequences that result in nonfunctioning protein products or epigenetic alteration. Many of these diseases are marked by **anticipation**, where the disease presents more severely or earlier than in the previous generation.

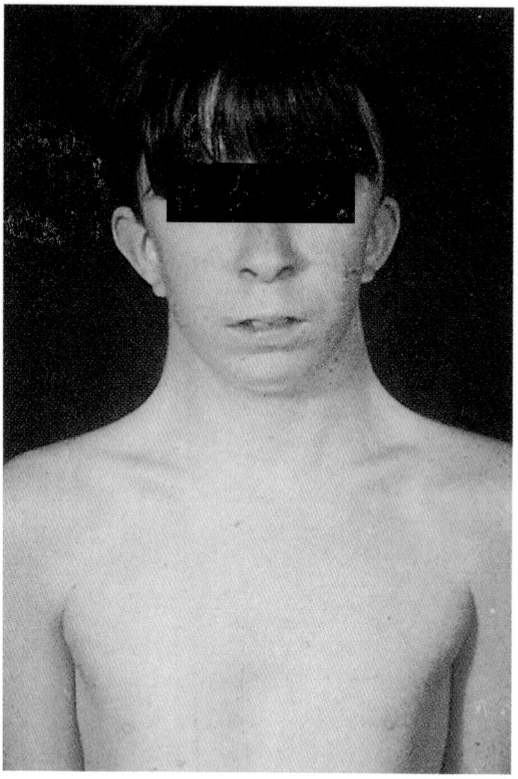

Fig. 2.32 Turner syndrome with the characteristic webbed neck. The "shield" chest can also be seen. (*From Epstein O, Perkin DG, Cookson J, et al.* Clinical Examination, *4th ed. Philadelphia: Elsevier; 2008.*)

Huntington disease is an autosomal dominant disorder of CAG repeats in the huntingtin (*HD)* gene. The increased number of glutamine (CAG codes for glutamine) amino acids in the protein leads to aggregation of the huntingtin protein, most notably in the neostriatum of the brain. The disease exhibits paternal anticipation, where number of CAG repeats increases if the affected gene is passed to the offspring by the father. The disease presents with choreiform (dance-like) movements, dementia, and psychiatric symptoms. The disease is progressive and uniformly fatal, and the age of onset is correlated to the number of CAG repeats.

Fragile X syndrome is an X-linked disorder caused by greater than 200 CGG repeats in the FMR1 (fragile X mental retardation 1) gene, which result in the methylation and subsequent silencing of the gene. The Fragile X phenotype is characterized physically by large ears, a long narrow face, and large testes (macroorchidism) in males and neurologically by developmental delay, intellectual disability, and autism. The prevalence is higher in males than females, and it is the most common inherited cause of intellectual disability.

Genetic Imprinting Diseases

Genetic imprinting occurs when a certain allele of a gene is inactivated (by methylation) depending on the parent of origin. Disease can result when there is a mutation or deletion of the remaining, nonimprinted allele. There are two relevant diseases associated with this phenomenon: Prader-Willi syndrome and Angelman syndrome. Both diseases are associated with imprinting of certain genes on chromosome 15q11-13. **Prader-Willi syndrome** is caused by loss of **paternal** genes, by either mutation or deletion, that are normally maternally imprinted. The disease is characterized by infantile hypotonia, hypogonadism, intellectual disability, hyperphagia, and obesity. Alternatively, this disease results from maternal uniparental disomy in approximately one fourth of cases (both alleles are from the mother and subsequently inactivated). In contrast, **Angelman syndrome** is caused by **maternal** loss of paternally imprinted genes on the long arm of chromosome 15. Most patients with Angelman syndrome have seizures, intellectual disability, ataxia and, interestingly, a persistently and inappropiately happy demeanor.

REVIEW QUESTIONS

(1) A patient presents with a headache and abdominal pain, and labs show anemia and basophilic stippling of red blood cells. Blockage of which two enzymes is causing this patient's anemia?

(2) An asymptomatic newborn is found to have PKU on routine neonatal screening. What amino acid was found to be elevated and why? What is the treatment?

(3) A 5-day-old male is brought in by his mother for poor feeding and lethargy. On review of systems, she mentions that his urine smells unusually sweet. Studies reveal an inborn error of metabolism. Which amino acids may be found in elevated levels in this child's urine?

(4) A 35-year-old male with schizophrenia presents to your clinic because of concerns from his caregiver that for many months he has absolutely refused to eat fruits and vegetables. On physical examination you note poor dentition with gingival bleeding, corkscrew hairs with perifollicular hemorrhage, and several large bruises on his skin. What vitamin deficiency may be causing this condition, and what is the mechanism of action?

(5) How do K_m and V_{max} differ for competitive and noncompetitive inhibitors?

(6) A patient is anemic and has high levels of orotate in her urine. What is the best treatment for this patient?

(7) What is the mechanism of action of allopurinol?

(8) What disorder is caused by defective nucleotide excision repair?

(9) An infant with vomiting, diarrhea, and jaundice is diagnosed with a deficiency of galactose-1-phosphate uridyltransferase. How should this infant be treated?

(10) An older male patient of Middle Eastern descent was treated for a urinary tract infection with trimethoprim-sulfamethoxazole. He then developed anemia and jaundice. What will his red blood cells look like on a smear?

(11) After a meal, what happens to levels of fructose 2,6-bisphosphate?

(12) A man with Leber hereditary optic neuropathy comes to your clinic and wants to know what the odds of his condition being passed down to his sons or daughters are. What is your response?

(13) A man comes to your clinic and states that his father has cystic fibrosis. He is concerned because this man's wife has a father who also has cystic fibrosis. What are the odds that the man and his wife will have a child with cystic fibrosis? Neither the man nor his wife have cystic fibrosis, and it is assumed that neither of their mothers are carriers.

(14) A man comes to your clinic with hemophilia A. He is concerned that he will have children with the same condition. What is the likelihood of having a son with hemophilia A? What is the likelihood of having a daughter with hemophilia A? Assume the mother is not a carrier.

3 DERMATOLOGY

Thomas E. Blair

HISTOLOGY AND PHYSIOLOGY

The skin is divided into the dermis and the overlying epidermis. The cellular component of the dermis consists of fibroblasts, adipocytes, and macrophages. The majority of the dermis, however, is acellular connective tissue composed primarily of type 1 collagen (for strength), elastin (for flexibility), and glycosaminoglycans. The dermis is mechanically responsible for cushioning the body and is also the site of the skin's adnexal structures (such as hair follicles), lymphatics, nerve fibers, and blood vessels. The superficial location of these blood vessels is particularly important in thermoregulation because vasodilation allows for increased heat loss to the environment, whereas vasoconstriction helps retain heat.

Layers of epidermis:
Stratum corneum
Stratum granulosum
Stratum spinosum
Stratum basale

The epidermis is the most superficial layer of skin and consists primarily of keratinocytes arranged as stratified squamous epithelium. Melanocytes, Langerhans cells, and Merkel cells can also be found in the epidermis (see later). The deepest epidermal layer is the **stratum basale,** which contains keratinocyte stem cells resting on a basement membrane. These cells divide and migrate upward to populate the **stratum spinosum,** where keratinization begins. The cells continue to migrate superficially as they mature. After they have reached the **stratum granulosum,** cross-linking of keratin continues, organelles begin to disappear, and the keratinocytes produce lamellar bodies (lipid-containing secretions that form a hydrophobic membrane). The granular appearance of these lamellar bodies gives this layer its name. In areas with thick skin, such as the palms and soles, the next layer is called the **stratum lucidum** (clear layer). It consists of densely packed cells that appear transparent under the microscope. Lastly, cells become part of the **stratum corneum,** where their nuclei are completely absent and keratin has formed a watertight barrier (Fig. 3.1). From superficial to deep, the skin layers are <u>c</u>orneum, <u>l</u>ucidum (in thick skin), <u>g</u>ranulosum, <u>s</u>pinosum, <u>b</u>asale. Mnemonic: <u>C</u>alifornian <u>l</u>adies <u>g</u>ive <u>s</u>uperb <u>b</u>ackrubs.

The skin can increase heat loss through arteriolar vasodilation and evaporation from eccrine sweat glands.

The skin has two major functions: thermoregulation and protection. **Thermoregulation** is accomplished through vasodilation or vasoconstriction of superficial arterioles (i.e., in hot conditions, arterioles dilate and shunt blood toward the skin surface, allowing for heat loss to the environment). Eccrine glands also promote heat loss through evaporation of sweat. The **barrier function** of skin is not only mechanical (keratinization) and immunologic (Langerhans cells) but also chemical because ultraviolet (UV) light is converted to harmless heat using melanin.

Melanocytes: Epidermal cells that produce melanin and package them within melanosomes, which can be phagocytosed by surrounding keratinocytes. By the process of internal conversion, melanin converts mutagenic UV radiation into harmless heat. It is also responsible for the color of an individual's skin. Those with darker skin tones, however, do not have more melanocytes; they produce melanosomes in greater number and size with greater distribution among keratinocytes. Melanocyte activation is under neurohormonal control of melanocyte-stimulating hormone (MSH), a cleavage product of adrenocorticotropic hormone (ACTH). It is not surprising, then, that the elevated ACTH in patients with Addison disease causes them to have darker skin. Melanoma arises from a malignant proliferation of melanocytes.

Individuals with darker skin have more melanosomes, not more melanocytes.

- Of note, melanin is synthesized from the amino acid tyrosine. It is not just responsible for coloring the skin but also the iris, the hair, and the substantia nigra of the brainstem (neuromelanin is a metabolite of dopamine and norepinephrine, which are also synthesized from tyrosine) (Fig. 3.2). Therefore melanoma can arise in any of these areas.

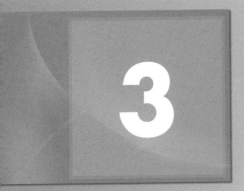

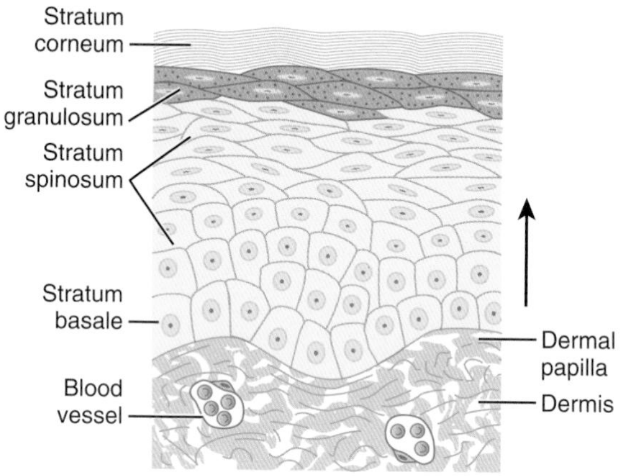

FIG. 3.1 Layers of the epidermis. In thick-skinned areas such as the palms and soles, the stratum lucidum separates the stratum corneum and stratum granulosum. (*From Burns ER, Cave MD.* Rapid Review Histology and Cell Biology. *2nd ed. Philadelphia: Elsevier; 2007.*)

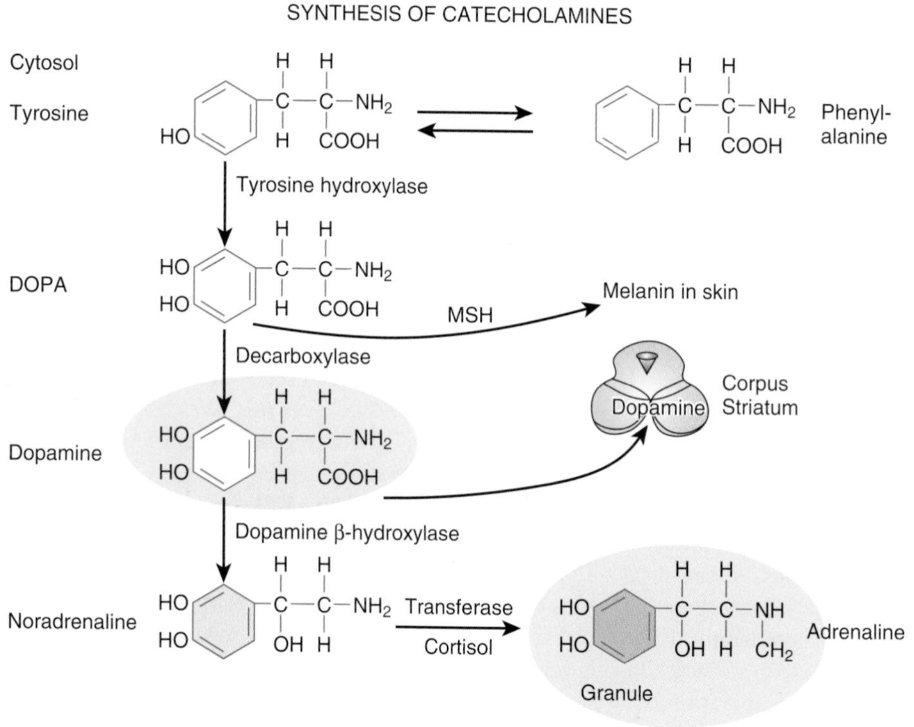

FIG. 3.2 Synthesis of catecholamines.

Langerhans Cells: Dendritic antigen-presenting cells that populate the dermis and epidermis (essentially the macrophage of the skin). After they have taken up antigen, they become active and migrate to lymph nodes, where they can interact with T and B cells. In this way, they act as a link between innate immunity and adaptive immunity. Of note, Langerhans cells in the mucosa of the vagina and foreskin are thought to be the initial target of human immunodeficiency virus (HIV).

Langerhans cells act as the macrophage of the skin.

Merkel Cells: Sensory neuroendocrine cells found in the stratum basale of the epidermis that communicate with large, myelinated sensory afferents. They are responsible for fine touch (see Chapter 13).

Adnexal Structures

Eccrine Glands: Sweat glands that cover the majority of the human body and participate in thermoregulation by secreting **hypotonic** NaCl for evaporation. They are stimulated by cholinergic fibers in the sympathetic nervous system.

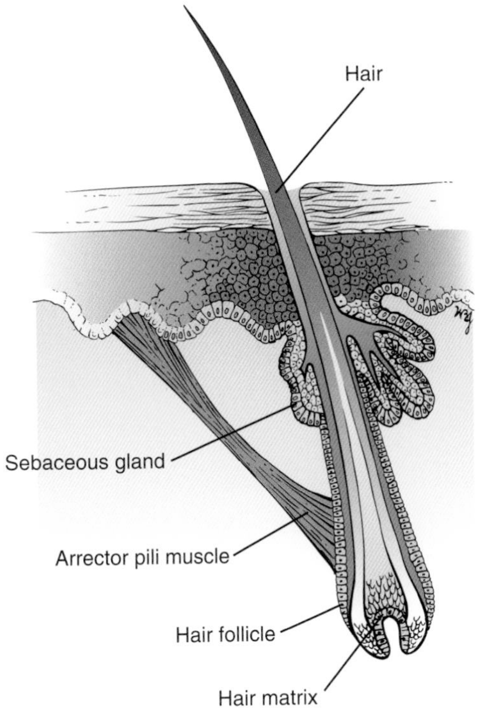

FIG. 3.3 The pilosebaceous unit. (*From Swartz MH. Textbook of Physical Diagnosis. 4th ed. Philadelphia: Elsevier; 2001.*)

- Of note, anticholinergic medications and toxins such as atropine inhibit cholinergic stimulation of eccrine sweat glands and produce vasodilation of peripheral vessels, leaving the patient **dry as a bone** and **red as a beet** (see toxicology section of Chapter 7).

Anticholinergic medications cause vasodilation and inhibition of eccrine sweat glands.

Apocrine Glands: Sweat glands that are found only in the axillae, genitoanal region, and areolae. They are activated at puberty and produce a viscous, protein-rich fluid that takes on its characteristic odor when metabolized by local bacteria. These are vestigial remnants of the mammalian sexual scent gland and serve no apparent function.

Pilosebaceous Unit: The hair fiber is composed of keratin that grows directly from the hair matrix (Fig. 3.3). The arrector pili muscle is responsible for piloerection ("goose bumps," a vestigial response to cold). The sebaceous glands produce sebum, which oils the skin and hair, preventing them from drying. Furthermore, sebum is somewhat toxic to bacteria. Sebaceous glands are activated by hormones during puberty and are important in the pathogenesis of acne vulgaris.

Describing Lesions

A standard terminology has been defined to describe dermatologic findings. These can be divided into primary lesions (Table 3.1 and Fig. 3.4A) and secondary lesions (Table 3.2 and Fig. 3.4B). Secondary lesions derive from primary lesions and are caused by trauma, evolution, or other modification of the primary lesion. Table 3.3 explains common histologic terms that describe dermatologic lesions.

PATHOLOGY

Common Dermatologic Conditions

Acne Vulgaris: The formation of a comedone occurs in a four-step process:

1. Hyperproduction of sebum within a sebaceous gland.
2. Formation of a plug blocking the pilosebaceous unit.
3. Inflammatory reaction to *Propionibacterium acnes,* an anaerobic bacterium and a component of skin flora.
4. Follicular wall rupture and spread of perifollicular inflammation.

Table 3.1 Primary Lesions

NAME	DESCRIPTION	EXAMPLE
Macule	Flat lesion < 0.5 cm	Ephelides (freckles)
Patch	Flat lesion > 0.5 cm	Vitiligo Melasma
Papule	Raised lesion < 0.5 cm	Acne vulgaris Rosacea
Plaque	Raised lesion > 0.5 cm	Psoriasis
Vesicle	Fluid-filled blister < 0.5 cm	Herpes simplex
Bulla	Fluid-filled blister > 0.5 cm	Bullous pemphigoid Pemphigus vulgaris
Pustule	Pus-filled lesion	Acne vulgaris Rosacea
Nodule	Firm or indurated lesion usually located in the dermis or subcutaneous fat. May or may not be raised	Erythema nodosum
Wheal	Dermal edema leading to a raised, erythematous, pruritic lesion lasting < 24 hr	Urticaria (hives)

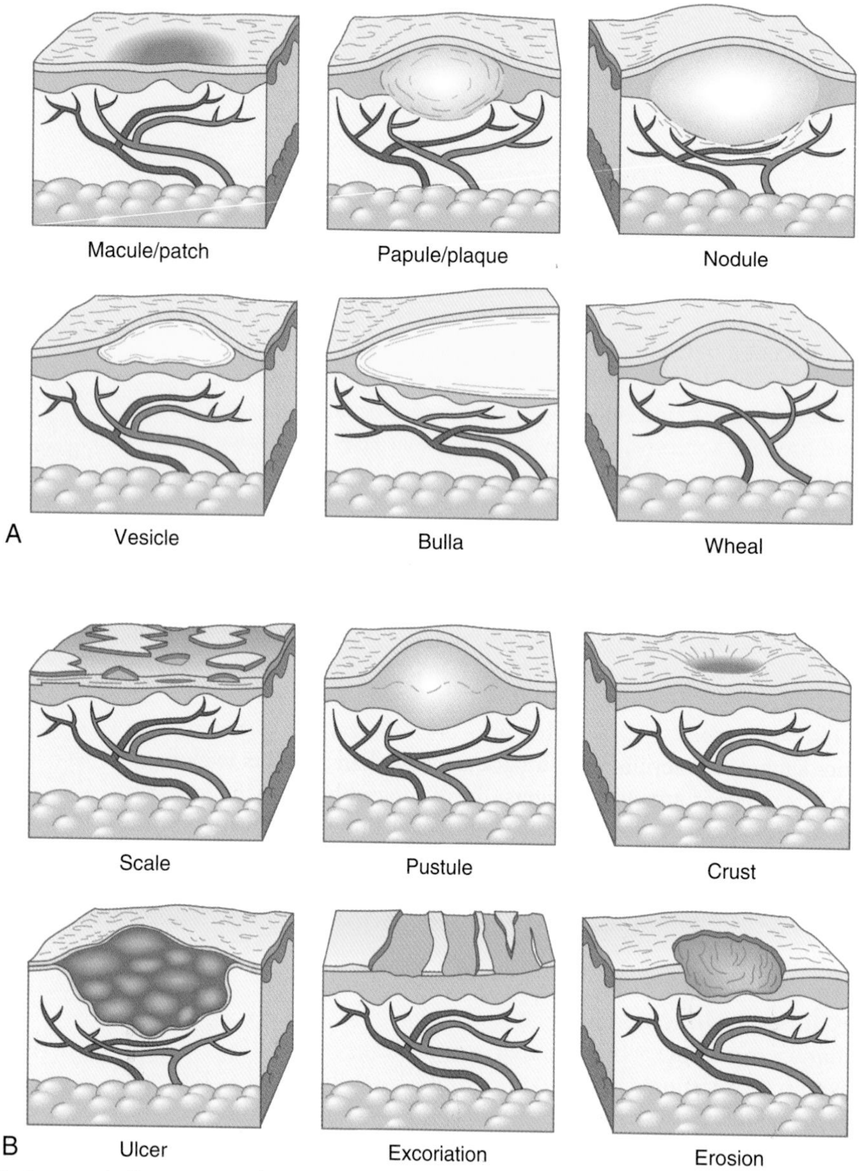

Fig. 3.4 **A,** Primary skin lesions. **B,** Secondary skin lesions. (*From Dieckmann R, Fiser D, Selbst S.* Pediatric Emergency and Crucial Care Procedures. *St. Louis: Mosby; 1997.*)

TABLE 3.2 Secondary Lesions

NAME	DESCRIPTION	EXAMPLE
Excoriation	Trauma to skin caused by scratching. Characterized by linear breaks in the epidermis	Scabies
Lichenification	Thick, rough area with accentuated skin lines; usually the result of repeated trauma or scratching	Eczema
Crust	Dried collection of serum, blood, pus, epithelial cells, and/or bacteria	Impetigo (honey-colored crust)
Scale	Fragment of stratum corneum (keratin) atop or peeling from the rest of the epidermis. Often secondary to rapid epidermal turnover	Psoriasis (silvery scale)
Erosion	Incomplete loss of epidermis causing shallow, moist, and well-circumscribed lesion	Pemphigus vulgaris (secondary to ruptured bullae)
Ulceration	Complete loss of epidermis with or without destruction of subcutaneous tissue and fat	Basal cell carcinoma (may have central ulceration)

TABLE 3.3 Histologic Terms

NAME	DESCRIPTION	EXAMPLE
Hyperkeratosis	Thickening of the stratum corneum	Callus
Parakeratosis	Thickening of the stratum corneum with persistence of nuclei (normally absent at this layer)	Psoriasis
Acanthosis	Thickening of stratum spinosum	Acanthosis nigricans
Acantholysis	Separation of keratinocytes caused by loss of intercellular cohesion	Pemphigus vulgaris

Sebum's exposure to air causes oxygenation of sebum and an **open comedone** (blackhead). Persistent occlusion leads to accumulation of sebum and a **closed comedone** (whitehead). Treatment often begins with topical retinoids and/or topical antibiotics, including benzoyl peroxide. Oral doxycycline or tetracycline may be used for moderate acne. Isotretinoin (Accutane) is reserved for nodulocystic acne. Treatments for hormonal acne (which is characterized by flares related to menstrual cycles and a jawline distribution) include oral contraceptive pills and spironolactone.

> Compared with acne, rosacea occurs in an older population. Telangiectasias, rhinophyma, and a lack of comedones also help distinguish the two.

Rosacea: Clinically and on Step 1, your job often will be to distinguish this condition from acne vulgaris. Like acne, rosacea may cause red papules and pustules on the face; however, the age group is generally an easy clue for rosacea because it is more likely to occur *de novo* in patients older than 30 years, whereas it is rarer to see new-onset acne in these patients (Fig. 3.5). Distinguishing features also include telangiectasias (which blanch), rhinophyma (a bulbous erythematous nose), and a lack of comedones. A trigger is often associated with the condition; such triggers include extreme temperatures or winds, strenuous exercise, severe sunburn, and certain foods such as alcohol, caffeinated beverages, and spicy foods. Usual treatment is with topical antibiotics such as **metronidazole** or oral antibiotics such as tetracyclines. In a patient older than 30 years with new-onset papules and pustules with strong environmental triggers, think rosacea before acne vulgaris. The etiology of rosacea is unclear, but it is thought to be from a pathologic interaction between the innate immune system and skin microbes.

> 6 Ps of lichen planus: purple, polygonal, pruritic planar, plaques and papules

Lichen Planus: Inflammatory lesions of the skin of unknown etiology but sometimes associated with hepatitis C infection. This condition is remembered and recognized by the **6 Ps** mnemonic: **p**urple, **p**olygonal, **p**ruritic, **p**lanar, **p**laques, and **p**apules (Fig. 3.6). Treatment usually involves high-potency topical steroids. It may be associated with **Wickham's striae** (whitish lines visible in the papules commonly seen on the oral mucosa) and **Koebner phenomenon** (new lesions that appear along lines of trauma, usually in linear patterns after scratching).

> Koebner phenomenon: skin lesions that develop along lines of trauma

Pityriasis Rosea: Thought to be secondary to a virus, this dermatologic condition may begin with a viruslike prodrome and a **herald patch**—a raised oval, pink patch with central clearing (Fig. 3.7). It appears on the trunk and may be confused with tinea corporis. The herald patch is followed 7 to 14 days later by multiple lesions similar in appearance but smaller. They form on the back and follow skin cleavage lines in a **"Christmas tree" pattern.** No treatment is necessary because the condition is usually

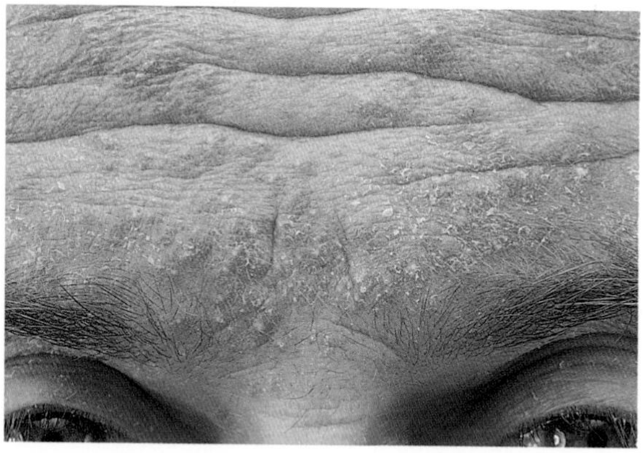

Fig. 3.5 Rosacea. Note papules and pustules in a middle-aged male. (*From Kumar P, Clark M. Clinical Medicine. 2nd ed. Philadelphia: Elsevier; 2002.*)

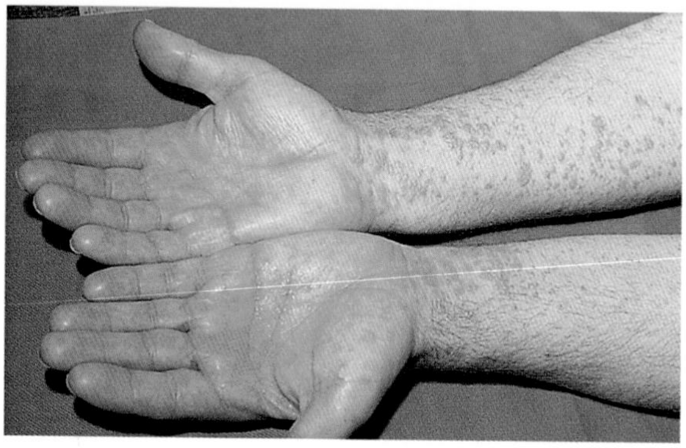

Fig. 3.6 Purple, polygonal, pruritic papules of lichen planus. (*From Douglas G, Nicol F, Robertson C. MacLeod's Clinical Examination. 11th ed. Philadelphia: Elsevier; 2005.*)

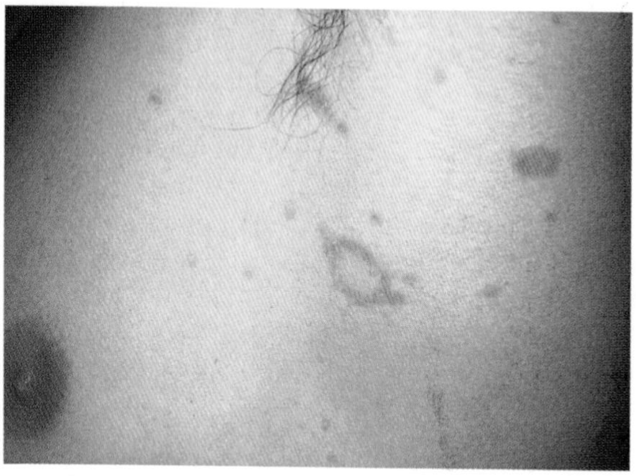

Fig. 3.7 Herald patch of pityriasis rosea. (*From Swartz MH.* Textbook of Physical Diagnosis. *6th ed. Philadelphia: Elsevier; 2009.*)

self-limited. The characteristic morphologic pattern described earlier and the lack of scale found on the lesions can distinguish pityriasis rosea from tinea corporis.

Keloid: Firm, shiny nodule of scar tissue (type 1 collagen) as a result of granulation tissue (type 3 collagen) overgrowing the boundaries of a wound. Keloids **overgrow the boundaries** of the initial injury, unlike hypertrophic scars, which are raised scars that respect wound margins. Keloids are common in African American individuals. They classically arise over scars but can also develop at sites of piercings or tattoos.

Contact Dermatitis: A delayed (type IV) hypersensitivity reaction in which contact with an antigen recruits previously sensitized T cells to initiate local inflammation. The sensitization can occur at any time after the initial exposure, even years later. Lesions are well-circumscribed, erythematous

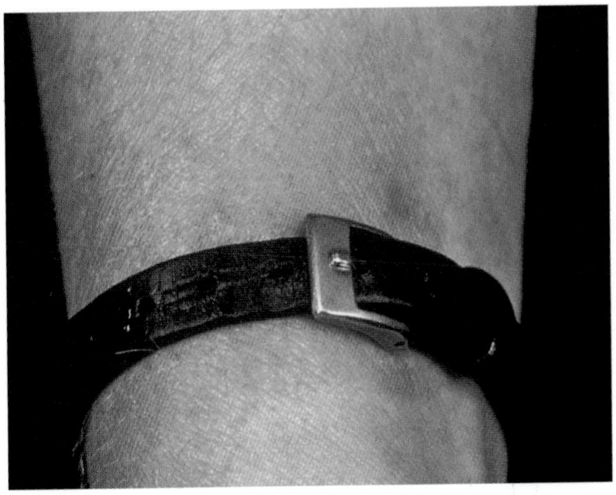

FIG. 3.8 Nickel contact dermatitis from a watchband. (*From Lim EKS, Loke YK, Thompson AM.* Medicine and Surgery. *Philadelphia: Elsevier; 2007.*)

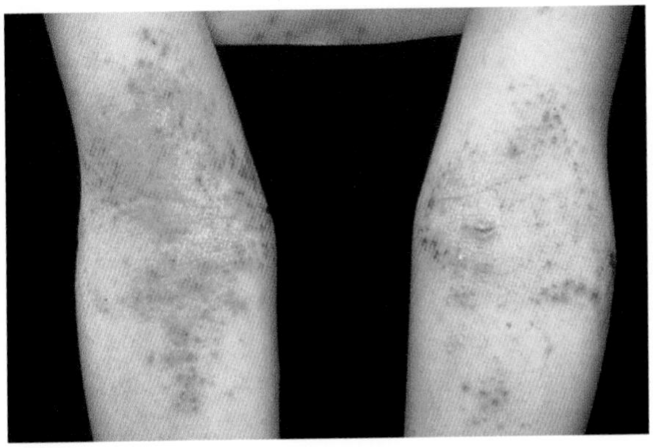

FIG. 3.9 Flexural distribution of atopic dermatitis. (*From Lim EKS, Loke YK, Thompson AM.* Medicine and Surgery. *Philadelphia: Elsevier; 2007.*)

plaques that may have vesicles or bullae over the area of exposure (Fig. 3.8). Common allergens include poison ivy, rubber, and nickel. Nickel can be found in jewelry and buttons, and the distribution of rash matches the area of contact. Treatment involves avoidance of the culprit allergen and topical steroids applied to any affected area. Systemic steroids may be needed in severe cases. After an exposure, contact dermatitis often takes days to develop. Consider a type 1 immunoglobulin E (IgE)–mediated reaction if development of rash (often urticaria) immediately follows an exposure (e.g., latex).

Contact dermatitis is a delayed (type IV) hypersensitivity reaction. Sensitized T cells initiate local reaction after an initial exposure.

Atopic Dermatitis (Eczema): Known as "the itch that rashes" because symptoms begin as **itching** that erupts into an erythematous, scaling lesion (Fig. 3.9). Vesicles may be present early, and lichenification occurs if the area is aggressively scratched. In adults, the distribution is in flexural areas (antecubital and popliteal fossae) and on the hands. The face and body may be affected in children. The etiology involves an overlap among genetics, environment, and the immune system. The terms *atopic march* and *atopic triad* describe the other hypersensitivity comorbidities that patients may later develop: eczema → asthma → allergic rhinitis. Treatment of eczema involves protecting the skin from excessive drying, avoiding irritants, and applying **topical steroids** and moisturizers (emollients).

The atopic march: eczema → asthma → allergic rhinitis

Urticaria (Hives): Pruritic wheals caused by mast cell degranulation spilling histamines and other inflammatory mediators into the surrounding tissue. Acute urticaria (<6 weeks) is often secondary to an environmental allergy, whereas chronic urticaria is thought to be an autoimmune condition. Initial treatment is with second-generation H1-antagonists (antihistamines). The lesions will be described as raised, erythematous, and intensely pruritic.

Urticaria is caused by mast cell degranulation.

Psoriasis: This disorder is caused by an interaction between the environment and genetics (HLA-B27) that causes a local inflammatory reaction and hastens the growth cycle of the epidermis, leading to thickened skin from keratinocyte accumulation in the stratum corneum at affected sites. Histologic examination reveals hyperkeratosis and parakeratosis. Clinically, psoriasis presents as red papules with **silvery scales** that coalesce into well-defined plaques, often on **extensor** surfaces (elbows and knees) (Fig. 3.10). Lesions may develop on sites of previous trauma (Koebner phenomenon). Removal of the scale will reveal pinpoint bleeding (**Auspitz sign**). Psoriasis can also affect nail beds (**pitting**) and joints (**psoriatic arthritis**). Treatment of skin lesions involves topical steroids. Systemic steroids should be avoided because initial improvement is often followed by a rebound phenomenon upon tapering. Severe psoriasis may necessitate stronger agents such as methotrexate or tumor necrosis factor α inhibitors, including etanercept and infliximab. The rash of psoriasis is usually improved with sunlight exposure, and light therapy can also be therapeutic.

Psoriasis usually occurs on extensor surfaces (elbows and knees), whereas eczema usually occurs on flexor surfaces (antecubital and popliteal fossae).

Langerhans Cell Histiocytosis (Histiocytosis X): Abnormal proliferation of histiocytes. On the skin this condition presents as red papules on the scalp or trunk that may display crusting or scaling. Painful osteolytic bone lesions of the skull are also characteristic. Lung nodules may also occur, accompanied by cough. Skin **biopsy will reveal Langerhans cells,** which are very large (about four times larger than a lymphocyte). Although this is a confusing disease that may affect many organ systems, on Step 1 the key diagnostic feature is often the presence of **Birbeck granules** on electron microscopy—tennis racket–shaped organelles within the cell (Fig. 3.11).

Langerhans cell histiocytosis: Birbeck granules (tennis racket–shaped organelles) on electron microscopy. Bone, skin, and other organs may be involved.

Autoimmune Diseases

Pemphigus Vulgaris: A severe autoimmune bullous condition caused by IgG antibodies within the epidermis that attack **desmosomes** and lead to a loss of adhesion between keratinocytes (acantholysis). The clinical result is the formation of painful, superficial, **flaccid, intraepidermal bullae.** These bullae may expand on gentle stroking of normal-appearing adjacent skin (Nikolsky sign) and may rupture, leading to painful erosions (Fig. 3.12). Unlike with bullous pemphigoid (see later), there is often mucous membrane involvement (on Step 1, oral involvement of disease is the most common clue that this represents pemphigus vulgaris and not bullous pemphigoid). Immunofluorescence reveals **IgG deposits between keratinocytes.** Treatment includes use of systemic steroids and supportive measures to maintain homeostasis (often treated like severe burn patients).

Bullous Pemphigoid (BP): A **less severe** autoimmune condition in which antibodies attack **hemidesmosomes,** which connect epidermal basal cells to the basement membrane. Binding of

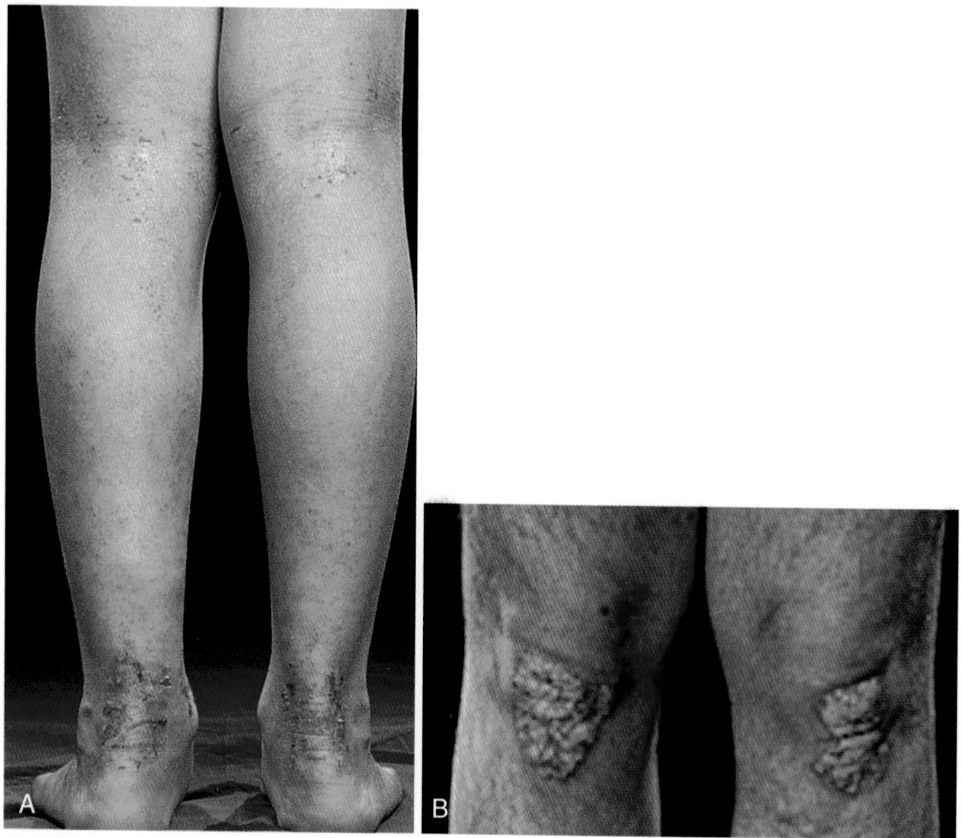

Fig. 3.10 A and **B,** Extensor rash of psoriasis. *(From Douglas G, Nicol F, Robertson C. MacLeod's Clinical Examination. 11th ed. Philadelphia: Elsevier; 2005.)*

complement leads to destruction of the basement membrane, separation of the dermoepidermal junction, and the formation of **subepidermal blisters.** Clinically this creates the appearance of **tense bullae** and subsequent erosions at the site of ruptured bullae (Fig. 3.13). BP typically presents in older adults (>60 years old), and unlike with pemphigus vulgaris, **mucous membranes are rarely involved** and **Nikolsky sign is negative.** The etiology of this condition is unknown, although it may

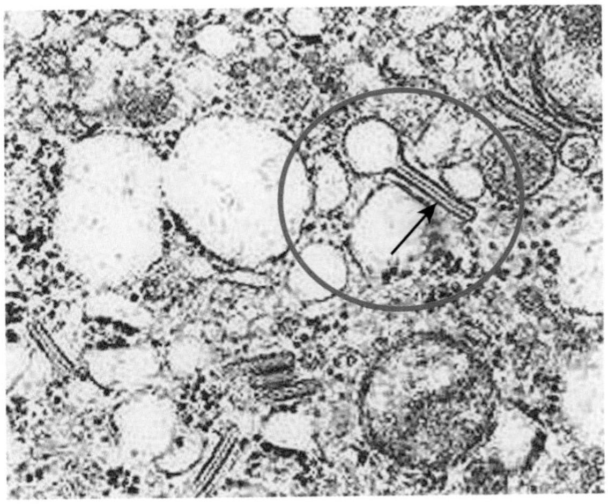

FIG. 3.11 Arrow pointing to Birbeck granule seen on electron microscopy of a Langerhans cell in Langerhans cell histiocytosis. (*From Goljan EF.* Rapid Review Pathology. *3rd ed. Philadelphia: Elsevier; 2009. Courtesy William Meek, Oklahoma State University, Center for Health Sciences, Tulsa, OK.*)

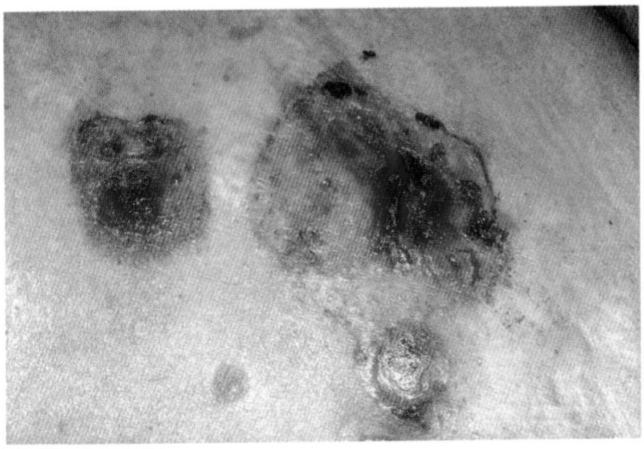

FIG. 3.12 Erosions from ruptured bullae in pemphigus vulgaris. (*From Lim EKS, Loke YK, Thompson AM.* Medicine and Surgery. *Philadelphia: Elsevier; 2007.*)

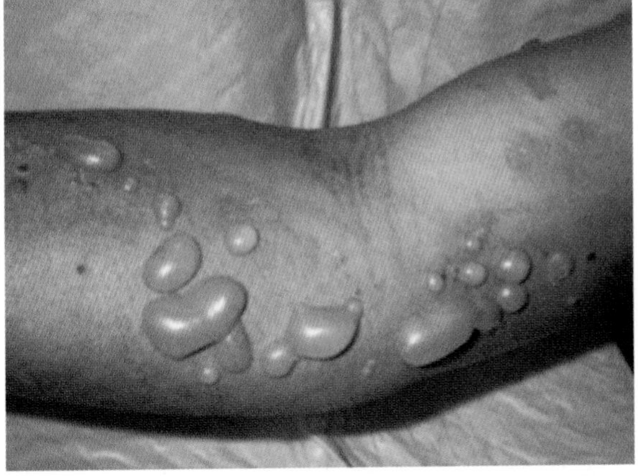

FIG. 3.13 Tense bullae of bullous pemphigoid. (*From Swartz MH.* Textbook of Physical Diagnosis. *6th ed. Philadelphia: Elsevier; 2009.*)

be triggered by initiation of culprit medications. BP is relatively mild compared with other bullous diseases and often responds to topical steroids alone. Mnemonic: antibodies in **bullous** pemphigoid line up **"bulow"** (below) the basement membrane and **bullous** pemphigoid is **"bulow"** pemphigus vulgaris in severity.

Antibodies in **bullous** pemphigoid line up **"bulow"** (below) the basement membrane and **bullous** pemphigoid is **"bulow"** pemphigus vulgaris in severity.

Conditions of Pigmentation

Vitiligo: An autoimmune condition in which antibodies target melanocytes within the epidermis. The subsequent absence of melanin leads to **depigmentation** in flat, well-circumscribed macules or patches. This condition may occur in any race but is more noticeable in dark-skinned individuals. Depigmented areas fluoresce under a Wood lamp (ultraviolet light), which can help detect depigmentation in light-skinned individuals. Vitiligo should not be confused with tinea versicolor, which causes hypopigmentation, not depigmentation. Key feature: **absent melanocytes.**

Albinism: Autosomal recessive inability to convert tyrosine into melanin (usually because of an inherited mutation in or deficiency of the tyrosinase enzyme). Patients have pale skin, white hair, and blue eyes. The risk for skin cancer is extremely high in these individuals. Key feature: **decreased melanin.**

Albinism: genetic inability to convert tyrosine into melanin

Solar Lentigo: Hyperpigmented patches seen in sun-exposed areas such as the face, chest, and arms, often seen in older patients who have had years of UV-light exposure. They are also known as lentigo senilis and "old-age spots." Although these lesions are benign, they can develop into a type of melanoma known as lentigo maligna. Key feature: **increased melanocytes.**

Melasma: Estrogen and progesterone stimulate melanocytes during pregnancy or oral contraceptive use to increase production of melanin. Hyperproduction of melanin causes formation of hyperpigmented macules and patches on sun-exposed areas. Also known as the "mask of pregnancy," this condition is only of cosmetic concern. Although it is much more commonly seen in women, men can also develop melasma. Treatment is with either makeup to darken surrounding skin, or topical hydroquinone to lighten the affected areas. Key feature: **increased melanin.**

Melanocytic Nevus (Common Mole): Benign neoplasms of melanocytes that need no intervention. There are several different types including junctional, intradermal, and compound nevi. These terms simply refer to their location in the skin: junctional nevi are found at the junction between the epidermis and the dermis, intradermal nevi are exclusively within the dermis, and compound nevi extend through both the dermal-epidermal junction and the dermis. Key feature: **increased melanocytes.**

Ephelis (Common Freckle): Contain normal numbers of melanocytes but increased concentrations of melanin. Key feature: **increased melanin.** Of clinical importance, freckles have similar histology to the café au lait spots of neurofibromatosis type 1.

Vitiligo: absent melanocytes
Albinism: decreased melanin
Melasma: increased melanin
Common mole: increased melanocytes
Ephelis: increased melanin
Melanoma: increased malignant melanocytes

Neoplasms, Dysplasias, and Malignancies

Basal Cell Carcinoma (BCC): The most common human malignancy. As the name implies, BCCs develop in the stratum basale, often as a result of UV-induced DNA damage. Patients present with lesions on sun-exposed areas that are characteristically **pearly nodules** with **rolled edges** (Fig. 3.14). **Central ulceration** and overlying **telangiectasias** also may be present. Diagnosis can be confirmed with biopsy, which reveals nests of basal cells demonstrating peripheral palisading. BCCs are treated with excision. The prognosis is extremely good because the risk of metastasis is vanishingly small. They are locally invasive, however.

BCC buzzwords:
Pearly
Rolled edges
Central ulceration
Telangiectasias
Peripheral palisading

Actinic Keratosis (AK): Precancerous, dysplastic lesion characterized by excessive keratin buildup forming crusty, scaly, **rough** papules and plaques. They tend to occur in sun-exposed areas such as the face and scalp and may progress to squamous cell carcinoma (SCC). Diagnosis is based on physical examination, although lesions suspicious for SCC should be biopsied. AKs are usually treated with cryotherapy or topical 5-fluorouracil.

Squamous Cell Carcinoma (SCC): Patients present with scaling plaques in sun-exposed areas (Fig. 3.15). Histologic examination reveals **keratin pearls.** Lesions are locally invasive and are more likely to metastasize than BCCs. Risk factors include sun exposure, immunosuppression, arsenic exposure, and chronic draining sinus tracts (e.g., from osteomyelitis). SCCs also have a tendency to grow on areas of scarring; an aggressive, ulcerative SCC that grows in an area of previous scarring or trauma is called a **Marjolin ulcer. Erythroplasia of Queyrat** is a specific term for SCC in situ on the glans penis, usually

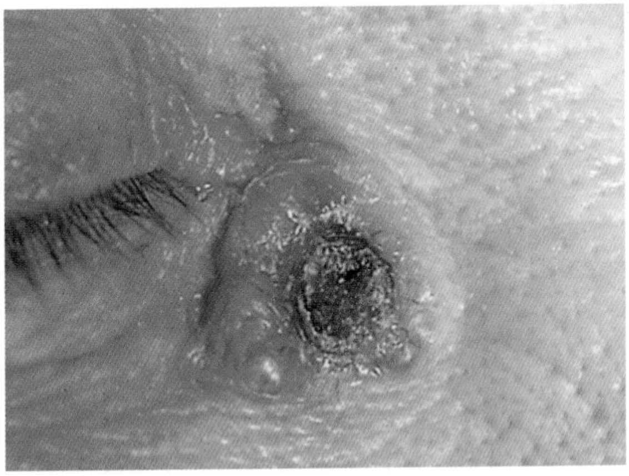

FIG. 3.14 Basal cell carcinoma. Note the rolled edges with central ulceration. (*From Savin JA, Hunter JAA, Hepburn NC.* Diagnosis in Color: Skin Signs in Clinical Medicine. *London: Mosby-Wolfe; 1997:104.*)

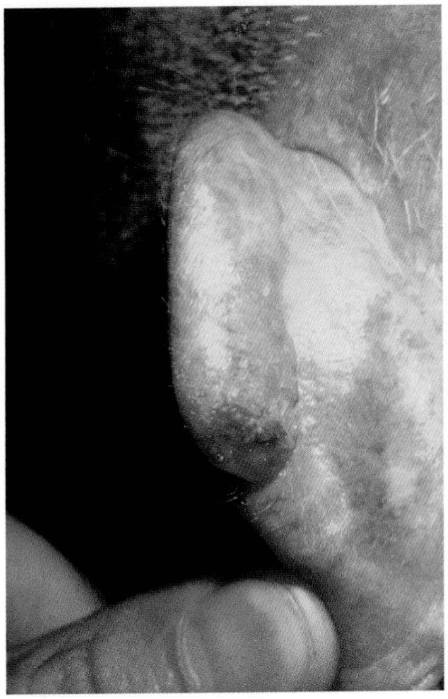

FIG. 3.15 Squamous cell carcinoma. (*From Talley NJ.* Clinical Examination. *Philadelphia: Elsevier; 2005.*)

secondary to infection with high-risk human papillomavirus serotypes 16 and 18. This subtype of SCC tends to present as a velvety-smooth, red plaque.

Keratoacanthoma: Controversially considered a subtype of SCC; this lesion is rapidly growing and forms a **dome** with a central **keratin plug** (Fig. 3.16). The lesion often grows so large so quickly that it outstrips its blood supply, necroses, and resolves with some scarring.

Melanoma: A malignant tumor of melanocytes recognized clinically by the ABCDEs: **a**symmetry, **b**orders (irregular), **c**olor (variance within the lesion), **d**iameter (>6 mm), and **e**volution (growing, changing color, becoming pruritic). Melanomas are most likely to metastasize if they enter a vertical phase of growth; therefore depth of invasion is correlated with mortality. Their precursor lesion is the **dysplastic nevus,** which may display some of the previously listed features and should be biopsied. This cancer has a positive **S-100 tumor marker,** which is consistent with melanocytes' derivation from neural crest cells. Although most melanomas are darkly pigmented, keep in mind that they can also lack this characteristic color and appear similar to the patient's skin tone; these are known as amelanotic melanomas.

There are several types of melanoma:

- Superficial spreading melanoma: the most common type of melanoma. It undergoes radial (lateral) growth before entering a vertical phase of growth, so prognosis is good.

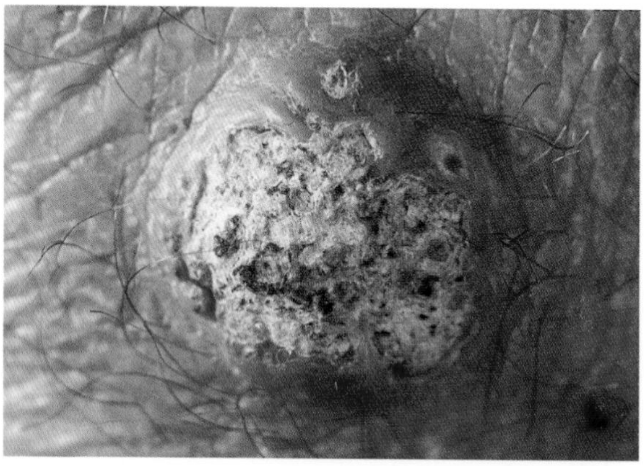

FIG. 3.16 Keratoacanthoma. Note the central keratin plug. (*From Lim EKS, Loke YK, Thompson AM. Medicine and Surgery. Philadelphia: Elsevier; 2007.*)

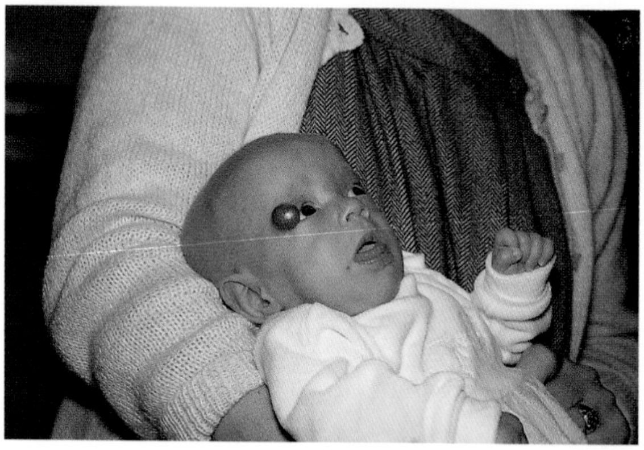

FIG. 3.17 Cherry hemangioma. (*From Fitzpatrick JE, Morelli JG. Dermatology Secrets in Color. 2nd ed. Philadelphia: Elsevier; 2000. Courtesy James E. Fitzpatrick, MD.*)

- Lentigo maligna melanoma: develop from benign lentigos (see earlier) in sun-exposed areas.
- Acral lentiginous melanoma: commonly occurs on the palms and soles, although can also occur under the nail (subungual). This type of melanoma is more common in dark-skinned individuals and is the least commonly observed type of melanoma overall.
- Nodular melanoma: enters a vertical phase of growth early on in its development, with a poor prognosis.

Melanomas arise from dysplastic nevi. Depth of invasion is highly correlated with mortality.

Seborrheic Keratosis (SK): Classically a **warty, stuck-on** appearing lesion formed by a benign proliferation of keratinocytes. SKs are tan to brown plaques and patches found on any part of the body (i.e., not correlated with sun exposure). They are very common in older individuals, and patients tend to acquire more as they age. The development of SKs is believed to be an inherited trait. Plugs of keratin are visualized on histologic examination, although these lesions need not be biopsied. Of note, the *sign of Leser-Trélat* refers to a paraneoplastic phenomenon with an eruptive presentation of multiple SKs, indicating an underlying malignancy (especially gastric adenocarcinoma).

Vascular Lesions

Cherry Hemangioma: A benign proliferation of capillaries that forms a small red macule. They are more common with age and require no treatment; however, they will not involute on their own (Fig. 3.17).

Strawberry Hemangioma: Benign vascular tumor that appears in the **neonatal** period and slowly **involutes** during childhood. No treatment is required unless it ulcerates or is near vital structures like the eye (Fig. 3.18), in which case the child is treated with a beta-blocker. Mnemonic: "Straw-baby" hemangioma occurs in childhood, whereas cherry hemangiomas develop later in life.

Nevus Flammeus: A vascular malformation consisting of dermal capillaries and postcapillary venules; also known as a port wine stain. They consist of blanchable pink, red, or purple patches that

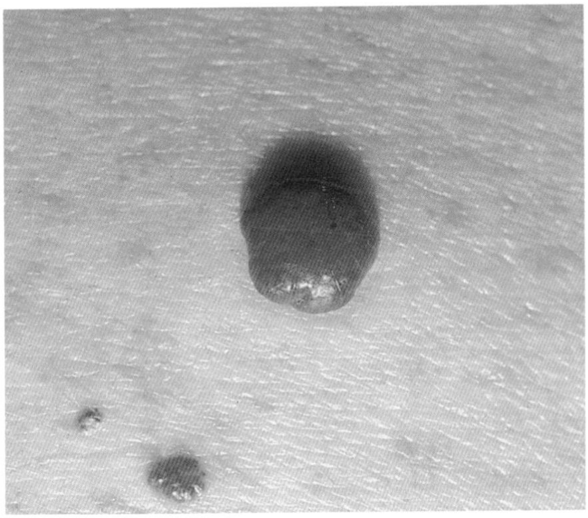

Fig. 3.18 Strawberry hemangioma. (*From Lissauer T, Clayden G. Illustrated Textbook of Pediatrics. 2nd ed. Philadelphia: Elsevier; 2001.*)

are present at birth and do not regress but usually grow with the child. Port wine stains are common on the face and usually do not cross the midline. They can be seen as part of Sturge-Weber syndrome.

Pyogenic Granuloma (PG): A benign erythematous papule that grows quickly and bleeds easily with a distinctive collarette of scale. PGs usually arise in young adults at sites of prior traumas but can also develop in children and during pregnancy. They do not usually spontaneously regress.

Angiosarcoma: A malignant proliferation of blood vessels or lymphatics that classically arises in the breast, scalp, or face after prior radiation exposure. They are blue to purple macules, papules, or nodules that bleed or ulcerate. Treatment is with complete resection and adjuvant radiotherapy if radiation is not believed to be a causative factor.

Skin Infections and Infestations

Cellulitis: Infection of deep dermal and subcutaneous tissue often caused by *Staphylococcus aureus* or *Streptococcus pyogenes*. Infection is often from direct penetration of bacteria into the skin. Cellulitis presents as a streaky, painful, warm, erythematous, edematous lesion with or without fever. Because the infection is deep, the margins of the infection are typically not well defined (which separates this from erysipelas, a more superficial infection with more well-defined borders). Treatment is with antibiotics. Distinguish cellulitis from chronic venous stasis by the bilateral nature of venous stasis changes.

Erysipelas: Similar to cellulitis, although infection is of the **superficial** dermis and lymphatics as opposed to deeper involvement. Erysipelas more commonly occurs in **children** and those with impaired lymphatic drainage. *S. pyogenes* is the most common pathogen. The lesion is **well circumscribed** with **raised borders** (Fig. 3.19A).

Streptococcal skin infections can cause poststreptococcal glomerulonephritis (PSGN) but not rheumatic fever. Antibiotics can prevent rheumatic fever but not PSGN.

Impetigo: ***S. aureus*** or, less commonly, ***S. pyogenes*** infection of the face, which begins as **vesicles** and **pustules** that later rupture, producing the characteristic **honey-colored crust** (Fig. 3.19B). Bullous impetigo is similar, but the initial lesions are flaccid bullae filled with transparent yellow fluid. Of note, if the causative organism is *S. pyogenes*, poststreptococcal glomerulonephritis (PSGN) is a potential complication but **not** acute rheumatic fever (which only appears after *S. pyogenes* pharyngitis). PSGN cannot be prevented with antibiotics, so treatment only affects the skin condition and does not prevent complications.

Staphylococcal Scalded Skin Syndrome (SSSS): A severe and generalized form of bullous impetigo. *S. aureus* skin infection produces exfoliative exotoxin, a protease that acts on desmoglein at the stratum granulosum to produce tense intraepidermal bullae followed by flaky, nonscarring desquamation over the entire body. This condition occurs predominantly in **neonates** and is often accompanied by fever. Note that the desmoglein of desmosomes is the target in both SSSS and pemphigus vulgaris.

Exfoliative exotoxin targets desmoglein and is responsible for the desquamation of SSSS.

Necrotizing Fasciitis: "Flesh-eating," rapidly progressive infection of subcutaneous tissue including fat and fascia that spreads along fascial planes. The cause may be either polymicrobial or

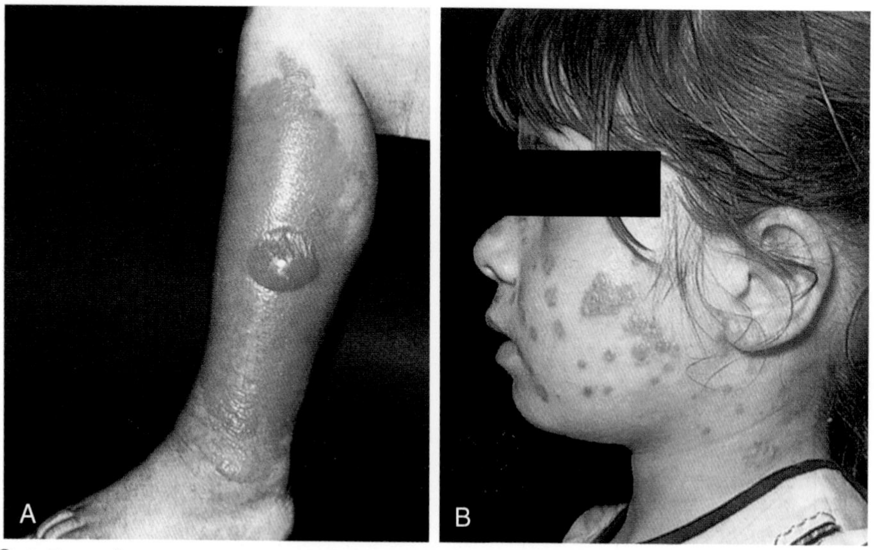

FIG. 3.19 **A,** Erysipelas. **B,** Impetigo. (*From Swash M, Glynn M. Hutchison's Clinical Methods. 22nd ed. Philadelphia: Elsevier; 2007.*)

monomicrobial. ***S. pyogenes*** is the most likely single organism. Necrotizing fasciitis often spreads from a site of local trauma or surgery. Clinically, it is similar to cellulitis but is characterized by extreme pain, fever, induration (hardening of skin), and **skip lesions** (noncontinuous islands of infected tissue with sparing of intervening tissue). Sepsis is common. Treatment involves intravenous antibiotics and surgical débridement. **Gas gangrene** is a similar condition caused by infection with *Clostridium perfringens*. In this infection, crepitus (crackling sensation on palpation) may also result from CH_4 and CO_2 production by the pathogen.

Gas gangrene occurs when infection with *C. perfringens* releases CH_4 and CO_2 gas into the tissue, which can be palpated as crepitus.

Dermatophytes: Superficial fungal infections of the skin or nails in which the fungus survives by metabolizing keratin. These infections are caused by *Epidermophyton*, *Microsporum*, and *Trichophyton* species. Infections are named for their location on the body (e.g., tinea capitis on the head, tinea pedis on the foot, tinea corporis on the body, and tinea cruris on the groin). Tinea corporis presents as a raised, erythematous, oval "ringworm." There is characteristic trailing scale that describes scale in the center of the lesion but not on the border; this feature can be used to distinguish tinea corporis from the herald patch of pityriasis rosea. KOH prep on microscopy can be confirmatory by demonstrating the presence of hyphae. Tinea pedis can present with scale along the sides of the feet in a moccasin pattern and can involve the nails (known as onychomycosis). Look for cracking between the toes, which can serve as a point of entry for bacteria and result in a superimposed cellulitis. Treatment is with topical antifungals, except onychomycosis, which requires systemic antifungals because of poor absorption of topicals through the nail. Topical steroids should be avoided because they can exacerbate the infection.

Tinea Versicolor: Superficial fungal infection with *Malassezia globosa* or *Malassezia furfur* that causes **hypopigmented** or hyperpigmented macules and patches with possible associated scaling (Fig. 3.20A). Lesions generally occur on the trunk and arms. Patients will note that it seems to get worse in the summer, which is usually because of sun-induced hyperpigmentation of surrounding normal skin, making the hypopigmented tinea versicolor lesions look even lighter. KOH prep reveals a **spaghetti and meatballs** appearance of the hyphae and yeast, respectively (Fig. 3.20B).

Scabies: A superficial infection with the parasite *Sarcoptes scabiei*, which burrows into the skin to live and reproduce. The mite is spread through person-to-person contact. The most profound feature of scabies is severe pruritus caused by a delayed (type IV) hypersensitivity reaction to the mites, their eggs, and their feces. The rash usually consists of erythematous papules with secondary excoriations; however, the **burrow** is pathognomonic and appears as a thin raised line along the skin (Fig. 3.21B). Crusted scabies (formally called Norwegian scabies) is a severe infestation that is associated with immunosuppression (e.g., from AIDS). Mineral oil prep may be confirmatory by direct visualization of the mites or eggs. Topical permethrin is the initial treatment of choice, and systemic ivermectin is used in severe or refractory cases.

In a patient with crusted scabies or oral hairy leukoplakia, investigate causes of immunosuppression (e.g., HIV test).

Oral Hairy Leukoplakia: White "hairy" plaque found on the side of the tongue caused by opportunistic infection of Epstein-Barr virus. The presence of leukoplakia should be **concerning for**

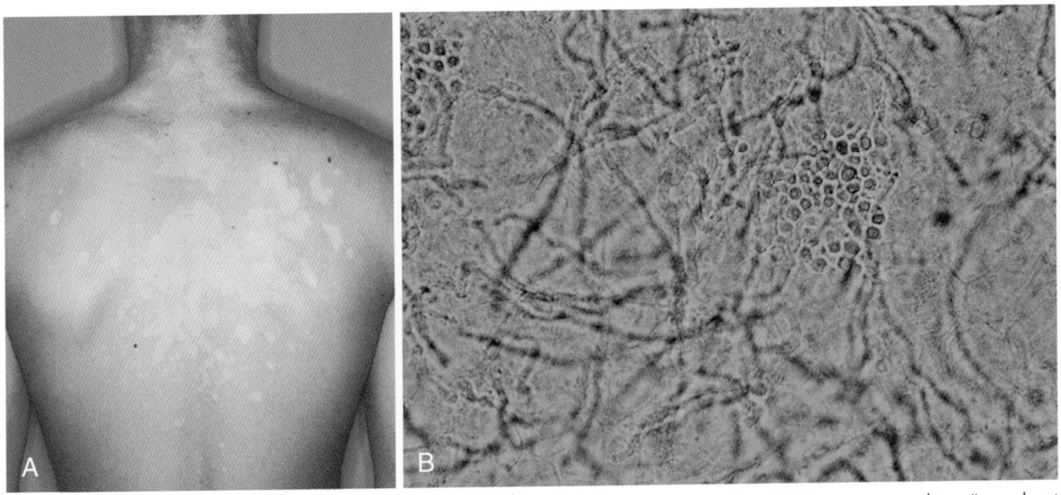

FIG. 3.20 **A,** Hypopigmented patches of tinea versicolor. **B,** Tinea versicolor KOH prep revealing "spaghetti and meatball" appearance of the hyphae and yeast. (**A** *from Swartz MH.* Textbook of Physical Diagnosis. *6th ed. Philadelphia: Elsevier; 2009.* **B** *from Habif TP.* Clinical Dermatology. *5th ed. Philadelphia: Elsevier; 2009.*)

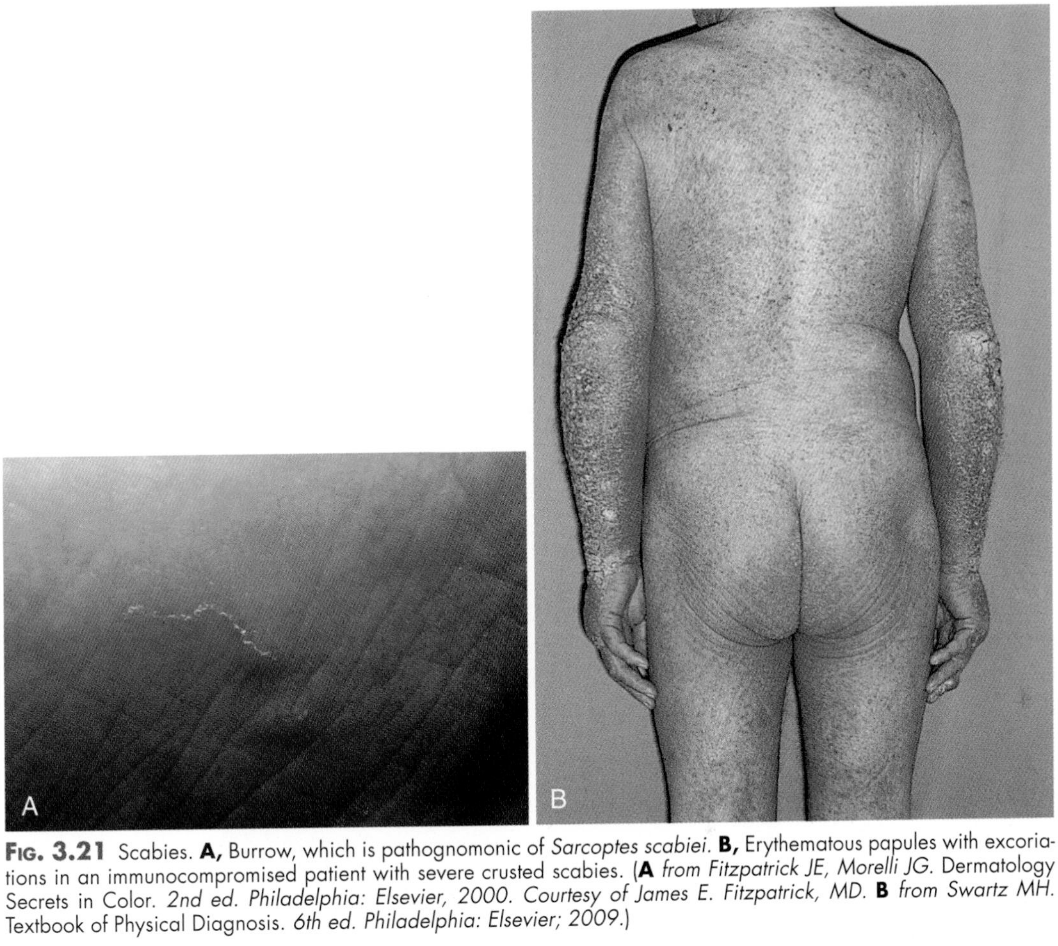

FIG. 3.21 Scabies. **A,** Burrow, which is pathognomonic of *Sarcoptes scabiei.* **B,** Erythematous papules with excoriations in an immunocompromised patient with severe crusted scabies. (**A** *from Fitzpatrick JE, Morelli JG.* Dermatology Secrets in Color. *2nd ed. Philadelphia: Elsevier, 2000. Courtesy of James E. Fitzpatrick, MD.* **B** *from Swartz MH.* Textbook of Physical Diagnosis. *6th ed. Philadelphia: Elsevier; 2009.*)

HIV. This lesion can be distinguished from **thrush/oral candidiasis** (caused by *Candida albicans*) because leukoplakia cannot be scraped off easily and tends to occur on the sides of the tongue. Oral candidiasis can occur in both immunocompetent and immunocompromised individuals. Esophageal candidiasis, on the other hand, is highly concerning for immunosuppression and is considered an AIDS-defining illness.

Leukoplakia: White patch on the tongue or oral mucosa secondary to squamous hyperplasia. Like oral hairy leukoplakia, this lesion will not scrape off. It is considered **precancerous** because some cases may progress to squamous cell carcinoma. It is highly associated with **tobacco use** (especially smokeless tobacco). Treatment is with cessation of any carcinogenic habits and/or surgical removal.

Oral hairy leukoplakia: EBV infection
Thrush: candidal infection
Leukoplakia: precancerous lesion

Verrucae (Warts):

Viral infection with human papillomavirus (HPV) causing acanthosis and hyperkeratosis. As in cervical infections with HPV, cells with enlarged, irregular nuclei (koilocytes) are present. Treatment is with cryotherapy.

- *Verruca vulgaris:* Common wart, often found on the hand. Presents as a raised, rough papule.
- *Verruca plantaris:* Smooth, flat wart, often found on the sole of the foot. Pinpoint bleeding is often present.
- *Condyloma acuminatum:* Genital warts caused by HPV subtypes 6 and 11 (low-risk strains).

HPV 2 and 7: common warts
HPV 6 and 11: genital warts
HPV 16 and 18: SCC

Dermatologic Manifestations of Internal Disease

Erythema Nodosum: Inflammatory condition of subcutaneous fat (panniculitis) resulting in tender erythematous nodules, often over the shins (Fig. 3.22). Associated especially with streptococcal infection, drugs, **sarcoidosis**, tuberculosis, inflammatory bowel disease, and fungal infections.

Erythema Multiforme: Multiple **target-shaped** lesions with "multiform" primary lesions (macules, papules, vesicles) (Fig. 3.23). Commonly a hypersensitivity reaction to drugs (usually antibiotics) leading to IgM deposition in the skin, but erythema multiforme may also be secondary to malignancies or infections such as herpes simplex virus (HSV) or *Mycoplasma.*

Stevens-Johnson Syndrome: Erythema multiforme but with more extensive and systemic symptoms, including **mucous membrane involvement,** fevers, diffuse erosions, and crusting. Lesions must cover less than 10% of the body surface area. It is associated with a high mortality rate.

Toxic Epidermal Necrolysis: A more severe form of Stevens-Johnson syndrome with lesions covering more than 30% of the body surface area. These conditions overlap when 10% to 30% of the body surface is involved.

Erythema multiforme, Stevens-Johnson syndrome, and toxic epidermal necrolysis are often considered on a continuum. They are commonly a result of drug hypersensitivity reactions.

Erythema Marginatum: Nonpruritic, erythematous, transient, ringed lesions of the trunk. This rash is one of the major criteria for **rheumatic fever.**

Erythema Chronicum Migrans: Expanding **bull's-eye**–shaped erythematous plaque at site of ***Ixodes* tick bite** and pathognomonic of early, localized **Lyme disease** (Fig. 3.24). Caused by localized infection with ***Borrelia burgdorferi*** (not hypersensitivity). Multiple lesions indicate the spirochete has spread hematogenously. Treatment is with doxycycline in teenagers and adults; ceftriaxone is preferred for children younger than 8 years old.

Dermatitis Herpetiformis: Pruritic vesicles and papules on an erythematous base (herpetiform), especially over extensor surfaces (elbows and knees). Caused by dermal IgA deposits in association with **celiac disease.** This condition is responsive to a gluten-free diet. (Fig. 3.25)

Acanthosis Nigricans: Velvety hyperpigmentation of skin overlying body folds associated with elevated insulin levels, which alter dermatologic growth factors (Fig. 3.26). Elevated insulin is most

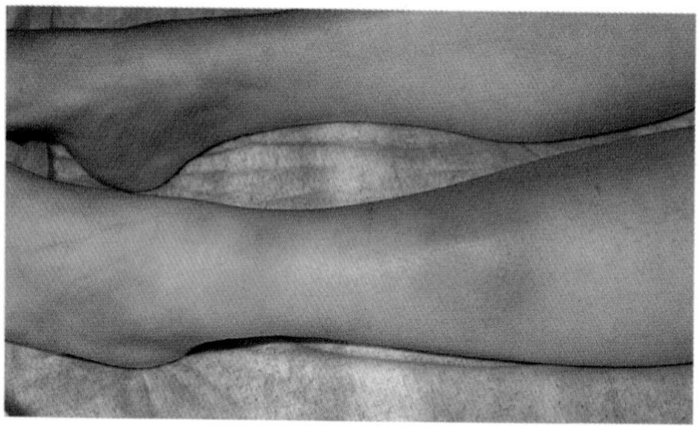

FIG. 3.22 Nodules of erythema nodosum. (*From Swartz MH. Textbook of Physical Diagnosis. 6th ed. Philadelphia: Elsevier; 2009.*)

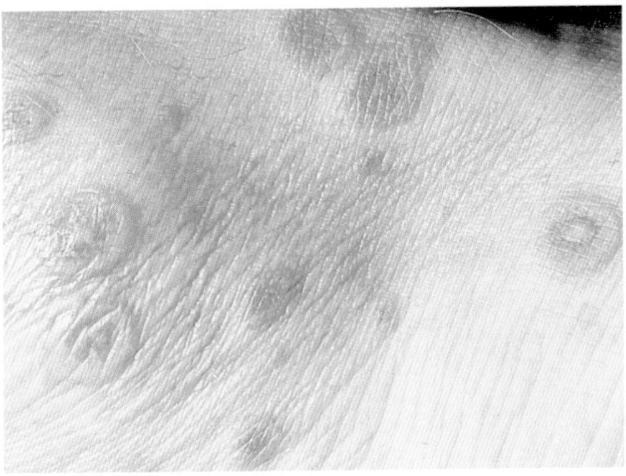

FIG. 3.23 Target lesions of erythema multiforme. (*From Stevens A, Lowe J, Scott I.* Core Pathology. *3rd ed. Philadelphia: Elsevier; 2008.*)

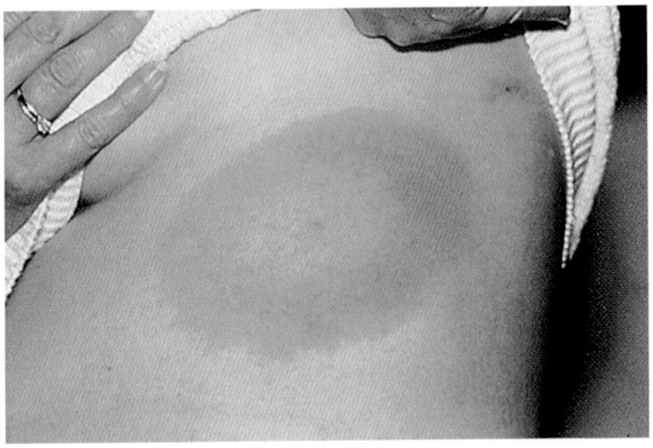

FIG. 3.24 Bull's-eye lesion of erythema migrans. (*Courtesy John Cook, MD. From Goldstein BG, Goldstein AO.* Practical Dermatology. *2nd ed. St. Louis: Mosby; 1997.*)

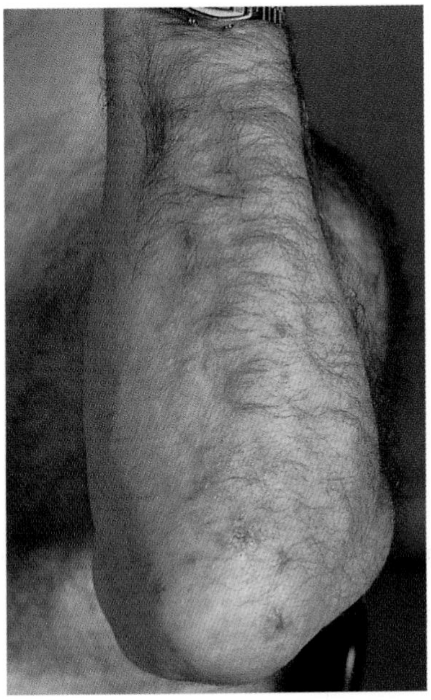

FIG. 3.25 Dermatitis herpetiformis. (*From Savin JAA, Hunter JAA, Hepburn NC.* Diagnosis in Color: Skin Signs in Clinical Medicine. *London: Mosby-Wolfe; 1997:92.*)

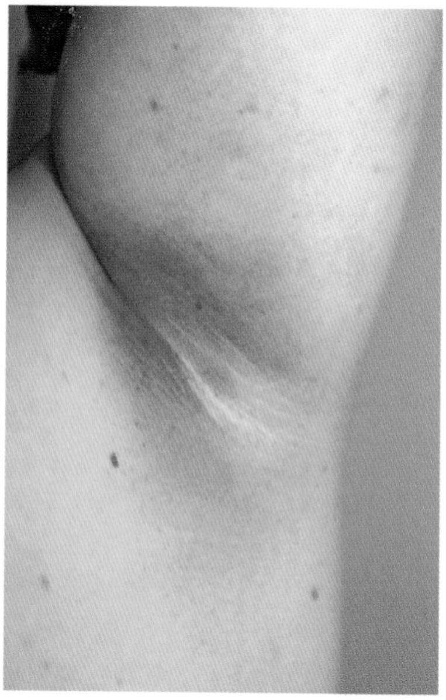

Fig. 3.26 Acanthosis nigricans. (*From Lissauer T, Clayden G. Illustrated Textbook of Pediatrics. 4th ed. Edinburgh: Elsevier; 2011.*)

commonly a result of insulin resistance in **type 2 diabetes.** Other endocrine disorders, such as polycystic ovary syndrome, may also be causative.

Stasis Dermatitis: Brawny discoloration of dependent areas (feet and ankles) caused by hemosiderin deposits from extravasation of erythrocytes as a result of venous hypertension (Fig. 3.27). Pedal edema is often present. The venous hypertension may simply be due to venous valve dysfunction, but heart failure producing peripheral edema may also be the underlying cause.

Dermatitis herpetiformis is caused by dermal IgA deposits in association with celiac disease.

PHARMACOLOGY

Retinoids: Vitamin A–related compounds that act as steroid hormones to alter gene transcription. These compounds bind nuclear retinoic acid receptors, which then activate promoter regions of DNA, leading to transcription of retinoid-sensitive genes. In the treatment of acne, the result is a decrease in size and sebum output of sebaceous glands. Topical retinoids are often used for the initial management of acne. Systemic isotretinoin, however, is reserved for nodulocystic acne as a result of its severe side effect profile, including hepatotoxicity and **teratogenicity** (causes embryologic and fetal malformations).

Retinoids activate promoter regions of DNA and increase transcription. Systemic retinoids are potent teratogens.

Permethrin: Antiparasitic agent used in the treatment of scabies and head lice *(Pediculosis capitis).* In arthropods, permethrin acts as a neurotoxin by prolonging sodium channel activation, thereby causing paralysis and death. It is poorly absorbed and easily inactivated in humans.

Topical Antifungals:

- Azoles: Inhibit an enzyme (14α-demethylase) responsible for formation of ergosterol (component of fungal membrane). Common agents for treatment of dermatophytes and tinea versicolor include clotrim**azole** (Lotrimin), micon**azole,** and ketocon**azole.**
- Terbinafine (Lamisil): Inhibits a different enzyme (squalene epoxidase) responsible for formation of ergosterol. Topically, terbinafine is a first-line agent for dermatophytes. It can also be used orally in the treatment of onychomycosis (fungal nail infection).

Antifungals often work by inhibiting the formation of ergosterol, an important component of fungal membranes.

Topical Steroids: Inhibit local inflammatory reaction by interfering with the production of inflammatory cytokines by phospholipase A_2. They are used in the treatment of lichen planus, atopic dermatitis, contact dermatitis, psoriasis, pemphigus vulgaris, and bullous pemphigoid, among others. Common topical steroids include hydrocortisone, triamcinolone, and clobetasol.

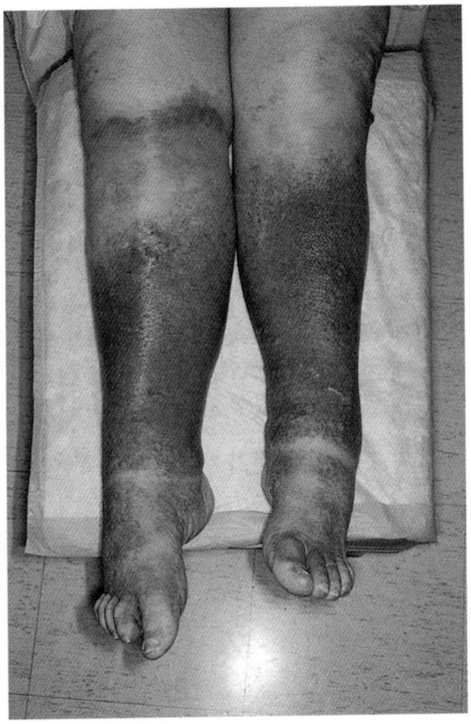

Fig. 3.27 Stasis dermatitis of dependent areas. (*From Swartz MH. Textbook of Physical Diagnosis. 4th ed. Philadelphia: Elsevier; 2001.*)

5-Fluorouracil (5-FU): Topical and systemic chemotherapeutic agent. 5-FU is a thymine (pyrimidine) analog that irreversibly inhibits thymidylate synthase, thus preventing DNA synthesis (see Chapter 11 for details). Used topically, it is one of the first-line therapies for actinic keratoses (cryotherapy is also a first-line treatment). 5-FU causes a local inflammatory response on the skin that may require interruption of treatment. Intravenously, it is used in the treatment of solid malignancies such as breast and colon cancer.

REVIEW QUESTIONS

(1) A 37-year-old man presents with fatigue, weight loss, and weakness for several months. He also notes that his skin has become much darker over the past few months despite rarely leaving the house. Labs reveal hyponatremia and hyperkalemia. Why has this patient's skin changed color?

(2) A 41-year-old man presents with joint pain in his ankles and knees. A thorough physical examination also reveals pitting of his nail beds. The patient states that during winter months he often has a rash, but since the weather turned warm it has resolved. Which HLA class is associated with this patient's condition, and what other autoimmune conditions are associated with this HLA class?

(3) A 71-year-old woman presents with several tense bullae over her arms. Immunofluorescence reveals linear IgG and C3 deposits along the basement membrane. What is the etiology of this patient's condition?

(4) A 44-year-old African American man presents with multiple hypopigmented patches with mild scaling on his chest and back. They are mildly pruritic and seem worse during hot, humid months. What is the likely etiology?

(5) A 20-year-old man presents with a 2-cm oval patch with central clearing on the trunk and is prescribed a topical antifungal by his physician. One week later, the patient returns to clinic with multiple pink oval plaques spread over his back. Why has this patient's rash worsened?

(6) A 61-year-old man with uncontrolled diabetes presents with a temperature of 40° C and rapidly progressing, severe pain of the lower extremity. Physical examination reveals induration and erythema from calf to thigh with islands of apparently unaffected tissue. What is the management of this patient?

(7) A 9-year-old girl presents to clinic with gross hematuria and is found to have hypertension. She has always been healthy; however, several weeks ago, she developed vesicles on her face that eventually crusted over and healed on their own. What is the most likely diagnosis in this patient?

(8) A 32-year-old African American woman presents with gradually worsening cough and shortness of breath. Chest radiograph reveals bilateral hilar lymphadenopathy. What dermatologic finding might be seen on the physical examination?

(9) A 25-year-old woman has required insulin since she was 10 years old and has had two previous admissions for diabetic ketoacidosis (DKA). She presents to the clinic for health care maintenance. Is this patient likely to have acanthosis nigricans on physical examination?

(10) All-*trans* retinoic acid is used in the treatment of acute promyelocytic leukemia (APL). Using the information given earlier about retinoids in the treatment of acne, what is the mechanism of action in the treatment of APL?

4 EMBRYOLOGY

Thomas E. Blair and Ryan A. Pedigo

DESCRIPTION OF ANATOMY

This chapter will make use of various anatomic terms, shown here. Familiarize yourself with them before beginning.

- **Cranial**: Toward the head (cranium), similar to the term **superior** (Fig. 4.1A).
- **Caudal**: Toward the tail, similar to the term inferior (Fig. 4.1A).
- **Medial:** Toward the midline (Fig. 4.1A).
- **Lateral:** Away from the midline (Fig. 4.1A).
- **Dorsal**: Toward the back of the body (Fig. 4.1B).
- **Ventral**: Toward the front of the body (Fig. 4.1B).
- **Sagittal, coronal, transverse**: Body planes that transect the body, each perpendicular to the others (Fig. 4.1C).

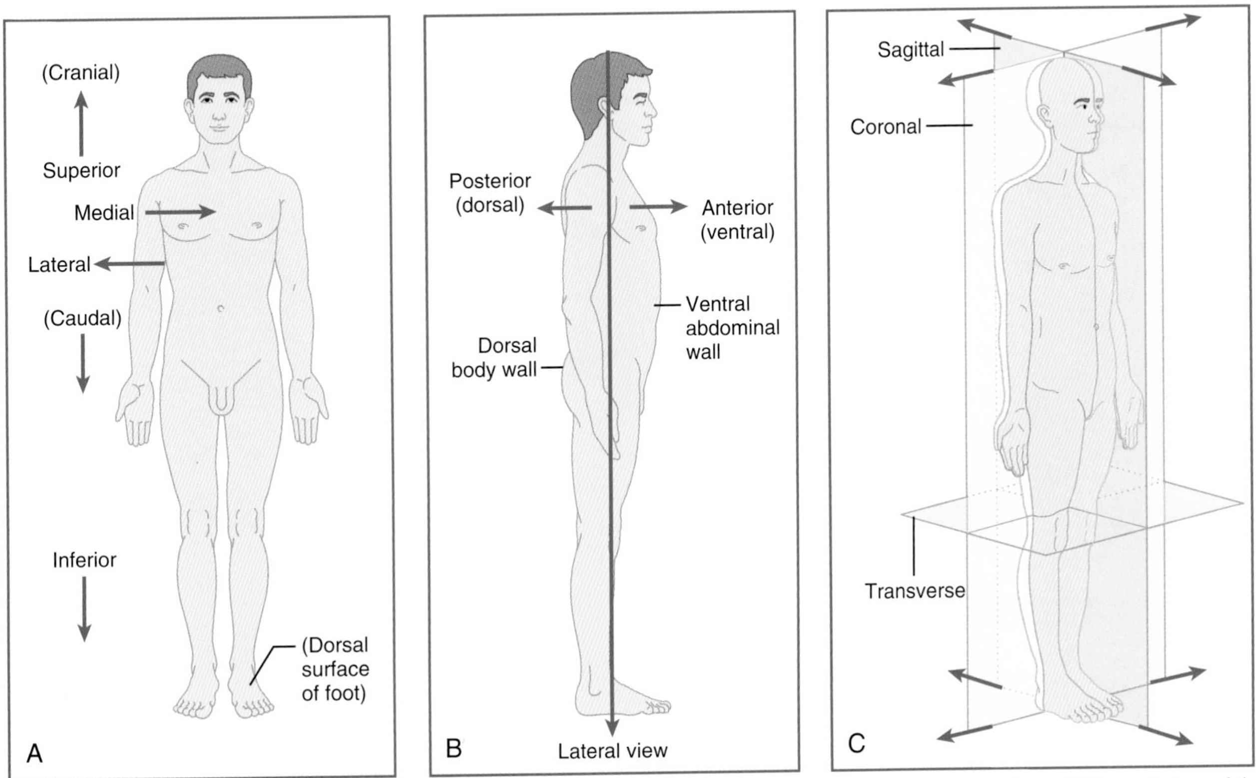

Fig. 4.1 Anatomic position and terminology. **(A)** Anterior view of the human body showing important terminology. **(B)** Lateral view of the human body. **(C)** The planes of section through the human body. (*From Bogart BI, Ort V. Elsevier's Integrated Anatomy and Embryology. Philadelphia: Elsevier; 2007.*)

EARLY EMBRYOLOGY: THE FIRST MONTH

The First Week: From Fertilization to Implantation

Day 0: Fertilization occurs when a sperm enters the egg, usually in the **ampulla of the fallopian tube.** The **acrosome reaction** occurs when a sperm meets the egg and releases enzymes that penetrate the zona pellucida (the outer "shell" of the egg).

Day 1: The single-cell **zygote** undergoes rapid mitotic cell divisions. Recall that the egg initially was arrested in metaphase II after ovulation but completes this division only after fertilization (see Chapter 16). There is no time for cell growth during this rapid dividing phase, so it is termed **cleavage** because the cells are cleaved into more numerous (but smaller) cells. Each cleavage doubles the cell number (as each individual cell participates).

Day 3: After there are 16 or 32 cells, it is now termed a **morula** (Latin for "mulberry" because there are now many cells resembling a berry).

Days 4 to 5: Na^+/K^+-ATPase pumps deliver sodium into the interior of the morula, creating an osmotic gradient and subsequently forming a fluid-filled cavity inside the morula. The **embryoblast** cells (inside, in a cluster) and the **trophoblast** cells (outside) are now distinct. Altogether, this is called the **blastocyst.** As can be seen in Fig. 4.2, the **embryonic pole** is the portion of the blastocyst in which the embryoblast cells are located. The **embryoblast** will go on to make the **embryo** (as expected), subsequently separating into the **epiblast** (dorsal) and **hypoblast** (ventral). The **trophoblast** will eventually make the **placenta,** including the **cytotrophoblast** and **syncytiotrophoblast** (see later).

Day 6: The blastocyst implants into the endometrium. If this implantation occurs in an abnormal location (e.g., the fallopian tube), it is termed an **ectopic pregnancy,** which is a medical emergency.

The blastocyst (consisting of embryoblast and trophoblast cells) implants into the endometrium on **day 6.** Abnormal implantation (usually into the ampulla of the tube): **ectopic pregnancy.** Scarring of tubes from pelvic inflammatory disease (PID) increases the risk of ectopic pregnancy.

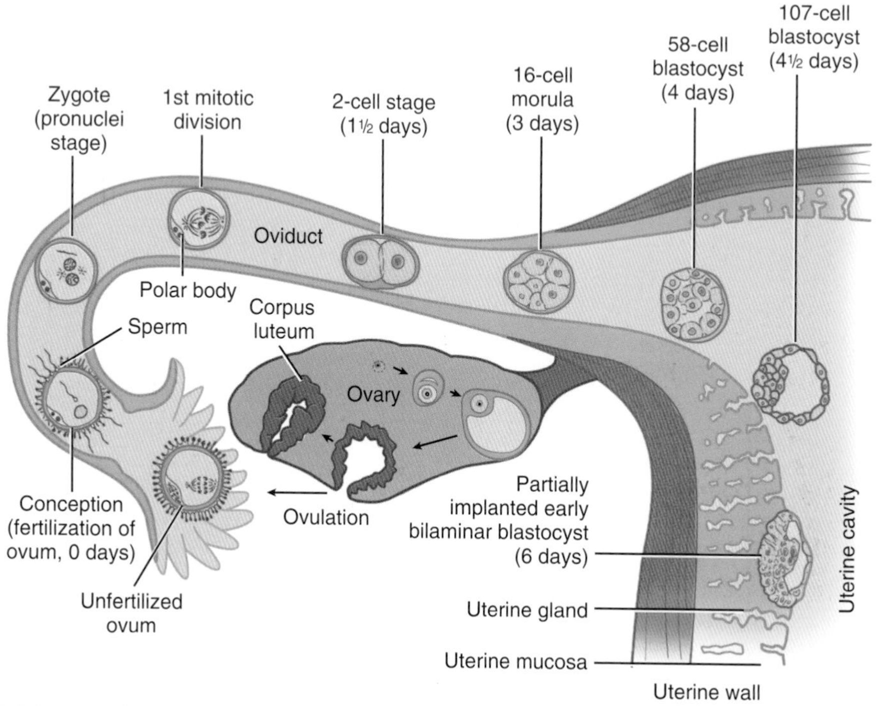

FIG. 4.2 Schematic showing the fertilization of an egg by a sperm (usually in the ampulla of the fallopian tube), creating a zygote. Over the next week, this zygote will divide while moving down the fallopian tube toward the uterus, finally implanting into the endometrium. Ovulation occurs 14 days before the onset of menses. Once ovulation occurs, the egg has a viable life of approximately 1 day. Therefore for pregnancy to occur, a viable sperm must fertilize the egg during this short window of time to form a zygote and begin embryogenesis. (*From Schoenwolf GC, Bleyl SB, Brauer PR, Francis-West PH. Larsen's Human Embryology. 4th ed. Philadelphia: Elsevier; 2008.*)

Twinning

Understanding twinning can be confusing because twinning is described in terms of the number of **zygotes** (monozygotic or dizygotic), the number of **chorions** (monochorionic or dichorionic), and the number of **amnions** (monoamniotic or diamniotic) (Fig. 4.3). The zygote part is easy: Recall that a zygote is made when an egg and sperm combine. Therefore when twins arise from one egg and one sperm, they are considered monozygotic. If two eggs were each fertilized by an individual sperm, the twins would be considered dizygotic. The chorion refers to a membrane that is formed by structures including both trophoblastic layers (cyto- and syncytiotrophoblast) and will eventually form the **placenta;** therefore monochorionic twins will share a placenta. The amnion refers to the amniotic sac; those that are monoamniotic will not be separated from one another (share the same "pool" of amniotic fluid) and could potentially be conjoined.

Because **dizygotic twins** are formed from two different eggs and two different sperm, they are **not** genetically identical and are called **fraternal** twins. **All dizygotic twins therefore have their own placenta (dichorionic) and amniotic sac (diamniotic),** and they each develop in the normal fashion independent of one another—they are simply two pregnancies simultaneously. The case with monozygotic twins can be more complicated.

Dizygotic twins: two eggs, two sperm—just two independent pregnancies at once; "fraternal" twins

Monozygotic twins: one egg, one sperm, cells broke off at some point; "identical" twins

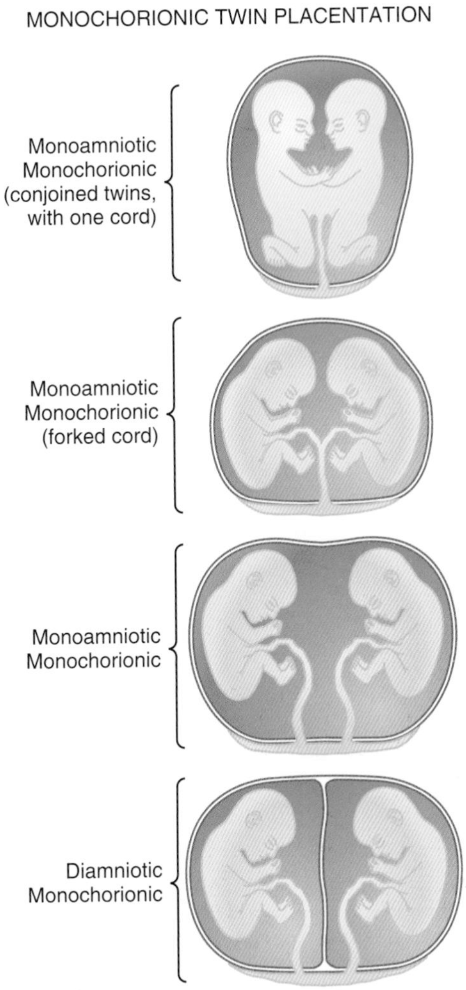

FIG. 4.3 Diagram showing different shared structures in twinning. (*Redrawn from Benirschke K, Driscoll SG.* Pathology of the Human Placenta. *New York: Springer-Verlag; 1974.*)

Monozygotic twins occur when a **single zygote splits and forms two embryos.** They are termed **identical** twins because each forms from the same zygote and therefore they have the same genetic makeup. However, depending on how early the split occurs, they may or may not share a chorion or amnion. **The later the embryo splits, the more structures will be shared**—imagine that the zygote had immediately split, that it had not started to form any structures yet and therefore each could do so on its own (dichorionic, diamniotic). If the split occurred later, structures would have already begun to form and therefore must be shared. The important landmarks to remember are that the **chorion** will form at **day 3** and the **amnion** will form at **day 8.** Splits that occur after these landmarks will share those structures. Remember that all of the following examples are only applicable to **monozygotic twins.**

- **Dichorionic, diamniotic:** The split must have occurred before day 3 to have two separate chorions. Because the amnion forms after the chorion, if the twin is dichorionic, it must also be diamniotic. Therefore these monozygotic twins will not share a placenta (dichorionic), nor will they share the same amniotic fluid sac (diamniotic).
- **Monochorionic, diamniotic:** The split must have occurred between days 3 and 8 because the chorion has formed (and is therefore shared) but the amnion has not. These fetuses therefore share a single placenta (monochorionic), but each has its own amniotic fluid sac (diamniotic), and they are spatially separated from one another.
- **Monochorionic, monoamniotic:** The split must have occurred after day 8 because both structures are shared. Therefore these fetuses will share a placenta (monochorionic) and amniotic fluid sac (monoamniotic) and will potentially be conjoined if the split was late enough. There is also a phenomenon called **twin-twin transfusion syndrome** that only occurs in monochorionic, monoamniotic twins in which, because of placental anastomoses, one twin gets proportionally more blood than the other. This leads to a large twin (that got most of the blood) and a small twin (that got less of the blood). It is usually a fatal condition for both twins.

Cytotrophoblast: cellular, will make chorionic villi
Syncytiotrophoblast: syncytium, makes hCG to maintain corpus luteum in early pregnancy

The Second Week: The Rule of Twos

The **second** week has the **rule of twos** (Fig. 4.4).

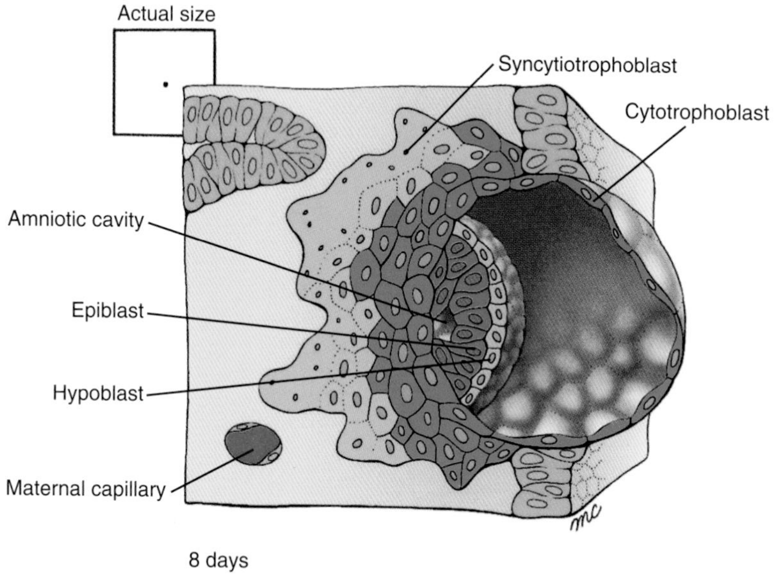

Fig. 4.4 The status of the embryo by the beginning of the second week. Note that the **trophoblast** (which makes placental tissue) has differentiated into **two layers**: the **cytotrophoblast** and **syncytiotrophoblast.** The **embryoblast** (which makes embryonic tissue) has differentiated into **two layers**: the **hypoblast** and **epiblast.** There are also **two cavities** that can be seen: the **amniotic cavity** (formed from the epiblast cells) and the **yolk sac** (formed from the hypoblast cells). The two sets of two layers and the two cavities are the basis for the rule of twos in week 2. *(From Schoenwolf GC, Bleyl SB, Brauer PR, Francis-West PH.* Larsen's Human Embryology. *4th ed. Philadelphia: Elsevier; 2008.)*

- The **trophoblast** (which will give rise to the placenta) has now differentiated into two layers: the **cytotrophoblast** (cellular) and the **syncytiotrophoblast** (a syncytium, in which the cells have fused together). The **cytotrophoblast** divides through mitotic division and will generate the chorionic villi; this has embryogenic importance because it allows maximal surface area of contact with maternal blood in the placenta. It also has clinical importance because chorionic villus sampling is a method to diagnose chromosomal or genetic disorders in the fetus. The **syncytiotrophoblast** does not divide through mitotic division; this generates human chorionic gonadotropin (hCG), which is used clinically. The beta subunit, β-hCG, is the substance that pregnancy tests detect. It is also important in the diagnosis of ectopic pregnancy (see Chapter 16).
- The **embryoblast** (which will give rise to the embryo) has now differentiated into two layers: the **epiblast** (dorsal structures) and **hypoblast** (ventral structures); together, the epiblast and hypoblast are known as the **bilaminar disk.**
- There are also two cavities now: the **amniotic cavity** (formed from the epiblast cells) and the **yolk sac** (formed from the hypoblast cells).

Lastly, at about day 10, the **syncytiotrophoblast** will begin to secrete hCG. As mentioned previously, β-hCG is used clinically to detect pregnancy and assess for an ectopic pregnancy as well. Because ovulation occurs 14 days before menses, by the time a patient is supposed to have menses, the pregnancy test should be accurate. **Dipstick** pregnancy tests are **qualitative,** meaning positive or negative (no numerical values). **Blood** tests can be **quantitative,** meaning they give an actual value. In early pregnancy, the β-hCG should **double every 48 hours;** this is used as a benchmark to determine whether an ectopic pregnancy is potentially present. This is because the syncytiotrophoblast, if not implanted into the endometrium (and implanted elsewhere, such as in a fallopian tube), would not have enough blood supply to increase the β-hCG twofold in 48 hours. This suggests an ectopic pregnancy or other nonviable pregnancy. Please refer to Fig. 4.5 for a summary of embryogenesis thus far.

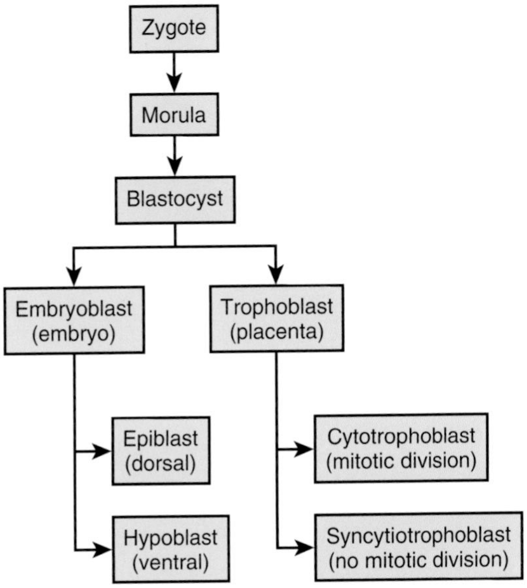

FIG. 4.5 Summary of embryogenesis thus far by the end of week 2. After fertilization, a **zygote** is formed, which subsequently undergoes multiple cleavages to become a morula, then later a blastocyst. The **blastocyst** differentiates into the **embryoblast** and **trophoblast.** These further differentiate by week 2.

The Third Week: Gastrulation and the Ectoderm, Endoderm, and Mesoderm

The **third** week has the **rule of threes** (three germ layers after gastrulation).

Gastrulation is the important step that produces the three **germ layers:** the ectoderm, endoderm, and mesoderm. Understanding the **ectoderm, endoderm, and mesoderm** and the organs they produce is helpful in understanding organogenesis and even development. This concept also becomes important in adult life because malignancies of tissues derived from the **mesoderm** (muscle, bone) are termed **sarcomas** (myosarcomas and osteosarcomas, respectively), whereas malignancies of tissues derived from **ectoderm** or **endoderm** are termed **carcinomas.**

The process of gastrulation begins with the formation of a **primitive streak,** which is essentially just a midline invagination (Fig. 4.6A). Subsequently, the epiblast cells migrate through the primitive streak: The bottom-most layer becomes **endoderm,** the middle layer becomes **mesoderm,** and the top layer of epiblast cells that did not migrate becomes **ectoderm** (Fig. 4.6B). These three germ layers will eventually give rise to various parts of the developing embryo.

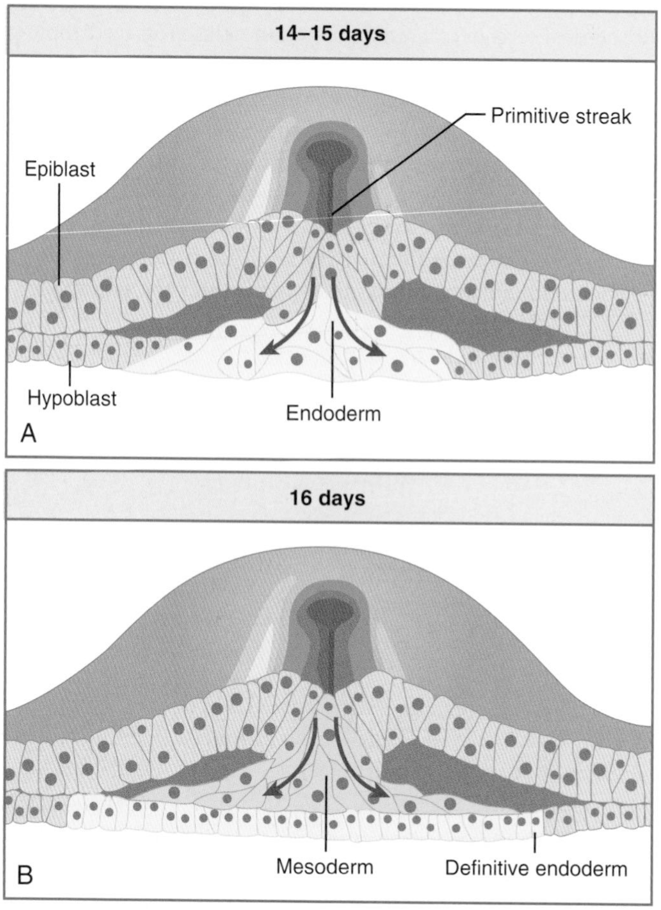

Fig. 4.6 The process of gastrulation, beginning with formation of the primitive streak **(A)**, and epiblast cells migrating inward **(B)**. *(From Bogart BI, Ort V. Elsevier's Integrated Anatomy and Embryology. Philadelphia: Elsevier; 2007.)*

Ectoderm

The ectoderm consists of surface ectoderm, neuroectoderm, and neural crest cells.

- **Surface ectoderm:** Makes the **surface layer** of many organs, including the **epidermis of the skin,** as well as sensory organ structures such as the olfactory epithelium and epithelium of the mouth. It also makes **glandular structures,** such as the adenohypophysis (which itself is an outpouching of the roof of the mouth, known as **Rathke pouch**) and other glands, including the mammary, sweat, and salivary glands.
- **Neuroectoderm:** Makes neural structures: essentially all **central nervous system** structures (brain and spinal cord) but also the **retina** because the retina is neural tissue.

- **Neural crest cells:** The neural crest cells create essentially all **peripheral nervous system** structures. This also includes melanocytes, parafollicular (C) cells of the thyroid, and chromaffin cells of the adrenal medulla, which become important in melanoma, medullary thyroid carcinoma, and pheochromocytoma, respectively. Neural crest cells also play an important role in the formation of **conotruncal endocardial cushions,** which are essential for the proper development of the heart (genetic disorders that involve problems in neural crest cell migration are often associated with cardiac abnormalities). Lastly, **many structures in the face** (including teeth and bony structures) are derived from neural crest cells. Therefore conditions such as **DiGeorge syndrome** (see later) involve both craniofacial abnormalities and cardiac defects.

Endoderm

The endoderm is mainly responsible for developing into structures of the **gut** (such as the liver, pancreas, and other organs of, or relating to, the gastrointestinal system) and some **endocrine glands** (thyroid follicles, parathyroid glands).

Mesoderm

The mesoderm further separates into **sclerotome, myotome, and dermatome,** which develop into bone, muscle, and skin structures, respectively. Although the skin is mostly of mesodermal origin, the epidermis is derived from surface ectoderm.

The rule of threes for week 3 also encompasses the formation of the **three body axes**: the cranial-caudal axis (the primitive streak is organized top to bottom, head to rump), the medial-lateral axis (because the primitive streak is midline), and the dorsal-ventral axis (front to back).

The end of the third week also marks the beginning of the **embryonic period,** during which organs begin to form. Before the end of the third week, teratogens typically have an **all-or-nothing** phenomenon, causing natural abortion of the embryo or no harm at all—there is nothing in between (such as birth defects). However, starting in the next week, with organogenesis, teratogens can cause errors in formation and lead to significant birth defects.

The Fourth Week: Neural Tube Closure and Beginning of Organogenesis

Week 4 also marks the **rule of fours** as organogenesis begins to take place:

- Four limb buds begin to grow.
- Four chambers of the heart have developed and begin to beat (heart begins to beat at 22 or 23 days, when it has grown to such a size that it cannot get adequate nutrition by diffusion alone).

Although the third week marked the beginning of neural plate development, which will give rise to the spinal cord, the **fourth week marks the closure of the neural tube.** This closure can be normal or abnormal: Abnormal cranial closure leads to **anencephaly,** whereas abnormal caudal closure leads to **spina bifida** in one of its three main forms.

Anencephaly occurs when the cranial (head) end of the neural tube does not close and leads to an absence of the forebrain and therefore is not compatible with life. Most patients with anencephaly die in utero or within hours to days of birth. Because there is no forebrain, there is no possibility to generate conscious thought, but because the brainstem is developed normally, primitive reflexes may be present.

Spina bifida occurs when the caudal (bottom) end of the neural tube does not close, usually near the L5–S1 area. This incomplete closure can lead to malformation of the vertebrae overlying the spinal cord and to a passageway for the spinal cord to protrude out of the back. The severity of the defect is related to the size of the opening. This can result in a spectrum of disease, ranging from completely asymptomatic to permanent paralysis.

- **Spina bifida occulta** (Fig. 4.7A): This defect usually does not have symptoms or signs because the incomplete closure is so minor that the spinal cord cannot protrude out of the defect (*occulta* is Latin for "hidden"). However, some common findings include a small tuft of hair or hyperpigmented skin over the affected area at the midline. Because there is a small vertebral fusion defect, this can be seen on lumbar spine radiographs.
- **Spina bifida with meningocele** (Fig. 4.7B): A meningocele occurs when the meninges (the three layers [dura mater, arachnoid mater, and pia mater] that surround the spinal cord) protrude through

Anencephaly: Failure of neural tube closure at the cranial end of the neural tube. Not compatible with life.

Spina bifida: Failure of neural tube closure at the caudal end of the neural tube. Spectrum of disease from asymptomatic (occulta) to paralysis (myelomeningocele).

a defect in the vertebrae, **but the spinal cord does not protrude.** Therefore the chance of neurologic dysfunction is still relatively low. A meningeal cyst (sac filled with cerebrospinal fluid [CSF]) may be visible at the site of the defect.

- **Spina bifida with myelomeningocele** (Fig. 4.7C): In this severe form, the defect is large enough that the **spinal cord and meninges** both protrude through the vertebral defect and are damaged. This leads to neurologic problems below the level of the cord damage, typically resulting in paralysis and loss of sensation of the legs. Associated with other structural neurologic defects such as Dandy-Walker syndrome and Chiari II malformation (see later).

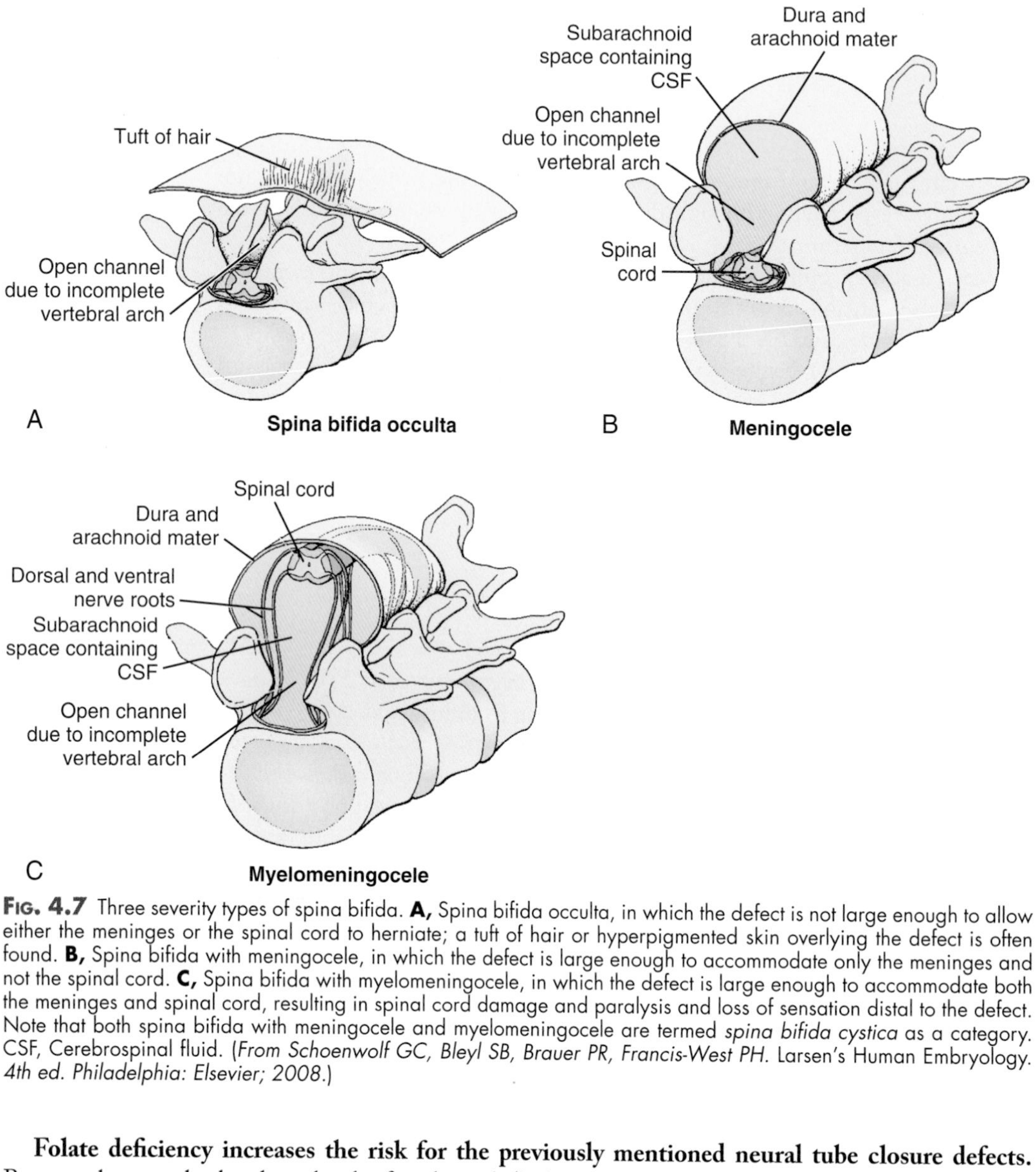

FIG. 4.7 Three severity types of spina bifida. **A,** Spina bifida occulta, in which the defect is not large enough to allow either the meninges or the spinal cord to herniate; a tuft of hair or hyperpigmented skin overlying the defect is often found. **B,** Spina bifida with meningocele, in which the defect is large enough to accommodate only the meninges and not the spinal cord. **C,** Spina bifida with myelomeningocele, in which the defect is large enough to accommodate both the meninges and spinal cord, resulting in spinal cord damage and paralysis and loss of sensation distal to the defect. Note that both spina bifida with meningocele and myelomeningocele are termed *spina bifida cystica* as a category. CSF, Cerebrospinal fluid. (*From Schoenwolf GC, Bleyl SB, Brauer PR, Francis-West PH.* Larsen's Human Embryology. *4th ed. Philadelphia: Elsevier; 2008.*)

Folate deficiency increases the risk for the previously mentioned neural tube closure defects. Because the neural tube closes by the fourth week (before many women even know they are pregnant), folate supplementation in women of reproductive age, especially during the prenatal period, is important in preventing both anencephaly and spina bifida. Anencephaly, myelomeningocele, and meningocele (but not spina bifida occulta) can be suspected in utero if high levels of **alpha-fetoprotein** (fetal albumin) are detected in maternal serum. This laboratory finding makes sense because alpha-fetoprotein will diffuse into the amnion. Polyhydramnios (excess amniotic fluid) may also be present as CSF leaks into the amnion through the defect.

EMBRYOLOGY: WEEK 5 AND BEYOND

The first month of embryogenesis is important to understand in detail. However, the rest of embryogenesis can be talked about in generalities.

Weeks 4 to 8: Organogenesis and Teratogenicity

Week 4 was described in detail because it marked the closure of the neural tube and the beginning of organogenesis (hence the rule of fours, with four cardiac chambers and four limb buds). Because this is a critical stage when the organs of the body begin to be constructed, **teratogen exposure in this period is especially deleterious** and can result in significant fetal malformations. Recall that the first 3 weeks marked the all-or-nothing period when an exposure to a teratogen would either cause abortion or nothing.

The most common teratogens are **alcohol, smoking, and medications.** Chapter 5 covers maternal infections that can lead to birth defects. High-yield teratogens are covered here.

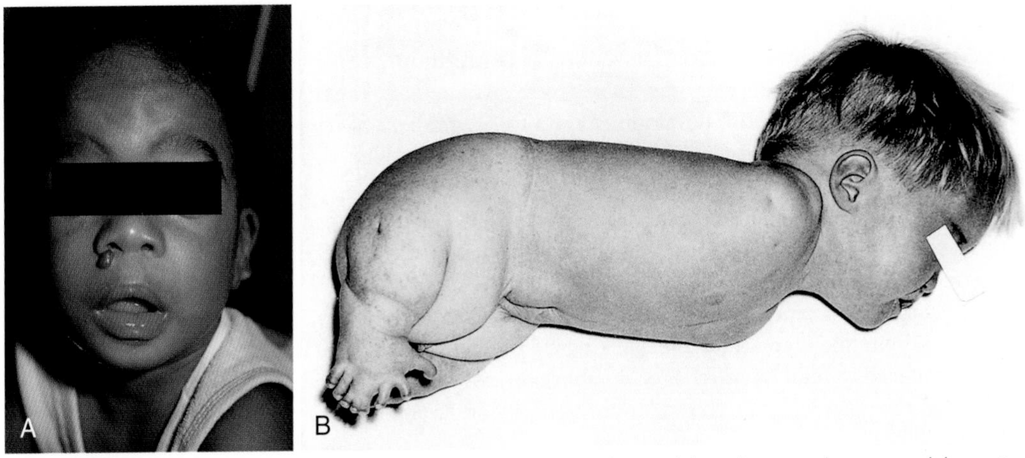

FIG. 4.8 A, Fetal alcohol syndrome, displaying the characteristic absent philtrum between the nose and the patient's characteristically thin upper lip. There is also a saddle-shaped nose and maxillary hypoplasia. **B,** Thalidomide causing amelia (agenesis of the limb) in the upper extremities and phocomelia (shortening) in the lower extremities. (**A** *from Lissauer T, Clayden G.* Illustrated Textbook of Paediatrics. *4th ed. Edinburgh: Elsevier; 2011.* **B** *from Turnpenny P, Ellard S.* Emery's Elements of Medical Genetics. *14th ed. Philadelphia: Elsevier; 2011. Courtesy R. W. Smithells, University of Leeds, UK.*)

Substances of Abuse

- **Alcohol:** Fetal alcohol syndrome represents the most common birth defect caused by a teratogen. Along with **developmental delay,** these patients have the classic smooth philtrum (Fig. 4.8A), a thin upper lip, a saddle-shaped nose, and maxillary hypoplasia.
- **Cocaine:** By preventing reuptake of catecholamines, cocaine is a potent sympathomimetic. This causes increased vasoconstriction (from α_1-agonist activity of catecholamines) and therefore decreased blood flow to the placenta, leading to hypoxia in the fetus. This can lead to **placental abruption** (abruptio placentae), or detachment of the placenta from the uterine wall before delivery, which is an obstetric emergency. Cocaine exposure in utero can also lead to generalized problems such as developmental delay and a number of birth defects, presumably also due to hypoxia in the fetus.
- **Smoking:** Smoking has not been shown to cause specific birth defects, but just as smoking causes damage to the endothelial cells in the rest of the body (predisposing the mother to heart attack and stroke), the placental vasculature is similarly damaged. This leads to a poorer blood supply to the fetus and can cause **intrauterine growth restriction** and **preterm labor.**
- **Note:** A common substance of abuse, opioids (e.g., heroin, prescription opioids) are **not** teratogenic, but opioid use in the mother can lead to neonatal opioid withdrawal.

Common Medications

Renal agenesis causes oligohydramnios, which is associated with Potter sequence.

- **Angiotensin-converting enzyme (ACE) inhibitors:** Recall that ACE changes angiotensin I to angiotensin II, which has effects on the renal system. Use of ACE inhibitors or angiotensin II receptor–blocking drugs during pregnancy has been linked to renal problems, including **renal agenesis.** Because amniotic fluid is essentially fetal urine, fetal renal dysfunction leads to **oligohydramnios** and Potter sequence (see Potter Sequence [Oligohydramnios Sequence] under Renal Embryology for details).
- **Antiepileptic medications:** Most antiepileptic medications are teratogenic to some degree. **Phenytoin** has a specific syndrome called **fetal hydantoin syndrome,** which consists of facial defects, nail hypoplasia, and developmental delay. Many antiepileptic medications have **folate antagonist** activity (such as **valproic acid**); therefore, as expected, many are associated with **neural tube defects.**
- **Aminoglycoside antibiotics:** Aminoglycoside antibiotics have ototoxicity and nephrotoxicity as side effects in adults; these side effects are amplified in the fetus if the mother takes these while pregnant. This can lead to **sensorineural (cranial nerve [CN] VIII) deafness** and **renal damage.**
- **Lithium:** Used in treatment of bipolar disorder, lithium is linked to a specific defect termed **Ebstein anomaly,** in which there is downward displacement of the tricuspid valve through "atrialization" of part of the right ventricle (right atrium becomes too large, right ventricle becomes too small).
- **Retinoic acid (vitamin A) and other retinoids:** Often prescribed as **isotretinoin,** a treatment for cystic acne, all retinoids in supraphysiologic amounts can cause severe birth defects. The developing embryo uses ***Hox* genes** to control anteroposterior development and uses a gradient of retinoic acid concentration to trigger development in the proper order. Large amounts of retinoids disrupt this and lead to **significant growth defects,** spontaneous abortion, and cleft palate.
- **Tetracycline antibiotics:** Most tetracycline antibiotics chelate calcium and therefore can deposit in developing bone. In the fetus and even in children, this can lead to discoloration of teeth from deposition and chelation of calcium.
- **Warfarin:** Warfarin has anticoagulant activity by blocking the vitamin K epoxide reductase enzyme, preventing the synthesis of active vitamin K and therefore blocking clotting factor synthesis. Therefore lack of fetal clotting factors can lead to **fetal hemorrhage** and **abortion,** as well as bone deformities. Heparin, which does not cross the placenta, is preferred for anticoagulation in pregnancy

Historical Medications

These medications are no longer prescribed but are commonly tested.

- **Diethylstilbestrol (DES):** Prescribed up until 1971 to supposedly prevent miscarriages (it did not), this drug was subsequently found to cause **clear cell carcinoma** of the vagina in female offspring and increased risk for cryptorchidism and sex hormone abnormalities in male offspring. The mothers who took DES are at increased risk for breast cancer as well.
- **Thalidomide**[1]: This medication was supposed to decrease morning sickness in pregnant women. However, it caused birth defects in the offspring, specifically **phocomelia,** which is a shortening of the limbs. Commonly, these patients were referred to as "flipper babies" because the shortened limbs had the appearance of flippers (Fig. 4.8B).

Weeks 9 to Birth: The "Fetal Period" of Organ Maturation

During this stage, all organs have at least begun to form. However, much development and maturation will still occur. Because the focus is now on growth, teratogens have less effect compared with during the period of organogenesis. However, teratogens can still have a significant impact on development.

FETAL CIRCULATION AND ERYTHROPOIESIS

Structure of the Placenta and Umbilical Cord

The **placenta** acts as the interface between the mother and fetus (Fig. 4.9). Through the placenta, oxygen and other nutrients are transferred, but so are potentially harmful things such as drugs,

[1] Thalidomide does still find use today in the treatment of multiple myeloma.

toxins, pathogens, and immunoglobulin G (IgG) antibodies (IgM pentamers are too large to traverse the placenta). The placenta is termed a **fetomaternal** organ because part of the placenta develops from the fetus (through trophoblastic cells) and part develops from the endometrium of the mother.

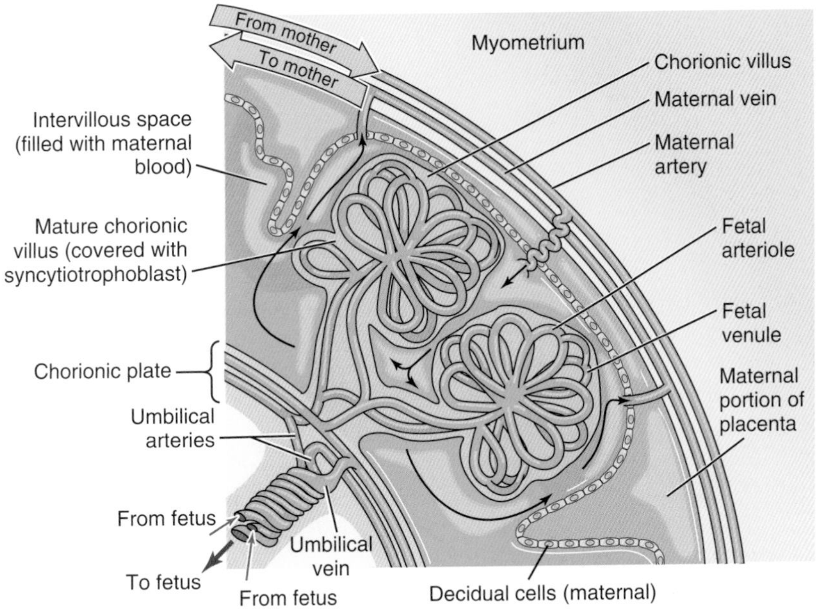

Fig. 4.9 The placenta. The maternal blood leaves through spiral arteries into the intervillous space; the maternal blood is no longer in an artery at this time. This blood bathes the fetal vessels and allows the fetal hemoglobin to "steal" oxygen from the maternal hemoglobin. (*From Boron WF, Boulpaep EL.* Medical Physiology. *2nd ed. Philadelphia: Elsevier; 2008.*)

The **umbilical cord** consists of **two umbilical arteries** and **one umbilical vein.** The **umbilical arteries** will become the **medial umbilical ligaments** when they close after birth. Do not confuse this with the **median** umbilical ligament that forms when the **urachus** closes (discussed later; logically the umbilical arteries, because there are two, could not be median because two things cannot be in the exact middle).

Overview of Fetal Circulation

The fetal circulation shares many similarities to the adult circulation but also has important differences. The main differences are in terms of **oxygen concentration** and the **presence of physiologic shunts.**

The oxygen in the fetus is transferred from maternal hemoglobin to fetal hemoglobin because fetal hemoglobin (HbF) has a higher affinity for oxygen than adult hemoglobin (HbA). Therefore at the interface of the maternal and fetal blood in the placenta, oxygen exchange occurs from mother to fetus. This newly oxygenated fetal blood **returns through the umbilical vein toward the fetal heart.** Therefore **oxygen tension is highest in the umbilical vein** because it was just oxygenated at the placenta (Fig. 4.10).

Ductus venosus: shunts half of blood away from liver

Foramen ovale: shunts blood from right atrium to left atrium (bypassing lungs)

Ductus arteriosus: shunts blood from pulmonary artery to aorta (bypassing lungs)

The first physiologic shunt is encountered in the **liver.** The **ductus venosus** shunts about half of the oxygenated blood away from the liver because the fetal liver does not need 100% of the blood to be adequately oxygenated. This blood moves into the inferior vena cava, subsequently moving into the right atrium. **The fetal lungs do not oxygenate blood** because they are not breathing air but rather are breathing amniotic fluid. The fetal lungs do not have a large oxygen requirement, so most of the blood will bypass the pulmonary circulation. It does so through the second and third shunts: the **foramen ovale** and the **ductus arteriosus.** The **foramen ovale** is a passageway between the right and left atria and allows blood to bypass the lungs and move directly to the left heart. The **ductus arteriosus** is a passageway between the pulmonary artery and aorta, allowing blood that

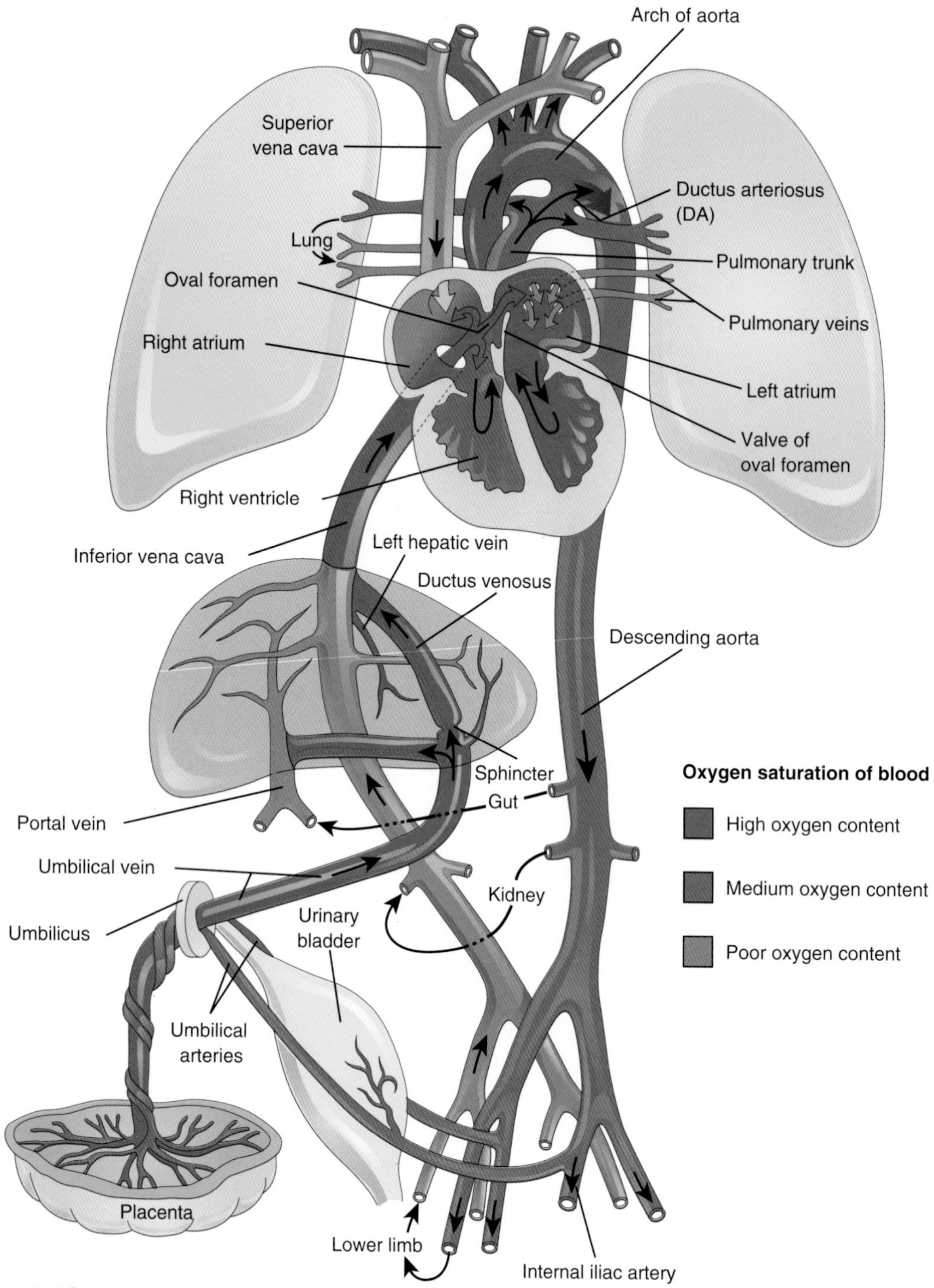

Fig. 4.10 The fetal circulation. Note that the **umbilical vein** has **high oxygen content** as it is taking blood that was oxygenated at the placenta back to the heart. The two umbilical arteries have low oxygen content. There exist three major shunts to help fetal circulation bypass the liver and lungs. (1) The ductus venosus to bypass the liver; (2) the foramen ovale, permitting passage of blood from the right atrium directly to the left atrium to bypass the lungs; and (3) the ductus arteriosus, permitting the passage of blood from the pulmonary artery to the aorta to bypass the lungs. (*From Moore KL, Persaud TVN.* Before We Are Born. *8th ed. Philadelphia: Elsevier; 2011.*)

did go into the right ventricle and pulmonary artery to again bypass the lungs by moving directly into the aorta.

The ductus arteriosus is distal to the aortic arch, so blood that moves through here will go into the descending aorta and to various end organs or back to the placenta for reoxygenation. On the other hand, the blood that went into the left ventricle can go into the aortic arch, oxygenating the upper limbs and brain. Interestingly, more deoxygenated blood returning from the brain through the superior vena cava will move into the right ventricle and then into the pulmonary artery, ductus arteriosus, and descending aorta to be reoxygenated. The oxygenated blood preferentially moves through the foramen ovale instead, helping to oxygenate the brain. In this way, **deoxygenated blood** is efficiently moved into either of the **two umbilical arteries** to be reoxygenated at the placenta.

Fetal Circulation Summary

- Fetal blood is oxygenated at the **placenta** and moves toward the right side of the heart through the **umbilical vein.**
- Fifty percent of this oxygenated blood bypasses the liver through the **ductus venosus.**
- Once at the right side of the heart, there are two possible shunts bypassing the lung: the **foramen ovale** and the **ductus arteriosus.**
- Oxygenated blood preferentially moves through the **foramen ovale** to allow the left side of the heart to pump oxygenated blood into the aortic arch and therefore the brain.
- Oxygen-poor blood returning from the superior vena cava preferentially moves into the right ventricle, pulmonary artery, and ductus arteriosus pathway to be placed into the descending aorta and to then move into either of **two umbilical arteries** to reoxygenate the blood at the placenta.

Changes to Fetal Circulation at Birth

At birth, changes occur that drastically change the fetal circulation and transition it to the adult circulation. Recall that in utero the fetus did not need to breathe for oxygenation because oxygen was provided through the placenta. (Note that the fetus in utero does "breathe" to cycle amniotic fluid containing growth factors through the lungs to promote development.) Once born, the baby now takes its first breath, causing multiple changes:

- **Reactive hypoxic vasoconstriction relieved:** Recall that low oxygen tension causes **vasoconstriction** in the pulmonary vasculature. Once the baby takes his or her first breath, the increased oxygen tension in the lungs causes significant **vasodilation** and subsequent dropping in pulmonary vascular resistance and therefore pressure.
- **Decreased pulmonary pressure:** Once born, the drop in pulmonary pressure causes a decrease in right-sided heart pressures; now the left-sided heart pressure is higher than the right, which **closes the foramen ovale.** Failure of this closure causes a **patent foramen ovale,** which is a type of atrial septal defect (ASD) and can cause a persistent left-to-right shunt (see Chapter 8 for details).
- **Beginning of closure of the ductus arteriosus:** The ductus arteriosus is no longer needed because there is no need to shunt blood away from the pulmonary vasculature. The ductus arteriosus will close functionally soon after birth and will subsequently close anatomically through fibrosis, becoming the **ligamentum arteriosum.** The closure occurs through a **decrease in prostaglandins,** which normally help keep the ductus open. In some congenital cardiac disease states, the presence of a **patent ductus arteriosus** is important, and **prostaglandin E_1** (alprostadil) is given to keep the ductus open. If the ductus arteriosus is improperly open, a nonsteroidal antiinflammatory drug such as **indomethacin** can be used to prevent prostaglandin production and close the ductus arteriosus.
- **Closure of the ductus venosus:** Because the neonate no longer needs to shunt blood away from the liver, the ductus venosus will close and subsequently become the ligamentum venosum.

Fetal Erythropoiesis

Now that the path of red blood cells and their oxygenation has been covered, the actual sites of synthesis and types of hemoglobin will be briefly discussed.

Fetal hemoglobin (HbF, $\alpha_2\gamma_2$) **binds oxygen with greater affinity** than maternal hemoglobin (i.e., the oxygen dissociation curve is shifted to the left). Normally, in adult hemoglobin, 2,3-diphosphoglycerate (2,3-DPG) is synthesized by red blood cells during breakdown of glucose. 2,3-DPG decreases the affinity of oxygen for hemoglobin. However, **fetal hemoglobin cannot bind 2,3-DPG,** and this results in fetal hemoglobin having a higher affinity for oxygen than adult hemoglobin. This allows fetal hemoglobin to preferentially bind oxygen over maternal hemoglobin to ensure oxygenation of the fetus.

The bone marrow does not synthesize red blood cells in the fetus until the 28th week. Before then, other sites provide that role because the bone marrow has not developed and matured enough to be the primary source of erythropoiesis. The way to remember where the fetus synthesizes red blood cells developmentally is that the **y**oung **l**iver **s**ynthesizes **b**lood (YLSB) in the fetus:

- **Y**olk sac: weeks 3 to 8
- **L**iver: weeks 6 to 30
- **S**pleen: weeks 9 to 28
- **B**one marrow: week 28+

CARDIAC EMBRYOLOGY

Formation of the Cardiac Loop

At about **22 to 23 days,** the fetal heart will begin to beat. It does this because it has now grown to a size at which diffusion alone does not meet the requirements for oxygen and nutrition delivery. Although

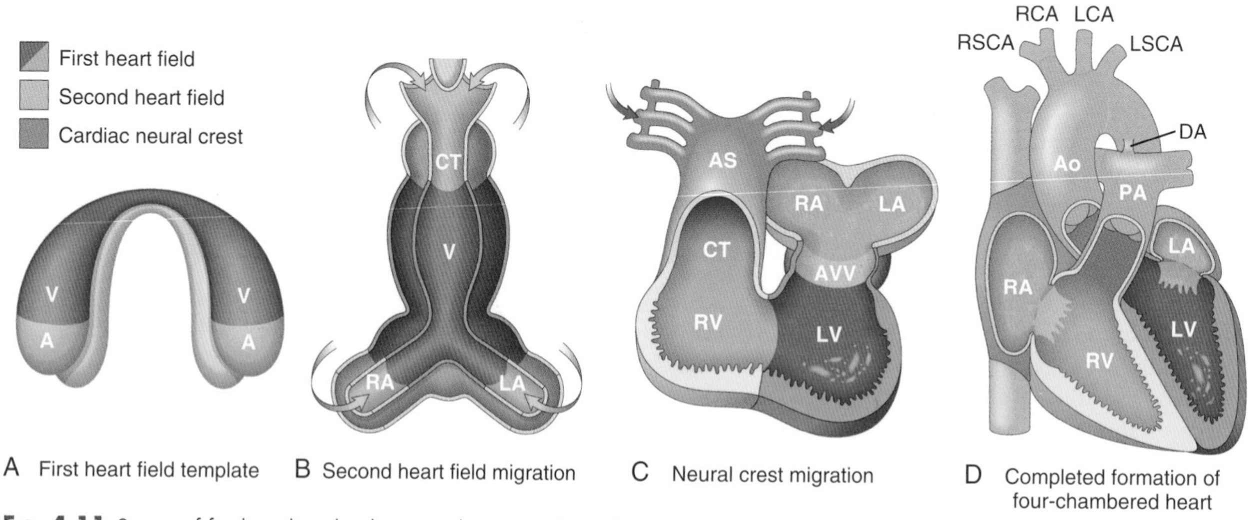

Fig. 4.11 Stages of fetal cardiac development; the image shown here ranges from **(A)** day 15, to **(B)** day 21, to **(C)** day 28, to **(D)** day 50. A, Atria; Ao, aorta; AS, aortic sac; AVV, atrioventricular valves; CT, conotruncus; DA, ductus arteriosus; LA, left atrium; LCA, left carotid artery; LSCA, left subclavian artery; LV, left ventricle; PA, pulmonary artery; RA, right atrium; RCA, right carotid artery; RSCA, right subclavian artery; RV, right ventricle; V, ventricle. (*From Kumar V, Abbas AK, Fausto N, Mitchell R.* Robbins Basic Pathology. *8th ed. Philadelphia: Elsevier; 2007. Modified by permission from Srivastava D. Making or breaking the heart: From lineage determination to morphogenesis.* Cell *2006;126:1037.*)

the heart is beating, the chambers are not yet in their proper orientation (Fig. 4.11); the "twisting" of the **cardiac loop** allows for the chambers to be moved into their rightful place. The proper movement of this is dependent on many **genes** and proper migration of **neural crest cells.** This is why there are many syndromes that include both **cardiac abnormalities** and **craniofacial abnormalities:** Proper migration of neural crest cells is required for both the heart and the jaw and face to form correctly. Specifically for the heart, the neural crest cells are important in the formation of "twisting" aorticopulmonary septa that **divide the truncus arteriosus** (common outflow tract of the right ventricle [RV] and left ventricle [LV]) into the **ascending aorta** and **pulmonary artery.** Failure of proper migration of neural crest cells to the truncus arteriosus region is implicated in **transposition of the great vessels** and **tetralogy of Fallot** (see Chapter 8).

Septation of the Heart: Interatrial Septum Formation

Understanding how the **interatrial septum** forms makes understanding atrial septal defects much easier. In the fetus, some passageway between the right and left atrium is always present to allow oxygenated blood to bypass the lungs by directly moving from the right to left atrium. Follow along with the explanation for Fig. 4.12:

A. The **foramen primum** is the first (primum) hole (foramen) between the two atria. The **septum primum** is the first septum to form, forming across the foramen primum to close it.
B. The **foramen primum** is now almost closed off by the **septum primum,** but the septum primum develops **perforations** in it. These perforations are now a new (second) set of holes.

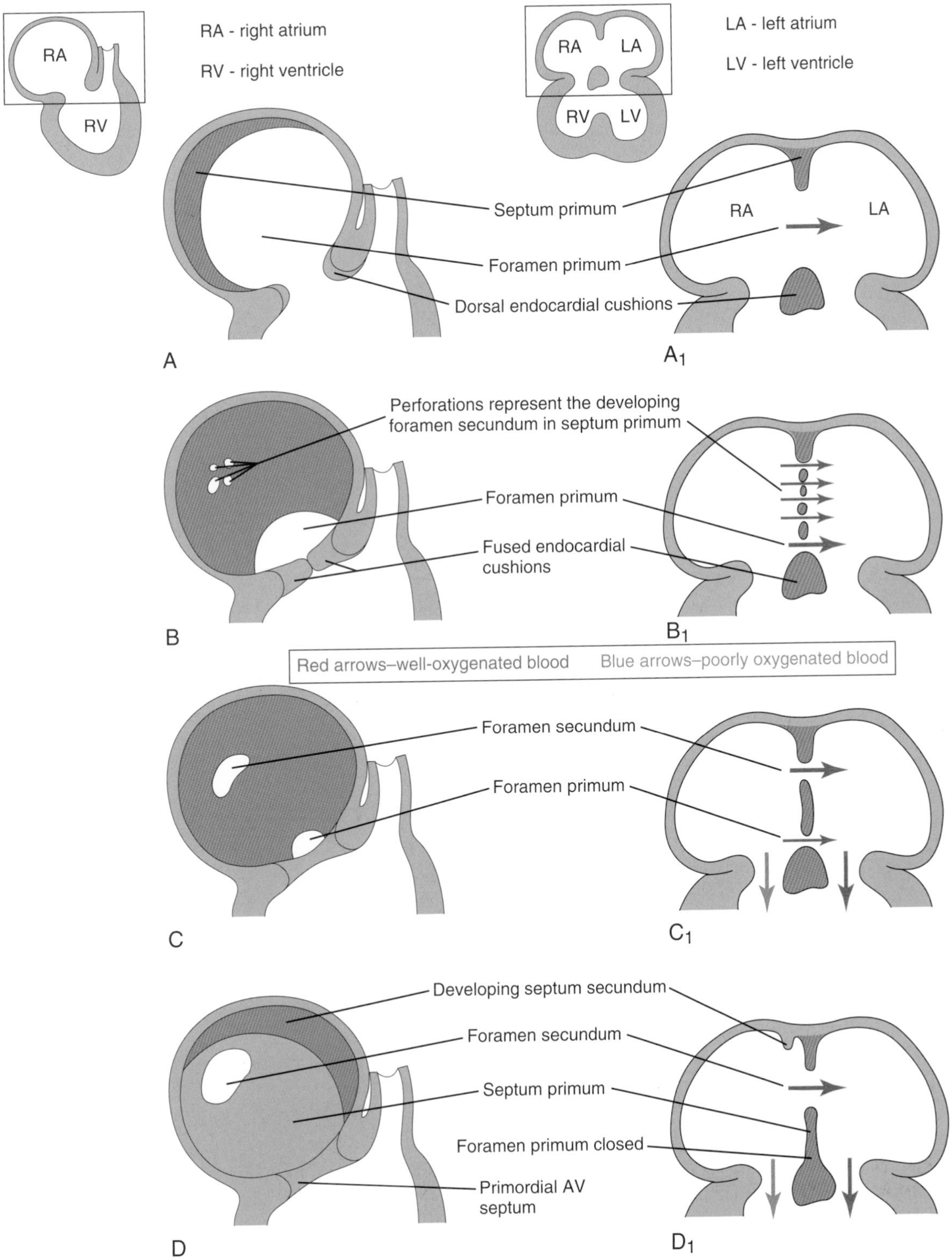

FIG. 4.12 Formation of the atrial septum (see text for explanation). (*From Moore KL, Persaud TVN. Before We Are Born. 7th ed. Philadelphia: Elsevier; 2007.*)

Continued

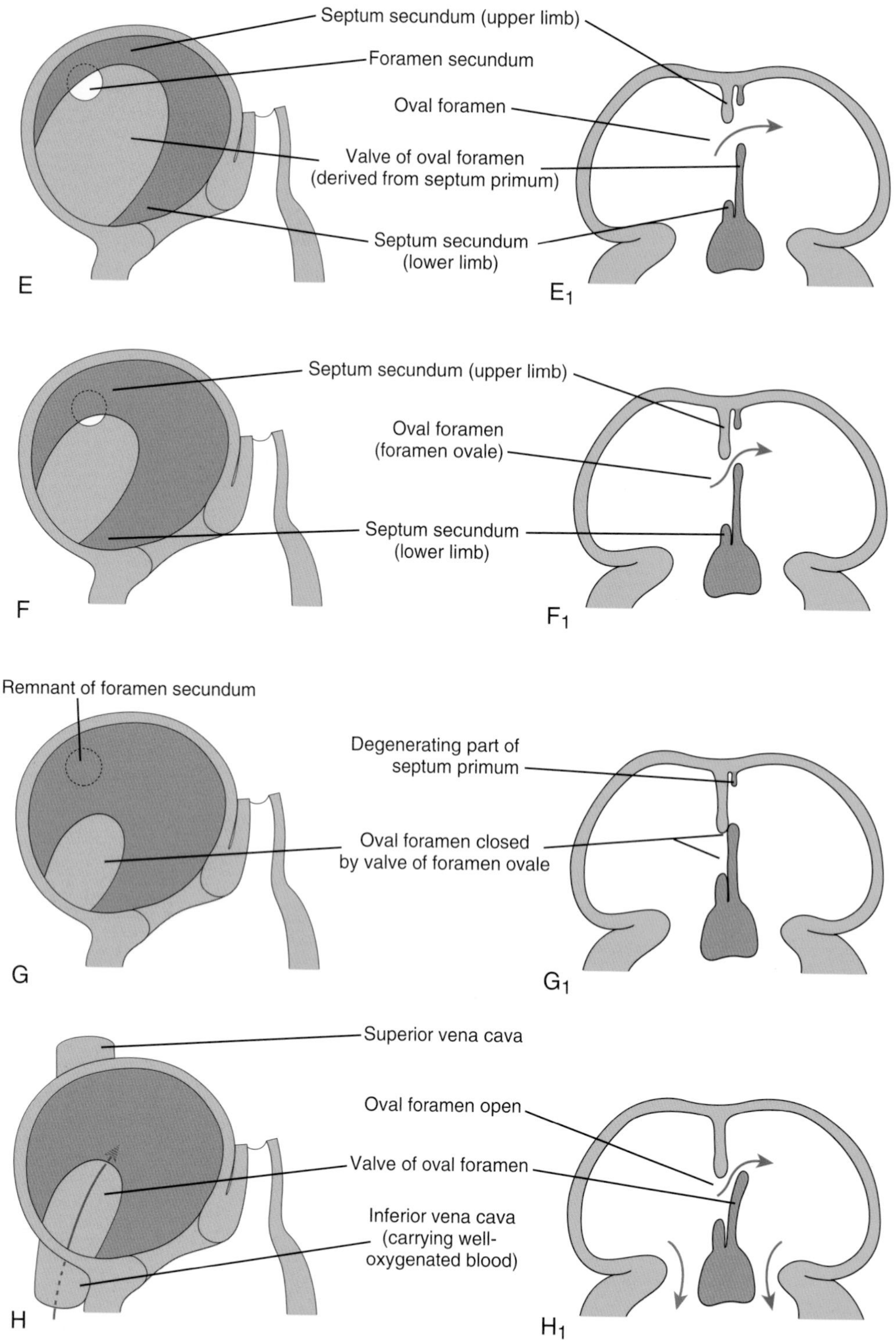

Fig. 4.12, cont'd

C. The perforations in the second set of holes coalesce, becoming the **foramen secundum.**
D. The **foramen primum** is now closed. The second septum, the **septum secundum,** can now be seen developing. Defects in the septum secundum are the most common type of ASD.
E. The **septum secundum** leaves a space between the atria, termed the **oval foramen** *(foramen ovale).*
F. The lower limb of the **septum primum** forms the valve of the oval foramen (which will later close the oval foramen when the baby is born because the left atrial pressure increase will shut the one-way valve).

G. Demonstration of the one-way valve: If left atrial pressure (as in a neonate) is higher than right atrial pressure, the valve should shut the oval foramen.
H. Failure of the oval foramen to close leads to a **patent foramen ovale,** a type of ASD.

Septation of the Heart: Interventricular Septum Formation

The fetal ventricle starts as a single chamber. The **muscular interventricular septum** begins by forming at the apex of the heart and grows upward. Because it has not yet fully formed, there is an **interventricular foramen** at this time. By the end of week 7, the foramen closes when the **membranous part of the interventricular septum** forms. This forms by the joining of nearby tissues, including the endocardial cushion and the bulbar ridges.

VASCULAR EMBRYOLOGY

Blood vessels develop through two separate processes: vasculogenesis and angiogenesis. Vasculogenesis involves angioblasts grouping to form the major vessels (e.g., dorsal aorta). Angiogenesis involves new vessels growing from existing ones and is the major source of vascular development.

The **aortic arches** (Table 4.1) are six paired embryologic arteries that supply their corresponding branchial arch and eventually form major adult vascular structures (Fig. 4.13). They emanate from the distal part of the truncus arteriosus.

TABLE 4.1 Aortic Arch Derivatives

FETAL ARTERIAL STRUCTURE	ADULT STRUCTURE	COMMENT
1st aortic arch	Maxillary artery	
2nd aortic arch	Hyoid artery Stapedial artery	
3rd aortic arch	**Common carotid artery** **Internal carotid artery**	"Carotid arch"
4th right aortic arch	Brachiocephalic artery	
4th left aortic arch	Arch of the aorta	
5th aortic arch	Not applicable	5th arch regresses early
6th right aortic arch	Right pulmonary artery	
6th left aortic arch	Left pulmonary artery **Ligamentum arteriosum**	
Truncus arteriosus	**Ascending aorta** **Pulmonary trunk**	Aorticopulmonary septum develops to divide the truncus

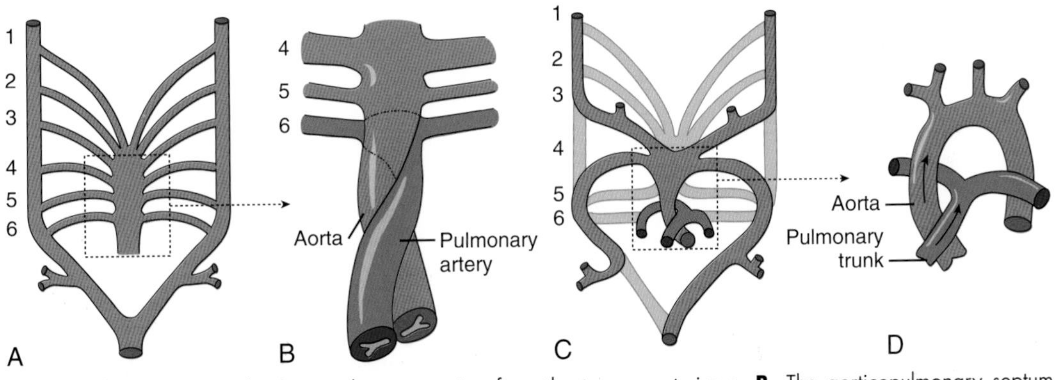

FIG. 4.13 A, Six paired aortic arches emanating from the truncus arteriosus. **B,** The aorticopulmonary septum divides the truncus arteriosus into the ascending aorta and pulmonary trunk. The sixth aortic arch contributes to the right and left pulmonary arteries. **C,** The third aortic arch forms the common carotid and internal carotid arteries. The left fourth arch forms the arch of the aorta. The right fourth arch forms the brachiocephalic artery. The fifth arch regresses early in development. **D,** Mature aortic arch. (*From Moore NA, Roy WA. Rapid Review Gross and Developmental Anatomy. 3rd ed. Philadelphia: Elsevier; 2010.*)

NEUROEMBRYOLOGY

The cephalic portion of the neural tube eventually dilates into three structures: the **forebrain (prosencephalon), midbrain (mesencephalon), and hindbrain (rhombencephalon).** The forebrain is further divided into the telencephalon (future cerebral hemispheres) and the diencephalon (future thalamus/hypothalamus). Logically, the fetal midbrain (mesencephalon) will develop into the adult midbrain. The hindbrain is also divided into two parts: the metencephalon (future pons and cerebellum) and the myelencephalon (future medulla) (Fig. 4.14).

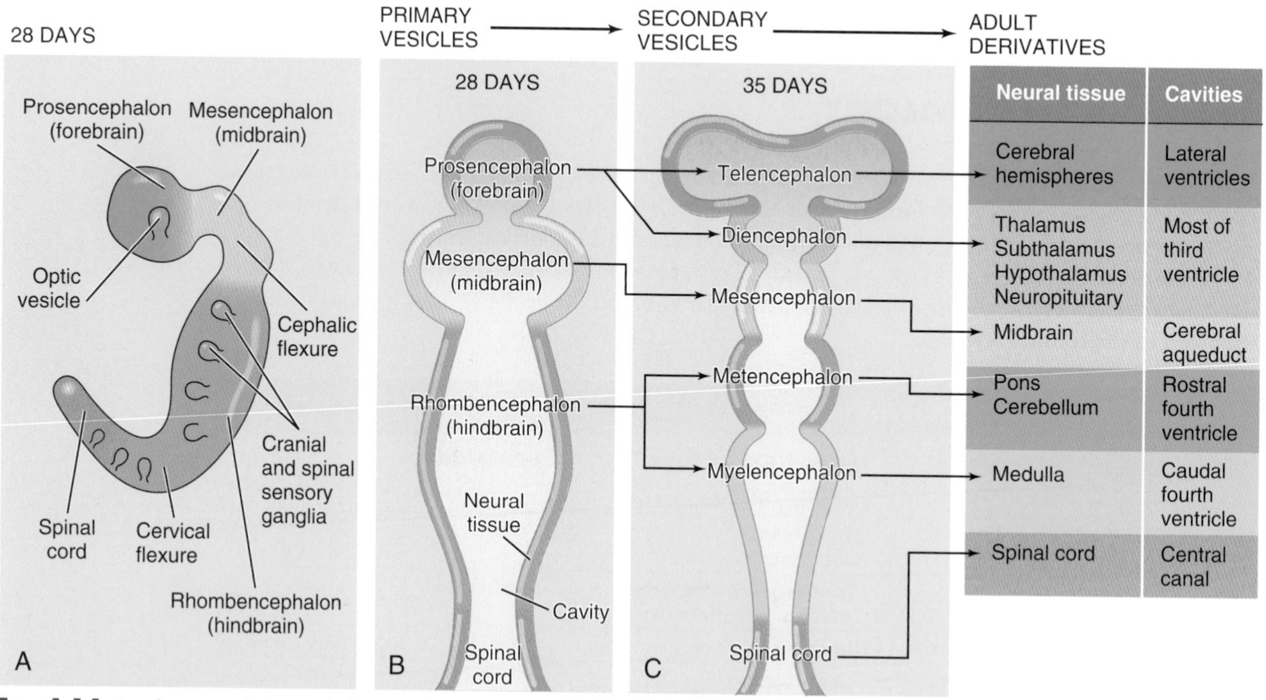

FIG. 4.14 Development of the cephalic neural tube into the adult brain. **(A)** The neural tube at 28 days. **(B)** Cross-sectional view of the neural tube at 28 days. **(C)** Cross-sectional view of the neural tube at 35 days. (*From Boron WF, Boulpaep EL. Medical Physiology. 2nd ed. Philadelphia: Elsevier; 2008.*)

Somites

Somites are primitive masses of mesoderm that flank the neural tube. This mesoderm is termed *paraxial mesoderm* because of its position lateral to the neural tube. Somites eventually form the **vertebrae** as well as some of the cartilage and musculature of the back.

Somites will later form the vertebrae and musculature of the back.

Pituitary Gland

The posterior pituitary is a neural structure formed from the downward growth of the diencephalon. The anterior pituitary, on the other hand, develops from an outpouching of the oral cavity called **Rathke pouch.** Persistence of Rathke pouch may lead to **craniopharyngiomas.** These benign suprasellar tumors may compress the pituitary, causing endocrine abnormalities or growth disturbances. They may also compress the optic chiasm, causing visual disturbance (e.g., bitemporal hemianopsia).

Notochord

Notochord is a longitudinal structure lying ventral to the neural tube that helps differentiate the ventral from dorsal axis of the spinal cord and body. It determines the **polarity of the spinal cord** with the help of the protein **sonic hedgehog homologue,** which induces the formation of motor neurons along the ventral aspect of the spinal cord. The notochord persists in the adult as the **nucleus pulposus** of the intervertebral discs.

The notochord uses sonic hedgehog homologue to differentiate the anterior from posterior spinal cord.

Holoprosencephaly

Holoprosencephaly is failure of development of midline structures as a result of incomplete cleavage of the prosencephalon into the telencephalon. In its most severe form, it is incompatible with life and results in cyclopia, absent nose, and fused cerebral hemispheres. In milder forms, midline structures may be affected, but two cerebral hemispheres develop. For example, a mildly affected individual may present with a single incisor. Holoprosencephaly may be associated with sonic hedgehog gene mutations.

Dandy-Walker Syndrome

Dandy-Walker syndrome is a spectrum of genetic conditions presenting as **loss of the cerebellar vermis** and eventually **dilation of the fourth ventricle.** Symptoms may be surprisingly absent at birth, although absence of the cerebellar vermis often causes ataxia. As dilation of the fourth ventricle progresses, a protuberance of the occiput can be seen on physical examination. Increased intracranial pressure may also result. A ventricular shunt can be used to drain the excess CSF, treat the hydrocephalus, and normalize the intracranial pressure.

Arnold-Chiari Malformation

Arnold-Chiari malformation is a congenital herniation of the cerebellar tonsils through the foramen magnum (Fig. 4.15). The cerebellar vermis also herniates in the Arnold-Chiari II malformation. This herniation may occlude the passage of CSF leading to hydrocephalus. It is almost always present in cases of spina bifida. Furthermore, this malformation is highly **associated with syringomyelia** because of altered CSF flow dynamics.

In syringomyelia, loss of the spinothalamic tract causes a capelike pattern of pain and temperature loss.

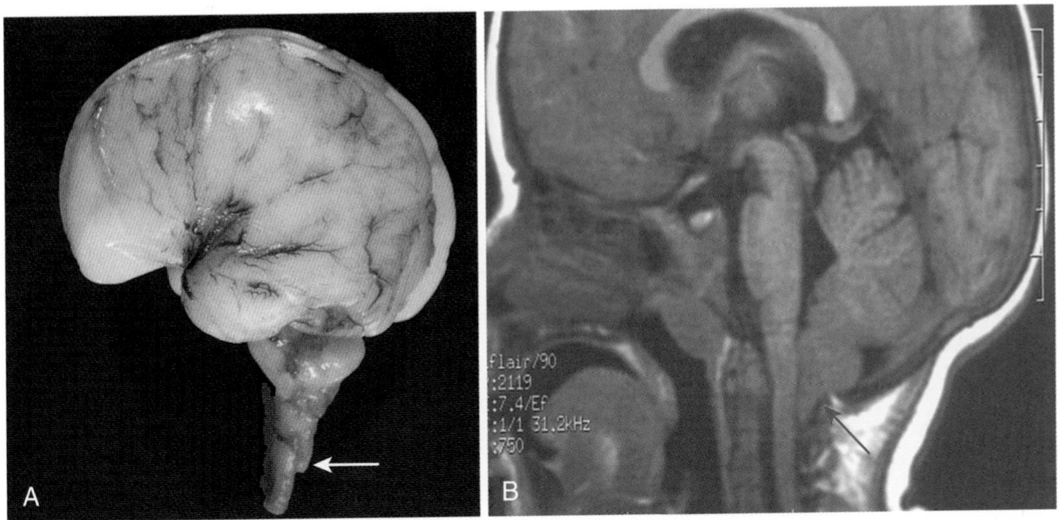

FIG. 4.15 The Arnold-Chiari malformation. The cerebellar tonsils *(arrow)* are inferior to the foramen magnum. (A) Gross specimen showing inferior deviation of the cerebellar tonsils. (B) MRI image showing cerebellar tonsils herniated through the foramen magnum. *(From Moore KL, Persaud TVN.* Before We Are Born. *7th ed. Philadelphia: Elsevier; 2007.* **A,** *Courtesy Dr. Marc R. Del Bigio, Department of Pathology [Neuropathology], University of Manitoba, Winnipeg, Manitoba, Canada.* **B,** *Courtesy Dr. R. Shane Tubbs and Dr. W. Jerry Oakes, Children's Hospital Birmingham, Birmingham, AL.)*

Syringomyelia

Syringomyelia is loss of pain and temperature sensation in a dermatomal **capelike** pattern around the back and arms as a result of cystic dilation of the **central canal compressing the spinothalamic tract** as it crosses the midline. Motor function (corticospinal tract) is initially spared but may be affected as the syrinx expands outward. Touch and vibration (dorsal columns) are unaffected.

GASTROINTESTINAL EMBRYOLOGY

Table 4.2 reviews the embryologic origins of the gastrointestinal structures as discussed in Chapter 10.

Table 4.2 Embryologic Divisions of the Gastrointestinal System*

DIVISION	ADULT STRUCTURES	ARTERIAL SUPPLY	NERVOUS SUPPLY
Foregut	Esophagus Stomach Proximal duodenum Liver Gallbladder Pancreas	Celiac trunk	PSNS: vagus nerve SNS: thoracic splanchnic nerves (T5–T9)
Midgut	Distal duodenum Jejunum Ileum Proximal transverse colon	Superior mesenteric	PSNS: vagus nerve SNS: thoracic splanchnics (T10–12).
Hindgut	Distal transverse colon Descending colon Sigmoid colon Rectum	Inferior mesenteric	PSNS: pelvic splanchnics (S2–S4) SNS: lumbar splanchnics (L1–L2).

PSNS, Parasympathetic nervous system; SNS, sympathetic nervous system.
*See Chapter 10 for details.

Allantois

Allantois is an outpouching of the hindgut that is nonfunctional in the human embryo and is obliterated early. It connects to the apex of the developing bladder at the proximal end and travels through the umbilical cord (Fig. 4.16). The proximal portion of the allantois is termed the **urachus,** which spans from the umbilicus to the bladder. Once obliterated, the urachus is termed the **median umbilical ligament.** It continues to have no physiologic use but may be used as a surgical landmark to indicate the midline of the abdomen.

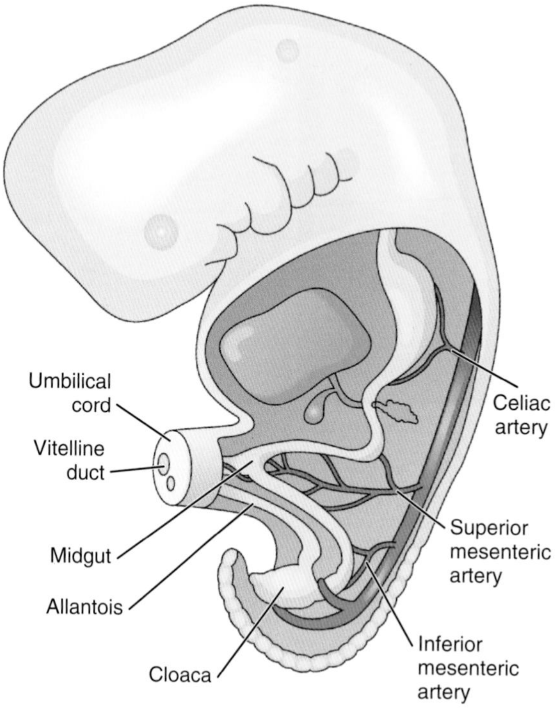

Fig. 4.16 An embryo at week 5. The urachus is the proximal portion of the allantois that connects to the developing bladder (cloaca). It will obliterate during the fetal period to form the median umbilical ligament. The vitelline duct connects the yolk sac to the midgut and provides nourishment to the embryo. (*From Becker J, Stucchi AF.* Essentials of Surgery. *Philadelphia: Elsevier; 2006.*)

Vitelline Duct (Omphalomesenteric Duct)

The vitelline duct (also known as the omphalomesenteric duct) is a tube that connects the embryologic yolk sac to the midgut and provides nourishment to the embryo. It is obliterated in the seventh week but may partially persist in the form of a **Meckel diverticulum** (see Chapter 10).

A persistent vitelline duct is termed a Meckel diverticulum.

Cloaca

The cloaca is the terminal portion of the hindgut, and the early embryologic cavity into which the gastrointestinal and genitourinary systems empty. The cloaca will later divide into the rectum and the **urogenital sinus.**

Congenital Diaphragmatic Hernia

In a congenital diaphragmatic hernia, an incomplete formation of pleuroperitoneal membrane of the diaphragm (usually in the left posterolateral portion) allows abdominal contents to herniate into the thorax. This herniation causes pressure on the lung buds and leads to pulmonary hypoplasia and pulmonary hypertension. Neonates will experience respiratory distress. This condition is associated with high perinatal mortality.

Omphalocele

Omphalocele is failure of the gastrointestinal viscera to enter the abdominal cavity after physiologic herniation during the early fetal period. The result is a **midline, peritoneal-covered** sac protruding through the umbilicus and containing abdominal organs (Fig. 4.17A). Although the condition is treatable, 40% of cases are associated with more severe problems, including heart defects, neural tube defects, and chromosomal abnormalities. Omphalocele can be distinguished by the common (and benign) umbilical hernia, which is covered by skin (not just peritoneum).

Omphalocele is associated with heart defects, neural tube defects, and chromosomal abnormalities.

Gastroschisis

Gastroschisis is incomplete fusion of the body wall leading to protrusion of gastrointestinal viscera. The protrusion is **lateral** to the umbilicus and is ***not*** **covered by peritoneum** (Fig. 4.17B). This condition is ***not*** **associated with chromosomal abnormalities** or other serious malformations.

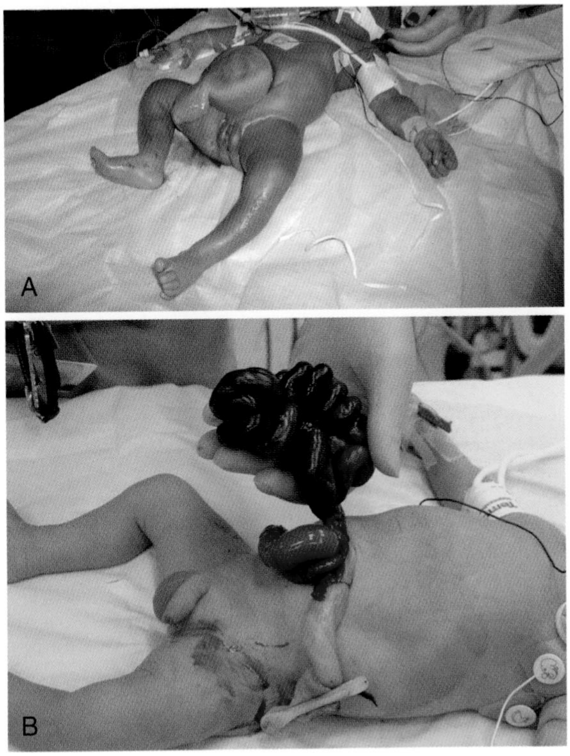

FIG. 4.17 A, Omphalocele. Note the midline protrusion of abdominal viscera surrounded by peritoneum. **B,** Gastroschisis. Note the lateral protrusion of viscera without surrounding peritoneum. *(From Schoenwolf GC, Bleyl SB, Brauer PR, Francis-West PH.* Larsen's Human Embryology. *4th ed. Philadelphia: Elsevier; 2008.)*

RENAL EMBRYOLOGY

Renal embryology has three distinct phases that chronologically occur in a cranial to caudal sequence (Fig. 4.18).

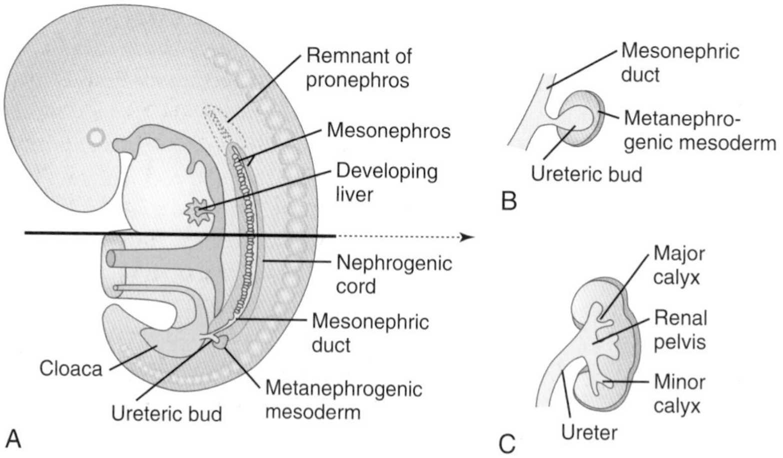

FIG. 4.18 The developing kidney. **A,** Renal development has three stages that progress in a cranial to caudal fashion. The pronephros regresses early. **B,** The ureteric bud of the mesonephros will form the collecting ducts, renal pelvis, and ureters of the adult kidney. **C,** The metanephros will form the majority of the adult kidney: Bowman capsules, proximal tubules, loops of Henle, and distal tubules. (*From Moore NA, Roy WA.* Rapid Review Gross and Developmental Anatomy. *3rd ed. Philadelphia: Elsevier; 2010.*)

Pronephros

In week 4, vestigial nephronlike units form and then regress without ever functioning.

> Renal parenchyma develops from the metanephros. The collecting system develops from the ureteric bud.

Mesonephros

The mesonephros system begins to develop nephronlike structures that also eventually regress. A structure persists, however, called the **ureteric bud,** which develops from the mesonephric ducts. This bud penetrates the metanephros to form the **renal pelvis, collecting duct system,** and **ureters**. Additionally, in males, the **mesonephric ducts (wolffian ducts)** persist and will later form the male reproductive tract.

Metanephros

The metanephros system will form the nephrons and parenchyma of the definitive kidney. Metanephric tissue, under the influence of the collecting duct system, begins to form into recognizable nephrons including Bowman capsules, proximal tubules, loops of Henle, and distal tubules. By the 12th week of gestation, distal tubules (metanephros) have connected with collecting ducts (ureteric bud), and glomeruli have formed. At this point, urine production can begin. Importantly, the placenta, not the fetal kidney, is responsible for clearing the body of waste. Fetal urine is excreted into the amniotic sac, where it is swallowed and recycled. This explains why **renal agenesis leads to oligohydramnios** because fetal urine is a major component of amniotic fluid.

Potter Sequence (Oligohydramnios Sequence)

A decrease in the volume of amniotic fluid (oligohydramnios) causes facial deformations (as a result of mechanical stress) and pulmonary hypoplasia (as a result of decreased nutrients and alveolar hydrostatic pressure). Oligohydramnios has many causes but usually is due to renal, ureteral, or urethral disease (classically bilateral renal agenesis). Knowing Potter sequence is high yield because it shows the importance of the fetal urologic system in producing amniotic fluid and the role of amniotic fluid as a mechanical cushion and promoter of growth.

REPRODUCTIVE EMBRYOLOGY

The reproductive system begins developing as paired gonadal ridges where primordial germ cells migrate and begin to form the primitive sex cords known as the **indifferent gonad.** The genetic determination of sexual differentiation begins at fertilization, when the ovum (X chromosome) is joined with a sperm containing either another X chromosome (XX) or a Y chromosome (XY). The **phenotypic determination** of sexual differentiation, however, begins with the gonads. The gonads will determine maturation of the duct system (wolffian or müllerian), external genitalia, and eventually secondary sexual characteristics.

The female phenotype is considered the default, and phenotypic "maleness" requires the presence of the **testis-determining factor,** the ***SRY* gene** (sex-determining region on Y).

The *SRY* gene causes the indifferent gonads to develop into the testes.

Male Embryology

The *SRY* gene encodes a transcription factor that causes the indifferent gonad to turn into the testes. The testes begin to produce testosterone, which influences the mesonephric duct (wolffian duct) to form the epididymis, vas deferens, and seminal vesicles. Testosterone is further converted into **dihydrotestosterone** (DHT) by the enzyme **5α-reductase.** This powerful androgen virilizes the **genital tubercle** and the rest of the male genitalia (Table 4.3). Meanwhile, **antimüllerian hormone** is produced by the Sertoli cells, which causes the regression of the müllerian ducts.

Testosterone develops the internal reproductive tract. DHT virilizes the external genitalia in addition to the prostate gland. 5α-Reductase inhibitors (such as finasteride) are used to treat benign prostatic hyperplasia by preventing DHT-dependent growth of the prostate.

TABLE 4.3 Female and Male Reproductive Embryology

FETAL STRUCTURE	MALE ADULT STRUCTURE	FEMALE ADULT STRUCTURE	COMMENT
Indifferent gonad	Testicle	Ovary	*SRY* determines whether ovaries or testes will form
Wolffian duct	Urinary collecting system Epididymis Vas deferens Seminal vesicles	Urinary collecting system	Male structures are formed under the influence of testosterone
Müllerian duct	Regress	Fallopian tubes Uterus Cervix Upper vagina	In males these ducts regress because of antimüllerian hormone
Genital tubercle	Penis	Clitoris	Virilized by DHT
Urogenital sinus	Bladder Proximal urethra Prostate gland Bulbourethral gland	Bladder Proximal urethra Bartholin glands Glands of Skene	The urogenital sinus is partitioned off from the cloaca
Labioscrotal swelling	Scrotum	Labia	Influenced by DHT or estrogen

DHT, Dihydrotestosterone.

Female Embryology

The absence of an *SRY* gene allows the indifferent gonads to turn into the ovaries by default. Absence of antimüllerian hormone in females allows the müllerian ducts to remain. The ovaries begin to produce estrogen, which influences the müllerian ducts to form the fallopian tubes, uterus, cervix, and upper vagina. Estrogen also causes the **genital tubercle** to form the lower vagina and the labioscrotal swelling to form the vulva.

Urogenital Sinus

By the end of the embryonic period (week 8), the ventral part of the cloaca has been partitioned off into the urogenital sinus, which will eventually form the **bladder** and **proximal urethra.** In men, it will also form the **prostate** and **bulbourethral glands,** whereas in women, it will form the **Bartholin glands** and **glands of Skene.**

Hypospadias

Hypospadias is incomplete fusion of the urethral folds leading to a urethral meatus on the inferior portion of the penis. Surgery can be curative.

Epispadias

Epispadias is a rare malformation in which defective migration of the genital tubercle results in a urethral meatus on the dorsum of the penis. It is highly associated with **exstrophy of the bladder,** in which epispadias is also a component. Only rarely can epispadias occur in isolation.

Exstrophy of the Bladder

Exstrophy of the bladder is an incomplete migration of the primitive streak mesoderm (abdominal wall) around the cloacal membrane leading to bladder mucosa extending outside the body. It is **always associated with epispadias.**

Undescended testicles are at risk for later development of testicular cancer.

Micropenis

Insufficient androgen stimulation from any part of the hypothalamic-pituitary-gonadal axis results in incomplete growth of the penis, known as micropenis. It is commonly seen in Klinefelter syndrome (genotype XXY).

Cryptorchidism

Three percent of males will be born with an undescended testicle, known as cryptorchidism. Most testicles will descend within the first months of life, and no treatment is indicated. Rarely, physiologic descent does not occur, and surgery is indicated before the age of 1 to prevent complications such as reduced fertility or testicular cancer. Most undescended testicles are located in the inguinal canal. Of note, any cause of an intraabdominal testicle (e.g., androgen insensitivity syndrome) puts a patient at increased risk for testicular cancer.

Uterine Anomalies

If the paired müllerian ducts fail to fuse, the result is a double uterus, double cervix, and double vagina **(uterus didelphys).** Partial fusion results in the more common **bicornuate uterus,** in which two uterine cavities share a single cervix and vagina (Fig. 4.19).

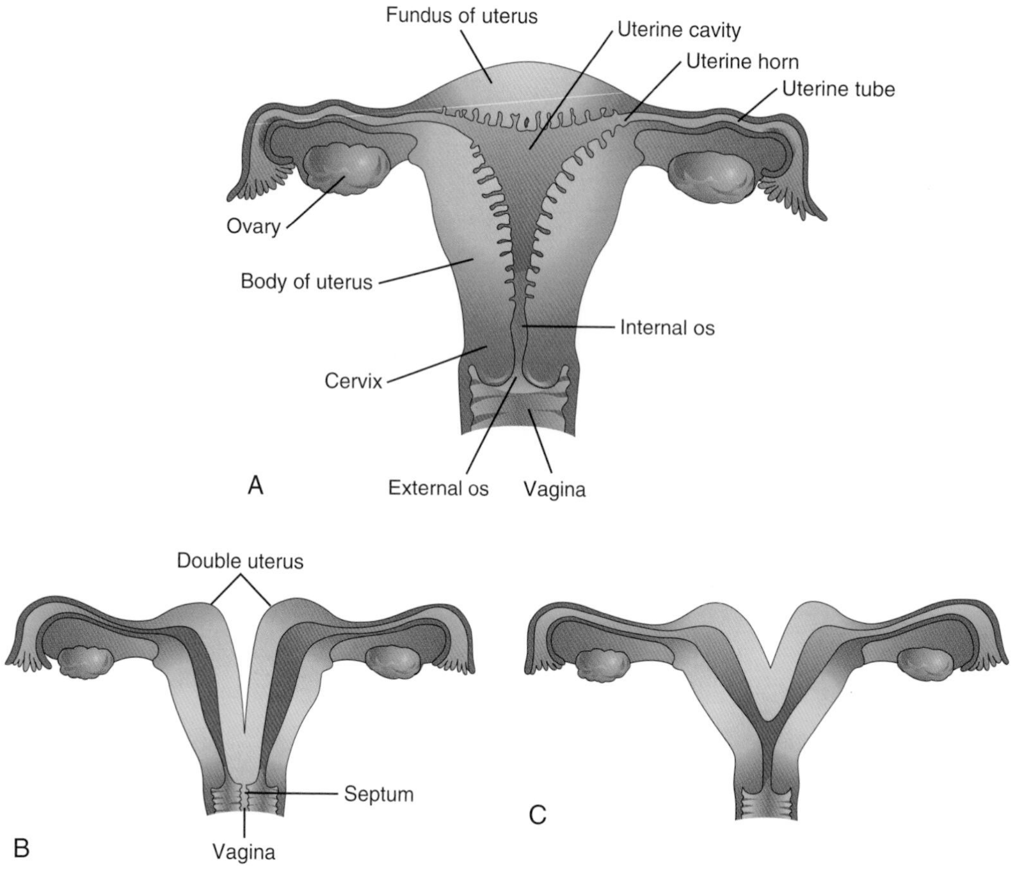

FIG. 4.19 Uterine embryologic anomalies. **A,** Normal female reproductive tract. **B,** Uterus didelphys. **C,** Bicornuate uterus. (*From Moore KL, Persaud TVN.* Before We Are Born. *8th ed. Philadelphia: Elsevier; 2012.*)

HEAD AND NECK EMBRYOLOGY

The most distinctive feature of head and neck embryology is the development of the branchial (pharyngeal) arches, which will develop into the musculoskeletal components of the region (Table 4.4). There are six paired arches composed of a "sandwich" with ectoderm on the outside, endoderm on the inside, and neural crest cells in the middle (Fig. 4.20). Each branchial arch is supplied by its numerically

Table 4.4 Branchial Arch Derivatives

BRANCHIAL ARCH	ADULT STRUCTURE	CRANIAL NERVE	COMMENT
1st arch	Muscles of **mastication** (temporalis, masseter, pterygoids) **Malleus** and **incus** bones (from "Meckel cartilage") Tensor tympani Maxilla Anterior tongue	V2 (maxillary) V3 (mandibular)	Simplified: "**chewing** and **listening** arch"
2nd arch	**Muscles of facial expression** Stapes Upper hyoid	VII (facial)	Simplified: "**facial expression** arch"
3rd arch	Lower hyoid Stylopharyngeus muscle	IX (glossopharyngeal)	Simplified: "stylopharyngeus arch"
4th arch	Laryngeal cartilage (thyroid, epiglottic) **Pharyngeal constrictors**	X (vagus) Superior laryngeal (swallowing)	Simplified: "**swallowing** arch"
5th arch	N/A	N/A	No significant contributions
6th arch	Laryngeal cartilage (cricoid, arytenoid, corniculate, cuneiform) **Intrinsic laryngeal muscles**	X (vagus) Recurrent laryngeal (speech)	Simplified: "**speaking** arch"

N/A, Not applicable.

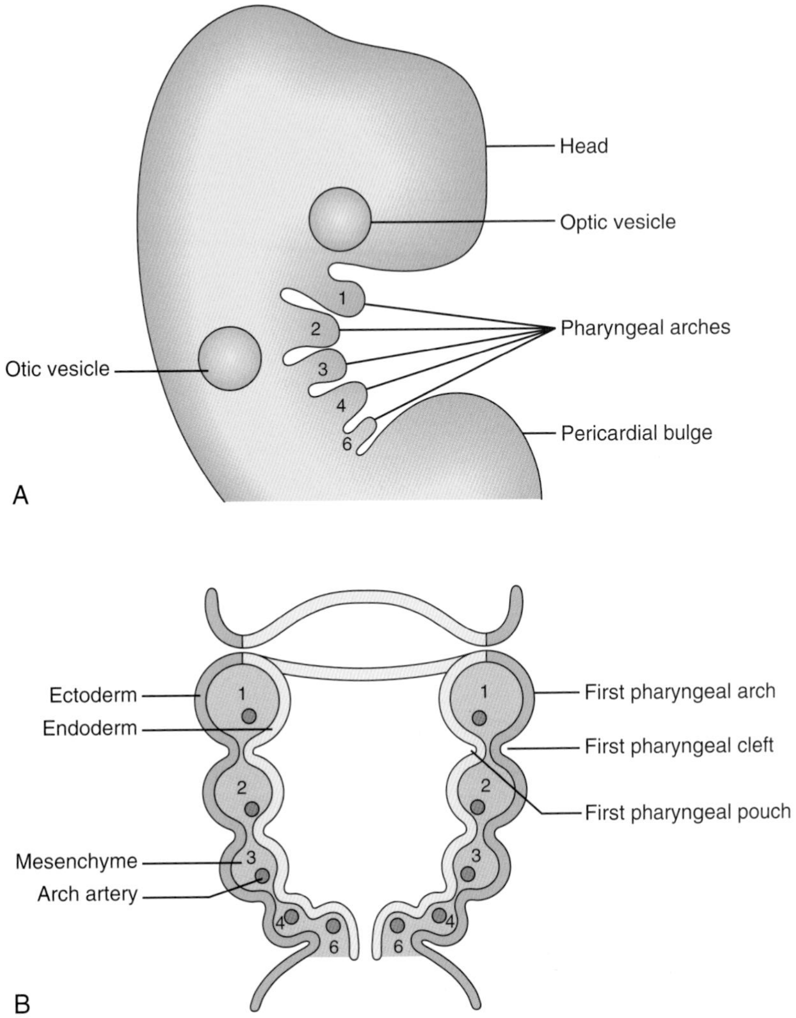

Fig. 4.20 Branchial apparatus including arches, clefts, and pouches. **A,** Lateral view. **B,** Cross-section. (*From Turnpenny P, Ellard S.* Emery's Elements of Medical Genetics. *14th ed. Philadelphia: Elsevier; 2011. Redrawn from Graham A, Smith A. Patterning the pharyngeal arches.* Bioessays *2001;23:54-61, with permission of Wiley-Liss Inc., a subsidiary of John Wiley & Sons, Inc.*)

corresponding aortic arch and a cranial nerve (which unfortunately does not correspond numerically). The branchial arches are separated from each other by branchial clefts. These clefts do not contribute to the adult structure, except for the first, which will form the external acoustic meatus (Table 4.5). On the endodermal side, between the pharyngeal arches, lie the pharyngeal pouches (Table 4.6). These pouches form many important structures of the head and neck.

Table 4.5 Branchial Cleft Derivatives

BRANCHIAL CLEFT	ADULT STRUCTURE	COMMENT
1st cleft	External auditory meatus	
2nd–4th cleft	Obliterated	Failure to obliterate these clefts leads to a branchial cleft cyst

Table 4.6 Branchial Pouch Derivatives

BRANCHIAL POUCH	ADULT STRUCTURE
1st pouch	Tympanic membrane Middle ear cavity Eustachian tube
2nd pouch	Palatine tonsil Tonsillar fossa
3rd pouch	Inferior parathyroid gland Thymus
4th pouch	Superior parathyroid gland
5th pouch	C cells of thyroid

Treacher Collins Syndrome

In Treacher Collins syndrome, lack of neural crest cell migration into the first branchial arch causes syndromic facial malformations, including micrognathia and **conductive hearing loss.** This can be remembered because Meckel cartilage develops from the first branchial arch. It forms the malleus and incus and also guides development of the mandible.

Pierre Robin Syndrome

In Pierre Robin syndrome, lack of neural crest cell migration into the first branchial arch causes syndromic facial malformations, including micrognathia and **cleft palate.** This can be remembered because the hard palate is made partially of the maxillary bone, a first arch derivative.

DiGeorge Syndrome

In DiGeorge syndrome, failure of differentiation of the third and fourth pharyngeal pouches leads to absent parathyroid glands (causing hypocalcemia) and thymic aplasia (causing T-cell immunodeficiency). This syndrome is accompanied by facial abnormalities (similar to first arch syndromes) and cardiac anomalies (especially tetralogy of Fallot). Mnemonic: **CATCH-22**—**C**ardiac anomalies, **A**bnormal facies, **T**hymic aplasia, **C**left palate, **H**ypoparathyroidism/**H**ypocalcemia as a result of a deletion on chromosome **22.**

DiGeorge syndrome: CATCH-22. **C**ardiac abnormalities, **A**bnormal facies, **T**hymic aplasia, **C**left palate, **H**ypocalcemia (caused by hypoparathyroidism) from a deletion on chromosome **22**.

Branchial Cleft Cyst

Failure of obliteration of one of the branchial clefts leads to a cystic structure of the **lateral neck** along the anterior border of the sternocleidomastoid (most commonly the second branchial cleft is implicated) called a branchial cleft cyst.

Tongue

The tongue receives contributions from branchial arches 1 to 4, which explains its complex innervation pattern (Fig. 4.21).

- **General Sensation:** The anterior two-thirds of the tongue (the body) derives from the first pharyngeal arch; therefore sensory innervation is through CN V3 (mandibular nerve). The posterior

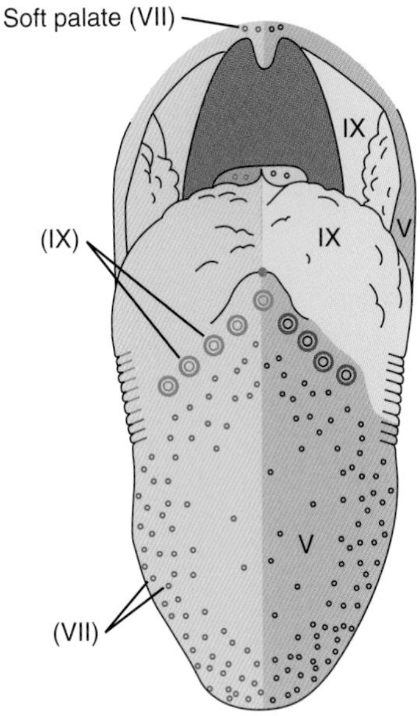

Fig. 4.21 Cranial nerve innervation of the tongue for taste *(left)* and general sensation *(right)*. (*From Nolte J.* The Human Brain. *6th ed. Philadelphia: Elsevier; 2008.*)

one-third of the tongue (the base) derives from the third (and partially the fourth) pharyngeal arch; therefore sensory innervation is through CN IX (glossopharyngeal).

- **Taste**: Taste to the anterior two-thirds of the tongue is through CN VII (**chorda tympani** branch), whereas taste to the posterior one-third, like general sensation, is through CN IX.
- **Motor:** The intrinsic and extrinsic musculature of the tongue (genioglossus, hyoglossus, styloglossus, and palatoglossus) is derived from occipital somites. Motor innervation is through CN XII (hypoglossal nerve) except for the palatoglossus muscle (innervated by CN X).

Thyroid

Thyroid tissue begins to proliferate on the pharyngeal floor and migrates down the midline of the anterior neck (Fig. 4.22). It remains connected to the base of the tongue by the thyroglossal duct, which will eventually be obliterated, leaving only the **foramen cecum,** a small indentation, at the base of the tongue.

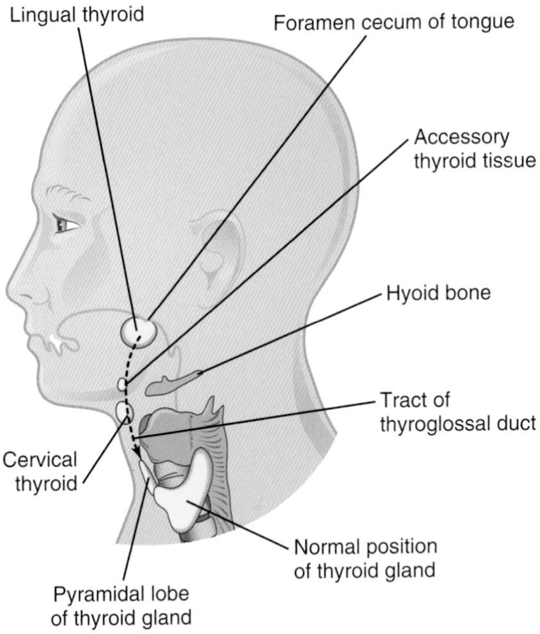

Fig. 4.22 The thyroid gland migrates from the foramen cecum (on the tongue) to its normal position inferior to the thyroid cartilage. Note the tract of the thyroglossal duct and the potential locations of ectopic thyroid tissue and thyroglossal duct cysts. (*From Moore KL, Persaud TVN.* Before We Are Born. *8th ed. Philadelphia: Elsevier; 2012.*)

Table 4.7 Apgar Score for Assessing the Health of Neonates

	0 POINTS	1 POINT	2 POINTS
Appearance	Blue/pale all over	Acrocyanosis (pink trunk with blue extremities)	Pink all over
Pulse	No pulse	<100 beats/min	≥100 beats/min
Grimace	No response to stimulation	Weak cry or grimace when stimulated	Cry, cough, pull away when stimulated
Activity	No movement	Some flexion of extremities	Active, flexed arms and legs that resist extension
Respirations	None	Irregular, weak, gasping	Strong cry, regular breathing

Thyroglossal duct cyst: Failure of obliteration of the thyroglossal duct causes a **midline** cystic dilation anywhere along the migratory pathway of the thyroid. This cyst will **move with swallowing,** unlike branchial cleft cysts.

Ectopic thyroid: Failure of descent of the thyroid tissue along the neck leads to ectopic tissue. Most commonly, the tissue is found on the base of the tongue, behind the foramen cecum; however, it can be anywhere along the migratory path. It is subject to the same disease states as the normal thyroid, including hyperthyroidism and thyroid cancer.

Ectopic thyroid tissue can be found anywhere along the migratory path of the thyroid.

Ear

It is worth reviewing the various pharyngeal apparatus contributions to the ear.

- Branchial arch 1: incus, malleus, tensor tympani muscle (dampens sound)
- Branchial arch 2: stapes, stapedius muscle (dampens sound)
- Pharyngeal pouch 1: middle ear cavity, eustachian tube
- Pharyngeal cleft 1: external auditory meatus
- Branchial membrane 1: tympanic membrane

The Apgar score is not necessarily indicative of long-term outcome. However, persistently low scores, such as ≤3 for more than 10 minutes of life, are associated with neurologic damage.

GROWTH AND DEVELOPMENT

Neonatal Medicine

Apgar Score

The Apgar score is a grading system, named for Dr. Virginia Apgar, to assess the general health of a newborn at 1 minute and 5 minutes of life (Table 4.7). For each of the five categories (each of which start with the letters of her name), 0 to 2 points may be given. Ten is a perfect score, but it is rarely given because most newborns will lose 1 point for acrocyanosis.

Low Birth Weight

Infants are typically born at around 40 weeks (full term) with a birth weight of approximately 2500 to 3800 g (5 lb, 8 oz to 8 lb, 6 oz). Infants who weigh **less than 2500 g** at birth are defined as **low birth weight,** and they are at risk for numerous complications. Because of the delicate vasculature in the **subependymal germinal matrix** of the cerebral ventricles, they are at risk for **intraventricular hemorrhage,** which can lead to neurologic devastation in some cases. They may have abnormal blood vessels in the retina, which can lead to scarring and blindness (called **retinopathy of prematurity**). With their suboptimally developed immune systems, they are susceptible to **infections,** which can be severe. Small infants are also at risk for **respiratory distress syndrome** because of **insufficient surfactant production.** They are at risk for **necrotizing enterocolitis,** a disease in which the bowel dies and may bleed and perforate. They are also more likely than babies of normal weight to have a persistently **patent ductus arteriosus,** which can lead to heart failure, as described in Chapter 8.

Infants may be low birth weight because of prematurity and/or growth restriction in utero.

Developmental Milestones

Unfortunately, developmental milestones can be difficult to commit to memory. The best strategy is usually to think of your own personal experience with normal infants and children and their abilities at certain ages. A list of testable milestones along with a few mnemonics are listed in Table 4.8. The rightmost column describes Jean Piaget's stages of cognitive development. He made these observations of how children's cognitive function develops by watching his own children.

Table 4.8 Developmental Milestones and Piaget's Stages of Cognitive Development

AGE	MOTOR MILESTONES	COGNITIVE, SOCIAL, AND LANGUAGE MILESTONES	PIAGET'S PERSPECTIVE
1 mo	Rooting reflex: turns toward cheek that is touched as if to eat (breastfeed) Moro reflex: startle reaction; head and legs extend, arms jerk up and out, then come together	Notices voices and orients to them	Sensorimotor stage Birth–2 yr Infant recognizes self and how self is different from external objects. Recognizes how to intentionally act on objects, such as shaking a rattle to make a noise. By 1 yr, toddler understands object permanence: objects that are hidden still exist and can be searched for. Often plays alone, exploring environment. Learns to trust parents.
2 mo	Can hold head up Eyes track objects to midline	Smiles spontaneously at nothing in particular Makes cooing noises; "coos at 2"	
4 mo	Disappearance of Moro and rooting reflexes Eyes follow objects across midline Can sit with support	Social smile: sees happy parents and smiles back Laughs	
6 mo	Sits without support Rolls from front to back Transfers a block from hand to hand	Stranger anxiety Babbling	
9 mo	Pincer grasp (between thumb and forefinger) Stands up with help, crawls May be starting to cruise (walk while holding onto furniture)	Can play pat-a-cake and peek-a-boo A few words: mama (think: it takes 9 mo to become a mama), dada, bye-bye	
1 yr	Walks! Can even walk up stairs Throws and kicks a ball Stack 3 blocks (= 1 yr × 3) Right or left hand dominance begins to become clear	Separation anxiety 10 words!	
2 yr	Walking down stairs is harder, but now can do it Stacks 6 blocks (= 2 yr × 3) Scribbles with crayons Can copy a line	About 200 words Put 2 words together to form little phrases, like "Daddy eat" Use pronouns: "My dolly" May have security objects, like a security blanket, called a transitional object Parallel play: playing independently alongside other kids, not interacting (think: 2 parallel lines)	
3 yr	Stacks 9 blocks (= 3 yr × 3) Rides a tricycle (3 wheels!) Can copy a circle Can cut paper with scissors Can catch a ball	Can play with others (think of 3 kids in a group playing together) Knows gender and full name Understands some gender roles Can take turns Now knows 900 words! Can repeat 3 digits back to you Can point to and count 3 objects	Preoperational stage 2–7 yr Learning language is a major accomplishment here. They can group objects together by one feature, such as red objects or square objects. Children are still egocentric and have trouble putting themselves in others' shoes.

Continued

Table 4.8 Developmental Milestones and Piaget's Stages of Cognitive Development—cont'd

AGE	MOTOR MILESTONES	COGNITIVE, SOCIAL, AND LANGUAGE MILESTONES	PIAGET'S PERSPECTIVE
4–5 yr	Can copy a cross and draw a stick person Hops on 1 foot (think: starting kindergarten and hopping to school)	Can count 10+ objects Can name 4+ colors Can tell stories Likes to sing and dance and act Can distinguish fantasy from reality	
6–12 yr	Can copy a triangle (6 yr) Learns to print letters, tie shoes, get dressed Rides a bicycle	Understands rules of games; can play organized group games and sports Play groups often separated by sex Not good with hypotheticals (if, then) Feels personal sense of right and wrong	Concrete operational stage 7–11 yr These elementary school children now have some logic. They understand conservation of number and mass. They can now group objects together by multiple features, such as red square hard objects.
12+ yr	Growth spurts and puberty: girls before boys	Importance of personal identity as well as conforming to others in peer group Interest in abstract ideas (e.g., positives and negatives of communism)	Formal operational stage: 11+ yr In contrast to younger children in concrete operations, these teens are able to think more abstractly. They can make hypotheses and test them. They think about hypothetical situations and what might happen in the future.

REVIEW QUESTIONS

(1) Describe the location of the T3 vertebral body in relation to the location of the left clavicle, using cranial/caudal, medial/lateral, and dorsal/ventral.

(2) When an egg is released from the ovary during ovulation, which stage of the cell cycle is it in? What must occur for the cell cycle to continue?

(3) If a set of monozygotic twins shares both a placenta and the same amniotic fluid sac, what is this termed? When must the split have occurred?

(4) From what germ layer do the following originate: (a) epidermis of the skin, (b) the gastrointestinal (GI) tract, (c) muscles?

(5) Why is it important to supplement folate for reproductive-age women who may become pregnant?

(6) What is the term for spina bifida when the defect is large enough to allow protrusion of the spinal cord and meninges? What is a potential problem these fetuses may have?

(7) A woman who is planning on becoming pregnant is currently taking levothyroxine for her hypothyroidism, lisinopril for her hypertension, and lithium for her bipolar disorder. Which of these are teratogenic, and what are the possible outcomes if she continues these medications during pregnancy?

(8) A woman says that she read online that there was a problem with diethylstilbestrol. Her mother took DES when she was pregnant with her, and she is curious as to whether she is at increased risk for any conditions because of this. Is she?

(9) What are the three main shunts in the fetus to bypass the liver and/or lungs? What occurs after birth with these shunts?

(10) If a neonate has a type of congenital heart disease that benefits from keeping the patent ductus arteriosus open, how can that be accomplished? How can it be closed medically?

(11) A neonate is found to have a midline abdominal wall defect. Examination reveals abdominal viscera filling a peritoneal covered sac. What is the diagnosis?

(12) A mother brings in her 9-year-old son because she recently noticed a "bump" in his neck. Examination reveals a midline cyst just inferior to the cricoid cartilage. It moves when the patient swallows. What is the likely diagnosis?

(13) A patient is born with the chromosomal anomaly XXXY. Will this patient have testicles or ovaries? Why?

(14) During a well-child examination, a 4-year-old boy is found to have a cyst on the lateral side of his neck along the border of the sternocleidomastoid. What is the embryologic origin of this condition?

(15) A child is able to walk up and down stairs and scribble with a crayon. She carries a security blanket with her much of the time. She is not yet able to catch a ball and does not appear to understand the concept of taking turns. What age is she, assuming she is meeting all developmental milestones?

5 MICROBIOLOGY

Lauren Sanchez, Will Babbitt, and John H. Baird

BACTERIA

Introduction to Bacterial Structure

The **Gram stain** is used to tell whether a bacterium is **gram negative** or **gram positive** (Fig. 5.1). To understand the Gram stain you must understand the structure of bacteria. All bacteria have a **peptidoglycan cell wall** (Fig. 5.2). In gram-positive bacteria it is thick, whereas in gram-negative bacteria it is thin. Importantly, gram-negative bacteria have an *additional* membrane outside the cell wall, consisting mainly of **lipopolysaccharide (LPS).** It is this LPS layer that prevents the blue dye applied during a Gram stain from being trapped in the cell wall, unlike gram-positive bacteria, which take up the blue dye. The process of Gram staining consists of applying the blue (crystal violet) dye, washing away the excess with alcohol, then applying a red (safranin) counterstain, which will adhere to anything not already stained by the blue dye (i.e., gram-negative bacteria). Hence, gram-positive bacteria appear blue, and gram-negative bacteria appear red.

Gram stain positive: blue; Gram stain negative: red.

Besides being important for Gram staining, the LPS layer of gram-negative bacteria can activate a cytokine-mediated immune response in a host, one of the major causes of septic shock. Specifically, the component of LPS called **lipid A** is an **endotoxin** ("endo" because it is found on the innermost portion of the LPS membrane). When our immune system lyses these bacteria in the blood, lipid A activates the cytokine cascade. Gram-positive bacteria and fungi can also cause septic shock.

"The lipid A component of LPS is a major cause of septic shock."

Importantly, the peptidoglycan cell wall consists of glycoproteins covalently bonded together by the enzyme **transpeptidase,** also called **penicillin-binding protein** because it is the enzyme inhibited by penicillin.

Bacterial **shape** is also important for distinguishing among the various species. They can be **cocci** (spherical), **bacilli** (rods), **coccobacilli** (short rods), **spiral** (comma shaped, S shaped, spiral shaped), or **pleomorphic** (lacking a characteristic shape and thus varying in shape).

Metabolic characteristics also help to distinguish the various species. Oxygen can be toxic through the formation of superoxide radicals, and only bacteria containing enzymes to break these down (**catalase, peroxidase, or superoxide dismutase**) can survive in oxygen. **Obligate aerobes** require oxygen to survive; **facultative anaerobes** prefer oxygen but can live without it through fermentation; **microaerophilic bacteria** can tolerate low amounts of oxygen but prefer to ferment their energy; and **obligate anaerobes** can't live in the presence of oxygen.

Finally, there is a category of bacteria that are **obligate intracellular organisms.** These bacteria cannot make their own adenosine triphosphate (ATP) and must rely on the host cell metabolism for survival. These bacteria only live within other cells, providing us with challenges for detection and treatment. **Facultative intracellular organisms** don't need to live in cells but have the ability to survive and replicate in macrophages after being phagocytosed because of enzymes protecting them against superoxide radical digestion. These organisms are *Listeria monocytogenes, Salmonella typhi, Yersinia, Francisella tularensis, Brucella, Legionella,* and *Mycobacterium.*

Some bacterial structures are important to know about:

- **Flagella** are used for movement and come in a variety of shapes.
- **Capsules** are an additional protective sugar layer around some bacteria (*Bacillus anthracis* is the only bacterium with an amino acid capsule). The capsules aid in immune evasion, and encapsulated bugs

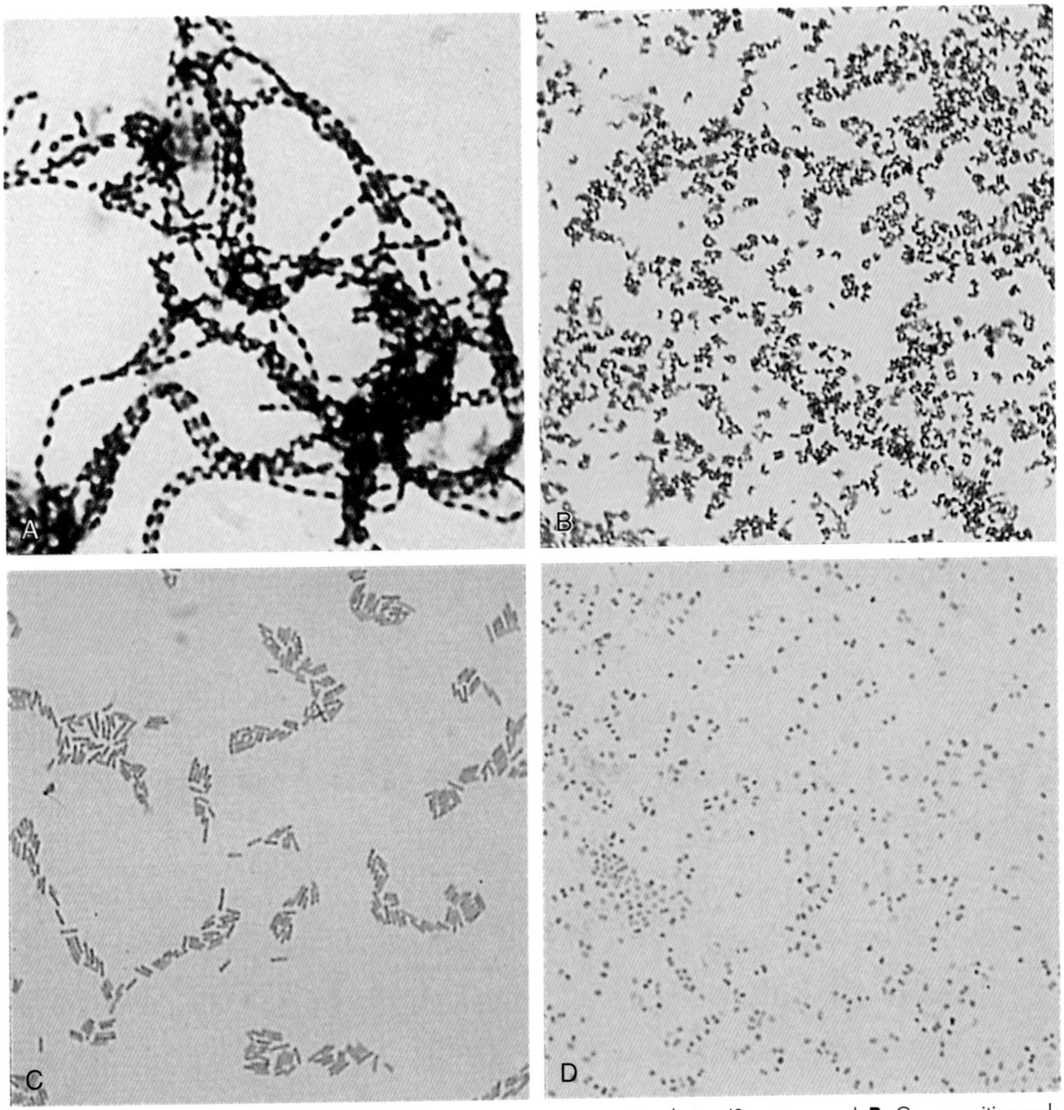

FIG. 5.1 Examples of Gram-stained bacteria. **A,** Gram-positive cocci in chains *(Streptococcus)*. **B,** Gram-positive rods *(Listeria)*. **C,** Gram-negative rods *(Escherichia coli)*. **D,** Gram-negative cocci *(Neisseria)*. (*From Goering R, Dockrell H, Wakelin D, et al.* Mims' Medical Microbiology. *4th ed. Philadelphia: Elsevier; 2007.*)

are particularly dangerous in individuals without working spleens (e.g., sickle cell disease) because that is where most phagocytosis of opsonized encapsulated bugs occurs. **Opsonization** is when a bacterium is coated with antibodies and therefore marked for phagocytosis and destruction. To detect an encapsulated bug, one must use either the **India ink stain** or the **Quellung reaction** (in which antibodies that bind to capsules are used to appreciate a swelling of the capsule under the microscope; Fig. 5.3).

- **Spores** are found in a few species of bacteria and are a protective form of the bacteria that allow them to survive harsh conditions until a host is found.
- **Biofilms** are similar to capsules in that they are made of a lattice of polysaccharides, in this case allowing groups of bacteria to bind to prosthetic devices (*Staphylococcus epidermidis* is notorious for doing this).
- **Toxins** are an important part of the disease-causing mechanisms of many bacteria. We can divide toxins into the organ system they infect (e.g., neurotoxins and enterotoxins), where they are found in the bacteria (**exotoxins** are released by all gram-positive bacteria except *Listeria,* which releases an endotoxin, and **endotoxins** such as **lipid A,** which was previously discussed) or by the effects they cause (**pyrogenic exotoxins** cause fever, **tissue invasive exotoxins** allow bacteria to tunnel through tissue, and **miscellaneous exotoxins** do various things tailored for certain bacteria).

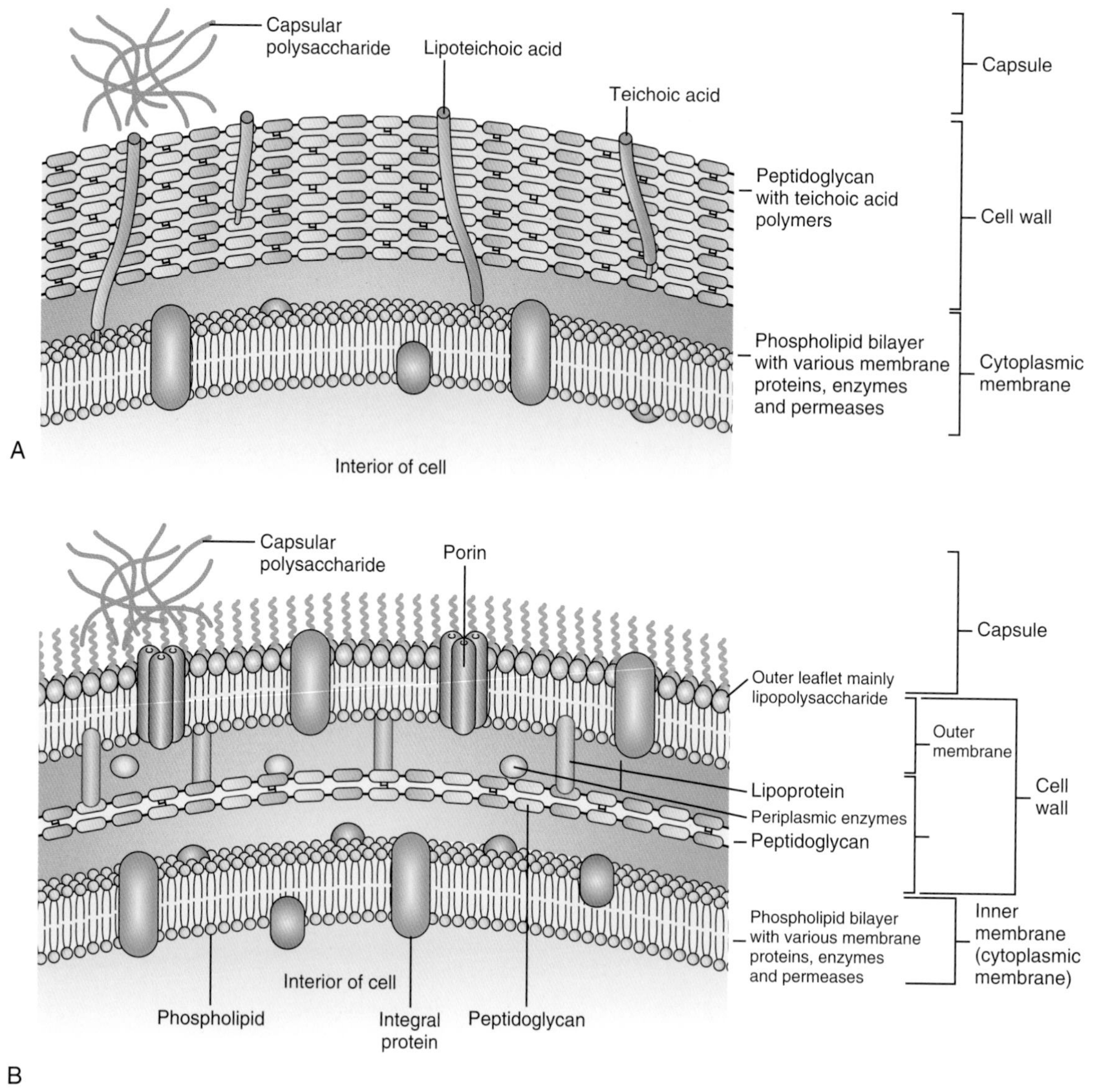

FIG. 5.2 Structure of gram-positive **(A)** and gram-negative **(B)** bacteria. (*From Greenwood D, Slack R, Peitherer J, Barer M. Medical Microbiology. 17th ed. Philadelphia: Elsevier; 2007.*)

Organization of the Rest of the Bacteriology Section

There are many ways to think about how to group and organize clinically important bacterial species. For the purposes of presenting several common species of disease-causing bacteria, we have chosen to organize by **shape** (or other defining physical characteristic) and **Gram stain.** The information is presented in 10 sections as follows:

- Gram-positive cocci
- Gram-negative cocci
- Gram-positive rods
- Gram-negative enteric rods
- Gram-negative nonenteric rods
- Gram-positive branching filamentous bacteria
- Gram-negative pleomorphic bacteria
- Gram-negative spirals
- Gram-positive acid-fast bacteria
- Gram-positive bacteria with no cell wall

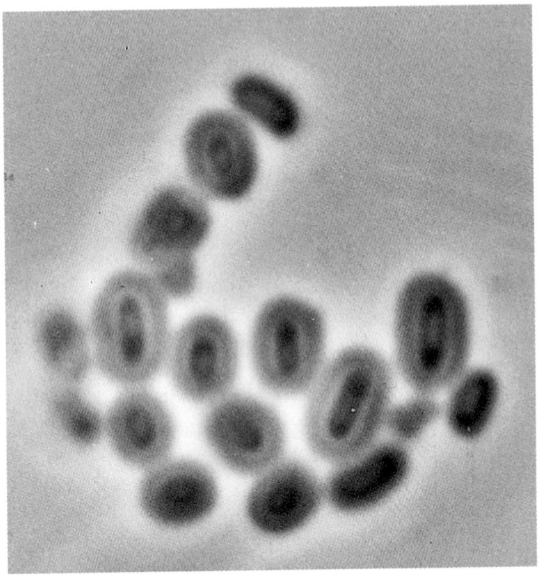

FIG. 5.3 Micrograph showing swelling of the capsule of *Klebsiella pneumonia* after antibody administration, demonstrating the Quellung reaction. (*From Greenwood D, Slack R, Peitherer J, Barer M. Medical Microbiology. 17th ed. Philadelphia: Elsevier; 2007.*)

Gram-Positive Cocci

Staphylococcus: *Staphylococcus* ("staph") species tend to form grapelike clusters. In the laboratory they can be distinguished from *Streptococcus* species by their formation of catalase; **all *Staphylococcus* species produce catalase,** whereas *Streptococcus* species do not. Staphylococci are subdivided into coagulase producing (*S. aureus*), and coagulase negative (*S. epidermidis* and *S. saprophyticus*) (Fig. 5.4).

Staphylococcus aureus is found on most surfaces, inhabiting the anterior nares of about 30% of individuals at any given time (good reason not to pick your nose), with higher rates among the ill and hospital personnel. Spread occurs through contact and is reduced by handwashing. *S. aureus* is the most virulent staph species in humans and can survive extreme conditions for long periods. A variety of surface adhesion proteins contribute to its virulence:

- **Coagulase** activates prothrombin, creating a fibrin shield (unique to *S. aureus*).
- **Protein A** binds the constant region (Fc) of immunoglobulin (protection from opsonization and phagocytosis).
- **Lipase, protease,** and **hyaluronidase** help *S. aureus* digest through connective tissue.

Staphylococcus aureus causes a variety of diseases, from self-limited skin infections, to toxin-mediated food poisoning or staph scalded skin syndrome (SSSS), to osteomyelitis and endocarditis, to life-threatening bacteremia in intravenous drug users and those with indwelling catheters (see Tables 5.1 and 5.2). A typical infection starts with colonization of the nares, anus, and/or skin. Local invasion of skin usually leads to a furuncle or other skin abscess as neutrophils come to the infectious site. Bacteria may then go on to directly invade other organs through lymphatics or blood (Table 5.1) and/or produce one of several potential toxins, which are then disseminated throughout the body (Table 5.2). Diagnosis of *S. aureus* is by culture on blood agar—colonies appear white with a golden pigment and have a clear halo as a result of hemolysis of red blood cells by hemolysins. A quicker test is to assess for coagulase

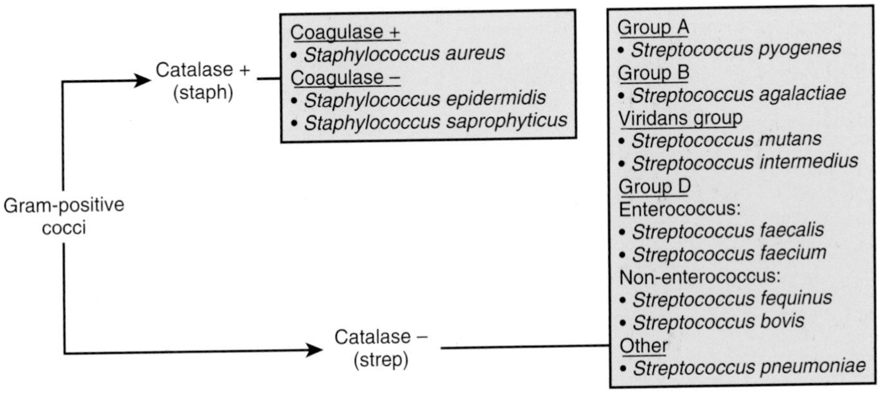

FIG. 5.4 Division of gram-positive cocci.

Table 5.1 Diseases Caused by Direct Invasion of *Staphylococcus aureus*

ORGAN/TISSUE	CLINICAL DISEASE	FEATURES
Skin: epidermis*	Impetigo (Fig. 5.5)	Area of erythema erupting into vesicles, which rupture to form characteristic **honey-colored crust.** Exposed areas most vulnerable (face, legs). Highly contagious.
Skin: hair follicles	Folliculitis (Fig. 5.6), furuncle, carbuncle	Folliculitis presents as raised red bumps at hair follicles. Furuncle (boil) is a deeper infection of a single hair follicle. Joining of multiple furuncles is a carbuncle.
Skin: dermis	Erysipelas	Geographically delineated zone of erythema on skin. Painful, raised, red, often presenting with fever/chills. More often caused by *Streptococcus pyogenes*.
Skin: subdermal	Cellulitis	No demarcated zone of redness as seen in erysipelas. Patient presents with severe pain and fever.
Skin: fascial layer	Necrotizing fasciitis	Starts as a swollen, red, hot area that soon becomes purple, then blue, with formation of large blisters. The muscle can become infected (myositis). Surgical emergency; amputation may be necessary.
Skin: breast	Mastitis	Common in breastfeeding mothers with newborns. Can develop into abscess; drain surgically.
Blood	Bacteremia	Approximately 22% of bacteremia is caused by *S. aureus*. Risk factors include prosthetic devices, indwelling catheters, surgical wounds, hemodialysis, intravenous (IV) drug use, HIV infection, diabetes, alcohol abuse, and *S. aureus* skin infections in healthy people.
Heart valve	Acute endocarditis	Acute sepsis (hypotension, tachycardia, fever). New-onset murmur (usually) from vegetation on valve. Complications occur from emboli to the brain (left-sided endocarditis) or lungs (right-sided endocarditis). IV drug users get acute tricuspid valve endocarditis. Endocarditis from *Streptococcus* sp. has a more gradual onset.
Lungs	Pneumonia	Common in hospitalized patients (especially intubated). Generally follows a viral upper respiratory infection (think influenza). Presents with fever, lobar consolidation, cavitary lesions, empyema.
Bone	Osteomyelitis	Common in children < 12 yr. Presents as a warm, swollen area overlying bone, fever.
Joint capsule	Septic arthritis	Common in children as well as adults > 50 yr. Acutely red, swollen, painful joint with decreased range of motion. Diagnosis by synovial fluid Gram stain and culture.
Brain/meninges	Meningitis, cerebritis, brain abscess	Presents with acute fever, stiff neck, headache, obtundation or coma, and/or focal neurologic signs.

**S. aureus* and *S. pyogenes* are often found inhabiting skin infections together. Antibiotics should be chosen to cover both.

Table 5.2 Diseases Caused by *Staphylococcus aureus* Toxins*

TOXIN	CLINICAL SYNDROME	FEATURES
Exfoliative toxin A or B	Scalded skin syndrome (SSS) in newborns Bullous impetigo in older children (acquired immunity helps protect from systemic spread of the toxin)	Skin desquamation, either systemically in SSS or locally around the primary infection in bullous impetigo. Important to distinguish SSS from toxic epidermal necrolysis (Lyell syndrome), which is more fatal. **Ritter syndrome** is the most severe form, resulting from infection of the cut umbilicus.
Toxic shock syndrome toxin 1 (TSST-1)	Toxic shock syndrome (Fig. 5.7)	TSST-1 is an example of a superantigen.† Famously associated with superabsorbent tampon use. Symptoms occur from massive cytokine release (hypotension, organ dysfunction, edema, desquamative rash). More likely to be fatal when caused by *Streptococcus*.
Enterotoxins	*Staphylococcus* food poisoning	Caused by contaminated food, in which toxin-producing *S. aureus* has been killed by cooking but preformed heat-stable toxin remains.

*Less than 10% of all colonies form any exotoxins, and those that do usually produce only one. The primary site of infection serves as a "base camp" for toxin production, even if the infection is small or clinically unapparent.
†Superantigens can activate the immune system without going through normal checkpoints.

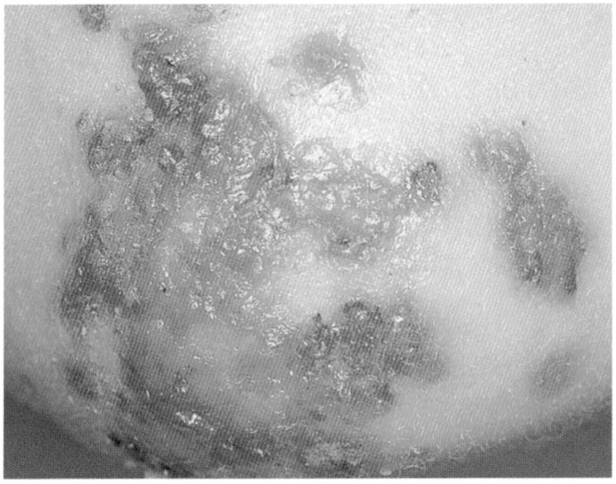

Fig. 5.5 Impetigo with its classic golden crust. (*From Stevens A, Lowe J, Scott I.* Core Pathology. *3rd ed. St. Louis: Mosby; 2008. Fig. 23.14.*)

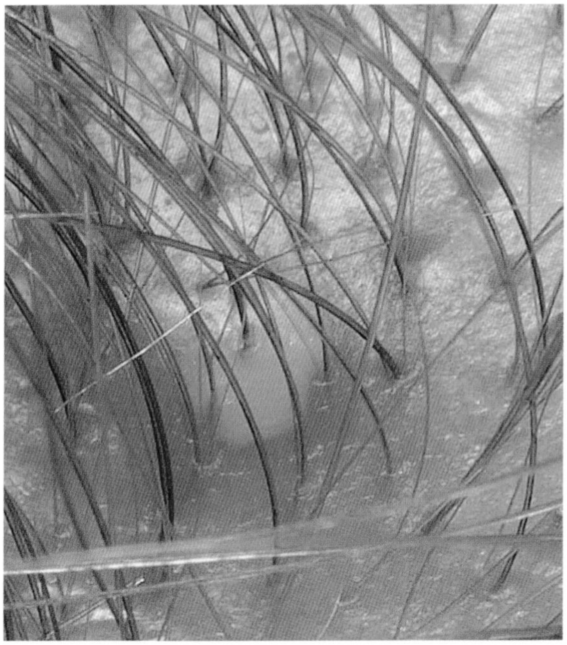

Fig. 5.6 *Staphylococcus aureus* folliculitis. (*From Colledge NR, Walker BR, Ralston SH.* Davidson's Principles and Practice of Medicine. *21st ed. London: Churchill Livingstone; 2010. Fig. 27.24.*)

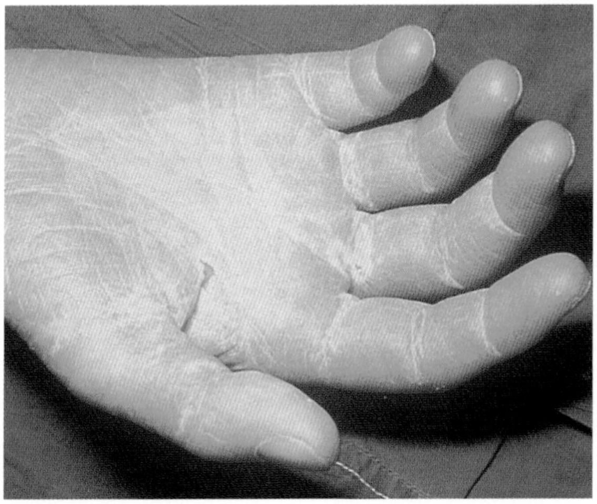

Fig. 5.7 *Staphylococcus aureus* toxic shock syndrome. (*From Goering R, Dockrell H, Wakelin D, et al.* Mims' Medical Microbiology. *4th ed. Philadelphia: Elsevier; 2007. Courtesy M. J. Wood.*)

production by observing whether the bacteria form clots when incubated in serum; this is the basis of the "slide clumping test."

Most staph species produce penicillinase and are resistant to penicillin. Some *S. aureus* strains have developed resistance to antibiotics that can bypass penicillinase (methicillin, nafcillin, and cephalosporins). These strains are now called MRSA (methicillin-resistant *S. aureus,* which is a misnomer because they are resistant to many other antibiotics). MRSA strains have acquired the *mecA* gene, which codes for **penicillin-binding protein 2A.** This protein can crosslink peptidoglycan when transpeptidase is inhibited (see "Introduction to Bacterial Structure" at the beginning of this chapter). Today, up to 70% of *S. aureus* is MRSA and is found in hospitals as well as the community. In the case of life-threatening MRSA infection, **vancomycin** (sometimes combined with an aminoglycoside, such as gentamicin or rifampin) is first-line treatment. Some newer antibiotics (linezolid and daptomycin) can treat serious MRSA infections, but these tend to be more expensive and are reserved for patients with intolerance to vancomycin. **Penicillins** remain the best drug for nonresistant strains, most commonly nafcillin (remember: for nonresistant strains, nafcillin is actually more bactericidal than vancomycin).

Cystitis in sexually active young women: think *E. coli* and *S. saprophyticus.*

Staphylococcus epidermidis inhabits the skin of normal individuals. It is a common contaminant of blood cultures (draw from two sites to be sure it's just a contaminant). Its ability to form a biofilm (polysaccharide scaffold) is what allows it to bind to synthetic materials and commonly infect Foley catheters, intravenous (IV) lines, and indwelling prostheses (mechanical heart valves, stents, prosthetic joints).

Staphylococcus saprophyticus is second only to *Escherichia coli* as the leading cause of urinary tract infections (UTIs) in women and girls. It is particularly prevalent in sexually active women.

Streptococcus: Streptococci are also gram-positive cocci, but unlike staph they do not produce catalase and are found in chains rather than clusters. Streptococci are usually subdivided by Lancefield antigen group or by degree of hemolysis on blood agar: complete (β-hemolytic), partial (α-hemolytic), or none (γ-hemolytic, also known as nonhemolytic).

Streptococcus pyogenes (Fig. 5.8) are Lancefield group A strep and are β-hemolytic. Virulence factors include the following:

- **Protein M** (antiphagocytic)

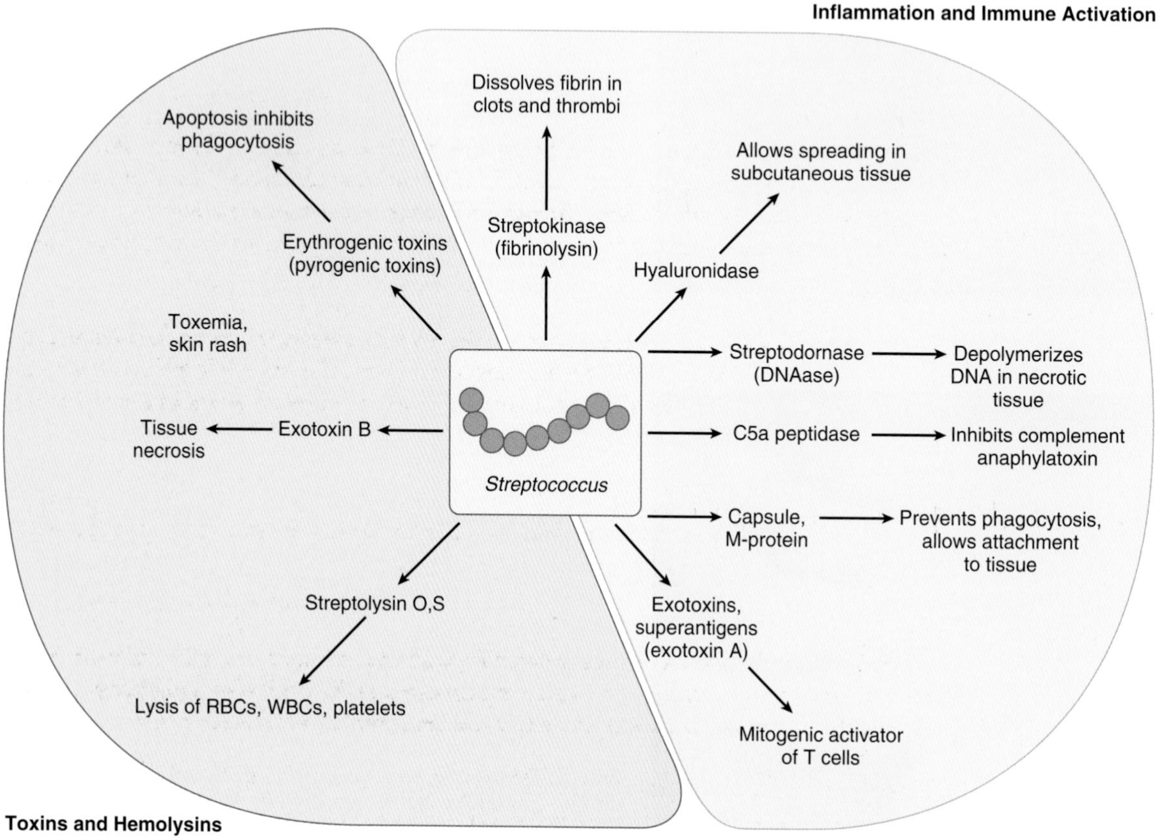

Fig. 5.8 Virulence factors of *Streptococcus pyogenes.* (From Actor JK. Elsevier's Integrated Immunology and Microbiology. *Philadelphia: Elsevier; 2006.*)

- **Streptolysin O and S** (lyse red blood cells [RBCs] and white blood cells [WBCs]); a test for **a**ntibodies to **s**treptolysin **O** (ASO) tells you if there was a recent strep infection
- **Streptokinase** (fibrinolysis through conversion of plasminogen to plasmin)
- Pyrogenic exotoxin (found only in a few strains; causes scarlet fever)
- Variety of destructive enzymes (e.g., hyaluronidase, DNAse, anti-C5a peptidase)

S. pyogenes can cause disease through direct invasion, toxin release, or delayed antibody response (Table 5.3). Treat *S. pyogenes* infections with penicillin.

TABLE 5.3 Diseases Caused by *Streptococcus pyogenes*

DISEASE	CAUSE	FEATURES
Pharyngitis "Strep throat" (Fig. 5.9)	Direct invasion of pharynx/ tonsils	Red, swollen tonsils and pharynx. Purulent exudate on tonsils. Fever. Diagnose with rapid antigen detection test (RADT) and throat culture. Treat with penicillin G (if not allergic).
Skin infections	Direct invasion of skin	The spectrum of skin disease caused by *S. pyogenes* is similar to that for *Staphylococcus aureus;* see Table 5.1.
Scarlet fever (Fig. 5.10)	Release of a pyrogenic toxin	Fever. Scarlet "sandpaper" rash starting on the trunk and neck, then spreading but sparing the face. "Strawberry" tongue. Later, the palms and soles desquamate.
Toxic shock syndrome (TSS) (Fig. 5.11)	Release of a pyrogenic toxin	Similar to TSS caused by *S. aureus* (see Table 5.1).
Rheumatic fever	Antibody mediated	Affects children 5–15 yr old and occurs 2–3 wk after group A strep pharyngitis. For symptoms, see Jones Criteria later. Can permanently affect heart valves (most often resulting in mitral stenosis), making them susceptible to future infections and bouts of rheumatic fever. Prevent with antibiotics for the initial infection. ASO (anti–streptolysin O) antibodies reveal recent group A strep infection, if not obvious from the history.
Acute poststreptococcal glomerulonephritis	Antibody mediated	Occurs 1 wk after group A strep infection (pharyngitis or skin infection). Antibody–antigen complexes deposit in the glomerular basement membrane. Edema and hematuria are the main features. **Cannot** be prevented with antibiotics.

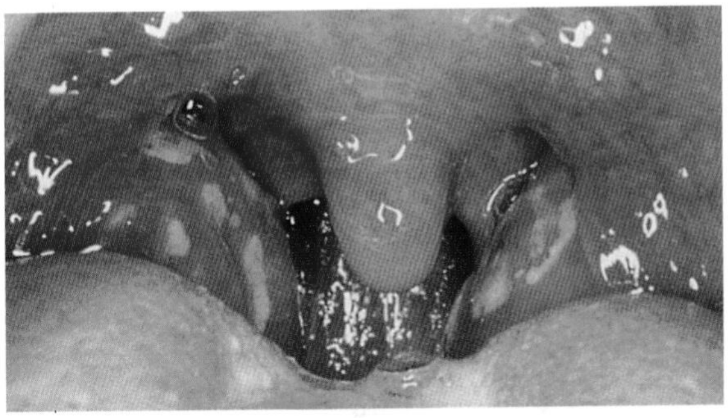

FIG. 5.9 *Streptococcus pyogenes* pharyngitis. (*From Goering R, Dockrell H, Wakelin D, et al.* Mims' Medical Microbiology. *4th ed. Philadelphia: Elsevier; 2007. Courtesy J. A. Innes.*)

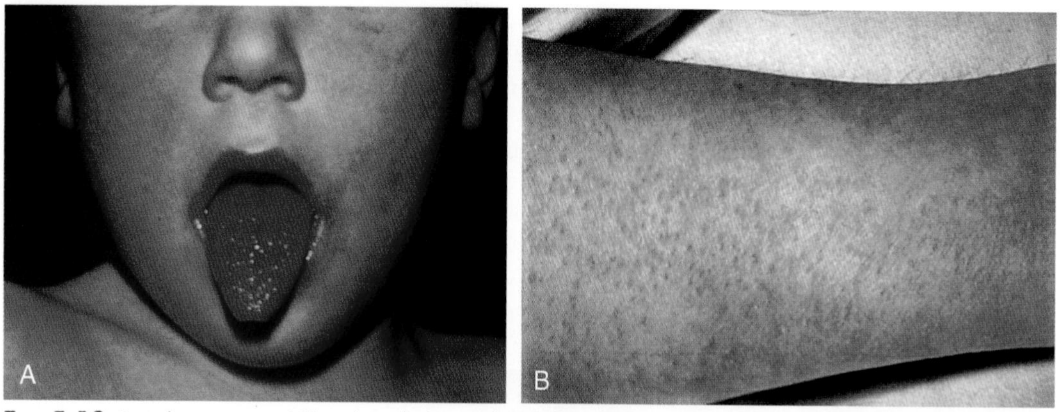

FIG. 5.10 Strawberry tongue **(A)** and sandpaper rash **(B)** of scarlet fever. *(From Greenwood D, Slack R, Peitherer J, Barer M. Medical Microbiology. 17th ed. Philadelphia: Elsevier; 2007.)*

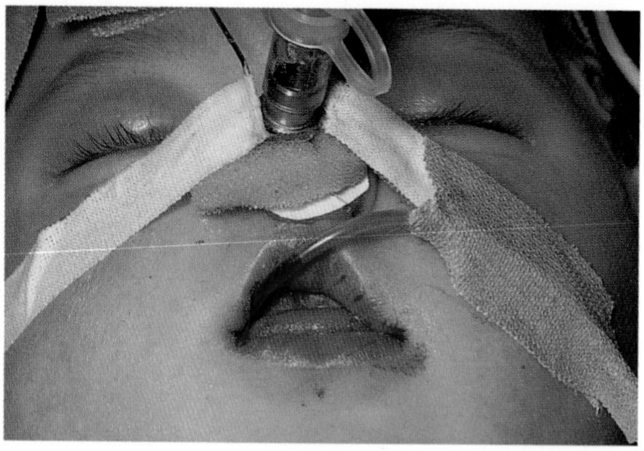

FIG. 5.11 *Streptococcus pyogenes* toxic shock syndrome. *(From Lissauer T, Clayden G.* Illustrated Textbook of Pediatrics. *4th ed. Philadelphia: Elsevier; 2011. Courtesy Professor Mike Levin.)*

Jones Criteria for Diagnosis of Rheumatic Fever

Evidence of prior strep infection, *and* two major criteria or one major + two minor criteria.

Major Criteria: JONES Mnemonic

- **J**oints: polyarthritis
- **O**bvious (heart!): carditis (peri-, myo-, or endo-)
- **N**odules: subcutaneous nodules
- **E**rythema marginatum rash
- **S**ydenham chorea

Minor Criteria

- Fever
- Arthralgia
- Elevated erythrocyte sedimentation rate or C-reactive protein
- Prolonged PR interval on electrocardiogram
- Positive streptococcal antibody

Streptococcus agalactiae is Lancefield group B streptococcus (group B strep, or GBS) and is also β-hemolytic. It lives in the vagina of 25% of women and is thus associated with serious infections of the newborn as they traverse the birth canal; neonatal meningitis, pneumonia, and sepsis are most common. Pregnant women are tested for GBS colonization at 35 to 37 weeks' gestation and receive prophylactic penicillin during labor if positive. GBS can also cause sepsis in pregnant women, leading to sepsis of the fetus and stillbirth. Patients with coexistent medical complications and older adults are also susceptible to infection. Group B strep infection in the neonate should initially be treated with penicillin G and an aminoglycoside.

Most common culprits in neonatal meningitis: *S. agalactiae, E. coli, Listeria monocytogenes.*

The **viridans group** is a heterogenous group of streptococci not defined by a single Lancefield antigen, but they are grouped together because they have certain things in common:

- They are normal inhabitants of the nasopharyngeal and gastrointestinal (GI) tract (found especially in saliva).
- They are α-hemolytic (incomplete hemolysis turns blood agar green; *viridans* is Latin for "green." Think "verde" = "viridans").
- They cause the following diseases:
  - Dental caries (especially *Streptococcus mutans*)
  - Subacute (slow-onset) bacterial endocarditis after a dental procedure, especially on previously damaged or prosthetic heart valves
  - Brain or abdominal abscesses (especially *intermedius* and *anginosus* groups—if these are found in the blood, use computed tomography [CT] to assess for abscess)

Endocarditis in a prosthetic heart valve: think *S. epidermidis* if < 60 days since surgery, Viridans group strep if > 60 days.

Group D strep comprises four species, two of which are enterococci (*Enterococcus faecalis* and *Enterococcus faecium*) and two of which are not (*Streptococcus bovis* and *Streptococcus equinus*). The enterococci have recently been given their own genus (*Enterococcus*) but will still be discussed here. ***Enterococcus faecalis*** and ***Enterococcus faecium*** are normal inhabitants of the bowel (grow well in bile) and commonly cause infections in hospitalized patients: UTIs, biliary tract infections, subacute bacterial endocarditis, wound infections, and bacteremia/sepsis from IV catheters. These species are resistant to many antibiotics. Beware of vancomycin-resistant enterococcus (VRE)! ***Streptococcus bovis*** bacteremia is highly associated with colon cancer—if you find it in the blood, check for cancer.

Streptococcus pneumoniae has no Lancefield antigen, appears as lancet-shaped cocci in pairs (diplococci), and contains a **polysaccharide capsule.** These organisms are α-hemolytic, but so are the viridans group, so two tests can distinguish between the two:

- **Quellung reaction:** Detects the presence of the polysaccharide capsule.
- **Optochin sensitivity:** Viridans grows in the presence of the chemical optochin; *S. pneumoniae* doesn't.

Pneumonia in adults: *S. pneumoniae, H. influenzae, Legionella.*

Pneumonia in older adults: *S. pneumoniae*, gram-negative rods, *H. influenzae.*

S. pneumoniae is a common cause of pneumonia and meningitis in adults (like group B strep in babies) and of otitis media and conjunctivitis in children (Fig. 5.12). Pneumococcal pneumonia presents with sudden chills, fever, chest pain, dyspnea, and a lobar consolidation on chest radiograph. Sputum culture should reveal gram-positive diplococci. Unlike neonatal meningitis, pneumococcal meningitis in adults typically presents with the classic stiff neck. The pneumococcal vaccine should be given to immunocompromised patients, older adults with chronic diseases, those with HIV, those with cochlear implants, and those without spleens (or who are functionally asplenic) because asplenic patients can't protect themselves against encapsulated bugs. Penicillin is still first-line treatment for *S. pneumoniae* infections, although intermediate resistance may require high-dose penicillin, and high-level resistance will require other antibiotics. Even with the introduction of the PCV7 and PCV13 vaccines, some strains are still not covered by the vaccine.

Meningitis in adults: *S. pneumoniae*, gram-negative rods, *Listeria.*

Purulent conjunctivitis: think *H. influenzae, S. pneumoniae*, or *S. aureus.*

Gram-Negative Cocci

- *Neisseria*
  - *N. meningitidis*
  - *N. gonorrhoeae*

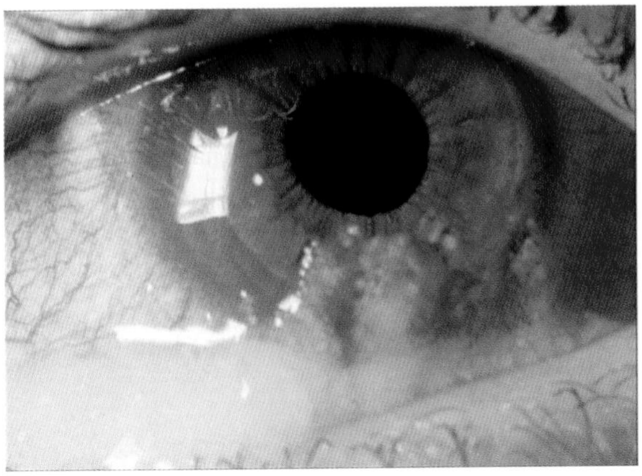

FIG. 5.12 *Streptococcus pneumoniae* conjunctivitis. (*From Soukiasian S, Baum J. Bacterial conjunctivitis. In: Krachmer JH, Mannis MJ, Holland EJ, eds.* Cornea. *3rd ed. Edinburgh: Elsevier; 2010.*)

- *Moraxella catarrhalis*
- *Kingella*
- *Acinetobacter*

Neisseria: Two *Neisseria* species cause disease in humans: *N. meningitidis* (meningitis and bacteremia/sepsis) and *N. gonorrhoeae* (gonorrhea). Both appear under the microscope as diplococci that look kidney shaped.

***N. meningitidis* ("meningococcus")** has a **polysaccharide capsule** (protects against phagocytosis). Infants 6 months to 2 years are at particular risk for infection (the time between acquiring protective antibodies from breastfeeding and being able to make their own). Groups living in close quarters (army recruits, dorm dwellers) are also at risk. Meningococcus lives in the nasopharynx and causes disease when it invades the bloodstream, causing meningitis or sepsis **(meningococcemia).** As the bacteria multiply, they release endotoxin (LPS), causing vascular hemorrhage (seen as a **petechial rash**), an acute inflammatory response (seen as spiking fever, chills, arthralgia, and muscle pain), and hypotension. Adrenal hemorrhage can also occur, known as fulminant meningococcemia or **Waterhouse-Friderichsen syndrome,** leading to adrenal insufficiency. More commonly, however, meningococcus causes meningitis (remember meningitis in infants may present merely as fever, lethargy, vomiting, or irritability, although older children may have classic stiff neck and Brudzinski and Kernig signs). A presumptive diagnosis may save a life. Confirmation of the diagnosis comes from cultures of blood, cerebrospinal fluid (CSF), or petechial scrapings grown on **Thayer-Martin VCN media** (which only grows *Neisseria* species). Penicillin G is the treatment of choice, and ceftriaxone is used for penicillin-allergic patients. Give prophylaxis (rifampin, ceftriaxone, or ciprofloxacin) to all close contacts and to anyone who came into close contact with the patient's oral secretions (the physician who intubated the patient, for example). Remember to be more aggressive with vaccinations in those at risk for serious meningococcus infections (asplenic/functionally asplenic patients, or those with complement deficiency). Anyone with meningococcemia should later be tested to see if they have a complement deficiency—up to 20% will!

Meningitis in a patient aged 6 to 60 years: think *N. meningitidis, Enterovirus, S. pneumoniae.*

***N. gonorrhoeae* ("gonococcus")** causes **gonorrhea,** the second-most common sexually transmitted infection (STI) after chlamydia. Specialized pili on the bacterial surface bind to epithelial cells. In men, it causes urethritis (dysuria, urethral discharge) but can extend to epididymitis or prostatitis. Women can also develop urethritis but more commonly develop endometritis (infection of the uterus), which is often asymptomatic but can present with abdominal pain, dyspareunia (painful intercourse), and cervical discharge. Endometritis can progress to salpingitis (inflammation of the fallopian tubes) or oophoritis (inflammation of the ovaries), called **pelvic inflammatory disease (PID),** which presents with abdominal pain, fever, discharge, irregular bleeding, and cervical motion tenderness. PID is also caused by *Chlamydia trachomatis.* Complications of PID include tuboovarian abscesses, peritonitis, and infection of the liver capsule **(Fitz-Hugh-Curtis syndrome).** Scarring of the fallopian tubes (especially with repeat infections) can lead to infertility and increases the risk for **fallopian ectopic pregnancy.** Those who have receptive anal sex from an infected partner can develop a rectal gonococcal infection (pruritus, tenesmus, rectal bleeding and discharge). Those who perform oral sex on an infected partner can develop oropharyngeal gonorrhea (this is in contrast to chlamydia, which cannot cause oropharyngeal infection).

Rarely, gonococcus may invade the bloodstream, causing fever, joint pains, and skin lesions. It is the most common cause of **septic arthritis** in someone who is sexually active; examination of synovial fluid may show gram-negative diplococci within WBCs. If you suspect gonococcal septic arthritis, swab the oral and genital mucosa for culture or nuclear acid amplification testing (NAAT). Neonates may acquire gonococcus from the birth canal, causing **ophthalmia neonatorum** (can cause blindness via corneal damage). Newborns receive erythromycin eye drops to prevent ophthalmic infection.

Diagnosis is by Gram stain (gram-negative kidney-shaped diplococci) and culture on Thayer-Martin VCN media. Treatment is with intramuscular [IM] or IV ceftriaxone (usually one dose is sufficient, unless there is systemic infection), and in the case of sexually transmitted gonorrhea, add azithromycin or doxycycline to cover chlamydia (common coinfection).

Other Gram-Negative Cocci: ***Moraxella catarrhalis*** causes about 20% of otitis media and sinusitis in children (third most common after *S. pneumoniae* and *Haemophilus influenzae*) and pneumonia in older adults and patients with chronic obstructive pulmonary disease (COPD). Moraxella produces β-lactamase. Therefore treat *M. catarrhalis* infections with a β-lactamase evading antibiotic such as amoxicillin-clavulanate (Augmentin). ***Kingella*** causes smoldering endocarditis in children and adults. Remember HACEK for culture-negative endocarditis (because they do not grow on standard culture medium): *Haemophilus, Actinobacillus, Cardiobacterium, Eikenella, Kingella. K. kingae* is also a common cause of osteomyelitis in children younger than 5 years old.

Acinetobacter baumannii is a soil bacterium that can colonize the skin, anything wet (even disinfectant!), and hospital equipment like ventilators. It causes **hospital-acquired infections:** burns and wound infection, urinary catheter UTI, ventilator-acquired pneumonia, and bacteremia. *Acinetobacter* infections can be severe and are notoriously difficult to treat because they can resist multiple classes of antibiotics.

Gram-Positive Rods

Spore Forming:

- *Bacillus*
  - *B. anthracis*
  - *B. cereus*
- *Clostridium*
  - *C. botulinum*
  - *C. tetani*
  - *C. perfringens*
  - *C. difficile*

Non–Spore Forming:

- *Corynebacterium diphtheriae*
- *Listeria monocytogenes*

There are four gram-positive bacillus groups, two of which are spore forming (*Bacillus* and *Clostridium*) and two of which are not (*Corynebacterium* and *Listeria*). Spores form a protective environment that helps bacteria remain dormant in harsh conditions.

Bacillus: ***Bacillus anthracis*** **(anthrax)** is the only bacterium with a **protein capsule.** It forms spores that live in the soil. Humans get infected from soil or from handling hides of infected animals. Spores germinate in open wounds, the lungs, or the GI tract. In all three cases, local release of **exotoxin** results in necrosis and hemorrhage of surrounding tissue: a black edematous lesion (eschar) in cutaneous anthrax, pulmonary and mediastinal hemorrhage in inhalation anthrax (**woolsorter's disease**), and bloody diarrhea in GI anthrax. In all three, hematogenous spread will occur without prompt diagnosis and treatment with **ciprofloxacin or doxycycline.**

> *Bacillus, Clostridium,* and *Coxiella* are spore-forming bacteria.

Bacillus cereus causes gastroenteritis by depositing spores in food (classically, reheated rice), which survive the cooking process then germinate and release enterotoxins into the food. When consumed, the toxin causes nausea, vomiting, and watery diarrhea. Because the syndrome is caused by toxins, antibiotics have no effect (Fig. 5.13). When infection is caused by the bacteria itself (IV catheter–related infections, eye infections in contact lens wearers, wound infections), treat with **vancomycin.**

Clostridium: ***Clostridium botulinum*** toxin blocks acetylcholine release at nerve synapses in the autonomic nervous system and motor endplates, causing rapid flaccid paralysis. Spores thrive in anaerobic environments (canned/jarred food) and release neurotoxin, which is then consumed. Spores can also be released from the soil by construction work. In infants, the spores germinate in the GI tract, releasing neurotoxin from there and causing **floppy baby syndrome** (the classic cause is jarred honey). Treatment involves antitoxin and intubation/ventilation. In adults, the GI tract is resistant to colonization, but rarely *C. botulinum* can infect deep wounds (called *wound botulism*) and release toxin, leading to flaccid paralysis, especially of cranial nerves.

Clostridium tetani spores are introduced into humans through a puncture wound, where they germinate under anaerobic conditions and release the toxin **tetanospasmin.** Tetanospasmin inhibits GABA and glycine release from Renshaw interneurons, which normally inhibit motor neuron activation. Inhibition of inhibition = activation; thus patients with tetanus have sustained muscle contractions, notably in the jaw **(trismus),** facial muscles **(risus sardonicus),** and sometimes the back, causing a severe arching of the back **(opisthotonus).** Treatment involves tetanus toxin immunoglobulin, a tetanus vaccine booster, débridement of the wound, antibiotics (metronidazole is preferred), and supportive therapy (muscle relaxants, ventilation).

Clostridium perfringens spores also enter the body through wounds. Once inoculated, they germinate and release toxins that digest local tissue. They also ferment carbohydrates to produce gas, hence the term *gas gangrene.* Additionally, spores can germinate in food (especially meat) and populate the

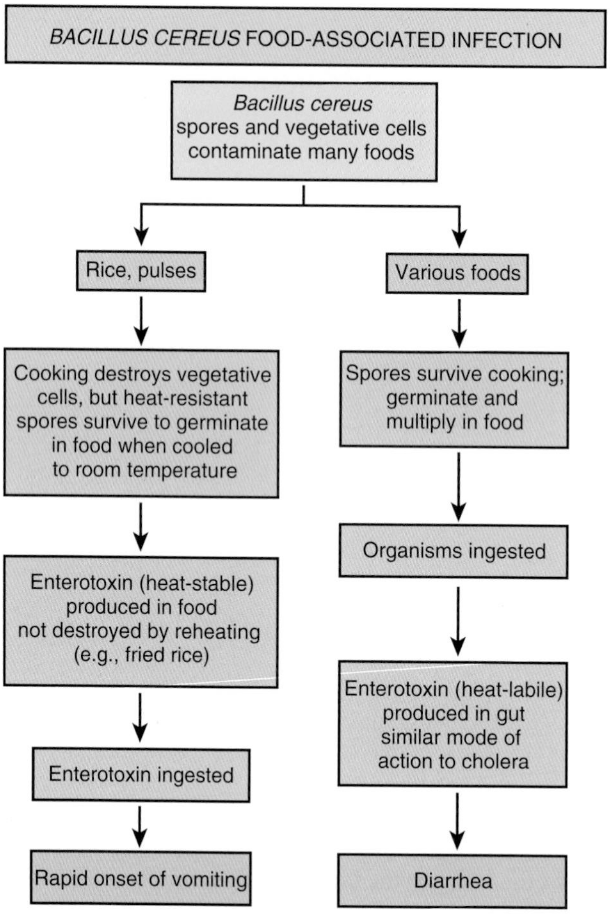

FIG. 5.13 The mechanisms of *Bacillus cereus* food poisoning. (*From Goering R, Dockrell H, Wakelin D, et al.* Mims' Medical Microbiology. *4th ed. Philadelphia: Elsevier; 2007.*)

gut when ingested, releasing enterotoxins and causing watery diarrhea. Severe gut infections can cause a necrotizing enteritis.

Clostridium difficile causes pseudomembranous enterocolitis (Fig. 5.14), usually within a month after broad-spectrum antibiotic use (e.g., clindamycin, ampicillin), which knocks out normal GI flora, allowing *C. difficile* to superinfect the colon. Patients experience abdominal cramps, diarrhea, and fever as a result of toxin release. Diagnosis is by **toxin detection** in the stool. Treatment is with **metronidazole** (oral or IV) or vancomycin (oral only; IV is ineffective in *C. difficile* colitis). For refractory cases, treatment with fidaxomicin or a fecal microbiota transplant can be considered.

Listeria: *Listeria monocytogenes* is introduced into the host through contaminated foods (usually unpasteurized soft cheeses and cold cuts). It causes gastroenteritis but can cause invasive infections in those with **compromised cell-mediated immunity** (the bacteria lives within macrophages): pregnant women (third trimester), neonates, older adults, and immunocompromised patients. Bacteremia/sepsis from *Listeria* during pregnancy can result in neonatal death or premature birth. Newborns can also acquire it during vaginal birth if the vaginal canal is colonized (mother is asymptomatic), resulting

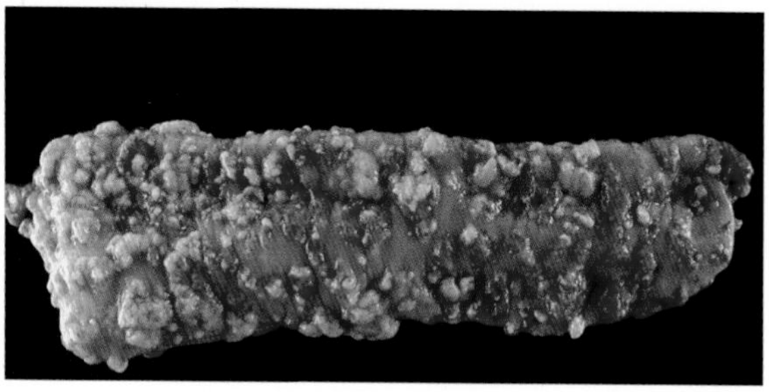

FIG. 5.14 Pseudomembranes on intestinal mucosa in *Clostridium difficile* colitis. (*From Kumar V, Abbas AK, Fausto N, et al.* Robbins and Cotran's Pathologic Basis of Disease. *8th ed. Philadelphia: Elsevier; 2009.*)

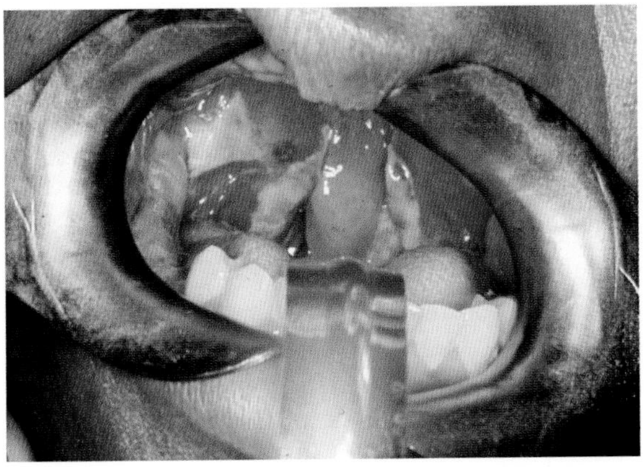

Fig. 5.15 *Corynebacterium diphtheria* pharyngitis. (*From Mandell G, Bennett J, Dolin R.* Principles and Practice of Infectious Diseases. *6th ed. Philadelphia: Churchill Livingstone; 2005.*)

in *Listeria* meningitis 2 weeks after birth (causes 20% of neonatal meningitis). People older than 50 years and immunocompromised patients (e.g., AIDS, transplant, corticosteroid use, lymphoma) are also at risk for *Listeria* meningitis. *Listeria* is the only gram-positive bacterium that produces **endotoxin.** Treat empirically with **ampicillin** with or without an aminoglycoside for serious infections or with trimethoprim-sulfamethoxazole (TMP-SMX) or vancomycin if the patient is penicillin allergic. Confirmation of diagnosis is by CSF analysis and culture.

Corynebacterium: ***Corynebacterium diphtheriae*** spreads by droplets and direct contact, colonizing the pharynx of children. Children rapidly develop gray pseudomembranes that are visible on examination (Fig. 5.15). From there, some strains can release a powerful toxin that damages the heart and neural tissue by inhibiting adenosine diphosphate (ADP) ribosylation of elongation factor-2 (EF-2), impairing translation and protein synthesis. Patients may present with stridor, hoarseness, respiratory compromise, and a swollen "bull neck." If **diphtheria** is suspected, take a throat swab (don't *scrape* the lesions!), then treat immediately with antitoxin immunoglobulin, antibiotics **(penicillin or erythromycin),** and TDaP (tetanus, diphtheria, and pertussis) vaccine to ensure future immunity. Confirmation of the diagnosis is by culture on potassium tellurite (forms gray-black cultures) and on Loeffler coagulated blood serum (reveals rod-shaped pleomorphic bacteria after staining with methylene blue).

Gram-Negative Enteric Rods

- *Escherichia coli*
- *Klebsiella pneumoniae*
- *Proteus mirabilis*
- *Shigella*
- *Salmonella*
  - *S. typhus*
  - *S. cholerae-suis*
  - *S. enteritidis*
- *Yersinia enterocolitica*
- *Vibrio*
  - *V. cholerae*
  - *V. parahaemolyticus*
- *Campylobacter jejuni*
- *Helicobacter pylori*
- *Pseudomonas aeruginosa*
- *Burkholderia cepacia*
- *Stenotrophomonas maltophilia*
- *Bacteroides*
- *Fusobacterium*

The enterics are gram-negative rods that either normally colonize the GI tract or cause GI disease (but *can* cause diseases elsewhere). Some cause GI disease by toxin release without cell invasion (watery diarrhea without fever); others cause disease by invasion of intestinal cells (bloody diarrhea with WBCs in stool and fever); and others cause disease by invading the lymph and the blood (bacteremia/sepsis). Enterics also cause diseases in other organ systems (e.g., UTIs, pneumonia), mostly in debilitated or hospitalized patients.

Escherichia: ***Escherichia coli*** normally lives peacefully in the GI tract. If it gains virulence factors through DNA exchange with other enterics, it can cause diarrhea in those who aren't immunized (infants in the developing world and adults in the developed world who travel to developing nations). Depending on the virulence factors, three types of diarrhea can result:

- **Enterotoxigenic *E. coli* (ETEC)** causes **traveler's diarrhea** (Montezuma's revenge). The bacteria bind to epithelial cells and release a cholera-like toxin, causing secretion of electrolytes into the intestinal lumen. Water follows electrolytes, so watery diarrhea results. It can be treated with ciprofloxacin or azithromycin in pregnant women.
- **Enterohemorrhagic *E. coli* (EHEC)** causes hemorrhagic colitis. The bacteria bind to epithelial cells, just like ETEC, but release a Shiga-like toxin that blocks protein synthesis in intestinal epithelia, causing cell death. Bloody diarrhea and abdominal cramps result. (Of note, the O157:H7 strain of EHEC can cause **hemolytic uremic syndrome (HUS)**—fever, anemia, thrombocytopenia, and uremia/renal failure.) EHEC is usually a foodborne illness, classically caused by undercooked and contaminated hamburger meat. Do NOT treat EHEC with antibiotics (has been found to stimulate HUS in some studies).
- **Enteroinvasive *E. coli* (EIEC)** has the ability to invade intestinal epithelia and also to release Shiga-like toxin, resulting in an inflammatory response that produces fever, cramps, and bloody diarrhea. WBCs will be found in the stool.

E. coli causes a number of other diseases in susceptible populations. *E. coli* is the most common cause of UTIs, especially affecting women and patients with Foley catheters. *E. coli* meningitis is common in neonates. It is the most common cause of gram-negative sepsis in hospitalized patients, and it commonly causes nosocomial (hospital-acquired) pneumonia.

Klebsiella: ***Klebsiella pneumoniae*** causes nosocomial sepsis (second most common after *E. coli*), Foley catheter–associated UTIs, and pneumonia in those susceptible to aspiration of stomach contents (**alcoholic patients,** intubated patients, and debilitated hospitalized patients). This is a violent form of pneumonia that forms cavitations; sputum is classically **currant jelly** colored. Most *Klebsiella* are resistant to ampicillin.

Proteus: ***Proteus mirabilis*** also causes nosocomial infections and is a cause of UTIs. Urine will be alkaline because of *Proteus'* ability to cleave urea into ammonia and CO_2 with urease. The alkalinized urine creates favorable conditions for enormous struvite renal stones. These are called **staghorn calculi** because they can fill the entire calyceal system, resembling the horns of the male deer (Fig. 5.16). Unique features of *Proteus* include its motility and its cross-reactivity with some rickettsial antigens, making it a useful tool to determine whether someone has a rickettsial infection. This is the **Weil-Felix** test (see later section, "Rickettsia-Like Infections").

Shigella: ***Shigella*** species (of which there are four) cause **dysentery** by the same mechanism as EIEC. Transmission is fecal–oral (usually by contaminated water or hand-to-hand contact by someone who hasn't washed properly) and occurs most often in preschools and nursing homes. Bacteria latch

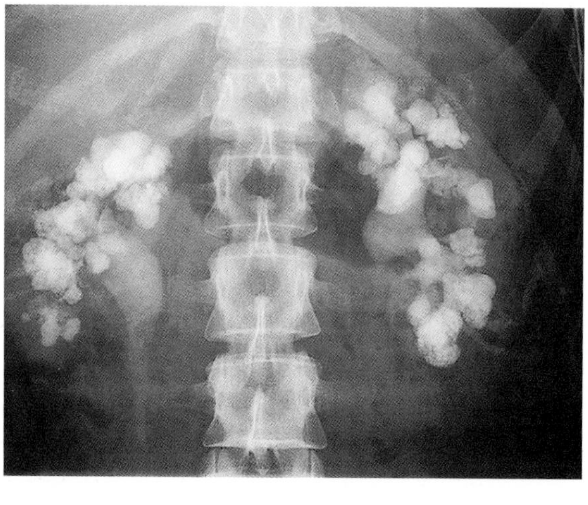

Fig. 5.16 Intravenous pyelogram demonstrating bilateral staghorn calculi. This patient had urinary infection with the urease-producing bacteria *Proteus*. The alkaline urinary conditions were favorable for the formation of struvite stones. (*From Colledge NR, Walker BR, Ralston SH.* Davidson's Principles and Practice of Medicine. *21st ed. London: Churchill Livingstone; 2010.*)

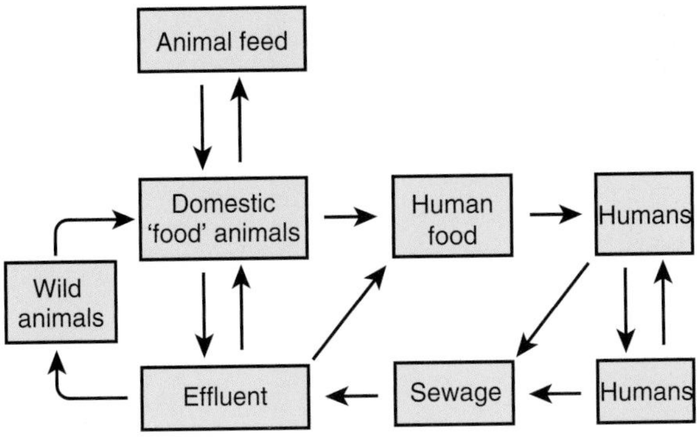

Fig. 5.17 The cycling of *Salmonella* through animals and humans (exception: *S. typhi*, which is only found in humans). (*From Goering R, Dockrell H, Wakelin D, et al. Mims' Medical Microbiology. 4th ed. Philadelphia: Elsevier; 2007.*)

onto the intestinal epithelium, invade cells, and release Shiga toxin (the same toxin used by EIEC), which inhibits protein synthesis and causes cell death. The result is an inflammatory response with blood-and-pus–speckled diarrhea and abdominal pain. Treat with ceftriaxone and not with antidiarrheal medications.

Salmonella: There are three clinically important species of *Salmonella: S. typhi, S. cholerae-suis,* and *S. enteritidis.* The first is only found in humans; the latter two live in animal GI tracts and infect humans through food or water contaminated with animal feces (they are examples of zoonoses; Fig. 5.17).

S. typhi, like EIEC and *Shigella,* invades intestinal epithelium, but then goes on to invade lymph and seeds multiple organs. Look for a history of exposure to animal products or live reptiles. The resulting **typhoid fever** includes fever, diarrhea, headache, abdominal pain, and inflammation of involved organs (e.g., the spleen). Light-skinned people may show a transient pink-spotted (salmon-colored "rose spots") rash on the belly. Diagnosis is through culturing blood, urine, or stool; and treatment is with ciprofloxacin or ceftriaxone. Some may go on to become chronic carriers (colonization of gallbladder—think of the famous Typhoid Mary, a cook who in the early 1900s unknowingly infected 51 people).

Most nontyphoidal *Salmonella* species cause diarrhea along with nausea and abdominal pain, sometimes fever, and self-resolve within 1 week. Do NOT treat nontyphoidal *Salmonella* diarrhea (increases the likelihood of becoming a chronic carrier), unless it is a child younger than 3 months of age or a patient with an immunocompromised state. ***S. choleraesuis*** is the most common cause of *Salmonella* sepsis and is particularly hard to clear in those without spleens (*Salmonella* is an encapsulated bug—antibody-coated [opsonized] encapsulated bacteria normally get caught in the spleen and are then phagocytosed and destroyed by macrophages).

Yersinia: Yersinia has two medically important species: ***Y. pestis* (bubonic plague)** and ***Y. enterocolitica* (acute gastroenteritis).** *Y. pestis* is discussed later. *Y. enterocolitica* is introduced by contaminated foods or focally contaminated water. It invades lymph and blood through the gastrointestinal mucosa and causes fever, diarrhea, and abdominal pain usually in the right lower quadrant because of ileal ulceration (this can mimic appendicitis and is therefore referred to as **pseudoappendicitis**). Look for exposure to **chitterlings or raw pork.**

Vibrio: Vibrio has two medically important species: ***V. cholera* (cholera)** and ***V. parahaemolyticus.*** *V. cholera* is transmitted via the fecal–oral route. Although adults in endemic areas become immune, all children (endemic area or not) and adults traveling to endemic areas are susceptible. Like ETEC, the bacteria bind to the epithelium and release a toxin that causes oversecretion of sodium chloride into the lumen (by increasing concentrations of cyclic adenosine monophosphate [cAMP]). Water and other electrolytes follow, classically in copious **rice-water diarrhea;** Fig. 5.18. Notably, patients are not febrile and the bowel is not directly injured. Death can result from dehydration, so the mainstay of treatment is hydration and electrolyte replacement. *V. parahaemolyticus* causes gastroenteritis, usually from uncooked fish (commonly in sushi).

Campylobacter: *Campylobacter jejuni* is one of the three leading causes of gastroenteritis worldwide (the other two are *Rotavirus* and ETEC), affecting mostly children. Its reservoir is animals, and it is acquired by the fecal–oral route or unpasteurized milk. A prodrome of fever and headache gives way in half a day to bloody diarrhea and abdominal cramps (because it invades the intestinal

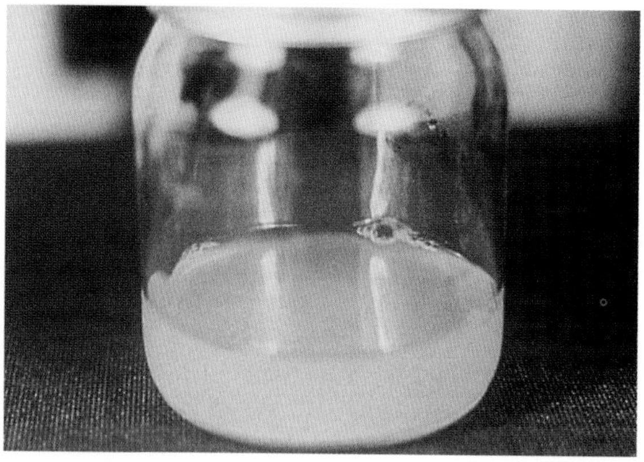

FIG. 5.18 Rice-water stool in *Vibrio cholerae* infection. (*From Goering R, Dockrell H, Wakelin D, et al. Mims' Medical Microbiology. 4th ed. Philadelphia: Elsevier; 2007. Courtesy of A.M. Geddes.*)

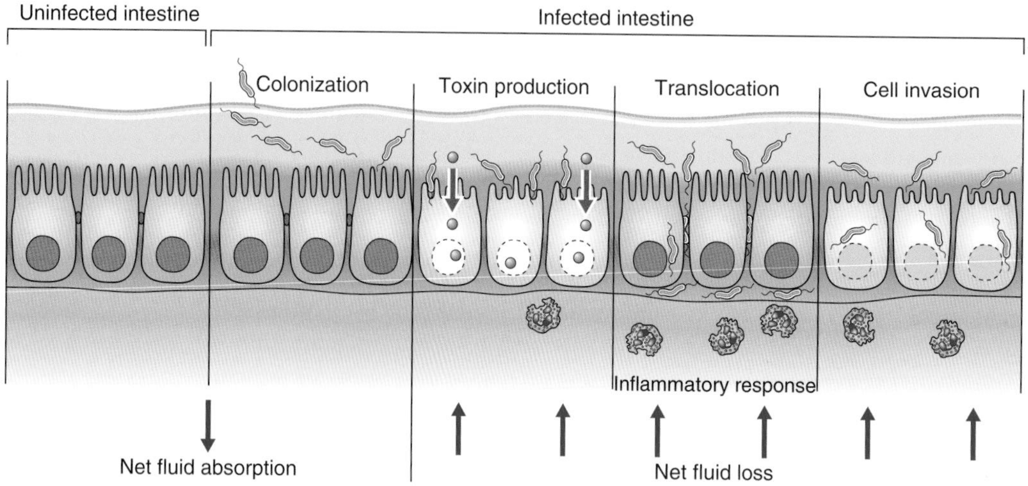

FIG. 5.19 Pathophysiology of *Campylobacter jejuni* infection. Bloody diarrhea results from invasion of the bacteria and subsequent inflammatory response. (*From Greenwood D, Slack R, Peitherer J, Barer M. Medical Microbiology. 17th ed. Philadelphia: Elsevier; 2007.*)

epithelium; Fig. 5.19). This infection is also associated with the development of Guillain-Barré syndrome, which is characterized by ascending paralysis (usually, but not always, reversible).

Helicobacter: ***Helicobacter pylori*** inhabits the stomach and is the leading cause of **duodenal** ulcers (second leading cause of gastric ulcers after nonsteroidal antiinflammatory drugs, including aspirin). It produces urease, which neutralizes the gastric pH.

Pseudomonas: ***Pseudomonas aeruginosa*** is a water- and soil-dwelling bacterium that generally does not infect healthy people (except when it causes **hot tub folliculitis**), but it does infect sick and immunocompromised patients and is very resistant to antibiotics. When visible, it looks blue-green and smells like sweet grapes. Important infections can be remembered by the mnemonic BE PSEUDO:

- Burns: burns infected with *Pseudomonas* lead to sepsis
- Endocarditis: especially right-sided heart valve endocarditis in IV drug users
- Pneumonia: prevalent among immunocompromised patients, ventilator-dependent patients, and **cystic fibrosis** patients
- Sepsis
- External otitis/otitis media: *Pseudomonas* that burrows into the mastoid from the external ear; elderly **diabetic patients** particularly susceptible
- UTIs, including pyelonephritis: often by Foley catheter infections (think hospitals, nursing homes)
- Diabetic Osteomyelitis: bone infections in diabetic patients (from foot ulcers), IV drug users (vertebrae, clavicle), and children (from soil entering puncture wounds through a rubber-soled shoe)

In neutropenic patients, pseudomonal bacteremia can lead to **ecthyma gangrenosum,** which is a round black lesion that is ulcerated in the center. These patients are also at risk for pseudomonal typhlitis (infection of the cecum).

Burkholderia and Stenotrophomonas: Like *Pseudomonas,* ***Burkholderia cepacia*** and ***Stenotrophomonas maltophilia*** also cause hospital-acquired infections, especially in burn patients and cystic fibrosis patients. Also like *Pseudomonas,* they are very resistant to antibiotics and antiseptics.

Bacteroides and Fusobacterium: *Bacteroides and Fusobacterium* species make up 99% of the normal gut flora. They are both gram-negative anaerobic rods. *Bacteroides fragilis* normally lives in peace in the intestine until the intestine perforates (e.g., trauma, iatrogenic, appendicitis, ischemia), at which point it forms abdominal abscesses. Because *B. fragilis* also lives in the vagina, it can cause abscesses in situations such as septic abortion, pelvic inflammatory disease (PID; tuboovarian abscess), or use of an intrauterine device. *B. melaninogenicus* also lives in the intestine, vagina, and mouth; it forms a black pigment (hence the name) and can cause necrotizing anaerobic pneumonia when aspirated (e.g., during a seizure or drunken state) as well as periodontal disease. *Fusobacterium* is similar to *B. melaninogenicus* (periodontal disease and aspiration pneumonia) and also causes abdominal abscesses and otitis media. *Fusobacterium necrophorum* is implicated in **Lemierre syndrome;** this is when a sore throat caused by the bacteria spreads from the tonsils to the jugular vein and causes a blood clot to form, which the bacteria then infects (thrombophlebitis).

Other Enterics: Remember that viridans group streptococci (already discussed) are also part of the normal GI flora and can be found coinhabiting abscesses. Also worthy of mention are ***Peptostreptococcus*** (gram-negative cocci in chains) and ***Peptococcus*** (gram-negative cocci in clusters), which are often found coinhabiting abscesses and aspiration pneumonias.

Gram-Negative Nonenteric Rods

- *Haemophilus*
  - *H. influenzae*
  - *H. ducreyi*
- *Gardnerella vaginalis*
- *Bordetella pertussis*
- *Legionella pneumophila*
- *Yersinia pestis*
- *Francisella tularensis*
- *Brucella*
- *Pasteurella multocida*

Haemophilus: *Haemophilus* species are usually acquired through the lungs. There are encapsulated (typed) and nonencapsulated (nontypeable) forms. In the past, encapsulated ***Haemophilus influenzae*** (types a through f), especially type b, invaded lung epithelium of children aged 6 months to 3 years as a result of a lack of immunoglobulin to *H. influenzae* type b (Hib). Since routine vaccination with purified type b capsule protein began, the incidence of Hib meningitis, acute epiglottitis, and septic arthritis has significantly decreased in the United States. Still, one should be aware of the clinical presentations for the various infections caused by *H. influenzae*—for example, epiglottitis usually presents in children aged 2 to 7 with fever, drooling, stridor, and "tripoding," with the classic "thumbprint sign" on lateral neck radiograph. Nonencapsulated *H. influenzae* mostly causes otitis media in children and sinusitis and upper respiratory infections (URIs) in adults with previous lung disease (e.g., COPD). Lack of the capsule limits invasiveness. *H. influenzae* infections should be treated with third-generation cephalosporins (i.e., ceftriaxone or cefotaxime for serious infections, cefdinir for mild infections such as otitis media).

There are other disease-causing *Haemophilus* species that are not acquired through the respiratory system. ***H. ducreyi*** causes an STI known as **chancroid** (Fig. 5.20), a **painful** genital ulcer sometimes accompanied by unilateral lymph node enlargement (the painfulness of the lesion can be remembered by the common mnemonic "with *Haemophilus ducreyi* you do-cry"). The inguinal lymph nodes are matted, accumulate pus, and will ulcerate. This disease should be distinguished from syphilis (*Treponema pallidum*), which causes a **painless chancre** with bilateral nonsuppurative lymphadenopathy; from herpes (herpes simplex virus [HSV] types 1 and 2), which has more vesicular lesions and includes systemic symptoms such as fever and arthralgias; and from lymphogranuloma venereum *(Chlamydia trachomatis),* in which the chancroid appears well before the matted lymphadenopathy.

Finally, a group of slow-growing *Haemophilus* species can cause smoldering endocarditis. A patient with persistent low-grade fever or heart valve vegetations but negative cultures should be worked up for

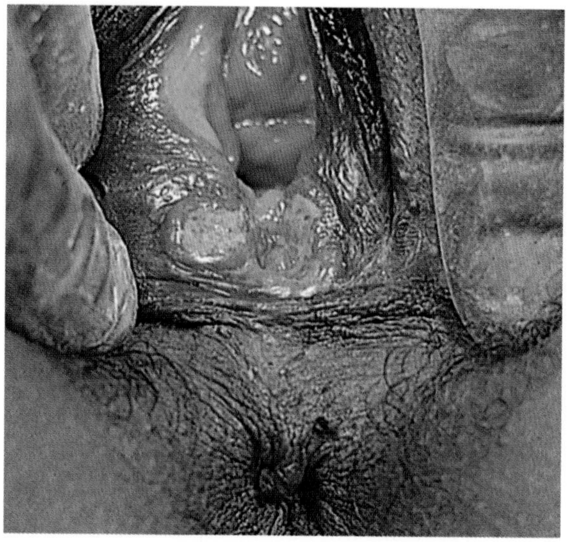

FIG. 5.20 Ulcers seen on a female patient with chancroid caused by *Haemophilus ducreyi*. (*From Swartz MH.* Textbook of Physical Diagnosis. *6th ed. Philadelphia: Elsevier; 2010.*)

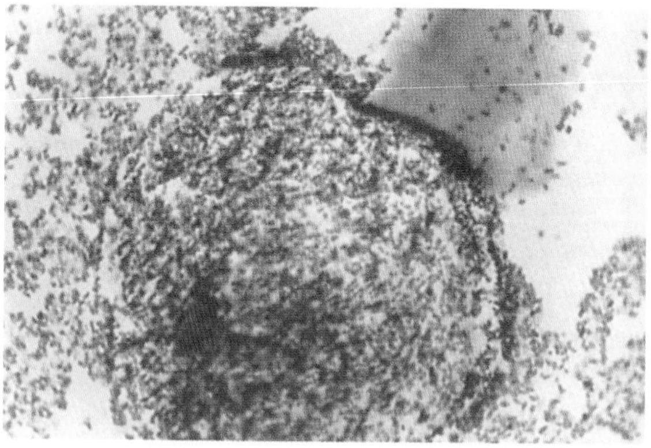

FIG. 5.21 Wet mount showing a "clue cell" from a patient with bacterial vaginosis. Note the obscured margin of the vaginal epithelial cell as a result of the numerous bacteria surrounding it. (*From Colledge NR, Walker BR, Ralston SH.* Davidson's Principles and Practice of Medicine. *21st ed. London: Churchill Livingstone; 2010.*)

the HACEK organisms, which involves growing specialized cultures for 2 weeks (normal cultures are negative because these organisms have special growth requirements, and therefore this is also referred to as *culture-negative endocarditis*).

Gardnerella: ***Gardnerella vaginalis*** is a common cause of vaginitis and should be distinguished clinically from vaginal candidiasis (caused by *C. albicans*) and trichomonas. Symptoms include dysuria, itching and burning of the labia, and foul-smelling discharge (fishy odor). Diagnosis is by examination of cells on a slide (can be done in clinic), showing the presence of more than 20% "clue cells" (normal epithelium with bacilli in cytoplasm; Fig. 5.21). Treat with metronidazole.

Bordetella: ***Bordetella pertussis*** is a particularly virulent organism that causes whooping cough. In the postvaccination era, whooping cough affects mostly unimmunized infants and young adults (as a result of waning immunity). Transmission is through respiratory secretions. After inoculation, a 1- to 2-week *catarrhal stage* ensues (low-grade fever, runny nose, cough, sneezing), followed by the *paroxysmal stage* characterized by several episodes per day of violent coughing followed by an inspiratory "whoop" (gasp of air through a narrowed epiglottis). Those with partial immunity may not have the whoop and will present with chronic cough. Laboratory tests may show leukocytosis with an absolute lymphocytosis.

B. pertussis doesn't invade the body; rather, it attaches to tracheal and bronchial (ciliated) epithelia and mediates disease through toxin release, which destroys epithelial cells, among other effects. Throat swabs must be done with calcium alginate (because the organism won't grow on cotton), then cultured on **Bordet-Gengou medium (polymerase chain reaction [PCR] testing is also available).** Treatment is mostly supportive (hospitalization may be required to provide oxygen in severe cases, especially to infants). A macrolide antibiotic such as **azithromycin or erythromycin** can prevent the paroxysmal stage if given in the catarrhal stage and reduces bacterial shedding in the paroxysmal stage. Household contacts should also be given erythromycin or azithromycin for prevention.

Legionella: ***Legionella pneumophila*** (named for an outbreak at the American Legion conference in Philadelphia in 1976) lives in water (including air conditioning units, whirlpools, and mist machines) and is usually acquired in the lungs through aerosolized droplets. These bacteria are *intracellular parasites,* replicating inside lung macrophages. *L. pneumophila* causes two diseases: the milder **Pontiac fever** (named for an outbreak in Pontiac, Michigan, the culprit being an air conditioner), in which a flulike illness (fatigue and muscle aches followed by fever and chills) self-resolves in 1 week; and **Legionnaire disease,** characterized by high fevers and lobar consolidative pneumonia. Legionnaire disease may be hard to distinguish from pneumococcal pneumonia except for a few unusual features: **relatively low heart rate** (usually fever is associated with tachycardia, except in this case), flulike symptoms that may precede lung findings, symptoms of gastroenteritis, and some unusual laboratory test results like elevated liver enzymes, hyponatremia, and hypophosphatemia. The electrolyte abnormalities are due to *Legionella* organisms' ability to damage the juxtaglomerular cells of the kidney and lead to a type IV renal tubular acidosis with a hyporeninemic hypoaldosteronism. If sputum is acquired, Gram stain will show many neutrophils but few to no organisms (requires silver stain), but a urine test for *Legionella* can be positive. Because it is intracellular and cannot be killed by penicillin, it is an "atypical" pneumonia and requires atypical coverage: **macrolides, tetracyclines, or certain quinolones.** Other atypical pneumonias (discussed later) include those caused by *Chlamydia* and *Mycoplasma.*

The next three organisms have the following in common: They are zoonoses (infections acquired from animals), they are so virulent as to be able to infect any tissue they come into contact with, they are facultative intracellular parasites (inhibit phagocytosis and therefore replicate within macrophages), and they are treated with an aminoglycoside (gentamicin or streptomycin).

Yersinia: *Yersinia enterocolitica* was previously described. Here we discuss ***Yersinia pestis*** **(bubonic plague).** It is carried by rats, prairie dogs, and squirrels (particularly in the Southwest United States) and transmitted by flea bites. As a facultative intracellular organism, it resists phagocytosis and multiplies within phagocytes, then moves to lymph nodes, *usually* (but not always!) causing the nodes of the groin or axilla to swell and become red and hot. Fever and headache are also seen. Hematogenous spread leads to organ involvement and hemorrhages under the skin that look black (hence "black death"). Spread to the lungs can causes hemorrhagic pneumonia (pneumonic plague) that can transmit from person to person. Untreated, there is a 75% mortality rate, so have a high index of suspicion and treat immediately with gentamicin or streptomycin.

Francisella: ***Francisella tularensis*** (**tularemia**) causes a bubonic plague–like illness. Transmission occurs through direct contact with rabbits or through bites of deer flies or ticks. Ulceroglandular tularemia occurs after a bite, in which a skin ulcer with a black base develops, followed by fevers, headaches, red swollen lymph nodes, and eventually hematogenous spread with organ involvement. Besides the skin ulcer, it is almost identical to bubonic plague but has a much lower mortality rate (5% if untreated). Tularemia can also cause pneumonia from inhaling aerosols while skinning an infected animal or from bacteremia after ulceroglandular tularemia. The eyes and GI tract can also be the primary source of infection. Because it is so virulent, culturing is dangerous, so diagnosis rests on the presence of antibodies to *Francisella* or a test for cellular immunity. Treat tularemia with gentamicin and doxycycline.

Brucella: *Brucella* species (of which there are many) are contracted from handling meat or milk from an infected animal. A classic patient is someone who works with animals or in the meat-packing industry, or a traveler to countries where milk isn't pasteurized or animals aren't immunized. Unlike *Yersinia* and *Francisella,* it doesn't cause buboes (red swollen lymph nodes) but rather causes chronic systemic symptoms (fever, chills, sweats, backache, headache). The fever can be *undulating* (rising throughout the day then normal in the morning). It is implicated in culture-negative endocarditis, sacroiliitis, and infections of various other organ systems. Diagnosis is by culture (which can take 4 weeks to grow) or serologic testing (antibodies indicate current infection, whereas subdermal testing for cellular immunity only indicates exposure). Treat with doxycycline plus an aminoglycoside, or TMP/SMX in children.

Pasteurella: ***Pasteurella multocida*** is zoonotic (mostly in cats and birds), but unlike the three bacterial species described earlier, it is not a facultative intracellular parasite. Infection usually follows a cat or dog bite or scratch with rapid-onset cellulitis. Don't close the wound! *P. multocida* likes this. Leave it open and treat with penicillin or doxycycline (although most bite wounds will be treated with amoxicillin-clavulanate because of the presence of mixed flora, including *S. aureus*).

The genera *Bartonella, Coxiella,* and *Ehrlichia* are nonenteric gram-negative bacteria but are discussed in the later section "Pleomorphic Bacteria" because of their similarity to rickettsial infections.

Gram-Positive Branching Filamentous Bacteria

Actinomyces and ***Nocardia*** behave like fungi in the sense that they grow like mycelia (the branching hyphae part of fungi), live in water and soil, and are saprophytes (digest organic matter extracellularly). All of these characteristics are usually attributed to fungi.

Treatment is a **SNAP:** **S**ulfa for ***N**ocardia*, ***A**ctinomyces* use **P**enicillin.

Actinomyces: ***Actinomyces israelii*** is a gram-positive anaerobe with a beaded, filamentous appearance. *A. israelii* is part of the normal oral flora and causes **actinomycosis,** a slowly growing abscess that erodes into the skin to create draining **sinus tracts.** Actinomycosis occurs in patients with poor dental hygiene or after trauma to the oral or GI mucosa (such as dental extraction). The pus from an abscess, when viewed under the microscope, has yellow granules called *sulfur granules* that are actually microcolonies of *A. israelii.* Treatment is with penicillin G and drainage of the abscess.

Nocardia: ***Nocardia asteroides*** is not part of the oral flora but rather lives in the soil (it has the scent of wet dirt). When inhaled, it causes pneumonia with lung abscesses and cavitations, much like tuberculosis. In fact, because the bacteria are *acid fast* (a feature unique to *Nocardia* and *Mycobacterium*), *Nocardia* infection is often misdiagnosed as tuberculosis (Fig. 5.22). Dissemination into the bloodstream can lead to abscesses elsewhere, notably in the brain. Immunocompromised and transplant patients are at particular risk. In healthy patients, *Nocardia* can cause cutaneous pustule (mycetoma) after minor trauma in the outdoors. Treatment is with TMP-SMX.

Pleomorphic Bacteria

- *Chlamydia*
  - *C. trachomatis* (A-C, D-K, L1-L3)
  - *C. psittaci*
  - *C. pneumoniae*
- *Rickettsia*
  - *R. rickettsia*
  - *R. akari*
  - *R. prowazekii*
  - *R. typhi*
- *Bartonella*
  - *B. quintana*
  - *B. henselae*
- *Coxiella burnetii*
- *Ehrlichia chaffeensis*

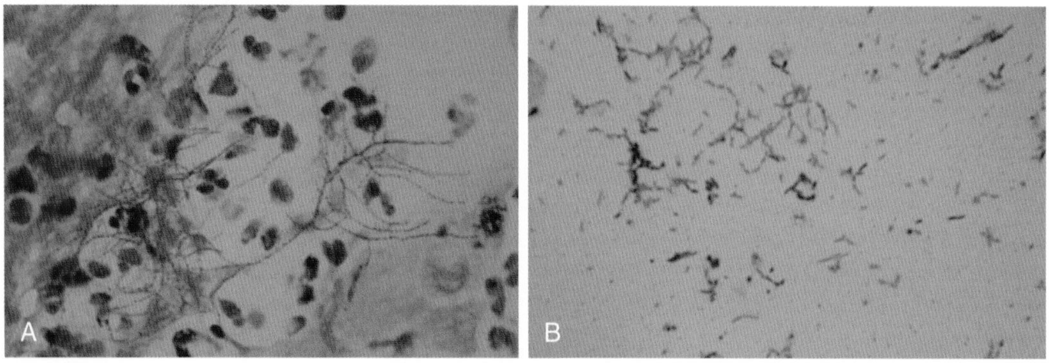

FIG. 5.22 *Norcardia* as seen by Gram stain **(A)** and acid-fast stain **(B).** (*From Nath SK, Revankar SG,* Problem-Based Microbiology. *Philadelphia: Elsevier; 2005. Courtesy Dr. Paul Southern, University of Texas Southwestern Medical Center, Dallas, TX.*)

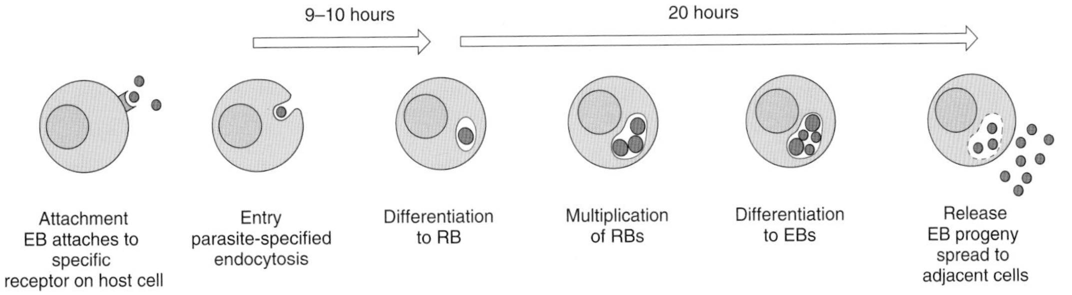

Fig. 5.23 Life cycle of chlamydia. EB, Elementary body; RB, reticulate body. (*From Goering R, Dockrell H, Wakelin D, et al. Mims' Medical Microbiology. 4th ed. Philadelphia: Elsevier; 2007.*)

Pleomorphic in this context refers to these bacteria's ability to alter their size and shape in response to their environment.

Chlamydia: *Chlamydia* species are obligate intracellular parasites (can only survive briefly outside of a host cell) that infect mucous membranes (e.g., eyes, genitourinary tract, lungs). They are extremely small (a little bigger than a large virus), and exist in two forms. As an *elementary body,* they are metabolically inert and very small but are *infectious.* Once inside a host cell, they grow, inhibit destruction by lysosomes, and divide to form the *reticulate body,* which can make its own proteins but requires ATP from the host cell (Fig. 5.23).

Chlamydia trachomatis can cause several human diseases depending on the serotypes. Serotypes A to C cause **trachoma,** a chronic conjunctivitis in children spread by contact that is the leading cause of preventable blindness worldwide. It is seen mostly in developing nations. Treat with azithromycin. Serotypes D to K cause several diseases:

- **Inclusion conjunctivitis:** Newborns can pick up *C. trachomatis* from the birth canal, causing yellow mucopurulent discharge and swelling of the eyelids 5 to 14 days after birth (gonococcal conjunctivitis presents sooner, in 2 to 5 days). In the United States all newborns receive prophylactic erythromycin eye drops, but if disease develops, treat with oral erythromycin solution. Adults can also get this—treat with doxycycline or a macrolide. Diagnosis is made by observing inclusion bodies (groups of elementary bodies) in cells scraped from the eyelids.
- Infants can also acquire **pneumonia** from the birth canal, which presents 4 to 11 weeks after birth. Treat with oral erythromycin.
- **Urethritis** can be contracted sexually. Urethritis caused by *C. trachomatis* often occurs in tandem with *N. gonorrhea* urethritis, and the two together cause most cases of urethritis (third is *Ureaplasma urealyticum*). Symptoms, if present, include dysuria and white discharge. Empiric treatment should cover all three organisms mentioned—usually ceftriaxone and a single dose of azithromycin; in the meantime, PCR on a urine sample will determine which organisms are present.
- **Cervicitis** can result from infection by *C. trachomatis* or *N. gonorrhea.* The cervix appears red and swollen, with yellow purulent discharge. The bacteria can travel up to infect the uterus, fallopian tubes, and ovaries, causing **PID,** which presents with lower abdominal pain, cervical discharge and bleeding, fever, nausea, vomiting, and dyspareunia (pain with sex). On examination there is cervical motion tenderness ("chandelier sign" because the patient jumps to the ceiling when the cervix is moved). PID can damage the fallopian tubes, leading to infertility, increased risk for ectopic pregnancy, and chronic pelvic pain (even after only a single episode). *C. trachomatis* is particularly harmful because it can cause asymptomatic PID (hence it is often left untreated too long). Treat with a shot of ceftriaxone (to cover for gonorrhea) and 2 weeks of doxycycline or a single dose of azithromycin (to cover for chlamydia).
- **Epididymitis** caused by *C. trachomatis* can develop in men with urethritis and causes unilateral scrotal swelling, tenderness, pain, and fever.
- Complications of infection with *C. trachomatis* include **reactive arthritis** (previously known as Reiter syndrome), which presents with the triad of an inflammatory arthritis, urethritis, and conjunctivitis or uveitis (can be caused by other infections as well); and **Fitz-Hugh-Curtis syndrome,** an infection of the capsule surrounding the liver (previously mentioned in the section "*Neisseria*").

Finally, serotypes L1, L2, and L3 cause **lymphogranuloma venereum** (LGV), an STI characterized by a *painless* genital ulcer that disappears, followed by slow bilateral enlargement of the inguinal lymph nodes. These nodes become suppurative and can ulcerate. Treat LGV with doxycycline.

Chlamydophila psittaci is carried by birds and can cause an atypical pneumonia called psittacosis in those exposed (usually bird breeders, veterinarians, pet shop workers, etc.), occurring 1 to 3 weeks after exposure (be careful, it looks a lot like *Histoplasma* pneumonia, which is caused by bird or bat droppings). Treatment is with doxycycline. *Chlamydophila pneumoniae* (TWAR strain) can also cause atypical pneumonia but is spread from human to human rather than contracted from animals and classically occurs in neonates with a "staccato cough." Treat walking pneumonia with a macrolide or doxycycline.

Rickettsia: *Rickettsia* species, like chlamydia, are extremely small and rely on host ATP (and hence are intracellular parasites). Unlike chlamydia, they require an arthropod vector and prefer endothelial cells in blood vessels (chlamydia prefers columnar epithelium of mucous membranes). Because most *Rickettsia* species have similar surface antigens to *Proteus* (coincidentally), diagnosis of rickettsial infection can be performed by the **Weil-Felix reaction,** in which patient serum is mixed with beads coated with *Proteus* antigens and observed for crystal formation (although it is not terribly accurate). Antibody titers are more reliable and help differentiate subspecies. Treatment of all rickettsial infections is with doxycycline (even in children younger than 8 years old, which we normally don't do, but doxycycline is so superior to other alternatives in this case).

Rickettsia rickettsii causes **Rocky Mountain spotted fever** (RMSF). Despite the name, this disease is most common in the Southeast United States. A week after being bitten by a dog tick *(Dermacentor variabilis)* or wood tick *(Dermacentor andersoni),* patients present with fever, conjunctival redness, severe headache, myalgias, and an ascending rash that becomes petechial (starts at the palms/wrists and soles/ankles, then moves to the trunk; Fig. 5.24). The organism proliferates in the endothelium of blood vessels, causing hemorrhage and thrombi (explaining the rash and conjunctival redness). Recognition and empiric therapy is important because, if untreated, RMSF can progress to disseminated intravascular coagulation and death.

Rickettsia akari causes **rickettsialpox.** After a bite from a mite that usually lives on house mice, patients develop a red vesicular skin lesion that becomes a black eschar. A few days later, the organism disseminates and causes fever, headache, and multiple vesicular lesions that look like chickenpox. The vesicles do not occur on the palms and soles. It's self-limited but responds to doxycycline.

Rickettsia prowazekii causes **epidemic typhus.** *Epidemic* refers to the sudden spread of an infection, whereas *endemic* refers to a disease that exists constantly in a population. Another rickettsial species, *Rickettsia typhi,* causes **endemic typhus.** The diseases are similar, and infection with one gives immunity to the other. *Rickettsia prowazekii* is carried by lice or fleas, and the vector in the United States is flying squirrels. Generally, the infection occurs in areas of poverty and overcrowding. After a bite, the patient has sudden onset of fever and headache, followed by a 2-week incubation period during which small pink macules appear on the trunk and then spread outward to the rest of the body (but sparing the palms, soles, and face, unlike Rocky Mountain spotted fever). Endothelial damage is responsible for the rash and can cause fatal thrombosis, but usually the disease self-resolves if untreated. All patients, when possible, should be treated to avoid (1) having them become reservoirs, and (2) developing a reactivated, but milder, form of the disease known as **Brill-Zinsser disease** caused by latent infection.

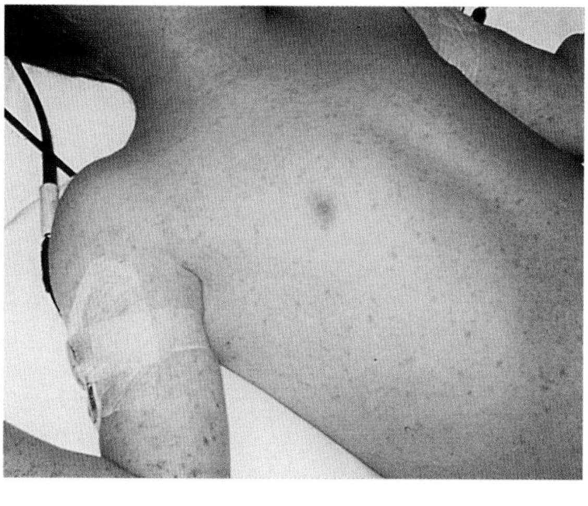

FIG. 5.24 Generalized maculopapular rash of Rocky Mountain spotted fever. (*From Goering R, Dockrell H, Wakelin D, et al. Mims' Medical Microbiology. 4th ed. Philadelphia: Elsevier; 2007. Courtesy T. F. Sellers, Jr.*)

Rickettsia typhi causes endemic typhus. The reservoir is rodents, it is transmitted by the rat flea (*Xenopsylla cheopis*), and it causes a milder (but still serious) disease than *R. prowazekii. Rickettsia tsutsugamushi* is carried by the larvae of mites living in the soil mostly in Asia and the South Pacific. Two weeks after a bite, the patient experiences fever, headache, a scab at the bite, and sometimes a widespread rash. *Rickettsia parkeri* causes fever, headaches, eschars, and regional lymphadenopathy (discovered in 2002 in the southeast coastal United States). *Rickettsia africae* causes **African tick-bite fever,** which has become a common cause of unexplained fever in travelers returning from Africa.

Rickettsia-Like Infections: *Bartonella quintana* causes **trench fever,** so named because it affected World War I soldiers in trenches. It is carried by the body louse, causing high fevers, headache, and back and leg pain. An erythematous rash develops on the trunk and abdomen. Soldiers would appear to recover and then relapse every 5 days (hence the species name *quintana*). Like epidemic typhus, this infection is prominent in unsanitary, overcrowded conditions (e.g., war, homelessness). It is not classified as *Rickettsia* because it is not an obligate intracellular parasite (the similarities are clinical only).

Bartonella henselae causes **cat scratch disease,** in which fever and malaise develop, with swollen lymph nodes after a cat scratch or bite. Treat cat scratch disease with azithromycin (although it will resolve even without treatment). Both *Bartonella* species can also cause bacteremia, endocarditis, and an AIDS-related condition known as **bacillary angiomatosis** in which small blood vessels proliferate and look like red raised lesions on the skin and visceral organs (can be confused with Kaposi sarcoma).

Coxiella burnetii causes **Q fever,** usually in **slaughterhouse workers** and those exposed to an infected animal's products of conception. The bacteria are unique from other rickettsial diseases in that they form endospores, conferring several unique properties: ability to survive (though not replicate) outside a host cell, resist heat and drying, and transmit by aerosolized tick/cow feces instead of by an arthropod vector. Because of this mode of infection, *C. burnetii* causes a mild atypical pneumonia along with fever and sweats 2 to 3 weeks after infection (the only rickettsial infection to cause pneumonia), without rash. *C. burnetii* can also cause granulomatous hepatitis and culture-negative endocarditis. Diagnosis is made with serologies or PCR. Though most cases are self-limited, doxycycline can be given.

Ehrlichia chaffeensis is transmitted by the Lone Star *(Amblyomma americanum)* tick and causes **ehrlichiosis,** which is similar to Rocky Mountain spotted fever (look for a patient with pancytopenia and tick exposure). There is **no rash** because these bacteria infect WBCs and not endothelial cells. *E. ewingii* can also cause ehrlichiosis, and *Anaplasma phagocytophilum* causes anaplasmosis. Smears will show morulae (berrylike inclusions) in monocytes (ehrlichiosis) or granulocytes (anaplasmosis). Diagnosis is confirmed by PCR. Doxycycline is the drug of choice.

Gram-Negative Spirals

- *Treponema pallidum*
  - Subspecies *endemicum*
  - Subspecies *carateum*
- *Borrelia burgdorferi*
- *Leptospira interrogans*

Spirochetes are very small, spiral-shaped bacteria that spin to achieve propulsion. Because they are so small, special techniques are used to view them (i.e., dark-field microscopy).

Treponema: *Treponema pallidum* causes **syphilis.** It is usually sexually transmitted, although contact with an infected ulcer (e.g., by a doctor not wearing gloves) can cause spread. Untreated, syphilis progresses through three stages (Fig. 5.25). In **primary** syphilis, a painless chancre develops 3 to 6 weeks after initial contact at the site of infection (a painless ulcer with a punched-out base) along with regional lymphadenopathy. This resolves over 4 to 6 weeks (but this doesn't mean it's cured!). Within a few weeks, patients go into **secondary** syphilis, in which hematogenous spread of the bacteria leads to a global, red, macular rash that *includes* the palms, soles, and oral mucosa. Also, condyloma lata develop (wartlike lesions in moist areas like the groin) that are extremely contagious! Virtually any organ system can be involved at this stage, so many different presentations are possible. The disease then enters the latent stage, in which the symptoms of secondary syphilis may wax and wane. Patients who don't progress to tertiary syphilis for 4 years are considered noninfectious (except pregnant women, who can still transmit to the fetus). One-third of patients progress to **tertiary** syphilis, which takes three forms:

Rash on the palms and soles: think syphilis, Rocky Mountain spotted fever, or hand-foot-and-mouth disease (Coxsackie A virus).

- **Gummatous syphilis** (3–10 years after primary infection) consists of gummas—local granulomatous lesions that necrose and fibrose—on the skin (painless) and bones (painful).

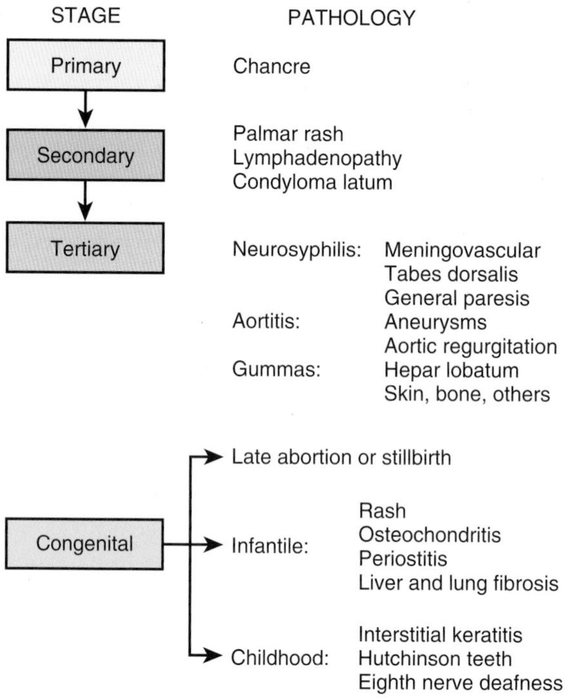

FIG. 5.25 The many manifestations of primary, secondary, tertiary, and congenital syphilis. (*From Kumar V, Abbas AK, Fausto N, et al.* Robbins and Cotran's Pathologic Basis of Disease. *8th ed. Philadelphia: Elsevier; 2009.*)

- **Cardiovascular syphilis** (10+ years after primary infection) results from inflammation of the small vessels supplying the aorta (the vasa vasorum), causing the tissue to weaken and eventually forming an aortic aneurysm in the *ascending aorta* or aortic arch. This can lead to aortic valve insufficiency. Although gummas are reversible with antimicrobials, these vascular changes are not.
- **Neurosyphilis** can present in a few different ways: asymptomatically (but with spirochete-positive CSF); as subacute meningitis (fever, stiff neck, and headache with CSF showing *high lymphocytes,* high protein, low glucose, and positive syphilis test); as meningovascular syphilis (damage to the small blood vessels of the brain and spinal cord, leading to multiinfarct dementia and a constellation of symptoms); tabes dorsalis (damage to the posterior column and dorsal root ganglia, causing ataxia and loss of reflexes, pain sensation, and temperature sensation); and general paresis (deterioration of brain cells leading to mental status changes and psychiatric problems). In both tabes dorsalis and general paresis, the **Argyll-Robertson pupil** may be present, caused by a midbrain lesion that leads to a pupil that constricts during accommodation (normal) but not to light (abnormal). This is sometimes referred to as the "prostitute's pupil" because the pupil accommodates but does not react.

Because *T. pallidum* crosses the placenta, fetuses of infected mothers acquire syphilis in utero. This confers a high risk for spontaneous abortion, stillbirth, or neonatal death. Those that survive will manifest with either early or late congenital syphilis. **Early congenital syphilis** presents within the first 2 years of life and looks like severe adult secondary syphilis (rash, condyloma lata, bone infection). **Late congenital syphilis** looks more like tertiary syphilis (except without cardiovascular involvement)—periosteal inflammation leads to characteristic changes in the cartilage of the nasal septum (saddle nose), tibia (saber shins), and teeth (Hutchinson teeth and mulberry molars). Corneal inflammation is also common. Congenital syphilis develops after the fourth month of gestation and can be prevented if the mother is treated in the first trimester.

Diagnosis of syphilis can be made by visualizing helical organisms moving in a corkscrew fashion under dark-field microscopy from *active* lesions (chancre, condyloma lata, macules), but when no active lesions are present, we rely on serologic tests. Nonspecific treponemal tests rely on the presence of antibodies against cardiolipin and lecithin, which are lipids released into the bloodstream during infection with *T. pallidum.* The two tests used to detect these antibodies are the VDRL (Venereal Disease Research Laboratory) and RPR (rapid plasma reagin) tests. False-positive results can occur, so these tests are used for screening—a confirmatory test (the FTA-ABS test, which looks for *Treponema*-specific antibodies) must then be performed. Treat syphilis with penicillin (including pregnant women).

Those with allergies to penicillin can be treated with erythromycin and doxycycline (*not* including pregnant women because doxycycline is harmful to the fetus). Pregnant women with penicillin allergies must be desensitized to penicillin and treated. Rarely, patients may experience flulike fevers, chills, myalgias, and headaches after treatment as a result of release of a pyrogenic toxin by the killed bacteria; this is called the **Jarisch-Herxheimer reaction.**

There are three important subspecies of *T. pallidum* that, although similar to *T. pallidum,* are regional and not sexually transmitted. They do manifest in three stages (skin ulcer, then widespread disease, then a tertiary stage), but the tertiary stage does not involve the cardiovascular or nervous system. *T. pallidum* subspecies *endemicum* causes **endemic syphilis (Bejel),** most commonly in Africa and the Middle East. It produces oral lesions similar to condyloma lata after sharing cups or utensils with someone with open ulcers, causing wartlike papules that can be disfiguring; later, skin and bone gummas develop. *T. pallidum* subspecies *carateum* causes **Pinta,** a disease of rural Latin America spread by direct contact that starts with a slowly expanding papule followed by an eruption of red lesions that turn blue in the sun, then white over time (there is no bone involvement in Pinta). *T. pallidum* subspecies *pertenue* causes **Yaws,** a tropical infection of the skin, bone, and joints. These nonvenereal syphilis can be treated with penicillin or azithromycin.

Borrelia: These are larger spirochetes that can be viewed under light microscopy with Giemsa or Wright stains.

Most common diseases in the United States spread by vectors: Lyme disease, Rocky Mountain spotted fever, and tularemia.

Borrelia burgdorferi causes **Lyme disease.** It is carried by rodents and white-tailed deer in the U.S. Northeast, Midwest, and Northwest and transmitted by the *Ixodes* tick. Infection requires about 24 hours of attachment to the host, so regular tick checks can prevent disease, especially after time spent in wooded areas. Like syphilis, Lyme disease has three stages:

- The early localized stage begins about 10 days after the bite and consists of regional lymphadenopathy, flulike symptoms, and a characteristic red, annular, expanding rash at the site of infection that leaves blue or necrotic tissue in its wake. This is called **erythema chronicum migrans** (ECM; Fig. 5.26) and represents the bacteria multiplying and spreading outward.
- Weeks later, in the *early disseminated stage,* the disseminated spirochetes multiply, and the immune response causes inflammatory damage in skin (ECM-like but with multiple smaller lesions), nervous system (meningitis, cranial nerve palsies, peripheral neuropathies), heart (atrioventricular node block, myocarditis), and joints (migratory arthritis).
- In the late stage, chronic arthritis and encephalopathy can develop (10% of untreated patients progress to the late stage). Skin atrophy can occur **(acrodermatitis chronicum atrophicans).**

Diagnosis can be made by culturing *Borrelia* from the leading edge of the ECM rash. If this isn't present, serum titers for anti-*Borrelia* antibodies by enzyme-linked immunosorbent assay (ELISA) or Western blot are effective (culturing the blood or CSF can be difficult). However, erythema migrans is pathognomonic for the disease, so in a patient with tick exposure and this rash, you can treat without checking serology. Treat with doxycycline or amoxicillin (stage 1) or ceftriaxone for late stages.

Several *Borrelia* species cause **relapsing fever,** including *B. recurrentis.* They are transmitted from human to human by the body louse or *Ornithodoros* tick. After infection, the bacteria disseminate and cause high fever, headache, muscle aches, and possible rash and meningeal signs. Symptoms resolve over 3 to 6 days, then recur about every 8 days but become progressively less severe. The relapses are due to the bacteria's ability to change the surface protein **VMP** after each antibody

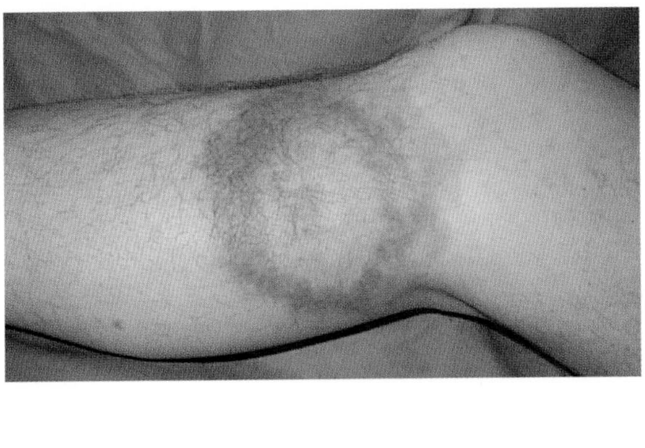

FIG. 5.26 Erythema chronicum migrans as seen in Lyme disease. (*From Swartz MH.* Textbook of Physical Diagnosis. *6th ed. Philadelphia: Elsevier; 2010.*)

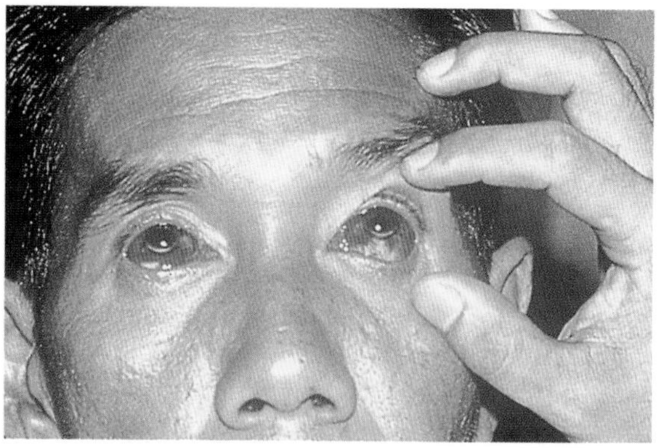

Fig. 5.27 Conjunctival hemorrhage and jaundice in a patient with leptospirosis. (*From Goering R, Dockrell H, Wakelin D, et al. Mims' Medical Microbiology. 4th ed. Philadelphia: Elsevier; 2007. Courtesy D. Lewis.*)

response. Diagnosis is by blood smears or culture during a fever (cultures can be negative between fevers). As with syphilis, treatment (doxycycline, penicillin) during a febrile episode can cause a Jarisch-Herxheimer reaction.

Leptospira: ***Leptospira interrogans*** causes **leptospirosis.** The organism is shed in animal urine and infects humans through contaminated water or soil (look for a recent history of swimming in open water or regional flooding). The first phase of the illness occurs when bacteria invade the blood and CSF, causing flulike symptoms, along with **red conjunctiva** (Fig. 5.27) and **photophobia.** Myalgias may be present, usually in the calves. A short afebrile period is followed by a second phase during which symptoms recur as a result of the host immune response. In the mild form, aseptic meningitis occurs. The more severe version **(Weil disease)** involves renal failure, hepatitis with jaundice, mental status changes, and hemorrhages in many organs. Given its rapid progression, make the diagnosis based on history, examination, and initial laboratory test results (elevated liver function tests, protein in the urine). Confirmation of the diagnosis is made by culturing blood or CSF during febrile phases, but treatment with **penicillin or doxycycline** should begin immediately and before cultures come back. Doxycycline can be used as prophylaxis (e.g., during a flood).

Gram-Positive Acid-Fast Bacteria

Both *Mycobacterium* and *Nocardia* species are called acid fast (*Nocardia* is "weakly" acid fast) because they resist decolorization by acid after staining with carbolfuchsin. This is due to the high lipid content of their cell walls. *Nocardia* species were discussed earlier; only *Mycobacterium* species are discussed here.

Mycobacterium: ***Mycobacterium tuberculosis*** causes **tuberculosis (TB)**, a worldwide pandemic that kills 2 million people per year. In the United States it is seen mostly in older adults and immunocompromised patients (e.g., AIDS patients, who lack the cellular immunity necessary to combat this bug). Although *M. tuberculosis* can infect any organ, it is famously associated with lung disease because it is usually acquired through inhalation.

Primary Tuberculosis: After inhalation, neutrophils and macrophages attempt to destroy the bacteria but are unsuccessful because **mycolic acid** in its cell wall prevents phagocytosis. During this period of *facultative intracellular growth,* bacteria spread through lymph and blood. Cellular immunity then kicks in, and helper T cells recruit macrophages to the site of infection in the lungs, resulting in local tissue destruction that looks like granular cheese and hence is called **caseous necrosis.** These granulomas often calcify, forming **tubercles** (Fig. 5.28). Tubercles usually form in the lungs (a Ghon focus, see later) but can form anywhere in the body the bacteria has managed to invade. At this point, the bacteria are contained, although still viable. Most patients are asymptomatic during primary infection; children, older adults, and immunocompromised people can experience symptoms of a more overt infection. Symptoms include cough, sometimes with sputum or blood, and constitutional symptoms (fever, chills, fatigue, night sweats, weight loss).

A **purified protein derivative (PPD)** test will tell you whether the patient has developed immunity to *M. tuberculosis.* It is positive for active, latent, *and* past infections, demonstrating only the presence of a type IV hypersensitivity (cell-mediated response) to TB antigens; *active* infections can only be diagnosed by demonstrating acid-fast bacteria in sputum. A subdermal injection of proteins is read 48 to 72 hours later (latency time for a type IV hypersensitivity reaction). A 15-mm induration indicates a positive test in a low-risk patient (10 mm in moderate risk individuals and 5 mm in the

Treat a positive PPD with 9 months of isoniazid (or 6 months of rifampin if they come from an area with high isoniazid resistance). Treat tuberculosis with RIPE therapy: **r**ifampin, **i**soniazid + B_6, **p**yrazinamide, and **e**thambutol. All cause hepatotoxicity, except ethambutol, which causes decreased visual acuity and color perception.

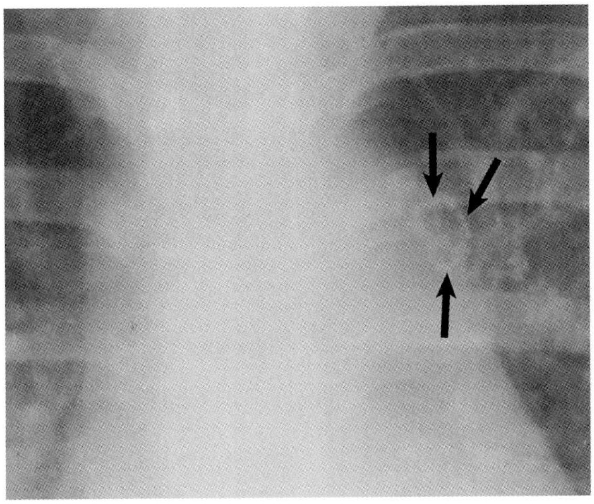

Fig. 5.28 Calcified nodule in a patient with primary tuberculosis. (*From Lawlor MW.* Rapid Review USMLE Step 2. *Philadelphia: Elsevier; 2006.*)

immunocompromised). False positives can result if the patient *recently* had a bacille Calmette-Guérin (BCG) vaccine, and false negatives are seen with compromised immune systems (called anergy) or if the patient was exposed to TB less than 10 weeks before the test. Another test is the interferon-γ release assay, which tests T cells *in vitro* to respond to bacterial antigens. This is more specific and is accurate in those with prior BCG vaccination. Radiologic findings in a patient who has recently experienced primary tuberculosis include calcified pulmonary lesions in the middle and lower lobes **(Ghon focus)** and hilar lymphadenopathy (Ghon focus + hilar lymphadenopathy = **Ghon complex**). Those who are experiencing symptomatic primary TB may show large cavitary lung lesions with air–fluid levels.

Secondary (Reactivation) Tuberculosis: Secondary TB usually occurs when a tubercle containing dormant bacteria weakens during an immunocompromised state (e.g., HIV patients with a history of primary TB have a 10% chance per year of developing secondary TB) but can also occur with reinfection. Reactivation TB is usually pulmonary, presenting with cough (sometimes with blood), fever, night sweats, and weight loss. The infection usually occurs in the apical areas of the lungs near the clavicles because oxygen tension is highest and these are obligate aerobes. As macrophages and T cells fight to wall off the bacteria, lesions form that follow the same pattern as the lesions in primary TB: They caseate (cheeselike), liquefy (air–fluid levels), and cavitate. Although pulmonary TB is most common, bacteria can spread from the lungs to other parts of the body, and tubercles in extrapulmonary sites can themselves reactivate. Hence, reactivation TB can take many forms:

- Lymph node infection is the most common extrapulmonary site of reactivation, usually in cervical lymph nodes. This is also called **scrofula** and manifests as large, matted lymph nodes.
- Pleural and pericardial infection presents as fluid in the pleural or pericardial space.
- Kidney infection presents with RBCs and WBCs (but no bacteria) in the urine. Because there are WBCs but no bacteria, this is known as **sterile pyuria.**
- Skeletal infection usually affects the spine **(Pott disease).**
- Joint infection presents as chronic inflammation of one joint.
- Central nervous system (CNS) involvement presents as subacute meningitis, and granulomas can be seen in the brain.
- **Miliary TB** presents as seed-sized granulomas all over the body. In fact, seeding to the adrenal glands is a common cause of adrenal insufficiency worldwide.

Several atypical species of *Mycobacterium* cause mild pneumonia. ***M. avium-intracellulare*** is a well-known opportunistic infection in AIDS patients with low T-cell counts (typically <50 cells/mm^3). The bacteria spread, leading to a wasting illness involving multiple organs (although it is rarely the cause of death in these patients). *M. avium-intracellulare* also causes nontender cervical lymphadenitis—treat by excising (not incising) the lymph node. *Mycobacterium marinum* causes "fish tank bacillus," an ulcerative skin lesion in people who work with fish tanks.

Mycobacterium leprae causes **leprosy.** The bacteria are transmitted through respiratory secretions or skin lesions of an infected individual, although it seems that not everyone is susceptible to infection (for unknown reasons). The bacteria prefer to grow in the cooler body areas (skin, peripheral nerves, eyes, nose, scrotum). Like *M. tuberculosis, M. leprae* is acid fast and is a facultative intracellular organism,

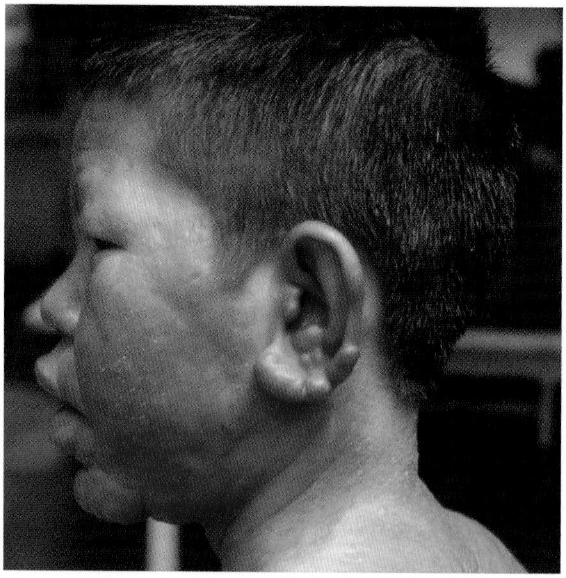

Fig. 5.29 Leonine facies of lepromatous leprosy. Note the enlarged earlobes and facial swelling. (*From Greenwood D, Slack R, Peitherer J, Barer M. Medical Microbiology. 17th ed. Philadelphia: Elsevier; 2007.*)

resisting destruction by macrophages (with mycolic acid) and dividing within them. Hence, the host must mount a cellular immune response (T cells) in order to destroy the bacteria. The severity of disease is dependent on the degree of this host response:

- **Lepromatous leprosy** is the most severe, in which the host mounts *no* cellular immune response. Although the bacterium can be found everywhere in the body, the infection produces lesions mostly on the skin (hairless lumps and thickening, including **leonine facies;** Fig. 5.29), peripheral nerves (**glove-and-stocking** distribution of sensory loss leading to repeated trauma, infections, and eventual deformities), nasal cartilage **(saddle nose deformity),** testes **(infertility),** and eyes **(blindness).**
- **Tuberculoid leprosy** occurs when the host *can* mount an effective cell-mediated immune response. These patients generally have a self-limited, noninfectious, mild form of leprosy with some damage of peripheral nerves (one or two palpable nerves, sensory loss in those areas). The lesions are macules or flattened plaques without sensation.
- Other severities can be seen between lepromatous and tuberculoid leprosy: borderline lepromatous, borderline, and borderline tuberculoid. The lepromin skin test (like a PPD) can be used to determine where the patient falls on this spectrum in order to determine prognosis. Other diagnostic tests include a skin/nerve biopsy (granulomas in tuberculoid, acid-fast bacteria in lepromatous) or cultures in a mouse footpad (can't grow *in vitro*).
- Treatment is with **dapsone** and rifampin, adding clofazimine for lepromatous disease. Patients may develop a hypersensitivity to sudden destruction of the bacteria; treat with prednisone. Erythema nodosum leprosum may also present after starting treatment (immune complex deposition in the skin); treat with thalidomide and *don't* stop treating for leprosy.

Gram-Positive Bacteria with No Cell Wall

- *Mycoplasma pneumoniae*
- *Ureaplasma urealyticum*

Mycoplasma: *Mycoplasma* species are tiny organisms without cell walls, so antibiotics targeting cell wall integrity (penicillin, cephalosporins) are ineffective, whereas those attacking ribosomes (azithromycin, tetracycline) are effective.

Mycoplasma pneumoniae is spread by respiratory droplets and causes tracheobronchitis and a mild, **"walking" or "atypical" pneumonia** with slow onset of fever, malaise, sore throat, and dry hacking cough, mostly in young adults and teens. The organism binds to respiratory epithelia (but does not invade), inhibiting ciliary motion and destroying mucosal cells. Radiographs may show a streaky infiltrate, and although most symptoms resolve in 1 week, the infiltrate and dry cough may persist for months. Infection can cause formation of anti-RBC antibodies, leading the blood to clump on ice (this is the **cold agglutinin test**) and causing anemia. Antibodies may form to other organ systems, leading

Atypical pneumonias: think *Legionella, Chlamydia, Mycoplasma,* or viruses.

to systemic symptoms like arthritis. Other diagnostic tests look for the presence of *Mycoplasma* itself (PCR, DNA probe, sputum cultures that look like **fried eggs** grown on **Eaton agar**). Treat with *atypical coverage* (macrolides, tetracyclines, or quinolones).

Ureaplasma urealyticum is actually a species of *Mycoplasma*. It is named *urealyticum* because it cleaves urea into ammonia and carbon dioxide using urease enzyme. It is a normal colonizer of the genitourinary tract but can cause postpartum bacteremia in neonates.

Urethritis: think *C. trachomatis, N. gonorrhoeae*, or *U. urealyticum*.

VIRUSES

Introduction to Viruses

Structure: All viruses are composed of a core of **nucleic acid** (either DNA or RNA) covered by a protective protein coat (**capsid**). Viruses are classified into groups by (1) the type of nucleic acid they use, (2) the shape of their capsid, and (3) the presence or absence of an outer membrane, called an envelope.

The **envelope** present on some viruses is derived from the host cell's plasma or nuclear membrane, as the virus progeny buds outward for release. Compared with naked viruses, enveloped viruses are more sensitive to inactivation or destruction by heat, drying, and detergents. Naked viruses are often transmitted by **outside environmental exposure** routes such as fecal–oral, whereas enveloped viruses are often transmitted by **direct contact** routes such as blood or respiratory secretions.

Replication: All viruses undergo these same general steps to replicate:

1. **Attachment** to specific host cell receptors. The specific receptors a virus can bind determine what type of cell can become infected **(tropism).**
2. **Penetration** using receptor-mediated endocytosis, coated pits, or fusion of the viral envelope to the host cell membrane.
3. **Uncoating** or release of the viral nucleic acid.
4. **Replication**:
   - Early mRNA and protein synthesis, including proteins to shut off host cell functions and proteins to replicate the viral genome;
   - Replication of the viral genome from template;
   - Late mRNA and protein synthesis, including structural and capsid proteins.
5. **Assembly** of the new viral particles within capsids.
6. **Release** from the host cell via lysis (causing host cell death) or budding (leaving the host cell alive).

General Principles:

- All DNA viruses are double-stranded DNA (dsDNA) **except** for Parvovirus (single-stranded DNA [ssDNA]).
- The DNA viruses can be remembered by the mnemonic HHAPPPy: **H**epadna, **H**erpes, **A**deno, **P**ox, **P**arvo, **P**apova.
- All DNA viruses have linear genomes **except** for Papillomavirus, Polyomavirus, and Hepadnavirus, which are circular genomes.
- All DNA viruses replicate in the nucleus and are icosahedral **except** for poxviruses (cytoplasm; complex shape).
- All RNA viruses replicate in the cytoplasm **except** for retroviruses and the influenza virus (nucleus).
- All RNA viruses are single-stranded RNA (ssRNA) **except** for reoviruses (dsRNA).
- All viruses are haploid (one copy of DNA or RNA) **except** for retroviruses (diploid; two identical ssRNA).

DNA Viruses

Herpesviridae

- **Capsid:** icosahedral
- **Envelope:** enveloped
- **DNA structure:** double-stranded, linear
- **Viruses of clinical significance:** cytomegalovirus (human herpesvirus [HHV] 5), herpes simplex virus types 1 and 2 (HHV-1 and -2), Epstein-Barr virus (HHV-4), varicella-zoster virus (VZV; HHV-3), roseolovirus (HHV-6), and Kaposi sarcoma–associated herpesvirus (HHV-8).

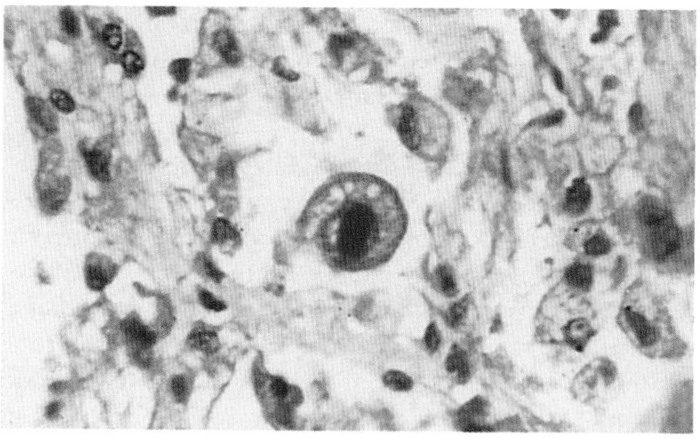

Fig. 5.30 Owl's eye inclusion bodies in a giant cell during cytomegalovirus infection. (*From Goering R, Dockrell H, Wakelin D, et al. Mims' Medical Microbiology. 4th ed. Philadelphia: Elsevier; 2007. Courtesy I. D. Starke and M. E. Hodson.*)

Cytomegalovirus

Cytomegalovirus (CMV; HHV-5) is transmitted through close contact (body fluid, organ transplant, transplacental) and infects a variety of cells. Unlike other herpesviruses that affect the skin, CMV causes visceral disease. Most infections (80%), but not all, are asymptomatic:

- CMV is one of the ToRCHeS infections (mnemonic for infections that cross the placenta). Congenital CMV occurs in mothers with a primary CMV infection. Fetal infection with CMV causes microcephaly, sensorineural deafness, seizures, hepatomegaly, purpuric rash (**"blueberry muffin"** from extramedullary hematopoiesis), and other birth defects. It is the leading *viral* cause of mental retardation. Look for intracranial calcifications that line the ventricles (CMV = "**C**oat **My** **V**entricles").
- It typically causes a mononucleosis-like disease (flu symptoms with abnormal lymphocytes).
- **AIDS patients** with low T-cell counts develop CMV **retinitis,** colitis, and viremia. Treat CMV retinitis with **ganciclovir.**
- Bone marrow transplant recipients develop CMV pneumonitis, esophagitis, colitis, and viremia (but not retinitis).

ToRCHeS infections that cross the blood–placenta barrier: **To**xoplasmosis, **R**ubella, **C**ytomegalovirus, **He**rpes simplex/**H**IV, **S**yphilis.

Help with diagnosis can be accomplished by observing tissues or urine for giant cells ("megalocytes") with **"owl's eye" intranuclear inclusion bodies** (Fig. 5.30). Culture of the buffy coat (WBC portion of blood) is confirmatory. In cases of mononucleosis-like symptoms, there should be a negative Monospot (see Epstein-Barr virus).

Herpes Simplex Virus

Herpes simplex virus types 1 and 2 (HSV-1, HSV-2) are transmitted by direct contact of mucocutaneous surfaces.

- **Primary infection:** Initial contact can lead to formation of multiple vesicular (fluid-filled) lesions with an erythematous base at the site of inoculation—skin, oral mucosa (gingivostomatitis), genitals, eyes (keratoconjunctivitis; Fig. 5.31)—with systemic symptoms like fever and malaise. However, most primary infections are asymptomatic.

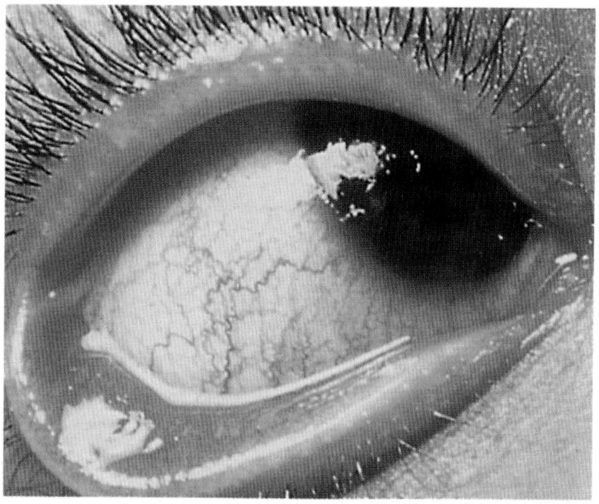

Fig. 5.31 Herpes simplex keratoconjunctivitis, with dendritic ulcers on the cornea. (*From Goering R, Dockrell H, Wakelin D, et al. Mims' Medical Microbiology. 4th ed. Philadelphia: Elsevier; 2007. Courtesy M. J. Wood.*)

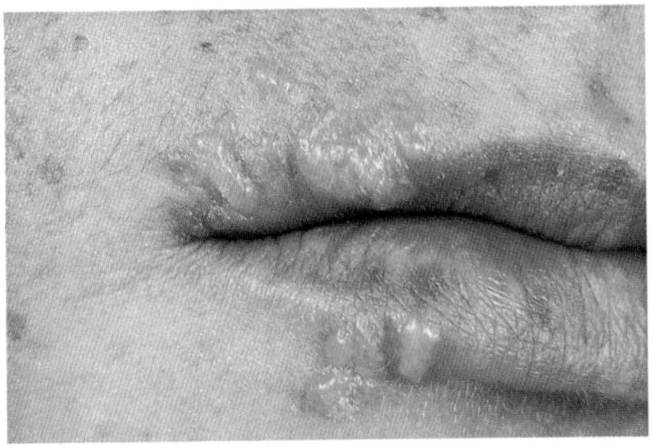

FIG. 5.32 Herpes labialis. (*From Swash M, Glynn M. Hutchison's Clinical Methods. 22nd ed. Edinburgh: Elsevier; 2007.*)

- **Reactivation infection:** The virus lives in a latent state in neural ganglia and reactivates under conditions of immune suppression or stress, leading to a few vesicular lesions at the site of primary infection, usually without systemic symptoms. **Herpes labialis** ("cold sores"; Fig. 5.32) and **genital herpes** are common reactivation infections, but recurrent gingivostomatitis and keratoconjunctivitis (common cause of blindness in the United States) are also possible.

HSV-1 typically prefers oral mucosa, whereas HSV-2 prefers the genitals, but both viruses can infect both anatomic areas. Special clinical situations include the following:

- Because HSV crosses the placenta, it is one of the ToRC**H**eS infections. Specifically, fetal infection with HSV leads to birth defects, intrauterine death, or neonatal encephalitis (typically HSV-2).
- HSV can infect the cornea (keratoconjunctivitis), which presents with painful red eye. Fluorescein staining will show a branching, dendritic ulceration that is vision threatening.
- Immunocompromised patients may experience more disseminated infections, either with extensive mucocutaneous lesions or infection of other organ systems (liver, lungs, GI tract).
- Occasionally, HSV-1 may cause encephalitis that usually starts in the temporal lobe. It is the most common *viral* cause of encephalitis in the United States, and it's treatable, so don't miss it. Patients often present with altered mental status, behavioral changes, focal neurologic signs, and evidence of **temporal lobe seizures** (behavior changes, smelling rubber, etc.). Electroencephalography and magnetic resonance imaging can be diagnostic, as well as PCR of the spinal fluid.
- **Herpetic whitlow** is infection of a finger by HSV. This used to occur in health care workers (especially dentists) after contact with an infected patient's saliva, before the routine use of gloves. The lesions can be pustular and mistaken for bacterial infection.

The **Tzanck smear** is a scraping of the base of a herpetic ulcer and can be used to detect **multinucleated giant cells** for the detection of HSV (and VZV). This test is no longer routinely used but may show up on the USMLE. Skin biopsy can also be performed to observe for eosinophilic nuclear inclusions, also called **Cowdry bodies** (again, for HSV and VZV). The gold standard is detection of viral DNA by PCR, but other detection methods such as culture and direct fluorescent antibody testing are nearly as good. Treat all HSV infections with **acyclovir** or one of its analogs, such as **valacyclovir.** For resistant infections, use **foscarnet.**

Epstein-Barr Virus

Epstein-Barr virus (EBV; HHV-4) causes **infectious mononucleosis** and can lead to cancers of lymphoid organs (commonly Burkitt lymphoma and nasopharyngeal cancer). The virus is transmitted by saliva (e.g., kissing) and infects oropharyngeal epithelium. It can then invade the bloodstream, where it infects B cells through the C3d complement receptor. EBV then causes a transformation in B cells, allowing them to evade normal growth and division controls. The result is massive proliferation of transformed B cells that contain latent viral DNA, and occasionally viral replication occurs within the cells until lysis releases them into the bloodstream. The immune response against these transformed B cells leads to the classic clinical picture of mononucleosis: lymph node and spleen enlargement,

Quick fact:
85% of patients with infectious mononucleosis develop an antibody-mediated rash when treated with ampicillin or penicillin.

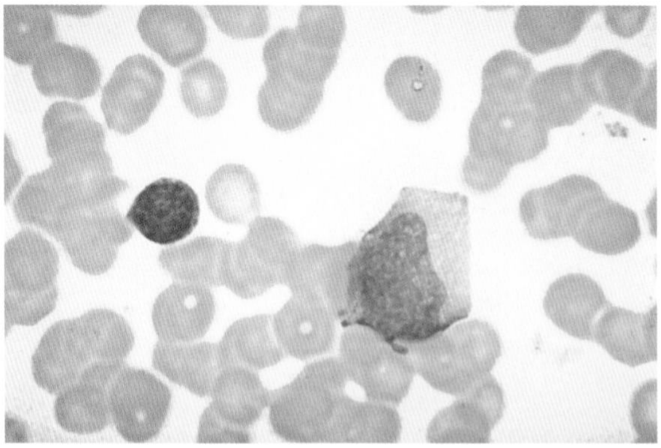

Fig. 5.33 Atypical lymphocytes in infectious mononucleosis—peripheral blood smear. The cell on the *left* is a normal small resting lymphocyte with a compact nucleus and scant cytoplasm. By contrast, the atypical lymphocyte on the *right* has abundant cytoplasm and a large nucleus with dispersed chromatin. (*From Kumar V, Abbas AK, Fausto N, et al.* Robbins and Cotran's Pathologic Basis of Disease. *8th ed. Philadelphia: Elsevier; 2009.*)

flulike symptoms, and painful pharyngitis. Patients with active mononucleosis are at **risk for splenic rupture**—no contact sports! If you give a patient with EBV amoxicillin thinking it is strep throat, they will break out into a macular rash.

Testing for EBV can be done with the Monospot test, which tests for the **heterophile antibody** (sensitive but not specific). Confirmation of the diagnosis is by **anti-EBV immunoglobulin M (IgM). Atypical CD8$^+$ cytotoxic lymphocytes** can also be seen on blood smear (Fig. 5.33).

If transformed B cells are not well controlled by the immune system and are allowed to proliferate, they will accrue mutations that can eventually lead to lymphoid cancers. EBV-associated Burkitt lymphoma is common in African children. EBV can also cause non-Hodgkin lymphoma and oral hairy leukoplakia in HIV-infected patients. Nasopharyngeal carcinoma in southern Chinese populations has also been highly associated with EBV infection.

Varicella-Zoster Virus

Varicella-zoster virus (HHV-3) causes **chickenpox** (primary infection) and **shingles** (reactivation infection). Transmission occurs through exposure to respiratory droplets or by direct contact with a varicella skin lesion. After inoculation, there is a 2-week incubation period followed by a viremic phase with fever, malaise, and pharyngitis, followed 24 hours later by the classic **"dew drops on rose petals"** vesicular rash that spreads outward in crops from the trunk and face (Fig. 5.34). The lesions rupture and crust over in 1 week, at which point the patient is no longer contagious. The entire process is relatively mild in immunocompetent children, whereas adolescents, adults, and immunocompromised patients generally experience more severe disease (**pneumonia and encephalitis** are common complications in these groups). Since the introduction of the VZV vaccine in 1995, the rate of hospitalization for these patients has declined significantly.

Because VZV can cause birth defects (microcephaly, limb hypoplasia, skin scarring), pregnant women must be especially protected. If a pregnant woman is exposed to someone with active VZV lesions (either chicken pox or shingles), she should receive **varicella-zoster immune globulin.** Do not give pregnant women the varicella vaccine because it is a live vaccine (pregnancy is a contraindication for live vaccines).

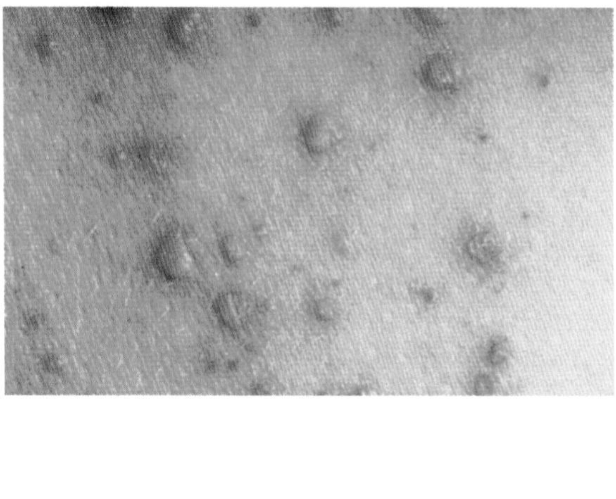

Fig. 5.34 Classic vesiculopapular rash of varicella chickenpox. (*From Goering R, Dockrell H, Wakelin D, et al.* Mims' Medical Microbiology. *4th ed. Philadelphia: Elsevier; 2007. Courtesy M. J. Wood.*)

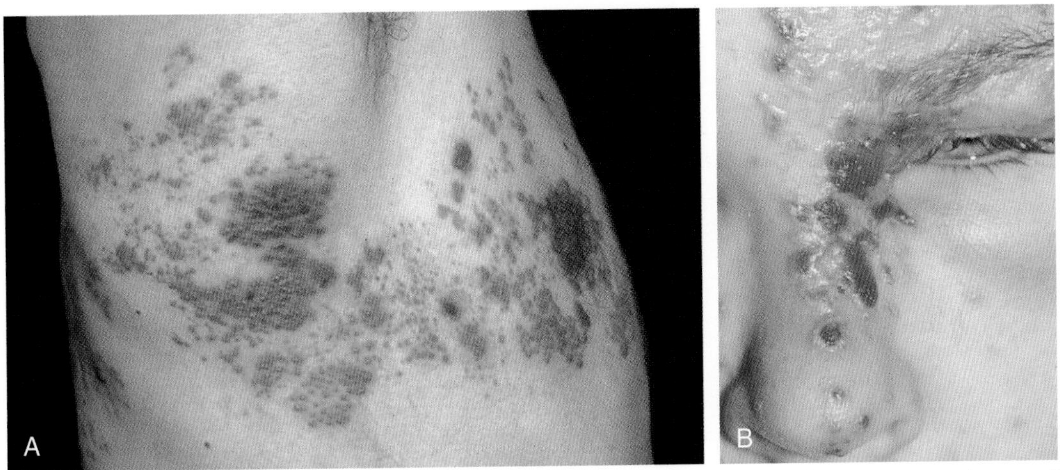

FIG. 5.35 **A,** Shingles affecting the chest of a patient. **B,** Herpes zoster ophthalmicus, demonstrating involvement of the V1 branch of the trigeminal nerve. Hutchison's sign is present, where the rash involves the tip of the nose; this is indicative of V1 involvement. (***A,*** *from Lim E, Loke YK, Thompson A. Medicine and Surgery. Edinburgh: Elsevier; 2007.* ***B,*** *from Dennis M, Bowen WT, Cho L. Mechanisms of Clinical Signs. Sydney: Elsevier; 2011.*)

VZV remains latent in sensory ganglia and can reactivate in times of stress or immune suppression. The reactivation is called "shingles" and consists of a painful burning prodrome overlaying a **specific dermatome** followed by a vesicular rash (*hint:* Remember that dermatomes don't cross the midline, so the rash of shingles doesn't either; Fig. 5.35). As with HSV, diagnosis of VZV can be accomplished with Tzanck smear (multinucleated giant cells), skin biopsy (Cowdry bodies), direct fluorescence antibody testing, and viral PCR. Treat with **high-dose acyclovir** to decrease duration and risk of postherpetic neuralgia.

Other Herpes Viruses: Human herpesvirus 6 (HHV-6) causes **roseola,** or **exanthem subitum,** consisting of a 3- to 5-day high fever followed by a 1- to 2-day rash on the trunk (the key is that *the rash occurs after the fever has resolved*). It is transmitted by saliva and occurs mostly in infants. HHV-8 is the cause of **Kaposi sarcoma** in AIDS patients and is transmitted sexually (see section on AIDS-related infections).

Hepadnaviridae

- **Capsid:** icosahedral
- **Envelope:** enveloped
- **DNA structure:** double-stranded, circular
- **Viruses of clinical significance:** hepatitis B virus

Orthohepadnavirus

Orthohepadnavirus (hepatitis B virus) is the only member of the orthohepadnavirus family. The other hepatitis viruses are RNA viruses (the "hepatitis" viruses are a heterogenous group, clumped together because they primarily infect the liver). Orthohepadnavirus is extremely contagious, existing in all body fluids of an infected person. Transmission occurs by contact with fluids, through sexual encounters, transplacentally, by accidental needle sticks, or by needle sharing. The hepa**DNA**virus uses DNA, not RNA.

Under electron microscopy, one can see the intact virus particle **(Dane particle),** which looks like a sphere. One can also see strands of capsid and envelope proteins that have broken off; these are called the hepatitis B surface antigen (HBsAg; Fig. 5.36). Antibodies to this antigen (anti-HBsAg) confer immunity to the virus. A patient can also develop antibodies to the **core antigens** (HBcAg), but these are not protective. During active viral replication, another antigen is released called HBeAg, which is a marker for active disease.

The serology of hepatitis B is complicated, but worth memorizing:

- HBsAg = disease (chronic, acute, carrier)
- Anti-HBsAg = immunity, after either resolved infection or immunization. Appearance of anti-HBsAg corresponds to the disappearance of HBsAg

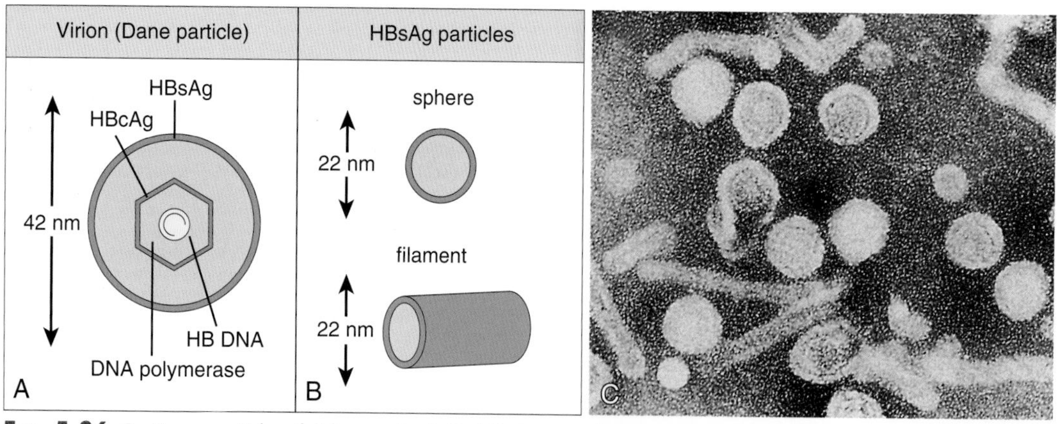

FIG. 5.36 A, Dane particles (full intact virus). **B,** HBsAg particles. **C,** Dane particles and HBsAg under electron microscopy. *(From Goering R, Dockrell H, Wakelin D, et al.* Mims' Medical Microbiology. *4th ed. Philadelphia: Elsevier; 2007. Courtesy J. D. Almeida.)*

- Anti-HBcAg IgM = new infection
- Anti-HBcAg IgG = old infection
- HBeAg = high infectivity
- Anti-HBeAg = low infectivity

There are several different disease states that can result from HBV infection:

- Asymptomatic carriers harbor the virus but never develop anti-HBsAg antibodies and never develop liver damage. Often, these patients are immunocompromised because it's the immune reaction that does most of the liver damage.
- Chronic persistent hepatitis: a low-grade smoldering hepatitis
- Chronic active hepatitis: an acute hepatitis that just doesn't resolve
- Fulminant hepatitis: acute hepatitis with rapid destruction of the liver

Complications of chronic HBV infection include **primary hepatocellular carcinoma** and **cirrhosis.** Diagnosis is by detection of HBsAg. Anti-HBcAg serology (IgM vs. IgG) is a marker of the length of disease in both acute and chronic states. HBeAg and anti-HBeAg tell you how infectious the patient is (Table 5.4).

Parvoviridae

- **Capsid:** icosahedral
- **Envelope:** nonenveloped (naked)
- **DNA structure:** single-stranded, linear
- **Viruses of clinical significance:** parvovirus B19

Parvovirus

Parvovirus B19 is a small, nonenveloped virus with single-stranded DNA (the only DNA virus with ssDNA). The virus inoculates the nasal cavity, leading to viremia and fever. It has a special preference

TABLE 5.4 Patterns of HBV Serology in Different Stages of Infection

	HBsAg	ANTI-HBsAg	ANTI-HBcAg IgM	ANTI-HBcAg IgG	HBeAg	ANTI-HBeAg
Acute infection	√		√		√	
Chronic infection—more contagious	√			√	√	
Chronic infection—less contagious	√			√		√
Resolved infection		√		√		√
Immunized		√				

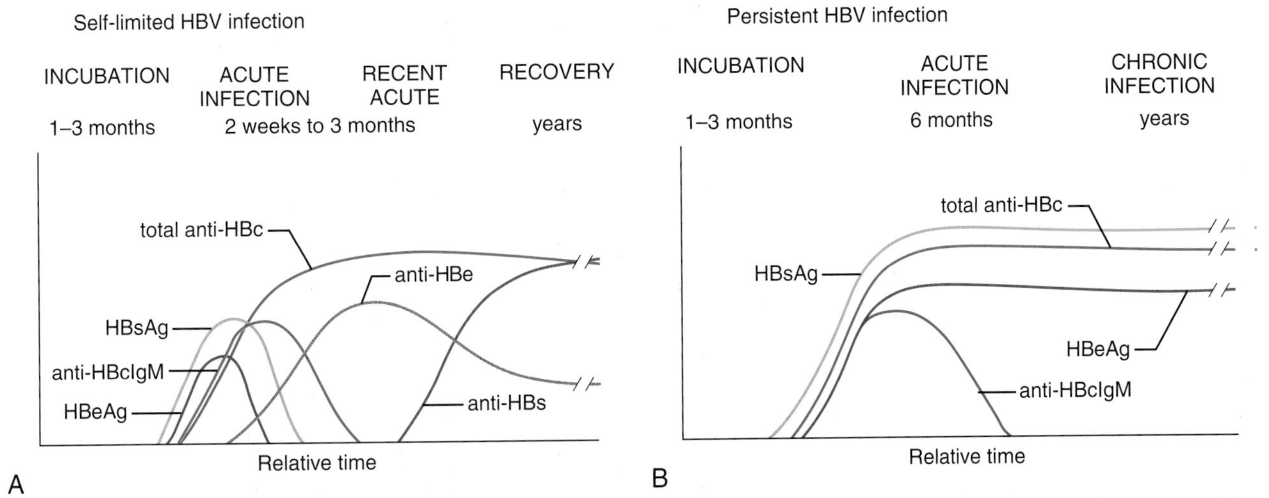

FIG. 5.37 A, Clinical and virologic course of hepatitis B, with recovery. **B,** Clinical and virologic course in a carrier of hepatitis B. (*From Goering R, Dockrell H, Wakelin D, et al. Mims' Medical Microbiology. 4th ed. Philadelphia: Elsevier; 2007. Redrawn from Farrar WE, Wood MJ, Innes JA, et al.* Infectious Diseases. *2nd ed. London: Mosby International; 1992.*)

for erythrocyte precursor cells, lysing them as the virus replicates. Normal individuals can tolerate this lack of erythropoiesis, but those with chronic hemolytic disorders (sickle cell anemia, thalassemia) or HIV/AIDS can experience a **transient aplastic anemia crisis.** In children with normal erythropoiesis, immune complex deposition in the skin and joints leads to a classic rash with a "slapped cheek" appearance and arthralgias for several days, called **erythema infectiosum** or "fifth disease." Other clinical syndromes include hydrops fetalis in a fetus infected in the first half of pregnancy and chronic anemia in an immunocompromised patient.

Papovaviridae

- **Capsid:** icosahedral
- **Envelope:** nonenveloped (naked)
- **DNA structure:** double-stranded, circular
- **Viruses of clinical significance:** human papillomavirus, polyomaviruses (BK virus and JC virus)

Human Papillomavirus

Human papillomavirus (HPV) is the most common STI in the United States. It infects the basal layer of squamous epithelium of the skin and mucosa. The virus uses **E6** and **E7** proteins to turn off replication checkpoints (p53 and Rb, respectively) in basal cells. This causes proliferation of cells, which we see as warts **(condyloma acuminata).** Strains **6 and 11** are the most highly associated with benign warts (both genital and nongenital). Other strains, particularly strains **16 and 18,** cause the development of cervical cancer, anal cancer, and oropharyngeal cancer. Figs. 5.37 and 5.38 show common clinical presentations of HPV.

Special clinical situations include the following:

- Patients with **epidermodysplasia verruciformis,** an autosomal recessive disorder, have a particular susceptibility to HPV and present with many flat warts all over their body in childhood. They are at particular risk for squamous cell carcinomas in adulthood.
- Infants born to mothers with genital warts can get laryngeal warts that cause airway obstruction.

Currently, screening recommendations are for women to begin having Papanicolaou (Pap) smears at age 21 years for detection of HPV (by PCR) and looking for evidence of dysplastic cells. A positive Pap smear may warrant further evaluation with colposcopy, in which 1% acetic acid is used to visualize any neoplastic lesions (they turn white). Any visualized lesions can then be biopsied. The advent of HPV vaccines has significantly reduced the incidence of HPV-caused cancers and warts (Gardasil protects against strains 6, 11, 16, 18, whereas Cervarix only protects against strains 16 and 18).

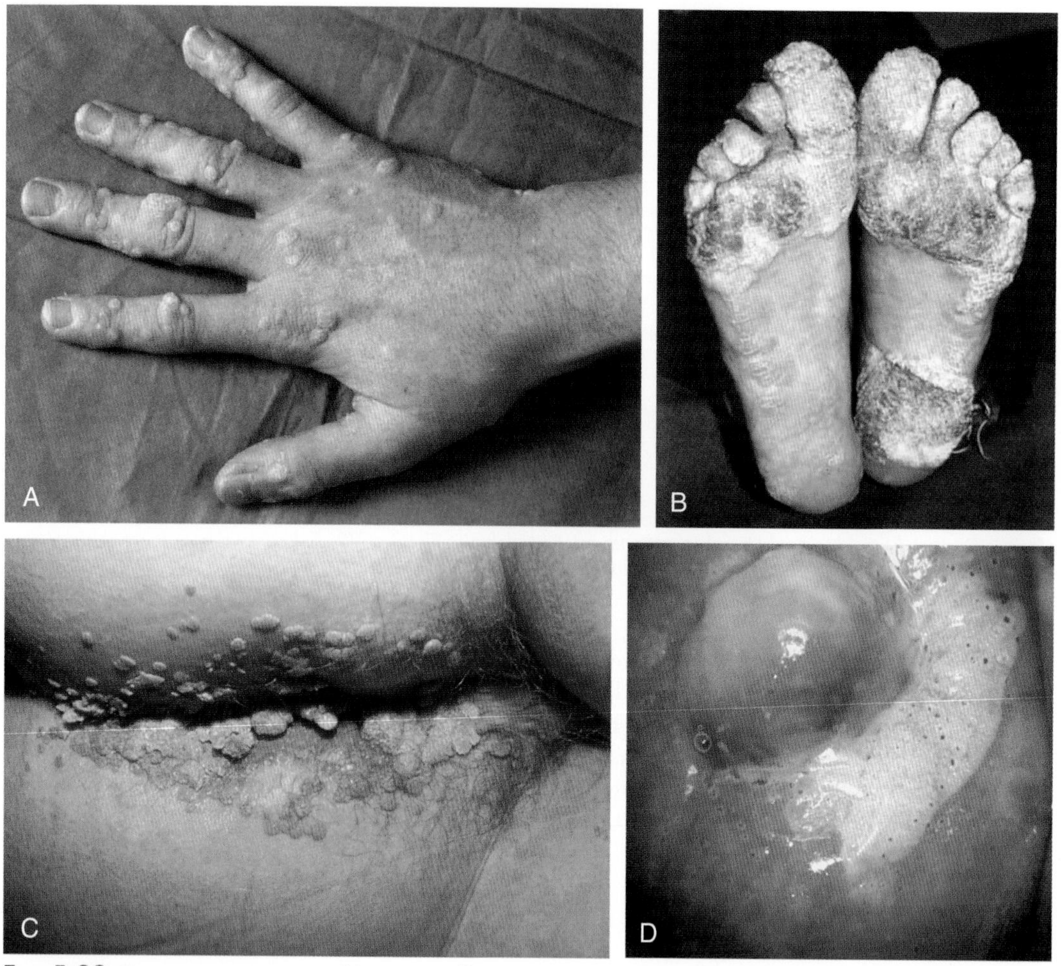

FIG. 5.38 Common presentations of human papillomavirus. **A,** Hand warts on a child. **B,** Plantar warts in a renal transplant recipient. **C,** Genital warts (condyloma acuminata). **D,** Cervical wart after application of acetic acid. (*From Greenwood D, Slack R, Peitherer J, Barer M. Medical Microbiology. 17th ed. Philadelphia: Elsevier; 2007. Courtesy Drs. M. H. Bunney and E. C. Benton.*)

Polyomaviruses

Polyomaviruses are ubiquitous and have two clinically important members: BK virus and JC virus. Both cause mild primary disease in an immunocompetent host and then lie dormant, causing disease during immunocompromise. In particular, BK virus has a tropism for genitourinary epithelium and can cause nephropathy and hemorrhagic cystitis in the immunocompromised host (classically, it causes allograft nephropathy after kidney transplantation). JC virus prefers to infect oligodendrocytes of the CNS, causing **progressive multifocal leukoencephalopathy (PML)** in an immunocompromised host, characterized by impaired coordination, speech, and memory.

Remember: **PA**pillomavirus and **PO**lyomavirus are **PAPO**vaviridae.

Causes of the common cold: rhinovirus, coronavirus, adenovirus, influenza C virus, and coxsackievirus.

Adenoviridae

- **Capsid:** icosahedral
- **Envelope:** nonenveloped (naked)
- **DNA structure:** double-stranded, linear
- **Viruses of clinical significance:** adenoviruses (50 subtypes)

Most common causes of conjunctivitis: *H. influenzae*, adenovirus, *S. pneumoniae*.

Adenoviruses are a group of 50 different subtypes that are an important cause of febrile illness, especially in preschools and in households with small children. Spread occurs by aerosol droplets, fecal–oral route, or direct contact. The virus binds through **hemagglutinin** entering and lysing epithelial cells of the following:

Respiratory tract: rhinitis, pharyngitis, and occasionally atypical pneumonia

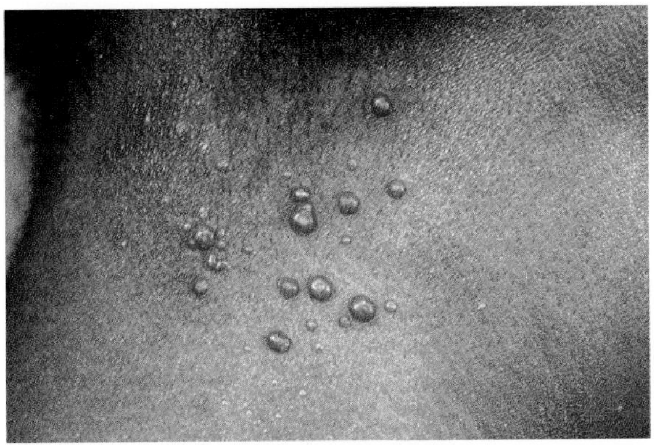

FIG. 5.39 Molluscum contagiosum. (*From Lim E, Loke YK, Thompson A. Medicine and Surgery. Edinburgh: Elsevier; 2007.*)

Conjunctiva: conjunctivitis
Bladder: hemorrhagic cystitis
GI tract: gastroenteritis with nonbloody diarrhea

A vaccine has been developed but is only used by the military. Immunocompromised individuals with severe adenoviral infections can be treated with **cidofovir.**

Poxviridae

- **Capsid:** complex
- **Envelope:** enveloped
- **DNA structure:** double-stranded, linear
- **Viruses of clinical significance:** smallpox (variola) virus, molluscum contagiosum

Variola virus was the cause of smallpox (fever, rash, high mortality) but was eradicated in 1979, and no cases have been reported since. ***Molluscum contagiosum*** is spread by skin-to-skin contact and causes pearly, umbilicated, dome-shaped papules (Fig. 5.39). It can be thought of as a chronic, localized, mild version of smallpox. Widespread disease can occur in immunocompromised patients (consider HIV). The palms and soles are spared in this case. Diagnosis can be made clinically, with confirmation by hematoxylin and eosin (H&E) staining of a lesion showing eosinophilic inclusion bodies ("molluscum bodies").

RNA VIRUSES

RNA viruses are presented in two sections: naked RNA viruses (lacking an envelope) and enveloped RNA viruses. Naked viruses are resistant to heat, drying, and detergents, allowing for prolonged survival, whereas viral envelopes are sensitive to these exposures.

Naked RNA Viruses

Picornaviruses

- **Capsid:** icosahedral
- **Envelope:** nonenveloped (naked)
- **RNA structure:** single-stranded, linear, positive sense
- **Viruses of clinical significance: p**oliovirus, **e**chovirus, **r**hinovirus, **c**oxsackievirus, **h**epatitis A virus **("PERCH")**

Most common causes of aseptic meningitis in the United States: echovirus, coxsackievirus, mumps virus.

The **picornavirus** (meaning "small RNA virus") family consists of nonenveloped, single-stranded, positive-sense RNA viruses. Clinically important members of this viral family cause enteric disease (the so-called **enteroviruses: poliovirus, echovirus, the "numbered" enteroviruses,** and **coxsackievirus**), hepatitis **(hepatitis A),** and the common cold **(rhinoviruses).**

Poliovirus has been nearly eradicated worldwide with the advent of vaccination and improved sanitation. The Sal**k** (**"K" = killed**) vaccine consists of formalin-killed, inactivated poliovirus (IPV). The Sabin oral polio vaccine (OPV) consists of a live attenuated strain. Before total use of the IPV, a rare complication of the OPV was vaccine-associated paralytic poliomyelitis (discussed later).

The virus is spread by the fecal–oral route, replicates in the tonsils and Peyer patches of the intestinal tract, and spreads through blood and lymph to the brain and spinal cord. There are three forms of the disease: **subclinical or mild illness** (febrile illness lasting 72 hours or less), **aseptic meningitis** (fever, neck pain and stiffness, skin rash, vomiting lasting 1–2 weeks), and **paralytic poliomyelitis.** Paralytic poliomyelitis is caused by viral infection of the **motor neurons of the anterior horn.** This causes muscle spasms and **asymmetric descending paralysis** (proximal muscles first, then distal) of the extremities. When bulbar nerves are involved, the diaphragm may be affected, leading to the need for respiratory support. Muscle tone and reflexes are eventually lost. Normal sensory nerve function is retained. Recovery of motor neuron function occurs over up to 6 months.

Echovirus is a common enterovirus, most common in the summer and fall. It can cause a spectrum of disease, from febrile illness, to URI symptoms, to petechial or purpuric rashes (serotype 9), to **maculopapular rash** (nonpruritic, salmon-pink macules of the face and upper chest). It mostly affects children and is the **most common cause of aseptic meningitis and encephalitis in children younger than 1 year.**

Rhinovirus (100+ species) is responsible for symptoms of the common cold (rhinorrhea, nasal congestion, cough, sore or scratchy throat). Most serotypes of rhinovirus bind to ICAM-1 on the epithelial cells that line the nasopharynx. It is easily transmissible from person to person through nasal secretions or by aerosolized droplets (cover your cough!). Unlike other picornaviruses, it does not transmit by fecal–oral routes because it degrades in gastric acid.

There are two groups of ***coxsackieviruses:*** **Coxsackie A** and **Coxsackie B**. Both Coxsackie A and B viruses can cause a nonspecific febrile illness, symptoms of the common cold, diffuse rash, and aseptic meningitis. **Coxsackie A** causes **herpangina** (febrile illness, small red vesicles at the back of the mouth) and **hand-foot-and-mouth disease** (febrile illness, small red vesicles of the mouth, *and* rashes of the palms and soles, Fig. 5.40). **Coxsackie B** can affect the heart (**myocarditis** or **pericarditis**) and the lungs **(pleurodynia)** and can also cause hepatitis and pancreatitis.

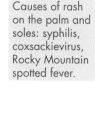

Causes of rash on the palm and soles: syphilis, coxsackievirus, Rocky Mountain spotted fever.

The **numbered enteroviruses** cause a multitude of symptoms. Enterovirus 71, for example, can cause hand-foot-mouth disease, encephalomyelitis or other severe neurologic disease, pulmonary hemorrhage, and cardiovascular collapse. Importantly, patients who lack robust antibody production (e.g., those with Bruton agammaglobulinemia) are particularly susceptible to severe enteroviral infections.

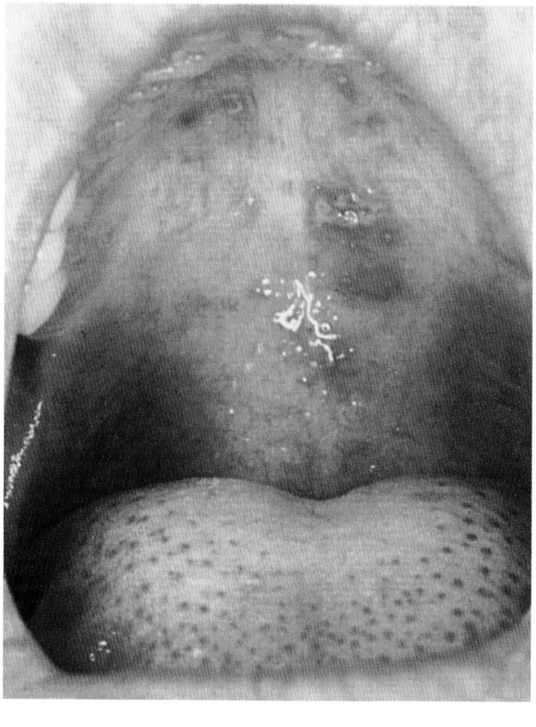

FIG. 5.40 Mouth lesions in hand-foot-and-mouth disease caused by Coxsackie A virus. (*From Goering R, Dockrell H, Wakelin D, et al.* Mims' Medical Microbiology. *4th ed. Philadelphia: Elsevier; 2007. Courtesy J. A. Innes.*)

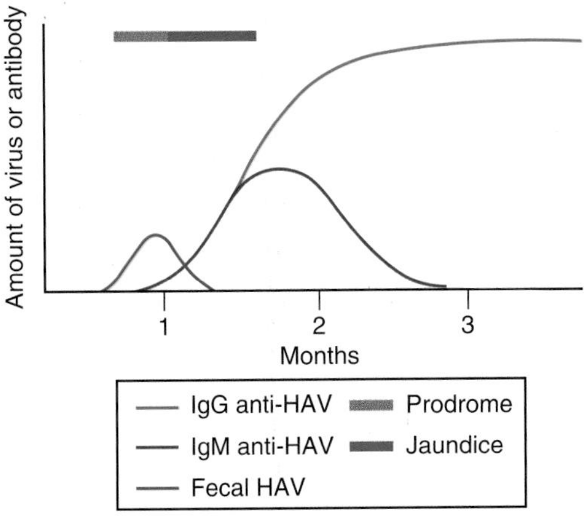

FIG. 5.41 Clinical course of hepatitis A infection. (*From Greenwood D, Slack R, Peitherer J, Barer M. Medical Microbiology. 17th ed. Philadelphia: Elsevier; 2007.*)

Hepatitis A virus (HAV) can cause a spectrum of disease from **asymptomatic** subclinical disease in young children to self-limited acute hepatitis with jaundice, and, in very rare cases (1% of individuals), to fulminant hepatic failure (Fig. 5.41). It is transferred by the fecal–oral route and is often associated with food- or waterborne outbreaks. Prodromal symptoms include fatigue, malaise, nausea, vomiting, anorexia, fever, and **right upper quadrant pain.** Diagnosis is by anti-HAV IgM. **Anti-HAV IgG indicates old disease and protects against future infection.** Vaccination against HAV is now included as a routine pediatric vaccine and is recommended for travelers to endemic countries.

Hepeviruses

Capsid: icosahedral
Envelope: nonenveloped (naked)
RNA structure: single-stranded, linear, positive sense
Viruses of clinical significance: hepatitis E virus

The most medically important member of the **Hepeviridae** family is the **hepatitis E virus** ("**E**" for **e**nteric). Clinical presentation is similar to that of **hepatitis A** and usually causes a self-limited viral hepatitis in immunocompetent individuals. Hepatitis E can cause **fulminant hepatic failure in pregnant women** and a chronic infection in immunocompromised patients (e.g., transplant recipients). It is endemic to the Indian subcontinent and Southeast Asia. Outbreaks are common after heavy flooding because the virus is spread by the fecal–oral route or through food- or waterborne outbreaks. A common mnemonic to help remember that hepatitis A and hepatitis E both have fecal–oral transmission is "the vowels (A and E) go through your bowels."

HAV and HEV (unlike HBV, HCV, and HDV) have oral transmission, no carrier state, no cirrhosis, and no hepatocellular carcinoma.

Caliciviruses

- **Capsid:** icosahedral
- **Envelope:** nonenveloped (naked)
- **RNA structure:** single-stranded, linear, positive sense
- **Viruses of clinical significance:** Norwalk virus

The calicivirus family has several genera, of which ***noroviruses*** are the most relevant to human disease. The ***Norwalk virus*** and other **noroviruses** are a major cause of acute viral gastroenteritis in individuals of all ages. Noroviruses cause vomiting and diarrhea and may be accompanied by fever, myalgia, and headache. Symptoms are usually self-limited (48–72 hours) and resolve with supportive care. Noroviruses are highly contagious and spread by the fecal–oral route, aerosolized droplets, contaminated food (often shellfish), and surfaces. Outbreaks in enclosed communities are common (**daycare centers, schools, cruise ships).** As with other naked viruses, norovirus infections are best prevented with diligent handwashing and thorough cleaning of affected surfaces with bleach.

Reoviruses (Respiratory Enteric Orphan Viruses)

- **Capsid:** icosahedral
- **Envelope:** nonenveloped (naked)

- **RNA structure:** double-stranded (only double-stranded RNA viruses), segmented (10–12)
- **Viruses of clinical significance:** reovirus (Colorado tick fever), rotavirus

Reoviruses are nonenveloped, double-stranded, and segmented RNA viruses. Their genetic material is divided into 10 to 12 **segments.** As naked viruses, the Reoviridae are resistant to drying and to detergents, which allows for prolonged survival in the environment outside of a host. They are easily transmissible between host (i.e., respiratory secretions, saliva, fecal–oral route) or by fomites. Naked viruses such as the Reoviridae are, however, sensitive to cleaning agents such as chlorine, bleach, and high heat, which is fortunate because outbreaks of highly contagious diarrheal illness are caused by members of the Reoviridae family.

Rotavirus causes gastroenteritis and is the **most common worldwide cause of fatal diarrhea in children.** Rotavirus is also to blame for epidemics of diarrheal illness in daycare centers. After an incubation period of about 2 days, symptoms may start with vomiting and fever, followed by **nonbloody diarrhea (watery or yellow stools).** The virus causes villous atrophy and impairs gut absorption of sodium and water (Fig. 5.42). Minimal to moderate fecal leukocytes are visualized. Treatment is supportive and is centered on preventing dehydration. Oral vaccination for infants and children (live, attenuated virus) is recommended. A previous rotavirus vaccine, withdrawn from the market in 1999, was associated with an increased risk for **intussusception.**

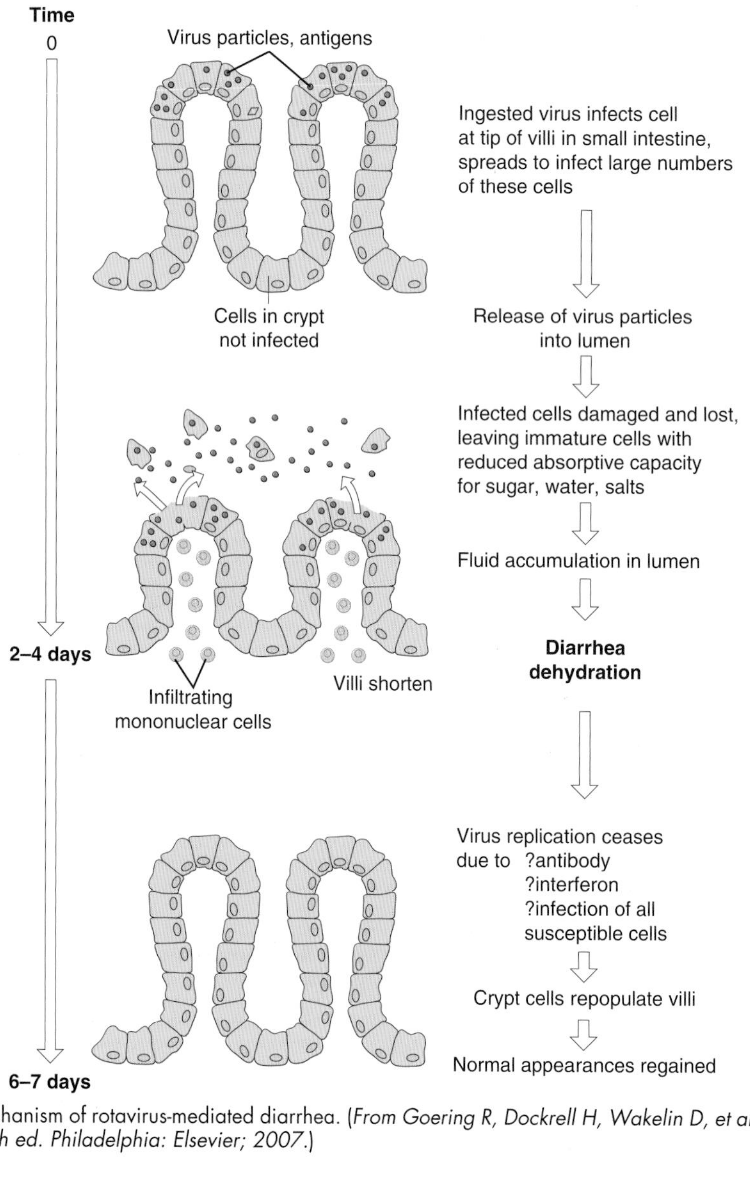

FIG. 5.42 Mechanism of rotavirus-mediated diarrhea. (*From Goering R, Dockrell H, Wakelin D, et al.* Mims' Medical Microbiology. *4th ed. Philadelphia: Elsevier; 2007.*)

Another type of reovirus causes ***Colorado tick fever,*** which is transmitted by the wood tick (*Dermacentor*) and is geographically limited to the Western United States. As a bloodborne infection, it has also been known to be transmitted by blood transfusion. Peak incidence is in the months of April to June. Illness is characterized by fever/recurrent fevers, chills, myalgia, petechial or maculopapular rash, and/or leukopenia 3 to 6 days after a tick bite.

Enveloped RNA Viruses

Flaviviruses

- **Capsid:** icosahedral
- **Envelope:** enveloped
- **RNA structure:** single-stranded, linear, positive
- **Viruses of clinical significance:** hepatitis C virus, yellow fever virus, dengue fever virus, West Nile virus, St. Louis encephalitis virus, Japanese encephalitis virus

Flaviviruses are single-stranded, positive-sense RNA viruses. This family includes hepatitis C, the most common worldwide cause of cirrhosis and the most common cause of hepatocellular carcinoma in the United States.

Many of the flaviviruses are arboviruses, or spread by the bite of an infected arthropod—a tick (i.e., tickborne encephalitis) or mosquito (e.g., yellow fever or West Nile virus). They can cause febrile illness (e.g., Dengue fever, yellow fever) and encephalitis (e.g., West Nile virus, St. Louis encephalitis virus, Japanese encephalitis virus).

Hepatitis C virus (HCV) is transmitted parenterally (IV drug use, blood transfusion, sexual contact, other bloodborne exposure). Initial infection is often asymptomatic or subclinical (fatigue, constitutional symptoms) but can present as acute hepatitis (i.e., fever, nausea, right upper quadrant pain). About 80% of hepatitis C infections become chronic, and 30% of these persistent infections progress to severe complications—cirrhosis and hepatocellular carcinoma. Cirrhosis from hepatitis C is second only to cirrhosis resulting from alcohol consumption in the United States. HCV mutates easily, and adaptive immune to rapidly changing antigens can form autoantibodies and immune complexes that can cause vasculitis from mixed cryoglobulinemia, as well as glomerulonephritis. Treatment until recently consisted of pegylated interferon alfa plus ribavirin and was effective with significant side effects. Newer antiviral therapies exist and regimens are tailored to the patient's HCV genotype. For genotype 1a HCV (the most common genotype in North America), sofosbuvir with simeprevir or ledipasvir can achieve a sustained virologic response in a vast majority of patients.

Yellow fever virus is transmitted by the bite of the *Aedes aegypti* mosquito and is endemic to South America and sub-Saharan Africa. Vaccination (live attenuated strain) is required for travelers to these endemic areas. Most people infected with yellow fever are asymptomatic. In those who develop illness, initial presentation is a febrile illness with malaise, headache, myalgia, nausea, and vomiting lasting a few days. After a brief 1- to 2-day remission of symptoms, 15% of affected individuals progress to jaundice ("yellow" fever), renal failure, and hemorrhagic fever (coagulopathy, cutaneous, mucosal, or GI bleeding ["black vomit"]).

Dengue fever virus is also transmitted by the *A. aegypti* mosquito and is found worldwide, including the southern United States. It causes a painful febrile illness ("break-bone fever"), with headache and severe muscle and joint pains for up to 1 week. Treatment is supportive. Repeat infection, especially with serotype 2, causes a severe immunologic response that results in dengue hemorrhagic fever, characterized by fever and severe hemorrhage (petechiae, spontaneous bleeding, thrombocytopenia) and leading to shock and possibly death (Fig. 5.43).

West Nile virus (WNV) is among a group of flaviviruses that cause fever, meningitis, and encephalitis. WNV, St. Louis encephalitis, and Japanese encephalitis virus are transmitted by the bite of the *Culex* mosquito. They are appropriately named for the region in which they were first endemic. **St. Louis encephalitis virus** was first identified in St. Louis, Missouri; **Japanese encephalitis virus** is the most common cause of viral meningitis in Southeast Asia.

West Nile virus is endemic worldwide, causing outbreaks in **North America,** Europe, Africa, West Asia, the Middle East, and Australia. It is asymptomatic in most people infected with the virus. In symptomatic individuals, the milder manifestation is West Nile fever, characterized by fever, malaise, myalgia, and in one out of two individuals, a maculopapular rash. More severe manifestations are meningitis or encephalitis with muscle weakness or **acute asymmetric flaccid paralysis.**

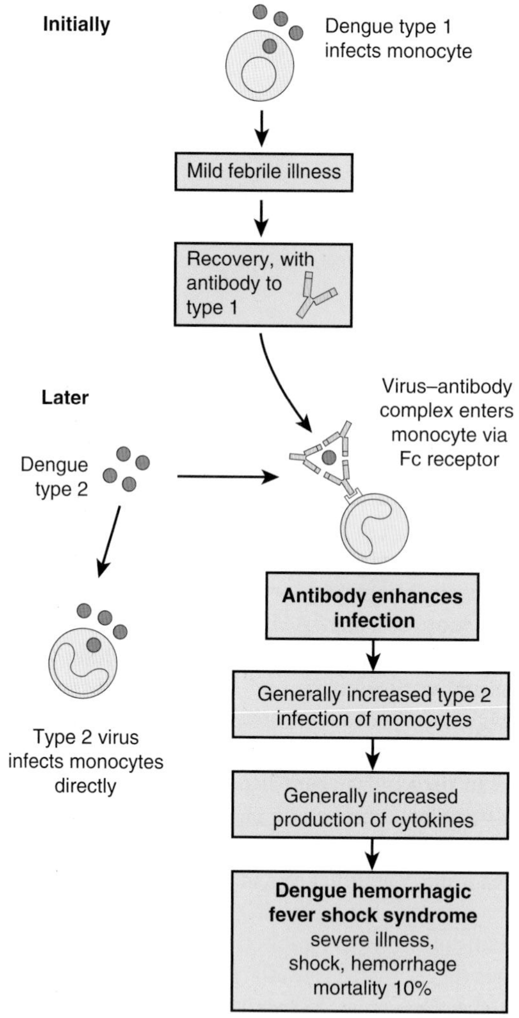

Fig. 5.43 Pathophysiology of dengue hemorrhagic fever. (*From Goering R, Dockrell H, Wakelin D, et al. Mims' Medical Microbiology. 4th ed. Philadelphia: Elsevier; 2007.*)

Immunocompromised individuals and older adults are at greater risk for developing severe disease or complications.

Togaviruses

- **Capsid:** icosahedral
- **Envelope:** enveloped
- **RNA structure:** single-stranded, linear, positive
- **Viruses of clinical significance:** rubella virus, Eastern equine encephalitis, Western equine encephalitis

The **togavirus** family is composed of **alpha viruses** and **rubivirus.** Alpha viruses (**Eastern equine encephalitis virus** and **Western equine encephalitis virus**) are **arboviruses** (discussed earlier) and cause **encephalitis** (as you probably guessed). Rubivirus (Rubella virus) causes the febrile illness **rubella.**

Eastern equine encephalitis (EEE) virus is found in the eastern United States and is so named because it was first isolated from horse brains. It is transmitted by the bite of an infected mosquito (such as the pesky *Aedes* mosquito). In infected humans, EEE virus causes encephalitis with a mortality rate of about 35%. The closely related arbovirus ***Western equine encephalitis (WEE)*** virus is endemic to the western United States and causes less severe encephalitis than EEE. Mortality rates from WEE are lower (about 4%). Treatment is supportive, and vaccination is available for horses only.

The five most common pediatric diseases with rash: measles, rubella, scarlet fever, roseola, erythema infectiosum.

Rubella virus is transmitted through the respiratory secretions of infected individuals. In children and adults, rubella virus causes **rubella** (German measles), a febrile illness followed by acute onset of pink, maculopapular rash (Fig. 5.44) that spreads from the head, to trunk, and to the extremities. This rash lasts 3 days (**"3-day rash"**) and can be accompanied by joint pains. In contrast to the rash of rubeola (measles), **the**

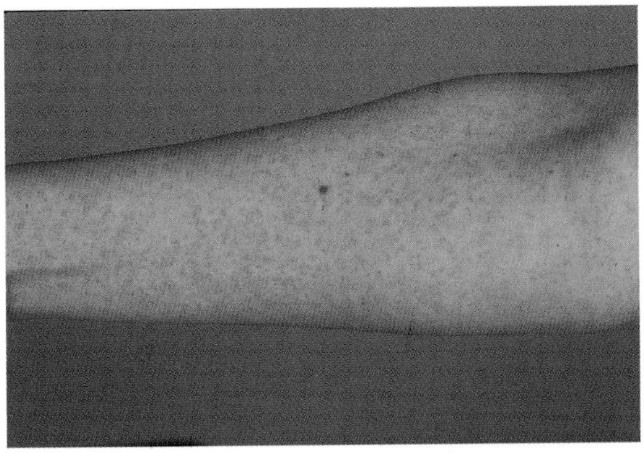

FIG. 5.44 Maculopapular rash of rubella. (*From Greenwood D, Slack R, Peitherer J, Barer M. Medical Microbiology. 17th ed. Philadelphia: Elsevier; 2007.*)

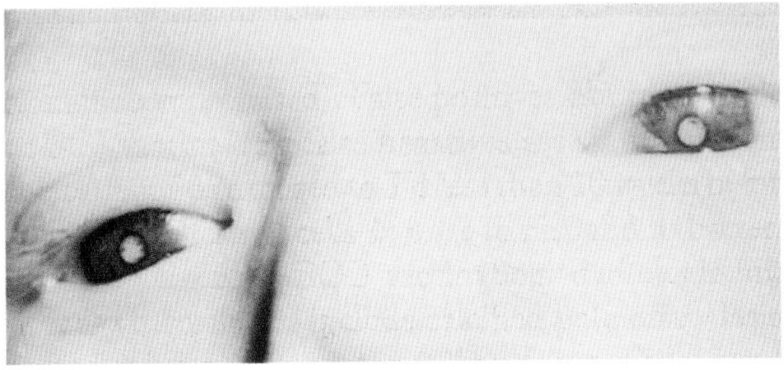

FIG. 5.45 Bilateral congenital cataracts as a result of congenital rubella infection. (*From Moore KL, Persaud TVN. The Developing Human. 8th ed. Philadelphia; Elsevier: 2007. Courtesy Dr. Richard Bargy, Cornell-New York Hospital, New York.*)

rubella rash is distributed similarly but spreads more rapidly and does not darken or coalesce. Whereas measles causes Koplik spots on the buccal mucosa, rubella may produce red petechiae on the soft palate (Forchheimer spots). In addition, the posterior cervical and occipital lymph nodes enlarge in rubella.

All children are vaccinated against rubella as part of the MMR (measles-mumps-rubella) vaccine. Pregnant women should not receive the MMR vaccine because of the theoretical risk for transplacental infection with the live, attenuated strain of rubella used in the vaccine. *In utero* infection with rubella causes congenital rubella, which affects the CNS (sensorineural hearing loss, microcephaly), eyes (congenital cataracts leading to blindness; Fig. 5.45), and heart (patent ductus arteriosus, pulmonary artery stenosis).

Retroviruses

- **Capsid:** icosahedral
- **Envelope:** enveloped
- **RNA structure:** single-stranded, linear, positive
- **Viruses of clinical significance:** human T-cell lymphotropic virus (HTLV), human immunodeficiency virus (HIV)

Retroviruses carry an enzyme called **reverse transcriptase**, an **RNA-dependent DNA polymerase.** In a retrograde fashion, it transcribes DNA from its own RNA genome. Another enzyme, known as **integrase,** integrates the viral DNA into the host genome.

Human T-cell lymphotropic virus type 1 (HTLV-1) is endemic to the Caribbean, parts of Japan, parts of the Pacific Islands, and parts of Africa. HTLV-1 is transmitted vertically and by contact with body fluids. Two diseases have been associated with HTLV-1: **adult T-cell leukemia/lymphoma (ATL)** and **tropical spastic paraparesis. ATL** is a neoplasm with circulating lymphocytes known as "flower cells" or "clover leaf cells" because of their abnormally convoluted nuclei. It presents with lymphadenopathy, hepatosplenomegaly, and **bone and skin findings.** Dermatologic findings may include **skin infiltrates** on biopsy (**Pautrier microabscess**). **Tropical spastic paraparesis** is a demyelinating infection of the spinal cord that causes slowly progressive lower extremity weakness and spasticity.

Human immunodeficiency virus (HIV) is one of the great public health challenges for the current generation of doctors, the pandemic of our time. The history of its discovery and understanding is steeped in science, politics, and culture, but this is a review book, and we digress! Remember that there are two HIV viruses. This section discusses HIV-1, the cause of **acquired immunodeficiency syndrome (AIDS).**

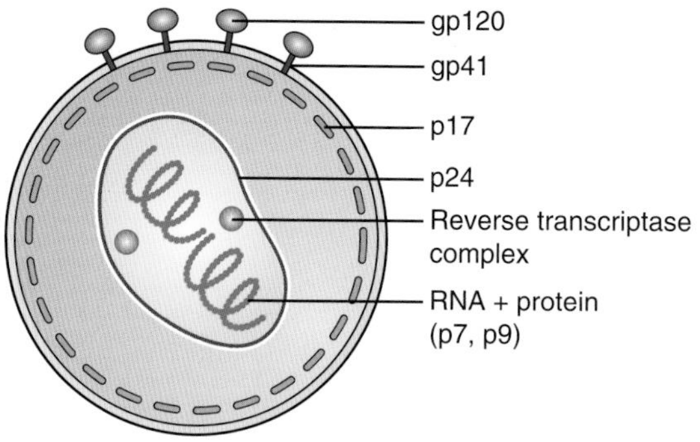

Fig. 5.46 HIV viral structure. (*From Greenwood D, Slack R, Peitherer J, Barer M. Medical Microbiology. 17th ed. Philadelphia: Elsevier; 2007.*)

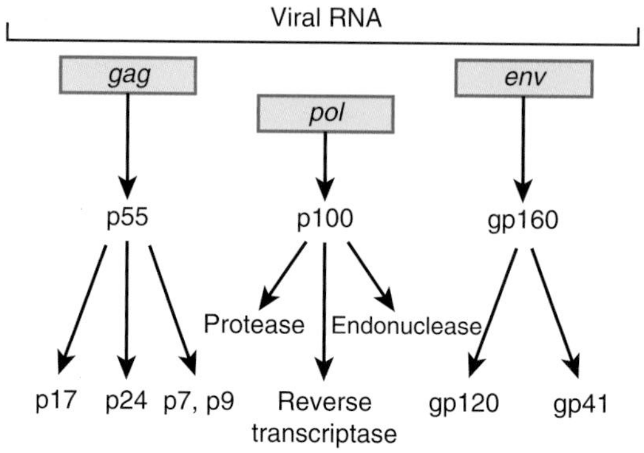

Fig. 5.47 HIV viral RNA genes and the proteins they code. (*From Greenwood D, Slack R, Peitherer J, Barer M. Medical Microbiology. 17th ed. Philadelphia: Elsevier; 2007.*)

At the center of the virion are two identical strands of ssRNA, associated with the nucleocapsid proteins **protease, reverse transcriptase, and integrase.** Surrounding these central components is the capsid shell, the most important protein of which is **p24.** The whole kit and caboodle is surrounded by a lipid bilayer with the matrix proteins **gp41** and **gp120,** which are essential for viral attachment and entry into the host cell (Figs. 5.46 and 5.47).

Much like hepatitis B, HIV is spread by the parenteral route (fluid–fluid):

- Sexual contact: Higher risk for transmission in women, in receptive anal intercourse, and with concomitant STIs because of greater mucosal injury.
- Blood product transfusion: Precautionary measures have reduced the incidence to 1 in 500,000 transfusions.
- IV drug use with needle sharing: Increased incidence in U.S. urban areas.
- Mother to child: There is a 30% incidence for pregnancies without prophylaxis (can occur transplacentally, during delivery, or from breastfeeding). HIV is one of the few absolute contraindications to breastfeeding in developed countries (although in developing countries, the risk for dehydration and death is potentially higher than the risk for HIV transmission).
- Needlestick injury among health care workers: Rate of transmission is only about 0.3% (compared with 3% for hepatitis C and 30% for hepatitis B after needlestick injuries).
- It is *not* spread by mosquito bites, casual contact (kissing, sharing food), or certain body fluids (tears, sweat, saliva, urine).

Once in the bloodstream, the matrix proteins gp41 and gp120 bind to the **CD4** protein found on **helper T cells** and a few other cells (macrophages, monocytes, CNS dendritic cells). The coreceptor **CCR5** is also required for cell entry, and rare individuals lacking this receptor appear to be resistant to HIV infection. Once the RNA and associated proteins are in the cytoplasm, the RNA is copied into DNA by **reverse transcriptase.** The DNA is transported to the nucleus and integrated into host DNA, where it may lie dormant or begin transcription and replication of new virions immediately, which bud from and kill the T cell (Fig. 5.48).

With exceptions, the usual course of infection occurs in three stages (Figs. 5.49 and 5.50): (1) an acute flulike illness, (2) a latent period, and finally (3) AIDS.

- **The acute illness phase** occurs about 1 month after infection. The virus replicates quickly in macrophages and lymph nodes, causing fever, malaise, generalized lymphadenopathy, and pharyngitis.

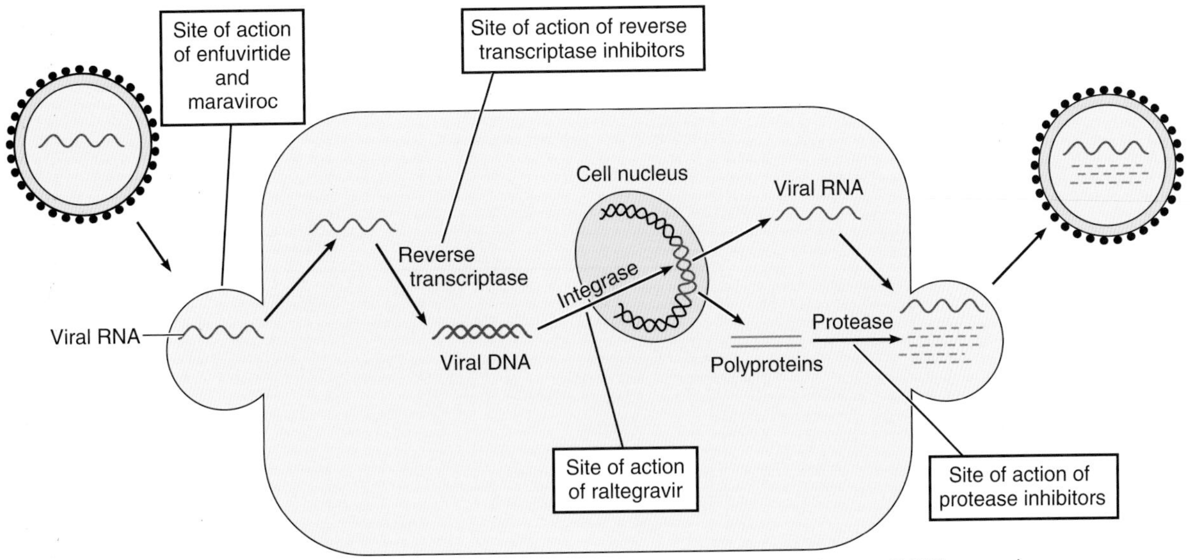

FIG. 5.48 Replication cycle of HIV and the drugs that act on key steps. (*From Brenner GM, Stevens CW.* Pharmacology. *3rd ed. Philadelphia: Elsevier; 2009.*)

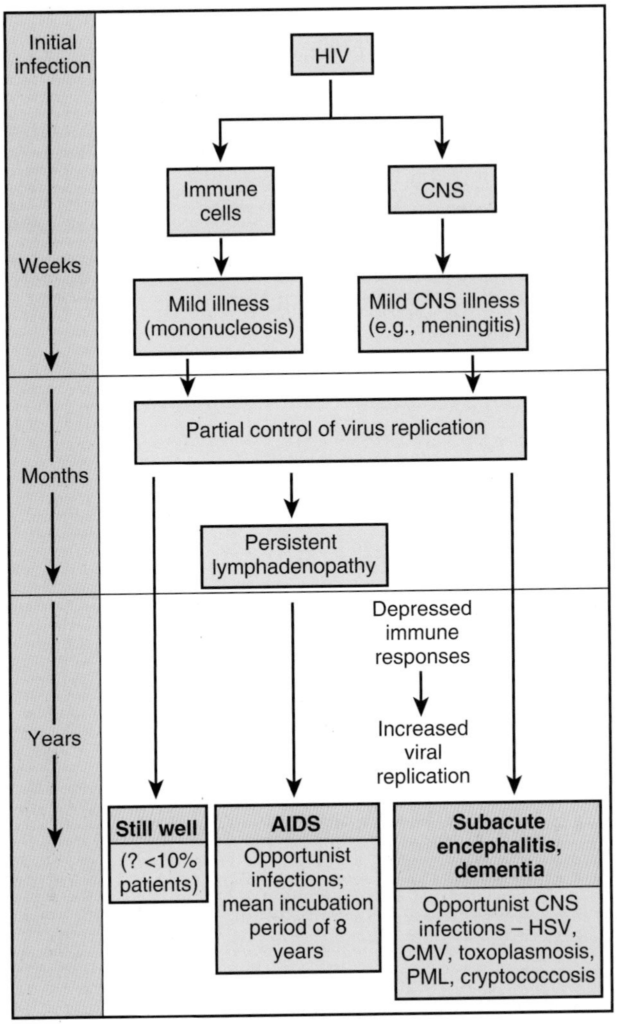

FIG. 5.49 HIV timeline of symptoms. (*From Goering R, Dockrell H, Wakelin D, et al.* Mims' Medical Microbiology. *4th ed. Philadelphia: Elsevier; 2007.*)

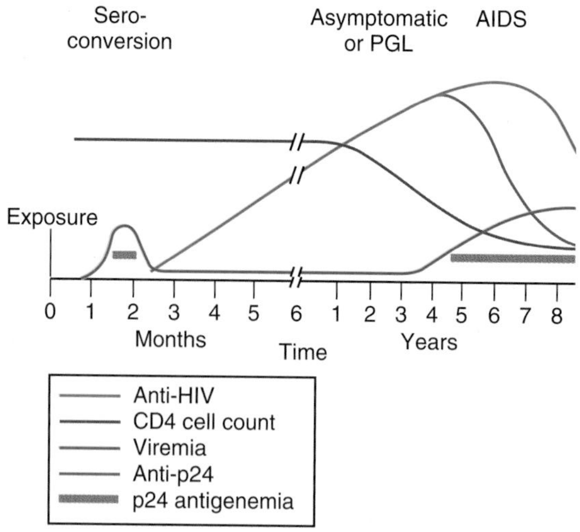

FIG. 5.50 Timeline of HIV showing levels of antigens and antibodies. (*From Greenwood D, Slack R, Peitherer J, Barer M. Medical Microbiology. 17th ed. Philadelphia: Elsevier; 2007.*)

Viral load is high. Antibodies may not yet have formed. This syndrome can resemble influenza or mononucleosis. Once the immune response kicks in, the symptoms dissipate and the viral load in the blood falls. The virus will continue to replicate in cells of the lymph nodes.

- **Latency** can last from 1 to 20 years (median, 8 years) and is not characterized by symptoms (except occasional lymphadenopathy, presumably from an immune response). The virus continues to replicate, and the CD4 cell count slowly decreases. Toward the end of latency, particularly when the CD4 count drops to less than 400, patients are more susceptible to skin infections (athlete's foot, oral thrush, shingles) and bacterial infections (*M. tuberculosis*) and develop constitutional symptoms (fever, weight loss, night sweats, adenopathy).
- **AIDS** is defined as having a **CD4 count less than 200** with clinical evidence of HIV infection **or by having one of the AIDS-defining illnesses** (Table 5.5). The diseases in Table 5.5 are organized by system, but another way to organize them is to think about what diseases are commonly seen at CD4 counts < 400, < 200, and < 50 because your patient's CD4 count will help you decide the likely organisms on your differential diagnosis. The CD4 count tells you what your patient is at risk for, whereas the viral load (measured by RNA or DNA PCR) tells you how quickly the patient is progressing to death. The median time from diagnosis of AIDS to death is about 2 years.

Besides allowing opportunistic infections, HIV also causes its own symptoms, predominantly the constitutional symptoms already mentioned, as well as neurologic disease. HIV is carried across the blood–brain barrier by infected monocytes and macrophages and can cause aseptic meningitis, an encephalitis that leads to cognitive decline **(AIDS dementia complex),** and myelopathy (spinal cord infection). Peripheral nerve damage can also occur.

Diagnosis of HIV is done in two steps. An ELISA screening test to detect antibodies to HIV and for the HIV the p24 antigen (high sensitivity but can give false-positive results) is done first. If the ELISA is positive, a **Western blot** is performed, which is a more specific test looking for antibodies to HIV by applying the patient's serum to a piece of paper containing common HIV antigens.

Efforts to control this pandemic involve four strategies:

- **Prevention:** Education to avoid high-risk activities, and screening blood donations.
- **Vaccine:** Efforts to vaccinate are challenging because of the virus's ability to quickly mutate, its ability to transfer between cells without contacting the bloodstream (where antibodies live), and the fact that we don't have a good animal model to develop vaccines (because HIV only infects humans; the closest thing we have is simian immunodeficiency virus, which is more like HIV-2 than HIV-1).
- **Limiting viral growth** is the best treatment we have right now. The big categories of HIV antivirals are **nucleoside/nucleotide reverse transcriptase inhibitors,** such as zidovudine (previously known as AZT) and zalcitabine, and **protease inhibitors** such as indinavir and saquinavir. The former category has been very successful, for example, in reducing mother-to-child transmission of HIV

Table 5.5 Opportunistic Infections in AIDS Patients

ORGAN SYSTEM	OPPORTUNISTIC INFECTION	CAUSATIVE ORGANISM	CD4⁺ COUNT	ANTIBIOTIC PROPHYLAXIS AT CD4 COUNT
Central nervous system (CNS)	Meningitis	*Cryptococcus neoformans*	<50 cells/mm³	
	Encephalopathy	Cytomegalovirus (CMV)	<50 cells/mm³	
	Brain abscess	*Toxoplasma gondii*	<100 cells/mm³	TMP-SMX Dapsone plus pyrimethamine
	AIDS dementia	Unknown (HIV, hepatitis C virus?)	↑ risk at <200 cells/mm³	
	Progressive multifocal leukoencephalopathy (PML)	JC virus		
	Primary CNS lymphoma	Epstein-Barr virus (EBV)		
Eye	Retinitis: "**cotton-wool spots**"	CMV	<50 cells/mm³	
Skin	Shingles	Varicella-zoster virus (VZV)	<400 cells/mm³	If unvaccinated, give varicella-zoster immune globulin (VZIG) to those who are exposed to zoster/chickenpox
	Tinea pedis	*Microsporum*, *Trichophyton*, and *Epidermophyton* sp.	<400 cells/mm³	
	Bacillary angiomatosis/nonneoplastic vascular lesion	*Bartonella henselae*		
	Kaposi sarcoma/neoplastic vascular lesion	Human herpesvirus-8 (HHV-8)		
	Condylomata acuminata	Human papillomavirus (HPV)		
	Anal/cervical squamous cell carcinoma (SCC)	HPV		
Mucosa	Oral hairy leukoplakia	EBV	<400 cells/mm³	
	Oral/esophageal thrush	*Candida albicans*	Oral: <400 cells/mm³ Esophageal: <100 cells/mm³	Consider prophylactic fluconazole in HIV patients with recurrent candidiasis
	Oropharyngeal non-Hodgkin lymphoma (large cell type)	EBV		
	Ulcerations	*Histoplasma capsulatum*	<100 cells/mm³	
		Herpes simplex virus-1 (HSV-1)	<200 cells/mm³	Consider prophylactic acyclovir in HIV patients with recurrent HSV or zoster
	Esophagitis	CMV	<50 cells/mm³	
		HSV-1	<200 cells/mm³	Consider prophylactic acyclovir in HIV patients with recurrent HSV or zoster
Gastrointestinal (GI) tract	Diarrhea	*Mycobacterium avium-intracellulare* complex (MAC)	<50 cells/mm³	Azithromycin Clarithromycin Rifabutin
		Isospora belli	<200 cells/mm³	
		Cryptosporidium parvum	<200 cells/mm³	
		Salmonella sp.	<400 cells/mm³	
		Shigella sp.	<400 cells/mm³	
		Giardia lamblia		
	Colitis	CMV	<50 cells/mm³	
	GI non-Hodgkin lymphoma	EBV		
Lung	Pneumonia	MAC	<50 cells/mm³	Azithromycin Clarithromycin Rifabutin
		CMV	<50 cells/mm³	
		Pneumocystis jiroveci (**p**neumo**c**ystis **p**neumonia, PCP)	<200 cells/mm³	TMP-SMX Dapsone Atovaquone
		Mycobacterium tuberculosis	<400 cells/mm³	
	Invasive/systemic	*Histoplasma capsulatum*	<100 cells/mm³	
		Coccidioides immitis	<200 cells/mm³	
		Aspergillus fumigatus		
Reticuloendothelial system	Lymphadenopathy or splenomegaly	MAC	<50 cells/mm³	
		EBV		

to 8% when given to the mother before birth and to the infant for 6 weeks postpartum. The latter category inhibits protease, which is crucial for viral replication. The combination of zidovudine, zalcitabine, and saquinavir has been shown to prolong life and extend elevations in CD4 counts. A combination of drugs (usually three) taken together is required to prevent resistance; this is called **highly active antiretroviral therapy (HAART).** The common side effects of these drugs are relevant for the examination; see the antimicrobials section later in this chapter for an overview.

Coronaviruses

- **Capsid:** helical
- **Envelope:** enveloped
- **RNA structure:** single-stranded, linear, positive
- **Viruses of clinical significance:** coronaviruses, severe acute respiratory syndrome (SARS) coronavirus

Up to one-third of acute upper respiratory infections—the common cold—are caused by **coronaviruses.** They are spread by respiratory secretions, aerosolized droplets (cover your cough!), and direct contact with mucocutaneous secretions (wash your hands!). Symptoms of the common cold include nasal congestion, rhinorrhea, sore throat, and cough. Individuals are usually afebrile. Vaccination against coronaviruses is not possible because of antigenic variation.

Severe acute respiratory syndrome (SARS) coronavirus gained worldwide notoriety in 2003 after causing an epidemic affecting more than 20 countries and thousands of people. It begins with a prodromal syndrome of **fever,** malaise, headache, and myalgias (unlike symptoms of the common cold), and then progresses to nonproductive cough and dyspnea. Chest radiographs reveal **diffuse interstitial infiltrates.** Death may occur from **acute respiratory distress syndrome (ARDS)/respiratory failure.** Treatment is supportive.

Orthomyxoviruses

- **Capsid:** helical
- **Envelope:** enveloped
- **RNA structure:** single-stranded, linear, negative
- Viruses of clinical significance: influenza virus

The ***influenza viruses A and B*** cause **epidemic flu,** which we experience every year during the winter months: upper respiratory symptoms such as sore throat and dry cough are accompanied by headache, myalgias (muscle aches), malaise, fever, and shaking chills. The virus owes its success to its high infectivity, quick spread by aerosolized droplets, and the principles of **antigenic drift and antigenic shift** (discussed later and shown in Figs. 5.51 and 5.52). Influenza can cause a primary pneumonia, but most of the complications and cases in which death occurs are due to **secondary infection** (usually pneumonia and otitis media) by bacteria *(S. aureus, H. influenzae, S. pneumoniae),* particularly in immunocompromised patients and older adults. Worse still is **pandemic flu,** a worldwide outbreak caused by the rare strain to which there is zero immunity. The H1N1 outbreak in 2009 was an example of this.

The viral structure is crucial to understanding its virulence. Its membrane contains lipoprotein spikes, some of which have **hemagglutinin (HA) activity** and some of which have **neuraminidase (NA)** activity. HA attaches to sialic acid receptors, found on erythrocytes (hence causing heme-agglutination) and upper respiratory tract epithelium, which the virus binds to in order to dump its RNA into the epithelial cell. The spikes with NA activity cleave neuraminic acid, a component of host defense found in the mucus lining the respiratory tract, allowing the virus to both expose sialic acid receptors and allow budding viruses to escape from the cell.

Antibodies to HA and NA are protective, so why can we get infected with the flu again and again? This is due to two concepts:

- **Antigenic drift,** in which replication leads to small variations in the surface proteins. Individuals previously exposed to that strain will have partial protection, causing a milder disease.
- **Antigenic shift,** in which viruses that infect different species infect the same cell and create new viruses during replication with mixed HA and NA antigens. Of the three types of influenza virus (types A, B, C), only **influenza type A** infects multiple species and hence is the only type in which this occurs. The different HA and NA antigens are given a number subscript, for example **H5N1 (avian influenza, or "bird flu").** These new strains, to which no one is immune at first, are what cause pandemic flu.

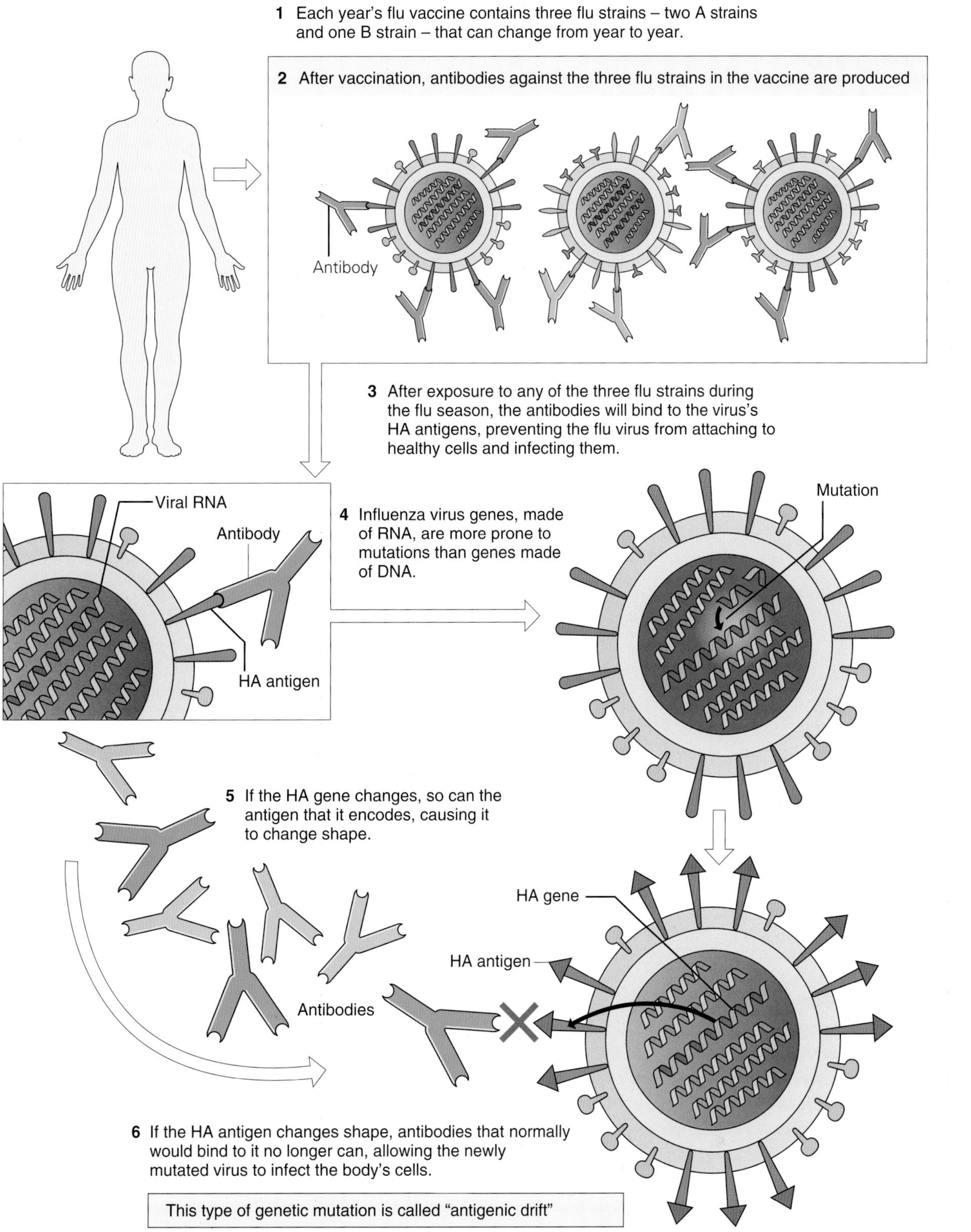
1 Each year's flu vaccine contains three flu strains – two A strains and one B strain – that can change from year to year.
2 After vaccination, antibodies against the three flu strains in the vaccine are produced
Antibody
3 After exposure to any of the three flu strains during the flu season, the antibodies will bind to the virus's HA antigens, preventing the flu virus from attaching to healthy cells and infecting them.
Viral RNA
Antibody
HA antigen
4 Influenza virus genes, made of RNA, are more prone to mutations than genes made of DNA.
Mutation
5 If the HA gene changes, so can the antigen that it encodes, causing it to change shape.
HA gene
HA antigen
Antibodies
6 If the HA antigen changes shape, antibodies that normally would bind to it no longer can, allowing the newly mutated virus to infect the body's cells.
This type of genetic mutation is called "antigenic drift"

FIG. 5.51 Antigenic drift. (*From Goering R, Dockrell H, Wakelin D, et al.* Mims' Medical Microbiology. *4th ed. Philadelphia: Elsevier; 2007. Data from Adegbola R, Secka O, Lahai G, et al. Elimination of Haemophilus influenzae type b (Hib) from the Gambia after the introduction of routine immunisation with a Hib conjugate vaccine: a prospective study.* Lancet *2005;366:144.*)

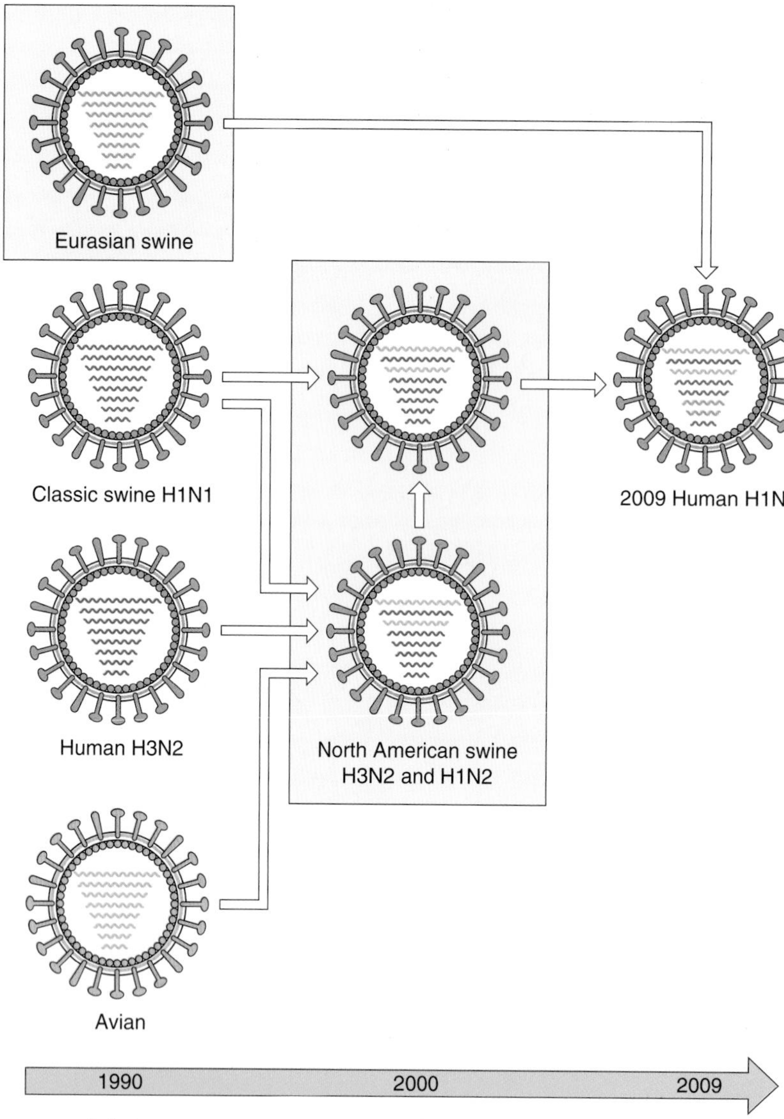

FIG. 5.52 Antigenic shift. (*From Goering R, Dockrell H, Wakelin D, et al. Mims' Medical Microbiology. 4th ed. Philadelphia: Elsevier; 2007. Reproduced from Male D, Brostoff J, Roth DB, Roitt I.* Immunology. *St. Louis: Mosby Elsevier; 2006, with permission.*)

Control of influenza involves "guessing" what strains will cause next year's epidemic flu and creating inactivated vaccines for the population—immunocompromised patients, older adults, and health care workers should be immunized first. A live-attenuated nasal spray vaccine is available for those who qualify. Drugs to treat influenza are most effective if given early or prophylactically. The **adamantanes (amantadine and rimantadine)** block the **M2 ion channel** of influenza **A** only, preventing acidification of the viral interior necessary for uncoating of the virion. The **neuraminidase inhibitors (zanamivir and oseltamivir)** are sialic acid mimics and prevent release of new viruses from cells by blocking neuraminidase from cleaving the sialic acid receptor, a crucial step for viral spread. Oseltamivir is currently considered first-line therapy, but to be effective, treatment should begin within 48 hours of symptom onset.

Paramyxovirus

- **Capsid:** helical
- **Envelope:** enveloped
- **RNA structure:** nonsegmented, single-stranded, linear, negative
- **Viruses of clinical significance:** parainfluenza virus, respiratory syncytial virus, rubeola virus, mumps virus

The paramyxoviruses are transferred by inhalation of respiratory secretions. They have a common **fusion ("F") protein** that causes infected cells (i.e., respiratory epithelial cells) to **fuse** together into multinucleated giant cells. **Palivizumab** is a monoclonal antibody against **F protein** and can be given to children at high risk for respiratory syncytial virus (RSV).

Parainfluenza virus can cause upper respiratory infection in healthy adults. In children and immunocompromised individuals, parainfluenza virus can cause lower respiratory infection—particularly **laryngotracheobronchitis**, or **croup**. Croup is characterized by a **barking, seal-like cough and stridor** as airway inflammation progresses. On chest radiographs, subglottic narrowing of the trachea is seen as a **"steeple sign."** Severe infections with respiratory distress are treated with glucocorticoids (usually dexamethasone) and racemic epinephrine.

Most common causes of pneumonia in young children: RSV, parainfluenza virus.

Respiratory syncytial virus is the **most common cause of lower respiratory tract infection in children younger than 1 year.** Outbreaks of RSV occur seasonally, with peaks in the winter season. Infants with RSV present with tachypnea or periods of apnea and signs of respiratory distress, including low O_2 saturation, intercostal/subcostal retractions, nasal flaring, grunting, and/or expiratory wheezing. Chest radiographs show patchy atelectasis and peribronchial thickening. Premature infants and infants with pulmonary disease are among those at higher risk for severe RSV infection.

The ***mumps virus*** causes low-grade fever, headache, malaise, and myalgia and is accompanied by painful swelling of the salivary glands (Fig. 5.53), particularly the **parotid gland** (other causes of parotid enlargement include Sjogren syndrome, *S. aureus* parotitis, and bulimia). About 30% of infected males will also develop **orchitis (swelling of the testes).** In rare cases, mumps-induced orchitis can lead to **fertility problems.** Rare complications include meningitis, hearing loss, and pancreatitis. Children are vaccinated against mumps with the MMR vaccine. Recently isolated outbreaks of mumps have affected unimmunized students on college campuses. Fig. 5.54 shows the pathophysiology of the disease.

Rubeola virus causes **measles,** which is highly contagious and is spread through respiratory secretions. After an incubation period of about 2 weeks, infected individuals have a **high fever with c**ough, **c**oryza, and **c**onjunctivitis ("the three Cs"). **Koplik spots** (Fig. 5.55), pathognomonic for measles, develop on the buccal mucosa. Koplik spots appear as small, red lesions with a white or bluish center and can take on a "grains-of-salt" appearance. The measles rash (Fig. 5.56) appears after the onset of fever and about 48 hours after the appearance of Koplik spots; it is an erythematous, maculopapular rash that starts on the head and spreads to the body; lesions can become confluent, especially on the face.

Children are vaccinated with a live, attenuated form of the virus as part of the MMR vaccine. Vaccination prevents against measles infection and its complications, including myocarditis and encephalitis. It also prevents against the serious late-onset complication **subacute sclerosing panencephalitis (SSPE),** which occurs 7 to 10 years after an initial measles infection and is a progressive and fatal neurodegenerative disease.

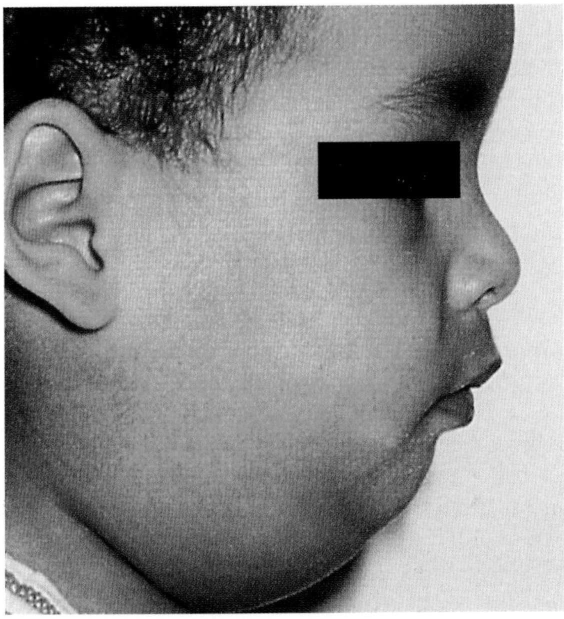

FIG. 5.53 Enlarged submandibular glands seen in mumps. (*From Goering R, Dockrell H, Wakelin D, et al. Mims' Medical Microbiology. 4th ed. Philadelphia: Elsevier; 2007. Courtesy J. A. Innes.*)

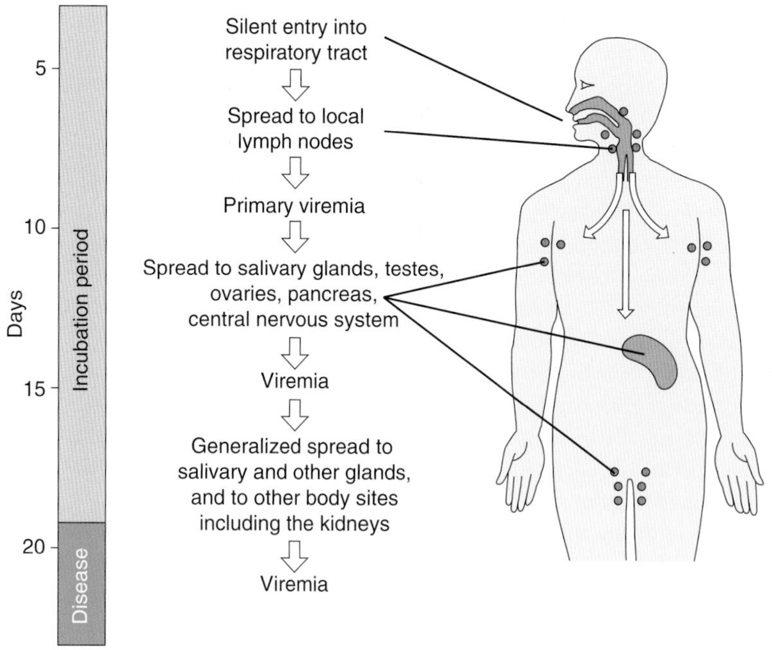

FIG. 5.54 Pathophysiology of mumps. (*From Goering R, Dockrell H, Wakelin D, et al.* Mims' Medical Microbiology. *4th ed. Philadelphia: Elsevier; 2007.*)

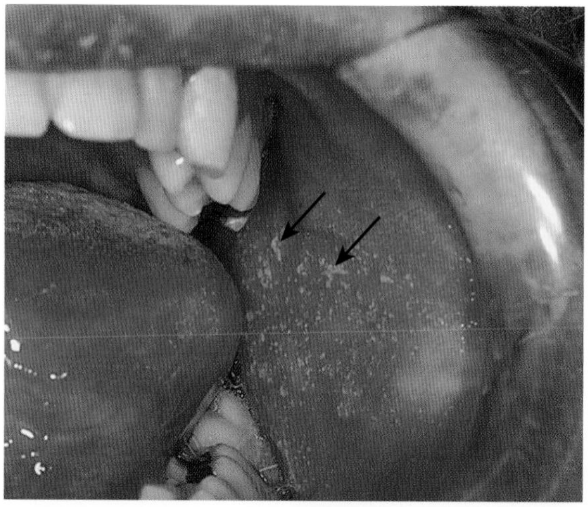

FIG. 5.55 Koplik spots. (*From Colledge NR, Walker BR, Ralston SH.* Davidson's Principles and Practice of Medicine. *21st ed. London: Churchill Livingstone; 2010.*)

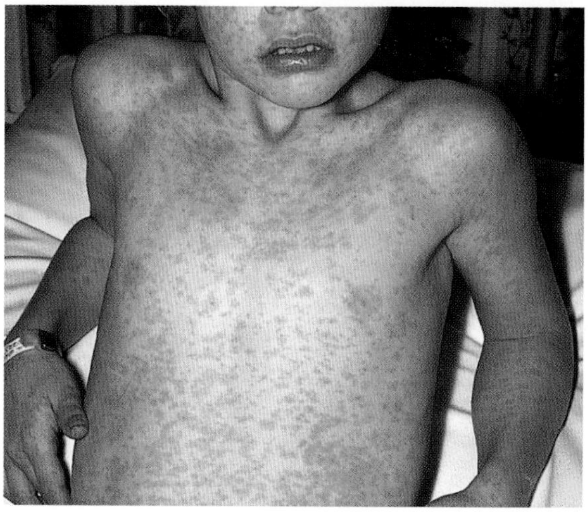

FIG. 5.56 Maculopapular rash seen in a child with measles. (*From Colledge NR, Walker BR, Ralston SH.* Davidson's Principles and Practice of Medicine. *21st ed. London: Churchill Livingstone; 2010.*)

Rhabdoviruses

- **Capsid:** helical
- **Envelope:** enveloped
- **RNA structure:** single-stranded, linear, negative
- **Viruses of clinical significance:** rabies virus

The ***rabies virus*** causes rabies and is transmitted by the bite of an infected mammal **(bat, dog, cat, skunk, raccoon, fox).** The virus replicates at the wound and then migrates in a **retrograde** fashion up **nerve axons** to the CNS. After a prodrome of fever, headache, and fatigue, an infected individual develops **encephalitis** marked by hyperactivity, agitation, and **painful pharyngeal or inspiratory spasms** incited by water **(hydrophobia)** or even air **(aerophobia).** Seizures and flaccid paralysis are also present. **Negri bodies** (collections of rabies virus; Fig. 5.57) are present in brain biopsy specimens of affected individuals.

A rabies vaccine is available for domesticated pets and animals. If an individual has been bitten by an animal whose rabies status is unknown and unable to be determined, the wound should be **washed and sterilized** as soon as possible for greatest risk reduction. The individual is vaccinated with **rabies immune globulin (RIG)** and a **rabies vaccine series.** Veterinarians and cave explorers get preexposure prophylaxis. If a patient wakes up and there's a bat in their room, they get RIG and the vaccine, regardless of whether a known bite has occurred (bat bites are notoriously very hard to find).

Filoviruses

- **Capsid:** helical
- **Envelope:** enveloped
- **RNA structure:** single-stranded, linear, negative sense
- **Viruses of clinical significance:** Marburg virus, Ebola virus

Marburg virus and ***Ebola virus*** cause a viral hemorrhagic fever, characterized by a prodromal flulike illness that progresses to coagulopathy and hemorrhage (i.e., maculopapular rash, purpura or petechiae, bleeding from mucosal surfaces, frank bloody vomit or stool). Death occurs from complications of capillary leak syndrome or shock. The virus is spread by direct contact with body fluids and may be potentially spread by aerosolized droplets. Treatment is supportive and is aimed at preventing further spread of disease. Ebola virus (Fig. 5.58) is likely acquired by the handling of infected wild animals.

Deltaviruses

- **Capsid:** helical
- **Envelope:** enveloped
- **RNA structure:** single-stranded, circular, negative sense
- **Viruses of clinical significance:** hepatitis D virus

Hepatitis D virus is transmitted parenterally (IV drug use, contact or transfusion with infected blood). It **requires previous infection or coinfection with hepatitis B virus to replicate.** HDV utilizes

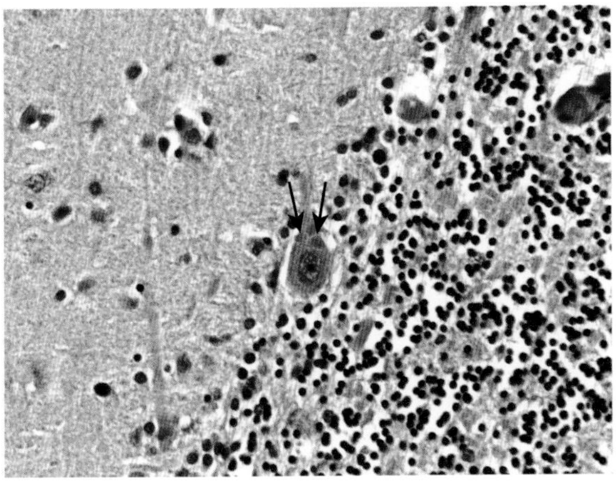

FIG. 5.57 A Negri body *(arrows)* in a patient with rabies. *(From Kumar V, Abbas AK, Fausto N, et al.* Robbins and Cotran's Pathologic Basis of Disease. *8th ed. Philadelphia: Elsevier; 2009.)*

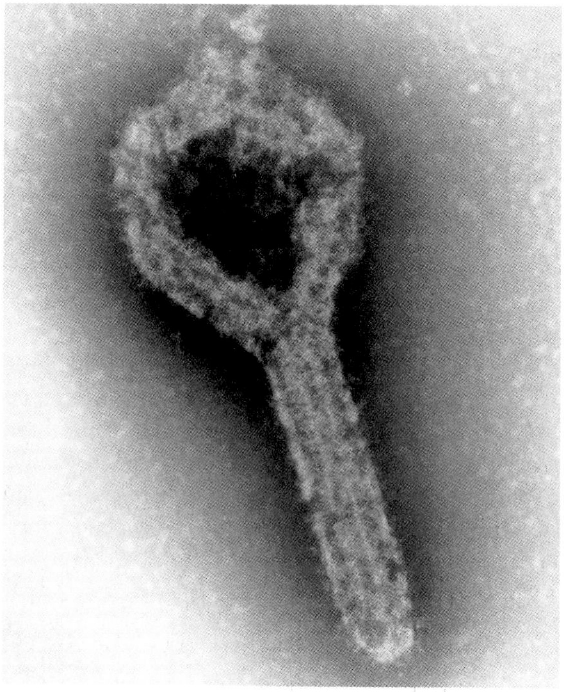

Fig. 5.58 Ebola virus visualized by electron microscopy. *(From Greenwood D, Slack R, Peitherer J, Barer M. Medical Microbiology. 17th ed. Philadelphia: Elsevier; 2007.)*

the HBV lipoprotein envelope. When HDV infects an individual with chronic HBV, coinfection results in an **acute on chronic hepatitis,** with risk for progression to **fulminant hepatitis.** Concomitant infection with HBV and HDV can accelerate cirrhosis or HCC progression. Vaccination against HBV prevents HDV infection.

Arenaviruses

- **Capsid:** helical
- **Envelope:** enveloped
- **RNA structure:** single-stranded, circular, negative, segmented (two)
- **Viruses of clinical significance:** lymphocytic choriomeningitis virus

Lymphocytic choriomeningitis virus (LCMV) is carried by the house mouse *(Mus musculus)* and other rodents. Humans acquire infection by exposure to infected mouse saliva or excrement (e.g., inhalation, eating affected food, direct exposure through an open cut). In symptomatic individuals, LCMV can cause a prodromal flulike illness followed by **meningitis or encephalitis.**

Bunyaviruses

- **Capsid:** helical
- **Envelope:** enveloped
- **RNA structure:** single-stranded, circular, negative, segmented (three)
- **Viruses of clinical significance:** hantavirus, Crimean-Congo hemorrhagic fever virus, Rift Valley fever virus, and California encephalitis

Bunyaviruses, with the exception of **hantavirus,** are arboviruses transmitted by the bite of infected mosquitos **(LaCross encephalitis virus, California encephalitis virus),** ticks **(Crimean-Congo hemorrhagic fever),** and sandflies (**Rift Valley fever,** a hemorrhagic fever).

Hantaviruses are carried by the **deer mouse and other rodents** (hantavirus is a "robovirus" for **ro**dent **bo**rne, whereas the others are "arboviruses" for **ar**thropod **bo**rne). Humans are infected by contact with rodent saliva (bites), urine, or feces. The disease has been reported across the United States but is more commonly reported in the **four-corners region (New Mexico, Colorado, Arizona, and Utah).** Suspect hantavirus in an individual who develops a flulike illness with severe respiratory symptoms after known exposure to rodents (e.g., rodent bite or sweeping out a barn with rodents and rodent feces present).

Hantavirus causes two severe illnesses: **hemorrhagic fever with renal syndrome (HFRS)** and **hantavirus pulmonary syndrome (HPS).** HFRS is endemic to China, the Korean peninsula, Russia, and Western Europe and causes a febrile illness with hemorrhage, hypertension, and acute renal failure. HPS is endemic to North and South America and causes a febrile illness with flulike symptoms and bilateral pulmonary interstitial edema.

California encephalitis virus causes encephalitis mostly in children. It is spread by forest rodents, with high risk for infection in Midwest forested areas. The disease has low mortality but can cause lasting cognitive effects.

Another bunyavirus, ***B. phleboviri,*** causes fever. In Africa, it is spread by mosquitos and causes **Rift Valley fever.** In Asia and South America, it is spread by the sandfly and causes **sandfly fever,** a classic 3-day fever with quick resolution.

PRION DISEASES

Prion diseases represent a unique and not fully understood set of infectious conditions. They are caused by prions, which are proteinaceous particles (no genetic material at all) that are able to convert normal proteins into prions. As a result, prion diseases have a slow incubation time, then cause rapid progression of symptoms and quick death once clinical signs become evident. Examples of prion diseases include **kuru, Creutzfeldt-Jakob disease (CJD),** and **mad cow disease** (which converts to **variant CJD** in the human host). Spread can occur by blood transfusion or ingestion of the meat of an infected host. On the USMLE, look for a patient from **England** (the epicenter of the mad cow epidemic) with **progressive psychiatric symptoms** followed by rapid neurologic deterioration, **dementia,** and **myoclonus.** Death occurs within months of symptom onset, and there is no treatment.

FUNGI

Introduction to Fungi

Most of the fungi among us are generally harmless and in some aspects even beneficial: We eat edible mushrooms, drink beer fermented by yeast, and eat cheese flavored with mold. There are, however, pathogenic fungi that have the potential to cause serious disease in humans. Although we come into contact with fungi and breathe in fungal spores constantly, in only rare instances do fungi cause serious disease.

Some antifungal drugs target ergosterol: ketoconazole inhibits its synthesis, amphotericin B and nystatin bind to it and bore holes through it.

Fungi are eukaryotic, aerobic organisms. They reproduce both sexually and asexually through budding. All fungi have a polysaccharide cell wall composed of chitin, mannan, and glucan and a cell membrane containing ergosterol. These components are not found in animal cell membranes, making **ergosterol** an excellent specific antifungal target. Fungi can exist in multiple forms (Fig. 5.59). Fungi can exist as unicellular **(yeast)** and multicellular **(mold)** organisms. Fungi that switch between the yeast and mold forms are termed **dimorphic.** In the vegetative phase, fungal cells divide by mitosis and bud; incomplete budding results in **pseudohyphae** (no true septa). **True hyphae** remain connected but have septa between them. In the reproductive phase, fungal cells produce spores (conidia). Conidia enclosed within a sporangium sac are known as **endospores.**

Mycotic diseases can be categorized into three types: superficial/cutaneous (Fig. 5.60), subcutaneous, and systemic infections.

Superficial and Cutaneous Mycoses

- Superficial infection
  - Tinea versicolor
  - Tinea nigra
- Cutaneous infection
  - Tinea barbae (barber's itch/folliculitis)
  - Tinea capitis

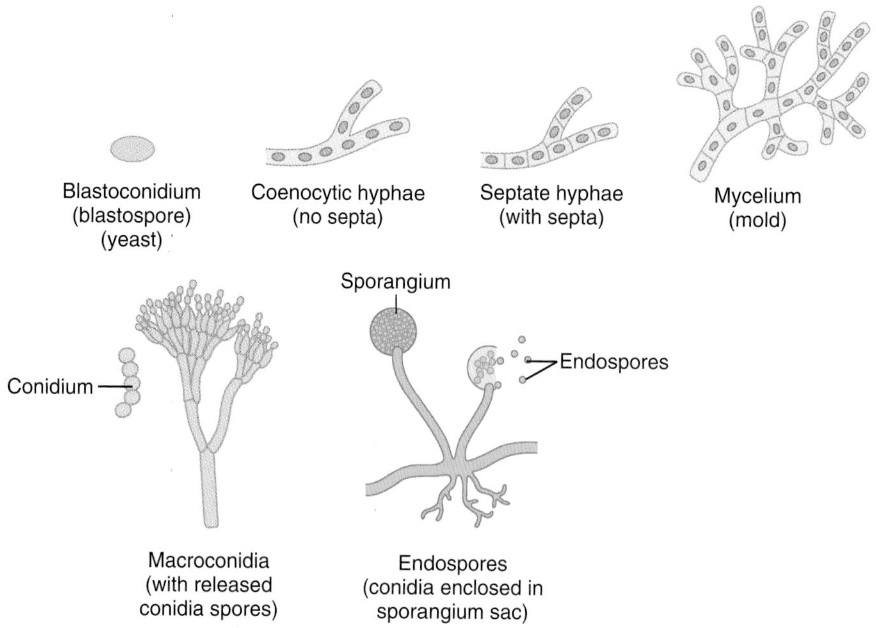

FIG. 5.59 Cartoon showing various forms of fungal phenotypes. (*From Actor JK.* Elsevier's Integrated Immunology and Microbiology. *Philadelphia: Elsevier; 2006.*)

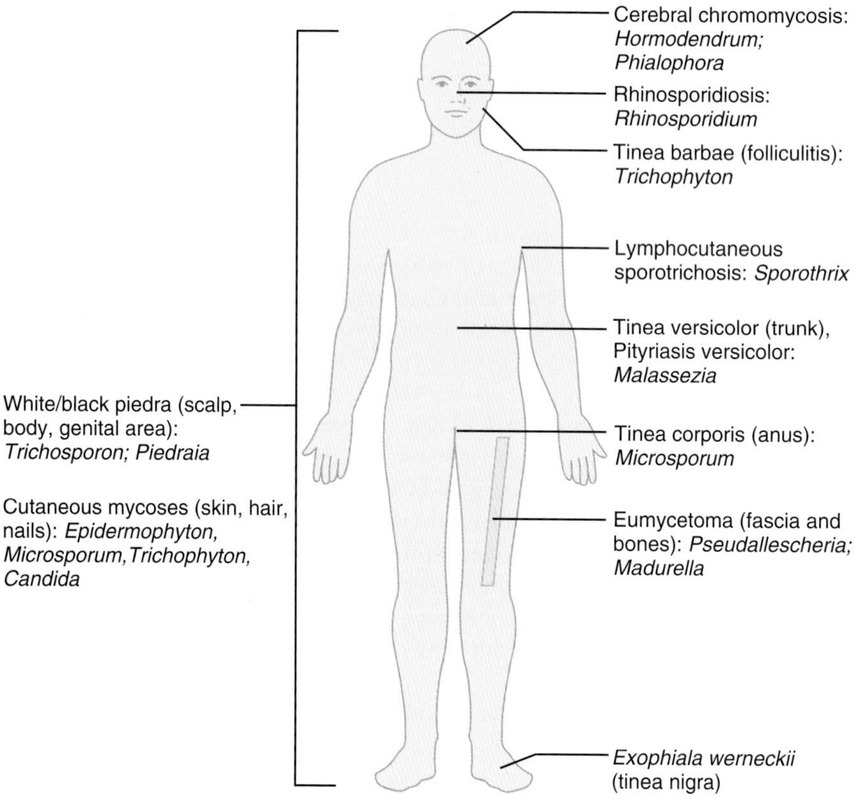

FIG. 5.60 Location of some of the more common superficial/cutaneous mycoses. Not all shown here are discussed in text. (*From Actor JK.* Elsevier's Integrated Immunology and Microbiology. *Philadelphia: Elsevier; 2006.*)

- Tinea corporis (ringworm)
- Tinea cruris (jock itch)
- Tinea pedis (athlete's foot)
- Tinea unguium (onychomycosis)

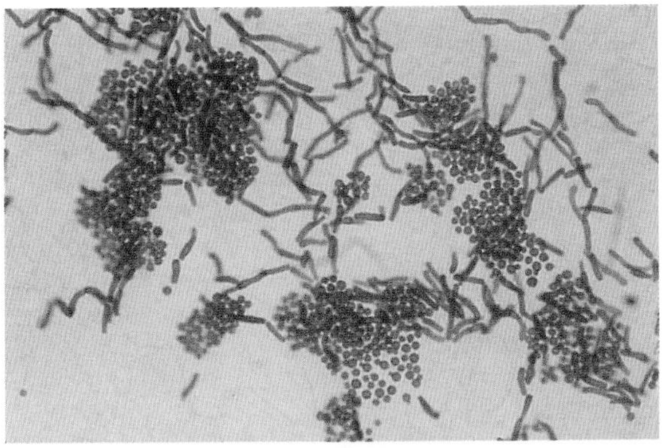

Fig. 5.61 "Spaghetti and meatballs" appearance of *Malassezia furfur* showing yeast forms and hyphae from a KOH prep of a skin sample from someone with tinea versicolor. (*From Goering R, Dockrell H, Wakelin D, et al.* Mims' Medical Microbiology. *4th ed. Philadelphia: Elsevier; 2007. Courtesy Y. Clayton and G. Midgley.*)

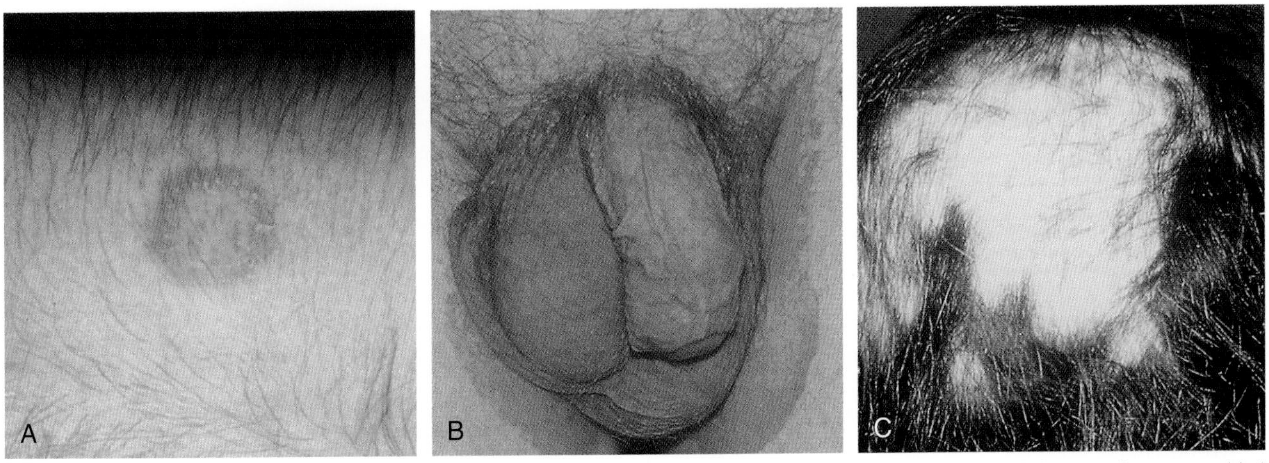

Fig. 5.62 **A,** Tinea corporis, or "ringworm." **B,** Tinea cruris, or "jock itch." **C,** Tinea capitis. (***A,*** *courtesy A. E. Provost.* ***B,*** *courtesy M. J. Wood.* ***C,*** *from Goering R, Dockrell H, Wakelin D, et al.* Mims' Medical Microbiology. *4th ed. Philadelphia: Elsevier; 2007. Courtesy M. H. Winterborn.*)

Most common in children: tinea capitis. In adults: tinea cruris and tinea pedis.

Tinea versicolor and **tinea nigra** are superficial infections that cause damage of melanocytes, manifesting as discoloration of the skin. Tinea versicolor presents as hypopigmented or hyperpigmented macular lesions. This is caused by benign infection with ***Malassezia furfur.*** Tinea nigra is caused by ***Exophiala werneckii*** and causes black or darkly pigmented macular lesions of the palms and soles. Both tinea versicolor and tinea nigra are diagnosed by **skin scraping with KOH prep.** *Malassezia furfur* appears as "spaghetti and meatballs" (Fig. 5.61). Both are treated with topical selenium sulfide or ketoconazole.

Cutaneous infections of the hair (**tinea barbae** and **tinea capitis**), skin (**tinea corporis, tinea cruris,** and **tinea pedis**), and nails **(tinea unguium)** are most commonly caused by various species of ***Trichophyton, Microsporum, Epidermophyton,*** and occasionally ***Candida.*** These fungi feed off keratin of the hair, nails, and skin, resulting in hair loss (tinea capitis); brittle, thickened, yellowish nails (tinea unguium); and chronic, scaly patches of skin (tinea corporis, tinea cruris, tinea pedis). Tinea corporis is also known as **ringworm** because of its appearance (Fig. 5.62).

Skin scraping with KOH prep shows **branched hyphae.** First-line treatment is topical imidazole (e.g., ketoconazole or clotrimazole). For infections of the **nail,** use oral **terbinafine.** For more involved skin infections, oral azoles (fluconazole or itraconazole) are used.

***Candidal* species** can exist as yeast forms, as hyphae, or as a variety of in-between forms called **pseudohyphae.** This is a relatively unique feature of *Candida.* Examples of superficial candidal infections include **oral thrush** (Fig. 5.63), vulvovaginitis **(yeast infection),** and diaper rash. **Chronic mucocutaneous candidiasis** is usually a sign of underlying immunocompromised state or primary immunodeficiency. Treat superficial candidal infections with **nystatin.**

Invasive candidiasis occurs in immunocompromised individuals. Oral thrush can extend to the esophagus, causing a painful **candidal esophagitis.** When *Candida* is disseminated hematogenously, it can cause serious disseminated disease (e.g., retinitis, endocarditis, pneumonitis). Treatment of candidal fungemia in neutropenic patients is with an echinocandin (caspofungin, micafungin, etc.) or lipid

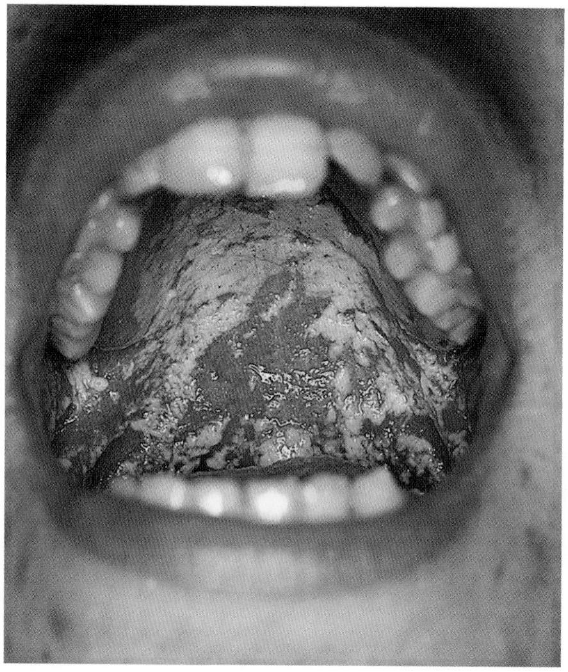

Fig. 5.63 Oral thrush caused by *Candida*. (*From Glynn M, Drake WM. Hutchison's Clinical Methods. 23rd ed. Oxford, UK: Elsevier; 2012.*)

amphotericin B (safer than nonlipid amphotericin B). Special care should be taken to find the source of infection (e.g., consider removing central lines, doing a CT scan to look for a focus of infection, and looking carefully at the skin and the retinas).

Subcutaneous Fungal Infections

- Chromoblastomycosis
- Mycetoma
- Sporotrichosis

Subcutaneous fungal lesions are caused by **saprophytes,** fungi that normally live in the soil and subsist on rotting matter. They are usually harmless unless they find their way into an unsuspecting individual's skin or tissue (e.g., a thorn prick or splinter).

Chromoblastomycosis occurs after fungi from soil or rotting wood enters the skin through a cut or puncture wound. A violaceous, wartlike lesion pops up at the site of the initial wound. Untreated, more subcutaneous warty lesions pop up in the distribution of lymphatics. **Skin scraping with KOH prep shows "copper pennies" or copper-colored sclerotic bodies.** Curative treatment is difficult. Standard treatment is itraconazole and/or lesion excision.

Mycetoma (Madura foot) is endemic to parts of Asia, Africa, and South America, occurring when an individual steps on a sharp object and the wound is inoculated with fungal spores. The fungi cause deep tissue infection, sinus tract formation, and swelling of the affected limb (Fig. 5.64).

Sporotrichosis *(Sporothrix schenckii)* is an example of a **dimorphic saprophytic fungus.** For the purposes of Step 1, remember that *Sporothrix* lives in the soil and rose thorns. A classic presentation involves an unsuspecting gardener who pricks himself on **a rose thorn.** A pustule or nodule-turned-ulcer appears at the site of the lesion. Left untreated, subcutaneous nodules **track up the arm in a lymphatic distribution,** called ascending lymphangitis (Fig. 5.65). This is rarely a systemic illness. Treat with **potassium iodide** or itraconazole. *Mycobacterium marinum* causes a similar-looking lesion in people who work with fish tanks, so look at the history—is the patient a gardener or a fish fancier?

Systemic Mycoses

Systemic Mycoses in Normal Individuals

- Blastomycosis
- Histoplasmosis

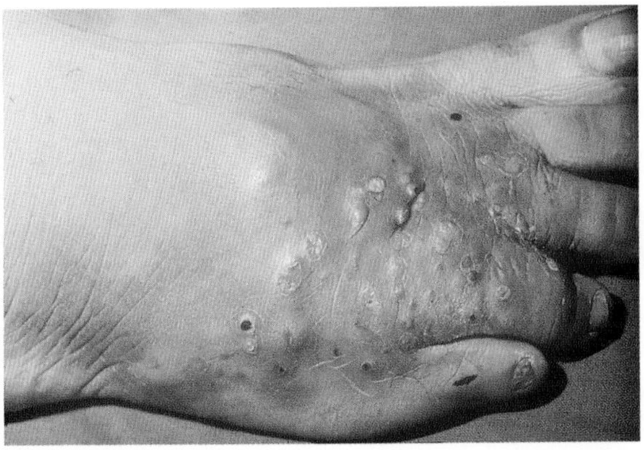

FIG. 5.64 Mycetoma of the foot. (*From Greenwood D, Slack R, Peitherer J, Barer M. Medical Microbiology. 17th ed. Philadelphia: Elsevier; 2007.*)

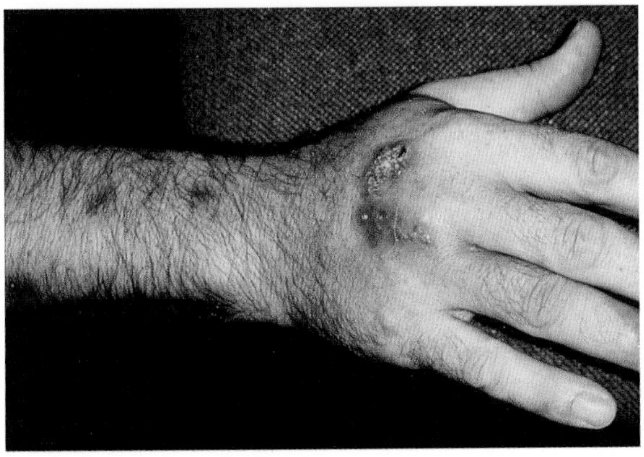

FIG. 5.65 Sporotrichosis spreading lymphatically from a primary infection in the nailbed of the third finger. (*From Greenwood D, Slack R, Barer M, Irving W. Medical Microbiology. 18th ed. Oxford, UK: Elsevier; 2012.*)

- Coccidioidomycosis
- Paracoccidioidomycosis

The systemic mycoses are caused by dimorphic fungi. Infection is usually acquired by the inhalation of mold spores from the soil. At elevated temperatures (i.e., in the lungs), the dimorphic fungi morph into yeast forms. Blastomycosis, histoplasmosis, and coccidioidomycosis are considered endemic infections in the United States, whereas paracoccidioidomycosis is primarily found in Central and South America. Dimorphic fungi can cause disease in normal, healthy individuals. Usually, primary infection starts in the lung, and secondary infection results from invasive spread to other organ systems. Most inhaled fungal infections are asymptomatic. Of symptomatic individuals, most develop a self-limited pneumonia. Very rarely does infection progress to chronic pneumonia or disseminated infection, which usually occurs in the setting of immunodeficiency or other immunocompromised states.

Blastomycosis is caused by inhalation of the mold spores of *Blastomyces dermatitidis.* It is endemic to the region of the Mississippi River valley and eastward. Diagnosis is made by visualization of *Blastomyces* yeast forms with **broad-based buds** (Fig. 5.66) in sputum, skin scrapings, or pus.

Acute pulmonary infection presents with nonspecific, flulike symptoms. In immunocompromised individuals, infection evolves into a tuberculosis-like chronic pulmonary disease with fever, weight loss, night sweats, and dissemination. Skin is involved in 70% of disseminated infections, causing characteristic raised granulomatous skin lesions, hence the name *Blastomyces* ***dermatitidis*** (Fig. 5.67). Bone infection is present in 30% of patients. Signs of systemic infection can occur in the absence of lung disease. **Treat all forms of blastomycosis** (it's rare, but it's severe). The drug of choice is either itraconazole for mild infection or amphotericin for serious infection.

Histoplasmosis is caused by *Histoplasma capsulatum,* **endemic in the Ohio and Mississippi River valleys as well as Central and South America.** *Histoplasma* is especially prevalent in soil with high nitrogen content (read: bird or bat droppings), hence its other names: **caver's disease** and **spelunker's lung.**

Again, most individuals (and cave explorers) exposed to *Histoplasma* will not develop symptoms. If the burden of exposure is high enough, an individual can develop an acute pulmonary infection with flulike symptoms. **Most acute pulmonary infections are self-limited** and do not require antifungal

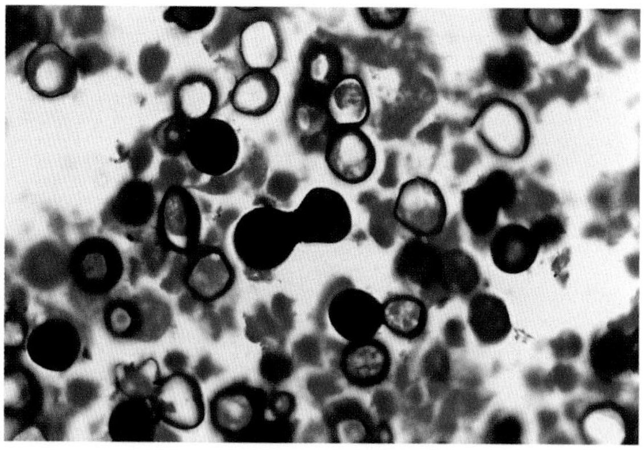

FIG. 5.66 Blastomyces showing broad-based budding. (*From Greenwood D, Slack R, Peitherer J, Barer M. Medical Microbiology. 17th ed. Philadelphia: Elsevier; 2007.*)

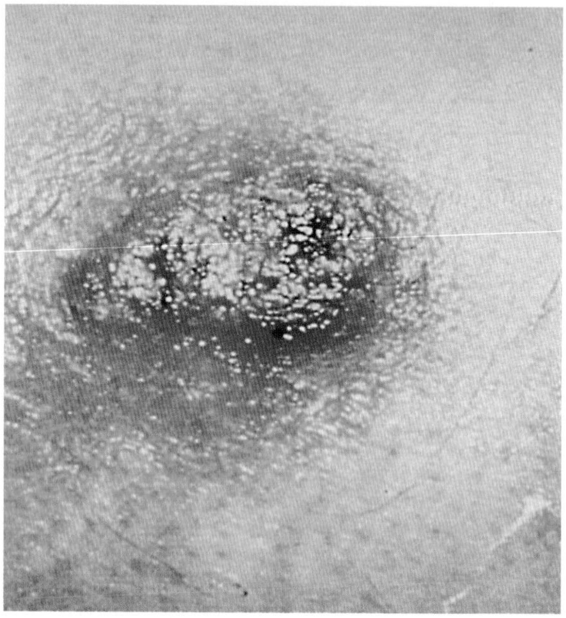

FIG. 5.67 Characteristic skin lesion of blastomycosis. These often occur in systemic infection, despite the lungs being the primary site of infection. (*From Goering R, Dockrell H, Wakelin D, et al. Mims' Medical Microbiology. 4th ed. Philadelphia: Elsevier; 2007. Courtesy K. A. Riley.*)

treatment. Dissemination occurs hematogenously or through the lymphatic system, with infection of the reticuloendothelial system (causes hepatosplenomegaly). Dissemination is rare and usually occurs in immunocompromised individuals (e.g., those with AIDS). Diagnosis is made by visualization of **yeast forms in macrophages and giant cells** (macrophage = histiocyte, hence *Histoplasma*). Urine *Histoplasma* antigen may also be used. Severe or chronic infections are treated with **itraconazole or amphotericin B.**

High yield: For the purposes of Step 1, systemic mycoses are extremely region dependent. In the Southwest United States, think cocci; in the Mississippi and Ohio River basins, think histo; and east of Mississippi and in Central America, think blasto.

Coccidioidomycosis is caused by *Coccidioides immitis.* Known as **valley fever** or **San Joaquin Valley fever,** it is endemic to the southwestern United States (southern California, Arizona, Nevada, New Mexico). Outbreaks of coccidioidomycosis in the southwest United States are often preceded by new construction projects, farming projects, or earthquakes.

In symptomatic individuals, *Coccidioides* usually causes a mild flulike illness, joint pains, and pneumonia. In less than 1% of individuals, *Coccidioides* causes chronic, disseminated infection that has a predilection for the CNS (meningitis). Patients may develop erythema nodosum ("desert bumps"), tender red nodules on both shins from inflammation of subcutaneous fat (not specific). Certain ethnic groups may be predisposed to disseminated infection (Filipino, African American, Native American). Diagnosis is made by visualization of **yeast forms with the appearance of large spherules** in tissue (Fig. 5.68). Treat non-CNS infections with **itraconazole.** For disseminated disease, use **amphotericin B.** For CNS infection, use **fluconazole.**

Paracoccidioidomycosis is caused by *Paracoccidioides brasiliensis.* This disease is endemic to South America. In symptomatic individuals, it causes a mild pneumonia and flulike illness similar to that in histoplasmosis and coccidioidomycosis. Diagnosis is made by visualization of a **"captain's wheel"** in tissue (Fig. 5.69).

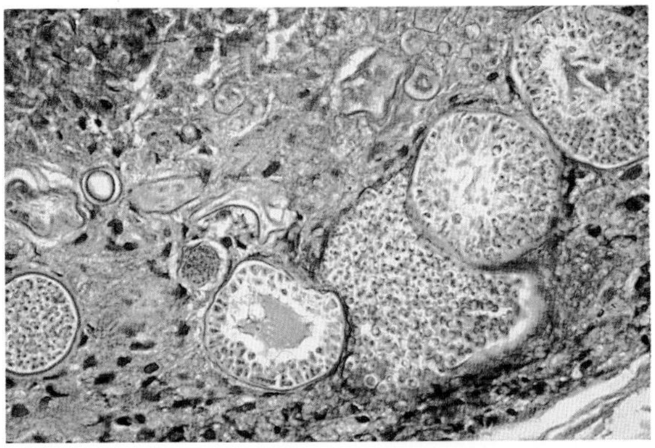

Fig. 5.68 *Coccidioides immitis* spherule with endospores. (*From Greenwood D, Slack R, Peitherer J, Barer M. Medical Microbiology. 17th ed. Philadelphia: Elsevier; 2007.*)

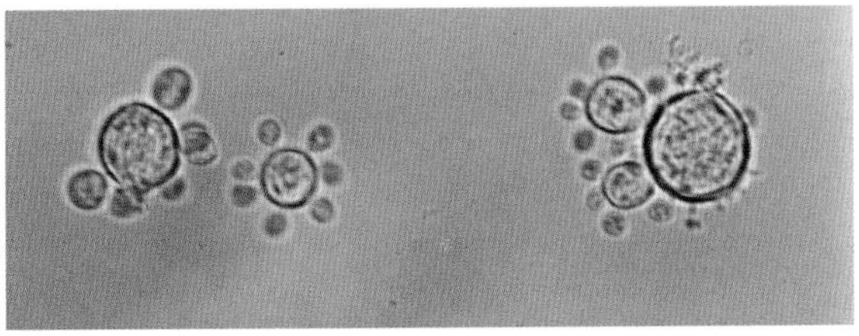

Fig. 5.69 *Paracoccidiomycosis brasiliensis* demonstrating "captain's wheel" multipolar budding. (*From Greenwood D, Slack R, Peitherer J, Barer M. Medical Microbiology. 17th ed. Philadelphia: Elsevier; 2007.*)

Systemic Mycoses in Immunocompromised Individuals

- Aspergillosis
- Cryptococcosis
- *Pneumocystis jirovecii*

***Aspergillus* species** are ubiquitous mold found in the environment and *usually* cause disease by inhalation of spores. In immunocompetent individuals, *Aspergillus* can cause **allergic bronchopulmonary aspergillosis (ABPA).** This condition manifests as an allergic, IgE-mediated hypersensitivity reaction to inhaled *Aspergillus,* causing peripheral eosinophilia, bronchospasm, and, if left untreated, irreversible lung changes. Anywhere from 5% to 20% of steroid-dependent asthmatic patients may have underlying ABPA. **Aspergilloma,** a literal "fungus ball" of *Aspergillus,* may take up residence in preexisting cavitary lung lesions in individuals with previous tuberculosis infections or other cavitary lung disease.

Aspergillus usually causes invasive disease in immunocompromised individuals, particularly those taking **immunosuppressive medications, neutropenic patients** (such as after bone marrow transplant), and those with **chronic granulomatous disease.** Invasive disease may manifest as rapidly invasive **acute fungal sinusitis** that can spread to the brain or as **disseminated invasive aspergillosis,** which is fatal without treatment with potent antifungals such as voriconazole, caspofungin, or amphotericin B.

Mucor and *Rhizopus* are also branching filamentous fungi, but they branch at 90 degrees and mainly affect diabetic patients.

Diagnosis is made by visualization of the characteristic mold forms in tissue biopsy or sputum (Fig. 5.70). Aspergillus hyphae are septated and branch at acute angles of 45 degrees (Fig. 5.71).

Cryptococcus neoformans cases occur mainly in immunocompromised individuals. Individuals acquire *Cryptococcus* through inhalation of **yeast forms** from the environment (particularly, **pigeon and bird droppings**). Cryptococcus is most notorious for causing **meningitis** that presents with fever, headache, and confusion (it is the *most common cause of fungal meningitis*). It also causes pneumonia and skin infections that manifest as cutaneous pustules and abscesses. Diagnosis is made by lumbar puncture with visualization of **encapsulated yeast forms by India ink stain** (Fig. 5.72). Diagnosis can also be made by measurement of cryptococcal antigen level in serum or CSF. Treat with **fluconazole** for mild infection and **amphotericin B/5-flucytosine** for meningeal or other severe infections. Those with cryptococcal meningitis who are immunosuppressed may need suppressive therapy with fluconazole after initial treatment.

Pneumocystis jirovecii (previously *Pneumocystis carinii,* or PCP) is a yeast that causes pneumonia among immunocompromised patients, although it silently infects most immunocompetent individuals (hence making it a perfect **opportunistic infection,** the most common opportunistic infection among AIDS patients in developing nations). Although the name has changed, you will still hear many physicians refer to *P. jiroveci* pneumonia as PCP. Suspect this disease when an HIV patient presents with symptoms of pneumonia and a CD4 cell count less than 200 (and *especially* if <100). Diagnosis

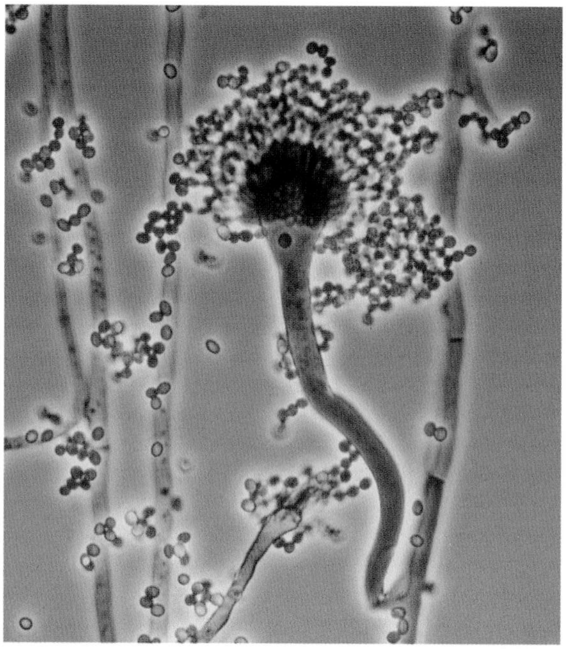

FIG. 5.70 "Rod and scepter" of *Aspergillus*. (*From Greenwood D, Slack R, Peitherer J, Barer M.* Medical Microbiology. *17th ed. Philadelphia: Elsevier; 2007. Reproduced with permission from Richardson MD, Warnock DW, Campbell CK.* Slide Atlas of Fungal Infection: Systemic Fungal Infections. *Oxford, UK: Blackwell Science; 1995.*)

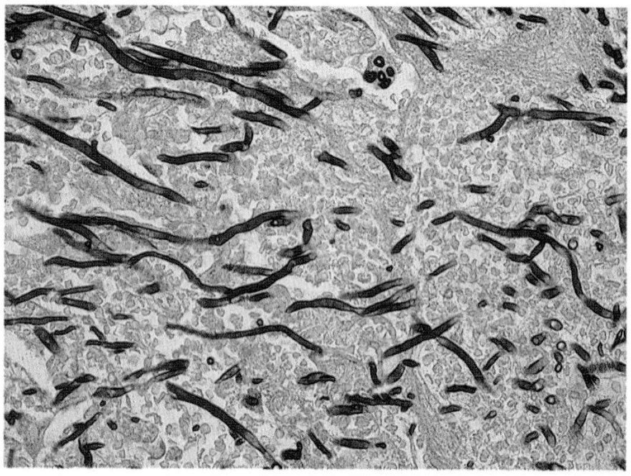

FIG. 5.71 *Aspergillus* in a biopsy of a blood vessel demonstrating septate hyphae with occasional 45-degree angle branching. (*From King T.* Elsevier's Integrated Pathology. *Philadelphia: Elsevier; 2006.*)

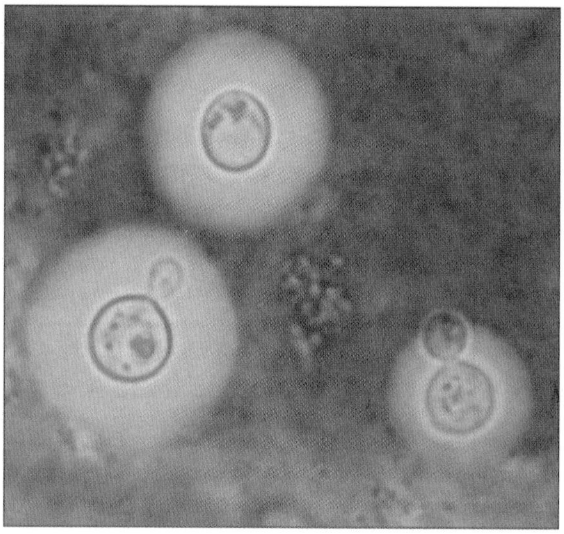

FIG. 5.72 *Cryptococcus* visualized by India ink stain in the cerebrospinal fluid of a patient with meningitis. (*From Goering R, Dockrell H, Wakelin D, et al.* Mims' Medical Microbiology. *4th ed. Philadelphia: Elsevier; 2007. Courtesy A. E. Prevost.*)

is by antibody staining of sputum, or by bronchoalveolar lavage if the sputum sample is inconclusive. Prophylaxis should begin with a CD4 count less than 200 in all AIDS patients (first choice: TMP-SMX; second choice: dapsone; don't forget to test for glucose-6-phosphate dehydrogenase [G6PD] deficiency first!). Prophylaxis in developing nations has significantly reduced the incidence of pneumocystis pneumonia, but breakthrough cases do occur. Treatment choices are the same as for prophylaxis but in IV form.

PARASITES

Parasites are eukaryotic organisms that require a **host** for survival. Human disease–causing parasites come in two forms: the single-celled **protozoa** and the multicellular **helminths (cestodes, nematodes, and trematodes).** Humans are **not** the primary host for parasites; rather, infection is acquired by **ingestion, insect bite, or penetration of the mucous membranes or skin.**

Parasites undergo different life stages, which determine both the route of entry for infection and the disease manifestations. Protozoa, for example, exist in both **trophozoite** form (the reproducing/feeding form) and as **cysts** (the protective/dormant form that even asymptomatic carriers may shed for years depending on the organism). In this section we discuss protozoa by mechanism of disease (CNS disease, GI disease, bloodborne disease, and STI) and then discuss helminths.

PROTOZOA

Protozoa That Cause Central Nervous System Infections

- *Acanthamoeba* sp.
- *Naegleria fowleri*
- *Toxoplasma gondii* (toxoplasmosis)

Acanthamoeba are free-living amoebae that cause infection through the skin, inhalation, or hematologic spread. Infection has been associated with **granulomatous amebic meningoencephalitis** in **immunocompromised patients.** In normal individuals, *Acanthamoeba* cause **keratitis** in **contact lens wearers** after use of contaminated lens-cleaning fluid.

Naegleria fowleri is also a free-living amoebae that takes residence in warm bodies of fresh water. Trophozoite forms of *Naegleria* swim through the **olfactory mucosa** and **cribriform plate** of the unsuspecting **swimmer** and into the brain, causing a **rapid-onset, acute meningoencephalitis** 1 to 14 days after exposure. Survival is rare. Diagnosis is made by confirmation of *Naegleria* in CSF.

Toxoplasma gondii can be found in all animals but is especially endemic to the intestinal tract of cats. Humans acquire infection by ingestion of **cysts** in infected undercooked meat (e.g., pork or lamb) or cat feces (e.g., cleaning a litter box). The organisms decyst once consumed, and eventually **sporozoites** released from the small intestine move into macrophages (Fig. 5.73). Infected, circulating macrophages eventually burst, allowing the organism to move into other host cells, including nerve cells.

Primary symptomatic infection is rare in normal individuals. In immunocompetent individuals, infection may manifest as a flulike illness with lymphadenopathy. **Immunocompromised** individuals are at risk for disseminated disease, including involvement of the brain and lung. **HIV/AIDS patients** may present with mental status changes or encephalitis, leading to brain imaging that reveals **ring-enhancing lesions** on CT or magnetic resonance imaging (Fig. 5.74). Lesions tend to occur in the basal ganglia. Prophylaxis is warranted in AIDS patients with CD4 T-cell counts less than 100/μL with TMP-SMX or sulfadiazine and pyrimethamine.

> Differential diagnosis of a ring-enhancing lesion in an AIDS patient: CNS lymphoma, toxoplasmosis.

Transplacental infection is possible. For this reason, **pregnant women are strongly encouraged to avoid cleaning litter boxes.** When *Toxoplasma gondii* (the T in ToRCHeS) causes intrauterine infection, it may cause stillbirth or severe congenital abnormalities **(chorioretinitis, hydrocephalus, and intracranial calcifications).** Diagnose by **IgM antibodies** against *T. gondii* or biopsy of brain lesions. Treat with **sulfadiazine and pyrimethamine.**

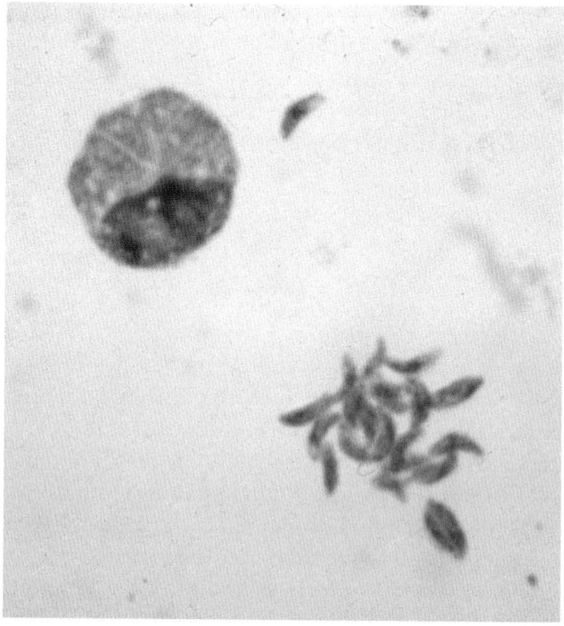

FIG. 5.73 Tachyzoites of *Toxoplasma gondii* in a macrophage *(top left)* and free *(bottom right)*. (*From Greenwood D, Slack R, Peitherer J, Barer M. Medical Microbiology. 17th ed. Philadelphia: Elsevier; 2007.*)

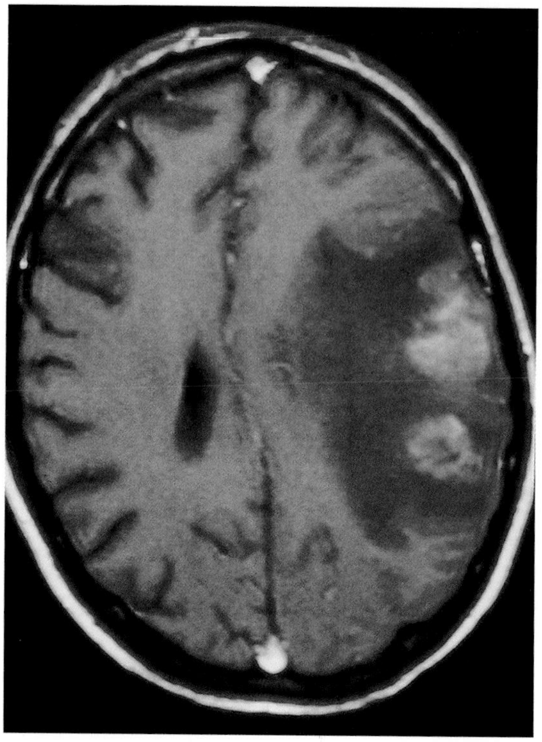

FIG. 5.74 Ring-enhancing lesions of toxoplasmosis. (*From Colledge NR, Walker BR, Ralston SH.* Davidson's Principles and Practice of Medicine. *21st ed. London: Churchill Livingstone; 2010.*)

Protozoa That Cause Gastrointestinal Infections

- *Cryptosporidium parvum*
- *Entamoeba histolytica* (amebiasis)
- *Giardia lamblia*

Diarrhea caused by protozoa:
Bloody → *Entamoeba histolytica*
Fatty → *Giardia lamblia*
Watery → *Cryptosporidium parvum*

Cryptosporidium parvum cysts can be found in unfiltered water and can be responsible for **"community outbreaks"** of watery diarrhea. When ingested, *C. parvum* **cysts** cause a mild, self-limited form of diarrhea in immunocompetent individuals. They may cause profuse, life-threatening diarrhea in immunocompromised individuals (HIV/AIDS patients). Diagnosis is made by detection of **partially**

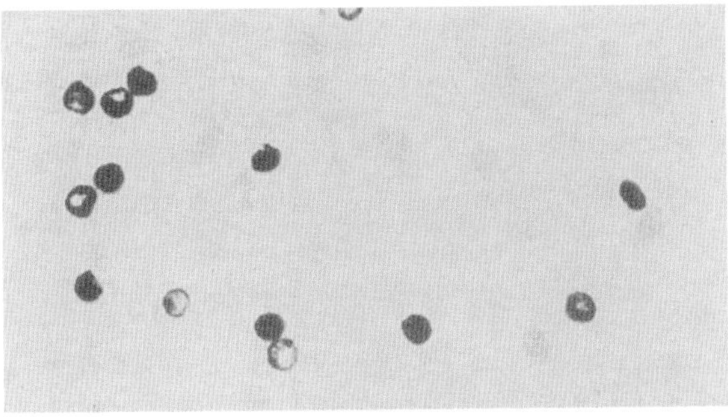

Fig. 5.75 *Cryptosporidium* cysts in a fecal sample. (*From Goering R, Dockrell H, Wakelin D, et al. Mims' Medical Microbiology. 4th ed. Philadelphia: Elsevier; 2007. Courtesy S. Tzipori.*)

acid-fast cysts in the stool (Fig. 5.75). Treatment is generally supportive. Patients with normal immune systems can be given nitazoxanide.

Entamoeba histolytica causes amebiasis, or amebic dysentery. Ingestion of **cysts** (Fig. 5.76) in contaminated water leads to infection and ulceration of the intestinal epithelium by the amoebae. This results in **abdominal pain and bloody diarrhea.** Biopsy of colonic tissue shows classic **flask-shaped ulcers.** Without treatment, *E. histolytica* can disseminate to other organs, leading to abscess formation in the lung (right-sided empyema as a direct extension from the liver), liver, colon, and brain (rarely). Aspiration of a liver abscess reveals **anchovy paste–like** material. Diagnosis is made by visualization of trophozoites or cysts forms in stool, colonoscopy with tissue biopsy, or antigen testing against *E. histolytica.* Treat colonization with **iodoquinol or paromomycin**; invasive disease should be treated with **metronidazole.**

***Giardia lamblia* infection (giardiasis)** is acquired through the fecal–oral route by ingestion of *Giardia lamblia* **cysts** in contaminated water. In the intestine, *Giardia* trophozoites (Fig. 5.77) attach to brush border enterocytes, causing injury to the microvilli and villous atrophy and subsequent **chronic, watery diarrhea.** Fat absorption is altered, leading to **foul-smelling, fatty diarrhea** with symptoms of chronic abdominal pain and bloating. **IgA** is important for prevention/clearance of *Giardia* infection, so **suspect IgA deficiency in an individual with recurrent giardiasis.**

Suspect giardiasis in an individual with chronic diarrhea with a **history of hiking or camping** and use of untreated spring or river water. Beavers, among other animals, are thought to be natural reservoirs of *Giardia.* Outbreaks of giardiasis also occur in daycare centers and schools. Diagnosis is made by visualization of cysts in stool (from three different stool samples) or detection of *Giardia* antigen in a single sample. Drugs approved for the treatment of *Giardia* include nitazoxanide and tinidazole, although metronidazole is most commonly used.

Protozoa That Cause Bloodborne Infections

- *Babesia microti*
- *Leishmania* spp. (leishmaniasis)

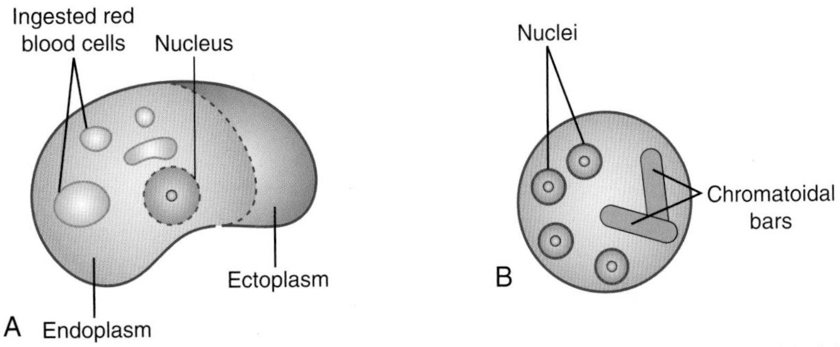

Fig. 5.76 A, Trophozoite of *Entamoeba histolytica* in acute stage of disease, with ingested red blood cells. **B,** Mature cyst of *E. histolytica*, showing classic four nuclei. (*From Greenwood D, Slack R, Peitherer J, Barer M. Medical Microbiology. 17th ed. Philadelphia: Elsevier; 2007.*)

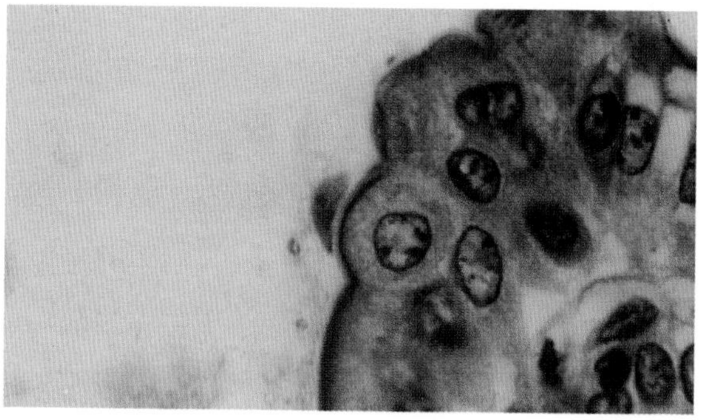

FIG. 5.77 Trophozoite of *Giardia lamblia* attached to the mucosal surface of the small intestine. (*From Goering R, Dockrell H, Wakelin D, et al.* Mims' Medical Microbiology. *4th ed. Philadelphia: Elsevier; 2007. Courtesy R. Muller and J. R. Baker.*)

- *Plasmodium* spp. (malaria)
- *Trypanosoma* spp.

***Babesia microti* (babesiosis)** is a protozoan transmitted by the bite of the infected ***Ixodes* tick.** It is a relative of malaria in the northeastern United States. *Babesia* sporozoites are introduced into the human bloodstream and infect RBCs. Babesiosis may also be transmitted by blood transfusion. Diagnosis is made by visualization of *Babesia* trophozoites (**"ring forms"**) and merozoites (**"Maltese crosses,"** Fig. 5.78). In symptomatic individuals, disease is similar to malaria and manifests as **fever, myalgia, fatigue, and hemolytic anemia.** Disease is more severe in immunocompromised individuals. Treat with **atovaquone** and **azithromycin; quinine** and **clindamycin** is considered second-line therapy. Exchange transfusion may be necessary for severe infections.

The *Ixodes* tick also carries *Borrelia burgdorferi*. In endemic areas (northeastern United States), rule out Lyme disease in patients in whom you suspect babesiosis.

***Leishmania donovani and Leishmania* species (leishmaniasis)** are found in more than 80 countries, most in the tropical and subtropical regions (Mexico, South America, southern Europe, Asia, Middle East, and North and East Africa). Leishmaniasis is spread by the bite of the infected **sandfly.** Diagnosis is made by visualization of **amastigotes** within macrophages and tissues (Fig. 5.79). Disease manifestation depends on *Leishmania* species and the host immune response.

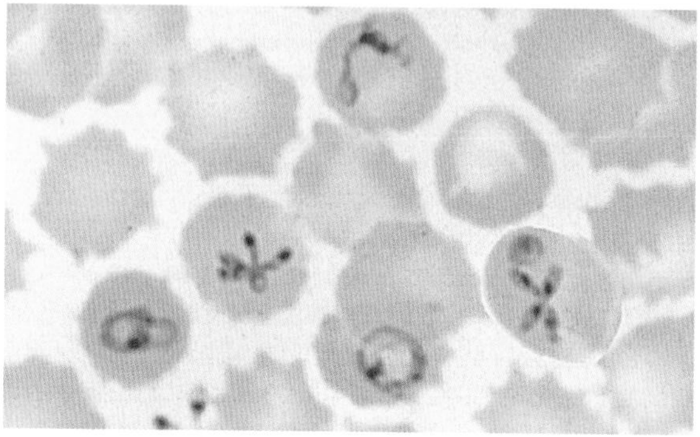

FIG. 5.78 Red blood cells infected with *Babesia* showing both ring form and Maltese cross form. (*From Kumar V, Abbas AK, Fausto N, et al.* Robbins and Cotran's Pathologic Basis of Disease. *8th ed. Philadelphia: Elsevier; 2009. Courtesy Lynne Garcia, LSG and Associates, Santa Monica, CA.*)

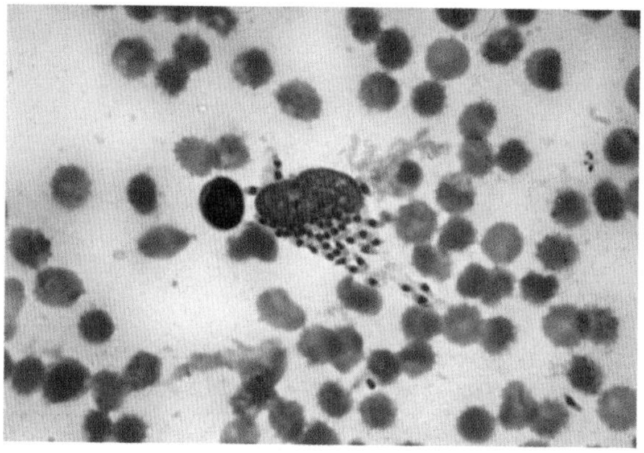

FIG. 5.79 Amastigotes of *Leishmania tropica* in a ruptured macrophage from a cutaneous lesion. (*From Greenwood D, Slack R, Peitherer J, Barer M.* Medical Microbiology. *17th ed. Philadelphia: Elsevier; 2007.*)

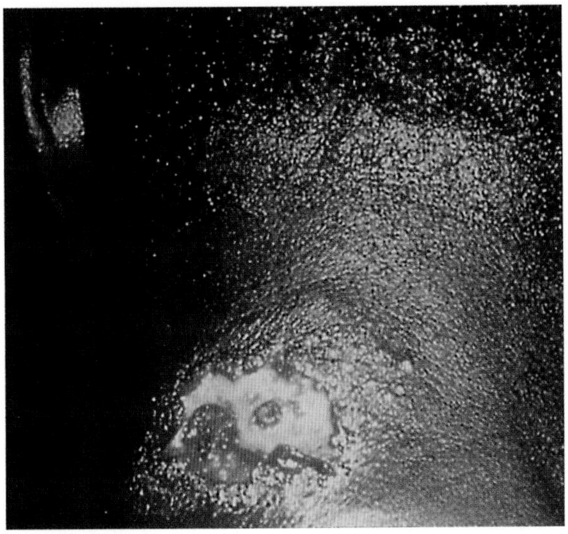

FIG. 5.80 Cutaneous lesion on the neck in *Leishmania braziliensis* infection. (*From Goering R, Dockrell H, Wakelin D, et al.* Mims' Medical Microbiology. *4th ed. Philadelphia: Elsevier; 2007. Courtesy P. J. Cooper.*)

- **Cutaneous leishmaniasis** *(L. tropica, L. Mexicana)*: A slowly healing skin ulcer at the site of the sandfly bite.
- **Diffuse cutaneous**: Disseminated infection leading to subcutaneous nodules lasting up to 20 years in individuals with impaired immune function.
- **Mucocutaneous leishmaniasis** *(L. braziliensis)*: Destructive ulcers of the skin and mucous membranes leading to disfiguring scarring (Fig. 5.80).
- **Visceral leishmaniasis** (**kala-azar,** which means "black-illness," named for the hyperpigmented skin lesions) *(L. donovani)*: The parasite disseminates in macrophages to the liver, spleen, lymph nodes, bone marrow, and other organs. Visceral leishmaniasis manifests with fevers, weight loss, hepatosplenomegaly, lymphadenopathy, and pancytopenia with dark granulomatous skin lesions.

Protective factors against malaria:
- Sickle cell trait
- RBCs lacking Duffy antigens a/b
- Thalassemia
- G6PD deficiency

Treat with sodium stibogluconate or amphotericin B.

Plasmodium species *(P. falciparum, P. vivax, P. ovale, P. malariae)* cause malaria. The infection is transmitted by the *Anopheles* mosquito. Different species are endemic to different regions; *P. falciparum* and *P. malariae* are found predominantly in Africa and Asia but can be found worldwide. *P. vivax* is concentrated in Latin America and the Indian subcontinent, whereas *P. ovale* is endemic to Africa. For travelers to foreign countries, consult with the Centers for Disease Control and Prevention (CDC) travel guide for appropriate malarial chemoprophylaxis.

The bite of an infected *Anopheles* mosquito introduces *Plasmodium* sporozoites into the bloodstream, which infect and mature into schizonts in liver cells. (*P. vivax* and *P. ovale* may persist in the liver, causing relapsing infection without appropriate treatment). Mature merozoites emerge and infect RBCs. Diagnosis of malarial infection can be made by blood smear by visualization of the ring trophozoite or the mature schizont and merozoites (Fig. 5.81). If the USMLE gives you "banana gametocytes" on the blood smear, it's *P. falciparum*.

Thick blood smear: used to screen for presence of malarial infection.
Thin blood smear: used to identify specific *Plasmodium* spp.

Malaria is characterized by recurrent fevers with severe chills, headache, nausea, muscle and joint pain, splenomegaly, and anemia. Between fevers, the patient is asymptomatic. Fevers correlate with emergence of new merozoites from infected RBCs. Periodicity of fevers is determined by the species-specific life cycle of *Plasmodium. P. vivax* and *P. ovale* cause fevers every 48 hours (tertian fevers). *P. malariae* cause fevers every 72 hours (quartan fevers). *P. falciparum,* the most severe form of malarial infection, causes recurrent fevers at irregular intervals (Fig. 5.82). Intravascular hemolysis may occur in *P. falciparum* infection, called blackwater fever because of the dark color hemoglobin gives the urine.

P. vivax and *P. ovale* infect young RBCs.
P. malariae affects old RBCs.
P. falciparum affects both (most severe).

Left untreated, *P. falciparum* infection leads to death. RBCs infected with *P. falciparum* stick to vessels, causing capillary congestion and infarction of the brain **(cerebral malaria),** lung **(pulmonary edema),** and kidney **(renal failure).**

Treatment is dependent on the region where the infection was acquired. Treatment resistance is also dependent on geographic location. **Chloroquine** is first-line treatment, but treatment resistance is now common. Use **mefloquine,** other quinine derivatives, or atovaquone-proguanil for chloroquine-resistant

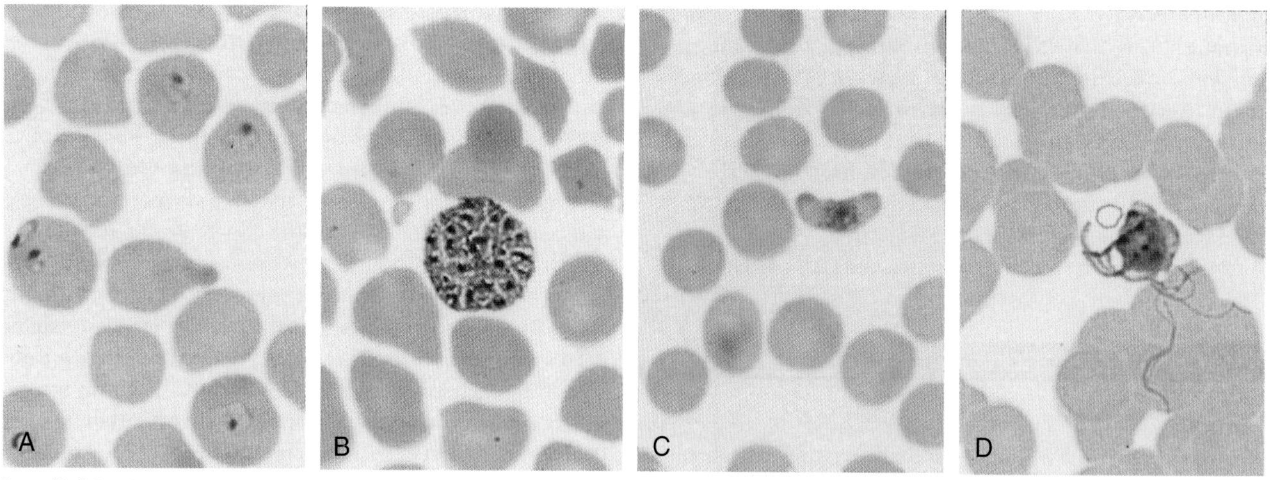

Fig. 5.81 Blood smears demonstrating different stages of malarial infection. **A,** *Plasmodium falciparum* ring forms in red blood cells. **B,** *Plasmodium vivax* erythrocytic schizont. **C,** *P. falciparum* female gametocyte. **D,** *P. vivax* male gametocytes exflagellating to form microgametes. (*From Goering R, Dockrell H, Wakelin D, et al.* Mims' Medical Microbiology. *4th ed. Philadelphia: Elsevier; 2007.*)

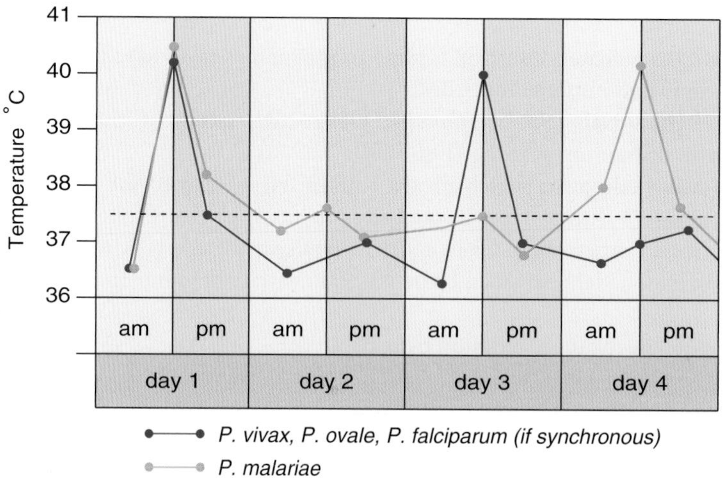

Fig. 5.82 Chart showing periodicity of fevers by malarial species. *Plasmodium falciparum* is often irregular, although sometimes synchronous as shown. (*From Goering R, Dockrell H, Wakelin D, et al.* Mims' Medical Microbiology. *4th ed. Philadelphia: Elsevier; 2007.*)

infections (remember that patients who are G6PD deficient can't receive quinine-derived medications). Infections with *P. vivax* or *P. ovale* should be treated with the addition of **primaquine** to eradicate persistent liver infection.

Romaña sign: unilateral periorbital swelling, conjunctivitis and preauricular lymph node enlargement from ocular exposure to "kissing bug" feces.

Trypanosoma cruzi causes American trypanosomiasis **(Chagas disease)** and is carried by the **reduviid bug, or "kissing bug."** An infected kissing bug feeds on a human and deposits feces nearby the site of the bite **(chagoma).** *T. cruzi* trypomastigotes, present in the feces, enter the blood through the bite wound or through mucous membranes, and infect various organs. If bitten near the eye, patients may have periorbital swelling **(Romaña sign).** Acute infection may manifest as fever, lymphadenopathy, hepatosplenomegaly, and myocarditis. Acute infection will resolve; however, without treatment, it will evolve into underlying chronic infection. Chronic Chagas disease may not manifest until months or years after initial infection. Although asymptomatic, carriers can transmit disease through blood transfusion or even transplacentally. Chronic Chagas disease causes **dilated organs: dilated cardiomyopathy, megaesophagus, megacolon.** The disease is endemic to Central and South America. Diagnosis is made by visualization of trypanosomes in the blood during acute infection. Treat with **benznidazole or nifurtimox.**

African trypanosomiasis, or **sleeping sickness,** is caused by ***Trypanosoma brucei gambiense*** (West Africa) and ***Trypanosoma brucei rhodesiense*** (East Africa) and transmitted by the bite of the **tsetse fly.** The East African form is more severe. Trypomastigotes are hematogenously disseminated through the body and replicate in the blood, lymphatics, and spinal fluid. Disease manifestation occurs in three stages:

1. Chancre: The painful tsetse fly bite leaves a large, itchy chancre that resolves within 1 to 2 weeks.
2. Hematologic/lymphatic dissemination: Recurrent fever, fatigue, and lymphadenopathy.

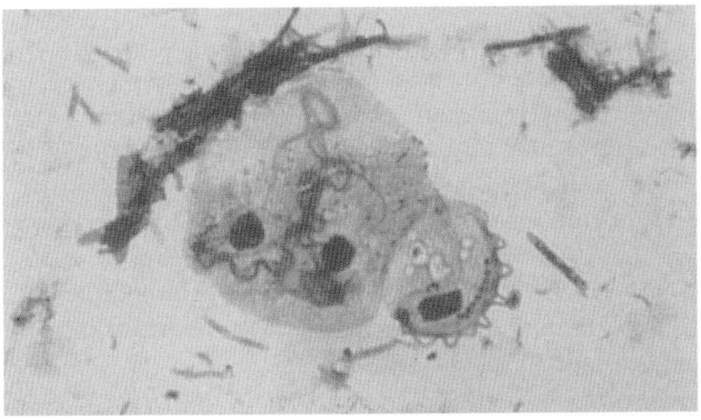

Fig. 5.83 Motile trophozoite in vaginal discharge in *Trichomonas vaginalis* infection. (*From Goering R, Dockrell H, Wakelin D, et al.* Mims' Medical Microbiology. *4th ed. Philadelphia: Elsevier; 2007. Courtesy R. Muller.*)

3. CNS changes: Meningoencephalitis causes headaches, changes in behavior, focal neurologic deficits, and excessive somnolence leading to eventual coma and death.

Treat with **suramin** (bloodborne infection) or **melarsoprol** (for CNS involvement).

Protozoa That Are Sexually Transmitted

❍ *Trichomonas vaginalis*

Trichomonas vaginalis causes **trichomoniasis** and is a motile, flagellated protozoan that does not form cysts. Infection is acquired by **sexual transmission** of *Trichomonas* trophozoites. In women, it causes a **vaginitis** characterized by **itching, burning, dysuria,** and a **frothy malodorous discharge** that can be clear, white, yellow, or green in color. In men, it may cause a mild urethritis. Diagnosis is made by visualization of **motile trophozoites** on wet mount (Fig. 5.83). Treat the patient and partner with **metronidazole.** Interestingly, *Trichomonas* is the only protozoan that does not exist in cyst form because it never leaves the host environment (it is sexually transmitted and therefore has no need for a protective/dormant form).

HELMINTHS

Helminths are divided into two major groups: **nematodes (roundworms)** and **platyhelminths (flatworms).** Flatworms are further divided into **cestodes (tapeworms)** and **trematodes (flukes).**

> Eosinophilia is a common finding in parasitic infection. Rule out parasitic infection in an individual with unexplained peripheral eosinophilia.

Nematodes

Nematodes that cause intestinal infections include the following:

❍ Hookworms *(Ancylostoma duodenale, Necator americanus)*
❍ Threadworm *(Strongyloides stercoralis)*
❍ Roundworm *(Ascaris lumbricoides)*
❍ Dog roundworm *(Toxocara canis)*
❍ Whipworm *(Trichuris trichiura)*
❍ Pinworm *(Enterobius vermicularis)*

Hookworms *(Ancylostoma duodenale, Necator americanus)* are commonly found in tropical and subtropical regions of the world. Hookworm eggs hatch in the soil; larvae are able to penetrate the soles of bare feet. They migrate through the bloodstream to the lung. They mature in the lung and are coughed up and swallowed into the intestine. Hookworms attach to the small intestinal mucosa and feed on human blood. Clinical manifestations of hookworm infection include **local reaction** at the site of parasite entry (Fig. 5.84), **pneumonitis** (in the lung phase), abdominal pain, and **iron deficiency anemia** as a consequence of parasitic feeding. Peripheral eosinophilia may be present. Diagnosis is made by stool ova and parasite testing (O&P). Treat with **pyrantel pamoate or albendazole.**

> Both hookworm and roundworm cause lung infection. Hookworm enters the body through the foot. Roundworm enters the body through the GI tract.

Threadworm *(Strongyloides stercoralis)* is also more commonly found in tropical and subtropical regions of the world. It can also be found in the **southeastern United States.** Much like hookworms, *Strongyloides* larvae in the soil penetrate the soles of bare feet and migrate to the lung, and then to the intestine when

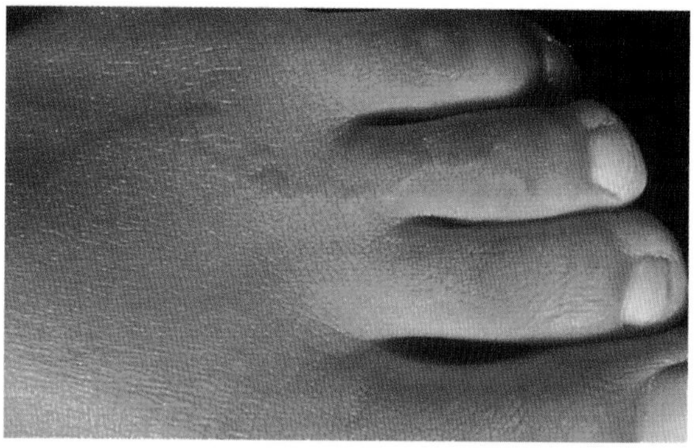

Fig. 5.84 Hookworm infection showing cutaneous larval migrans (raised inflammatory track left by invading hookworm larvae). (*From Goering R, Dockrell H, Wakelin D, et al.* Mims' Medical Microbiology. *4th ed. Philadelphia: Elsevier; 2007. Courtesy A. du Vivier.*)

coughed up and swallowed. *Strongyloides* are able to lay eggs that hatch directly into the intestine, perpetuating infection. ***Strongyloides* is the only helminth that is able to multiply within the human body (it is "strong").** This is the reason that (1) *Strongyloides* infection can be diagnosed by visualization of **larvae** (not eggs) in the stool, and (2) *Strongyloides* infection can persist for years. Clinical manifestations of *Strongyloides* infection include pruritic rash at the site of parasite entry, **pneumonitis,** abdominal pain, and diarrhea. Individuals who are immunocompromised, especially after receiving high-dose corticosteroids, may have severe, disseminated *Strongyloides* infection. They may also be at risk for sepsis because the *Strongyloides* larvae track gut bacteria into the bloodstream as they invade. Treat with **ivermectin.**

Roundworm (*Ascaris lumbricoides*) eggs are present in soil. When ingested, *Ascaris* eggs hatch in the intestine. Emergent larvae breach into the bloodstream through the intestinal mucosa. They undergo further development in the lung, after which they are coughed up and swallowed back into the intestine. *Ascaris* may present with **pneumonitis** (in the lung phase) or with **malnutrition or bowel obstruction** (in the gut phase). Diagnosis is made by visualization of *Ascaris* eggs in stool. Treat with **pyrantel pamoate, ivermectin, or albendazole.**

Ascariasis is the most common helminthic infection.

Dog roundworm *(Toxocara canis)* is a parasite usually found in dogs, but it may occasionally cause disease in humans. The eggs are passed in dog feces. When ingested by humans, the hatched eggs are unable to undergo a lung phase and embed in the organs instead. The complications of *Toxocara canis* include **visceral larva migrans** (causing hepatitis, myocarditis, seizures) and **ocular larva migrans** (retinal lesions, strabismus). Look for a patient with fever, hepatosplenomegaly, and **eosinophilia.**

Whipworm *(Trichuris trichiura)* is so named for its distinctive shape (Fig. 5.85). Whipworm infection is found worldwide but is especially endemic to tropical regions. Whipworm eggs are ingested, hatch in the small intestine, and **parasitize the large intestine.** It is different from the roundworm in that it does not need to migrate to the lung to mature. Especially severe infections are associated with **bloody diarrhea** and **rectal prolapse.** Diagnosis is made via stool O&P. Treat with **mebendazole.**

Pinworm *(Enterobius vermicularis)* infection is the most common helminthic infection in the United States. Infection is particularly common in children. Pinworm eggs are swallowed (found in contaminated food). Mature pinworms hatch and live in the large intestine. At night, female worms crawl to the anus and lay their eggs (Fig. 5.86) in the perianal area, causing **nighttime anal pruritus.** Diagnosis is made by the **Scotch tape test,** where eggs can be visualized on adhesive tape after being applied to the perianal area. Treat with **albendazole or pyrantel pamoate.**

Nematodes that cause other tissue infections include the following:

- Guinea worm *(Dracunculus medinensis)*
- Loa loa
- *Onchocerca volvulus*

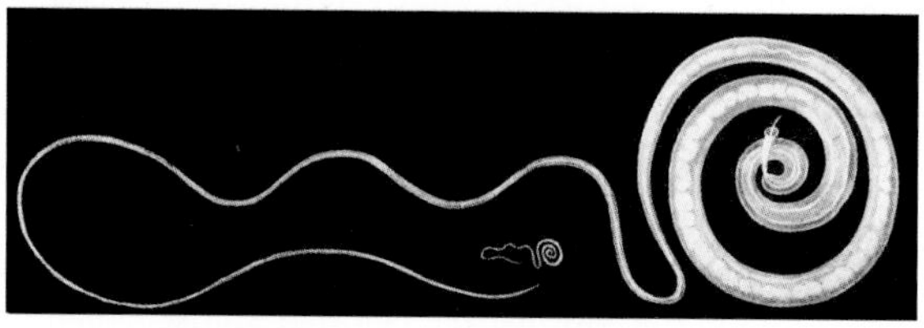

Fig. 5.85 Whipworm. (*From Wikipedia. Trichuris trichiura. Available at: http://en.wikipedia.org/wiki/File:Trichuris_trichiura.jpg. Accessibility verified July 26, 2017.*)

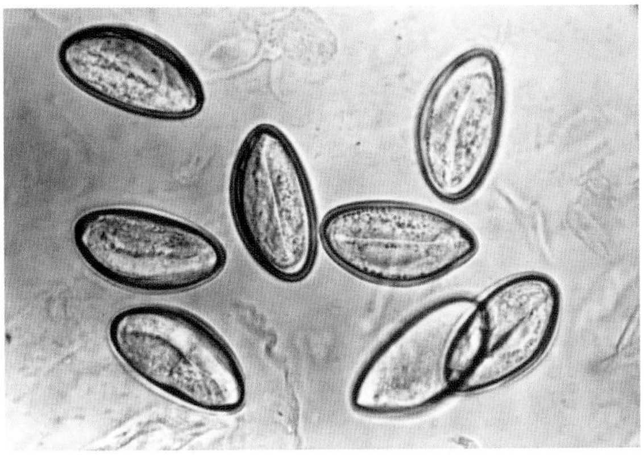

FIG. 5.86 Pinworm eggs, often described as "D-shaped" eggs. (*From Wikipedia. Eggs of Enterobius vermicularis. Available at: https://commons.wikimedia.org/wiki/File:Eggs_of_Enterobius_vermicularis_5229_lores.jpg. Image courtesy Centers for Disease Control and Prevention, Atlanta, GA. Accessibility verified July 11, 2017.*)

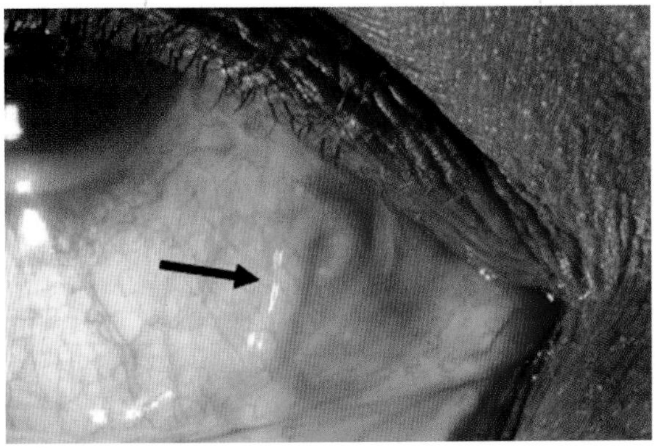

FIG. 5.87 *Loa loa* conjunctivitis with worm (*arrow*) moving in the inferior fomix. (*From Jain R et al, Subconjunctival loa loa worm, International Journal of Infectious Diseases, 2008;12(6): e133–e135.*)

❍ *Trichinella spiralis*
❍ *Wuchereria bancrofti*

Guinea worm *(Dracunculus medinensis)* larvae take residence in the **water flea** and are transmitted to humans by **contaminated drinking water.** As a result of preventive measures such as filtering water, the guinea worm is endemic only to certain regions of Africa. Larvae migrate from the gut to the subcutaneous tissues; adult females emerge from the skin to give birth to larvae, causing painful skin ulceration.

Loa loa is transmitted to humans by **biting flies** (i.e., **horse fly**). Adult worms parasitize the subcutaneous tissue. Their migration through the skin is marked through reactions called ***Calabar swellings.*** They are most notable for their appearance in the **conjunctivae of the eye** (Fig. 5.87). Treat with **diethylcarbamazine.**

Onchocerca volvulus is transmitted by the **female blackfly.** Worms live in the skin, causing pruritus. Chronic skin infection can manifest as subcutaneous nodules, **hyperpigmented skin lesions,** or **skin lichenification.** Worms may affect the eye causing corneal and retinal lesions (**"river blindness"**). Treat with **ivermectin.**

Trichinella spiralis **(trichinosis)** larvae take residence in the skeletal muscle of infected animals and lie dormant as **cysts.** Humans acquire *Trichinella* infection by **eating raw or undercooked meat** (particularly **pork**). Larvae excyst in the stomach and migrate from the intestine to the muscle. Their migration causes **muscle pain and weakness** and, occasionally, **periorbital edema.** Diagnosis can be made by rising serologic titers or visualization of cysts on muscle biopsy. Treat with mebendazole or albendazole, corticosteroids, and supportive therapy during the migratory phase, which can be life threatening.

Wuchereria bancrofti (filariasis) is found in tropical and subtropical countries and transmitted by the bite of the **female mosquito.** *Wuchereria* parasitize the lymphatics. Chronic, untreated infection leads to **lymphedema** and **elephantiasis,** particularly of the lower limbs (Fig. 5.88). The drug of choice is **diethylcarbamazine.**

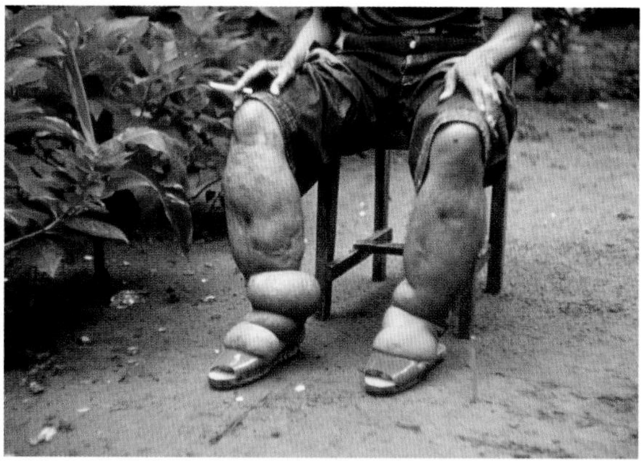

Fig. 5.88 *Wuchereria* elephantiasis. (*Centers for Disease Control and Prevention Public Health Library image no. 373.*)

Platyhelminths

Cestodes (tapeworms) include the following:

- *Taenia* spp. *(T. saginata, T. solium)*
- *Diphyllobothrium latum*
- *Echinococcus granulosus*

Diphyllobothrium latum **(fish tapeworm)** is acquired by the consumption of **raw, freshwater fish.** It infects the ileum and is usually asymptomatic but may cause macrocytic anemia from **vitamin B_{12} deficiency** (as a result of parasite competition for dietary B_{12}). Treat the B_{12} deficiency and give **praziquantel.**

Echinococcus granulosus **(dog tapeworm)** is carried by dogs as well as its usual intermediate host, sheep. Humans may acquire infection after the consumption of eggs in contaminated food or exposure to sheep or dog feces. Newly hatched larvae migrate to the liver, where they grow and form a cystic cavity **(hydatid cyst).** Diagnosis is usually made when the cyst becomes symptomatic (causing right upper quadrant pain). The contents of the cyst may cause **anaphylaxis,** so echinococcal antigens are first neutralized with hypertonic saline or ethanol before surgical removal of the cyst. Treat with albendazole.

Taenia **species *(T. saginata, T. solium)*** cause intestinal infection and are acquired by the consumption of larvae in **cysticerci** in infected beef *(T. saginata)* or pork *(T. solium).* Intestinal infection is manifested by abdominal pain and rarely may cause intestinal obstruction. When a human consumes *T. solium* **eggs,** however, the eggs hatch in the intestine and form **cysticerci** in human tissue, causing **cysticercosis** (cysts in muscle, eye, internal organs) or **neurocysticercosis** if they migrate to the brain (Fig. 5.89). Neurocysticercosis may present as seizures. First-line treatment is with **praziquantel.** For neurocysticercosis, use albendazole with antiepileptics and steroids and supportive therapy.

Trematodes (Flukes)

All trematodes develop in two intermediate hosts before definitive infection in humans. Almost all trematodes first infect **snails.** Humans acquire trematode infection from the second host (fish, shellfish, the environment).

Trematodes that cause gastrointestinal infections include the following:

- *Clonorchis sinensis*
- *Paragonimus westermani*
- *Schistosomiasis*

Clonorchis sinensis **(Chinese liver fluke)** is acquired by eating cysts present in **raw or undercooked fish.** The worms mature in the **bile ducts,** causing inflammation and fibrosis in particularly heavy infections. Long-term consequences of clonorchiasis include biliary obstruction and **gallstones,** bacterial cholangitis, and **cholangiocarcinoma.** Treat with **praziquantel.**

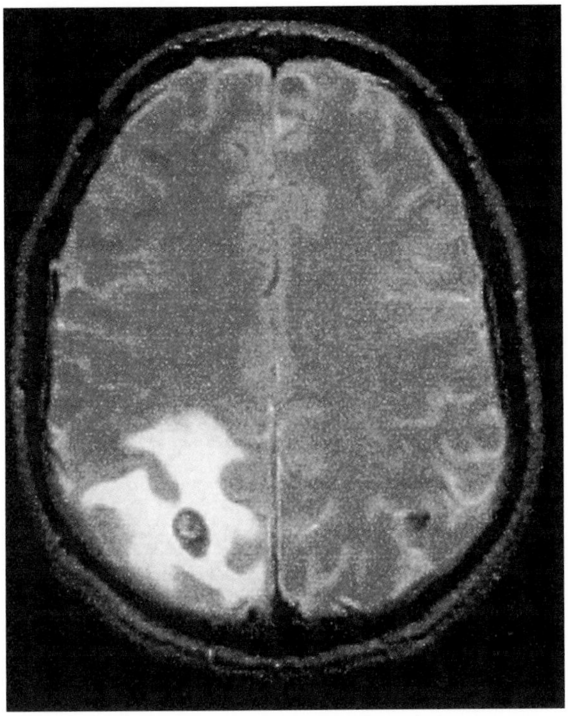

Fig. 5.89 Cerebral cysticercosis on magnetic resonance imaging showing a cyst containing developing larva. (*From Goering R, Dockrell H, Wakelin D, et al.* Mims' Medical Microbiology. *4th ed. Philadelphia: Elsevier; 2007. Courtesy J. Curé.*)

Paragonimus westermani **(lung fluke)** is acquired by eating **raw or undercooked** freshwater crab or crayfish. Larvae migrate from the gut to the lung, which causes pulmonary inflammation and **hemoptysis.** Diagnosis is made by visualization of parasite eggs in the sputum or stool. Treat with **praziquantel.**

Schistosomiasis **(blood flukes)** species are found in tropical and subtropical regions worldwide. *S. mansoni* can be found in Africa and South America. *S. haematobium* is endemic to Africa, whereas *S. japonicum* is endemic to parts of Asia. Schistosomes start their life cycle in water snails. Humans acquire schistosomiasis infection by swimming in snail-infested waters; free-living larvae penetrate the skin (**"swimmer's itch"**), migrate to the lung, and mature in the liver. Acute infection may be marked by fever with urticarial rash (Katayama fever). Adult worms migrate in the portal system (hence blood flukes) to submucosal venules to lay eggs. *S. haematobium* has a predilection for the bladder and may cause dysuria, hematuria, and eventually **squamous cell carcinoma of the bladder.** *S. mansoni* and *S. japonicum* favor the intestines but can lay eggs into the portal veins, leading to **portal hypertension, hepatosplenomegaly, and fibrosis of the liver and spleen.** Treat with **praziquantel.**

ANTIMICROBIALS

In this section we cover antibiotics, antivirals, and antifungals. Antiprotozoals and antihelminthic agents are not covered because they are not generally considered high yield for Step 1.

Antibiotics

Antibiotic agents can be broadly classified as either **bacteriostatic (inhibit the replication and growth of bacteria without killing them)** or **bacteriocidal (kill bacteria).** Whether or not an agent is able to kill bacteria outright is usually determined by how it acts on the bacteria, such that families of antibiotics that share a similar mechanism of action can be broadly classified as shown in Table 5.6.

β-Lactam Antibiotics

- Penicillin family
  - Penicillins
  - Aminopenicillins

Table 5.6 Bacteriostatic and Bacteriocidal Antibiotics

BACTERIOSTATIC AGENTS	BACTERIOCIDAL AGENTS
Macrolides	Vancomycin
Clindamycin	Penicillins
Sulfonamides	Cephalosporins
Trimethoprim	Carbapenems
Tetracyclines	Monobactams
Chloramphenicol	Fluoroquinolones
Spectinomycin	Aminoglycosides
	Metronidazole
	Daptomycin
	Trimethoprim-sulfamethoxazole

- Penicillinase-resistant penicillins
- Antipseudomonal penicillins

○ Cephalosporins
○ Monobactams
○ Carbapenems

Penicillins: Penicillin G (IV); Penicillin V (Oral):

○ **Mechanisms:** (1) Bind penicillin-binding proteins (PBPs), which synthesize peptidoglycan in bacterial cell walls (Fig. 5.90). (2) Competitively inhibit transpeptidase cross-linking of cell wall. (3) Activate autolytic enzymes.

○ **Coverage:** Gram-positive organisms including *S. pneumoniae,* group A strep such as *S. pyogenes, Actinomyces,* and syphilis.

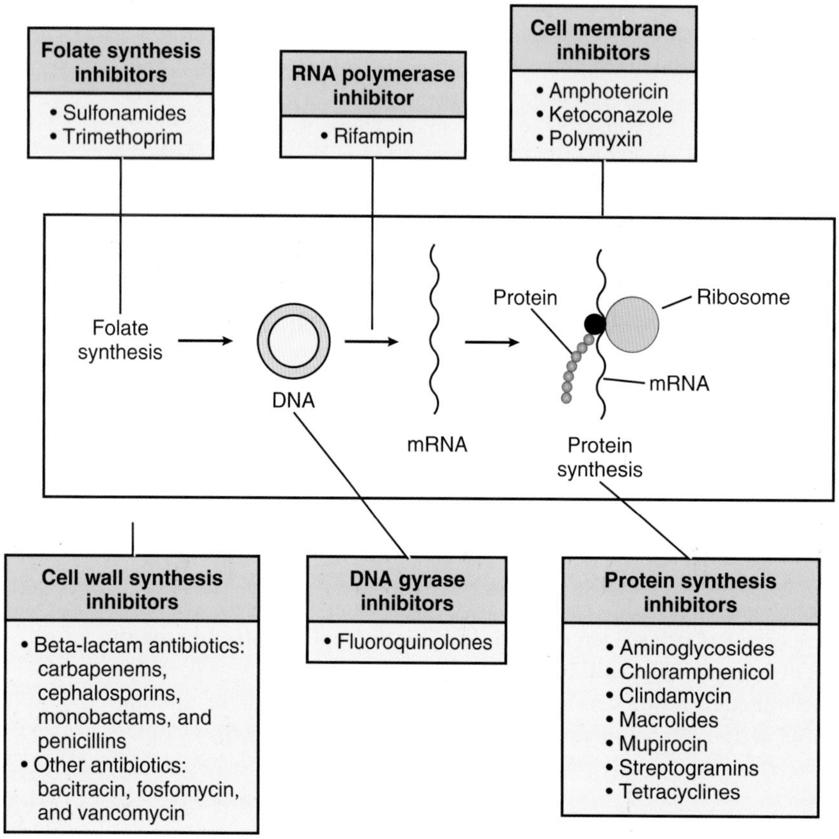

Fig. 5.90 Sites of action of antimicrobials. (*From Brenner GM, Stevens CW. Pharmacology. 3rd ed. Philadelphia: Elsevier; 2009.*)

- **Resistance:** Broad because of penicillinase (β-lactamase), altered porins (gram-negative only), and altered PBPs.
- **Toxicity:** Hypersensitivity reaction, hemolytic anemia. Penicillin (or β-lactam) allergies are mediated by type 1 hypersensitivity reactions directed against penicillin-derived hapten–protein complexes. There is a **5% to 10% chance of cross-reactivity with cephalosporins and carbapenems** as a result of their similar β-lactam ring structures.

Aminopenicillins: Ampicillin (IV, Oral); Amoxicillin (Oral):

- **Mechanisms:** Same mechanisms as penicillin.
- **Coverage:** Same as penicillin plus some gram-negative rods, including *H. influenzae, E. coli, Listeria monocytogenes, Proteus mirabilis, Salmonella,* and enterococci.
- **Resistance:** Penicillinase (β-lactamase), altered porins (gram-negative only), altered PBPs.
- **Toxicity:** Hypersensitivity reaction, pseudomembranous colitis, ampicillin rash (especially when given to a patient with **infectious mononucleosis**).

Penicillinase-Resistant Penicillins: Methicillin, Nafcillin, Oxacillin (IV); Cloxacillin, Dicloxacillin (Oral):

- **Mechanisms:** Same mechanisms as penicillin.
- **Coverage:** Same as penicillin plus coverage for methicillin-sensitive *Staphylococcus aureus* (MSSA).
- **Resistance:** Altered porins (gram-negative only), altered PBPs (MRSA).
- **Toxicity:** Hypersensitivity reaction; methicillin—interstitial nephritis.

Antipseudomonal Penicillins: Ticarcillin, Piperacillin (IV); Carbenicillin (Oral):

- **Mechanism:** Same mechanisms as penicillin.
- **Coverage:** Same as penicillin plus coverage for *Pseudomonas aeruginosa,* gram-negative rods, and anaerobes such as *Bacteroides fragilis.*
- **Resistance:** Penicillinase (β-lactamase), altered porins (gram-negative only), altered PBPs.
- **Toxicity:** Hypersensitivity reaction.

β-Lactamase inhibitors (clavulanic acid, sulbactam, tazobactam) are used in combination with β-lactam antibiotics to extend their coverage by inhibiting β-lactamases. Combinations include:

- amoxicillin + clavulanic acid = Augmentin (oral)
- ticarcillin + clavulanic acid = Timentin (IV)
- ampicillin + sulbactam = Unasyn (IV)
- piperacillin + tazobactam = Zosyn (IV)

Cephalosporins:

- **Mechanisms:** (1) Inhibit cell wall synthesis similar to penicillin. (2) β-Lactam ring modified to be resistant to penicillinases (Table 5.7).
- **Coverage:** Gram-positive coverage diminishes, whereas gram-negative coverage improves with each generation.
- **Resistance:** Cephalosporinases, altered porins (gram negative only), altered PBPs.
- **Toxicity:** Hypersensitivity reactions, increases nephrotoxicity of aminoglycosides; impaired vitamin K–dependent clotting factor synthesis and **disulfiram-like reaction** with alcohol use (only cephalosporins containing methylthiotetrazole [MTT] side chain).

Drugs that can cause disulfiram-like reactions include metronidazole, cefamandole, cefmetazole, cefotetan, cefoperazone, first-generation sulfonylureas, and griseofulvin.

Monobactams—Aztreonam (IV, IM):

- **Mechanism:** Inhibit cell wall synthesis by binding to PBP3.
- **Coverage:** Gram-negative aerobic bacteria *only.* No activity against gram-positive bacteria or anaerobes.
- **Resistance:** Does not bind PBPs of anaerobes or gram-positive bacteria.
- **Toxicity:** GI upset, *no* cross-hypersensitivity with penicillins or cephalosporins.

Table 5.7 Cephalosporins

	MEMBERS	COVERAGE
First generation	Cephalothin Cephapirin Cephradine **Cephalexin** **Cefazolin** Cefadroxil	Gram-positive cocci *Proteus mirabilis* *Escherichia coli* *Klebsiella pneumoniae*
Second generation	Cefamandole Cefaclor Cefuroxime **Cefoxitin** **Cefotetan** Cefmetazole Cefonicid Cefprozil Loracarbef Cefdinir	< Gram-positive cocci *Haemophilus influenzae* *Enterobacter aerogenes* *Neisseria* spp. *Proteus mirabilis* *E. coli* *Klebsiella pneumoniae* *Serratia marcescens*
Third generation	**Ceftriaxone** Ceftazidime* Cefotaxime Ceftizoxime Cefixime Cefoperazone* Cefpodoxime Ceftibuten	Gram-negative > > gram-positive coverage
Fourth generation	**Cefepime***	Broad gram-positive and gram-negative coverage *Pseudomonas aeruginosa*
Fifth generation	**Ceftaroline**† **Ceftolozane*** **Ceftobiprole***†	Broad gram-positive and gram-negative coverage

Bold type indicates anaerobes.
*Antipseudomonal.
†Anti-MRSA.

Aztreonam is often used in patients with a penicillin allergy who cannot tolerate β-lactam antibiotics or in patients with renal insufficiency who cannot tolerate aminoglycosides.

Carbapenems—Imipenem/Cilastatin, Meropenem, Ertapenem, Doripenem (IV, IM):

- **Mechanisms:** (1) Inhibit cell wall synthesis similar to penicillin. (2) Structure modified to be highly resistant to β-lactamases. (3) Cilastatin inhibits renal tubular dehydropeptidase I, which breaks down imipenem to toxic metabolites; thus when administered together, imipenem's half-life is increased and its nephrotoxicity is reduced.
- **Coverage:** Broad-spectrum gram-positive, gram-negative, and anaerobic coverage. Do *not* cover MRSA. Ertapenem does *not* cover *Pseudomonas aeruginosa.*
- **Resistance:** Carbapenemases (metallo-β-lactamases such as New Delhi metallo-β-lactamase-1 [NDM-1]).
- **Toxicity:** GI upset when infused rapidly, skin rash, CNS toxicity (seizures) at high plasma levels (reduced risk with meropenem), hypersensitivity reaction.

Antiribosomal Antibiotics

- Aminoglycosides
- Tetracyclines
- Macrolides
- Amphenicols
- Lincosamides
- Oxazolidinones
- Streptogramins

Aminoglycosides—Gentamicin, Amikacin, Streptomycin (IV); Neomycin (Topical, IV, Oral), Tobramycin (IV, Inhaled), Neosporin:

- **Mechanisms:** (1) Irreversibly bind to 30S subunit and inhibit formation of initiation complex. (2) Cause errors of RNA reading and translocation with premature termination. (3) Require oxygen for uptake into bacteria, limited by diffusion across cell wall. (4) Complete renal excretion. Crosses into CNS only if meninges are inflamed.
- **Coverage:** Gram-negative aerobic bacteria. Active against gram-positive bacteria and synergistic with β-lactam antibiotics, but limited use because alternatives are less toxic. *No* activity against anaerobes or abscesses because uptake is through an oxygen-dependent mechanism. Neomycin given orally to kill bowel flora (poorly absorbed, useful in hepatic encephalopathy and before bowel surgery). Nebulized tobramycin used in cystic fibrosis because of activity against *Pseudomonas aeruginosa.*
- **Resistance:** Ribosomal binding site alteration, decreased membrane permeability, aminoglycoside inactivating enzymes by acetylation/phosphorylation/adenylation.
- **Toxicity:** Nephrotoxicity, vestibular and ototoxicity (especially in combination with loop diuretics), neuromuscular blockade, teratogen.

Tetracyclines—Tetracycline, Doxycycline, Minocycline, Demeclocycline (PO, IV, Topical), Tigecycline (IV):

- **Mechanisms:** (1) Reversibly bind to 30S subunit and prevent aminoacyl-tRNA binding to the ribosome–RNA complex, causing inhibition of protein residue elongation. (2) Oral tetracyclines chelated by divalent cations: cannot take with food, milk, antacids or iron, calcium, or magnesium-containing supplements. (3) Undergo enterohepatic recirculation; only doxycycline is eliminated in stool and is thus safe in renal disease.
- **Coverage:** Intracellular pathogens including *Rickettsia* and *Chlamydia;* spirochetes including *Borrelia burgdorferi, Leptospira,* and *Treponema pallidum;* and specific pathogens including *Mycoplasma pneumoniae, Helicobacter pylori, Entamoeba histolytica, Brucella, Nocardia,* and *Propionibacterium* in inflammatory acne. **Tigecycline** is an IV-only glycylcycline derivative with broad-spectrum coverage even against **MRSA** and **VRE.**
- **Resistance:** Drug efflux pumps, ribosomal binding site alteration/accommodation, tetracycline inactivating enzymes through acetylation.
- **Toxicity:** Pill esophagitis, GI upset, phototoxic dermatitis, Fanconi syndrome with expired drugs. Discoloration of teeth and inhibited bone growth in children; teratogen.

Macrolides—Erythromycin, Azithromycin (PO, IV); Clarithromycin (PO):

- **Mechanisms:** (1) Reversibly bind to 23S rRNA of the 50S subunit and block translocation, causing inhibition of protein synthesis. (2) Undergo enterohepatic recirculation and are metabolized by the cytochrome P-450 system (CYP450). (3) Potent inhibitors of CYP450 system, leading to many drug–drug interactions.
- **Coverage:** Atypical organisms including *Legionella, Mycoplasma, Chlamydia,* and some gram-positive cocci (mainly *Streptococcus*).
- **Resistance:** Methylation of 23S rRNA binding site, macrolide-inactivating enzymes through esterification/phosphorylation, drug efflux pumps.
- **Toxicity:** GI upset, QT interval prolongation, acute cholestatic jaundice and hepatitis, eosinophilia, skin rashes; CYP450 inhibitor, therefore increases serum concentrations of some chemotherapeutics, theophylline, warfarin, clopidogrel (azithromycin does not have major interactions).
- **Erythromycin** (and to a lesser degree other macrolides) is an **agonist of motilin receptors** in the GI tract that stimulate peristalsis and gastric emptying, making it useful in the treatment of gastroparesis or during esophagogastroduodenoscopy. **Telithromycin** is an oral ketolide derivative with coverage similar to the macrolides plus improved activity against *S. pneumoniae* but may be hepatotoxic.

Amphenicols—Chloramphenicol (PO, IV):

- **Mechanisms:** (1) Irreversibly bind to 50S subunit and inhibits peptidyltransferase activity. (2) Metabolized and completely inactivated by glucuronidation in liver; metabolites and IV form excreted by kidneys. (3) Lipid soluble, with excellent tissue penetration including the CNS.

- **Coverage:** Broad-spectrum activity against gram-positive, gram-negative, and anaerobic organisms. Low cost, but limited use outside of developing countries because of high toxicity.
- **Resistance:** Reduced membrane permeability, inactivating enzyme (chloramphenicol acetyltransferase), ribosomal binding site alteration.
- **Toxicity:** Dose-dependent bone marrow suppression and anemia/pancytopenia, dose-independent aplastic anemia, gray baby syndrome (ashen gray skin discoloration, cyanosis, vomiting, vasomotor collapse; caused by drug accumulation in infants because they lack sufficient levels of liver UDP-glucuronyl transferase to metabolize).
- Chloramphenicol is still the drug of choice in these scenarios: (1) bacterial meningitis in a patient known to have allergies to penicillins and/or cephalosporins; (2) *Rickettsia* infections in children and pregnant women, where tetracyclines should be avoided; (3) brain abscesses caused by *Staphylococcus* or mixed flora.

Lincosamides—Clindamycin (PO, IV, Topical):
- **Mechanism:** Irreversibly bind to 50S subunit and block peptide bond formation and translocation, causing inhibition of protein synthesis.
- **Coverage:** Anaerobes including *Bacteroides* and *Clostridium perfringens,* some aerobic gram-positive organisms including *Streptococcus* spp. and *Staphylococcus* (including MRSA, but not *Enterococcus* spp.).
- **Resistance:** Methylation of 23S rRNA binding site, ribosomal structural alteration, lincosamide inactivating enzymes by adenylation, intrinsic resistance because of poor permeability through outer membrane (gram-negative only).
- **Toxicity:** Pseudomembranous colitis, diarrhea, rash.
- Because clindamycin is ineffective against enterococci and most aerobic gram-negative bacteria, it is often more effective when used to treat anaerobic infections originating *above* the diaphragm (e.g., aspiration pneumonia, lung/dental/skin abscesses), whereas metronidazole is often more effective when used to treat anaerobic infections originating *below* the diaphragm (e.g., pseudomembranous colitis, bacterial vaginosis, abdominal penetrating wounds).

Oxazolidinones—Linezolid (PO, IV):
- **Mechanisms:** (1) Irreversibly binds to 50S subunit and prevents formation of the initiation complex. (2) Bioavailability is equivalent between PO and IV forms.
- **Coverage:** Gram-positive bacteria including methicillin- and vancomycin-resistant organisms. *No* activity against most gram-negative organisms.
- **Resistance:** Point mutation in 23S rRNA, intrinsic resistance as a result of drug efflux pumps (gram negative only).
- **Toxicity:** Bone marrow suppression and thrombocytopenia/pancytopenia, headache, GI upset, serotonin syndrome in combination with monoamine oxidase inhibitor (MAOI) or selective serotonin reuptake inhibitor (SSRI, because of weak MAO inhibition).
- Both linezolid and clindamycin are often used in the treatment of exotoxin-producing *Streptococcus* and *Staphylococcus* infections (e.g., toxic shock syndrome, group A strep infections) because they inhibit the production of exotoxin.

Streptogramins—Quinupristin/Dalfopristin (IV):
- **Mechanisms:** (1) Dalfopristin irreversibly binds to 23S rRNA of the 50S subunit, inhibiting peptidyltransferase activity and causing a conformational change allowing quinupristin to bind more avidly to a nearby site of the 50S subunit. (2) Quinupristin reversibly binds to the 50S subunit, blocks polypeptide elongation, and causes premature termination and release.
- **Coverage:** Gram-positive organisms including group A strep, *Staphylococcus* (including MRSA), and *Enterococcus* (including VRE, but only *E. faecium, not E. faecalis*).
- **Resistance:** Streptogramin-inactivating enzymes by acetylation, methylation of 23S rRNA binding site, drug efflux pumps.
- **Toxicity:** GI upset, myalgia/arthralgia, rash, hyperbilirubinemia, thrombophlebitis.

Miscellaneous Antibiotics

- Glycopeptides
- Lipopeptides
- Antimetabolites
- Quinolones
- Nitroimidazoles/nitrofurans
- Polymyxins
- Monoxycarbolic acids

Glycopeptides—Vancomycin (IV, PO):

- **Mechanisms:** (1) Inhibits cell wall synthesis by binding D-alanine, the substrate of the enzyme that penicillin antibiotics inhibit. (2) IV-administered drug is excreted renally, whereas PO administered drug is not absorbed by the GI tract and attains high stool concentrations.
- **Coverage:** Gram-positive bacteria including MRSA. PO form can be used to treat *Clostridium difficile* pseudomembranous colitis; the large molecular structure of vancomycin means it cannot be systemically absorbed from the gut.
- **Resistance:** Terminal mucopeptide amino acid alteration to D-lactate or D-serine, outer membrane impermeable to glycopeptides (gram negative).
- **Toxicity:** "Red man syndrome," idiosyncratic reaction to rapid IV infusion causing histamine release; reversible hearing loss, nephrotoxicity, thrombophlebitis at infusion site; *no* cross-hypersensitivity with penicillins or cephalosporins.

Lipopeptides—Daptomycin (IV):

- **Mechanisms:** (1) Inhibits bacterial DNA, RNA, and protein synthesis by forming ion channels in the cell membrane that sap the membrane potential. (2) Is 92% protein bound, not extensively metabolized, and renally excreted. (3) Binds avidly to pulmonary surfactant; does not penetrate lung tissue well.
- **Coverage:** Gram-positive bacteria including methicillin- and vancomycin-resistant organisms. *Cannot* be used to treat pneumonias.
- **Resistance:** Uncommon; mechanism is unknown.
- **Toxicity:** Rash, constipation, nausea, headache, insomnia, rash or injection site reaction, rarely myopathy or rhabdomyolysis (increased risk with concurrent statin use).

Antimetabolites—Trimethoprim/Sulfamethoxazole (IV, PO); Dapsone, Sulfoxone, Sulfadiazine (PO):

- **Mechanisms:** (1) Sulfonamides are paraaminobenzoic acid (PABA) antimetabolites that act as competitive inhibitors of dihydropteroate synthetase to inhibit dihydrofolate (DHF) synthesis. (2) Trimethoprim inhibits dihydrofolate reductase (DHFR) to block conversion from DHF to tetrahydrofolate (THF; Fig. 5.91). (3) THF is crucial cofactor in the synthesis of purine nucleotides; animal cells require folate from the diet rather than relying on DHF synthesis.
- **Coverage:** Gram-positive and gram-negative for wide range of pathogens, notably *S. pneumoniae, H. influenzae, Shigella, Salmonella, E. coli, Neisseria gonorrhoeae, Chlamydia, Nocardia,* and some fungal infections, including *Pneumocystis jirovecii* (formerly *carinii*), *Toxoplasma gondii,* and *Isospora belli.*
- **Resistance:** Mutations in the enzymes that the antimetabolites bind to.
- **Toxicity:** Marrow suppression with megaloblastic anemia, leukopenia, granulocytopenia (all can be alleviated with folinic acid supplementation [leucovorin rescue]); hypersensitivity reactions, tubulointerstitial nephritis, photosensitivity, skin rash including severe reactions (Stevens-Johnson syndrome, toxic epidermal necrolysis, erythema multiforme); hemolysis with G6PD deficiency; displaces albumin-bound molecules, causing hyperbilirubinemia and kernicterus in infants, and increasing plasma concentrations of warfarin, phenytoin, and methotrexate.
- Sulfa drug allergies are mediated by type 1 hypersensitivity reactions against the common sulfonamide functional groups shared by a number of drugs: sulfonamide antibiotics, sulfasalazine, sulfonylureas, thiazide diuretics, acetazolamide, furosemide, celecoxib, and probenecid.

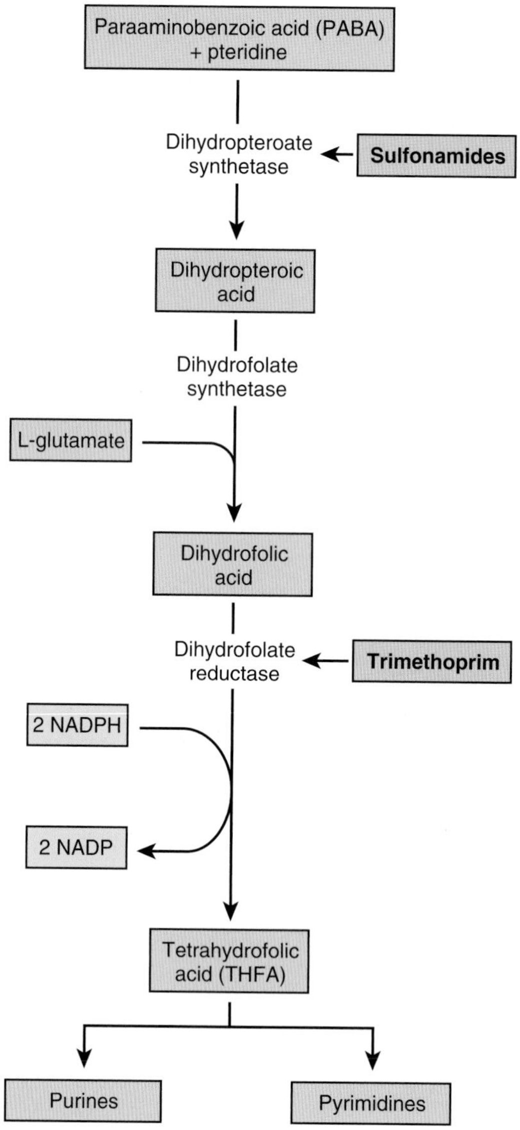

Fig. 5.91 Sulfonamides and trimethoprim inhibit in series the steps in the synthesis of tetrahydrofolic acid by interacting with key enzymes in the pathway. (*From Goering R, Dockrell H, Wakelin D, et al.* Mims' Medical Microbiology. *4th ed. Philadelphia: Elsevier; 2007.*)

Quinolones: Ciprofloxacin, Levofloxacin, Moxifloxacin (PO, IV, Some Ophthalmic):

- **Mechanism:** (1) Inhibit DNA gyrase (topoisomerase II), causing DNA double-strand breaks. (2) Fourth-generation fluoroquinolones also inhibit topoisomerase IV, causing additional inhibition of DNA replication in gram-positive bacteria. (3) Enterohepatic circulation results in high stool concentrations. High tissue penetration and renally excreted, resulting in high urine concentrations.
- **Coverage:** Spectrum of activity determines generation, with higher generations having expanded coverage (Table 5.8).
- **Resistance:** Mutations in topoisomerase II or IV, drug efflux pumps, protective DNA gyrase-binding proteins (gram-negative only).
- **Toxicity:** GI upset, tendonitis or tendon rupture, cramps and myalgias, headache, tremor, insomnia, superinfections with *C. difficile* or MRSA, QT interval prolongation (most often moxifloxacin), cartilage damage in animal studies (contraindicated in pregnant women and children for this reason). Specific reactions such as hyper- and hypoglycemia (mostly gatifloxacin, now ophthalmic only), hepatotoxicity (most often trovafloxacin) have removed their systemic forms from the market.

TABLE 5.8 Quinolones and Their Coverage Spectrum

	MEMBERS	COVERAGE
First generation (quinolones)	Nalidixic acid	Narrow gram-negative coverage Enterobacteriaceae, e.g., *Salmonella, Shigella, Campylobacter, Escherichia coli*
Second generation (fluoroquinolones)	Ciprofloxacin* Norfloxacin Lomefloxacin Ofloxacin	Same as first generation, plus coverage for: Atypical (*Legionella, Mycoplasma, Chlamydia*) Brucella Atypical *Mycobacteria*
Third generation (fluoroquinolones)	**Levofloxacin** Grepafloxacin Temafloxacin	Same as second generation, plus moderate coverage for: *Streptococcus* spp. (including *S. pneumoniae*)
Fourth generation (fluoroquinolones)	**Moxifloxacin** **Gatifloxacin** **Gemifloxacin** **Trovafloxacin**	Same as third generation, plus coverage for: Anaerobes

Bold type indicates methicillin-sensitive *Staphylococcus aureus* (MSSA).
*Antipseudomonal.

Nitroimidazoles/Nitrofurans—Metronidazole (PO, IV, Topical); Nitrofurantoin (PO):

- **Mechanisms:** (1) Nonenzymatically reduced intracellularly to form nitroso intermediates and thioester linkages that deactivate/damage numerous enzymes. (2) Reactive drug metabolites combine with DNA to create unstable molecules and cause oxidative damage.
- **Coverage:** Nitrofurantoin—*E. coli* and *S. saprophyticus.* Metronidazole—*Giardia, Entamoeba, Trichomonas, Gardnerella vaginalis, H. pylori,* enteric anaerobes including *Bacteroides* and *C. difficile.*
- **Resistance:** Multistep reduction in pathways responsible for cellular uptake of drug (Fig. 5.92).
- **Toxicity:** Disulfiram-like reaction with alcohol use, headache, metallic taste, sensory neuropathy; thrombophlebitis with IV form. Nitrofurantoin can trigger hemolysis in G6PD deficiency (oxidative stress) and can cause pulmonary fibrosis with prolonged use.
- Nitrofurantoin does not achieve sufficient concentrations for bactericidal activity in any body tissues or fluids except for the urine, so it can only be used to treat lower UTIs. It is often used in pregnant women who are unable to use fluoroquinolones or trimethoprim for this purpose.

Helicobacter pylori is treated using one of three protocols: triple therapy (proton pump inhibitor [PPI]), amoxicillin, and clarithromycin) is usually first line; quadruple therapy (PPI, bismuth, metronidazole, tetracycline) or sequential therapy (PPI and amoxicillin, then PPI, clarithromycin, tinidazole) if clarithromycin resistance is suspected.

Polymyxins—Polymyxin B, Colistin/Polymyxin E (IV, Inhaled, Topical):

- **Mechanisms:** (1) Binds to lipopolysaccharide (LPS) and causes detergent-like outer and inner membrane disruption. (2) Not absorbed from the GI tract.
- **Coverage:** Gram-negative bacteria *only.* Use is limited to resistant organisms such as multidrug-resistant *Pseudomonas aeruginosa* and carbapenemase-producing Enterobacteriaceae because of high toxicity.
- **Resistance:** Modification of LPS binding site.
- **Toxicity:** Neurotoxicity, acute tubular necrosis leading to renal failure.

Monoxycarbolic Acids—Mupirocin (Topical):

- **Mechanism:** Reversibly binds to isoleucyl-tRNA synthetase, resulting in inhibition of ligase activity and protein synthesis (see Fig. 5.90).
- **Coverage:** Gram-positive skin flora, *Streptococcus* and *Staphylococcus* (including MRSA).
- **Resistance:** Modification of isoleucyl-tRNA synthetase binding site, acquisition of *mupA* isoleucine synthetase gene.
- **Toxicity:** Rash, pain at application site.

Table 5.9 outlines treatment options for resistant organisms.

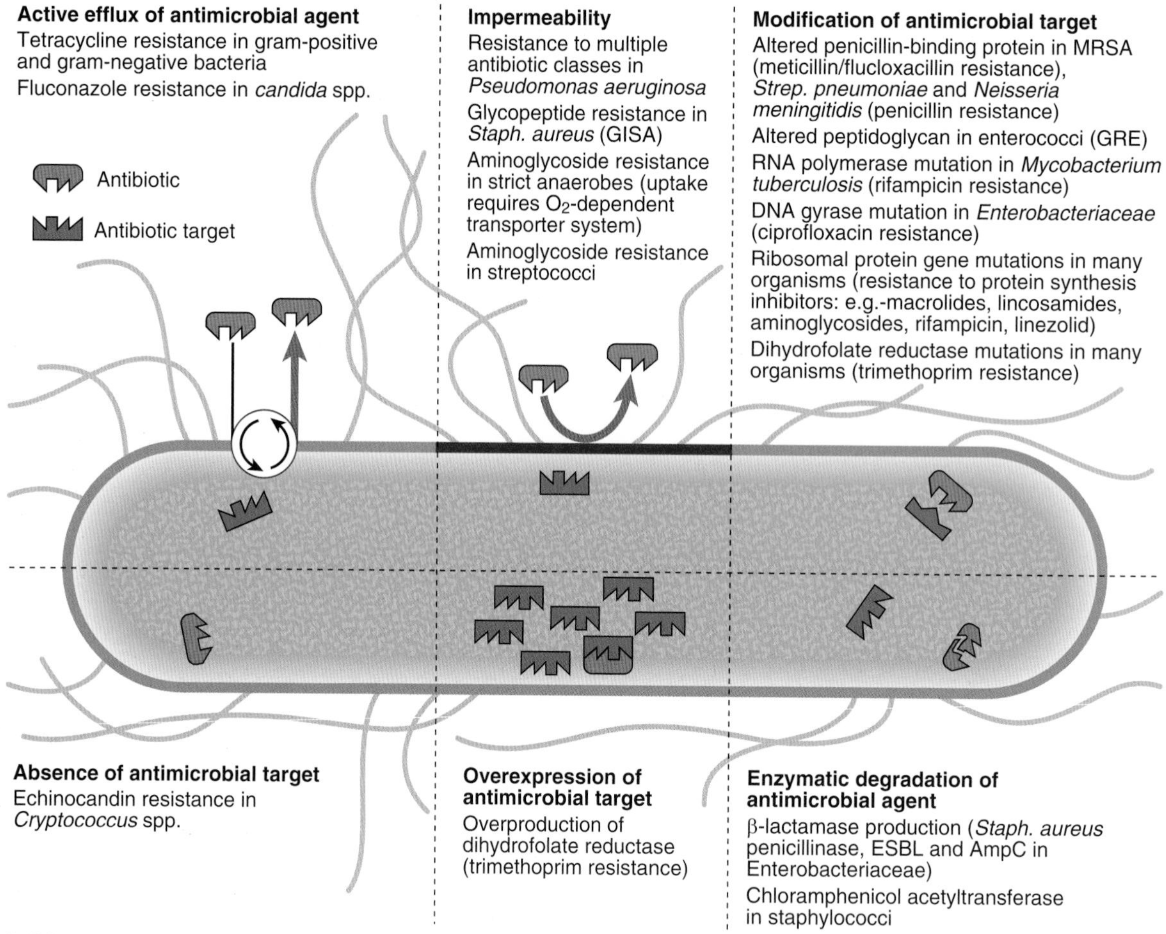

FIG. 5.92 Mechanisms of antimicrobial resistance. (*From Colledge NR, Walker BR, Ralston SH.* Davidson's Principles and Practice of Medicine. *21st ed. London: Churchill Livingstone; 2010.*)

Antimycobacterial Drugs

Refer to Table 5.10.

- Isoniazid
- Rifamycins
- Pyrazinamide
- Ethambutol

Isoniazid (INH)—PO, IM, IV

- **Mechanisms:** (1) Inhibits the synthesis of mycolic acid required for mycobacterial cell wall. (2) Requires bacterial catalase-peroxidase to convert INH to active metabolite. (3) Metabolized in the liver through acetylase enzymes that are also involved in alcohol metabolism.
- **Coverage:** Intracellular and extracellular *Mycobacterium tuberculosis, most* nontuberculous mycobacteria are resistant.
- **Resistance:** Loss or alteration of bacterial catalase-peroxidase, overexpression or structural alterations in mycolic acid pathway targets.
- **Toxicity:** Neurotoxicity (peripheral neuropathy and CNS disturbances including seizures, depression, ataxia, nystagmus), hepatotoxicity, drug-induced lupus, sideroblastic anemia, anion gap metabolic acidosis, pellagra skin rash.

Table 5.9 Treatment of Resistant Organisms

RESISTANT ORGANISM	TREATMENT OPTIONS (DEPENDING ON *IN VIVO* SUSCEPTIBILITY TESTING)	
Pseudomonas aeruginosa	Ticarcillin ± clavulanic acid Piperacillin ± tazobactam Carbenicillin Ceftazidime Cefoperazone Cefepime Ceftobiprole Ceftolozane + tazobactam	Imipenem Meropenem Doripenem Aztreonam Ciprofloxacin Gentamicin Tobramycin Amikacin
Anaerobes (*Bacteroides, Prevotella, Fusobacterium, Peptostreptococcus, Clostridium* spp.)	Amoxicillin + clavulanic acid Ampicillin + sulbactam Ticarcillin + clavulanic acid Piperacillin + tazobactam Cefoxitin Cefotetan Cefmetazole Imipenem	Meropenem Ertapenem Doripenem Chloramphenicol Clindamycin Metronidazole Moxifloxacin Tigecycline
Methicillin-resistant *Staphylococcus aureus* (MRSA)	Vancomycin Daptomycin Linezolid Quinupristin/dalfopristin Ceftaroline Ceftobiprole Tigecycline	
Vancomycin-resistant Enterococcus (VRE)	Ampicillin ± sulbactam Above ± gentamicin or streptomycin Linezolid Daptomycin Tigecycline Quinupristin/dalfopristin	
Acinetobacter baumannii	Ampicillin + sulbactam Ceftazidime Cefepime Imipenem Meropenem Doripenem	Gentamicin Tobramycin Amikacin Ciprofloxacin Colistin* Tigecycline*
Carbapenemase-producing Enterobacteriaceae (KPC or NDM)	Tigecycline Polymyxin B ± rifampin Colistin Aztreonam	

KPC, *Klebsiella pneumoniae* carbapenemase; NDM-1, New Delhi metallo-β-lactamase-1.
*Multidrug-resisten *Acinetobacter*.

Table 5.10 Treatment of Mycobacterial Infections

SPECIES	TREATMENT REGIMENS (DEPENDING ON *IN VIVO* SUSCEPTIBILITY TESTING)
M. tuberculosis complex (also *M. bovis, M. africanum, M. microti, M. canetti*)	INH Rifampin Ethambutol ± Pyrazinamide RIPE therapy for active TB (rifampin, isoniazid, pyrazinamide, ethambutol) can be remembered by the "4 for 2, 2 for 4" mnemonic: all 4 drugs required for 2 months, then isoniazid and rifampin only (2 drugs) for 4 months.
M. leprae (Hansen disease)	Dapsone or Rifampin or Clofazimine
M. avium complex (MAC) (*M. avium, M. intracellulare*)	Clarithromycin or azithromycin Rifampin or rifabutin Ethambutol ± Streptomycin
M. kansasii	Isoniazid Rifampin Ethambutol ± Clarithromycin (moxifloxacin, streptomycin, TMP-SMX)
Slowly growing NTM (>1 wk to culture) *M. marinum, M. ulcerans, M. terrae* complex, *M. szulgai, M. xenopi, M. simiae,* and *M. malmoense*	Optimal regimen unknown
Rapidly growing NTM (<1 wk to culture) *M. fortuitum* complex, *M. smegmatis, M. abscessus, M. chelonae, M. mucogenicum,* and *M. massiliense*	Optimal regimen unknown

NTM, *Non-tuberculous mycobacteria.*

Isoniazid demonstrates a bimodal population distribution in plasma half-life because of the different metabolic rates of the two predominant acetylase enzyme isoforms (slow vs. fast acetylators). INH can cause a functional pyridoxine (vitamin B_6) deficiency by binding to pyridoxine and inhibiting the formation of the active cofactor. Side effects during treatment with INH as a result of B_6 deficiency (including peripheral neuropathy, seizures, metabolic acidosis, rash, and sideroblastic anemia) can be prevented or ameliorated by **supplementing vitamin B_6.**

Rifamycins—rifampin, rifabutin (PO, IV); rifaximin (PO)

- **Mechanisms:** (1) Inhibit DNA-dependent RNA polymerase. (2) Metabolized in the liver through CYP450 system. Act as a potent inducer of this system, causing increased metabolism of both itself and other drugs sharing the same elimination pathway.
- **Coverage:** *M. tuberculosis* and atypical mycobacteria, variable resistance among *Mycobacterium avium* complex (MAC); wide gram-positive and gram-negative coverage, though not often used to treat these infections.
- **Resistance:** Structural modification of RNA polymerase (resistance develops predictably and rapidly, so *cannot* use as monotherapy).
- **Toxicity:** Urine/sweat/tears have **red-orange discoloration** (like the sweat in Gatorade ads), hepatotoxicity can range from asymptomatic jaundice to hepatitis. Decreases half-life of other drugs (warfarin, corticosteroids, oral contraceptives, oral hypoglycemic, digoxin, methadone).

Rifampin can also be used as prophylaxis after exposure to *Neisseria meningitides* or *H. influenzae* (especially type B), or as an add-on agent for the treatment of complicated MRSA infections including prosthetic valve endocarditis. Rifaximin can be given for traveler's diarrhea and to prevent hepatic encephalopathy in cirrhosis by killing ammonia-producing bacteria.

Pyrazinamide (PZA)—PO

- **Mechanisms:** (1) Unknown, metabolized to active form by intracellular pyrazinamidase; posited to inhibit fatty acid synthase I (FASI) of *M. tuberculosis.* (2) Metabolite active in acidic pH (i.e., inside macrophage phagolysosomes containing intracellular *M. tuberculosis*).
- **Coverage:** *M. tuberculosis* and *M. africanum only.*
- **Resistance:** Mutations in gene encoding pyrazinamidase (resistance develops predictably and rapidly, so *cannot* use as monotherapy).
- **Toxicity:** Hepatotoxicity, hyperuricemia (competes with uric acid for renal excretion).

Ethambutol (EMB)—PO

- **Mechanism:** Unknown, posited to inhibit arabinosyl transferase required for carbohydrate polymerization of mycobacterial cell wall.
- **Coverage:** *M. tuberculosis* and atypical mycobacteria, variable resistance among MAC.
- **Resistance:** Arabinosyl transferase overexpression, random spontaneous genetic mutations.
- **Toxicity:** Optic neuropathy (red-green color blindness, optic neuritis, central scotoma).

Specific Antiviral Agents

Amantadine, Rimantadine—PO:

- **Mechanisms:** (1) Target M2 protein ion channel and block viral penetration and uncoating. (2) Through unknown mechanisms, cause increased release of dopamine from intact nerve terminals.
- **Coverage:** Influenza A *only.*
- **Resistance:** Alteration of M2 protein (90% of influenza A, all influenza B strains are resistant).
- **Toxicity:** Ataxia, dizziness, slurred speech (fewer CNS effects with rimantadine, which does not cross blood–brain barrier).
- The **dopaminergic activity** of amantadine is used as a short-term treatment option to alleviate the akinesia, rigidity, and tremor associated with **Parkinson disease.**

Zanamivir, Oseltamivir—PO, Inhaled:

- **Mechanisms:** Inhibit viral neuraminidase and decrease the release of progeny virus.
- **Coverage:** Influenza A and B.

- **Resistance:** Alteration of neuraminidase.
- **Toxicity:** Bronchospasm (zanamivir, because it is an inhaled powder).

Ribavirin—PO:

- **Mechanism:** Competitively inhibits inosine monophosphate (IMP) dehydrogenase, causing decreased synthesis of guanine nucleotides for viral replication.
- **Coverage:** RSV (severe neonatal infections), HCV (monotherapy and combination therapy).
- **Toxicity:** Hemolytic anemia, teratogenic.

HCV Nucleotide Analogs (-Buvir): Sofosbuvir (PO):

- **Mechanism**: Nucleotide analog that causes chain termination in RNA-dependent RNA synthesis.
- **Coverage:** HCV in combination therapy only; not used in monotherapy.
- **Toxicity:** Fatigue, headache, nausea.

HCV Protease Inhibitors (-Previr): Simeprevir, Telaprevir, Paritaprevir (PO):

- **Mechanism:** Inhibit HCV protease to prevent maturation of virions.
- **Coverage:** HCV in combination therapies only; not used in monotherapy.
- **Toxicity:** Photosensitivity, rash.

Interferons (IFN-α, -β, -γ) (IV, Subcutaneous):

- **Mechanisms:** (1) Glycoproteins that are normally produced by infected cells have far ranging immunomodulatory, inflammatory, and cellular growth effects. (2) Cytokine activity blocks replication and enhances clearance of both RNA and DNA viruses through upregulation of antiviral gene transcriptional activity.
- **Coverage:** Interferon α (IFN-α)—chronic HBV and HCV infections, Kaposi sarcoma. IFN-β—acute flares in multiple sclerosis. IFN-γ—NADPH oxidase deficiency and chronic granulomatous disease.
- **Toxicity:** Neutropenia, flulike symptoms, depression.

Acyclovir, Valacyclovir, Famciclovir, Ganciclovir, Valganciclovir (PO, IV, Topical):

- **Mechanisms:** (1) Guanine analogs that require initial 5′-monophosphorylation by HSV/VZV thymidine kinase (and CMV viral kinase for ganciclovir). Cellular kinases then create triphosphate nucleotide analog. (2) Guanosine triphosphate (GTP) analogs preferentially inhibit viral DNA polymerase, causing chain terminations and disruption of viral replication.
- **Coverage:** HSV (acyclovir; active mucocutaneous lesions and encephalitis), VZV (famciclovir; herpes zoster), EBV, CMV (ganciclovir; retinitis, colitis, pneumonitis).
- **Resistance:** Loss of viral thymidine kinase, altered CMV DNA polymerase.
- **Toxicity:** Neutropenia, thrombocytopenia (both more common with ganciclovir); crystal-induced renal toxicity (IV hydrate aggressively!).

Foscarnet (IV):

- **Mechanisms:** (1) Pyrophosphate analog that competitively binds to viral DNA polymerase and inhibits viral replication in a similar manner to acyclovir and ganciclovir. (2) Does not require activation by viral kinases.
- **Coverage:** Ganciclovir-resistant CMV, acyclovir-resistant HSV.
- **Resistance:** Altered DNA polymerase.
- **Toxicity:** Nephrotoxicity, hypocalcemia, hypokalemia, and hypomagnesemia.

HIV Therapeutics/Highly Active Antiretroviral Therapy (HAART)

- Protease inhibitors
- Nucleoside reverse transcriptase inhibitors
- Nonnucleoside reverse transcriptase inhibitors
- Fusion inhibitors
- CCR5 receptor antagonists
- Integrase inhibitors

Protease Inhibitors—Atazanavir (ATV), Darunavir (DRV), Lopinavir (LPV), Ritonavir (RTV), Indinavir, Nelfinavir, Amprenavir (PO):

- **Mechanisms:** (1) Inhibit HIV-1 protease (*pol* gene product) and prevent cleavage of polypeptide product from mRNA translation into functional subunits. (2) Prevent viral maturation and budding of viral progeny. (3) Many protease inhibitors (PIs), in particular ritonavir, are potent inhibitors of hepatic microsomal enzyme CYP3A4, the primary metabolic pathway for all protease inhibitors.
- **Resistance:** Multiple genetic mutations, multifactorial.
- **Toxicity:** GI upset (diarrhea, nausea, vomiting), lipodystrophy, hyperglycemia, hyperlipidemia, crystal nephrolithiasis (indinavir).

Because of its severe dose-limiting GI side effects, **ritonavir** is rarely used as a monotherapy to treat HIV infection. However, because of its strong inhibitory effect on the **CYP3A4 microsomal system,** it is often used to "boost" the plasma levels of other coadministered PIs by inhibiting their metabolism. These dual-PI–boosted regimens are often used as an alternative first-line drug regimen for HAART (Table 5.11). The proteases end in –navir: "navir **tease** a pro**tease**." CYP inducers, especially rifampin, can decrease protease inhibitor concentrations.

Nucleoside Reverse Transcriptase Inhibitors (NRTIs; PO)—Lamivudine (3TC), Emtricitabine (FTC), Zidovudine (ZDV/AZT), Tenofovir (TDF), Didanosine (ddI), Abacavir (ABC), Stavudine (d4T):

- **Mechanisms:** (1) Nucleoside analogs that require intracellular phosphorylation to create triphosphate nucleotide analogs. (2) Nucleotide analogs preferentially inhibit viral reverse transcriptase, causing chain terminations and disruption of viral replication.
- **Resistance:** Multiple genetic mutations, multifactorial.
- **Toxicity:** Mitochondrial toxicity (manifested as peripheral neuropathy, pancreatitis, lipoatrophy, hepatic steatosis), lactic acidosis, bone marrow suppression. Didanosine is notable for pancreatitis.

Nonnucleoside Reverse Transcriptase Inhibitors (NNRTIs; PO)—Efavirenz (EFV), Nevirapine (NVP), Delavirdine (DLV), Etravirine (ETV), Rilpivirine (RPV):

- **Mechanism:** Allosteric inhibitors of viral reverse transcriptase, causing decreased affinity for nucleosides and disruption of viral replication.
- **Resistance:** Multiple genetic mutations, multifactorial.
- **Toxicity:** Rash including erythema multiforme, Stevens-Johnson syndrome, and toxic epidermal necrolysis (common to all); sleep disturbances (EFV); hypersensitivity reaction, hepatotoxicity (NVP). Delavirdine and efavirenz are teratogenic.

TABLE 5.11 HAART Regimen Options in Therapy-Naïve Patients

REGIMEN	COMMON EXAMPLES
NNRTI + 2 NRTI	Recommended: EFV + TDF/(FTC *or* 3TC) Alternatives: EFV + (ABC *or* ZDV)/(FTC *or* 3TC) RPV + TDF/(FTC *or* 3TC) RPV + ABC/(FTC *or* 3TC)
PI + 2 NRTI	Recommended: ATV/(± RTV) + TDF/(FTC *or* 3TC) DRV/(± RTV) + TDF/(FTC *or* 3TC) Alternatives: ATV/(± RTV) + (ABC *or* ZDV)/(FTC *or* 3TC) DRV/(± RTV) + ABC/(FTC *or* 3TC) LPV/(± RTV) + (ABC *or* ZDV)/(FTC *or* 3TC)
INSTI + 2 NRTI	Recommended: RAL + TDF/(FTC *or* 3TC) Alternative: RAL + ABC/(FTC *or* 3TC)
Preferred in pregnancy	LPV/(± RTV) + ZDV/(FTC *or* 3TC)

3TC, Lamivudine; ABC, abacavir; efavirenz; EFV, efavirenz; FTC, emtricitabine; INSTI, integrase inhibitor; NNRTI, nonnucleoside reverse transcriptase inhibitor; NRTI, nucleoside reverse transcriptase inhibitor; RAL, raltegravir; RPV, rilpivirine; TDF, tenofovir; ZDV, zidovudine.

Fusion Inhibitors (Subcutaneous)—Enfuvirtide (ENF):
- **Mechanism:** Binds to viral gp41 subunit expressed on outer envelope, prevents conformational change required for binding with CD4 during fusion and entry into $CD4^+$ cells.
- **Resistance:** Mutations in *gp41;* no cross-resistance with NRTIs or NNRTIs, relatively low barrier to resistance (so must use as combination therapy).
- **Toxicity:** Hypersensitivity reactions, GI upset, increased risk for bacterial pneumonia.

CCR5 Receptor Antagonists (PO)—Maraviroc (MVC):
- **Mechanism:** Reversibly inhibits binding to coreceptor CCR5 required simultaneously with CD4 binding during fusion and entry into $CD4^+$ cells.
- **Resistance:** Use of CXCR4 as coreceptor; no cross-resistance with NRTIs or NNRTIs.
- **Toxicity:** Rash, hepatotoxicity.

Integrase Inhibitors (INSTI; PO)—Raltegravir (RAL):
- **Mechanism:** Inhibits activity of integrase enzyme, prevents viral cDNA complex from integrating with host cell DNA.
- **Resistance:** Multiple genetic mutations; no cross-resistance with NRTIs and NNRTIs; low barrier to resistance (so must use as combination therapy).
- **Toxicity:** Generally well tolerated in limited clinical experience. May cause myopathy with elevated creatine kinase.

ANTIFUNGALS

This section is divided into three parts: systemic antifungals for systemic infections, oral antifungals for mucocutaneous infections, and topical antifungals for mucocutaneous infections.

Systemic Antifungals for Systemic Infections
- Amphotericin B
- Flucytosine (5-FC)
- Azoles
- Echinocandins

Amphotericin B
For a long time, **amphotericin B** was the only antifungal agent used for systemic treatment. It is now falling out of favor because newer agents are less toxic. Like many antifungals, amphotericin B exploits the fact that the lipid composition of fungi cell membranes differs from mammalian cells: They contain **ergosterol** instead of cholesterol. Amphotericin B binds ergosterol and forms permeable pores in the cell membrane.
- **Mechanism:** Forms ergosterol-associated pores in cell membranes.
- **Coverage:** Broad coverage, including the clinically significant yeasts *(Candida albicans, Cryptococcus neoformans),* endemic mycoses *(Histoplasma, Blastomyces, Coccidioides),* and pathogenic molds (*Aspergillus,* agents of mucormycosis). However, because of its toxicity, it is generally reserved for life-threatening infections, particularly for susceptible patients (i.e., immunosuppressed), to reduce fungal load. Once that is accomplished, patients are usually switched to a less toxic substitute for maintenance and prevention of relapse.
- **Resistance:** Only a few organisms are resistant, because of either reduced or modified ergosterol.
- **Toxicity:** Immediate effects (with infusion) include fever, chills, dyspnea, muscle spasms, vomiting, headache, and hypotension. These can be prevented with slow infusion or premedication. Long-term effects include renal damage (including irreversible renal tubular damage), hepatotoxicity, anemia (as a result of low erythropoietin from renal damage), and neurotoxicity if administered intrathecally.

Flucytosine
- **Mechanism:** 5-FC is taken up by the fungal enzyme cytosine permease, then metabolized into its active forms, which inhibit RNA and DNA synthesis (human cells are unable to convert 5-FC to its active forms and thus are protected).

- **Coverage:** *Cryptococcus neoformans,* some *Candida* spp., chromoblastomycosis. It is always used in combination because of its synergistic effects, usually with amphotericin B for cryptococcal meningitis or itraconazole for chromoblastomycosis.
- **Toxicity:** Human intestinal flora can convert 5-FC to the antineoplastic agent 5-fluorouracil (5-FU), which is toxic to bone marrow (anemia, thrombocytopenia, leukopenia) and less so to the liver and intestines.

Azoles

- **Mechanism:** Inhibition of fungal CYP450 enzymes, which inhibits production of ergosterol. Each of the azoles has a varying degree of inhibition of mammalian CYP450 enzymes, which determines toxicity (the highest being **ketoconazole,** which is no longer used systemically for that reason).
- **Coverage:** Broad coverage as a group. **Itraconazole** is the drug of choice for infections caused by dimorphic fungi *(Histoplasma, Blastomyces, Sporothrix)* and for dermatophytoses and onychomycosis. **Fluconazole** has less interaction with mammalian CYP450 enzymes, so it can be tolerated in higher doses; it also has higher bioavailability and CSF penetrance than itraconazole; it is therefore the drug of choice for cryptococcal meningitis (treatment *and* prophylaxis). It is also used for coccidioidal meningitis and mucocutaneous candidiasis. **Voriconazole** has similar coverage to itraconazole, can penetrate CSF, and is the drug of choice for invasive aspergillosis. **Posaconazole** is the newest of the triazoles and has the broadest coverage, including being the only one with activity against the agents of mucormycosis. Currently it is only licensed as salvage therapy for invasive aspergillosis and prophylaxis of fungal infections in induction chemotherapy for leukemia.
- **Resistance:** Resistance is rising to azole drugs.
- **Toxicity:** As a group, GI upset and hepatotoxicity are the main side effects. Itraconazole has less bioavailability when taken with rifamycins (e.g., rifampin). Voriconazole is an inhibitor of mammalian CYP3A4, so certain medications must be reduced in dosage when starting voriconazole (cyclosporine, tacrolimus, and HMG-CoA reductase inhibitors); rash and visual disturbances are also common.

Echinocandins

These are the newest class of antifungal agents.

- **Mechanism:** Disruption of fungal cell wall through inhibition of synthesis of β-(1,3)-glucan, similar to β-lactam antibiotics in bacteria.
- **Coverage: Caspofungin** is licensed for *Candida* infections (disseminated and mucocutaneous), antifungal prophylaxis for neutropenic fever, and salvage therapy for disseminated aspergillosis. **Micafungin** and **anidulafungin** can also be used for *Candida* and is licensed for anticandidal prophylaxis in bone marrow transplants.
- **Toxicity:** Minor GI upset and flushing. Don't give with cyclosporine (elevated liver function tests).

Oral Antifungals for Mucocutaneous Infections

- Griseofulvin
- Terbinafine

The drugs in this category are useful because they are **keratophilic;** that is, they preferentially deposit in tissues containing keratin (skin, hair, nails).

Griseofulvin

- **Mechanism:** Deposits in the skin where it binds to keratin, protecting the skin from new infection, so it must be administered for several weeks to allow new hair/skin to grow. It interferes with microtubule function needed for mitosis.
- **Coverage:** Only used for dermatophytoses (not first-line treatment because of toxicities).
- **Toxicity:** Serum sickness–like allergy, hepatitis, interactions with warfarin and phenobarbital. It is a CYP450 inducer and is teratogenic.

Terbinafine

- **Mechanism:** Keratophilic like griseofulvin, but unlike griseofulvin it is fungicidal through inhibition of squalene epoxidase (leads to buildup of squalene, which is toxic to the cell). All **allylamine** antifungals have this mechanism.

- **Coverage:** Used for dermatophytoses, especially onychomycosis.
- **Toxicity:** Hepatic toxicity, GI upset, and headache.

Topical Antifungals for Mucocutaneous Infections

- Nystatin
- Topical azoles
- Topical allylamines

Replication stage	Drugs available
1 Adsorption	Fusion inhibitors, e.g., T-20*
2 Penetration and uncoating	Amantadine
3 Viral DNA/RNA synthesis	Examples include: acyclovir zidovudine lamivudine nevirapine ribavirin
4 Viral protein synthesis	Interferons
5 Assembly	Protease inhibitors
6 Release	None available

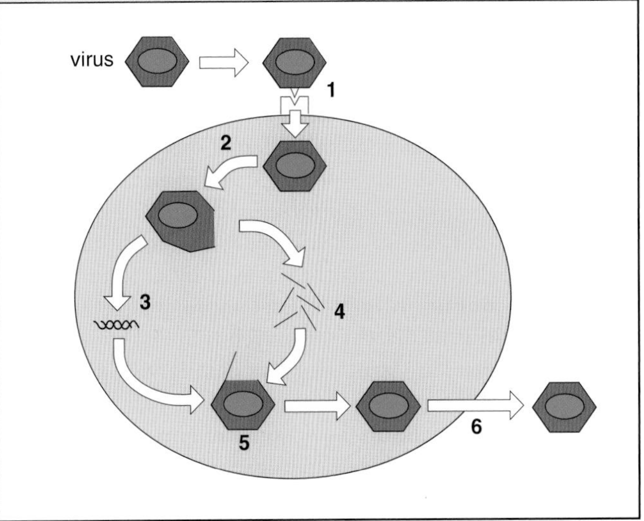

FIG. 5.93 The site of action of antiviral agents. (*From Goering R, Dockrell H, Wakelin D, et al.* Mims' Medical Microbiology. *4th ed. Philadelphia: Elsevier; 2007.*)

Nystatin

- **Mechanism:** Like amphotericin B, nystatin binds to ergosterol and forms pores in fungal cell membranes (Fig. 5.93).
- **Coverage:** Used mostly for *Candida* infections, especially **oral thrush, vulvovaginal candidiasis,** and **intertriginous candidal infections.**
- **Toxicity:** Extremely toxic if used parenterally (so not used parenterally), but because it isn't well absorbed across skin or mucous membranes, when used topically it has few side effects. It can be taken orally but has a foul taste (clotrimazole is a better-tasting alternative; see later).

Topical Azoles

Azoles were previously discussed. The two used for mucocutaneous infections are **clotrimazole** and **miconazole.** These are mostly used for vulvovaginal candidiasis, oral thrush (can take orally, not as foul tasting as nystatin), and dermophytic infections when applied as a cream (tinea corporis, tinea cruris, tinea pedis). A shampoo form of **ketoconazole** is available for seborrheic dermatitis and tinea versicolor.

Topical Allylamines

The mechanism of allylamines was previously discussed with **terbinafine.** Both terbinafine and **naftifine** can be used topically for tinea cruris and tinea corporis.

REVIEW QUESTIONS

(1) List some differences between gram-positive and gram-negative bacteria.
(2) What is an (a) obligate aerobe; (b) obligate anaerobe; (c) facultative anaerobe; (d) microaerophilic bacterium; (e) obligate intracellular organism; (f) facultative intracellular organism?

(3) For whom do encapsulated organisms cause significant problems, and why? How do we detect encapsulated organisms?
(4) What are the two ways *Staphylococcus aureus* causes disease? By what additional mechanism can *Streptococcus pyogenes* cause disease? Name some examples for each mechanism.
(5) What are the similarities and differences among erysipelas, cellulitis, and necrotizing fasciitis?
(6) A girl is brought to the clinic by her parents with a complaint of a few days of sore throat, fever, and a rough rash that started on her trunk and spread to her arms: (a) What is the most likely diagnosis, (b) what is the organism responsible, (c) what laboratory tests will confirm the diagnosis, (d) what is the appropriate treatment, and (e) what should you tell the parents to expect clinically?
(7) What is the most likely organism responsible for pneumonia in a 50-year-old with no recent hospitalization? What are you likely to see on Gram stain?
(8) List the different disease states caused by *Neisseria* spp.
(9) How are *Neisseria* species detected? How are they treated?
(10) What are the HACEK organisms?
(11) What disease states are caused by *Bacillus* species? What is unique about *B. anthracis*?
(12) By what mechanisms do the different species of *Clostridium* cause disease?
(13) Who is at risk for infection by *Listeria monocytogenes*? What is unique about this species?
(14) How is *Corynebacterium diphtheriae* detected? How is it treated?
(15) What gram-negative enteric rods commonly cause the following disease states: (a) watery diarrhea, (b) bloody diarrhea caused by a toxin, (c) bloody/inflammatory diarrhea caused by bacterial invasion, (d) nosocomial pneumonia, (e) urinary tract infections, (f) duodenal ulcers, (g) external otitis media, (h) osteomyelitis in diabetics, (i) hemolytic uremic syndrome.
(16) What diseases are gram-negative enteric rods known for causing in hospitalized patients (i.e., nosocomial infections)?
(17) What species make up the majority of normal GI flora, and when do they cause disease?
(18) What are the major disease states caused by *H. influenzae* in immunized individuals? Unimmunized?
(19) What are some of the main clinical features of the diseases caused by (a) *G. vaginalis,* (b) *B. pertussis,* and (c) *L. pneumophila*? What clues either aid in or confirm the diagnosis?
(20) For each of the following cases, what is the most likely causative organism: (a) 45-year-old man who recently returned from camping in New Mexico presenting with fever, dark skin patches, and painful, enlarged inguinal lymph nodes; (b) 45-year-old woman from Arkansas who owns a rabbit farm and presents with a black ulcer on her arm and tender axillary lymphadenopathy.
(21) What features make *Nocardia* and *Actinomyces* unique in the bacteria world?
(22) How are infections caused by *Nocardia* and *Actinomyces* diagnosed? How are they treated?
(23) Describe the life cycle of *C. trachomatis.* What disease states are caused by which serotype groups?
(24) What are some similarities and differences between *Chlamydia* and *Rickettsia* species?
(25) A 30-year-old woman who returned from visiting relatives in Georgia about a week ago presents with headache, bloodshot eyes, fever, and a rash on her palms and soles. She does not recall any insect bites. A Weil-Felix reaction is positive. What is the most likely causative organism?
(26) A pregnant woman in her third trimester presents with an ulcerated lesion on her labia. (a) What is on your differential diagnosis (three answers)? (b) An RPR test is positive; what is your confirmatory diagnostic test? (c) What is the appropriate treatment if the patient is allergic to penicillin? (d) In what stage of syphilis is the patient? (e) In what stages is risk for transmission to the fetus greatest? (f) In what trimester(s) of pregnancy is transmission risk greatest? (g) If treatment were begun now on this patient, would the fetus be protected?
(27) A middle-aged man who recently returned from visiting his brother in Connecticut and had a flulike illness with rash 2 weeks later now presents with an irregular heartbeat and joint pain. (a) What is the likely causative organism? (b) What did the primary rash most likely look like? (c) What stage is the disease in now? (d) What organ systems are affected in this stage?
(28) A public health worker who was doing water quality research in the slums of Mexico City presents with jaundice and conjunctival hemorrhage. What should you do while you are waiting for blood cultures to come back?
(29) What are the two groups of acid-fast bacteria? What about them makes them "acid fast"?

(30) A 40-year-old recent immigrant from Mexico presents with 3 months of chronic coughing that recently became blood tinged, weight loss, and night sweats. A PPD test shows an 18-mm indurated lesion. (a) What is the most likely diagnosis? (b) What is the confirmatory test? (c) In what stage is the disease most likely? (d) What is the appropriate treatment?
(31) Why does it take 48 hours to determine whether a protein derivative skin test for TB or leprosy is positive or negative?
(32) What areas of the body are usually affected in lepromatous leprosy, and why?
(33) What diagnostic tests are performed in suspected cases of *Mycoplasma* pneumonia?
(34) What diagnostic tests confirms *Ureaplasma* spp. UTI?
(35) Why do DNA viruses replicate in the nucleus, and which family is the only exception to this rule?
(36) How are enveloped and naked (nonenveloped) viruses transmitted differently?
(37) A 30-year-old nurse develops fever and jaundice after an accidental needlestick injury. A physician tests her blood for HBs antigen and anti-HBs antibody, both of which are negative. Why? What additional test could be the cause of her illness?
(38) A 24-year-old woman has had a fever and a sore throat for the past week. On physical examination, she has moderate to severe pharyngitis and bilateral cervical lymphadenopathy. What are possible infectious causes for this woman's illness?
(39) Several children in a second grade class have developed a lacy erythematous rash on their cheeks and upper chest over the past week, and some of their parents have complained of joint pain and stiffness during that same period. Which two groups of people should be the most concerned about these developments?
(40) Which naked viral genomes are infectious?
(41) What are the classic presentations for rubella and rubeola (measles) infection and how are they different? Which long-term problems are each associated with?
(42) Despite receiving his yearly influenza vaccination, a 35-year-old man develops the flu. What are two possible explanations for the apparent failure of his vaccine?
(43) What are risk factors for infection with hepatitis A, B, C, D, and E viruses?
(44) A 28-year-old man diagnosed with HIV infection 5 years ago and subsequently lost to follow-up is brought to the emergency department with confusion and lethargy. A CT scan performed in the emergency department demonstrates multiple ring-enhancing lesions within his brain. What are the two feared complications these lesions could represent? What if the lesions were nonenhancing instead?
(45) What distinguishes fungal cell membranes from animal cell membranes, and how is this difference used in antifungal therapy?
(46) What is the difference between hyphae and pseudohyphae?
(47) An otherwise healthy 18-year-old man notices small, white, blotchy patches on his chest after a day of surfing at the beach. It is not painful or pruritic. What is the most likely diagnosis, and how is the diagnosis confirmed?
(48) A 25-year-old man newly diagnosed with HIV develops white sores on the tongue and mouth. His physician is able to scrape off white exudate from his tongue. What is the most likely diagnosis, and how is the diagnosis confirmed?
(49) The patient in the previous question develops pain with swallowing. What is the most likely diagnosis?
(50) A 42-year-old landscaper pricks her finger while pruning her client's rosebushes. One week later, a mildly painful papule develops on her affected finger. Several more ulcerative lesions appear on her forearm days later. What is the most likely diagnosis, and how is it treated?
(51) What are dimorphic fungi?
(52) Name systemic mycoses found in the United States and the regions to which they are endemic.
(53) Name the most likely diagnosis: (a) A 21-year-old woman from Los Angeles develops a fever and persistent cough after construction starts near her home. A chest radiograph shows a right-sided infiltrate and ipsilateral hilar adenopathy. Silver staining of respiratory sputum reveals spherules. (b) A 21-year-old woman from Arkansas develops a fever and persistent cough after camping. A chest radiograph shows right-sided infiltrate. Examination of sputum for fungal elements reveals large, broad-based buds. (c) A 21-year-old woman from Ohio develops a fever

and persistent cough after a spelunking trip. A chest radiograph shows right-sided cavitary lesion. Silver staining of respiratory sputum reveals yeast forms with narrow based buds, some within macrophages.

(54) Name one way in which *Aspergillus* may cause disease in healthy individuals.

(55) What are some risk factors for *Aspergillus* infection?

(56) What are some risk factors for *Mucor* infection?

(57) A 30-year-old man with known HIV presents with a 1-week history of fever and chills, with increasing headache and neck stiffness. His current CD4 count is 75. Examination of his CSF reveals encapsulated yeast forms with India ink stain. What is the most likely diagnosis, and how is it treated?

(58) What is the most likely diagnosis of the following patients: (a) a 43-year-old man with known HIV who presents with a 2-day history of fever, chills, and cough, a CD4 count of 50, oxygen saturation within normal limits, and a chest radiograph showing right-sided lobar consolidation; (b) a 43-year-old man with known HIV who presents with a 5-day history of worsening fever, chills, and productive cough; a CD4 count of 50; needing oxygen via nasal cannula; and a chest radiograph showing diffuse bilateral interstitial infiltrates.

(59) A 32-year-old woman with known HIV presents with headache and progressive mental status changes over the past few days. Her CD4 count is 72. CT imaging of the brain shows intracranial ring-enhancing lesions. What is the most likely infectious cause, and how is it treated?

(60) A 1-day-old girl born at 37 weeks of gestation is witnessed to have a seizure. Physical examination reveals microcephaly and yellow-white, fluffy patches of the retina. CT imaging of the head shows hydrocephalus and intracranial calcifications. What is the most likely diagnosis?

(61) Name the most likely infectious cause: (a) A 39-year-old woman with a diagnosis of AIDS presents with a several-day history of severe, watery diarrhea. Acid-fast cysts are present in the stool. (b) A 32-year-old man from Mexico presents with a 5-day history of fever and severe right upper quadrant pain. He has a history of bloody diarrhea in the last year. (c) A 29-year-old man develops persistent watery and foul-smelling diarrhea after camping with his friends. He admits to drinking freely from a mountain stream.

(62) A 9-year-old boy presents to his physician with his third episode of *Giardia lamblia* diarrhea in the past 2 years. He has a childhood history of recurrent otitis and sinusitis. What is a likely underlying etiology?

(63) Name the parasite and vector that underlie the following hematologic parasitic infections: (a) babesiosis, (b) malaria, (c) leishmaniasis, (d) Chagas disease, (e) sleeping sickness.

(64) Name the acute and chronic manifestations of Chagas disease.

(65) Thick and thin peripheral blood smears are used to diagnose malarial infection. What is the purpose of a thick versus thin smear?

(66) Characterize the approximate periodicity of fevers in the following: (a) *P. vivax, P. ovale;* (b) *P. malariae;* (c) *P. falciparum.*

(67) Why is infection with *P. falciparum* especially serious?

(68) An 18-year-old woman presents to her physician with a few days' history of a thin, foul-smelling, vaginal discharge. She complains of vaginal itching and pain with urination and sex. Cervical examination reveals a bright red "strawberry cervix." What is the most likely diagnosis, and how is it treated?

(69) A 3-year-old girl is brought to the clinic for an itchy rash of her lower extremities. Her mother states she played in the local playground sandbox barefoot recently. On physical examination, she has intensely pruritic, erythematous, and serpiginous lesions between her toes and the dorsum of her feet. What immunoglobulin subset is likely to be elevated in this patient?

(70) A 5-year-old boy complains of anal itching. His mother notices that his itching is worse at night and prevents him from sleeping. How is this condition diagnosed and treated?

(71) How is trichinosis acquired?

(72) Match the keyword or key phrase to the relevant parasite or parasitic infection:

A. Vitamin B_{12} deficiency	a. *Wuchereria bancrofti*
B. Hepatic hydatid cyst	b. *Onchocerca volvulus*
C. Neurocysticercosis	c. *Loa loa*
D. Cholangiocarcinoma	d. *Taenia* spp.

E. Consumption of raw crayfish	e. *Paragonimus westermani*
F. Squamous cell carcinoma	f. *Echinococcus granulosus*
G. Parasitic visible in conjunctivae	g. Hookworm (*Ancylostoma* spp.)
H. Iron deficiency anemia	h. *Clonorchis sinensis*
I. Elephantiasis	i. *Schistosoma* spp.
J. "River blindness"	j. *Diphyllobothrium latum*

(73) A 20-year-old man presents to your clinic after a 1-week history of a sore throat and a fever. On physical examination, he has a maculopapular rash over his palms and soles of his feet. On further questioning, he reports having multiple sexual partners within the past 3 months and no drug allergies. After the diagnosis is confirmed with laboratory testing, you proceed with giving him a dose of intramuscular penicillin. Before he leaves your office, he begins to develop an erythematous blanching rash associated with a headache, muscle aches, and chills. Is this an allergic reaction?

(74) Two patients arrive to your emergency department. One is a man treated 1 week ago for a case of lower extremity cellulitis who presents with intermittently bloody diarrhea. The other is a woman presenting with intense vaginal pruritus and motile flagellated organisms on wet prep. What treatment can you use for both?

(75) A 55-year-old man with alcohol-induced cirrhosis and recurrent episodes of large-volume ascites develops a fever, confusion, and agitation. On physical examination, his abdomen is distended and diffusely tender to palpation. A fluid sample taken from his abdomen contains many white blood cells. What are the most likely causes of infection in this patient, and how would this guide your choice of antibiotic therapy?

(76) A 38-year-old man who underwent liver transplantation 2 years ago develops intense pain on swallowing liquids and solids. Esophagogastroduodenoscopy identifies extensive ulcerations throughout the length of the esophagus, and a biopsy taken from one contains mucosal cells with large eosinophilic nuclei surrounded by a clear halo. What medication should be started, and which should be avoided?

(77) A 26-year-old man from Arkansas who enjoys exploring caves as a hobby complains of a chronic cough for the past 3 months. A chest radiograph shows several large calcified lung nodules and cavitary lesions in the upper lobes. Induced sputum samples contain budding yeast forms. What would be the appropriate treatment? How would this change if the man was from an earthquake zone in California? What if the man was found to be neutropenic?

6 IMMUNOLOGY

Brenton Bauer

LYMPHOID STRUCTURES

Anatomy of the Immune System

Primary lymphoid organs are organs that function as "housing" for immature progenitor cells to generate, mature, and educate new lymphocytes in an antigen-**independent** manner. The main examples of these organs include the **B**one marrow for **B** cells and the **T**hymus for **T** cells.

- **Bone marrow** is a critical primary lymphoid organ. It consists of two primary types: red marrow and yellow marrow. Red marrow is the bone marrow parenchyma and contains the hematopoietic stem cells, which function in the formation of **all blood cell lines,** including B and T cells. Yellow marrow is the bone marrow stroma (supportive tissue) and contains mostly fat.
- The **thymus** is the other primary lymphoid organ. Its embryologic origin is the epithelium of the third branchial pouch. Structurally, it is an encapsulated, bilobed organ situated in the anterior mediastinum. During early childhood, the thymus is large and is easily seen on a chest radiograph. However, as the individual ages, there is a natural regression and atrophy of the thymic tissue, and it becomes "invisible" on a chest film. The main physiologic immune function of the thymus is to act as the **T-cell classroom** for differentiation and maturation, which occur as cells go from the outer cortex to the inner medulla of the thymus.
    - **Cortex:** High cellular density with packed immature T cells awaiting positive (functional) selection. Positive selection ensures that the T cells will have the bare minimum functionality of binding the cell surface proteins major histocompatibility complex class I (MHC I) or II. Of note, most immature T cells that undergo this process never make it past this step and subsequently undergo apoptosis. It is of critical importance that these thymocytes are able to bind MHC. When mature, they will bind MHC I if they differentiate into $CD8^+$ T cells and MHC II if they differentiate into $CD4^+$ T cells.
    - **Corticomedullary junction:** In this region, T cells undergo negative selection. Negative selection destroys cells that see the body's own normal antigens as foreign invaders. Negative selection is highly important in preventing autoimmune disease by destroying T cells that could potentially start an attack on the body's own cells. A T cell that has made it through positive selection is presented with self-antigen. If the specificity of binding is too strong, an apoptotic signal will be given to that particular T cell. Of note, some autoreactive T cells are able to make it through the negative selection phase but are eliminated by peripheral mechanisms (e.g., anergy, regulatory T cells). However, if peripheral mechanisms also fail, then this sets the stage for potential predisposition to autoimmunity.
    - **Medulla:** Pale, low cellular density, with mature T cells having already gone through positive and negative selection.

Secondary lymphoid organs are sites where lymphocytes undergo differentiation (increased specificity) and clonal expansion (increased number) in an antigen-**dependent** fashion (meaning differentiation and expansion occurs when an invader is thought to be present). Examples of secondary lymphoid organs include lymph nodes, spleen, tonsils, adenoids, and mucosa-associated lymphoid tissue (MALT).

At birth most bone marrow is of the red type and is gradually replaced by fatty yellow marrow with time. This is important because older adults with long bone fracture (e.g., a femoral fracture), which contains a lot of yellow marrow, are at risk for developing a fat embolism.

Remember that tumors of the thymus (thymomas) can be a reason to see a mass in the anterior mediastinum on radiography, and these thymomas are often associated with myasthenia gravis. Removal of the thymus is associated with better prognosis.

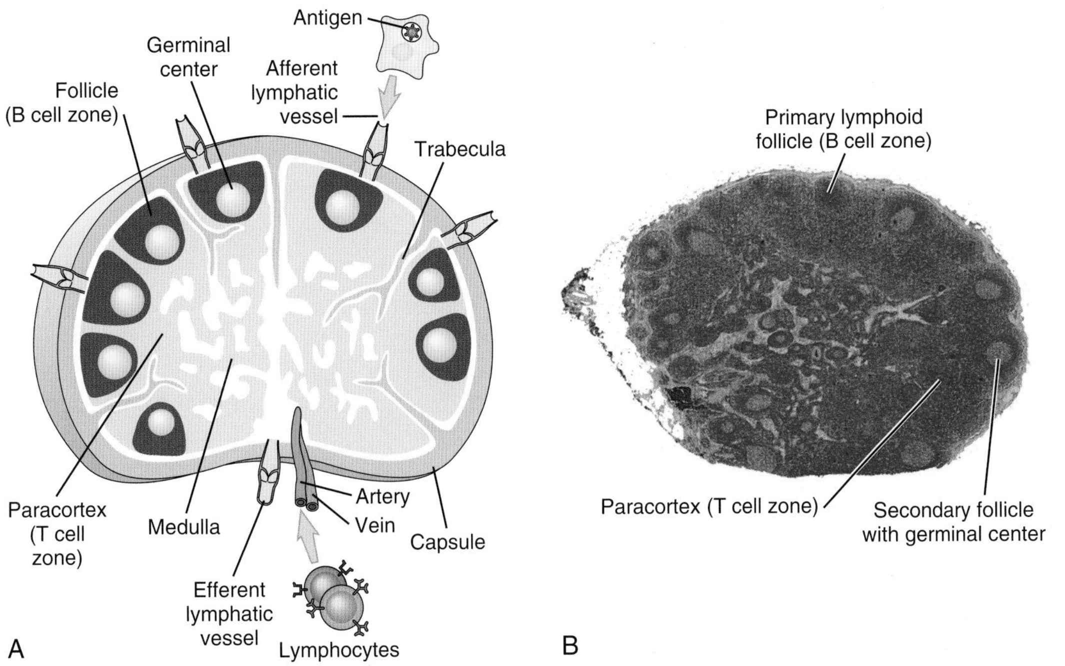

FIG. 6.1 A, Lymph node illustration, showing the outer portion (cortex) with follicles containing B cells, the paracortex where B and T cells enter from the blood, and the innermost portion (medulla). **B,** Histologic staining of a lymph node showing primary lymphoid follicles, paracortex, and germinal centers in secondary follicles. (*From Abbas A, Lichtman A.* Basic Immunology Updated Edition. *3rd ed. Philadelphia: Elsevier; 2010.*)

Lymph nodes (Fig. 6.1) are encapsulated and trabeculated secondary lymphoid organs with many afferent vessels and single or few efferents ("many ways in and only one way out!"). The specific functions are determined by anatomic position within the node (cortex, medulla, and paracortex areas).

Flow Through a Lymph Node: Afferent lymphatic vessel → subcapsular sinus → trabecular sinus → medullary sinus (filtration by macrophages) → efferent lymphatic vessel.

- **Medulla:** The medulla of the node consists primarily of cords (densely packed lymphocytes) and sinuses (reticular cells and macrophages/histiocytes).
- **Paracortex:** The area in the deep cortex containing the high endothelial venules where both B and T cells enter from the blood. T cells are concentrated within the paracortex; hence, when a cellular adaptive immune response occurs (T-cell mediated), the paracortex enlarges.
- **Cortex:** The area where B cells migrate and arrange in **follicles.** The primary follicles are densely packed and dormant, whereas the secondary follicles (after activation by antigen response) are large and have pale germinal centers.

> Bite cells on peripheral blood smear, which appear as if a macrophage took a bite out of them, are formed from the splenic macrophages removing Heinz bodies in such diseases as G6PD deficiency.

The **spleen** is a critical component of the reticuloendothelial system in hematology and immunology. The spleen is structurally and functionally divided into two "pulp" divisions. The **red pulp** contains long vascular channels and a fenestrated basement membrane allowing for filtration of red blood cells (RBCs). Older senescent RBCs are filtered into the sinusoids but are unable to reenter the circulation and are phagocytosed by splenic macrophages. The **white pulp** contains the periarterial lymphatic sheath (PALS), which contains T cells and follicles that contain B cells.

> Patients with infectious mononucleosis (Epstein-Barr virus infection) get splenomegaly and are at risk for rupture.

Remember some of the findings after a splenectomy: modest thrombocytosis (the spleen can store one-third of total body platelets, so removal allows more to circulate in the blood), Howell-Jolly bodies (nuclear remnants in RBCs), poorer response to some vaccines, and higher risk for infection by encapsulated organisms (***S****treptococcus pneumoniae*, ***H****aemophilus* ***i****nfluenzae*, ***N****eisseria meningitidis*, ***S****almonella*—"***SHiNS***").

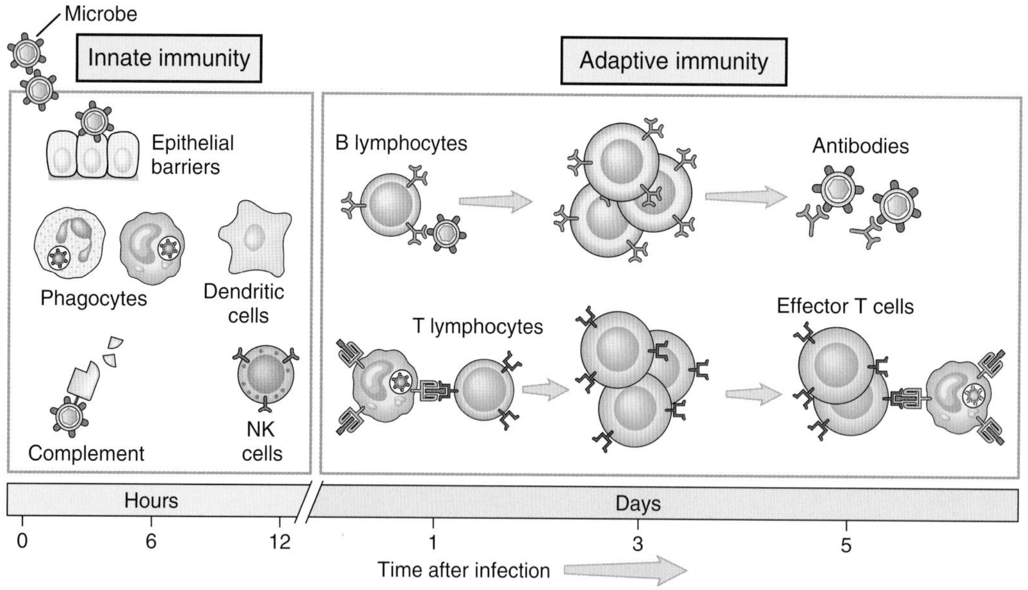

FIG. 6.2 The innate immune system has a fast and nonspecific response to infection. The adaptive immune system has a slower initial response but a robust and specific response during subsequent exposures. *(From Abbas A, Lichtman A. Basic Immunology Updated Edition. 3rd ed. Philadelphia: Elsevier; 2010.)*

OVERVIEW OF INNATE VERSUS ADAPTIVE IMMUNITY

Basic Versus Learned Responses

The **innate immune system** (Figs. 6.2 and 6.3) is characterized by its fast and nonspecific response to infection as well as its lack of immunologic memory. It allows for an individual to have basic immunity before developing adaptive immunity (have a "baseline" immune system before learning to fight specific pathogens that are encountered). The innate immune system recognizes foreign antigens that are highly conserved over time and across pathogenic species. For example, lipopolysaccharide (LPS) is a component of the cell wall conserved between gram-negative bacteria. Toll-like receptors are able to recognize LPS and, once bound, activate the release of inflammatory cytokines.

- Constituents of innate immunity include phagocytes (neutrophils, macrophages, dendritic cells), natural killer (NK) cells, and the complement system. Epithelial barriers (e.g., skin) also prevent microbes from ever entering the body and are considered part of the innate immune system.

The **adaptive immune system** (see Figs. 6.2 and 6.3) is characterized by its slow initial response to a first-time antigen exposure and a more rapid and robust response during subsequent exposures secondary to "immunologic memory." The adaptive immune system is able to generate a large diversity of antigen-specific responses. The adaptive immune system can be further divided into humoral immunity (circulating antibodies) and cell-mediated immunity (Fig. 6.4).

> The property of self-renewal is important because bone marrow transplants are fundamentally the allogeneic transplantation of hematopoietic stem cells from one person to another to repopulate a new normal set of blood cell lines after myeloablative therapy (radiation and/or chemotherapy).

CELLS OF THE IMMUNE SYSTEM

Workhorses of Immunity

To begin, we'll start with an overview of the various lineages that give rise to the cell types of the immune system. The cells of the immune system all originate from hematopoietic stem cells found within the marrow of long tubular bones. These hematopoietic stem cells are multipotent (can form all blood cell types) and have the capacity of self-renewal. These cells will differentiate to commit a cell down the path of either **myeloid** or **lymphoid** cell lines (see Fig. 11.1 in Chapter 11 for details).

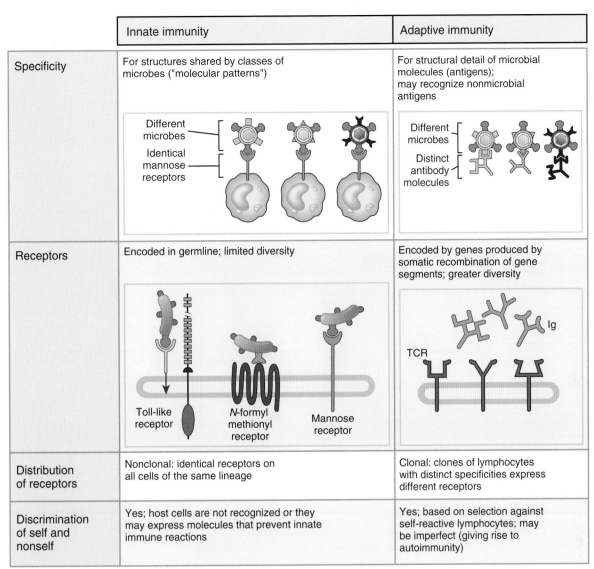

	Innate immunity	Adaptive immunity
Specificity	For structures shared by classes of microbes ("molecular patterns") 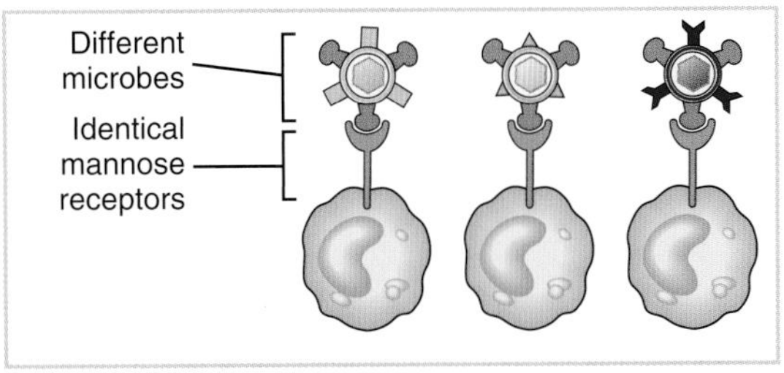	For structural detail of microbial molecules (antigens); may recognize nonmicrobial antigens 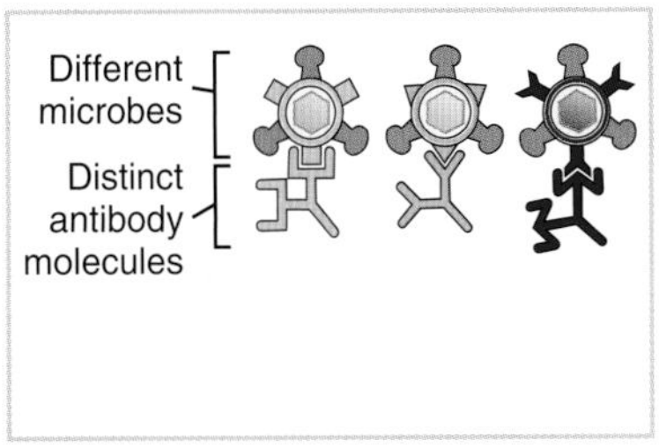
Receptors	Encoded in germline; limited diversity 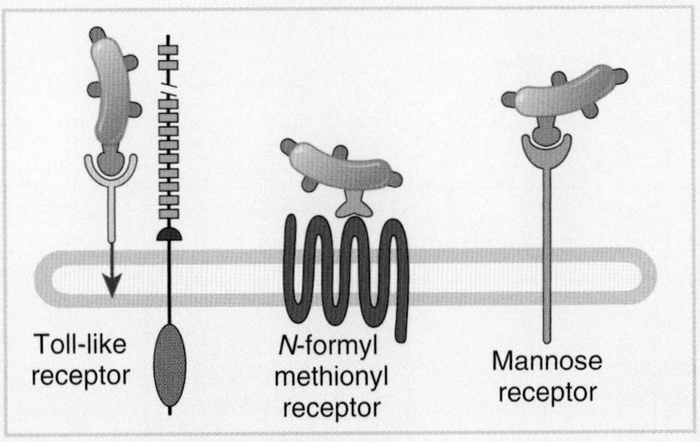	Encoded by genes produced by somatic recombination of gene segments; greater diversity 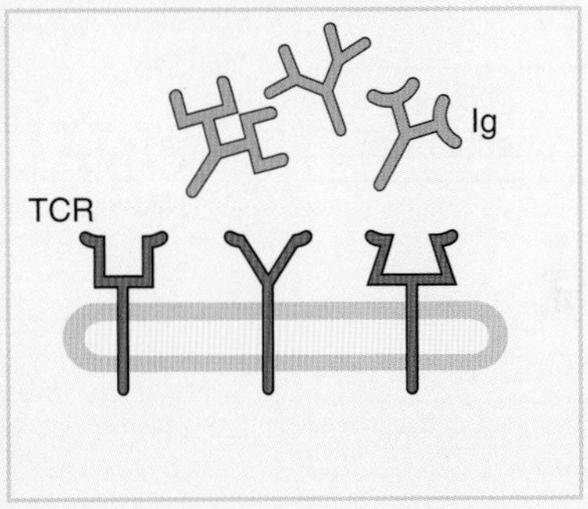
Distribution of receptors	Nonclonal: identical receptors on all cells of the same lineage	Clonal: clones of lymphocytes with distinct specificities express different receptors
Discrimination of self and nonself	Yes; host cells are not recognized or they may express molecules that prevent innate immune reactions	Yes; based on selection against self-reactive lymphocytes; may be imperfect (giving rise to autoimmunity)

Fig. 6.3 Comparison between innate immunity and adaptive immunity. (*From Abbas A, Lichtman A.* Basic Immunology Updated Edition. *3rd ed. Philadelphia: Elsevier; 2010.*)

Neutrophils should be multilobular, but a "hypersegmented" neutrophil (six or more lobes) suggests vitamin B_{12} or folate deficiency.

Myeloid Lineage

Monocyte: Phagocytic cells located in the bloodstream that will differentiate into tissue macrophages once stimulated.

Macrophage: Tissue histiocyte (differentiated monocyte) capable of phagocytosis and synthesis and secretion of various cytokines (e.g., interleukin 1 [IL-1], tumor necrosis factor α [TNF-α], IL-6, IL-8, and IL-12). Also considered an antigen-presenting cell (APC).

Dendritic cell: Cell with long cytoplasmic arms capable of efficient antigen presentation to lymphocytes ("professional antigen-presenting cell [APC]").

Neutrophil: Mature cell that has a multilobed nucleus and contains toxic cytoplasmic granules with potent bactericidal capability.

Eosinophil: Mature cell that has a bilobed nucleus with large pink granules containing major basic protein. Major basic protein functions in attack against parasitic and helminthic infections.

Basophil: Mature cell that has a bilobed nucleus with large blue granules.

The drug cromolyn sulfate works as a mast cell stabilizer for conditions such as allergic rhinitis and allergen-induced asthma.

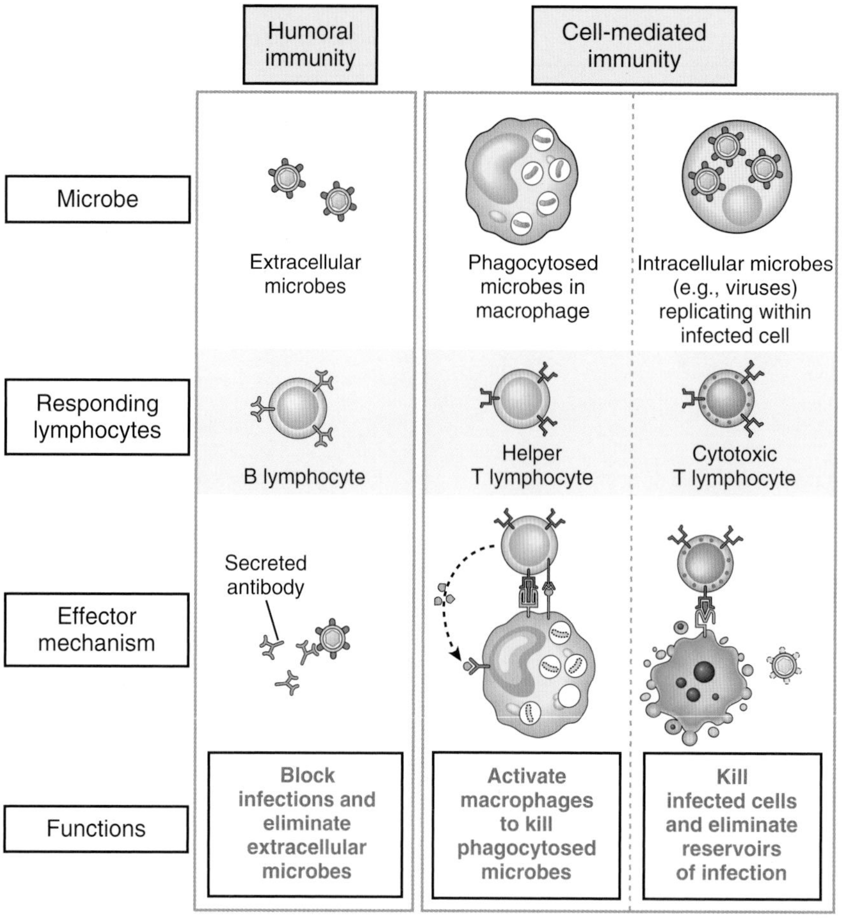

Fig. 6.4 Overview of humoral immunity versus cell-mediated immunity. (*From Abbas A, Lichtman A.* Basic Immunology Updated Edition. *3rd ed. Philadelphia: Elsevier; 2010.*)

Mast cell: Cell with a small nucleus and large cytoplasmic granules containing histamine and other preformed allergic mediators, which play a role in allergies, hives, and anaphylaxis.

Lymphoid Lineage

Lymphocytes:

- B cells undergo further differentiation into either memory B cells or plasma cells (which produce antibodies).
- T cells further differentiate into either $CD4^+$ helper T cells, $CD8^+$ cytotoxic T cells, regulatory T cells, or memory T cells.

Natural Killer Cells: $CD56^+$ lymphocytes that contain cytoplasmic toxic granules (such as granzymes) and are able to kill malignant cells, virus-infected cells, or antibody-coated (opsonized) cells.

MAJOR HISTOCOMPATIBILITY COMPLEX I AND II

How We Differentiate Ourselves from Everything Else

The MHC is a critical portion of the immune system's ability to discern self from nonself as well as detect when the body's own cells are either infected or have undergone malignant change. There are two major classes of MHC involved in the human immune system; these two classes are both structurally and functionally distinct from one another (Fig. 6.5).

Feature	Class II MHC pathway	Class I MHC pathway
Composition of stable peptide-MHC complex	Polymorphic α and β chains, peptide 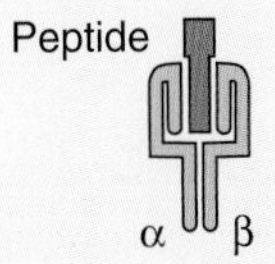	Polymorphic α chain, β_2-microglobulin, peptide 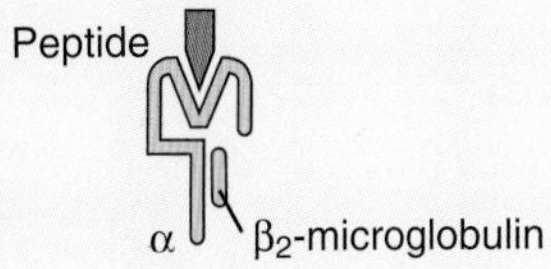
Types of APCs	Dendritic cells, mononuclear phagocytes, B lymphocytes; some endothelial cells, thymic epithelium	All nucleated cells
Responsive T cells	$CD4^+$ T cells (helper T cells) 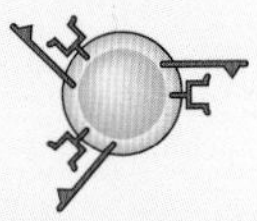	$CD8^+$ T cells (CTLs) 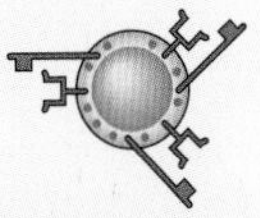
Source of protein antigens	Endosomal/lysosomal proteins (mostly internalized from extracellular environment)	Cytosolic proteins (mostly synthesized in the cell; may enter cytosol from phagosomes)
Enzymes responsible for peptide generation	Endosomal and lysosomal proteases (e.g., cathepsins)	Cytosolic proteasome
Site of peptide loading of MHC	Specialized vesicular compartment	Endoplasmic reticulum
Molecules involved in transport of peptides and loading of MHC molecules	Invariant chain, DM	TAP

Fig. 6.5 Comparison of MHC I versus MHC II. (*From Abbas A, Lichtman A.* Basic Immunology Updated Edition. *3rd ed. Philadelphia: Elsevier; 2010.*)

Table 6.1 Specific Diseases with an HLA Subtype Association

HLA Subtype*	Associated Disease(s)
A3	Hemochromatosis
B27	**P**soriasis, **a**nkylosing spondylitis, **i**nflammatory bowel disease, **r**eactive arthritis (**PAIR**)
B8	Graves disease
DR2	Goodpasture disease
DR3	Diabetes mellitus type 1
DR4	Diabetes mellitus type 1, rheumatoid arthritis
DR5	Hashimoto thyroiditis, pernicious anemia

*Certain HLA subtypes are linked with autoimmune disease. These associations are occasionally tested on Step 1.

MHC class I is **present on all nucleated cells** in the body in addition to platelets (platelets don't have a nucleus because they are cytoplasmic fragments of megakaryocytes, which are nucleated). MHC class I is encoded by human leukocyte antigen genes *HLA-A, HLA-B,* and *HLA-C* (Table 6.1). MHC is a cell surface protein that displays peptide fragments from inside the cell on the outside. Functionally, antigen is loaded onto the MHC I in the rough endoplasmic reticulum before the MHC I is inserted into the cell membrane. Normally the antigen that is loaded onto MHC I is self-antigen, and cytotoxic

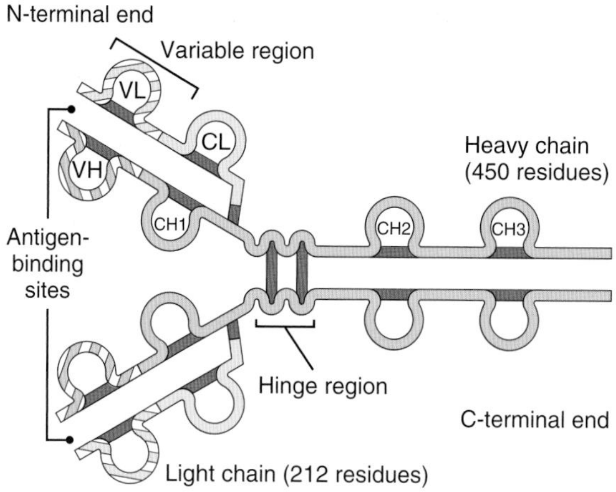

Fig. 6.6 The structure of an antibody. The antigen-binding region (Fab) is on the *left* of the diagram. The constant region (Fc) is on the *right*. Note that the antibody is composed of two light chains and two heavy chains connected by disulfide bonds (shown in *red*). (*From Male D, Brostoff J, Roth D, Roitt I.* Immunology. *7th ed. Philadelphia: Elsevier; 2007.*)

T cells (CD8+ T cells) will not react to it. If a virus infects a cell, however, the virus produces viral proteins using the host's cellular machinery. These viral proteins will also be loaded onto MHC I. This is how cytotoxic T cells confer immunity to viral infection. They recognize MHC I with loaded viral antigen and target it for cytotoxic destruction if the proper costimulatory signal is present (discussed later in the chapter).

MHC class II is **present only on antigen-presenting cells** such as macrophages and dendritic cells. It is encoded by human leukocyte antigen genes *HLA-DP, HLA-DQ,* and *HLA-DR.* Structurally, it is composed of two α- and two β-subunits. After APCs phagocytose microbes, they process and load these antigens onto MHC II. Then the MHC II is inserted into the cell membrane for binding and recognition by helper T cells (CD4+ T cells). Helper T cells can then activate B cells and/or trigger local inflammation.

B CELLS, ANTIBODIES, AND HUMORAL IMMUNITY

B Cell Is King

Humoral immunity is responsible for synthesizing soluble serum proteins called antibodies (or immunoglobulins), which have a variety of functions involved in eradicating infectious agents. Antibodies are composed of two light chains and two heavy chains that form a Y shape. The trunk of the Y is the **c**onstant fragment (F**c**) and the two branches are **a**ntigen-**b**inding fragments (F**ab**) (Fig. 6.6). The chains are linked together by disulfide bonds. The **Fc region** is the constant region (containing the carboxy terminal and various carbohydrate side chains) and is important in both complement factor binding and determining the **isotype** of the immunoglobulin (e.g., immunoglobulin M [IgM], IgG, IgA, IgE, or IgD). The **Fab region** contains two antigen-binding fragments (at the amino terminal side) that are important in determining the **idiotype** of the immunoglobulin (uniqueness of the site and specificity for only one antigen).

Certain disease states result from the inability of isotype class switching to occur. Specifically, hyper-IgM syndrome occurs as a result of a defective CD40L on Th cells. This prevents activation of antibody class-switching. Selective immunoglobulin deficiency occurs from a specific genetic defect preventing expression of a particular isotype (most commonly IgA).

Antibody formation is accomplished by mature plasma B cells, which synthesize and release antibodies after they have been activated by appropriate mechanisms after antigen stimulation. There are nearly unlimited antigens; therefore there are a number of mechanisms in place to ensure that there will be a B cell that can make the required antibody when needed. This process is called **antibody diversity** and consists of four main processes:

1. Random recombination of VJ (light chain) or V(D)J (heavy chain) genes
2. Random combination of various heavy chains with light chains
3. Somatic hypermutation (in germinal centers after antigen stimulation)
4. Terminal deoxynucleotidyl transferase (TdT) addition of DNA nucleotides to the heavy and light chains

At baseline, a mature B cell will either express IgM or IgD isotypes on its cell surface. **Isotype switching** occurs after antigen stimulation and appropriate activation of a mature B cell, resulting in alternative splicing of mRNA. The resultant posttranslational modification of messenger RNA (mRNA) dictates the isotype of plasma cell (i.e., IgA, IgE, or IgG).

- **IgD:** Found on the cell surface of mature B cells. Its function in serum is otherwise unclear.
- **IgM:** Also found on the surface of mature B cells. As a serum immunoglobulin, it is produced in the primary (fast) antigenic response and is found as either a monomer or more commonly as a pentamer (five IgM molecules linked) for more efficient antigen trapping and complement fixation/activation. **The pentamer is very bulky and therefore <u>does not</u> cross the placenta!**
- **IgG:** The main immunoglobulin in the secondary (delayed/slow) antigenic response. Occurs as a monomer with functions to fix complement, cross the placenta to provide passive immunity to a developing fetus, opsonize bacteria, and neutralize various toxins and viruses. **IgG does not make multimers and therefore <u>does</u> cross the placenta!**
- **IgA:** Occurs as a monomer in the bloodstream and as a dimer when secreted (linked by the secretory component attained from epithelial cells before secretion). IgA is secreted onto mucosal surfaces (gastrointestinal, genitourinary, and respiratory) to block attachment of pathogens to mucous membranes.
- **IgE:** Implicated in the allergic response (type 1 hypersensitivity) because it binds both mast cells and basophils and undergoes cross-linking after exposure to appropriate antigen.

When the immune system generates antibodies against an antigen (via plasma B cells), memory B cells are also produced. These memory B cells can lie dormant for long periods but can respond quickly to produce antibodies if the same antigen is encountered in the future.

Now, how does the B cell become activated and become an antibody-secreting **plasma cell**? Resting B cells have a high level of expression of surface immunoglobulin (IgM or IgD) and MHC II, but they do not secrete immunoglobulin. If they encounter their matching antigen, they will engulf it, digest it, and present it on their MHC II. A helper T cell subtype 2 (Th2 cell) can then recognize the antigen on the MHC II with its T-cell receptor (TCR). The Th2 cell will then secrete specific cytokines (IL-4, IL-5, and IL-6) to stimulate B-cell proliferation, hypermutation, and isotype switching. Once a B cell becomes a plasma cell, it is no longer able to proliferate because it is designed for maximal immunoglobulin secretion. Of note, it actually takes two signals to make a Th2 cell secrete B-cell activating cytokines: (1) the TCR–MHC II antigen interaction, and (2) CD40–CD40 ligand interaction.

There is also a **T-cell–independent** way to activate B cells. Nonpeptide antigens cannot be presented to T cells, but it is often important for the immune system to recognize these antigens. B cells' response to these antigens is solely IgM release. No isotype switching or immunologic memory is established after the encounter.

Active and Passive Immunity: The way that a host develops or obtains antibodies to a specific antigen can also be classified as active or passive immunity, both of which can be further subcategorized.

- **Active immunity** signifies that the host's immune system came directly in contact with an antigen and developed its own immunity. There is a subcategorical breakdown of active immunity into naturally acquired active immunity (i.e., direct pathogen exposure) and artificially acquired active immunity (i.e., exposure through vaccination).
- **Passive immunity** occurs when the host was given its supply of antibodies by an outside source. This can also be naturally or artificially acquired. Naturally acquired passive immunity occurs most commonly when a mother transfers her actively formed antibodies to her offspring both transplacentally (IgG) and through breast milk (IgA). In contrast, artificially acquired passive immunity occurs when antibodies are administered as medication, which is the case in tetanus antitoxin, antivenoms, digitalis antibody fragments, or intravenous immunoglobulin (IVIG).

B-Cell Deficiency and Immunoglobulin Deficiency Syndromes:

- **X-linked agammaglobulinemia (Bruton agammaglobulinemia):** Results from a mutation in the receptor tyrosine kinase (BTK). This prevents the maturation of B cells, thereby halting immunoglobulin production.
- **Common variable immunodeficiency:** Most common form of primary B-cell deficiency, with characteristically low levels of measurable IgG and IgA (occasionally IgM) resulting in immunodeficiency; associated with higher rates of lymphomas and gastric cancer.

- **Hyper IgM syndrome:** Normal level of B cells but with diminished levels of IgG and IgA and with high levels of IgM; associated with higher risk for *Pneumocystis* infection. This condition usually results from an inability to undergo isotype class switching secondary to deficiency in CD40 ligand on Th2 cells.
- **Selective IgA deficiency:** Most common immunoglobulin deficiency; associated with increased respiratory, gastrointestinal, and genitourinary infections. Risk for anaphylaxis with blood product transfusions.

T CELLS, CELL-MEDIATED IMMUNITY, IMMUNE SYSTEM REGULATION

Regulators and Educated Assassins

T cells are critical in regulation, activation, and action of the adaptive immune system. As previously discussed, the T cells stem from the lymphoid lineage of hematopoietic differentiation. They are "born" in the bone marrow but "educated" in the thymus. Within the thymus both positive and negative selection occurs, resulting in specialized T cells with different clusters of differentiation (CD) on their cell surface; the main cell types are $CD4^+$ and $CD8^+$ T cells.

$CD4^+$ T cells: These "helper T cells" will undergo further differentiation after appropriate stimulation by interleukins to become either Th1 or Th2 cells with specific functions to help regulate both the humoral and cell-mediated immune system.

- **Th1:** These cells are involved in the regulation of the **cell-mediated response.** They are activated by APCs by the secretion of IL-12 and secrete interferon γ (IFN-γ), which activates APCs for efficient killing. They also secrete IL-2, which activates $CD8^+$ (cytotoxic T cells) to kill virally infected cells.
- **Th2:** These cells are activated by secretion of IL-4. They **activate B cells** and enhance isotype switching by secreting IL-4, IL-5, and IL-6. They are also involved with recruiting eosinophils for parasite defense.
- **Regulatory T cells** (Tregs; formerly known as suppressor T cells): These cells maintain specific immune tolerance by decreasing activity of CD4 and CD8 T cells. They are activated by antiinflammatory signals such as IL-10 and TGF-ß.

Anergy is the process of T lymphocytes becoming completely nonreactive when the TCR is activated but no costimulatory signal is received (e.g., B7, IL-2). Remember: It takes at least two signals to be approved!

$CD8^+$ T cell: Otherwise known as cytotoxic T cells, these cells are responsible for seeking out and eliminating virus- or parasite-infected cells, cancer cells, and other foreign cells.

It is important to understand the main steps involved when viral antigen is taken up by an APC to the point at which $CD8^+$ T cells are "seeking and destroying" the infected cells.

1. When an APC (mainly dendritic cell or macrophage) is exposed to viral antigen, it will load the antigen onto an MHC II for presentation to a CD4+ T cell. It will also express a costimulatory signal on its cell membrane (e.g., B7). The TCR can then interact with the antigen-positive MHC II on the APC.
2. A single signal is not enough for activation. The immune system's checks and balances require a second signal for appropriate activation to occur. The B7 costimulatory signal on the APC must interact with CD28 on the $CD4^+$ T cell while the TCR–MHC II interaction is occurring. If these conditions are met, the $CD4^+$ T cell will release IFN-γ to stimulate the APC to efficiently kill its pathogen. The $CD4^+$ T cell will also release IL-2 to (1) cause activation and proliferation of $CD8^+$ cytotoxic T cells to kill virally infected host cells and (2) cause $CD4^+$ T-cell proliferation and differentiation in an autocrine manner (Fig. 6.7).
3. What happens when a TCR recognizes and binds to host antigens (self-reactivity)? In health, the way the immune system tackles this issue is by ***anergy,*** deactivating that self-reactive T cell. If this process fails, it could potentially lead to the development of an autoimmune disease.

High-Yield Cytokines/Interleukins

- **IL-1:** An acute phase reactant synthesized by macrophages contributing to the acute inflammatory response, including **fever,** leukocyte recruitment, adhesion molecule activation, and stimulation of further chemokine production.
- **IL-2:** Interleukin secreted by Th cells that enables growth, maturation, and proliferation of $CD4^+$ and $CD8^+$ T cells.

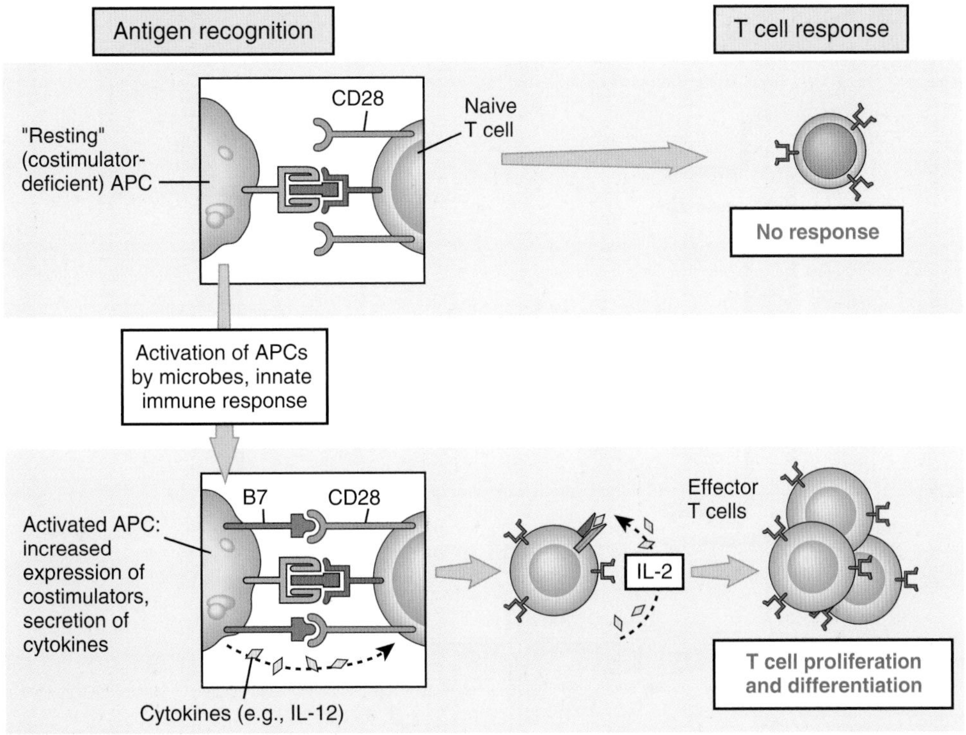

FIG. 6.7 Top row, A resting APC will not stimulate a $CD4^+$ T cell even if the T-cell receptor binds MHC II. In fact, this causes anergy in the T cell to prevent autoimmune disease. **Bottom row,** B7 acts as a costimulatory signal that binds CD28 on the $CD4^+$ T cell while the TCR–MHC II interaction is occurring. Now the T cell will be activated. It will secrete IL-2 to cause activation and proliferation of itself and $CD8^+$ cytotoxic T cells. (*From Abbas A, Lichtman A.* Basic Immunology Updated Edition. *3rd ed. Philadelphia: Elsevier; 2010.*)

- **IL-3:** Interleukin that stimulates bone marrow.
- **IL-4:** Interleukin secreted by Th2 cells to further B-cell development as well as enhance immunoglobulin class type switching to IgG.
- **IL-5:** Interleukin secreted by Th2 cells that enhances immunoglobulin class type switching to IgA and increases production of eosinophils.
- **IL-6:** Like IL-1, an acute phase reactant produced by Th cells and macrophages to further the acute inflammatory response. Also stimulates antibody production and fever.
- **IL-8:** Neutrophil chemotactic factor.
- **IL-10:** Secreted by regulatory T cells in order to suppress cell-mediated immunity and stimulate humoral immunity.
- **IL-12:** Secreted by macrophages with functions to enhance NK cells and T cells.

T-Cell Deficiency Syndromes:

- **Severe combined immunodeficiency (SCID):** The most common form is X-linked SCID, followed by adenosine deaminase deficiency; results in susceptibility to numerous pathogenic infectious diseases (e.g., diarrhea, pneumonia, otitis, sinusitis).
- **Acquired immunodeficiency syndrome (AIDS):** The final stage in the decremental quantity and quality of T-cell immunity (particularly $CD4^+$ cells); caused by infection with human immunodeficiency virus (HIV).
- **DiGeorge syndrome:** 22q11.2 deletion syndrome resulting in CATCH-22 (**C**ardiac defects, **A**bnormal facies, **T**hymic hypoplasia, **C**left palate, and **H**ypocalcemia).
- **Ataxia telangiectasia:** T-cell deficiency along with ataxia (cerebellar dysfunction) and increased risk for various cancer types (impaired double-stranded DNA repair).
- **Hyper IgE (Job) syndrome:** Has an unclear pathophysiology, but likely secondary to impaired IFN-γ leading to impaired neutrophil chemotaxis. Remember FATED mnemonic: coarse/leonine **F**acies, cold *Staphylococcus* **A**bscesses, retained primary **T**eeth, elevated levels of Ig**E**, and **D**ermatologic conditions.

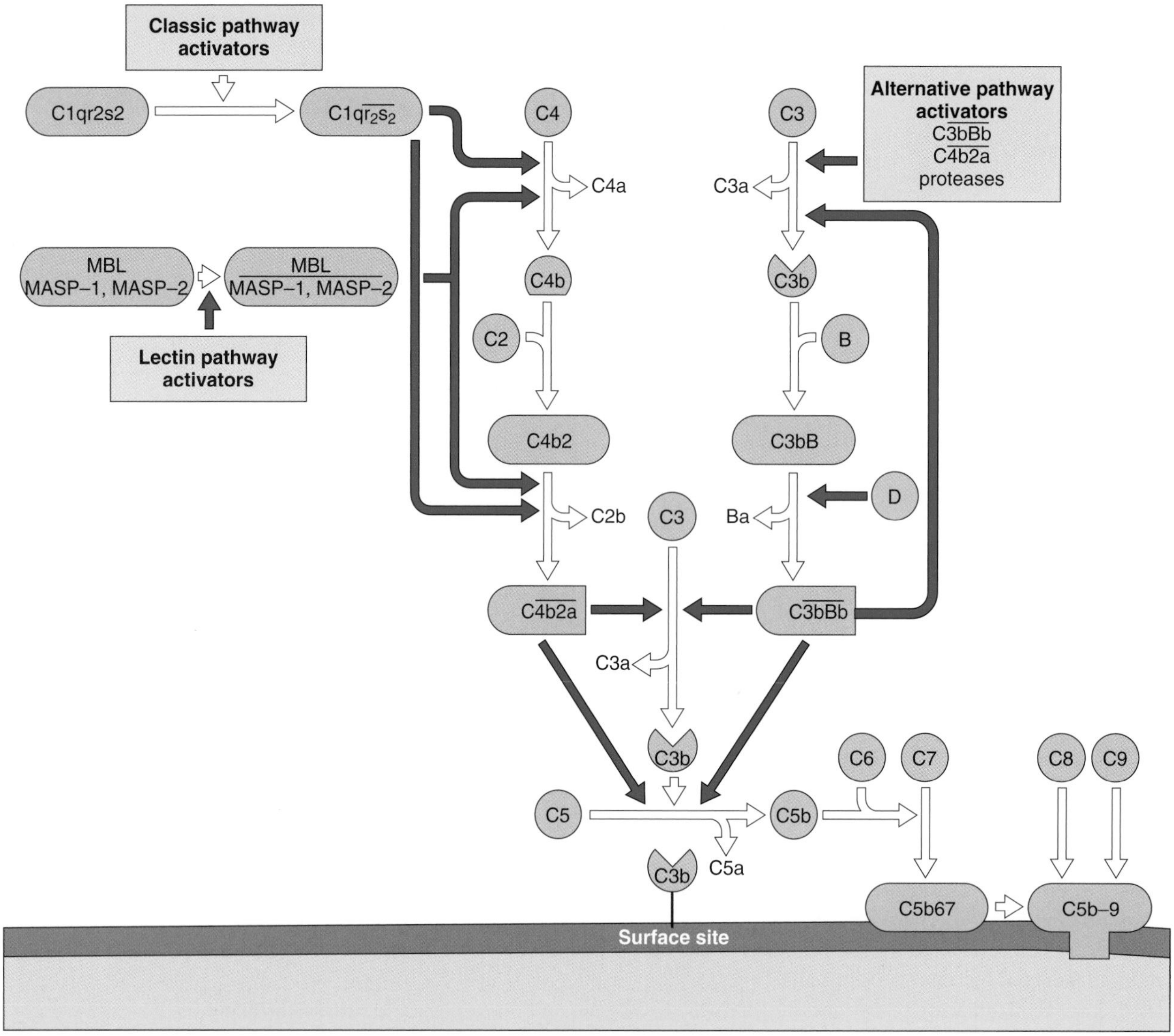

Fig. 6.8 The complement system and the formation of the membrane attack complex. (*From Male D, Brostoff J, Roth D, Roitt I.* Immunology. *7th ed. Philadelphia: Elsevier; 2007.*)

- **Wiskott**-Aldrich syndrome: X-linked recessive condition caused by a mutation in the WAS gene, resulting in T cells' inability to reorganize actin cytoskeleton. Remember the WATER mnemonic: **W**iskott-**A**ldrich, **T**hrombocytopenic purpura, **E**czema, **R**ecurrent infections.

COMPLEMENT SYSTEM

The Confusing Cascade of Complement Simplified

Complement is a system of liver-derived serum proteins that, once activated, triggers a cascade of proteolytic cleavage reactions to further the cascade and convert proproteins into functionally active immune system constituents. There are three main initial pathways that may be taken to ultimately activate C5 and initiate the final common pathway—the formation of the membrane attack complex (MAC) (Fig. 6.8).

1. Classical pathway → antigen–antibody complexes
2. Mannan-binding lectin pathway → microbial lectin particles
3. Alternative pathway → microbial surfaces such as LPS/endotoxin

Main Functions of the Complement System:

1. Opsonization → C3b
2. Neutrophil chemotaxis → C5a
3. Viral neutralization → C1, C2, C3, C4
4. Lysis (membrane attack complex) → C5b-9
5. Anaphylactic reaction → C3a, C5a

Complement Deficiencies and Associated Conditions

- C1 esterase inhibitor deficiency → hereditary angioedema; cannot take angiotensin-converting enzyme inhibitors
- Decay-accelerating factor (CD55) deficiency → paroxysmal nocturnal hemoglobinuria
- Protectin (CD59) → paroxysmal nocturnal hemoglobinuria
- C3 deficiency → propensity to develop severe, recurrent pyogenic infections of the sinus and respiratory tracts
- MAC (C5-C9) deficiency → propensity to develop *Neisseria* bacteremia

HYPERSENSITIVITY RESPONSE

Immunity Gone Wild!

Type I (Allergy): Type I reactions occur when presensitized mast cells or basophils with antigen-specific IgE are exposed to a particular antigen. The antigen binds the Fab portion of IgE, resulting in cross-linking and subsequent immediate release of preformed vasoactive substances (e.g., histamine). Anaphylactic reactions occur in this fashion through a type I reaction resulting in fast and widespread vasodilation and subsequent shock (hypotension). Bee stings and peanuts are common causes of anaphylaxis.

- *Disorders:* Allergic rhinitis, atopic dermatitis (eczema), urticaria (hives), asthma, and anaphylaxis.
- *Testing:* The main test used by allergists is scratch testing, in which a positive test results in a wheal-and-flare reaction of the scratched skin site.

Type II (Antibody-Dependent Cytotoxic): Type II reactions occur when either IgM or IgG antibodies bind to a **cell surface antigen,** resulting in cytotoxic destruction by a few possible mechanisms. These mechanisms include opsonization for histiocytes/neutrophils, activation of complement, and interference of cellular functioning.

- *Disorders:* Autoimmune hemolytic anemia, idiopathic thrombocytopenic purpura (ITP), acute transfusion reactions with hemolysis, rheumatic fever, Goodpasture syndrome (antibasement membrane), bullous pemphigoid (antihemidesmosome), pemphigus vulgaris (antidesmoglein), Graves disease (anti–thyroid-stimulating hormone receptor), and myasthenia gravis (anti-Ach receptor).
- *Testing:* Examples include the direct and indirect Coombs test of RBCs for hemolytic anemia and direct immunofluorescence of the glomerular basement membrane for Goodpasture syndrome (see Chapter 15).

Type III (Immune Complex Disease): Type III reactions occur when antigen–antibody (mainly IgG) complexes **form and are deposited** in tissues, resulting in activation of the complement system and recruitment of neutrophils and leading to tissue injury. Historically, the Arthus reaction resulted from intradermal injection of antigen, which resulted in a type III reaction in the underlying skin, causing edema and necrosis.

- *Disorders:* Systemic lupus erythematosus (SLE), rheumatoid arthritis (RA), hypersensitivity pneumonitis, serum sickness, and poststreptococcal glomerulonephritis.
- *Testing:* The main mode of testing is immunofluorescent staining.

Type IV (Delayed-Type Hypersensitivity, Antibody-Independent Cytotoxicity): Type IV reactions are the only hypersensitivity reactions that are not antibody mediated and thus cannot be transferred through serum. These cell-mediated reactions occur in a delayed fashion after a previously

> For a type IV reaction to occur, prior exposure to the antigen of interest is required. Hence, if a patient has been exposed to tuberculosis (TB), and thus TB antigens, when exposed to the purified protein derivative (PPD) test there will be a localized induration of the skin testing site secondary to the previously exposed T lymphocytes interacting with antigen in the PPD test.

exposed T lymphocyte interacts with the same antigen, resulting in lymphokine production and subsequent activation of other immune system players (e.g., macrophages).

- *Disorders:* Contact dermatitis (e.g., nickel allergy, exposure to urushiol oil from poison ivy/oak), Mantoux skin test (purified protein derivative [PPD]) for tuberculosis (TB) testing, graft-versus-host disease (GVHD), multiple sclerosis (MS), and Guillain-Barré syndrome.
- *Testing:* The main clinical test using the type IV response as a tool to help diagnose exposure to TB is the PPD test.

TRANSPLANTATION IMMUNOLOGY

Immunology is a critical factor whenever transplanting material with foreign antigens into a patient, whether it is a blood transfusion, a bone marrow transplant, or a solid organ transplant.

Types of Tissue Transplants

- **Autograft:** Transplantation of tissue back to the same host in a different location. A common example would be skin grafting from one site to another.
- **Allograft:** Transplantation of tissue from one human to another, such as is commonly performed in solid organ transplantation (e.g., kidney, liver, lung).
- **Xenograft:** Tissue transplantation from a different animal species to a human.

Types of Rejection

- **Hyperacute rejection:** Very rapid form of rejection occurring within minutes to hours of transplantation as a result of host antibodies binding to donor tissue endothelium. This results in complement activation and neutrophil migration into the donor graft.
- **Acute rejection:** T-cell–mediated rejection occurring within weeks to months after transplantation. This is the primary form of rejection for which immunosuppressant medications are used. This is the only form of rejection that can be acutely reversed by increased immunosuppressant dosing.
- **Chronic rejection:** A long-term form of rejection in which there is progressive loss of function of the transplanted organ or tissue secondary to vascular fibrosis.

High-Yield Immunosuppressant Drugs

- **Azathioprine:** A prodrug converted enzymatically in vivo to 6-mercaptopurine (6-MP), which acts to inhibit purine metabolism. Inhibition of purine metabolism preferentially affects proliferating cells such as T and B cells. Used both in autoimmune disorders and in acute rejection.
- **Cyclosporine:** Binds to cyclophilin, which inhibits calcineurin and therefore prevents transcription of IL-2 in T lymphocytes. Used primarily in tissue transplantation.
- **Tacrolimus:** Binds to FK-binding protein, but otherwise inhibits calcineurin (and therefore IL-2) similarly to cyclosporine. Used primarily as an alternative to cyclosporine in renal and liver transplant recipients.
- **Sirolimus:** Binds to FKBP to block T-cell activation and B-cell differentiation by inhibiting IL-2 signal transduction. Acts on the same pathway as cyclosporine and tacrolimus. Also used in drug-eluting stents.
- Glucocorticoids: Suppress both B- and T-cell function by decreasing cytokine transcription.
- **Mycophenolate mofetil:** Inhibits inosine monophosphate dehydrogenase, which is the rate-limiting enzyme in guanosine monophosphate (GMP) synthesis in the de novo purine synthesis pathway (see Chapter 2). Inhibition of purine synthesis inhibits replication of T and B cells. Primarily used in renal, heart, and liver transplant recipients.

REVIEW QUESTIONS

(1) A young child is brought to the pediatrician because of recurrent infections and failure to thrive. On examination the patient is noted to have a cleft palate, and a murmur is heard on cardiac auscultation. Based on this array of symptoms and physical findings, the patient is diagnosed with

DiGeorge syndrome. He is found to have thymic aplasia. What blood cell line is deficient in this patient causing his recurrent infections?

(2) An adolescent African American male patient with sickle cell disease is brought in for a regular examination and laboratory studies. On review of the patient's peripheral smear, not only are sickle cells seen but also a number of RBCs with inclusions and large number of platelets. What is responsible for this patient's smear findings?

(3) A patient in the intensive care unit is found to be in septic shock. A Gram stain of the patient's blood reveals gram-negative rods. Is the innate or adaptive immune system most likely to be active at this time?

(4) A 10-year-old girl is brought into the emergency department by ambulance after suffering a bee sting. She is covered in a red rash and is having difficulty breathing, with audible wheezing. What cell type is involved in this patient's presentation and what is going on?

(5) What cell type in the human body does not express MHC class I?

(6) True/False: $CD8^+$ T cells bind to the virally infected somatic cell's MHC class II and trigger cell destruction.

(7) A patient who has suffered from recurrent viral and bacterial infections throughout her life had immunoglobulin typing that revealed a large fraction of one immunoglobulin isotype but none of the others. What condition does she most likely have and what is the defect involved?

(8) True/False: *Anti-Rh* IgM from an untreated Rh-negative mother can cause erythroblastosis fetalis of her second Rh-positive child.

(9) Which cytokine is a strong neutrophil chemotactic factor?

(10) What occurs when a T-cell receptor binds to an MHC, exposing a host antigen, but no costimulatory signal is provided?

(11) A patient with a complement disorder involving deficiency of the membrane attack complex should specifically receive which immunization?

(12) A 15-year-old female patient presents to the clinic complaining of an erythematous rash and significant pruritus over her earlobes after wearing a pair of new earrings she received for her birthday. What is the most likely diagnosis and what is the most likely etiology of the diagnosis?

7 PHARMACOLOGY AND TOXICOLOGY

Ryan A. Pedigo

PHARMACOKINETICS

Overview

Pharmacokinetics is the description of a drug's journey through a patient's body. This involves four main processes: (1) absorption, (2) distribution, (3) metabolism, and (4) excretion. Imagine this sequence logically: The patient takes a drug and absorbs it; then the drug distributes throughout the body, is metabolized by the body, and finally is excreted.

Pharmacokinetics: (1) absorption, (2) distribution, (3) metabolism, and (4) excretion

(1) Absorption is simply how the patient's body takes in (absorbs) the drug in question.

- **Enteral,** meaning absorbed through the intestines: oral and rectal.
- **Parenteral,** meaning absorbed without the intestines: intravenous (IV), intramuscular (IM), subcutaneous (SQ), inhaled, topical, or transdermal.

The term **bioavailability** describes how much of what is ingested makes it into the systemic bloodstream. Oral drugs often have a lower bioavailability because (1) not everything is absorbed (incomplete tablet breakdown, barriers to absorption across the gut mucosa, gastric acid or enzymatic destruction), and (2) after absorption through the intestines into the portal vein, the drug **first passes** through the liver, where some of the drug is metabolized before reaching the systemic bloodstream—termed **first-pass metabolism** (Fig. 7.1).

Bioavailability: always 100% for IV; variable for oral administration, depending on drug

IV administration always has 100% bioavailability because it goes directly into the bloodstream; all parenteral routes bypass first-pass metabolism, and rectal administration typically bypasses about half of first-pass metabolism (because some drug is absorbed through the portal system into the liver and some into the caval system [meaning through the vena cava] back to the heart).

First-pass metabolism: A drug is absorbed through the intestine and travels to the liver through the portal vein, where it may potentially be metabolized.

(2) Distribution is where the drug goes after it is absorbed and is usually discussed as the **volume of distribution (V_d).** The volume of distribution is defined as

$$V_d = \frac{\text{Amount of drug in body}}{\text{Plasma drug concentration}}$$

Conceptually, the volume of distribution is a way to indicate how much of a drug stays in the patient's bloodstream and is unbound to protein. If the volume of distribution is high, it indicates that the drug is somehow not in the free state in the bloodstream—either it is bound to protein in the bloodstream or has left the bloodstream, such as lipid-soluble drugs going into fat. The average adult has about 5 L of blood, and therefore a V_d of about 5 indicates that it distributes only in blood—higher volumes of distribution indicate that it distributes further, likely into tissues or fat.

(3) Metabolism is one of the two ways that the body can decrease the concentration of active drug in the bloodstream (the other being **excretion,** described later). The **liver is the primary site for metabolism of drugs;** this is the reason that first-pass metabolism exists—if people in the Stone Age ate something poisonous, the liver would have a chance to detoxify it before it killed them! Unfortunately, the body also sees the drugs we prescribe as potential toxins and attempts to metabolize them through a process called biotransformation. There are two phases of biotransformation: **phase I biotransformation** (oxidation) and **phase II biotransformation** (conjugation).

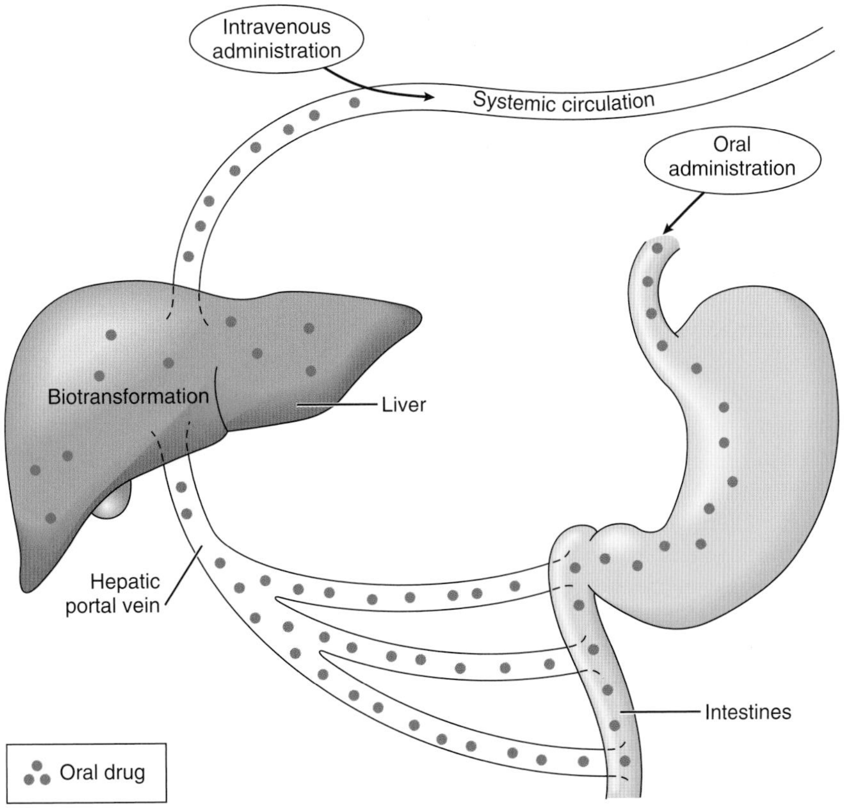

FIG. 7.1 First-pass metabolism. Any substance absorbed through the intestinal mucosa (except at the very end of the rectum) will drain into the portal system and be processed by the liver before reaching the systemic circulation. (*From Brenner GM, Stevens CW.* Pharmacology. *3rd ed. Philadelphia: Elsevier; 2009.*)

- **Phase I biotransformation:** Mediated by the microsomal cytochrome **P-450 (CYP)** monooxygenase system, with CYP3A4 being the most common subtype for these reactions. In general, these reactions are **oxidations** (by far the most common), reductions, or hydrolysis—the exact reactions are not important, but **the goal is to make the drug more polar (more water soluble) so that it can be excreted by the kidney.** The bioavailability of drugs is reduced by this step, but some drugs retain their activity after this process. In fact, some drugs (called **prodrugs**) are actually made active, rather than inactive, by this process—but this is the exception rather than the rule. Older adults have decreased phase I biotransformation ability, and this is one of the reasons that older adults often need smaller doses of medications for the same effect.
- **Phase II biotransformation:** In these reactions, a molecule is "strapped on" (conjugated) to the drug, such as an acetyl group, sulfide, or glucuronide. Again, the reactions are not important, but **this reaction almost always makes the drug inactive.**

Metabolism has many important clinical implications. For instance, the opioid analgesic codeine is metabolized into the more active morphine by CYP2D6—10% of whites have decreased CYP2D6 activity and will not get adequate pain relief with codeine administration. In addition, CYP2C19 activates the antiplatelet agent clopidogrel into the active form. Therefore those with poor CYP2C19 activity (more common in Asian populations) will not have therapeutic levels of the drug in their body, and this may have catastrophic consequences. Both drugs mentioned here are made active by the CYP enzymes in the liver—for review, is this a phase I or phase II reaction? Because the drugs are made active by this process, what are they called? If you did not get these answers immediately, revisit the previous paragraphs. These differences in CYP activity vary based on genetics; race and ethnicity are imperfect proxies for this but are sometimes tested on examinations and so are used as examples here.

Grapefruit juice, cimetidine, erythromycin: common CYP3A4 inhibitors
St. John's wort, phenytoin, rifampin: common CYP3A4 inducers

Another commonly tested and clinically relevant aspect of metabolism is that many drugs, herbs, and even foods can either inhibit or induce the CYP family of enzymes. Grapefruit juice inhibits CYP3A4 (recall this is the most common CYP for metabolizing drugs), and therefore patients may have higher drug levels if they take their medication with it. St. John's wort, an herbal treatment for depression, induces CYP3A4 and can "rev up" metabolism of drugs so that the level of active drug in the body will decrease.

Finally, the drug must be **(4) excreted** from the body, typically by the kidneys in the urine (but also through feces by biliary excretion). For renal excretion, the previous metabolism steps helped make the drug more polar to be water soluble to stay in the urine, and now the kidneys must excrete the drug. There are a few things to keep in mind when looking at renal excretion:

- **Glomerular filtration:** The drug must be delivered to the glomerulus if it is to be filtered. Therefore patients with a decreased glomerular filtration rate (GFR; i.e., renal disease) or those taking a drug that is bound to proteins (so it cannot be delivered to the glomerulus free and unbound) will have decreased renal clearance of the drug.
- **Active tubular secretion:** The kidney has channels called organic cation transporters and organic anion transporters for the active secretion of charged ions into the nephron. These can be blocked by medications such as probenecid, used in the treatment of gout.
- **Passive tubular reabsorption:** Uncharged, lipid-soluble molecules can be more readily absorbed through renal tubular cell membranes. The metabolic steps in phase I and phase II biotransformation reactions help keep the molecules water soluble and charged, facilitating excretion. Many drugs are weak acids or weak bases, and the pH of the soon-to-be-urine can determine how much of the acid or base stays inside the nephron to be excreted in the urine and how much will be reabsorbed. Therefore **if the drug is a weak acid, then alkalization of the urine will increase excretion** by making more of the drug in the charged A^- form rather than the uncharged HA form—this is referred to as **ion trapping** (Fig. 7.2) because the charged ions are "trapped" inside the lumen of the nephron. Conversely, if the drug is a weak base, then acidification of the urine to make more of the drug in the charged HB^+ form will facilitate excretion.

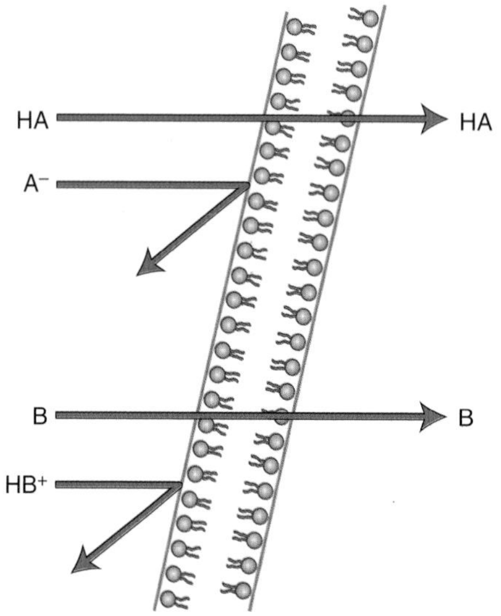

FIG. 7.2 Ion trapping. It can be seen that the uncharged molecules can move across the lipid cell membrane much more readily than ionized molecules.

A similar concept is found in the use of **lactulose** for patients with **hepatic encephalopathy.** Patients with liver failure have decreased urea cycle activity because the liver is the main site where the urea cycle takes place, and therefore toxic ammonia-containing compounds build up and can cause changes in mental status. Lactulose taken orally is broken up by the bacteria in the colon to make lactic acid and acetic acid, acidifying the colonic contents and changing the absorbable weak base ammonia NH_3 derived from dietary proteins into the charged, unabsorbable NH_4^+ ammonium ion. This ion-trapping mechanism is the same as in the kidney—the charged ion is not absorbed and is instead excreted.

Another form of **excretion** is through the **bile** to eventually be excreted in the stool. Many drugs that underwent conjugation (recall that this is a phase II biotransformation) with **glucuronate** can be excreted in this fashion. In fact, bilirubin (a byproduct of red blood cell breakdown) is excreted in this way through a phase II reaction with UDP-glucuronosyltransferase (which is deficient in patients with Gilbert disease and those with Crigler-Najjar disease). Now when you look at a patient's laboratory values for "unconjugated" and "conjugated" bilirubin (referred to as indirect and direct, respectively, in the laboratory values) you will understand what is occurring. However, because the intestines have so much surface area and absorptive capacity, as well as bacteria that can deconjugate the molecule, the drug has a "second chance" to be absorbed into the bloodstream yet again—termed **enterohepatic recycling or enterohepatic circulation.** If this occurs, the entire process of being absorbed and excreted in bile repeats.

Calculations and Kinetics

A basic understanding of the calculations in pharmacokinetics is important for both the USMLE Step 1 and also for clinical practice. First, it is important to talk about elimination of drugs in terms of **zero-order kinetics** versus **first-order kinetics.**

Zero-order kinetics: constant amount of drug eliminated per unit time
First-order kinetics: constant fraction of drug eliminated per unit time

- **Zero-order kinetics:** A **constant amount** of drug is eliminated per unit of time, so the rate of elimination is constant regardless of concentration of drug. Examples include **p**henytoin, **e**thanol, and **a**spirin **(PEA)**—use the following mnemonic: A **PEA** is round, just like the **0** of **zero**-order kinetics. The zero-order kinetics of ethanol is where the idea that the body can only metabolize one alcoholic drink (such as a beer) per hour comes from. Regardless of how many beers are consumed, the body can only metabolize one beer per hour. Therefore it exhibits zero-order kinetics because a **constant amount** of beer is removed from the body. Drinking more alcohol won't make the body remove alcohol from your body any faster—drink one beer, and your body will metabolize one beer per hour; drink 10 beers (don't test this, just take our word for it!), and your body will metabolize one beer per hour! The reason is that the elimination pathway becomes **saturated,** and there are only enough enzymes to clear one beer per hour.
- **First-order kinetics:** A **constant fraction** of drug is eliminated per unit time, so the rate of elimination is proportional to the drug concentration—this is a **much more common** method in which drugs are metabolized. Except for the drugs in the **PEA** mnemonic mentioned earlier, almost all drugs are eliminated by first-order kinetics. For example, if the body can eliminate half of a given drug per hour, and a patient has a blood concentration of 100 mg/mL of that drug, the concentration will halve each hour from 100 to 50 to 25 to 12.5, and so on. Note that a progressively smaller absolute amount of drug is being removed each hour (50 in the first hour, 25 in the second hour, and so on), whereas in zero-order kinetics, a constant amount is removed each hour.

Another important concept to learn is the **half-life** of a drug, which is the time it takes for half the drug to be metabolized. Recall in the zero-order kinetics model that a constant amount of drug is eliminated per unit time, so the **half-life of zero-order kinetics will change with the concentration of the drug.** For instance, if you drank 10 beers, it would take 5 hours at the rate of one beer per hour to metabolize half the beer (half-life of 5 hours). However, if you instead drank two beers, it would only take an hour to metabolize half the beer because after 1 hour, you would have one beer left in your body (half-life of 1 hour). On the other hand, because in first-order kinetics, a constant proportion is metabolized, the half-life is constant for a specific drug.

For a **first-order kinetics** drug, the half-life can be given by the equation

$$\text{Half-life} = \frac{0.7 \times V_d}{\text{Clearance}}$$

where V_d is the volume of distribution. This equation basically says that a higher volume of distribution will increase the half-life (because it is redistributing into fat or other body compartments and will not be available to be metabolized readily) and a faster clearance will cause a decreased half-life (which is intuitive because if the body gets rid of the drug faster, it will decrease the concentration of the drug faster). After a patient has taken a drug for a period of time (typically **4 to 5 times the half-life** of the drug), it reaches a **steady state** (Table 7.1 and Fig. 7.3), where the amount of drug taken equals the amount of drug leaving the body.

TABLE 7.1 Concentration of Drugs by Number of Half-Lives

NO. OF HALF-LIVES	1	2	3	4	5
Concentration	50%	75%	87.5%	93.75%	96.88%

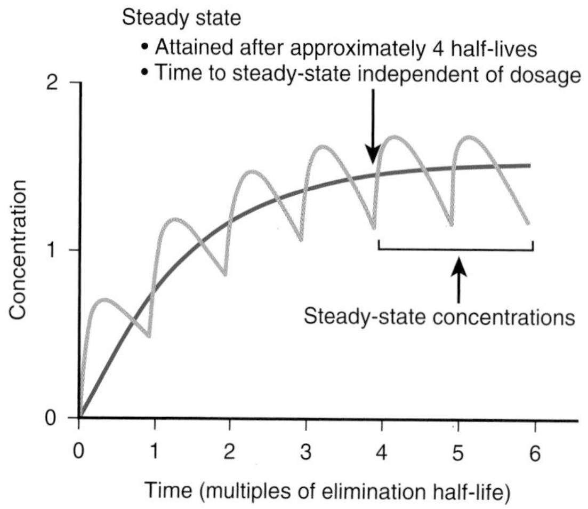

FIG. 7.3 The steady state of a drug is reached after 4 to 5 half-lives of that drug.

The concept of steady state also applies to clinical practice. For instance, in hypothyroidism, levothyroxine is given as replacement T_4 thyroid hormone and has a half-life of about 1 week. Therefore when a patient is started on this daily medication, it will take about 5 half-lives to come to a new steady state. This is the rationale for checking thyroid-stimulating hormone (TSH) 6 weeks after starting a patient on levothyroxine for hypothyroidism; any sooner and the drug would not have reached steady state, and the TSH would not be an accurate reflection of whether or not the dose was therapeutic. (Refer to Chapter 9 for details on thyroid hormone physiology.)

The last calculations that you are expected to know are the **loading dose** and **maintenance dose** for a medication. These calculations build on the information already presented in this chapter.

❍ The **loading dose** is given as

$$\text{Loading dose} = \frac{C_p \times V_d}{F}$$

where $\mathbf{C_p}$ is the target plasma concentration, $\mathbf{V_d}$ is the volume of distribution, and **F** is the bioavailability of the drug (remember this is always 1.0 [100%] for intravenous drugs). The loading dose is a larger one-time dose to get the patient up to the desired plasma concentration without having to wait for 5 half-lives because waiting isn't always feasible. For a large volume of distribution, a much larger loading dose may need to be given because such a small amount of the drug will stay inside the plasma—instead, those drugs may be redistributing into fat or other tissues outside of the bloodstream.

❍ The **maintenance dose** is given as

$$\text{Maintenance dose} = \frac{C_p \times \text{clearance}}{F}$$

where C_p is the target plasma concentration and F is the bioavailability of the drug. It represents the dose at which the net concentration of that drug in the bloodstream is unchanging. Therefore the elimination of the drug equals the rate of administration of the drug. Think of this as a leaking bucket—the water leaking out is the metabolism of the drug, and the water being poured into the bucket is the administration of the drug. The goal here is to equalize these two things so that the level of water in the bucket (the amount of drug in the patient) remains unchanged.

PHARMACODYNAMICS

> Agonists: activate receptor
> Antagonists: block receptor
> Partial antagonists: elicit a submaximal response

Overview

Pharmacodynamics is the study of how a given drug causes its effect. Pharmacodynamics includes, for example, the understanding of receptor activity, signal transduction pathways, and physiologic effects of a given drug. This section will highlight the fundamental concepts and some prototypical drugs that are instrumental to understanding this concept.

Fundamentally, drugs will interact with some form of receptor. When a drug interacts with a receptor, it can do so in many ways. Some drugs activate the receptor; these are called **agonists.** Some drugs block the receptor; these are called **antagonists.** Some drugs activate the receptors but are unable to do so fully; they are called **partial agonists** because they can only elicit a submaximal (partial) response.

To have an effect, the drug must bind to the receptor in question—it can either do this **reversibly** (noncovalent bonding, such as hydrogen bonding) or **irreversibly** (covalent bonding, such as with aspirin). Drugs will "like" to attach to different receptors more or less depending on their particular shape and size, referred to as the **affinity** of the drug for its receptor. We express this chemically by looking at the following equilibrium:

$$[\text{Drug}] + [\text{Receptor}] \leftrightarrow [\text{Drug - Receptor}]$$

If the drug has a high affinity for the receptor, most of this equilibrium will lie to the right as the drug–receptor complex. Only a small amount of the drug will be required to achieve the intended effect because it sticks to the receptor so well—this is called high **potency.** Potency is measured as the half maximal effective concentration **(EC50),** which is the concentration of the drug needed to elicit 50% of the maximal effect: If you need a lot of the drug to achieve that, the drug is a low-potency drug. For instance, benzathine penicillin, a long-acting antibiotic used in the treatment of syphilis, has a dose of 2.4 million units. Because a high dose of the drug is required to have the intended effect, it is a low-potency drug.

As an aside, because pharmacologists love to confuse medical students, sometimes the drug–receptor interaction will be described in terms of a K_D, or dissociation constant. This is tricky because a high dissociation constant (a high K_D) means that the drug–receptor complex **wants** to dissociate and come apart, and therefore it would have a low affinity. Conversely, a low K_D means the drug doesn't want to dissociate, and it would have a high affinity—don't get tricked by this.

The **efficacy** of a drug is the **maximum response achievable from a drug**—regardless of the amount of drug needed. Note that a drug can have great efficacy but not be potent if a drug has a high maximal response but requires a lot of the drug to do so. If an analgesic can take away 100% of a patient's pain, but requires 1,000,000 mg to do so, this would have a high efficacy but low potency. Conversely, a drug can have high potency (small amount of drug required to get 50% of the maximal response) but have low efficacy if the drug cannot ever achieve a maximal response regardless of dose given (i.e., a very potent **partial agonist**). Do not be confused by this concept. Remember, **potency and efficacy are independent of each other.** Refer to graphs A to C later in Fig. 7.4 to illustrate this concept.

Antagonists block receptor sites and try to prevent activation of that receptor. They can be either **competitive** (meaning they compete for the same active site as the normal agonist for that receptor) or **noncompetitive** (meaning they bind to a different site separate from that of the normal agonist for that receptor) (Fig. 7.5). This difference is important because if there are high levels of an agonist present, the **competitive** antagonist can be outcompeted, being "drowned out" by all the agonists competing for the same site. On the other hand, because noncompetitive antagonists and agonists do not compete for the same site, the noncompetitive antagonist cannot be outcompeted by high concentrations of agonists.

Take some time to familiarize yourself with Fig. 7.4.

A. The addition of a **competitive antagonist** does not decrease the efficacy (ability to achieve a maximal effect) of the agonist because adding more of the agonist overwhelms the competitive antagonist; however, because more drug is required to achieve 50% of the maximal effect, the agonist is **less potent.**

B. The addition of an **irreversible antagonist** causes decreased efficacy because regardless of how much of the agonist is added, it cannot outcompete the antagonist—it is irreversible and will not unbind. A **noncompetitive antagonist** would have the same effect because it does not bind to the same site as the agonist, so the high concentration of agonist cannot displace it.

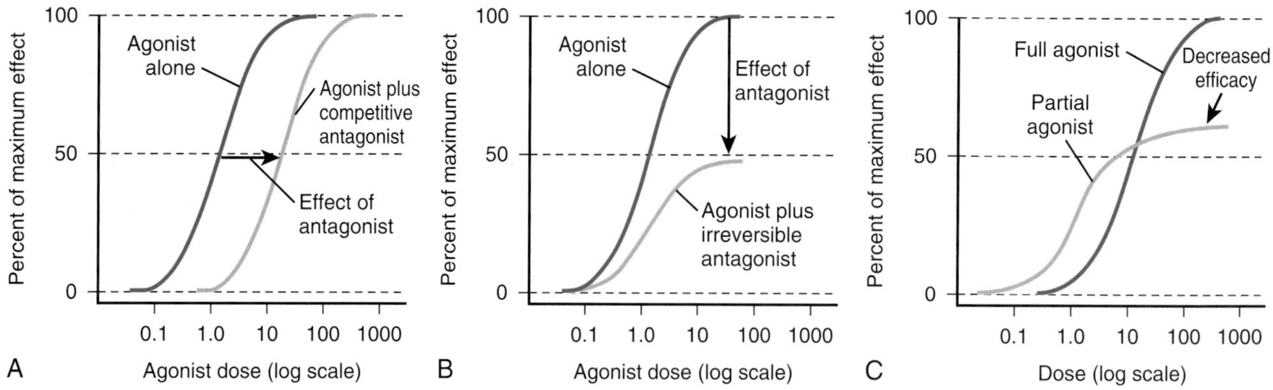

FIG. 7.4 A dose–response curve and the modifications with a competitive agonist **(A)**, an irreversible antagonist or noncompetitive antagonist **(B)**, and a partial agonist **(C)** added.

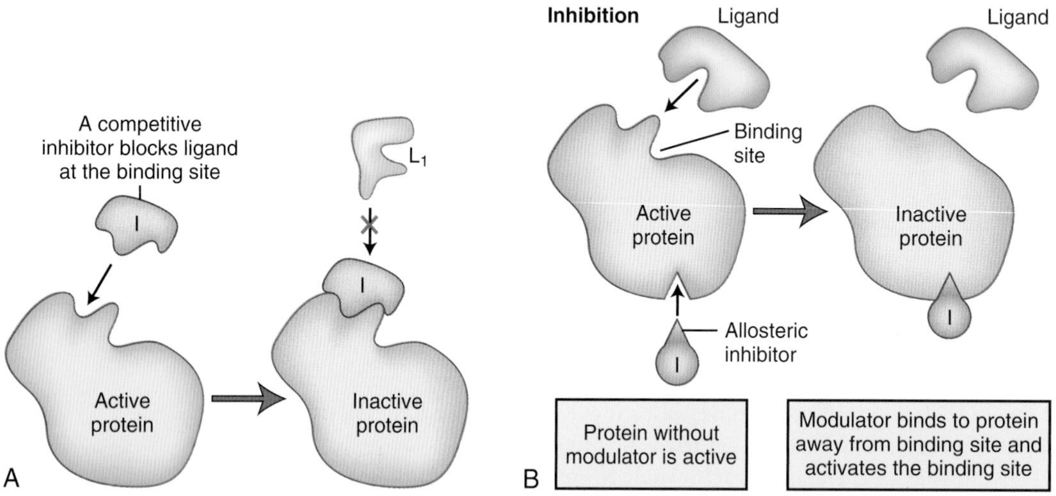

FIG. 7.5 A, A competitive antagonist, binding at the same active site as the normal agonist for that receptor. **B,** A noncompetitive antagonist, with the antagonist binding at a separate site from the normal agonist for that receptor.

C. A **partial agonist,** as mentioned earlier, is something that cannot have a maximal effect (less than 100% efficacy). Of note, in this particular case, the partial agonist is **more potent** than the full agonist because the EC50 is at a lower dose than the full agonist. Again, this demonstrates the idea that **efficacy and potency are independent of each other.**

Lastly, familiarize yourself with the idea of the **therapeutic index (TI),** a measurement of the margin of safety of a drug. It is calculated as

$$TI = \frac{\text{Median toxic dose}}{\text{Median effective dose}}$$

If the drug has a TI of 100, then the median toxic dose is 100 times greater than the median effective dose—a very safe medication. However, if the TI was 1.001, for example, the median toxic dose would be barely greater than the median effective dose, and toxic effects would be much more likely (i.e., chemotherapeutics).

AUTONOMIC NERVOUS SYSTEM AND SIGNAL TRANSDUCTION

Overview

The **nervous system** is broken down into the **central** (brain and spinal cord) and **peripheral** (everything else) nervous systems; the peripheral nervous system includes the **somatic** (voluntary) and **autonomic** (involuntary) nervous systems. The **autonomic** nervous system is further divided into the **sympathetic** and **parasympathetic** nervous systems (Fig. 7.6A). In this chapter, the autonomic nervous system is described because understanding the sympathetic and parasympathetic nervous systems is critically important to understanding their pharmacology.

Autonomic nervous system: includes sympathetic and parasympathetic nervous systems

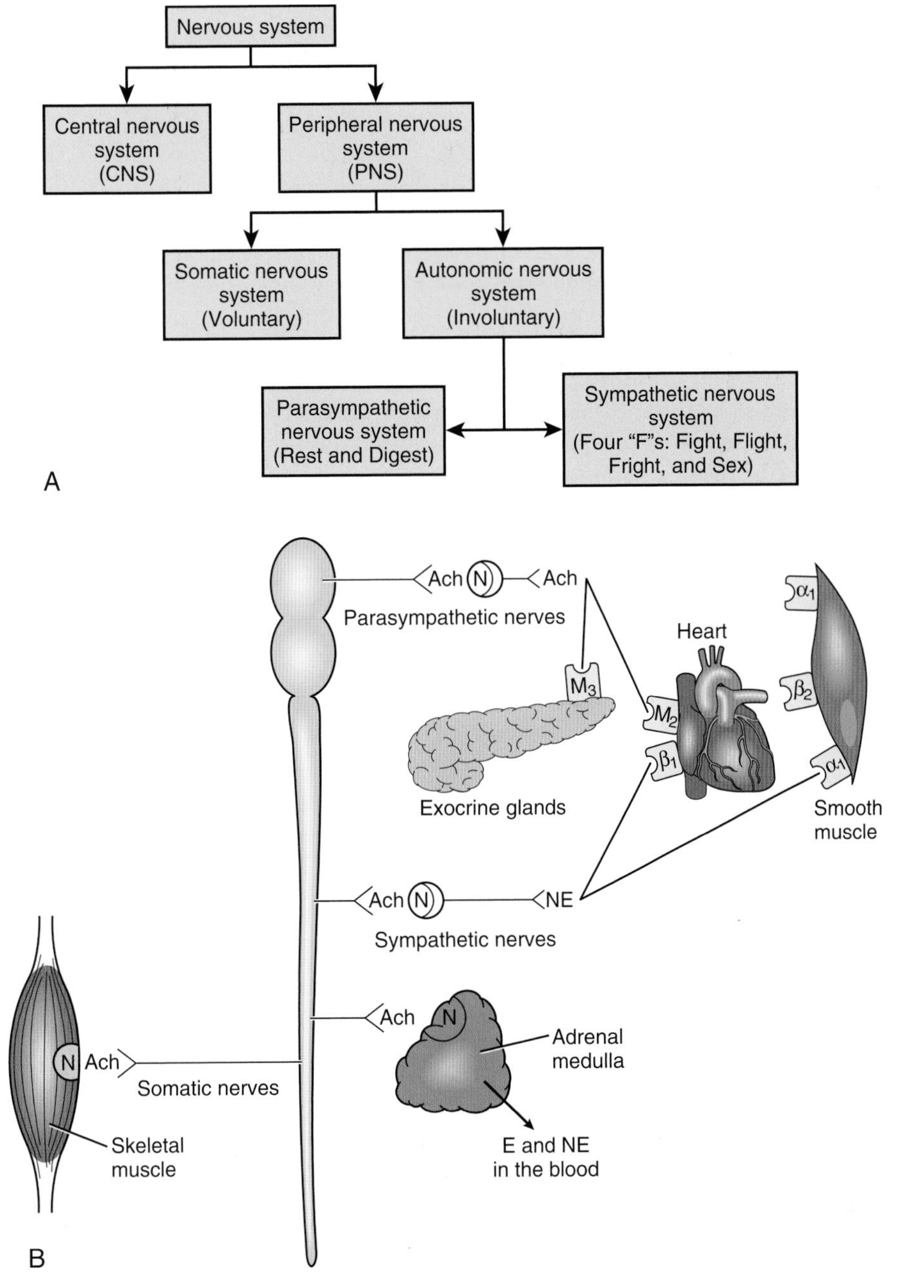

FIG. 7.6 **A,** A breakdown of the nervous system and its components. **B,** A schematic of the actions of the parasympathetic nervous system and sympathetic nervous system on various organs in the body. (**B,** *from Brenner GM, Stevens CW.* Pharmacology. *3rd ed. Philadelphia: Elsevier; 2009.*)

The **autonomic nervous system** is **automatic** (involuntary)—it involuntarily regulates the body's activities, such as the activity of the intestines, tone of blood vessels, heart rate, secretions, and more. Recall that the **sympathetic** and **parasympathetic** divisions make up the autonomic nervous system; the actions of each of them are mostly opposing. The **sympathetic** nervous system regulates the four Fs of life: fight, flight, fright, and sex. The goal of the sympathetic nervous system is to keep you alive in a dangerous situation or one that requires a lot of activity. The **parasympathetic** nervous system (Fig. 7.6B) mediates the "rest-and-digest" response when it is safe to be more sedentary, and promotes gastrointestinal (GI) motility, defecation, and urination—you wouldn't want to have to use the bathroom when running from an attacker!

SYMPATHETIC NERVOUS SYSTEM

The **sympathetic** nerves leave from the **thoracolumbar** (thoracic and lumbar) spinal cord. The primary neurotransmitter of the sympathetic nervous system is **norepinephrine,** but **epinephrine** is indirectly a key player because the adrenal medulla releases epinephrine into the bloodstream to further activate the sympathetic response. The sympathetic nervous system exerts its effect **through alpha (α) and beta (β) receptors.**

- **α_1 Receptors** act as **smooth muscle constrictors,** meaning that they tighten sphincters (again, don't want to use the bathroom when running from a tiger) and also contract the smooth muscles of arterioles in the circulatory system (vasoconstriction), increasing systemic vascular resistance and raising blood pressure. The goal of this vasoconstriction is to decrease blood flow to nonvital areas and redirect it to skeletal muscle to support activity. Those parts of the body that are less vital to be perfused during activity will have more of these receptors, causing more vasoconstriction in these areas. In addition, the pupillary dilator muscle in the eye has α_1 receptors, which cause dilation of the pupil to allow more light in during the fight-or-flight response. **Phenylephrine** is a pure α_1 agonist that clamps down blood vessels, often used to raise blood pressure in hypotensive patients in the operating room and also used to stop runny noses (constricting vessels in the nose to stop vascular congestion)!

α_1: smooth muscle constrictor
α_2: negative feedback; reduces sympathetic outflow
β_1: cardiac stimulant
β_2: smooth muscle relaxer

- **α_2 Receptors** act as **negative feedback** to keep the sympathetic response regulated. **Clonidine** is an **α_2 agonist** and therefore through negative feedback has the net effect of **decreasing sympathetic outflow,** which is beneficial in the treatment of hypertension but more commonly is used to manage the sympathetic nervous system activation surges that often accompany opiate withdrawal in patients attempting to quit their addiction.
- **β_1 Receptors** are found mostly on the heart and act as **cardiac stimulants.** They mainly increase the rate (chronotropy) and contractility (inotropy) of the heart, allowing for increased cardiac output and delivery of blood to tissues to support their increased activity during one of those four Fs. **Beta blockers** work by preventing activation of this receptor, which ensures that the heart doesn't work too hard (require more oxygen) in patients with heart disease. In patients with heart failure, prolonged sympathetic activation actually causes long-term remodeling and changes in the heart that are maladaptive—beta blockade also helps prevent this neurohumoral remodeling.
- **β_2 Receptors** act as **smooth muscle relaxers,** which seems counterintuitive when contrasted with α_1 receptors. However, it is the location of these receptors that is important—to increase blood flow to skeletal muscle, more β_2 receptors instead of α_1 receptors are found on arterioles feeding skeletal muscles. In addition, β_2 receptors are found on the bronchioles of the lung, and activation of these receptors relaxes smooth muscle in this area, allowing for better airflow during breathing—which is why the β_2 agonist **albuterol** is so effective in treating asthma. You have **1 heart** (β_1 works on the heart), and you have **2 lungs** (β_2 works on the lungs).

Signal Transduction Pathways

All of the aforementioned receptors (and all receptors) need to trigger some sort of signal transduction pathway to relay the message and start the cascade that eventually causes the intended effect of the receptor. The **most common pathway for this is through G-protein–coupled receptors (GPCRs),** which are also known as seven-transmembrane domain receptors because they cross the cell membrane seven times. There are many subtypes of GPCRs, each of which has a different downstream pathway; it is important to understand the **G_q, G_s, and G_i** pathways (only three!). Now that you understand what each receptor of the sympathetic nervous system does, it is time to move on to **how** it does it, through these GPCRs.

GPCRs have α, β, and γ subunits and are active when a signal molecule (e.g., a neurotransmitter or drug) attaches to the receptor and causes the α subunit to exchange its bound inactive guanosine diphosphate (GDP) for an active guanosine triphosphate (GTP)—this activates the α subunit to in turn activate the βγ complex, which will then go on to activate whatever downstream pathway is involved, depending on whether or not it goes through the G_q, G_s, or G_i pathway. The α subunit has a GTPase, which will eventually hydrolyze one of the phosphates off of GTP to change it back to inactive GDP, to ensure that the signal doesn't continue going on forever. (Note: These α and β are subunits of the GPCR—different from the α and β sympathetic nervous system receptors discussed previously!)

- **G_q:** The G_q pathway has the end result of increasing calcium levels in the targeted cells; in the case of the **α_1 receptors** on the arterioles of blood vessels, the calcium surge causes contraction of those muscles and therefore causes vasoconstriction. The exact mechanism of how calcium release allows muscular contraction is covered in detail in Chapter 12. Refer to the graphic that depicts the G_q pathway: The active βγ complex activates phospholipase C, cleaving the PIP_2 molecule into IP_3 and diacylglycerol (DAG). The IP_3 binds to a special channel on the sarcoplasmic reticulum (an organelle in smooth muscle cells that holds calcium to be ready for contraction) and releases that calcium. DAG, on the other hand, can be made into prostaglandins, which regulate pain and inflammatory responses, and also activates protein kinase C (PKC), which can phosphorylate other molecules and exert other effects (Fig. 7.7A).
- **G_s:** The G_s pathway has the end result of activating protein kinase A (PKA), which phosphorylates various proteins to modify their activity (**kinases** phosphorylate things, **dephosphorylases** remove phosphates from things). The active βγ complex activates adenylyl cyclase, causing cyclic adenosine monophosphate (cAMP) production, which activates PKA. Both β_1 and β_2 receptors work through this pathway—each phosphorylating proteins that in turn cause their intended effects (Fig. 7.7B).
- **G_i:** Luckily this one is easy—it **inhibits** adenylyl cyclase, preventing cAMP production and PKA activation. G_s **stimulates** cAMP production; G_i **inhibits.**

PARASYMPATHETIC NERVOUS SYSTEM

The **parasympathetic nervous system** has nerves that exit from the **cervicosacral spinal cord;** neurons that have parasympathetic activity are also found in some of the cranial nerves (specifically cranial

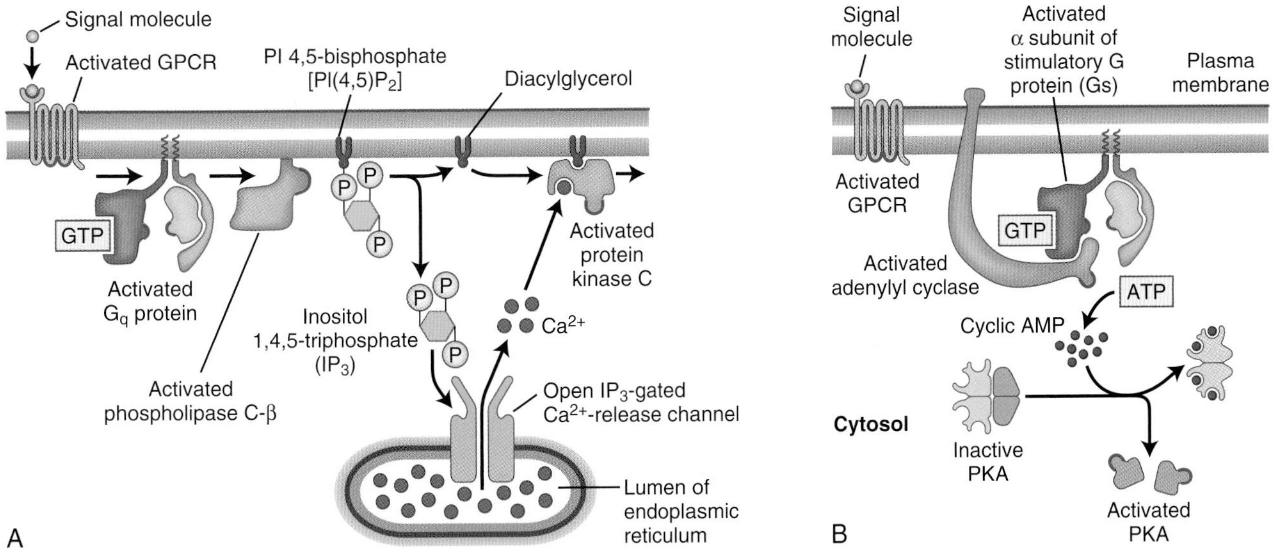

FIG. 7.7 G-protein–coupled receptor (GPCR) pathways, including Gq pathway **(A)** and Gs pathway **(B)**.

nerves III, VII, IX, X, discussed in detail in Chapter 13). The parasympathetic nervous system mediates the **rest-and-digest** response; when you are relaxed and sedentary, your body slows the heart rate, increases blood flow to the intestines and promotes digestion, and promotes urination and defecation—all of the "body maintenance" activities that the body previously put on hold while you were running from that tiger. In contrast to the sympathetic nervous system, which uses catecholamines such as norepinephrine and epinephrine, the parasympathetic nervous system uses **acetylcholine** to exert most of its effects on the body through **muscarinic receptors.**

- **M_1, M_3, and M_5 (odd) receptors:** Use the **G_q** pathway described previously. **M_3** receptors cause smooth muscle contractions at smooth muscles that **aren't** sphincters (because if your sphincters were tight, it would make urinating and defecating difficult!)—an example of this contraction is the detrusor muscle, the smooth muscle of the urinary bladder, promoting urination. The M_3 receptor also increases glandular secretions, important in the parasympathetic-mediated digestion response as well as in bronchial secretions, in which blocking this receptor is helpful to patients with asthma or chronic obstructive pulmonary disease (COPD). Again, the **G_q pathway causes a calcium surge,** leading to **smooth muscle contraction through calcium release** from the sarcoplasmic reticulum, but the receptors are in locations different from the sympathetic α_1 receptors that also mediate smooth muscle contraction. In general, the **odd-numbered muscarinic receptors are excitatory** (whereas the even-numbered muscarinic receptors are inhibitory). A way to remember this is **it's *odd* to be *excited* about muscarinic receptors.** (The M_1 and M_5 receptors are much less clinically important.)
- **M_2 and M_4 (even) receptors:** As you may guess from earlier, M_2 and M_4 receptors are inhibitory and therefore act through the G_i pathway. The most important inhibitory muscarinic receptor is the **M_2 receptor** found on the **atria of the heart**—the inhibitory actions on the **sinus node** (the pacemaker of the heart) cause a **decreased heart rate** as well as decreased contractility of the atria only. The ventricles do not have a high density of these receptors, and ventricular contractility is unaffected.

Muscarinic receptors: Odd-numbered receptors have excitatory function, whereas even-numbered receptors typically have inhibitory function.

PHARMACOLOGY

Adrenergic Pharmacology

Adrenergic pharmacology will address how drugs manipulate **catecholamines** such as norepinephrine and epinephrine and their G-protein–linked α_1, α_2, β_1, and β_2 receptors. Drugs modifying this system have a wide clinical application, from treating anaphylactic shock (the most severe allergic response) with epinephrine to helping people with benign prostatic hyperplasia (BPH) urinate. Just as with the cholinomimetics, the **sympathomimetics** can act either **directly** through receptor agonists or indirectly. The indirect sympathomimetics work either by **preventing reuptake of catecholamines** or by **increasing release** of them. Catecholamines are synthesized from tyrosine and subsequently undergo various modification steps (Fig. 7.8A).

Fig. 7.8B depicts an adrenergic **synapse.** The **presynaptic neuron** is stimulated to release norepinephrine into the **synaptic cleft,** the space between the presynaptic neuron and postsynaptic receptors, which may be located either on another neuron to carry the signal downstream or on the end organ to be affected. The acetylcholine binds to those receptors and activates them. Drugs act to potentiate or block this system.

Direct sympathomimetics act directly as agonists at an adrenergic receptor. The main direct sympathomimetics are **epinephrine, norepinephrine, isoproterenol, dopamine, dobutamine,** and **phenylephrine.** Epinephrine, norepinephrine, and dopamine are referred to as **endogenous** catecholamines because they are naturally found inside the body. The synthesis of these endogenous catecholamines begins with the amino acid tyrosine and then progresses to the active catecholamines dopamine, norepinephrine, and epinephrine, in that order.

- **Epinephrine:** Affinity for $\alpha_1 = \alpha_2$ and affinity for $\beta_1 = \beta_2$, with preference at low doses for β_1. Therefore because of the α_1 and β_1 agonist activity, epinephrine acts to **vasoconstrict** (increasing blood pressure) and **increase cardiac output,** respectively. The β_2 agonist activity causes **bronchodilation** and **increases blood flow to skeletal muscles.** All of these should be intuitive: These are all things that you might need to happen when you are fighting an attacker. Clinically, this is used in **anaphylaxis** when an allergic reaction has caused histamine release with subsequent bronchospasm as well as widespread

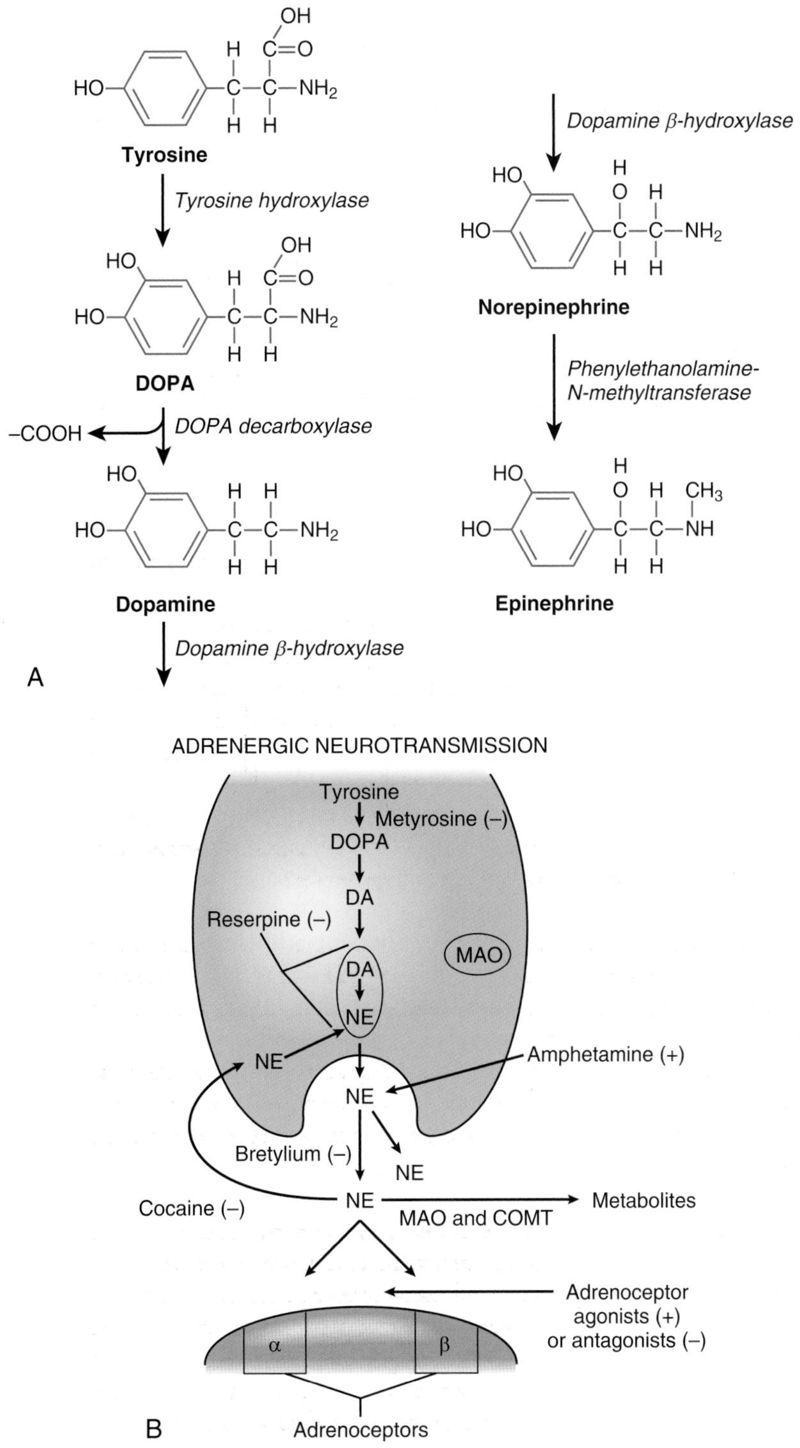

FIG. 7.8 A, Synthesis of catecholamines from tyrosine. **B,** Neurotransmission at a sympathetic nervous system neuron synapse. (**B** *from Brenner GM, Stevens CW. Pharmacology. 3rd ed. Philadelphia: Elsevier; 2009.*)

hypotension as a result of vasodilation; the epinephrine can help reverse these changes and save the patient's life. This drug is so important clinically that patients with a history of anaphylaxis carry an intramuscular epinephrine injector with them in case another anaphylactic reaction occurs. This drug is also used in severe **asthma** exacerbations to allow for bronchodilation and ease of breathing.

- **Norepinephrine:** Affinity for both α receptors is greater than for the β_1 receptor; it has no significant β_2 activity. Therefore norepinephrine is primarily an excellent **vasoconstrictor.** It is used as a vasopressor (a drug that constricts blood vessels) in septic shock.

- **Dopamine:** The immediate precursor to norepinephrine in the synthetic pathway, dopamine at low doses causes renal vasodilation through D_1 and D_2 dopamine receptors; at medium doses, it causes β_1 stimulation and increases cardiac output; at high doses, it causes α_1 activation and vasoconstriction. This is also used in treating the low blood pressure in septic shock.
- **Isoproterenol:** A pure β agonist, $\beta_1 = \beta_2$. Therefore the drug will cause increased cardiac output from β_1 activation as well as vasodilation and decreased blood pressure from β_2 activation. This is rarely used clinically.
- **Phenylephrine:** A pure α_1 agonist, phenylephrine is a potent vasoconstrictor that is used in various forms to decrease nasal congestion (nasal spray), increase blood pressure (IV), and even dilate pupils (eye drops) for eye examinations by activating the pupillary dilator muscle.
- **Albuterol:** A β_2 agonist, albuterol is inhaled and relaxes smooth muscles in the airways, helping asthmatic patients breathe better. Salmeterol is another agent commonly used; it is longer acting.
- **Terbutaline:** A β_2 agonist, terbutaline relaxes smooth muscles and has found its use in the treatment of premature labor as a tocolytic (something that decreases uterine contractions). It can also be used in asthma exacerbations as a bronchodilator.
- **Indirect sympathomimetics** work by either increasing release of catecholamines (such as amphetamine or ephedrine) or by preventing their reuptake into the presynaptic neuron (such as cocaine). These will generally increase sympathetic outflow, causing increased activity at all four adrenergic receptors, α_1, α_2, β_1, and β_2.
- **Amphetamine** is used in the treatment of attention-deficit/hyperactivity disorder (ADHD), narcolepsy, and obesity; it causes increased release of endogenous catecholamines. This is similar to **ephedrine,** which can be used as a decongestant.
- **Cocaine** blocks reuptake of catecholamines and leaves them in the synaptic cleft to continue to stimulate receptors.

In addition, there are many drugs that act to block these receptors or to reduce sympathetic outflow in general. These are called **sympathoplegics** or **sympatholytics.**

α_2 Agonists such as **clonidine** and **methyldopa** decrease sympathetic outflow because the α_2 receptor acts as **negative feedback. Clonidine** is used for the sympathetic surges that accompany opioid withdrawal, and **methyldopa** is used to treat hypertension in pregnancy because other blood pressure medications often have deleterious effects on the fetus.

α_1 Antagonists block the smooth muscle–constricting effects of the α_1 receptor.

- **Phenoxybenzamine:** This is an **irreversible** nonselective α antagonist (unlike **phentolamine,** which is reversible), which is used in the treatment of pheochromocytoma (a catecholamine-secreting tumor). The fact that it is irreversible is important because the high levels of catecholamines secreted by this tumor would displace reversible antagonists. By blocking vasoconstriction at the arterioles, hypotension is a common side effect.
- **Prazosin, terazosin, doxazosin:** These are α_1 antagonists that are primarily used for their prevention of smooth muscle constriction in the urinary tract to treat benign prostate hyperplasia. The enlarged prostate causes increased resistance to urinary flow out of the bladder; this medication helps relax the smooth muscle and aid in urination. Of course, the side effect is that it also would block vasoconstriction and has the potential to cause hypotension; **tamsulosin** is a newer medication that is specific for the subtype of receptors in the urinary system.

β Antagonists ("beta blockers") are commonly used in patients with high blood pressure, myocardial infarction, supraventricular tachycardia, and heart failure. Recall that β_1 stimulation causes the heart to increase in rate (positive chronotrope) and contractility (positive inotrope); beta blockade prevents these responses, causing a decreased oxygen demand for the heart, as well as slowing it in patients with fast heart rates. These drugs typically end in *-lol* (e.g., propranolol, atenolol, metoprolol) and can either be β_1 selective (atenolol, metoprolol) or nonselective for the β receptor (propranolol).

> Somatic nervous system: part of the peripheral nervous system; also uses acetylcholine, but uses nicotinic receptors instead of muscarinic receptors; is involved in voluntary movement

Cholinergic Pharmacology

Cholinergic pharmacology addresses how drugs manipulate **acetylcholine** and their G-protein–linked **muscarinic receptors** to have their intended effects on the body (Fig. 7.9). Before this is discussed, a concept that has not been introduced yet must be briefly mentioned—the **somatic** nervous system. The somatic nervous system is used for voluntary movement and also uses acetylcholine as a

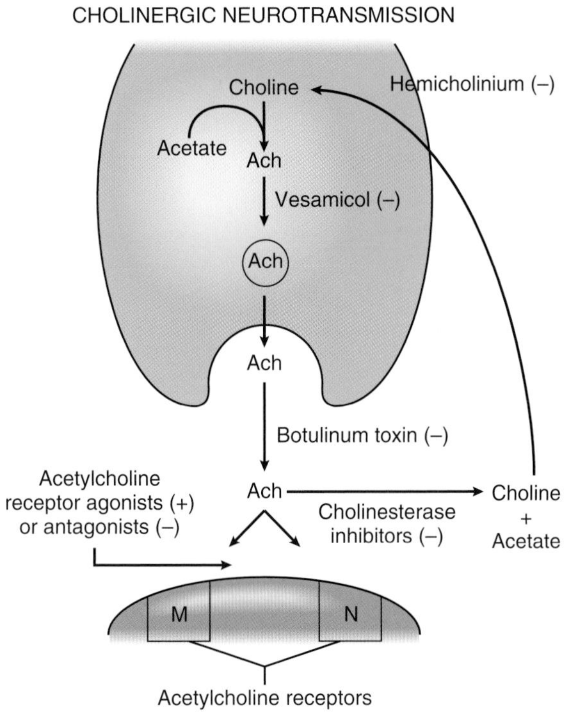

FIG. 7.9 Neurotransmission at a parasympathetic nervous system neuron synapse. (*From Brenner GM, Stevens CW. Pharmacology. 3rd ed. Philadelphia: Elsevier; 2009.*)

neurotransmitter to cause muscle contraction through **nicotinic** receptors that are linked to ion channels. Therefore drugs that act directly on muscarinic receptors will not affect the somatic nervous system, but drugs that increase the activity of acetylcholine will because they share the same neurotransmitter type. A description of exactly how nicotinic receptor activation leads to muscular contraction is covered in Chapter 12.

There are two ways to increase muscarinic cholinergic transmission: either **directly** through **muscarinic receptor agonists** or **indirectly** by **inhibiting acetylcholinesterase,** the enzyme that degrades acetylcholine by splitting it into choline and acetate for recycling into the neuron. Both of these would be called **cholinomimetic** agents because they mimic acetylcholine's activity.

The most commonly used example of a direct cholinomimetic is **pilocarpine,** given as eye drops (Fig. 7.10). Pilocarpine works on the M_3 muscarinic receptor on the pupillary sphincter muscle, causing contraction and miosis (constriction of the pupil). Study Fig. 7.10; the circular muscles of the iris sphincter will get smaller when contracted, causing pupillary constriction, whereas the dilator muscle under α-receptor control will stretch back the iris and cause mydriasis (my**D**riasis = pupillary **D**ilation). This drug is important in the treatment of **angle-closure glaucoma,** in which the aqueous humor of the eye builds to high pressures as a result of blockage of the canal of Schlemm. Angle-closure glaucoma is often precipitated in susceptible individuals by dilation of the pupil, which increases the contact between the iris and the lens as the iris becomes "scrunched up" by compacting and thickening during dilation. Pilocarpine will constrict the pupil, helping restore normal flow of aqueous humor.

There are also **indirect** cholinomimetics that function by blocking the breakdown of acetylcholine into acetate and choline. This prolongs the action of acetylcholine in the synapse. The indirect cholinomimetics include the reversible acetylcholinesterase inhibitors (edrophonium, pyridostigmine, and physostigmine) as well as pesticides, which are commonly irreversible acetylcholinesterase inhibitors. **Edrophonium** is a commonly tested medication because of it previously being a test for diagnosing **myasthenia gravis,** an autoimmune disease in which the body blocks and destroys the nicotinic receptors that the somatic nervous system uses for movement, leaving fewer functional nicotinic receptors and causing weakness. Edrophonium is a short-acting reversible acetylcholinesterase inhibitor, allowing more acetylcholine to attach to the nicotinic receptors that are still functioning, restoring strength. If the patient improved after administration, it was suggestive of the disease. Because the half-life of edrophonium is so short, treatment of myasthenia gravis is with **pyridostigmine,** which is longer

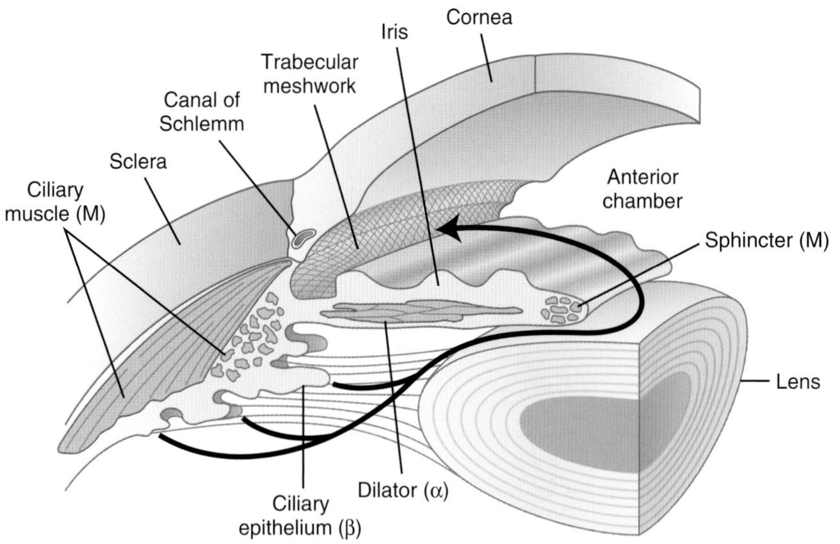

FIG. 7.10 The eye and its pupillary dilator muscle (α receptor, sympathetic) and pupillary constrictor muscle (M receptor, parasympathetic).

acting. Pyridostigmine does not cross the blood–brain barrier and therefore does not affect the brain. **Physostigmine** crosses the blood–brain barrier and is therefore less commonly used, except in overdoses of anticholinergics that cross the blood–brain barrier.

Too much activation of the parasympathetic nervous system as a result of cholinomimetics can lead to **SLUDGE** syndrome, a mnemonic toxidrome characterized by **S**alivation, **L**acrimation, **U**rination, **D**efecation, **G**astrointestinal upset, and **E**mesis—this is covered more in depth later in the section "Toxicology," but by now each of these symptoms should make sense given the activity of the cholinergic system. The parasympathetic nervous system through muscarinic receptors mediates the rest-and-digest response; salivation, urination, and defecation, as well as increased GI motility (GI upset), are all direct parts of that response. Additionally, because of the pupillary sphincter muscle discussed previously, increased cholinergic tone will cause miosis. **Pilocarpine** does not have these systemic effects because it is administered as eye drops, which are not absorbed in large quantities into the systemic circulation.

There are also **muscarinic antagonists** that are used to prevent activity at these receptors.

- **Atropine** is a common muscarinic antagonist that finds many uses—eye drops of atropine analogs cause mydriasis (because it blocks the iris constrictor muscle, blocking constriction). In addition, it is used in the treatment of symptomatic bradycardia because the M_2 receptor inhibits the sinus node, which is the pacemaker of the heart; inhibiting the inhibitory receptor causes an increase in heart rate.
- **Oxybutynin** is used to inhibit urination in individuals with urinary incontinence, allowing the patient to feel less urinary urgency and be more comfortable. This works because the parasympathetic nervous system promotes urination; oxybutynin blocks this response.
- **Ipratropium** is an inhaled muscarinic antagonist often used in the treatment of asthma and COPD. It decreases bronchial secretions and also opens the bronchi by blocking muscarinic-mediated bronchoconstriction.

TOXICOLOGY

When people think of **toxicology,** they think of **poisons.** However, the drugs that we use can be poisonous too, usually at higher doses than intended. Toxins can also be environmental exposures such as pesticides or lead. Many of these have antidotes, and an understanding of why each antidote works the way it does is important in treating these patients.

Acetaminophen: hepatotoxic; use *N*-acetylcysteine to help conjugate the toxic NAPQI metabolite and prevent liver damage in overdose

Common Drugs and Toxicology

Acetaminophen (Tylenol) is a common analgesic. Recent guidelines recommend no more than 3 g of acetaminophen daily, for fear of liver damage. The reason that acetaminophen hurts the liver is that during its metabolism, a fraction of the drug is turned into a compound that can cross-link and damage proteins called *N*-acetyl-*p*-benzoquinone imine (NAPQI) through a phase I biotransformation. NAPQI is normally immediately made harmless by conjugation with glutathione. In individuals who either consume a lot of acetaminophen or are alcoholic and have poor nutritional status, this pathway can be overwhelmed and cause liver failure. The treatment is ***N*-acetylcysteine.** This regenerates glutathione stores and allows detoxification of the NAPQI.

Aspirin (acetylsalicylic acid) and other salicylates in overdose can cause tinnitus (ringing in the ears), an anion gap metabolic acidosis (because it is an acid), and a respiratory alkalosis (because aspirin directly stimulates central chemoreceptors and stimulates respiration). Because the drug is an acid, alkalinization of the urine with sodium bicarbonate ($NaHCO_3$) will cause ion trapping in the kidney and increase excretion. In children, any administration of aspirin is considered unsafe because it can cause **Reye syndrome** (liver failure and encephalopathy), which potentially can be fatal. (An exception to the "never give kids aspirin" rule is in patients with **Kawasaki disease,** for which the treatment includes aspirin and intravenous immunoglobulin.)

Beta-blocker overdose is characterized by hypotension, bradycardia, and first-degree atrioventricular block as well as possible altered mental status. Treatment is with **glucagon,** which is not intuitive—glucagon activates myocardial adenylyl cyclase independently of the β receptor and therefore provides an alternative pathway to stimulate the G_s pathway in the face of complete beta blockade.

Digoxin is used as a positive inotrope, improving symptoms in congestive heart failure (although it unfortunately does not improve mortality rates). Digoxin works by blocking the Na^+/K^+-ATPase pump, leading to increased myocardial intracellular sodium concentration and therefore preventing use of a sodium–calcium exchanger that normally pumps calcium out of the cell; this inhibition of calcium efflux causes increased calcium concentration in the cell (Fig. 7.11). This increased calcium is now available to aid in contraction, increasing inotropy. Digoxin has a specific antidote: fragmented antibodies that bind to digoxin, called digoxin-specific Fab antibody fragments. Because digoxin competes for potassium at the Na^+/K^+-ATPase site, hypokalemia causes more digoxin to bind (less K^+ competing for binding site) and can promote toxicity.

Opioid pain medications and heroin are commonly abused and can lead to overdose. Clinical clues are history, presence of track marks on the arms at prior injection sites, miosis ("pinpoint pupils"), and respiratory depression because the μ-opioid receptor that most opioids use for analgesic effects also can cause significant respiratory depression. Treatment is straightforward: Use an opioid antagonist such as **naloxone.**

Benzodiazepines (alprazolam, lorazepam) are used in the treatment of anxiety, insomnia, seizures, and alcohol withdrawal. They are γ-aminobutyric acid (GABA) agonists; the GABA receptor is found in the central nervous system and when activated causes chloride influx into the cell, which hyperpolarizes it and therefore decreases neuronal excitability and causes sedation and anxiolysis. The treatment is also intuitive: **flumazenil,** a GABA antagonist. Caution in treatment of benzodiazepine overdose is warranted because blocking the inhibitory GABA receptors can lead to overexcitation and seizures in some patients.

Tricyclic antidepressants (TCAs) (amitriptyline, nortriptyline) are now rarely used as antidepressants; they have been supplanted by selective serotonin reuptake inhibitors (SSRIs) but now find use in treating chronic pain as well as other diseases. Toxicity is characterized by the **three Cs: cardiotoxicity, convulsions, and coma.** TCAs have actions on many receptors, including antihistamine (causing sedation), α_1 antagonism (hypotension), inhibition of catecholamine reuptake (accounting for its antidepressant efficacy), and sodium channel blockade (important in cardiotoxicity). The treatment is **sodium bicarbonate ($NaHCO_3$)** for two reasons: (1) It allows for ion trapping of the medication and increased renal excretion, and (2) it helps correct the sodium channel blockade of the TCA, preventing cardiac arrhythmias.

Heparin is an anticoagulant that is commonly used for patients with deep venous thrombosis (a clot in the deep veins of the leg) or pulmonary embolism (clot in the pulmonary arterial tree) because it prevents new blood clots from forming. It can also be used to prevent clot formation in patients who

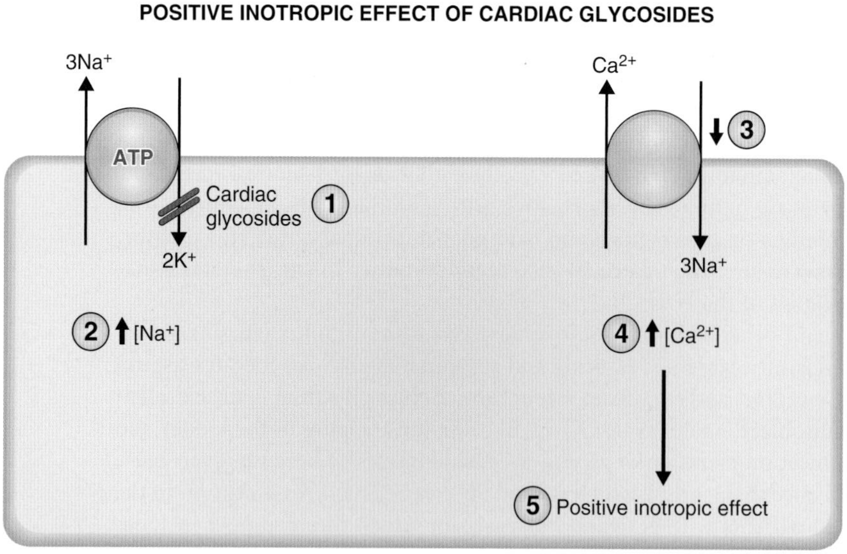

FIG. 7.11 A cardiac myocyte showing digoxin blocking the potassium site of the Na^+/K^+-ATPase pump, with subsequent decreased function of the Na^+/Ca^+ exchanger and increased cytosolic calcium. (*From Costanzo L. Physiology. 4th ed. New York: Elsevier; 2009.*)

are at risk. Heparin activates **antithrombin,** which, in turn, inactivates thrombin (factor IIa) and factor Xa. Supratherapeutic doses of heparin can lead to uncontrolled bleeding; **protamine sulfate** binds to heparin and is the antidote.

Warfarin is an oral anticoagulant that blocks vitamin K epoxide reductase to prevent the liver's synthesis of the vitamin K–dependent clotting factors II, VII, IX, X, C, and S. Because warfarin prevents synthesis of clotting factors, rather than blocking existing ones, the onset of action is delayed, and this is one reason that patients started on warfarin need to be "bridged" by being started on heparin first to give immediate anticoagulation (there is also a transient phase of warfarin that makes patients hypercoagulable, which is discussed in Chapter 11). Although giving **vitamin K** would treat an overdose, it would take hours to days to replenish all of the clotting factors by synthesizing new ones, so **fresh frozen plasma (FFP)** or prothrombin complex concentrate which has donor clotting factors is given for immediate reversal.

Warfarin: blocks synthesis of vitamin K–dependent clotting factors (II, VII, IX, X, C, and S). Give fresh-frozen plasma (or prothrombin complex concentrates) for immediate factor replacement. Give vitamin K to outcompete the blockade of vitamin K epoxide reductase enzyme to resume endogenous factor synthesis, which takes longer to take effect.

Tissue plasminogen activator (tPA), a thrombolytic, is used for **active** breakdown of blood clots (unlike warfarin and heparin, which prevent formation of new clot). It does this by turning the body's inactive plasminogen into active plasmin, which is the body's own natural pathway for breaking down clots. This is used acutely in ischemic stroke, myocardial infarction, and massive pulmonary embolism. In contrast, **aminocaproic acid** binds competitively to plasminogen, preventing transformation into active plasmin, and is therefore the antidote.

Heavy Metal Toxicity

- **Iron** is widely available as a supplement for individuals with iron deficiency anemia; most of the overdoses occur in children accidentally taking someone else's iron because the pills are often colorful and sugar coated. Iron, although important in the synthesis of hemoglobin and other enzymes, also is a **potent catalyst for free radical formation.** Overdose can cause high amounts of free radical formation in the intestines where the iron is passing through and cause **damage to the intestines,** leading to mucosal ulceration, GI bleeding, diarrhea, and vomiting. Normally, when the body has surplus iron, intestinal absorption of iron is inhibited—when the intestines become damaged, iron can enter in the bloodstream unimpeded and can cause **mitochondrial damage and subsequent lactic acidosis,** as well as liver damage from the high amounts of iron entering the liver through the portal vein. The treatment of iron overdose is **deferoxamine,** an iron-chelating agent. Mnemonic: Treat **Fe** (iron) overdose with de**FE**roxamine.
- **Lead** is a heavy metal that used to cause numerous cases of lead poisoning because of **lead-based paint** (patient history will usually describe an "old" house, built before 1974 when lead paint use was stopped). The mechanism of lead toxicity is complex, but in general it interferes with a multitude of

enzymes, especially δ-aminolevulinic acid dehydratase (leading to a buildup of aminolevulinic acid) and ferrochelatase, which both are important in heme synthesis, leading to a microcytic anemia. The buildup of aminolevulinic acid leads to increased vessel permeability, cerebral edema, and encephalopathy. Interference with **ribonuclease** leads to persistent ribosomes in the red blood cells that are made, leading to **basophilic stippling** (Fig. 7.12) on a peripheral blood smear. There are many treatments for lead poisoning, including **dimercaprol** (previously known as British anti-Lewisite, or BAL), CaEDTA, succimer, and penicillamine. A common mnemonic: When kids **succ** on lead paint chips, they need **succimer.** Dimercaprol and succimer are also effective in treating mercury, arsenic, and gold toxicity; a way to remember this is a **British** (BAL, dimercaprol) reading a **MAG**azine (**M**ercury, **A**rsenic, **G**old) that **succs (succimer).**

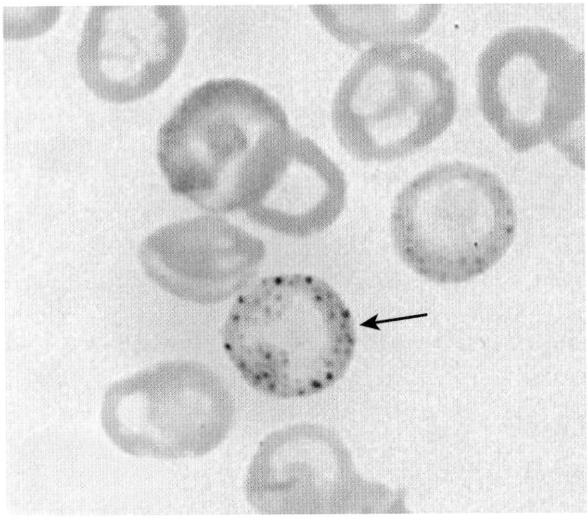

FIG. 7.12 Basophilic stippling, seen in lead poisoning as a result of denaturing of ribonuclease. Without ribonuclease, the ribosomes in the red blood cell are not degraded and cause the basophilic inclusion. (*From Naeim F. Atlas of Bone Marrow and Blood Pathology. Philadelphia: Saunders; 2001:27.*)

- **Copper** is only rarely ingested as an overdose, but those with **Wilson disease** (also known as hepatolenticular degeneration, for the damage it does to the **liver** and the **lenticular** nucleus of the brain) have an inability to excrete copper. The treatment is **penicillamine,** which chelates copper.

Environmental Exposures

- **Carbon monoxide** (CO) is a colorless and odorless gas, a byproduct of combustion; and toxicity is either intentional (e.g., a suicide attempt by leaving a running car in a closed garage) or unintentional (e.g., using combustion as a means of heating a cold house in winter, thinking it's a good idea to barbeque indoors). CO has an **affinity for hemoglobin more than 200 times greater than that of oxygen,** causing CO to take up spots on hemoglobin that should be taken up by oxygen, leading in turn to hypoxia and relative anemia (not that there is too little hemoglobin, it's just occupied by CO). History is usually suggestive, and symptoms include headache, vomiting, and confusion. **Treatment is to outcompete the CO with as much oxygen as possible**, either 100% oxygen or hyperbaric oxygen.
- **Cyanide** (CN^-), in addition to being a means of murder in movies, is also released when synthetic materials are burned, and therefore a house fire could cause not only CO poisoning but also cyanide poisoning. The antihypertensive medication **nitroprusside** has cyanide as part of its molecular structure and can cause cyanide poisoning as well. Cyanide binds highly to cytochrome oxidase in the mitochondria, halting the electron transport chain and stopping adenosine triphosphate (ATP) production. Anxiety, palpitations, dyspnea, and headache are common symptoms. Treatment is two step: (1) Administer **nitrites** (such as amyl nitrite inhaled or sodium nitrite IV) to oxidize the hemoglobin (Fe^{2+}) to methemoglobin (Fe^{3+}), which avidly binds cyanide, helping steer it away from the mitochondria, where it is poisonous. (2) Administer **sodium thiosulfate,** which changes cyanide to thiocyanate, a less toxic substance that is excreted by the kidneys. An alternative therapy is giving a form of vitamin B_{12}, **hydroxycobalamin,** because the cobalt can bind cyanide.

- **Methemoglobinemia** occurs when the Fe^{2+} in hemoglobin is oxidized to Fe^{3+} by oxidizing agents; this form cannot carry and deliver oxygen to the peripheral tissues. Common precipitating agents include sulfa drugs, local anesthetics such as benzocaine, and of course nitrates, as described earlier for the treatment of cyanide poisoning. **METH**emoglobinemia can be treated with **METH**ylene blue. Methylene blue is a potent reducing agent that changes the Fe^{3+} back into Fe^{2+}.
- **Organophosphate poisoning** is common in farm areas; the pesticide can be an acetylcholinesterase inhibitor and with exposure can cause symptoms of excessive cholinergic activation called **SLUDGE syndrome,** a mnemonic toxidrome characterized by **S**alivation, **L**acrimation, **U**rination, **D**efecation, **G**astrointestinal upset, and **E**mesis. The organophosphates **phosphorylate** acetylcholinesterase, leading to irreversible inhibition of the enzyme. However, there is a window period during which a medication called **pralidoxime** can be given, which can detach the organophosphate from the receptor—however, this is time dependent, and after hours have passed, the pralidoxime will no longer be able to unbind the organophosphate because a process called "aging" has occurred and the bond is unbreakable. Because the problem is overactive cholinergic signaling, the supportive treatment is an antagonist—**atropine** is a muscarinic antagonist that reverses the symptoms of overactive cholinergic drive. It does not, however, do anything to prevent the overactive acetylcholine at nicotinic receptors of the somatic nervous system, so it cannot treat the muscle weakness.
- **Atropine**, described earlier, is a muscarinic antagonist; too much atropine (or other anticholinergics) will cause symptoms consistent with shutting down the effects of acetylcholine at muscarinic receptors. The common way to remember these is **hot as a hare** (no sweating), **dry as a bone** (no sweating, no salivation, no urination), **red as a beet** (cutaneous vasodilation), **blind as a bat** (mydriasis), and **mad as a hatter** (disorientation). Treatment is the opposite of that described for organophosphate poisoning: Administer an **acetylcholinesterase inhibitor** that is **reversible,** such as **physostigmine.**

Ethanol, Methanol, and Ethylene Glycol

Ethanol, methanol, and ethylene glycol are all metabolized by the same enzymatic pathway but with different substrates at each step, causing different clinical symptoms (Fig. 7.13).

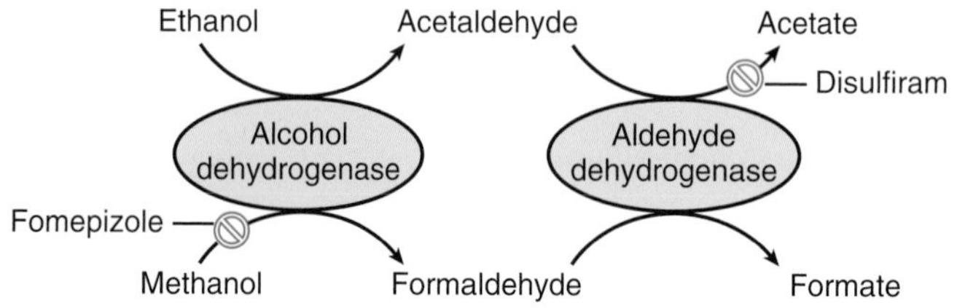

FIG. 7.13 Metabolic pathway for ethanol **(top)** and methanol **(bottom)**. Note that aldehyde dehydrogenase is commonly referred to as acetaldehyde dehydrogenase (because it dehydrogenates acetaldehyde), but it can also dehydrogenate other aldehydes (such as formaldehyde). (*From Brenner GM, Stevens CW. Pharmacology. 3rd ed. Philadelphia: Elsevier; 2009.*)

- **Ethanol** is the most common ingestion of the three; it is metabolized by alcohol dehydrogenase into acetaldehyde and then by acetaldehyde dehydrogenase to acetate. **Disulfiram,** a medication created to prevent alcohol abuse, blocks acetaldehyde dehydrogenase to cause a buildup of acetaldehyde when drinking; this leads to unpleasant side effects such as flushed skin, tachycardia, and nausea and vomiting. Some antibiotics such as metronidazole are said to have a "disulfiram-like" reaction because drinking alcohol while taking these antibiotics leads to similar symptoms as taking disulfiram. Also, the red flushing that some individuals (especially of Asian descent) experience while drinking alcohol is due to decreased acetaldehyde dehydrogenase activity.
- **Methanol,** found in windshield washer fluid and photocopying fluid, is highly toxic when ingested because of **formaldehyde generation** (the same stuff used to embalm your cadavers in anatomy laboratory) by alcohol dehydrogenase enzyme activity and **formic acid generation** from aldehyde dehydrogenase activity. Formic acid binds to cytochrome oxidase and blocks the electron transport chain, leading to lactic acidosis; formic acid also causes optic nerve damage and retinal damage, leading to permanent blindness. Because disulfiram only inhibits acetaldehyde dehydrogenase, it would be ineffective in treatment—an antagonist such as **fomepizole** at the **alcohol dehydrogenase**

enzyme must be used. Before fomepizole, physicians administered ethanol to compete for the alcohol dehydrogenase enzyme.

- **Ethylene glycol** is found in antifreeze and tastes sweet, making it appealing to children to drink. Again, like with methanol, the metabolism of the substance results in damaging byproducts. **Oxalic acid** is produced by alcohol dehydrogenase. Oxalic acid avidly binds calcium, leading to hypocalcemia and precipitation of calcium oxalate crystals in the urine and kidneys, leading to stone formation and renal damage, respectively. The classic findings are metabolic acidosis (as with methanol poisoning), altered mental status, and renal failure from calcium precipitation. Treatment is similar to methanol poisoning in that **fomepizole** is used because toxic products are formed by alcohol dehydrogenase, which fomepizole inhibits.

REVIEW QUESTIONS

(1) Why is the bioavailability of oral drugs not always 100%?

(2) If a drug were very fat soluble, would it be likely to have a very low or very high volume of distribution?

(3) A depressed woman who has been taking St. John's wort comes to your office with nausea and a missed period. She has a positive pregnancy test. When you tell her, she says in disbelief, "But I always take my birth control pills at the same exact time every day—I've never even missed one!" What is the most likely explanation for her pregnancy?

(4) A patient comes in to the emergency department with nausea, vomiting, and tinnitus (high-pitched ringing in the ears) and admits to having taken a bottle of aspirin in a suicide attempt (aspirin is a weak acid). Would making the urine more alkaline or more acidic cause the patient to excrete the aspirin more quickly?

(5) Name the three drugs that are metabolized through zero-order kinetics. Do these drugs get metabolized by having a constant amount removed per unit time or a constant fraction removed per unit time?

(6) How many half-lives before a drug reaches steady state?

(7) How can you reach steady state quickly without waiting for the number of half-lives in question 7?

(8) Describe what happens with regard to efficacy and potency to an agonist drug when (a) a competitive antagonist is added, and (b) a noncompetitive antagonist is added.

(9) Aspirin (acetylsalicylic acid) attaches an acetyl group to the cyclooxygenase enzyme of platelets, preventing expression of thromboxane and preventing platelet aggregation; this effect lasts the lifetime of the platelet even when the aspirin is metabolized away. What is the explanation for this?

(10) Which receptor would you want to activate if you wanted to constrict smooth muscle? What is the cell signal cascade that is activated, and how does it work?

(11) How does the G_s pathway generally work? What receptors in the sympathetic nervous system use this pathway?

(12) In anaphylactic shock, an immunoglobulin E–mediated reaction in which histamine release causes the patient to have hypotension as a result of vasodilation, also causing bronchospasm, which sympathetic receptor needs to be activated to reverse (a) the hypotension and (b) the bronchospasm? Why use epinephrine instead of norepinephrine? Bonus: What cell signaling pathway does each receptor in (a) and (b) use?

(13) Would the pupils of a patient who used cocaine be expected to be dilated or constricted? What receptor activation would cause this? What is the medical term for this change in pupil diameter?

(14) Why is too much acetaminophen toxic? What is the treatment?

(15) Why is iron overdose potentially lethal? What is the treatment?

(16) What are the effects of (a) methanol and (b) ethylene glycol intoxication? What is the treatment and how does it work?

8 CARDIOLOGY

Ryan A. Pedigo

HEART AND BLOOD VESSELS

Overview

The **heart** is responsible for pumping oxygen- and nutrient-rich blood to all the organs. If at any point in a person's life the heart stops doing this for more than a few minutes, irreversible organ damage can result. The heart, blood, and blood vessels make up the **cardiovascular** system.

The heart has **four chambers** that blood flows through: **right atrium, right ventricle, left atrium, and left ventricle.** It is important to understand the path that the blood takes through these chambers of the heart to understand how problems with each of these chambers will lead to symptoms. Each time blood leaves a ventricle, blood is leaving the heart through an artery. Therefore **arteries,** such as the aorta and pulmonary artery, take blood **away** from the heart **(A-A). Veins,** such as the superior and inferior vena cava, return blood back **to** the heart **(T-V).** Each time blood flows from an atrium to a ventricle or from a ventricle to an artery, blood passes through a valve, which if working correctly, ensures that blood flows only in the correct direction. Study the following steps of blood flow with the image of the circulatory system provided in Fig. 8.1.

Blood flow through heart: vena cava, right atrium, right ventricle, pulmonary arteries, pulmonary veins, left atrium, left ventricle, aorta

1. After the body's tissues and organs have taken up the oxygen from the blood and delivered their metabolic waste to the bloodstream, **deoxygenated** blood returns to the heart through the **superior and inferior vena cava** to the **right atrium.**
2. From the **right atrium,** the blood travels through the **tricuspid valve** into the **right ventricle.**
3. From the **right ventricle,** the blood travels through the **pulmonic valve** to the **pulmonary arteries,** which travels away from the heart to the **lungs** to drop off all of the CO_2 (a product of aerobic metabolism in tissues) and replenish the oxygen supply in the blood.
4. After gas exchange in the lung occurs, the **oxygenated** blood returns to the **left atrium** through the **pulmonary veins.**
5. From the **left atrium,** the blood travels to the **left ventricle** through the **mitral valve (also known as the bicuspid valve). Always "tri" something before you "bi" it; the tricuspid valve is before the mitral (bicuspid) valve!**
6. From the **left ventricle,** the blood travels to the **aorta** through the **aortic valve** to be distributed to the tissues, and the cycle repeats.

Anatomy of the Heart

The heart has three layers, from inside to out: the **endocardium, myocardium, and epicardium.**

- The **endocardium** is a single layer of endothelial cells that envelops the inside of the heart, including the valves, similar to the endothelial cells that line blood vessels. This is important in terms of talking about ischemia of the heart, which can be either transmural (across all layers of the heart including the endocardium) or subendocardial (just affecting the endocardium), as well as in **infective endocarditis,** which is an infection that takes hold at the endothelium covering the heart valves.
- The **myocardium** (myo = muscle) is the thick, striated muscular layer of the heart that is responsible for the pumping activity of the heart. These muscles are perfused by **coronary arteries,** and in a **myocardial infarction** (heart attack) the death of parts of cardiac muscle can cause the heart to fail.
- The **epicardium** is actually the **visceral pericardium,** which will be discussed next.

Pericardial effusion: If effusion occurs quickly or is large, it can cause cardiac tamponade, during which the pressure from the effusion prevents filling of the heart.

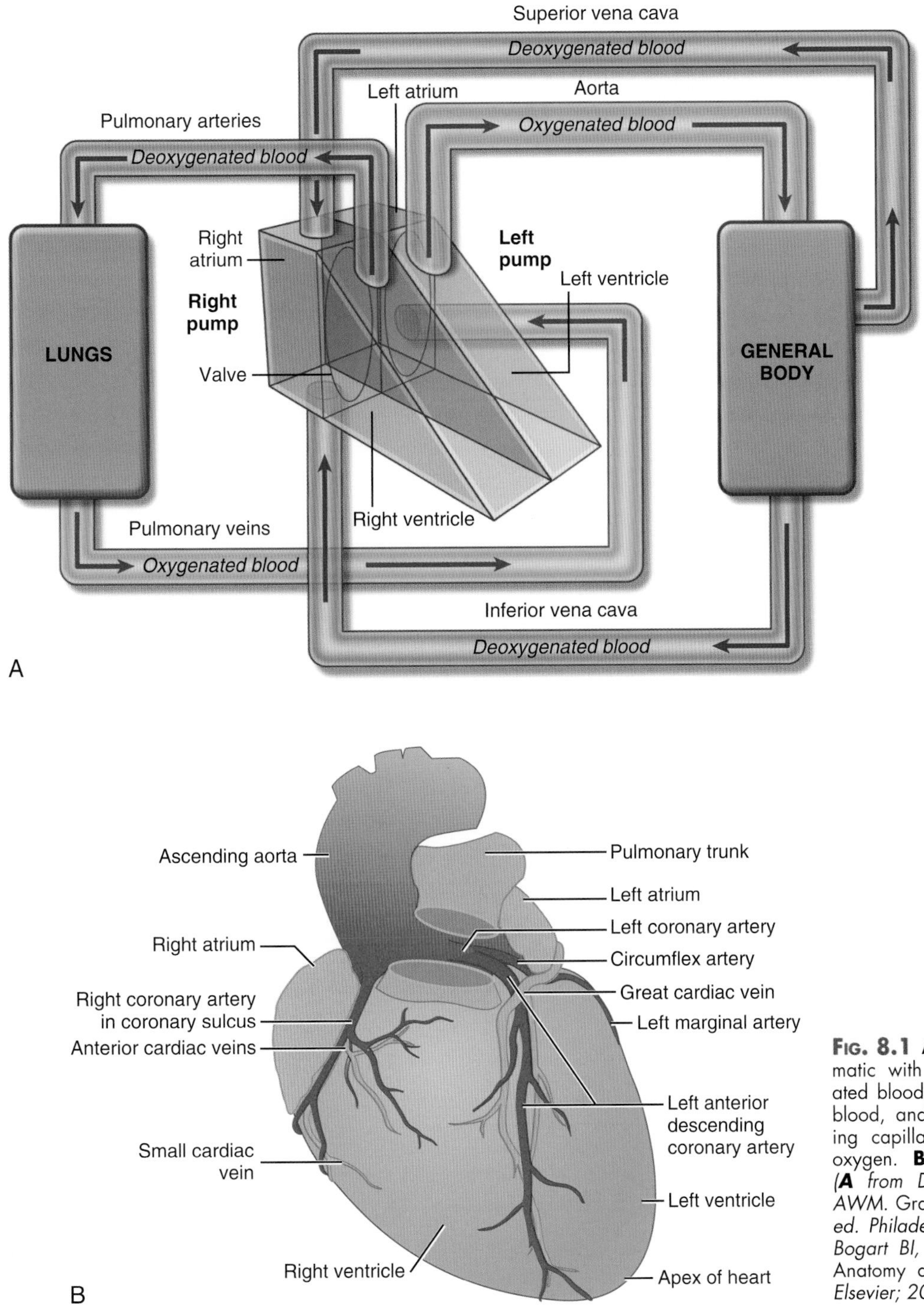

Fig. 8.1 A, Cardiovascular system schematic with *blue* representing deoxygenated blood, *red* representing oxygenated blood, and *red-blue* gradients representing capillary beds, which take up the oxygen. **B,** General cardiac anatomy. (***A*** *from Drake RL, Vogl AW, Mitchell AWM.* Gray's Anatomy for Students. *2nd ed. Philadelphia: Elsevier; 2009.* ***B*** *from Bogart BI, Ort VH.* Elsevier's Integrated Anatomy and Embryology. *Philadelphia: Elsevier; 2007.)*

The heart is surrounded by a **pericardium,** a double-walled sac that has a serosal **visceral** (inner) layer and a fibrous **parietal** (outer) layer; between the visceral and parietal pericardium there exists a minute amount of pericardial fluid, which allows the heart to beat with minimal friction, similar to how a car uses oil to decrease friction between moving parts. This becomes important clinically with **pericarditis,** which is inflammation of the pericardium, usually as a result of infection, uremia, or autoimmune disease. It is also important in **pericardial effusion** and **tamponade,** when too much fluid builds up between the two layers **(effusion)** and can even act to "strangle" the heart if enough fluid and pressure builds up such that the heart's ability to fill with blood is impeded **(tamponade).**

The heart relies on an **electrical conduction system** to ensure rapid, coordinated contraction of the heart (Fig. 8.2).

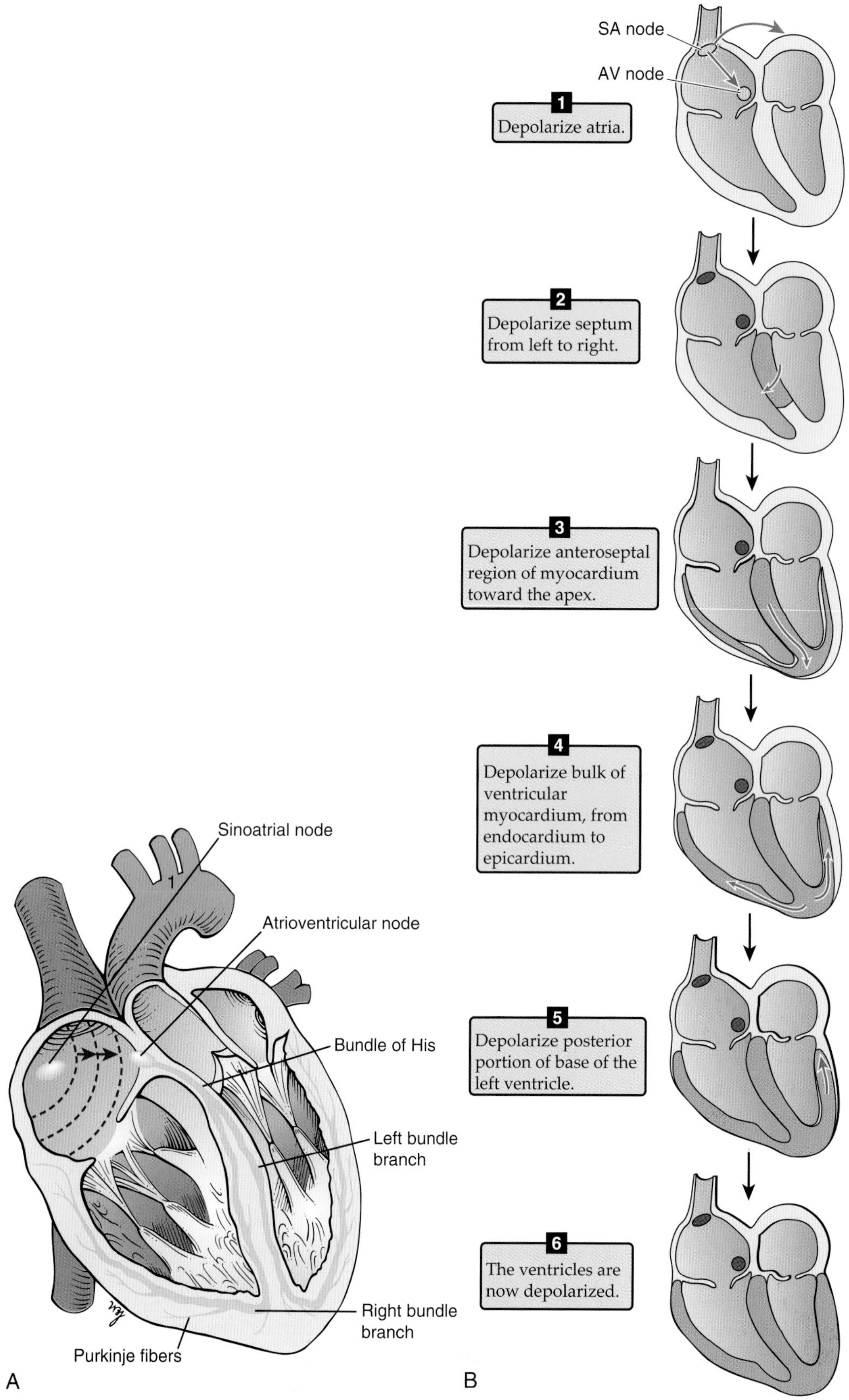

Fig. 8.2 **A,** The cardiac conducting system, in which the signal is normally generated in the sinoatrial (SA) node and travels through the atria to the atrioventricular (AV) node; it then transmits to the bundle of His and subsequently to the left and right bundle branches. **B,** Image depicting the normal sequence of depolarization of the heart: from the SA node to the AV node, to the bundle of His, with initial septal depolarization, and then moving through the right ventricle via the right bundle branch and left ventricle via the left bundle branch. (***A*** *from Moore NA, Roy WA.* Rapid Review Gross and Developmental Anatomy. *3rd ed. Philadelphia: Elsevier; 2010.* ***B*** *from Boron WF, Boulpaep EL.* Medical Physiology. *2nd ed. Philadelphia: Elsevier; 2008.)*

- **Sinoatrial (SA) node:** The "pacemaker" of the heart, which sets the normal heart rate by generating electrical signals. These electrical signals depolarize the atria and are conducted to the AV node.
- **Atrioventricular (AV) node:** Named because it lies between the atria and ventricles; in the normal heart this area is the **only** place where the electrical signal can be transmitted to the ventricles, through the **bundle of His,** which further branches into the **left and right bundle branches.** Malfunction of the AV node and bundle of His leads to various types of **AV block (heart block),** which are described later.
- **Left bundle branch:** Responsible for coordinated contraction of the **left ventricle.** If these fibers are damaged and lose conducting ability, a left bundle branch block results. (Although too detailed for the purposes of Step 1, the left bundle further separates into the **anterior, posterior,** and **septal** branches, and blockage of these can lead to anterior fascicular block [anterior branch] or posterior fascicular block [posterior branch].)
- **Right bundle branch:** Responsible for coordinated contraction of the **right ventricle.** Can be damaged and lead to a right bundle branch block, although a right bundle branch block can be normal in some individuals.

SA node: pacemaker of heart

AV node: normally the only conduit for action potentials from the atria to be transmitted to the ventricles

The **coronary arteries** are responsible for perfusion of the heart; narrowing (such as caused by atherosclerosis) and blockage of these vessels can lead to angina (chest pain) or myocardial infarction, respectively. The **left** and **right** coronary arteries come off the **aorta** at the aortic valve cusps (Fig. 8.3).

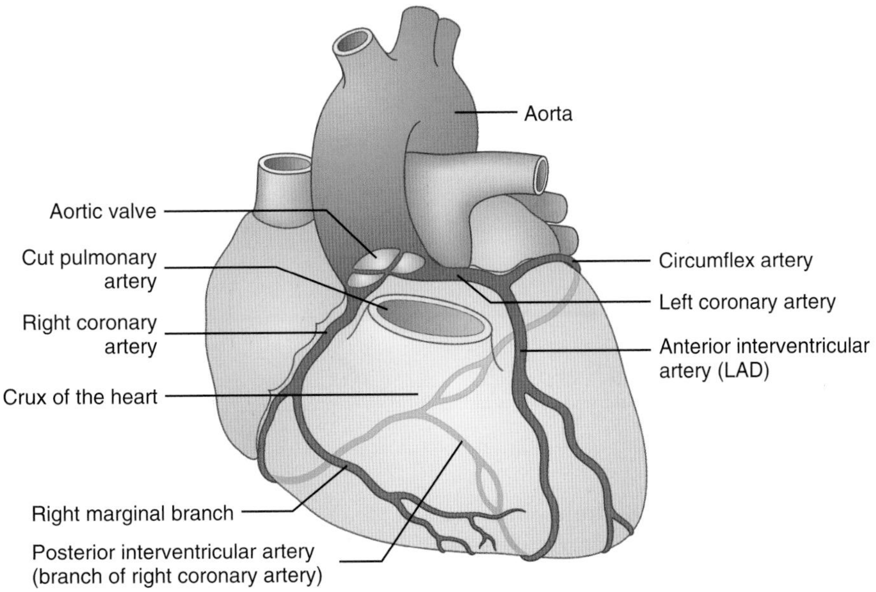

Fig. 8.3 Coronary arterial vasculature, anterior view. The right and left coronary arteries can be seen coming off of the aortic valve cusps. The right coronary artery supplies the sinoatrial node and most often the posterior aspect of the heart; the left coronary artery divides into the left anterior descending (LAD) and the circumflex arteries. *(From Bogart BI, Ort VH.* Elsevier's Integrated Anatomy and Embryology. *Philadelphia: Elsevier; 2007.)*

- **Left coronary artery (LCA):** Divides into the **left anterior descending (LAD) artery,** which supplies the anterior left ventricle, and the **circumflex** artery, which supplies the lateral and posterior left ventricle. The LAD is the most commonly occluded vessel in patients with myocardial infarction.
- **Right coronary artery (RCA):** Supplies the right ventricle. In most people (85%), the **posterior descending artery (PDA)** comes off of the right coronary artery, which perfuses the inferior and posterior ventricles; this is called right-dominant circulation. In the remainder of individuals the PDA comes off the circumflex (left-dominant) or both the circumflex and right coronary artery (codominant). The right coronary artery also supplies the SA node and AV node, which can lead to arrhythmias and heart block if damaged.

Anatomy of the Circulatory System

The circulatory system can be divided into two components: the **pulmonary circulation** and the **systemic circulation.**

- **Pulmonary circulation:** Made up of the right side of the heart, pulmonary arteries, capillaries feeding the lungs, and pulmonary veins. Responsible for taking deoxygenated blood from the right side of the heart to the lungs for oxygenation and then moving the newly oxygenated blood to the left side of the heart so that it may be pumped into the systemic circulation.
- **Systemic circulation:** Made up of the left side of the heart, systemic arteries, capillaries, and veins. The systemic circulation is everything outside of the pulmonary circulation; the goal of this circulation is to take oxygenated blood to the body to deliver oxygen and nutrients and return that newly deoxygenated blood to the right side of the heart.

The circulatory system uses **arteries, arterioles, capillaries, venules, and veins**—each serves a different purpose. Blood flows through these structures in the order written earlier (Fig. 8.4).

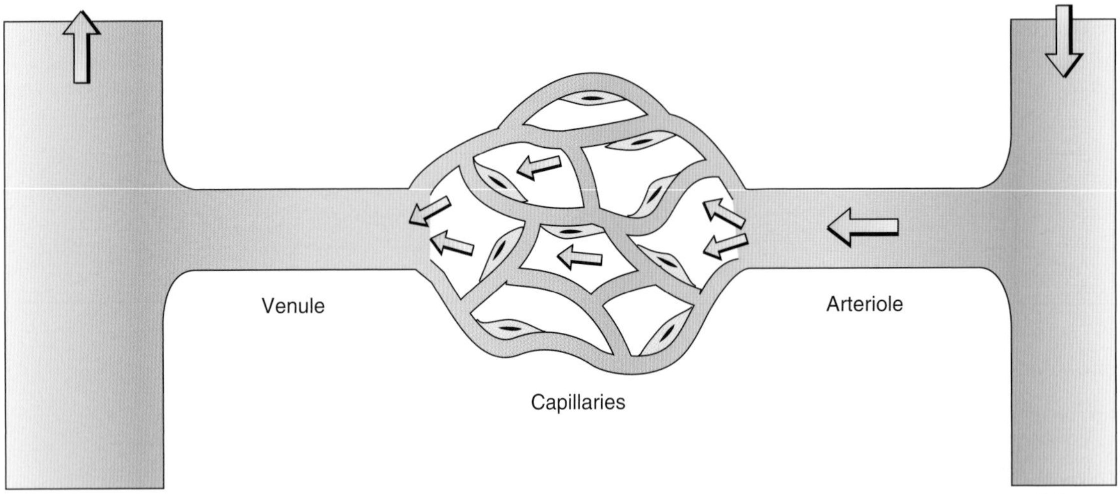

FIG. 8.4 In the systemic circulation, oxygenated blood from the arterial system enters a capillary bed, oxygen is extracted by the tissues, and deoxygenated blood enters the venous system and returns to the heart. *(From Costanzo LS.* Physiology. *4th ed. New York: Elsevier; 2009.)*

1. **Arteries** are thick walled because they **receive blood from ventricles** and therefore must withstand large changes in pressure. Examples include the pulmonary artery and aorta. The arteries have **three layers,** starting at the inside layer called the **intima** (intima—inside), which has a single layer of endothelial cells; the **media** (media—middle), a thick elastic and muscular layer; and the **adventitia,** the outer layer which houses the vasa vasorum ("vessel of vessels," blood vessels that nourish the artery itself), nerves, and lymphatics.
2. **Arterioles** are the site of **highest resistance** to blood flow and are regulated by **α_1 receptors** for constriction and **β_2 receptors** for dilation of their smooth muscle, helping the body regulate distribution of blood to various organs.
3. **Capillaries** have a **single layer** of endothelial cells, allowing for diffusion and exchange of gases, fluid, and nutrients between the blood and tissues. The amount of fluid exchange that occurs is dictated by **Starling forces,** which describe the net driving force for fluid to come into or out of capillaries. The Starling forces are determined by the hydrostatic pressure and the oncotic pressure of both the capillaries and the interstitium that surrounds them. The **oncotic** pressure is the osmotic pressure derived from proteins that cannot traverse the capillary–interstitium interface; the oncotic pressure of the capillaries (π_c) is mainly determined by **albumin,** the main plasma protein. Low albumin (hypoalbuminemia) therefore causes decreased capillary oncotic pressure and can promote fluid moving from capillary to interstitium as the osmotic drive keeping fluid in the capillary is lost.

Thus hypoalbuminemia can cause edema. Hydrostatic pressure is simply the pressure exerted by the fluid.

- **P_{net}** = (forces promoting fluid leaving capillary) – (forces promoting fluid returning to capillary)
- **P_{net}** = $[(P_c + \pi_i) - (P_i + \pi_c)]$
- P_c: hydrostatic pressure in capillaries—attempts to push fluid out of the capillary
- π_i: interstitial oncotic pressure—attempts to pull fluid out of the capillary
- P_i: hydrostatic pressure in interstitium—attempts to push fluid back into the capillary
- π_c: capillary oncotic pressure—attempts to pull fluid out of the interstitium
  - Positive P_{net}: fluids leave capillary
  - Negative P_{net}: fluids return to capillary

4. **Venules and veins** are also thin walled because they are meant to be **capacitance vessels,** meaning that they can hold a large amount of blood. The veins, like the arteries, have three layers (intima, media, adventitia) but have a thin, nonmuscular, media. Sympathetic tone can cause these veins to constrict, promoting venous return back to the heart to assist in increasing cardiac output. Veins have one-way valves that help ensure that blood can return to the heart even in the face of gravity.

PHYSIOLOGY

Cardiovascular Terminology and Formulas

- **Systole:** The phase during which the heart contracts, pumping the blood in the ventricles into the arteries through the pulmonic valve (right ventricle) and aortic valve (left ventricle).
- **Diastole:** The phase during which the heart relaxes and allows the ventricles to fill with blood from the atria through the tricuspid valve (right ventricle) or mitral valve (left ventricle). During exercise, the time spent in diastole is decreased to allow for a greater heart rate.
- **Mean arterial pressure (MAP):** $MAP = \frac{2}{3}$ (diastolic pressure) $+ \frac{1}{3}$ (systolic pressure). This is the average pressure in the artery. It is important to note that **because the heart spends more time in diastole (2⁄3) than systole (1⁄3), the mean arterial pressure is not a simple average of the two pressures.**
- **Stroke volume (SV):** SV = left ventricular end-diastolic volume - left ventricular end-systolic volume. The absolute amount of blood ejected from the heart; how much blood the heart started with after filling (left ventricular end-diastolic volume [LVEDV]) subtracted by how much it ended up with after contraction (left ventricular end-systolic volume [LVESV]).
- **Ejection fraction (EF):** $EF = \frac{SV}{LVEDV}$. This describes what percentage of blood was ejected from the heart. A normal EF is greater than or equal to 55%; in systolic heart failure, this number is significantly reduced.
- **Cardiac output (CO):** $CO = SV \times HR = \frac{\text{rate of } O_2 \text{ consumption}}{\text{arterial } O_2 \text{ content} - \text{venous } O_2 \text{ content}}$. The CO is the volume of blood being pumped per minute; this can increase considerably during exercise in the healthy heart and is decreased in heart failure. Initially in exercise, the stroke volume increases to augment cardiac output; as exercise continues, the heart rate increases to meet the increased demand. Increasing either the stroke volume or the heart rate can increase cardiac output. The second equation is more tricky. Imagine with a low cardiac output, the blood is moving more slowly through the tissues, giving them more time to extract oxygen, leading to a large arterial-venous oxygen content difference (large denominator). Conversely, with a high cardiac output, so much oxygenated blood is being circulated through the tissues that the tissues do not need to extract all the oxygen from the blood each time it passes through.
- **Total peripheral resistance (TPR):** $MAP = CO \times TPR$. The total peripheral resistance is the resistance in the entire systemic circulation (not the pulmonary circulation). This is largely determined by the **arterioles,** which constrict as a result of α_1-receptor activation to increase TPR and which dilate as a result of β_2-receptor activation to decrease TPR.

- **Poiseuille's equation:** Resistance $= \frac{8\eta L}{\pi r^4}$ where η is viscosity, L is length, and r is radius. This law describes how much resistance there is in a circuit; **radius is to the fourth power and is therefore the largest determinant of resistance.** Decreasing the radius of an arteriole by 2, for example, raises the resistance by 2^4, or 16 times. Increased viscosity can be seen if there are more red blood cells (polycythemia) or more protein (such as in multiple myeloma).
- **Preload:** Ventricular end-diastolic volume, based on how much blood has come back to the heart by venous return. Sympathetic tone increases venous return and preload; venodilators such as nitroglycerin decrease preload.
- **Afterload:** Mean arterial pressure—essentially how much pressure the heart has to work against to eject blood from the ventricles. Increased afterload, such as from hypertension, aortic stenosis, or vasoconstriction, causes the heart to work harder and consume more oxygen to eject blood.

Preload: how much blood is delivered to the ventricle (end-diastolic volume)

Afterload: how much resistance the ventricle has to pump against

ELECTROPHYSIOLOGY

The **electrical conducting system** described in the anatomy section is the basis for an organization of the electrical signal leading to a coordinated and effective contraction. The heart rate is set by the pacemaker that generates electrical signals, or **action potentials,** at the fastest rate. In a normally functioning heart this is the **SA node,** although the AV node and the bundle of His are the next quickest and will generate action potentials if the SA node is malfunctioning.

Pacemaker cells: Upstroke of depolarization (phase 0) occurs because of calcium.

Myocardium: Upstroke (phase 0) occurs because of sodium.

Pacemaker cells such as the **SA node** and AV node do not require outside stimuli to generate an action potential—they are self-depolarizing because of activity of the **funny sodium channels** ("funny" in that the channels are open **before** an action potential occurs, different from most sodium channels, which only open during an action potential). When the heart rate is slow, fewer of these channels will be open and the sodium current I_f will be lower, such as after parasympathetic stimulation by the vagus nerve (through inhibitory M_2 receptors); more channels will be open when the heart rate is fast (Fig. 8.5A).

- **Phase 0:** Once the funny sodium channels have leaked enough sodium to reach the **threshold potential,** voltage-gated calcium channels open to cause further depolarization. The upstroke of phase 0 in the AV node is slower than in myocytes, allowing the ventricles time to fill fully before the AV node transmits the signal to them.
- **Phase 3** (note that phases 1 and 2 are not present in pacemaker cells): The calcium channels close, and potassium channels open to repolarize the cell by causing potassium efflux.
- **Phase 4:** The funny sodium channels open, slowly depolarizing the cell until the threshold potential is reached, when the process will restart.

The **cardiac myocytes** are responsible for the contraction of the heart and normally depolarize when they have received the signal from the conducting system of the heart or nearby myocytes. The depolarization of myocytes is more complex, consisting of phases 0, 1, 2, 3, and 4 (Fig. 8.5B).

- **Phase 0:** Once the threshold potential has been reached, sodium channels open and cause a quick and transient influx of sodium, rapidly depolarizing the cell. Note that in cardiac myocytes, the ion causing the upstroke of depolarization is **sodium,** unlike in pacemaker cells, which use calcium.
- **Phase 1:** The sodium channels are now closed, and some potassium efflux occurs, leading to a small drop in voltage.
- **Phase 2: L-type calcium channels** (L for long-lasting) open, leading to a plateau where potassium efflux is balanced with calcium influx. This "trigger calcium" triggers release of stored calcium from within the sarcoplasmic reticulum in the cardiac myocyte and will lead to contraction.
- **Phase 3:** Calcium channels have inactivated and potassium efflux dominates, leading to repolarization of the cell.
- **Phase 4:** Resting state. Unlike the pacemaker cells such as the SA and AV node, these cells do not spontaneously depolarize under normal conditions and wait for another depolarizing signal before the process restarts.

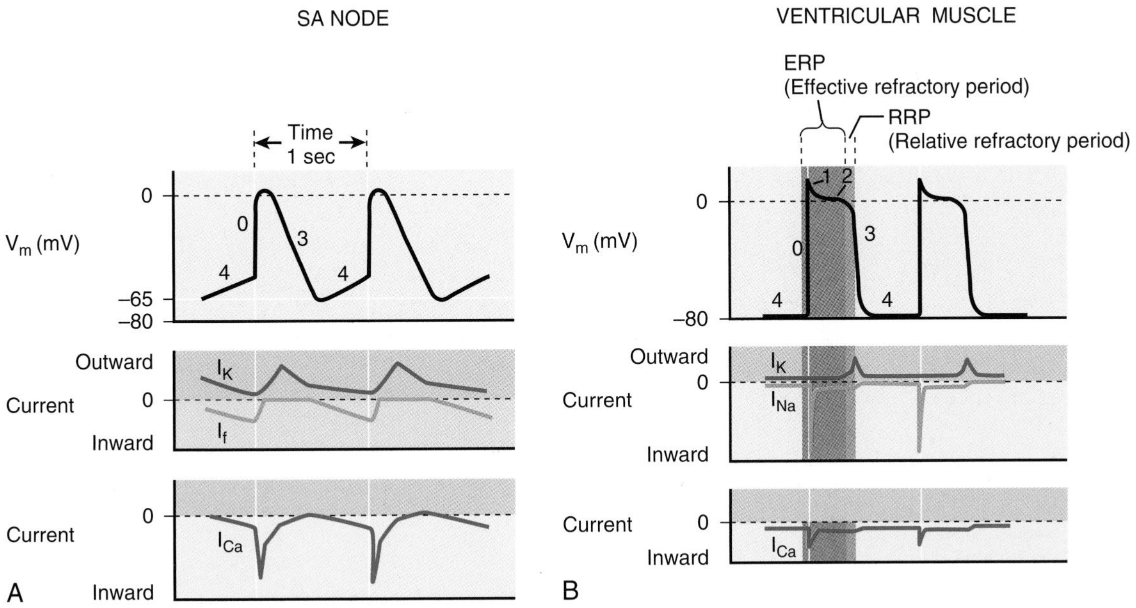

FIG. 8.5 A, Electrophysiology of the sinoatrial (SA) node, where "funny" sodium channels are open before an action potential occurs; the sodium leak causes an action potential when the threshold potential is reached. This then triggers calcium (not sodium) influx to depolarize the cell. **B,** Electrophysiology of ventricular myocytes; these are, in the normal state, not self-depolarizing and must have a depolarizing stimulus to cause an action potential. Like most cells (but unlike the pacemaker cells), the main cation entering to initially depolarize the cell is sodium via sodium channels. The depolarization is sustained by calcium from L-type calcium channels, and potassium efflux repolarizes the cell. I_K, I_{Ca}, I_{Na}, I_f, currents through potassium, calcium, sodium and "funny" sodium channels, respectively; Vm, membrane voltage. *(From Boron WF, Boulpaep EL.* Medical Physiology. *2nd ed. Philadelphia: Elsevier; 2008.)*

Cardiac Myocytes

The details of muscle contraction in general are covered in Chapter 12, but important points regarding cardiac myocyte contraction will be covered here.

> More calcium available to the myocytes during contraction = increased contractility.

- **Troponin** has three types: troponin T, troponin I, and troponin C. Troponin I **inhibits** contraction, and troponin C binds to **calcium** (I—inhibits, C—calcium). When calcium binds to troponin C, it stops troponin I's inhibition and allows for actin and myosin to interact and for contraction to occur. Therefore **more calcium** means **more actin and myosin interaction** and **increased strength of contraction (increased contractility, inotropy).**
- **Calcium** influx during phase 2 of myocyte depolarization causes stored calcium to be released from the **sarcoplasmic reticulum (SR),** in much greater amounts. This is referred to as **calcium-induced calcium release.** After this calcium release, myocytes pump calcium either (a) out of the cell or (b) back into the SR. Anything that increases calcium influx from the outside or increases calcium storage in the SR will increase contractility by providing more intracellular calcium to the myocytes. **Digitalis** prevents calcium efflux from the cell, causing increased retrieval into the SR and increased inotropy. **Sympathetic activation of β_1 receptors** causes increased **sarcoplasmic reticulum Ca^{2+} ATPase** activity (SERCA, the pump that pumps calcium back into the SR), leading to increased calcium stored in the sarcoplasmic reticulum and therefore increased contractility. Both of these will be covered in depth later, in the section "Pharmacology," but it is important to keep the concept in mind that **more calcium availability leads to increased contractility.**
- The actin (thin filaments) and myosin (thick filaments) overlap more favorably **when stretched;** therefore more blood returning to the heart (increased **preload**) will fill the heart more, causing the myocytes to stretch and in turn creating a stronger contraction. However, do not confuse this with **contractility,** which is ability to contract **at a given preload** and is dependent on intracellular calcium levels. More preload will lead to a stronger contraction but not increased contractility. This concept will be further explained in the next section.

Frank-Starling Curve

The Frank-Starling curve (Fig. 8.6) shows that the **force of contraction** of the myocytes is dependent on the **initial length of cardiac muscle fiber,** the degree of stretch, which is determined by the **preload.**

Contractility is defined as force of contraction **at a given preload.** Therefore although a contraction may be more forceful at a higher preload, there is not necessarily increased contractility.

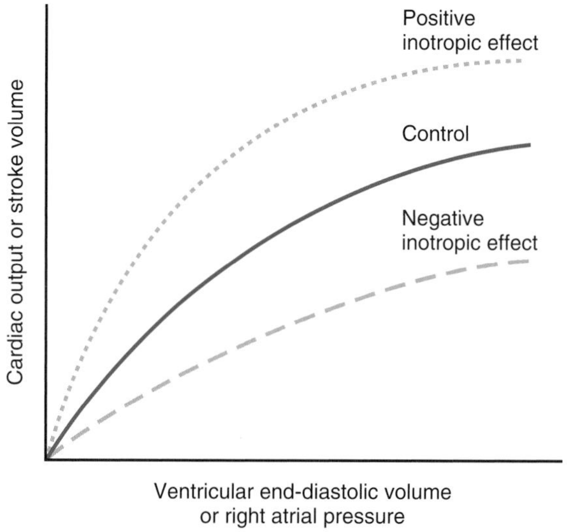

FIG. 8.6 Frank-Starling curve. The control curve shows the strength of contraction of the myocytes for a given preload (ventricular end-diastolic volume). When there is a change in contractility (inotropy), which is defined as strength of contraction for a given preload, a new curve occurs. *(From Costanzo LS.* Physiology. *4th ed. New York: Elsevier; 2009.)*

- More venous return = more preload → larger ventricular end-diastolic volume → more muscle fiber stretch → stronger contraction.
- Ensures that if more blood returns to the heart, the heart can pump that extra blood by increasing stroke volume.
- **Contractility** is the force of contraction at a given preload, and therefore increasing preload does **nothing** to contractility. Increased contractility would be a whole new curve (such as the positive inotropic effect curve shown in Fig. 8.6), **not** moving along the existing curve (with increased preload without change in contractility, it would move to the right on the same curve). Contractility, or the inotropic state, can increases with β_1 stimulation or positive inotropes (digitalis) and can decrease with negative inotropes (beta blockers), heart failure, or acid–base disturbances.

Cardiac Cycle

The **cardiac cycle** is described by one round of diastole and systole. During this time, the ventricle will fill (diastole) from the preload offered to it by the atrium by flowing through the respective AV valve (the **left atrial pressure** is shown by the **black** line at the bottom of Fig. 8.7A). The atrium will contract near the end of filling to help push more blood into the ventricle, called **atrial kick.** After filling, the AV valve will close and the ventricle will contract and eject the blood out of the pulmonic (right side of the heart) or aortic (left side of the heart) valve into the pulmonary artery or aorta, respectively. A closer look at the cardiac cycle and the heart sounds follows.

The **aortic pressure** is shown in the figure by the **light green** line on top of Fig. 8.7A. When the **left ventricular pressure** (shown by the **darker green** line in Fig. 8.7A) is higher than the aortic pressure, the aortic valve is pushed open by the pressure gradient; this valve remains open until the left ventricle has ejected the **stroke volume** for that beat. A similar waveform (but with lower pressures because the pulmonary circulation has lower pressure than the systemic circulation) would be present for the right side of the heart.

The **venous pressure** is depicted by the solid black line in Fig. 8.7B and will be described for the right side of the heart; this is usually shown as "jugular venous pressure," which is an estimation of right atrial pressure. A similar waveform occurs for the left side of the heart as well. The normal venous waveform has **a, c, and v waves** as well as **x and y descents.** The **a wave** represents the **atrial** kick (atrial contraction) for the right atrium, which helps fill the right ventricle, but also transmits some pressure back to the jugular veins. The **c wave** is the next upward deflection in pressure, corresponding to **contraction** of the right ventricle, causing the tricuspid to bow inward toward the right atrium, transiently

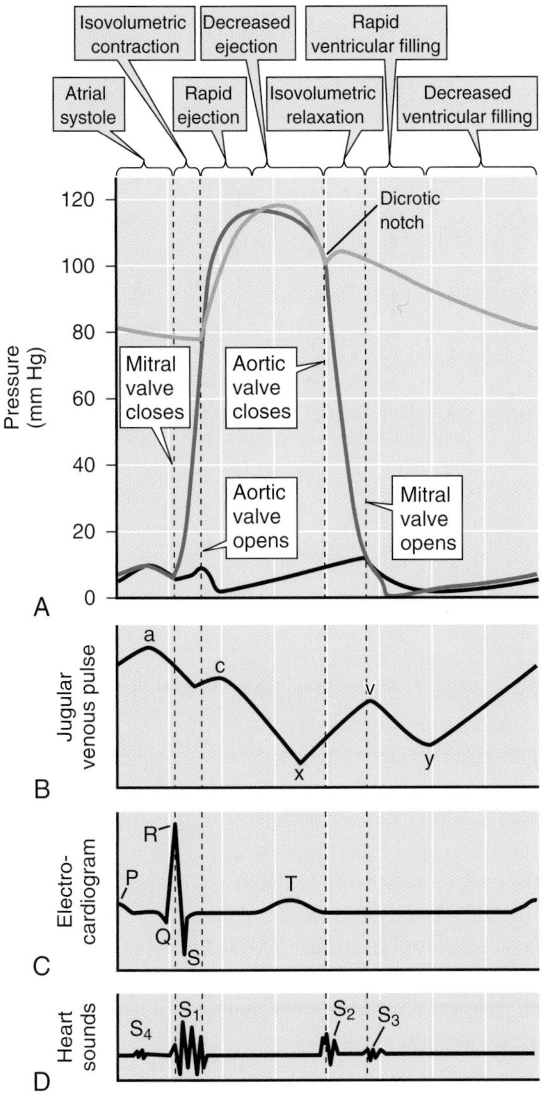

Fig. 8.7 Cardiac cycle. **A, Pressure:** showing left-heart tracing only, where the *dark blue* represents ventricular pressures, *light green* represents aortic pressure, and *black line* represents left atrial pressure (which is estimated by the pulmonary capillary wedge pressure). **B, Jugular venous pulse:** shows pressures in the jugular vein, which feeds into the superior vena cava and into the right atrium. The "a" wave rise in pressure is due to atrial kick; the "c" wave rise is due to the contraction of the ventricle; the following "x" descent represents blood refilling the relaxes and empty atria; the "v" wave represents venous filling (mnemonic: "villing" from the veins); the "y" descent represents ventricular filling once the tricuspid valve opens. **C, Electrocardiogram:** shows ECG findings of the cardiac cycle. "P" wave: atrial depolarization. "QRS" complex: ventricular depolarization. "T" wave: ventricular repolarization. **D, Heart sounds:** normal sounds include S_1, closure of tricuspid/mitral valves, and S_2, closure of aortic/pulmonic valves. *(From Boron WF, Boulpaep EL. Medical Physiology. 2nd ed. Philadelphia: Elsevier; 2008.)*

increasing pressure. The right atrium, having finished contracting, is now relaxing and filling, causing the **x descent** during relaxation (as blood moves from the venous system into the empty atrium). The **v wave** occurs during **venous** filling (v for "villing"). At first, it can be seen that atrial pressure decreases with relaxation (x descent) but subsequently rises as the atrium becomes full. Now the filled right atrium can move the blood into the right ventricle. During ventricular diastole, the tricuspid valve opens and the blood in the atrium will empty into the right ventricle, leading to the **y descent.**

- **Atrial fibrillation** leads to **loss of the a wave** because there is no coordinated atrial contraction. **Tricuspid stenosis** will lead to a **prominent a wave** because the atrium will be contracting against a valve that cannot open sufficiently, and the atrial kick will cause an increase in venous pressure because the blood cannot go into the ventricles.
- **AV regurgitation** (mitral or tricuspid) will show a **c-v wave** where there is a large upward deflection in pressure between the c and v waves. This is because during ventricular contraction, some of the blood will move back into the atrium, causing a large rise in pressure.
- A **stenotic aortic valve** would manifest by **larger ventricular pressures than aortic pressures** because the aortic valve, which cannot open fully, cannot receive all the blood that the ventricle is attempting to pump into it as a result of the increased resistance through the valve opening. (In Fig. 8.7A, this would manifest as the dark green line, which represents ventricular pressures, being significantly higher than the light green line, which represents aortic pressures.)

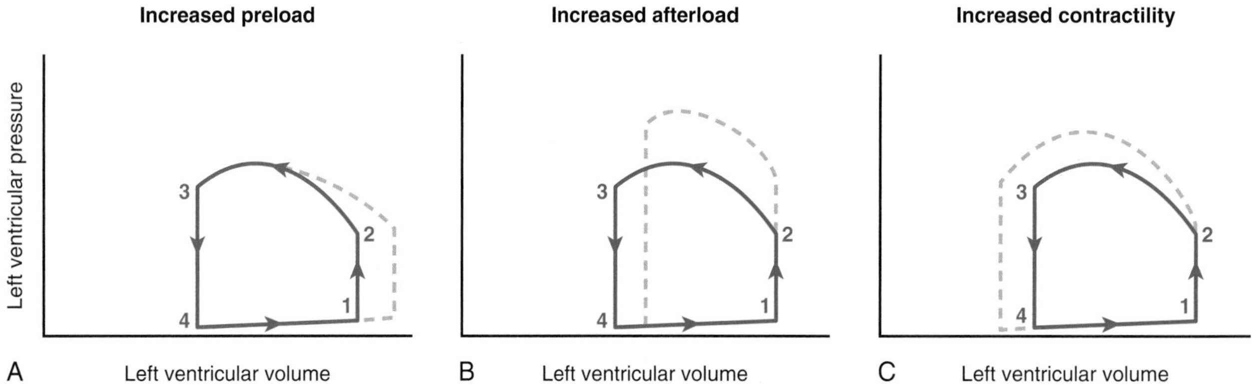

Fig. 8.8 A pressure-volume loop that demonstrates how left ventricular volume (x-axis) and left ventricular (y-axis) pressure are related in conditions of increased preload **(A)**, increased afterload **(B)**, such as in aortic stenosis or hypertension, and increased contractility **(C)**, such as in exercise. *(From Costanzo LS. Physiology. 4th ed. New York: Elsevier; 2009.)*

Fig. 8.8 demonstrates a **pressure-volume loop,** which occurs during each cardiac cycle. The loop shown represents the left ventricle only; follow each step described in Fig. 8.8 (dashed lines show how the pressure-volume loop would change with changes in physiology):

- **Isovolumetric contraction** (1 → 2): At the end of diastole (point 1), the ventricle is filled (end-diastolic volume) and the mitral valve closes (the aortic valve is already closed). The ventricle begins to contract against the closed mitral and aortic valves, increasing pressure but not changing volume (**iso**volumetric) because both valves are closed. When the ventricular pressure exceeds aortic pressure (point 2), the aortic valve will open.
- **Ventricular ejection** (2 → 3): The aortic valve opens (point 2), and blood leaves the ventricle into the aorta. Once the blood is ejected, the aortic valve will close (point 3) because the aortic pressure is now greater than the ventricular pressure. The blood remaining is the end-systolic volume. Recall from earlier that the stroke volume is simply the end-diastolic volume (filled ventricle) minus the end-systolic volume (emptied ventricle); therefore this curve also shows the stroke volume. With **increased afterload** the ventricle has to generate higher pressures to open the aortic valve (it is working harder, pushing against a higher pressure), causing a decreased stroke volume and increased myocardial oxygen demand (Fig. 8.8B). With **increased contractility,** the heart will generate a larger stroke volume; thus, even with the same end-diastolic (filling) volume, there will be a smaller end-systolic volume.
- **Isovolumetric relaxation** (3 → 4): The aortic valve is closed (point 3), and the mitral valve is still closed, and the ventricle now relaxes. Because there are no valves open, the volume inside the ventricle cannot change (**iso**volumetric).
- **Ventricular filling** (4 → 1): Once the pressure in the ventricle is lower than that of the left atrium (point 4), the mitral valve will open and fill the ventricle. The amount the ventricle fills (end-diastolic volume) is dependent on the **preload** (amount of blood in the left atrium waiting to fill the ventricle), the compliance of the ventricle (whether or not it is "stiff," e.g., from hypertrophy), and the presence of the **atrial kick.** Fig. 8.8A depicts a higher preload, leading to a higher end-diastolic volume.

Heart Sounds and Murmurs

Heart sounds are generated by the **closing** of valves. Understanding when valves normally open and close during the cardiac cycle will make it easy to understand how abnormal valve or heart function will cause abnormal heart sounds. Refer to the figure when various valves are mentioned to understand where they are heard best. A mnemonic commonly used to remember where to auscultate for each valve is **APT M** (apartment M) for **a**ortic, **p**ulmonic, **t**ricuspid, **m**itral (Fig. 8.9A).

S_1: This is the sound made normally by the **closure of the tricuspid and mitral valves.** This sound marks the end of diastole because filling of the ventricles is complete. These two events occur nearly simultaneously, so there is **never any splitting** of this sound.

S_2: This is the sound made normally by **closure of the pulmonic and aortic valves, referred to as P_2 and A_2, respectively.** This sound marks the end of systole because ejection of blood from the ventricle

Hearing the S_2 sound split during inspiration is normal. Not hearing an S_2 split on inspiration is also normal. Anything else is abnormal.

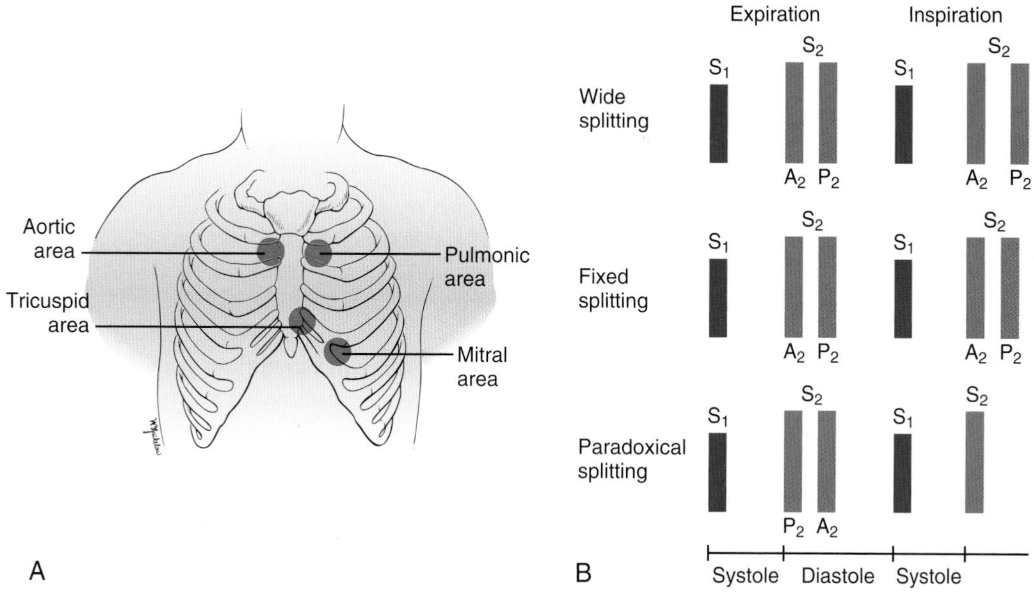

FIG. 8.9 A, Areas on the chest to auscultate to best hear sounds generated by each valve. **B,** S_1 sound (generated by mitral and tricuspid valve closure) and S_2 sound (generated by aortic and pulmonic valve closure) in pathologic condition. The S_2 sound can be normally split during inspiration only, but pathologic splitting such as wide, fixed, or paradoxical splitting can occur. *(**A** from Swartz M.* Textbook of Physical Diagnosis: History and Examination. *5th ed. Philadelphia: Saunders; 2006.* ***B*** *from Seidel HM, Ball JW, Dains JE, et al.* Mosby's Physical Examination Handbook. *6th ed. Philadelphia: Elsevier; 2006.)*

has now been completed. During inspiration, intrathoracic pressure becomes more negative, "sucking" more blood back into the right atrium from the vena cava, increasing venous return. This increases right ventricular preload, leading to a larger right ventricular stroke volume, prolonging the duration in which the pulmonic valve is open (needs more time to eject all that extra blood). This moves P_2 after A_2 and causes the S_2 sound to be split, termed **physiologic splitting** (a completely normal entity). On expiration, this does not occur and P_2 and A_2 occur at the same time, causing the S_2 sound to not be split. There are some examples of when splitting can be pathologic (Fig. 8.9B):

- **Fixed splitting:** Described when splitting occurs on both inspiration and expiration. This occurs with an **atrial septal defect (ASD)** because there is a hole between the two atria. Because there is always a left-to-right shunt present (because left atrial pressures are higher than right atrial pressures), the right ventricle always has increased preload and the pulmonic valve will always close after the aortic valve.
- **Wide splitting:** Described when the P_2–A_2 split is longer than usual, seen with anything that causes a delay in right ventricular emptying. With **pulmonic stenosis,** the valve is narrowed, and therefore it takes the blood longer to fully eject, leading to a delay in valve closure. In **right bundle branch block,** the fast His-Purkinje system to the right ventricle is blocked and right ventricular contraction is delayed, causing the pulmonic valve to close after the aortic valve because the left ventricle will contract and finish ejecting blood first.
- **Paradoxical splitting:** Described when the aortic valve paradoxically closes **after** the pulmonic valve, seen with anything that causes a delay in left ventricular emptying. This causes the split to paradoxically occur during expiration rather than inspiration. This is because the pulmonic valve is closing earlier than the aortic valve as a result of a pathologic condition, but during inspiration the increased volume moving through the pulmonic valve allows the valves to open for the same amount of time. As you may have guessed, **aortic stenosis** and **left bundle branch block** can cause this, for the same reason described with wide splitting, just now affecting the left ventricle.

Normally, there are **no other sounds** other than S_1 and S_2 during the cardiac cycle. However, there can be extra sounds, called S_3 and S_4 sounds (also called "gallops"). See Fig. 8.7D for the location of these heart sounds in relation to the S_1 and S_2 sounds.

S_3: Although this can be a normal finding in children, it is **always abnormal in adults** and usually signifies **volume overload.** When the tricuspid valve and mitral valve open during diastole, the extra volume rushes into the ventricle, tensing the chordae tendineae (tendons that tether the valve to the heart) of the affected valve (depending on which side of the heart is overloaded with volume), causing the extra sound. This sound is heard during the **rapid ventricular filling phase** in **early diastole** and is therefore positioned **after the S_2 sound.**

S_4: At the very end of diastole, the atria contract, called the **"atrial kick,"** to try to squeeze in the last bit of blood before the mitral and tricuspid valves close (S_1 sound). If the ventricle is stiff and noncompliant (such as from hypertrophy from hypertension), there will be no room for the extra blood, and the S_4 sound will be generated. Because the atrial kick occurs just before the end of diastole and closure of the AV valves, this sound is heard just **before the S_1 sound.**

Blood flow through the heart is normally laminar and silent. When there is **turbulent** blood flow through the heart, a **murmur** is heard (turbulent flow through a narrowed artery is instead called a **bruit**). Understanding the cardiac cycle and when valves should be opened or closed makes understanding murmurs easy. **Stenosis** is a problem with **opening** a valve because it has been narrowed, whereas **regurgitation** (or insufficiency) is a problem with keeping a valve **closed.**

During **systole,** the aortic and pulmonic valves should **open** to allow for ejection of blood from the ventricles, and therefore the murmur of aortic or pulmonic stenosis will be heard during systole. Because the tricuspid and mitral valves should be **closed,** the murmur of tricuspid or mitral regurgitation will also be heard during systole (Fig. 8.10).

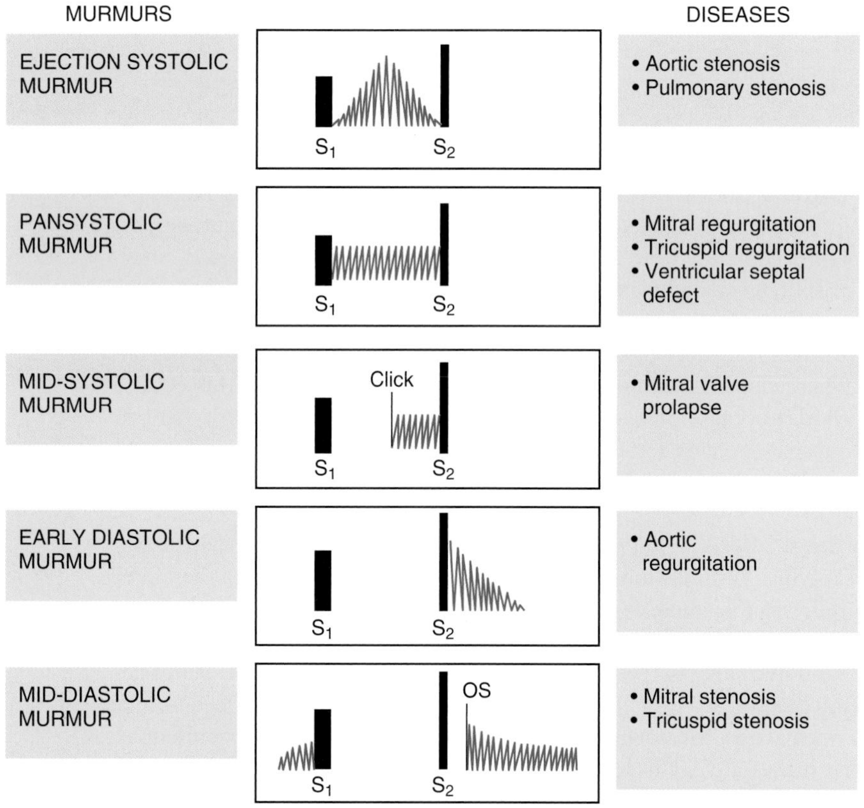

FIG. 8.10 Heart murmurs, their location during the cardiac cycle, and their characteristics. *OS*, opening snap, seen in stenosis. *(From Damjanov I. Pathophysiology. Philadelphia: Elsevier; 2008.)*

Aortic stenosis: crescendo–decrescendo murmur at the right second intercostal space, exertional syncope, angina, *pulsus parvus et tardus*

❍ **Aortic or pulmonic stenosis** (Fig. 8.11): The murmur is described as **"crescendo–decrescendo"** or "diamond shaped" because as the contraction of the heart progresses, the pressure builds up and drops again, leading to a murmur that increases and then decreases in intensity. Individuals with aortic stenosis will often complain of chest pain because of increased myocardial oxygen demand from the increased afterload. They may also experience exertional syncope because the demands for

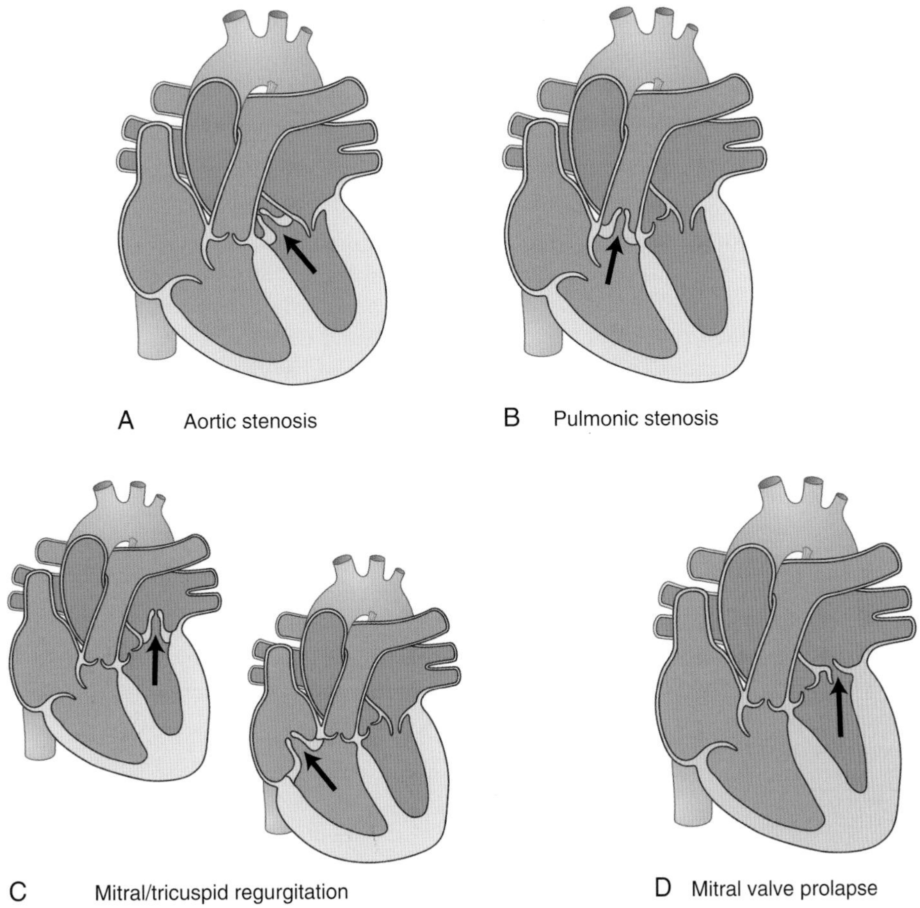

FIG. 8.11 A, Aortic stenosis. **B,** Pulmonic stenosis. **C,** Mitral/tricuspid regurgitation. **D,** Mitral valve prolapse. *(**A** and **B** from Lissauer T, Clayden G.* Illustrated Textbook of Pediatrics. *4th ed. Edinburgh: Elsevier; 2011.)*

increased cardiac output during exercise cannot be met with the high resistance through the aortic valve and will experience syncope as a result of cerebral hypoperfusion. Classically, on physical examination these patients will have *pulsus parvus et tardus,* which is Latin for a weak *(parvus)* and late *(tardus)* pulse. Predisposing factors to aortic stenosis include congenital bicuspid aortic valve (two cusps instead of three) and rheumatic heart disease causing damage to the aortic valve.

- **Mitral or tricuspid regurgitation:** The murmur is described as "holosystolic" or "pansystolic" because it occurs at the same intensity for the duration of systole. This is because the left and right atria have low pressure and can accept blood even at low pressures if the valve is incompetent.
- **Mitral valve prolapse:** The most common valvular lesion, in which an abnormally thickened valve "prolapses" into the left atrium during systole. The sudden tensing of the chordae tendineae that stops the movement of the valve causes a "click" to be heard, and an end-systolic murmur is present if there is regurgitant flow. This is most often a benign lesion and is associated with connective tissue diseases such as Marfan syndrome and Ehlers-Danlos syndrome.
- **Ventricular septal defect:** If there is a passage between the left and right ventricles, during systole the left ventricle (which has higher pressures) will eject blood into the right ventricle, leading to a left-to-right shunt. This leads to a holosystolic murmur, similar to that of mitral regurgitation. It is classically described as "harsh" sounding, whereas regurgitant murmurs are "high pitched."

During **diastole,** the tricuspid and mitral valves should be **open** to allow for ventricular filling through the atria, and therefore murmurs of tricuspid or mitral stenosis will be heard during diastole. Conversely, the aortic and pulmonic valves should be **closed** to prevent backward flow of blood from the arteries into the ventricles, and therefore the murmurs of aortic or pulmonic regurgitation will be heard during diastole. In contrast to systolic murmurs, which can be benign, **diastolic murmurs are always pathologic** (see Fig. 8.10).

- **Mitral or tricuspid stenosis:** The murmur is described as beginning with an opening "snap" when the stenotic valve finally opens, followed by a turbulent rumbling murmur. Most commonly this is caused by **rheumatic fever,** which most often affects the **mitral valve.**
- **Aortic or pulmonic regurgitation:** The murmur is described as early decrescendo because after the ventricles eject the blood, the valves should shut—failure to do so causes blood to crash back into the ventricle during diastole, leading to the murmur. Because in aortic regurgitation, the blood crashes back into the left ventricle instead of staying in the systemic circulation, there is a wide pulse pressure from decreased diastolic blood pressure. This drop in diastolic blood pressure leads to many clinical signs, including a large-volume pulse that collapses in diastole (termed a *Corrigan water-hammer pulse*); de Musset sign, in which the head bobs with the heartbeat; and Quincke sign, in which the capillary bed in the nail can be seen to be pulsating from the wide pulse pressure.

Aortic regurgitation: wide pulse pressure, early decrescendo murmur

Lastly, the murmur of a **patent ductus arteriosus (PDA)** is a **continuous** murmur (present in systole and diastole) and is described as "**machine-like**" (Fig. 8.12). See Chapter 4 for a detailed description, but briefly, the ductus arteriosus is normally open when the fetus is in utero to act as a bypass tract from the pulmonary artery to the aorta because the lungs did not need significant blood flow (the fetus can't breathe in utero). After birth, the increased oxygen tension in the lungs (because the baby now needs to breathe) causes constriction of the ductus arteriosus and eventually fibrosis, becoming the ligamentum arteriosum. Although a postnatal PDA is not normal, it may be beneficial to the baby if there are other congenital heart disease lesions present; vasodilating prostaglandins keep this open, and therefore medications that block prostaglandin synthesis (such as **indomethacin**) will promote closure, whereas giving prostaglandin E analogs such as **misoprostol** will help keep it open.

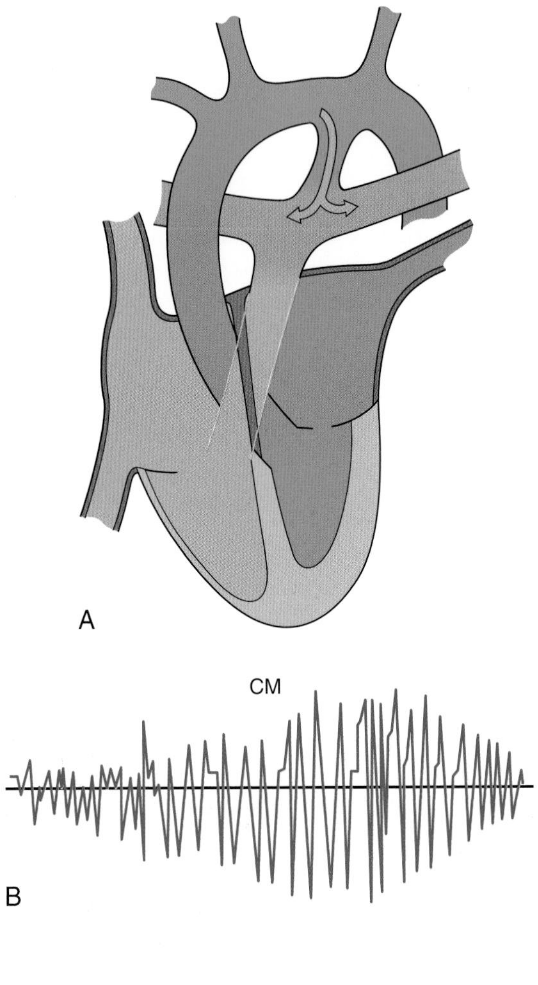

Fig. 8.12 A, Patent ductus arteriosus, connecting the aorta to the pulmonary artery, resulting in a left-to-right shunt (oxygenated blood being put back into the pulmonary circulation). **B,** Continuous machine-like murmur (CM) heard in patients with a patent ductus arteriosus. *(**A,** from Stevens A, Lowe J, Scott I.* Core Pathology. *3rd ed. Philadelphia: Elsevier; 2008.)*

Performing maneuvers that change afterload or preload can change the intensity or characteristic of certain murmurs and may allow the clinician to diagnose valvular disease from physical examination alone. For instance, right-sided lesions get louder with inspiration (because of increased right ventricular preload). Increasing afterload (such as clenching a fist) increases the intensity of aortic regurgitation, mitral regurgitation, and ventricular septal defect (VSD) murmurs. Decreasing preload (e.g., with Valsalva maneuver) will cause many murmurs to decrease in intensity and the mitral valve prolapse click to occur earlier, whereas increasing preload (squatting) will cause increased intensity of aortic stenosis (AS) murmur and the mitral valve prolapse (MVP) click to occur later.

Murmur Summary

Although it is good to know about all the murmurs, left-sided lesions are much more likely to be tested on Step 1 (or relevant clinically). Furthermore, right-sided murmurs will usually have a question stem that hints at intravenous drug use (tricuspid regurgitation). Mitral stenosis will often have a question stem that hints at rheumatic fever. Aortic regurgitation will usually be your diastolic murmur without other clues. The main goal will then be distinguishing the two left-sided systolic murmurs: aortic stenosis (crescendo–decrescendo, radiates to carotids) and mitral regurgitation (holosystolic, radiates to axilla).

Pressure in the Cardiovascular System

Pressures in the heart can be measured with a pulmonary artery (Swan-Ganz) catheter (Fig. 8.13) and can provide information about the clinical status of a patient.

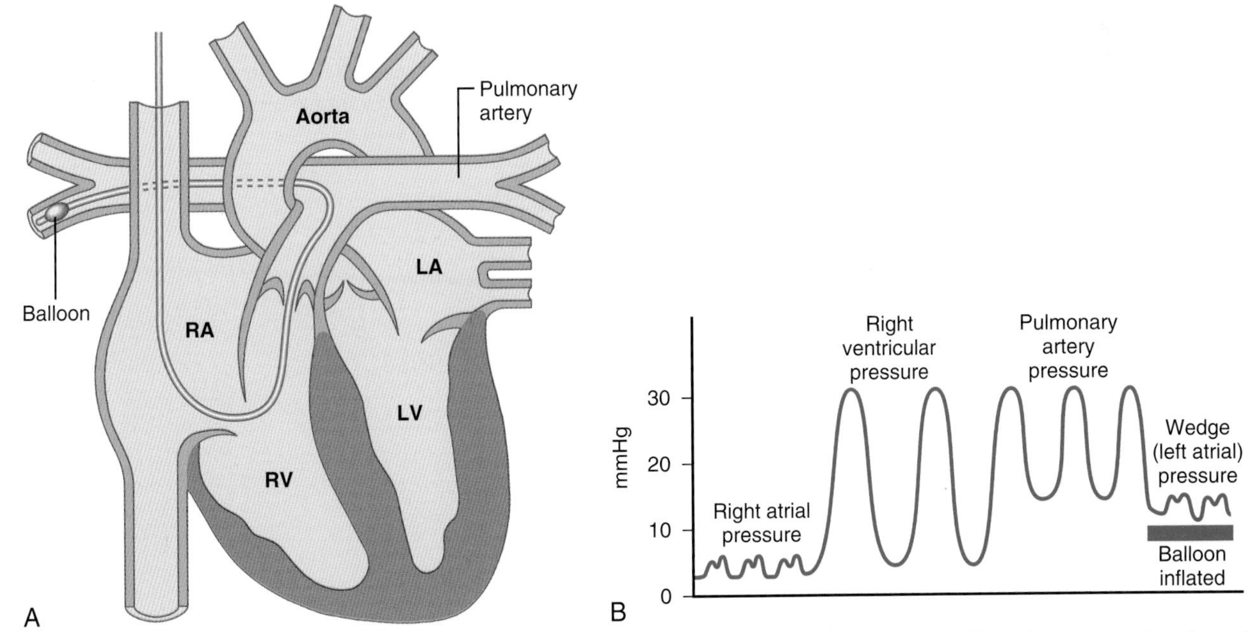

Fig. 8.13 A, A pulmonary artery (Swan-Ganz) catheter to assess pressures in the cardiovascular system. The catheter is introduced into the patient and can measure right atrial pressure, move into the right ventricle to measure right ventricular pressure, move into the pulmonary artery to measure pulmonary arterial pressure, and wedge into the distal pulmonary arteries to get a pulmonary capillary wedge pressure (PCWP), which approximates the left ventricular pressure. **B,** Schematic showing pressure outputs as the pulmonary artery catheter moves through the right atrium, right ventricle, and pulmonary artery, and finally with the balloon inflated in a distal pulmonary artery. LA, Left atrium; LV, left ventricle; RA, right atrium; RV, right ventricle. *(From Colledge NR, Walker BR, Ralston SH.* Davidson's Principles and Practice of Medicine. *21st ed. Philadelphia: Elsevier; 2010.)*

- **Right atrial pressure** is equal to **central venous pressure** because the central veins (the superior and inferior vena cava) feed the right atrium. This is a **low-pressure** area because the **veins are low-pressure vessels.** Right atrial pressure will be increased when there is too much volume in the veins or difficulty feeding that volume to the heart (such as in right ventricular failure, when the ventricle cannot pump the blood given to it).
- **Right (RV) ventricular pressure** is normally lower than left ventricular pressure because the **pulmonary circulation is normally a lower-pressure circuit than the systemic circulation.**

RV pressure can increase if it is pushing against a higher pressure (afterload), such as in **pulmonic stenosis** or **pulmonary hypertension.** Because the right side of the heart has lower pressures than the left, atrial or ventricular septal defects will result in a shunt (at least initially; see Eisenmenger syndrome later) from left side of the heart to right side of the heart (high pressure to low pressure).

- The **pulmonary artery pressure** can be increased in **pulmonary hypertension** (from lung disease or pulmonary vessel disease such as pulmonary embolism) or from **left-sided heart failure** (because the fluid will back up into the lungs if the left ventricle cannot pump it out).
- The **pulmonary capillary wedge pressure** (PCWP) is a way of measuring **left atrial pressure** because the catheter cannot fit through the small capillary beds of the lungs. This can be increased if the left atrial pressure is high, such as in left-sided heart failure, but also in problems with the mitral valve: stenosis because the left atrium cannot empty, regurgitation because blood will be forced back into the atrium from the ventricle.
- In **cardiac tamponade** (covered in depth later), essentially the heart is being strangled by fluid that is trapped in the pericardial sac. This leads to **equalization of pressure across all four chambers**—the high pressure exerted on the heart is from all sides because the pericardium surrounds the heart. This is rapidly fatal if not corrected.

ELECTROCARDIOGRAPHY

An electrocardiogram (Fig. 8.14; ECG, or often referred to as EKG from the German spelling) is a useful tool to assess the electrical activity of the heart. When the cardiac myocytes go from polarized (resting state) to depolarized from an action potential, an electrical current is generated that can be measured. The USMLE Step 1 will only test ECG basics, but it is worth your while to invest time in reading an ECG book to gain a deeper understanding—after you're done crushing Step 1.

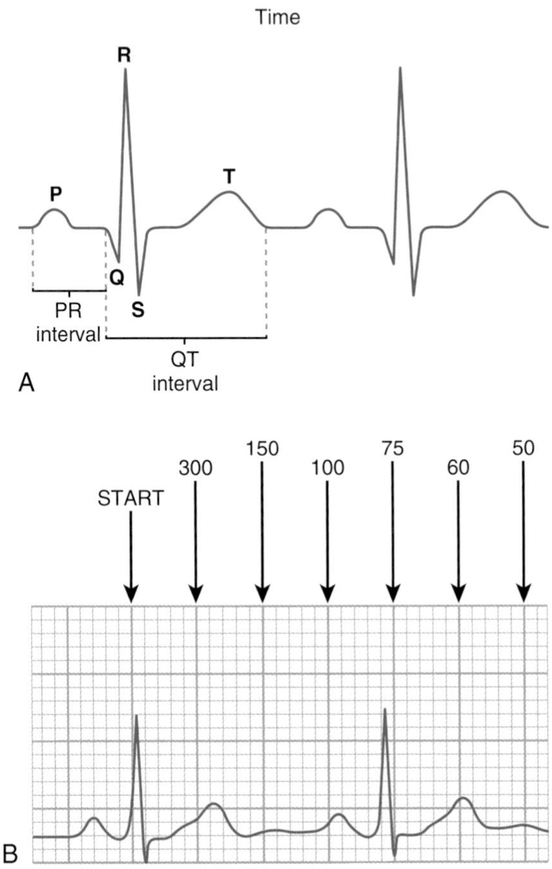

FIG. 8.14 A, ECG tracing from a single heartbeat with the output labeled. P wave: atrial depolarization; PR interval: time between atrial depolarization and ventricular depolarization; QRS complex: ventricular depolarization; ST segment: time after ventricular depolarization but before repolarization; T wave: ventricular repolarization. Note atrial repolarization is never found on the ECG tracing because it occurs during the QRS complex (ventricular depolarization). **B,** The 300-150-100-75 method of counting heart rate. Count the number of large boxes (denoted by the *thicker lines* on the tracing, comprising five smaller boxes) that occur from the R wave (peak of the QRS complex). If the amount of large boxes separating the two R waves is 1, the heart rate is 300; 2, the heart rate is 150, and so on. Each large box represents 0.2 second (200 msec) and each small box represents 0.04 second (40 msec). *(**A** from Pazdernik T, Kerecsen L. Rapid Review Pharmacology. 3rd ed. Philadelphia: Elsevier; 2010.)*

- **P wave:** Represents **atrial depolarization.** After the P wave, there is a **PR segment**—this is the conduction delay at the AV node, which allows the ventricles time to fill fully before contraction (normally 0.12 to 0.20 second). Therefore diseases of the AV node often manifest as PR-segment prolongation or abnormalities.
- **QRS complex:** Represents **ventricular depolarization.** The terminology of the QRS complex can be difficult, but basically, if the first deflection is downward, it is a Q wave; if the first deflection is upward, a Q wave is not present. The first upward reflection is always an R wave. Any downward deflection after the R wave is known as an S wave. The atria repolarize during the QRS complex but do not make a tracing because the ventricles have many more myocytes and dominate the ECG. Normally the QRS duration is less than 0.12 second, but if the fast His-Purkinje conduction system is malfunctioning, then the QRS complex becomes abnormally widened, such as in bundle branch blocks.
- **T wave:** After the ventricles depolarize during the QRS complex, there is a brief delay (ST segment) followed by repolarization, which is the T wave. There is sometimes a U wave that follows the T wave, which can be normal, but is not a common finding. It may also be seen in conditions such as hypokalemia or bradycardia.

An ECG printout has two main components: the 12-lead ECG, which looks at the heart from different vectors or angles, and the rhythm strip, which is useful for noting abnormalities in rhythm (arrhythmias) or rate. Basic rhythm strip abnormalities will be presented and explained. It is important to be able to assess the heart rate—each "little box" on the ECG strip is 0.04 second (40 msec), and each "big box" is made up of five "little boxes" and is therefore 0.20 second (200 msec). To assess the heart rate, count the number of "big boxes" between QRS complexes—and then remember 300-150-100-75-60-50. If there is one big box between beats, the rate is 300; two is 150, and so forth (see Fig. 8.13B).

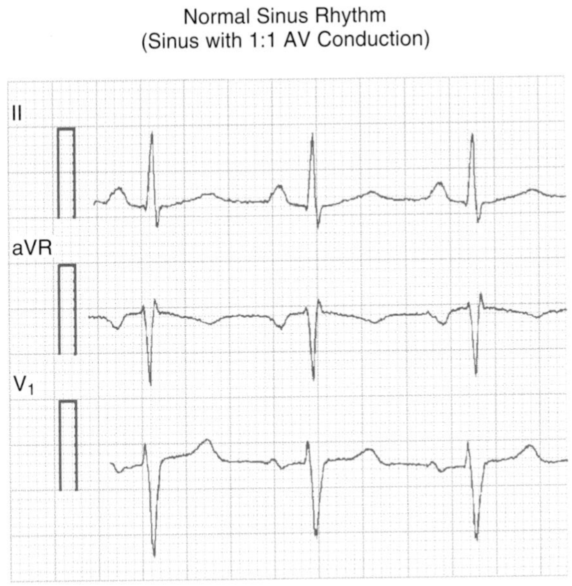

Fig. 8.15 Normal sinus rhythm. *(From Goldberger AL, Goldberger ZD, Shvilkin A. Clinical Electrocardiography: A Simplified Approach. 8th ed. Philadelphia: Saunders; 2012.)*

Atrial flutter: "saw tooth" pattern on ECG; atrial rate usually 300, but 2:1 block leads to ventricular rates of 150

Normal Sinus Rhythm: This is a normal ECG (Fig. 8.15). To be classified as sinus, a P wave (atrial contraction) must precede every QRS complex, denoting that the atria are conducting the impulse that was generated by the SA node through the AV node. In addition, it is "normal" because there is neither bradycardia nor tachycardia present: The heart rate is between 60 and 100. In this ECG, using the big box counting method, the heart rate is 75.

Sinus Tachycardia. This ECG is sinus because there are P waves before each QRS complex, but using the big box counting method, we see that the heart rate is 150 (Fig. 8.16). Therefore it is sinus tachycardia.

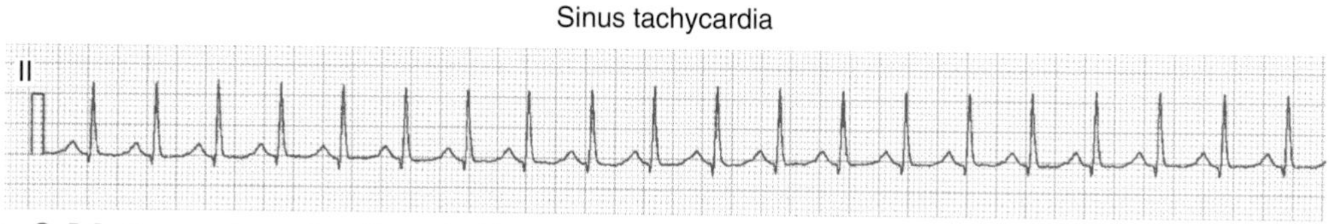

Fig. 8.16 Sinus tachycardia. *(From Goldberger AL, Goldberger ZD, Shvilkin A. Clinical Electrocardiography: A Simplified Approach. 8th ed. Philadelphia: Saunders; 2012.)*

Atrial Flutter: In atrial flutter (Fig. 8.17), there is an abnormal reentry of electrical activity around the tricuspid valve annulus, causing a self-sustaining loop of activity. This usually occurs at an atrial rate of 300, which is too fast for the AV node to conduct to the ventricles. Most commonly, the impulses have a 2:1 conduction block, meaning the ventricular rate is about 150 if the atrial rate is 300 because only half the impulses are conducted.

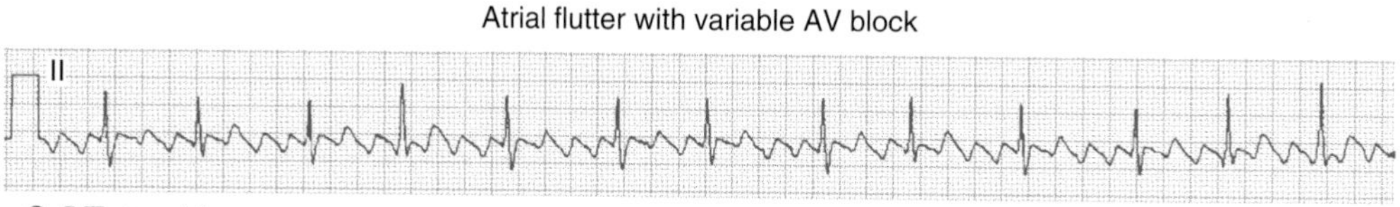

Fig. 8.17 Atrial flutter. *(From Goldberger AL, Goldberger ZD, Shvilkin A. Clinical Electrocardiography: A Simplified Approach. 8th ed. Philadelphia: Saunders; 2012.)*

Patients with atrial flutter most commonly have some form of structural heart disease. The flutter waves in the image are denoted with an F and often have a "**saw tooth**" appearance, and each wave should be nearly identical.

Atrial Fibrillation: In atrial fibrillation (Fig. 8.18), there is random activation of the atria that is unpredictable and chaotic, leading to **no discernible P waves** because there is no coordinated depolarization; the impulses that are transmitted through the AV node to the ventricles occur without a pattern, leading to an **irregularly irregular** rhythm. This is in contrast to a regularly irregular rhythm in which the irregularity is predictable and occurs at regular intervals (e.g., an irregular beat every fifth beat, which can occur with atrioventricular blocks). This is the most common chronic arrhythmia and can be dangerous because without a coordinated atrial contraction, stasis of blood can occur with resulting clot formation, potentially leading to strokes if the thrombi occur in the left atrium, with embolization of clots to the brain. Therefore these patients require anticoagulation with either aspirin or **warfarin/DOAC** (direct oral anticoagulants such as dabigatran), depending on their risk factors.

Atrial fibrillation: "irregularly irregular" pulse, risk for blood stasis from lack of coordinated atrial contraction leading to clots and embolization risk

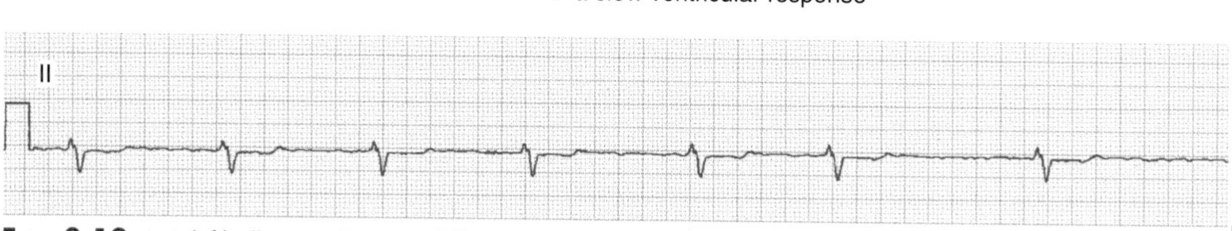

Fig. 8.18 Atrial fibrillation. *(From Goldberger AL, Goldberger ZD, Shvilkin A. Clinical Electrocardiography: A Simplified Approach. 8th ed. Philadelphia: Saunders; 2012.)*

Ventricular Tachycardia: In ventricular tachycardia (Fig. 8.19), there is an abnormality in the patient's ventricles, often an old scar from a myocardial infarction, that causes abnormal conduction and a reentry circuit in the ventricle leading to rhythmic depolarization of the ventricles. In the ECG tracing in Fig. 8.19, the patient's rhythm changes from sinus rhythm to ventricular tachycardia. Treatment is to "reset" the heart to normal sinus rhythm, which in the stable patient can be done either chemically (e.g., with procainamide or amiodarone) or electrically with cardioversion. Patients with ventricular tachycardia *without a pulse* should receive cardiopulmonary resuscitation (CPR) and early defibrillation.

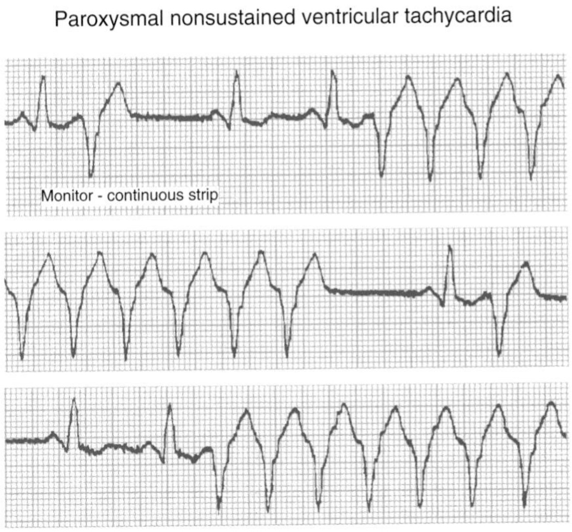

FIG. 8.19 Ventricular tachycardia. *(From Goldberger AL, Goldberger ZD, Shvilkin A. Clinical Electrocardiography: A Simplified Approach. 8th ed. Philadelphia: Saunders; 2012.)*

Torsades de Pointes: French for "twisting of the points," torsades de pointes (Fig. 8.20) is a specific type of **polymorphic ventricular tachycardia** (in contrast to the previous example of ventricular tachycardia, where each beat looked the same and was therefore monomorphic). Anything that **prolongs the QT interval** makes this more likely to occur—such as **congenital long-QT syndromes, hypocalcemia, hypomagnesemia, hypokalemia, or medications that prolong the QT interval.** In fact, treatment of torsades de pointes includes rapid intravenous infusion of magnesium. Medications associated with increased QT interval include certain antibiotics, antiarrhythmics, antipsychotics, antidepressants, and antiemetics.

Torsades de pointes: long QT interval risk factor, as triggered by R-on-T phenomenon. Give rapid infusion of magnesium.

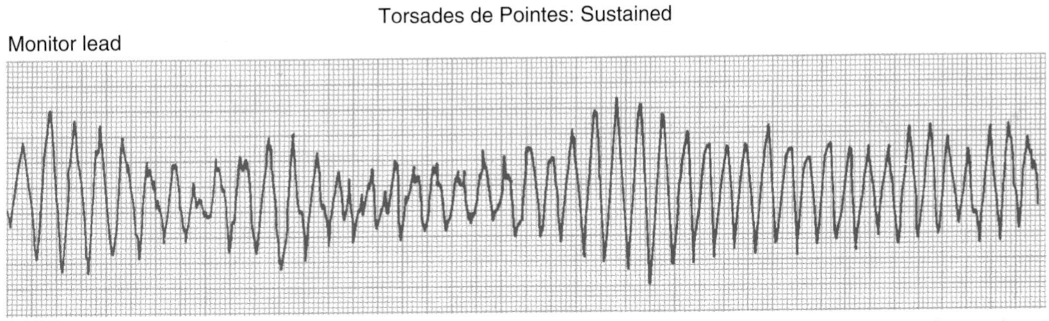

FIG. 8.20 Torsades de pointes. *(From Goldberger AL, Goldberger ZD, Shvilkin A. Clinical Electrocardiography: A Simplified Approach. 8th ed. Philadelphia: Saunders; 2012.)*

Ventricular Fibrillation: This disordered and rapid depolarization of the ventricles (Fig. 8.21) causes cardiac output to drop to essentially zero—making this rhythm life threatening and rapidly fatal if untreated. CPR and defibrillation in a rapid manner are lifesaving.

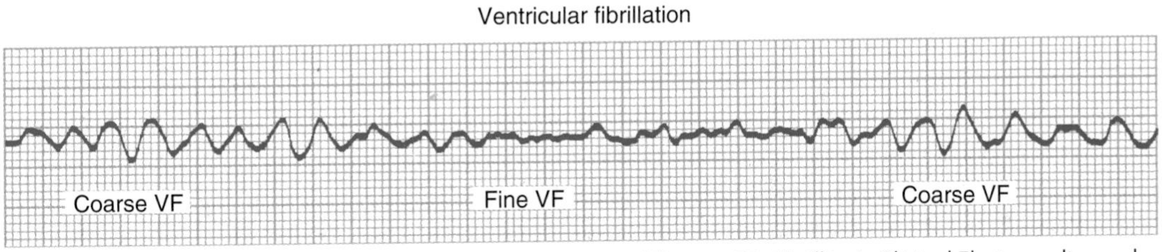

FIG. 8.21 Ventricular fibrillation (VF). *(From Goldberger AL, Goldberger ZD, Shvilkin A. Clinical Electrocardiography: A Simplified Approach. 8th ed. Philadelphia: Saunders; 2012.)*

Wolff-Parkinson-White Syndrome: Also known as **ventricular preexcitation syndrome,** Wolff-Parkinson-White (WPW) syndrome (Fig. 8.22) is caused by an accessory pathway (known as the bundle of Kent) between the atria and ventricles. Normally, the AV node is the only passageway for electrical conduction; these patients have an extra pathway. This extra pathway causes the ventricles to begin depolarizing before they normally would, leading to a premature upsloping in the QRS complex known as a **delta wave.** Because now there are two routes to transmit impulses through the ventricle, it is possible to

Wolff-Parkinson-White syndrome: "delta waves" on ECG as a result of early depolarization of ventricles through bypass tract (bundle of Kent); at risk for extremely fast arrhythmias and death

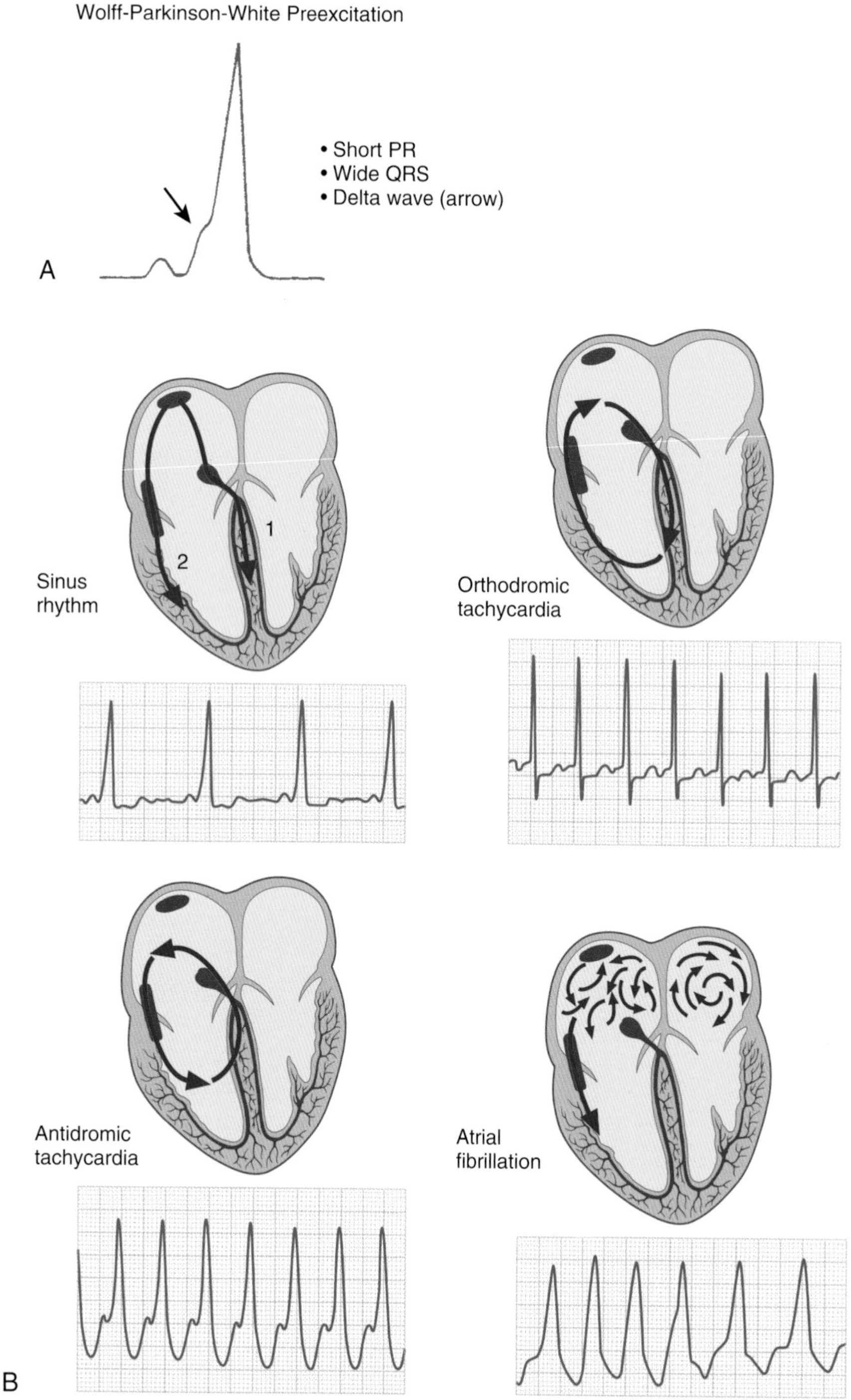

FIG. 8.22 Wolff-Parkinson-White (WPW) syndrome. **A,** ECG demonstrating "delta waves" where there is an upslope before the QRS complex as a result of premature ventricular depolarization by early transmission of the action potentials via the accessory pathway (bundle of Kent). **B,** Demonstration of the accessory pathway; recall that normally there is no other method for conducting impulses from the atria to the ventricles other than via the AV node. (**A** *from Goldberger AL, Goldberger ZD, Shvilkin A.* Clinical Electrocardiography: A Simplified Approach. *8th ed. Philadelphia: Saunders; 2012.* **B** *from Colledge NR, Walker BR, Ralston SH.* Davidson's Principles and Practice of Medicine. *21st ed. Philadelphia: Elsevier; 2010.)*

have a reentry circuit in which an electrical impulse can travel in a circuitous path in one of two directions: (1) orthodromic, meaning that the signal travels antegrade down the AV node (as normal), but then retrograde through the bundle of Kent; (2) antidromic, meaning the signal travels antegrade through the bundle of Kent and then retrograde through the AV node (Table 8.1). Orthodromic tachycardias generally have normal-appearing QRS complexes (because electrical signal travels normally down bundles of His), whereas antidromic tachycardias are characterized by widened QRS complexes.

TABLE 8.1 Atrioventricular Blocks ("Heart Blocks")

First degree (Fig. 8.23)	Prolonged PR interval (≥0.20 sec), **no dropped beats** (can be normal).
Second degree (two types, Fig. 8.24)	**Mobitz type I (Wenckebach):** progressive PR prolongation leading to dropped beat with subsequent resetting of PR interval. **Mobitz type II:** randomly dropped beats without progressive PR prolongation. At risk for degenerating to third-degree block; much more dangerous; treat with pacemaker.
Third degree (Fig. 8.25)	Complete AV dissociation: the atria and ventricles act independently of one another; treat with pacemaker.

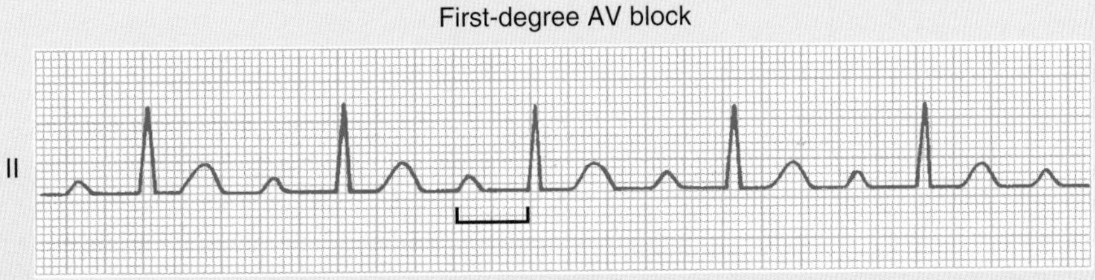

FIG. 8.23 First-degree AV block. *(From Goldberger AL, Goldberger ZD, Shvilkin A. Clinical Electrocardiography: A Simplified Approach. 8th ed. Philadelphia: Saunders; 2012.)*

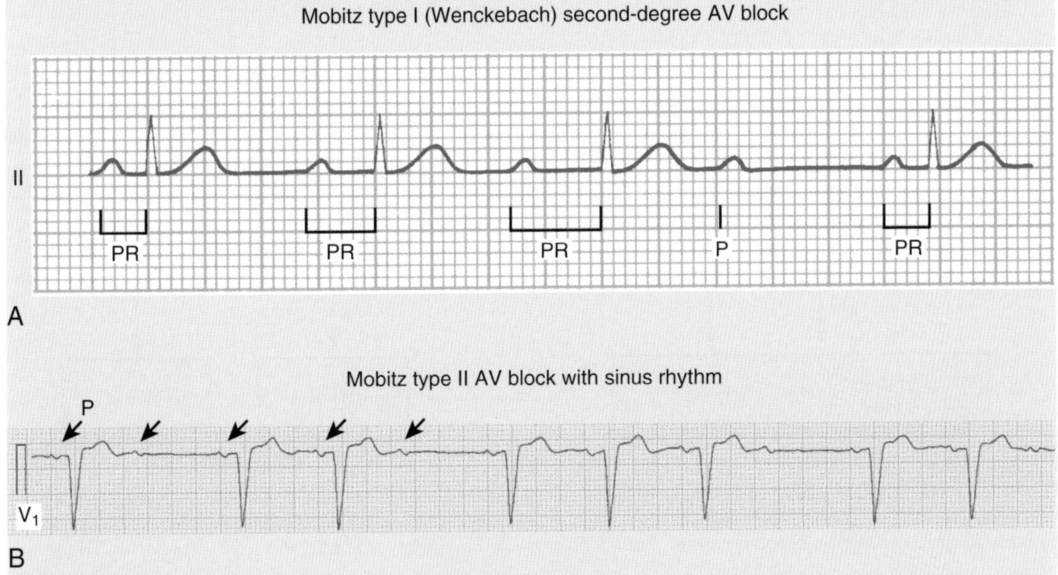

FIG. 8.24 Second-degree AV block. **A,** Mobitz type I. **B,** Mobitz type II. *(From Goldberger AL, Goldberger ZD, Shvilkin A. Clinical Electrocardiography: A Simplified Approach. 8th ed. Philadelphia: Saunders; 2012.)*

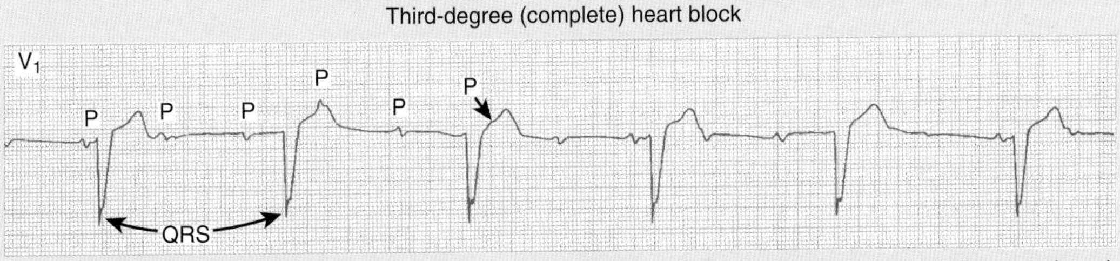

FIG. 8.25 Third-degree (complete) AV block. *(From Goldberger AL, Goldberger ZD, Shvilkin A. Clinical Electrocardiography: A Simplified Approach. 8th ed. Philadelphia: Saunders; 2012.)*

Regulation of Blood Pressure

Regulation of blood pressure occurs with two main mechanisms: (1) the **baroreceptor reflex** and (2) the **renin-angiotensin-aldosterone** axis.

The **baroreceptor reflex** uses pressure sensors (baro- = pressure) in both the aortic arch and carotid body to monitor blood pressure and modulate parasympathetic and sympathetic tone accordingly. These baroreceptors are constantly sending signals to the brainstem, but the rate of these signals will change with the pressure exerted on their receptors. With an increase in blood pressure, the rate of these parasympathetic signals will increase; with a decrease in blood pressure, the rate will decrease in an effort to normalize the blood pressure disturbance. The **carotid sinus** baroreceptors send their information to the brainstem using the **glossopharyngeal nerve** (cranial nerve [CN] IX), whereas the **aortic arch** baroreceptors use the **vagus nerve** (CN X) as their afferent nerve. Fig. 8.26 illustrates how a change in blood pressure leads to a reaction from the baroreceptors.

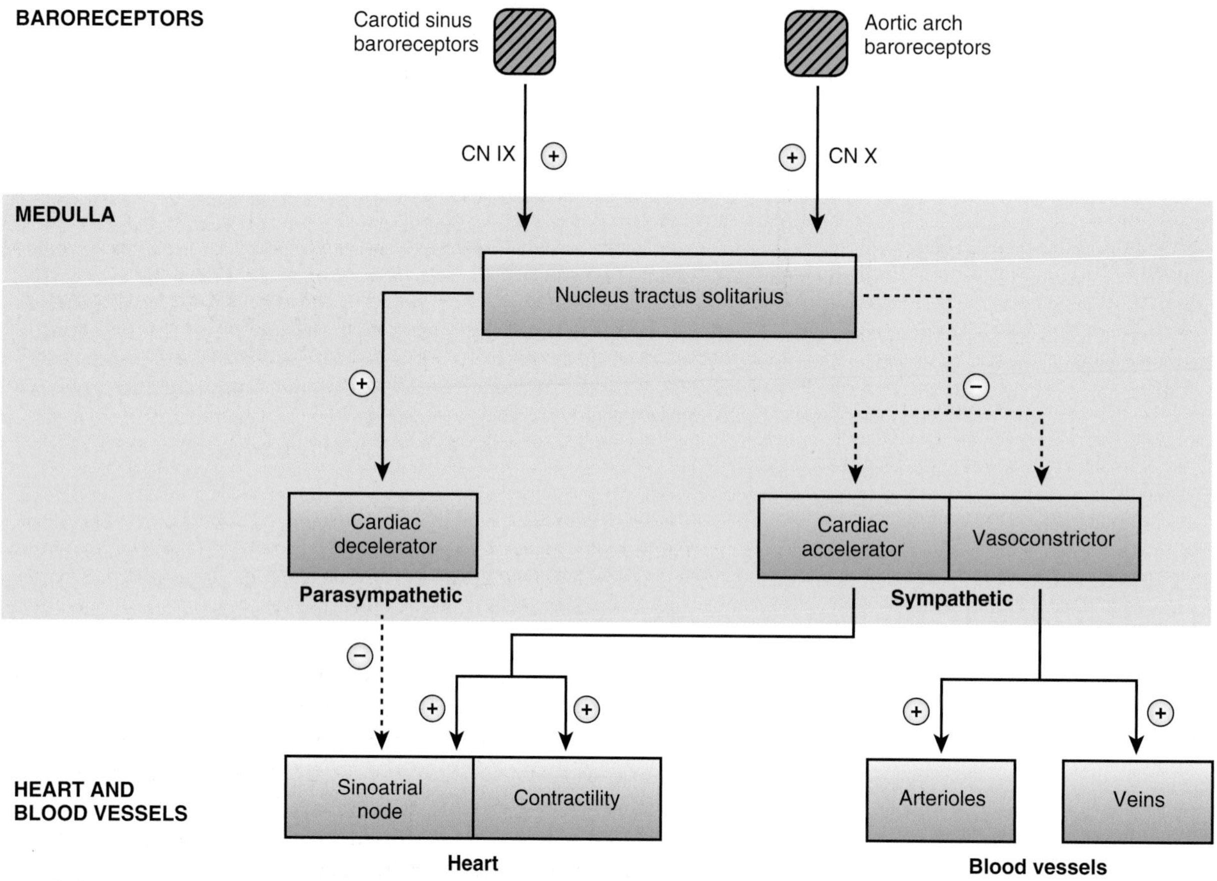

Fig. 8.26 Baroreceptor pathway. The **carotid sinus** sends its signals via the glossopharyngeal nerve (CN IX), whereas the aortic arch sends its signals via the vagus nerve (CN X) to the brainstem. In both cases, this signal is sent via the nucleus tractus solitarius, which distributes the signal to the body to effect changes in blood pressure. *(From Costanzo LS.* Physiology. *4th ed. New York: Elsevier; 2009.)*

- **Increase in blood pressure:** Causes more stretch on the pressure sensors because the arteries have more pressure to exert on the arterial wall. This causes the baroreceptors to enact changes that will decrease blood pressure. The **increased stretch** leads to **increased firing** of the baroreceptors, which (1) increase parasympathetic tone through the vagus nerve (CN X) on the SA node to decrease heart rate and also (2) decrease sympathetic tone.
- **Decrease in blood pressure:** Causes less stretch on the pressure sensors because the arteries have less pressure to exert on the arterial wall. This causes the baroreceptors to enact changes that will increase blood pressure. The **decreased stretch** causes **decreased firing** of the baroreceptors; this in turn causes (1) decreased vagal tone to the SA node, resulting in an increased heart rate, and (2) increased sympathetic tone to increase heart rate, contractility, and vasoconstriction. This helps mediate the body's response to acute decreases in blood pressure, such as what occurs during **hemorrhage.**

- **Carotid sinus massage** puts pressure on the baroreceptors in the carotid body, leading to the body "thinking" there is high blood pressure, causing increased parasympathetic tone (as well as decreased sympathetic tone) and therefore a decrease in heart rate. This was previously proposed as a treatment for supraventricular tachycardia (SVT) but is falling out of favor because of the risk for inducing embolic stroke by massaging cholesterol-laden carotid arteries. Similarly, Valsalva maneuver can also increase vagal tone and is a noninvasive treatment for SVT without risk of embolic stroke.

The **renin-angiotensin-aldosterone** axis is explained in detail in Chapter 9, but briefly, the juxtaglomerular (JG) cells of the kidney also sense blood pressure. Any decrease in blood flow to the kidney will cause the JG cells to secrete the enzyme **renin** into the bloodstream. The bloodstream always has angiotensinogen in it, and renin cleaves this angiotensinogen into angiotensin I. Angiotensin I gets cleaved into angiotensin II by **angiotensin-converting enzyme (ACE)**, which an ACE inhibitor blocks. **Angiotensin II is a potent vasoconstrictor,** increasing systemic vascular resistance (SVR) and therefore blood pressure, and also mediates **aldosterone release** from the zona glomerulosa of the adrenal gland. Aldosterone increases sodium reuptake from the kidney, leading to an expansion in blood volume and thus an increase in blood pressure.

PATHOLOGY

Congenital Heart Disease

There are many congenital heart diseases, classified broadly into two categories: (1) **cyanotic heart disease** and (2) **acyanotic heart disease.** Cyanotic heart diseases are characterized by right-to-left shunts, where deoxygenated blood is put into the systemic circulation with subsequent early cyanosis; acyanotic lesions have left-to-right shunts, causing oxygenated blood to be circulated back into the lungs and therefore not causing early cyanosis. Definitive treatment for cyanotic lesions is almost always surgical.

It is necessary to remember the **five cyanotic heart diseases** (Fig. 8.27); a common mnemonic is the **five Ts** of **T**runcus arteriosus, **T**ransposition of the great vessels, **T**ricuspid atresia, **T**etralogy of Fallot, and **T**otal anomalous pulmonary venous return (TAPVR). Another way to remember this is using the "five-finger method," as described next.

One Finger Up—Truncus Arteriosus: One finger because there is one common vessel.

- Embryologically, the **truncus arteriosus** should divide into the **pulmonary trunk** and **aorta;** failure to do so results in a single common artery leaving both ventricles.

Two Fingers Up, Fingers Crossed—Transposition of the Great Vessels: Fingers crossed because they are transposed.

- The **aorta** and **pulmonary artery** are transposed (switched!): The **aorta** comes off the **right ventricle,** whereas the **pulmonary artery** comes off the **left ventricle.** This causes **two completely separate circulations,** whereby the right ventricle is pumping deoxygenated blood to the body through the aorta, which returns to the right ventricle; the left ventricle is pumping oxygenated blood to the lungs through the pulmonary artery, which returns to the left ventricle.
- For the infant to survive, **a shunt that connects the two systems must be present** to bridge the two circulations, such as a **patent ductus arteriosus** or **patent foramen ovale (an opening between the right and left atria).**
- **Prostaglandin E** (misoprostol) can be given to ensure that the ductus arteriosus remains open.
- A commonly tested association of infantile transposition is maternal diabetes!

Three Fingers Up—Tricuspid Atresia: Three fingers for **tri**cuspid.

- **Absence** of the tricuspid valve, leading to **no connection between the right atrium and right ventricle.** Because the right ventricle is not receiving blood to pump, it is **hypoplastic** (very small, underdeveloped).
- **An atrial septal defect and a ventricular septal defect** must **both** be present to maintain blood flow—from the right atrium, the blood must flow through the ASD to the left atrium to the left ventricle and through the VSD to the right ventricle to allow access to the lungs!

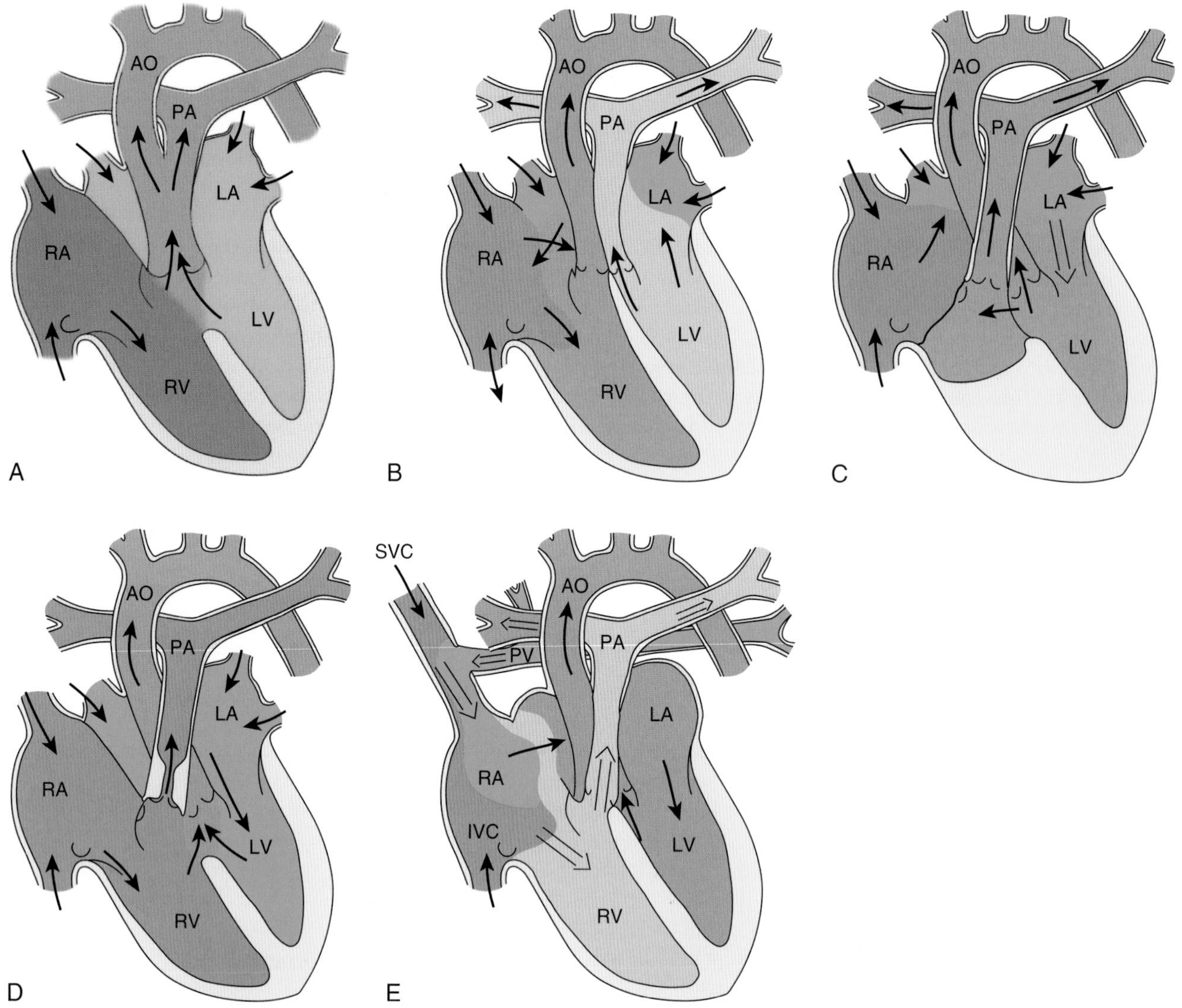

Fig. 8.27 Cyanotic congenital heart disease. **A,** Truncus arteriosus. **B,** Transposition of the great vessels. **C,** Tricuspid atresia with hypoplasia of the right ventricle. **D,** Tetralogy of Fallot. **E,** Total anomalous pulmonary venous return. AO, Aorta; IVC, inferior vena cava; LA, Left atrium; LV, left ventricle; PA, pulmonary artery; RA, right atrium; SVC, superior vena cava. *(From Marcdante KJ, Kliegman RM, Behrman RE, Jenson HB.* Nelson Essentials of Pediatrics. *6th ed. Philadelphia: Elsevier; 2010.)*

Four Fingers Up—Tetralogy of Fallot: Four fingers for **tetra**logy (tetra- means four, for four abnormalities).

- Developmental defect is **anterosuperior displacement of the infundibular septum** leading to **four abnormalities** that can be remembered with the **PROV**e mnemonic (**PROV**e that they have **tetralogy of Fallot**):
  - **P**ulmonary stenosis: Degree of stenosis correlates with prognosis.
  - **R**ight ventricular hypertrophy: A consequence of the high resistance against blood flow out of the right ventricle from the pulmonary stenosis. Leads to **"boot-shaped heart"** (coeur-en-sabot) on radiograph.
  - **O**verriding aorta.
  - **V**entricular septal defect.
- The **pulmonary stenosis** causes high resistance out of the right ventricle, causing **right ventricular hypertrophy** and deoxygenated blood to instead move **into the left ventricle through the VSD** but also directly from the right ventricle to the aorta because the **overriding aorta** often has connection to both ventricles.

- Patients suffer cyanotic spells called **"Tet spells"**—children learn to improve their cyanosis by **squatting,** which increases SVR (afterload) by putting pressure on the femoral arteries, leading to comparatively less resistance in the pulmonary circulation and therefore more blood going into the lungs through the stenotic pulmonary valve.
- This is the **most common** and **most commonly tested** cyanotic congenital heart disease.

Five Fingers Up—Total Anomalous Pulmonary Venous Return: Five fingers for the five words of **TAPVR.**

- Normally, the pulmonary veins drain into the left atrium; in TAPVR, the **pulmonary veins drain into the systemic venous circulation.** It is called **total** because **none of the pulmonary** veins correctly return to the left atrium.
- A shunt between the two atria such as an ASD or patent foramen ovale **must** be present or oxygenated blood will never reach the left side of the heart.

The **acyanotic** heart defects include **VSD** (most common), **ASD,** and **PDA** in descending order of frequency; these cause **left-to-right shunts,** whereby oxygenated blood is put back into the right side of the heart (Fig. 8.28). Although these do not typically cause problems in the neonate, eventually it can lead to **Eisenmenger syndrome.**

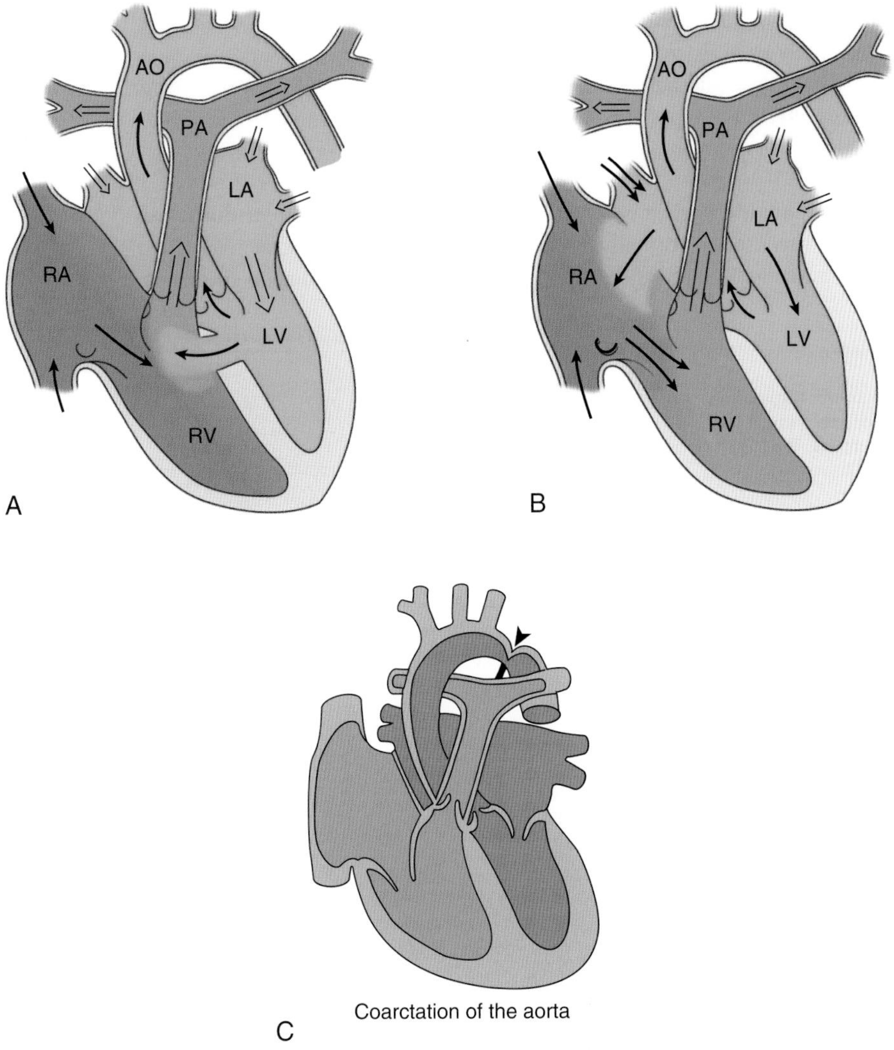

Fig. 8.28 A, Ventricular septal defect (VSD). **B,** Atrial septal defect (ASD). **C,** Coarctation of the aorta. AO, Aorta; IVC, inferior vena cava; LA, Left atrium; LV, left ventricle; PA, pulmonary artery; RA, right atrium. *(**A** and **B** from Marcdante KJ, Kliegman RM, Behrman RE, Jenson HB.* Nelson Essentials of Pediatrics. *6th ed. Philadelphia: Elsevier; 2010. **C** from Lissauer T, Clayden G.* Illustrated Textbook of Paediatrics. *4th ed. Edinburgh: Elsevier; 2011.)*

- **Eisenmenger syndrome:** With a left-to-right shunt, the right side of the heart receives additional blood, which is pumped through the pulmonary circulation. This additional flow causes hypertrophy of both the right side of the heart and the pulmonary vasculature. The hypertrophy and subsequent intimal narrowing of the pulmonary causes increased pulmonary resistance (recall resistance is proportional to $1/r^4$). Eventually, the pulmonary resistance increases enough that the left-to-right shunt now becomes a right-to-left shunt, leading to deoxygenated blood being shunted into the systemic circulation, with resulting cyanosis.

Lastly, **coarctation of the aorta** is a **narrowing** of the aorta most strongly associated with **Turner syndrome** (45,XO) and **bicuspid aortic valves** (see Fig. 8.28C).

In women with coarctation of the aorta, consider Turner syndrome.

- Narrowing causes **increased afterload** for the left ventricle, resulting in **left ventricular hypertrophy.** Because the narrowing is after the aortic arch vessels, there is no impediment to perfusing the "upper half" of the body (head and upper limbs).
- Long-standing coarctation can lead to **dilation of intercostal vessels** that act as collateral circulation, meaning that the blood flows in the reverse direction from intercostal vessels to aorta to allow blood to reach the legs; this causes a characteristic "rib notching" appearance on radiograph as a result of erosion of the ribs.
- Classic findings are **weak femoral pulses** and **differential cyanosis.** In neonates, the coarctation is "preductal," meaning the narrowing occurs before the ductus arteriosus; therefore, the lower half of the body can be cyanotic as a result of deoxygenated blood from the pulmonary artery being shunted through the ductus arteriosus into the aorta. Because the narrowing is after the aortic arch, the upper half of the body is perfused normally with oxygenated blood from the left ventricle: pink top, blue bottom = differential cyanosis. In children and adults, the diagnosis can also be made by measuring a systolic blood pressure difference between upper and lower extremities of more than 10 mm Hg.

Atherosclerosis

1. **Fatty streaks** (Figs. 8.29 and 8.30) are the beginning of atherosclerosis and start with **endothelial dysfunction.** The endothelium of the arteries normally makes vasodilating substances such as nitric oxide and also prevents fatty deposition. Chemical disruption such as toxins in **tobacco smoke** or

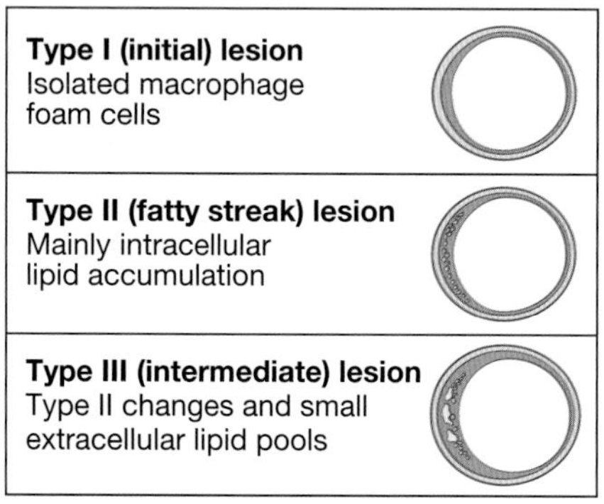
Type I (initial) lesion
Isolated macrophage foam cells
Type II (fatty streak) lesion
Mainly intracellular lipid accumulation
Type III (intermediate) lesion
Type II changes and small extracellular lipid pools

Fig. 8.29 Early atherosclerosis, demonstrating damaged, activated endothelium taking in monocytes (which become macrophages), which then phagocytose lipids, becoming foam cells. Atherosclerosis, often referred to as "hardened arteries" by lay people, causes roughly half of all deaths in developed countries by causing **cardiovascular disease** and **stroke.** Risk factors include **smoking, hypertension, diabetes, and dyslipidemia.** The most common site for atherosclerosis is the abdominal aorta, followed by the coronary arteries, popliteal arteries, and carotid arteries. The stages of plaque development include (1) fatty streak formation, and (2) atherosclerotic plaque progression and rupture. *(From Colledge NR, Walker BR, Ralston SH.* Davidson's Principles and Practice of Medicine. *21st ed. Philadelphia: Elsevier; 2010.)*

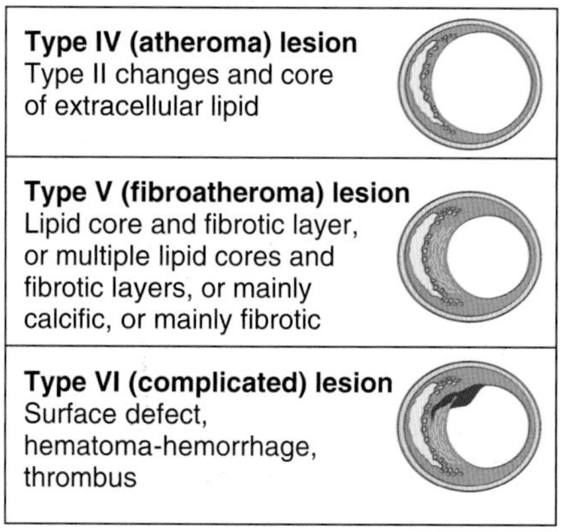
Type IV (atheroma) lesion
Type II changes and core of extracellular lipid
Type V (fibroatheroma) lesion
Lipid core and fibrotic layer, or multiple lipid cores and fibrotic layers, or mainly calcific, or mainly fibrotic
Type VI (complicated) lesion
Surface defect, hematoma-hemorrhage, thrombus

Fig. 8.30 Advanced atherosclerosis leading to significant stenosis (which in the coronary arteries can lead to stable angina), or complications such as plaque rupture with thrombus formation (which in the coronary arteries can lead to myocardial infarction if the thrombus occludes blood supply, or unstable angina if the thrombus is severe but nonocclusive). *(From Colledge NR, Walker BR, Ralston SH.* Davidson's Principles and Practice of Medicine. *21st ed. Philadelphia: Elsevier; 2010.)*

high levels of blood sugar in **diabetes** cause the endothelium to have lower defenses against lipid deposition. Physical disruption such as **high blood pressure** and turbulent flow such as at **arterial branch points** also promote lipid deposition. This endothelial damage allows low-density lipoprotein (LDL) cholesterol to slip under the endothelium. **Macrophages** then eat this LDL cholesterol, becoming **foam cells** that are too full to leave and are now stuck. **High cholesterol** exacerbates lipid deposition simply because there is more LDL cholesterol available in the blood.

2. **Plaque progression** occurs when the smooth muscle of the media migrates toward the intima, promoted by platelet-derived growth factor **(PDGF)** secreted by the resident foam cells. These smooth muscle cells produce extracellular matrix and lead to a fibrous plaque, which narrows the affected artery. Those plaques with large amounts of lipid, prolonged inflammation, or a thin fibrous layer are at risk for rupture. Plaque **rupture** exposes thrombogenic tissue (e.g., collagen) to coagulant factors in the blood that can generate **thrombi** with devastating consequences, such as a plaque rupturing in a coronary artery leading to myocardial infarction.

The main **complications** of this atherosclerotic process include **aneurysm formation** (especially in the abdominal aorta, where atherosclerosis is the main risk factor), **ischemia** (leading to angina in the coronary arteries, peripheral vascular disease, and claudication in the peripheral vasculature), and **clot formation** (leading to severe consequences such as myocardial infarction or stroke).

Hypertension

Known to the public simply as **high blood pressure,** hypertension is a major risk factor for numerous causes of morbidity and mortality, including **coronary artery disease, strokes, heart failure, and kidney failure** (Table 8.2). Because hypertension is often **asymptomatic,** it is termed the "silent killer." About 90% to 95% of hypertension is **essential (primary) hypertension,** and the remaining 5% to 10% is **secondary hypertension.**

Essential hypertension comes from a mix of genetic factors, obesity, lifestyle, and dietary factors. Secondary hypertension has discrete causes that are often curable if recognized, so the **causes of secondary hypertension** are important to keep in mind (note that most of these will be covered in detail in Chapter 9):

- **Renovascular hypertension:** In Chapter 9, the renin-angiotensin-aldosterone (RAA) system is explained in detail. Briefly, whenever the kidney's JG cells "see" less blood, they will think the blood pressure is low and act to increase it. If the renal arteries are stenotic, which in **older adults** occurs because of **atherosclerosis** and in **younger women** because of **fibromuscular dysplasia,** the JG cells will "see" less blood and secrete **renin** to **activate the RAA system** and increase the blood pressure. The increased **angiotensin II** causes vasoconstriction, and the increased **aldosterone** causes sodium retention. Diagnosis is by plasma renin activity; in the setting of high blood pressure, renin should be low, but it will be high in renovascular hypertension. Aldosterone levels will be high in both renovascular hypertension and primary aldosteronism, but renin levels will be low in the latter.
- **Primary aldosteronism (Conn syndrome):** Caused by an aldosterone-secreting (mineralocorticoid) tumor in the zona glomerulosa of the adrenal gland. Primary aldosteronism causes increased blood pressure by increased sodium retention by the kidney (see Chapter 9 for a description of other effects). Levels of aldosterone are high, but renin levels are low because the aldosterone is being secreted directly by the tumor.
- **Pheochromocytoma:** A catecholamine-secreting tumor most commonly found in the medulla of the adrenal gland (10%–15% are extraadrenal), causing paroxysmal hypertension and sporadic

Table 8.2 Stages of Hypertension

CLASSIFICATION	SYSTOLIC (mm Hg)	DIASTOLIC (mm Hg)
Normal	<120	<80
Prehypertensive	120–139	80–89
Stage I hypertension	140–159	90–99
Stage II hypertension	≥160	≥100

episodes of palpitations, diaphoresis, and headache as a result of intermittent release of epinephrine and norepinephrine.

- **Cushing syndrome:** Increased glucocorticoid levels as a result of (1) an exogenous cause, such as prescription steroids; (2) an adrenocorticotropic hormone (ACTH)–secreting tumor in the pituitary gland (Cushing disease); (3) an ectopic ACTH-secreting tumor (e.g., small cell carcinoma of the lung); or (4) a corticosteroid-secreting tumor of the zona fasciculata of the adrenal gland. ACTH stimulates corticosteroid secretion by the adrenal gland. The reason for increased blood pressure in Cushing syndrome is twofold: Glucocorticoids such as cortisol in high levels can attach to aldosterone receptors (thus functioning as mineralocorticoids) as well as cause increased sensitization to adrenergic agonists (α_1 stimulation vasoconstricts the peripheral vasculature, β stimulation increases cardiac output). Patients often have typical stigmata of Cushing syndrome such as moon facies (a round face), central obesity, hemorrhagic purple-red striae, and hirsutism.

Regardless of etiology, hypertension causes **increased afterload** on the left ventricle, potentially causing **heart failure** over time. In addition, direct arterial damage from the high pressures leads to **accelerated atherosclerosis,** which can promote myocardial infarction, stroke, and organ failure such as renal failure.

Ischemic Heart Disease

Ischemic heart disease occurs when there is an **imbalance of myocardial oxygen supply and demand,** leading to inadequate oxygenation of the myocardium. This can lead to **angina, myocardial infarction,** or **chronic ischemic heart disease.**

Angina is the squeezing or pressure-like sensation in the chest that patients have during myocardial ischemia. There are three types of angina that must be understood.

- **Stable angina:** Occurs during exertion, is relieved by rest, but is not worsening and is therefore stable. Typically secondary to stable nonocclusive atherosclerotic plaques in the coronary arteries (to be symptomatic, severity of stenosis typically must be at least 70%).
- **Unstable angina:** Angina that is worsening (such as with less exertion) or is occurring at rest. Unstable angina is often caused by nonocclusive coronary arterial thrombi, which could potentially become completely occlusive; therefore, this is a medical emergency because it may progress to a myocardial infarction.
- **Prinzmetal (variant) angina:** This angina usually occurs at rest and is not due to atherosclerosis but rather vascular spasm.
- **Chronic ischemic heart disease:** With chronic oxygen deprivation, progressive congestive heart failure (CHF) can be due to replacement of ischemic cardiac myocytes with noncontractile fibrous tissue over time.

Myocardial Infarction

Myocardial infarction (MI) is typically caused by thrombus formation from a disrupted atherosclerotic plaque in a coronary artery, resulting in **ischemia and death of myocardial tissue.** Whereas in stable and unstable angina no heart tissue dies from the ischemia, in MI there is coagulation necrosis. These MIs can either be a ST-elevation myocardial infarction (STEMI) or non–ST-elevation myocardial infarction (NSTEMI) (Fig. 8.31).

- STEMI: Ischemic and necrosis involving the entire thickness of myocardium as a result of occlusion of a coronary artery leading to ST-segment elevation on ECG. It is transmural because the coronary artery branches are responsible for perfusing all three layers of the heart; blockage causes cessation of blood flow to all these layers.
- NSTEMI: Ischemia and necrosis is usually involving only the innermost part of the heart. The subendocardial area is the farthest from the coronary arteries and therefore is the last to be perfused with the fewest collaterals supplying it; in addition, the contracting myocardium exerts high pressure in this area, reducing blood flow further. This usually is due to hypoperfusion from either generalized hypotension or a coronary artery that is not completely occluded but rather is narrowed enough to cause death of the most starved myocardial tissue. There is usually ST-segment depression on ECG.

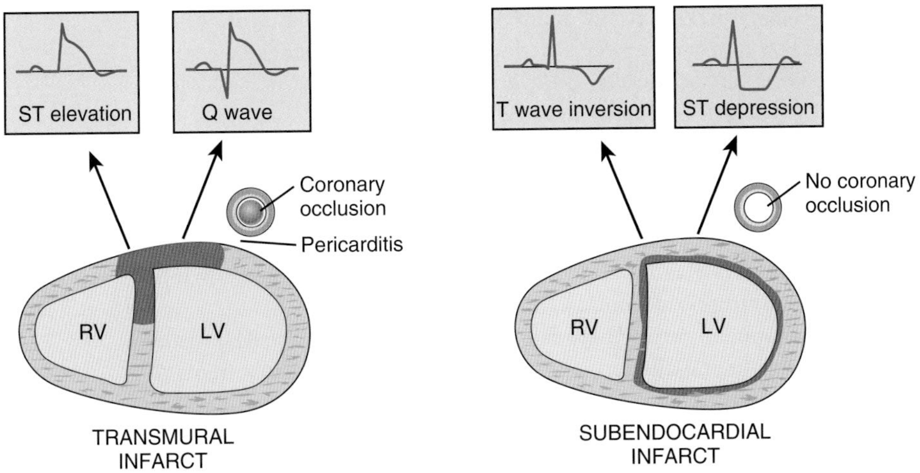

FIG. 8.31 Difference between transmural infarction and subendocardial infarction. The endocardium is the most oxygen-deprived area of the heart and is at risk for infarction with hypoperfusion. LV, Left ventricle. *(From Damjanov I.* Pathophysiology. *Philadelphia: Elsevier; 2008.)*

The **ECG** is very helpful and can show ST-segment changes as well as pathologic Q waves (Q waves more than one-third the height of the QRS complex; this can be a permanent change after an MI). The ECG is what is used to initially diagnose a STEMI; in the correct clinical setting, the patient should be treated with cardiac catheterization immediately (or, if unavailable, thrombolytics). When myocytes die, their cellular contents are released into the bloodstream and aid in the diagnosis of an MI. **Troponin I** rises within 4 hours and stays elevated for 1 week, whereas **CK-MB** (creatine kinase) rises essentially as fast as troponin (range of 3–8 hours) but normalizes after about 3 days. CK-MB is also less specific than troponin elevation because it may be released from cells other than just cardiac myocytes, such as skeletal myocytes. A positive troponin and/or CK-MB in the correct clinical setting establishes the diagnosis of an NSTEMI (as long as the ECG does not demonstrate a STEMI).

There are many **complications** of MI, from the second it happens to weeks afterward (Fig. 8.32).

- **Arrhythmia:** Fatal arrhythmias are a common cause of death before hospitalization (in the hospital, arrhythmias are usually immediately recognized and treated because of cardiac monitoring and access to defibrillation). Damaged cell membranes and sections of dead myocardium all promote abnormal conduction and arrhythmias. **Ventricular fibrillation** is the most common fatal arrhythmia in acute MI (see Fig. 8.21).

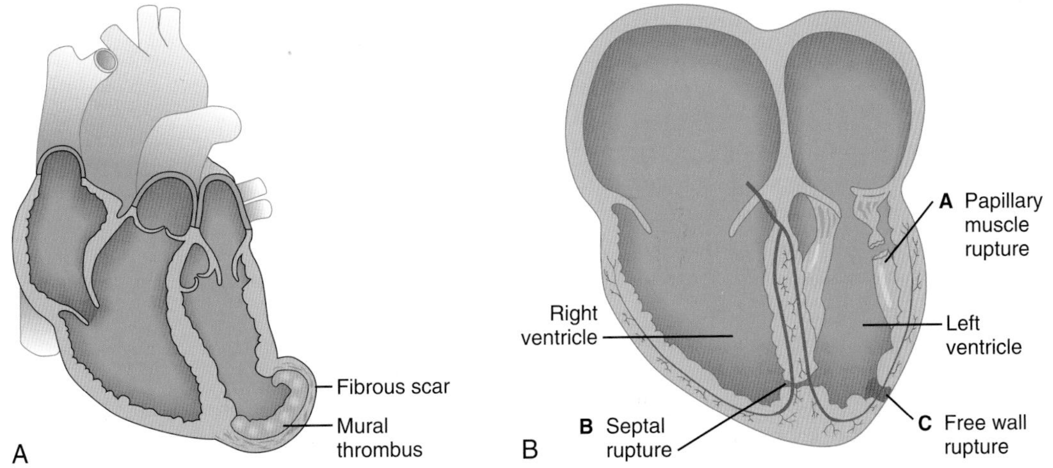

FIG. 8.32 Selected complications of myocardial infarction. **A,** Ventricular aneurysm without rupture, leading to stasis of blood in the aneurysm and mural thrombus formation. **B,** Papillary muscle rupture, septal rupture, and free wall rupture. *(From Damjanov I.* Pathophysiology. *Philadelphia: Elsevier; 2008.)*

- **Myocardial dysfunction:** With the death of myocardium and possible ongoing ischemia, the ability of the heart to function as a pump is compromised. With large MIs, cardiogenic shock can occur immediately, causing severely decreased cardiac output and hypotension, but delayed heart failure can also occur.
- **Papillary muscle rupture:** With some MIs involving the left ventricle, the papillary muscle can rupture, leading to acute mitral regurgitation because the chordae tendineae no longer function to prevent regurgitation.
- **Ventricular free wall rupture:** Usually occurs when macrophages begin to remove necrotic areas, causing a weakening, typically between days 3 and 7 after an MI. This leads to rapid bleeding into the pericardium, resulting in pericardial tamponade and death.
- **Ventricular aneurysm:** A late complication occurring between 1 and 2 months after the MI; weakening of the ventricular wall leads to fibrosis and dilation *without* rupture (unlike ventricular free wall rupture, which is a relatively early complication *with* rupture). This is a late complication because fibrosis takes time, just like scar formation. The fibrotic aneurysmal area cannot contract, leading to congestive heart failure and potential clot formation in the ventricle from stasis of blood (mural thrombus, like the mural on a wall, covered in clot).
- **Fibrinous pericarditis:** Early after an MI (within the first week), the inflammation caused by the necrosis of myocardium can cause increased vessel permeability and exudate formation. This is directly caused by inflammation, unlike Dressler syndrome.
- **Dressler syndrome (autoimmune fibrinous pericarditis):** When myocardium dies, it releases cellular contents that the immune system has not seen before (previously sequestered in cells); the body can see these as foreign and develop an autoimmune response to them. This leads to autoimmune pericarditis that usually occurs 1 to 2 months after the MI.

Heart failure is **inability of the heart to supply sufficient blood flow** to meet the demands of the body, causing specific symptoms and signs depending on which side of the heart is affected. Heart failure can occur from either (or both) of two types of dysfunction: **systolic dysfunction** and **diastolic dysfunction.**

- **Systolic dysfunction**: A problem with **ejection of blood during systole,** characterized by a **low ejection fraction** (normal, ≥55%). There is no problem in filling; the heart is full but cannot eject the blood that it needs to. This can be because the heart either cannot contract well (**poor contractility,** secondary to **ischemia or infarction** or **cardiomyopathy**) or is contracting against too great of an **afterload** (aortic stenosis, severe hypertension).
- **Diastolic dysfunction:** A problem with **filling in diastole,** typically with a **preserved** (normal or near-normal) **ejection fraction.** This typically is due to a **stiff ventricle** from hypertrophy, fibrosis, or restrictive diseases (restrictive cardiomyopathy, pericardial tamponade). In this case the stiff ventricle cannot relax enough to fill adequately, but the ventricle can eject the little blood it receives without difficulty.
- Heart failure can also be divided into **left-sided heart failure, right-sided heart failure, and biventricular failure.**

Systolic dysfunction: problem ejecting blood in systole (decreased EF)

Diastolic dysfunction: problem filling in diastole (normal EF)

Left-sided heart failure: pulmonary edema, orthopnea, paroxysmal nocturnal dyspnea, pulmonary hypertension

Left-sided heart failure occurs when the left ventricle cannot eject sufficient blood into the aorta, causing the blood to back up into the lungs, producing **pulmonary edema.** Systolic dysfunction from ischemia and myocardial infarction is a common cause of left-sided heart failure, although diastolic dysfunction can occur as well. The higher pressures in the pulmonary system lead to increased afterload for the right ventricle, which can subsequently lead to right-sided heart failure (Fig. 8.33). Most of the manifestations of left-sided heart failure are symptoms rather than signs.

- **Pulmonary edema:** Transudation of fluid into alveoli caused by increased hydrostatic pressure in the pulmonary capillaries because the left side of the heart can no longer pump that fluid out. This fluid also causes the physical examination finding of **bibasilar inspiratory crackles** because inspiration forces air into fluid-filled alveoli that are edematous. Often, there may be small hemorrhages, which is why patients with pulmonary edema often cough up a pink frothy liquid. Macrophages eat the blood hemorrhaged into the alveoli but retain the hemosiderin; microscopically, these hemosiderin-laden macrophages (siderophages) are called **heart-failure cells.**

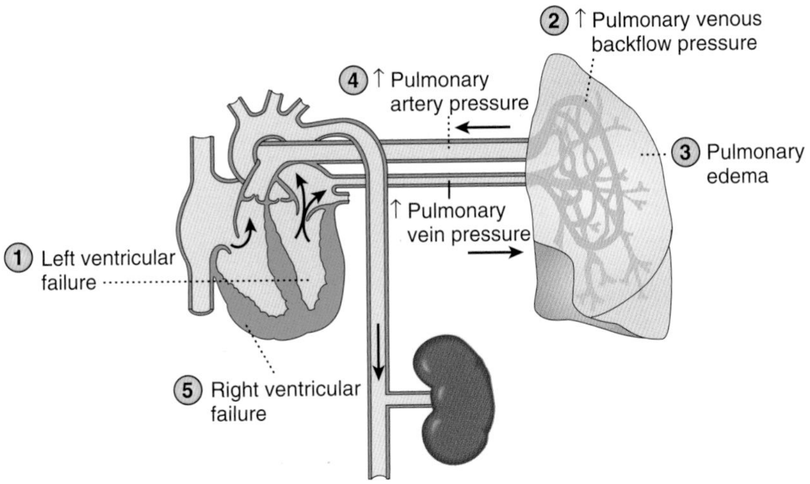

FIG. 8.33 Left-sided heart failure, demonstrating blood "backing up" into the lungs, causing pulmonary edema, pulmonary hypertension, and cor pulmonale (right-sided heart failure from pulmonary hypertension). *(From Damjanov I. Pathophysiology. Philadelphia: Elsevier; 2008.)*

- **Orthopnea:** Difficulty breathing while lying supine, as a result of **increased venous return** because gravity is no longer impeding blood from returning to the heart. This exacerbates the volume overload because the left ventricle cannot pump the added fluid, leading to worsening pulmonary edema. Often, patients will **sleep with multiple pillows,** propping themselves upright in an attempt to reduce venous return to the heart.
- **Paroxysmal nocturnal dyspnea (PND):** This also causes difficulty breathing while lying supine but **takes hours to occur,** usually after the patient has fallen asleep. Unlike in orthopnea, when blood already in the vasculature returns to the heart, in PND the interstitial edema outside of the vasculature reaccumulates into the vasculature and returns to the heart.
- **S_3/S_4 sound:** The S_3 sound, as previously discussed, occurs during the rapid-filling phase of diastole and is a marker for fluid overload. The S_4 sound occurs when the atrial kick attempts to force more blood into a stiff or overfilled ventricle. Both sounds can be present in left-sided heart failure.

Right-sided heart failure: jugular venous distention, congestive hepatomegaly, peripheral edema

Right-sided heart failure (Fig. 8.34) occurs when the right ventricle cannot eject sufficient blood into the pulmonary artery, causing blood to back up into the rest of the body (not the lungs). It is worth noting that **the most common cause of right-sided heart failure is left-sided heart failure.** Left-sided heart failure causes fluid overload in the lungs, increasing the afterload for the right ventricle, eventually contributing to the failure of the right ventricle. When the right ventricle fails as a result of pulmonary hypertension in the absence of left ventricular dysfunction, it is termed **cor pulmonale;** examples include increased pulmonary resistance (afterload) from destruction of pulmonary vasculature from lung diseases such as chronic obstructive pulmonary disease, obstructive sleep apnea, or blood clots blocking branches of the pulmonary artery (pulmonary embolism). Rather than symptoms, most of the manifestations of right-sided heart failure are signs.

- **Jugular venous distention (JVD):** Backup of blood from the right ventricle moves into the right atrium and the veins feeding it. The increased venous hydrostatic pressure can be measured at the internal jugular vein.
- **Edema:** The increased hydrostatic pressure also forces fluid out of the capillary beds into the interstitial tissue in the periphery (similar to how increased pulmonary hydrostatic pressure in left-sided heart failure causes pulmonary edema). Usually, the edema is **dependent,** meaning it occurs in the areas where gravity further increases hydrostatic pressure (ankles for those sitting or upright, sacrum for those supine).
- **Hepatomegaly:** Because the hepatic veins drain into the vena cava, blood will back up into the liver as well, causing liver congestion. In severe cases, this can cause ascites or even cirrhosis if the pressure in the liver impedes portal vein drainage into the liver. Because the now-congested liver holds much blood, the physical examination maneuver "hepatojugular reflux" can be used to accentuate the JVD in those with heart failure. This hepatomegaly can be painful.

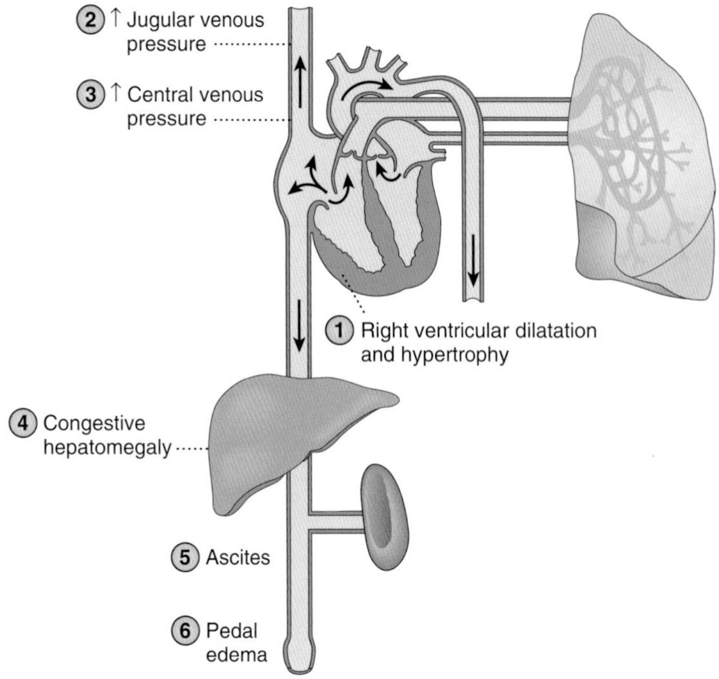

FIG. 8.34 Right-sided heart failure, demonstrating blood "backing up" into the body, including the jugular veins (jugular venous distension on physical examination), the liver (congestive hepatomegaly), and the capillary beds of the systemic circulation (dependent edema). *(From Damjanov I.* Pathophysiology. *Philadelphia: Elsevier; 2008.)*

Cardiomyopathies

There are **three cardiomyopathies** (Fig. 8.35): **dilated, hypertrophic, and restrictive** (in order of decreasing prevalence). Any of these can cause symptoms of **heart failure,** described previously.

Dilated cardiomyopathy is the **most common,** accounting for 90% of cases (see Fig. 8.35B).

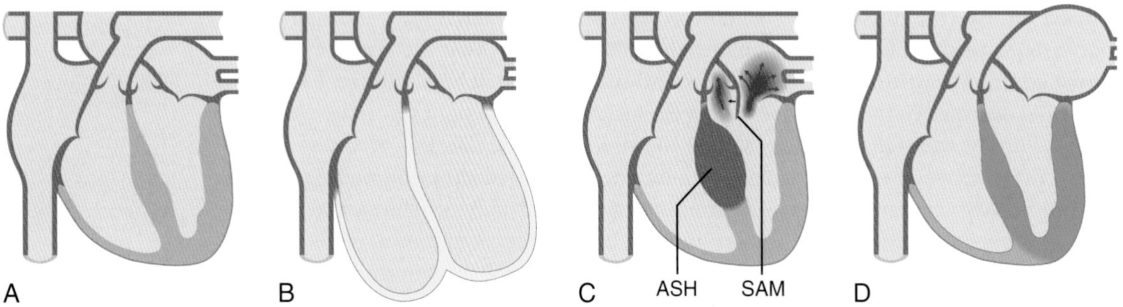

FIG. 8.35 Cardiomyopathies. **A,** Normal heart. **B,** Dilated cardiomyopathy. **C,** Hypertrophic cardiomyopathy. **D,** Restrictive cardiomyopathy. ASH, Asymmetric septal hypertrophy; SAM, systolic anterior motion (of the mitral valve). *(From Colledge NR, Walker BR, Ralston SH.* Davidson's Principles and Practice of Medicine. *21st ed. Philadelphia: Elsevier; 2010.)*

- **Etiology:** Most commonly **idiopathic** but also caused by **alcohol and drugs** (both illicit drugs such as cocaine and medications such as the chemotherapeutic agent doxorubicin); it can also occur during pregnancy and after **myocarditis** (most commonly viral myocarditis from **coxsackievirus** but also from Chagas disease, caused by the trypanosome *Trypanosoma cruzi*).
- **Findings:** A globally dilated heart (eccentric hypertrophy) with poor contractility leads to **systolic failure** (meaning low ejection fraction). Dilation of the valve ring seats causes valves to no longer line up correctly, leading to **mitral and tricuspid regurgitation.** Poor ejection leads to fluid overload leading to an **S_3 heart sound.** Typical symptoms of **heart failure** are present.
- **Treatment:** Medical therapy is similar to congestive heart failure, but cardiac transplantation may be necessary if refractory to treatment.

Hypertrophic cardiomyopathy (previously called idiopathic hypertrophic subaortic stenosis) is a common cause of syncope and sudden death in young athletes and in those with Friedreich ataxia (see Fig. 8.35C).

Hypertrophic cardiomyopathy: autosomal dominant, common cause of sudden death in young athletes

- **Etiology:** Most commonly this is familial, with autosomal dominant inheritance.
- **Findings:** There is asymmetric hypertrophy near the ventricular septum (concentric hypertrophy), leading to possible obstruction of flow out of the left ventricle. The narrowed outflow tract leads to a Venturi phenomenon, in which the high velocity of blood being ejected through the narrowed opening causes the anterior leaflet of the mitral valve to be pulled toward the septum during systole (termed systolic anterior motion [SAM] of the mitral valve), closing the outflow tract. The narrowing also causes a systolic crescendo–decrescendo murmur similar to that of aortic stenosis. An S_4 heart sound is also common in hypertrophic cardiomyopathy.
- The intensity of the murmur of hypertrophic cardiomyopathy is inversely related to the preload. Increased preload causes the ventricle to fill more, increasing the diameter of the outflow tract and therefore decreasing the intensity of the murmur. A poorly filled ventricle will have a much more narrow outflow tract and a louder murmur. The Valsalva maneuver (forcible exhalation against a closed glottis) causes a transient rise in intrathoracic pressure, which prevents venous return, causing decreased preload and a more harsh murmur. Squatting compresses lower extremity veins, increasing venous return and thus preload, decreasing the murmur intensity; standing will cause venous pooling from gravity and decreased preload. This concept is important because the murmur sounds similar to that of aortic stenosis; but in aortic stenosis, the increased preload leads to a louder murmur (more blood being ejected through the stenotic valve), whereas in hypertrophic cardiomyopathy, the increased preload leads to a softer murmur (larger ventricular volumes lead to a larger outflow tract and less obstruction).
- **Treatment:** Ensure that the ventricular chamber volumes are always relatively high to lessen the obstruction. Beta blockers or calcium channel blockers are used to ensure that the heart rate does not increase (which would decrease filling time and lead to smaller chamber volumes) and that the contractility does not increase (which would lead to smaller ventricular volumes from increased stroke volumes and worsening obstruction).

Restrictive cardiomyopathy is characterized by **rigid, noncompliant ventricles,** which may be able to contract normally (normal systolic function and therefore normal ejection fraction) but **cannot fill correctly** as a result of their rigidity **(diastolic dysfunction)** (see Fig. 8.35D).

- **Etiology:** Most commonly caused by **amyloidosis,** a systemic disease in which abnormal proteins are deposited in the body's organs and can be detected on biopsy with a **Congo red stain,** which demonstrates **apple-green birefringence.** In addition, **sarcoidosis, hemochromatosis,** and **postirradiation fibrosis** are common causes of this uncommon cardiomyopathy.
- **Findings:** Symptoms of **heart failure** are present. Fibrosis of the conduction system can lead to arrhythmias.
- **Treatment:** Unfortunately, there is no treatment for restrictive cardiomyopathy except to treat the condition responsible for it. Treatment of volume overload with diuretics can be beneficial for symptomatic relief.

Rheumatic Fever

Rheumatic fever (RF) occurs in about 1% of cases of untreated group A *Streptococcus* (GAS) pharyngitis ("strep throat"); with the advent of antibiotic treatment, RF has become rare in developed countries. (Note: Although poststreptococcal glomerulonephritis can occur after either a skin or pharynx infection with GAS and cannot be prevented with antibiotics, only a pharyngeal infection with GAS can cause RF, and this can be prevented with antibiotics.) This is primarily a disease of **childhood and adolescence** because children more often have strep throat. These bacteria have a protein called **M protein;** when the immune system makes antibodies to the M protein, they can cross-react with proteins on the heart, leading to symptoms (a type II hypersensitivity reaction). The criteria for diagnosis are called the **Jones criteria,** and the mnemonic **JONES** can help you remember the main parts of this:

- Joints: This is classically described as a **migratory arthritis** that affects many joints but **leaves no permanent damage.** Most patients with RF will have this symptom.
- Obvious (the heart!): Rheumatic fever affects the heart, so it can damage the heart. This can range from **endocarditis** leading to valve damage and risk for future infective endocarditis, to **myocarditis** (inflammation of the cardiac muscle itself, which can be fatal), to **pericarditis.** RF can thus easily become **rheumatic heart disease** (with permanent damage to the heart)!

- Nodules: Subcutaneous nodules that are painless and firm can appear, typically over bones or tendons.
- Erythema marginatum: An erythematous macular rash that spreads out, leaving a clearing in the middle.
- Sydenham chorea (St. Vitus dance): Chorea refers to involuntary abnormal movements (from the Greek word for "dance"); Sydenham chorea affects all limbs and can occur months after initial infection.

Infective Endocarditis

Endocarditis is inflammation of the endocardium, usually involving the **heart valves.** Although there are noninfectious causes of endocarditis, such as Libman-Sacks endocarditis (LSE) from immune complex deposition in autoimmune diseases such as systemic lupus erythematosus (SLE—remember SLE causes LSE!), infectious endocarditis is the most common endocarditis and the most highly tested on the USMLE Step 1.

Infectious endocarditis can be either **acute** or **subacute,** which is mostly dependent on the virulence of the organism causing the infection. Although damaged valves are easier for bacteria to latch on to because of irregularities in the surface, normal valves can be affected by virulent bacteria. Any time there is a patient with **fever** and a **heart murmur** (valve damaged from the infection), consider endocarditis.

- **Acute:** Usually caused by *Staphylococcus aureus,* which can infect normal valves and aggressively destroy them. This is characterized by large vegetations, rapid onset, and patients who are very sick. **IV drug use** is the most common etiology; unsterile injection technique seeds *S. aureus* from the skin directly into the veins. Because the veins bring blood back to the right atrium, the **tricuspid valve** is the first valve the *S. aureus* encounters and is the **most commonly affected valve** in acute infectious endocarditis in IV drug users.
- **Subacute:** Usually caused by less virulent bacteria such as viridans group streptococci, which are found as normal oral flora in humans and routinely find their way into the bloodstream during toothbrushing and dentist visits. Because they are low virulence, they require **damaged valves** to attach and cause progressive and less dramatic symptoms compared with acute endocarditis. The **most common valve affected** in **subacute** infectious endocarditis is the **mitral valve** because it is often damaged by **rheumatic fever,** followed by the aortic valve.
- Other bacteria deserve mention, although they are much less common. *Streptococcus bovis* endocarditis can be found in patients with **colorectal cancer.** *Staphylococcus epidermidis* is implicated in endocarditis involving **prosthetic valves** because of its ability to generate a **biofilm** on the prosthesis. There is a group of bacteria that do not grow on standard bacterial cultures (because they need a special environment to survive that is not provided by the culture medium) and therefore cause endocarditis with "negative" cultures, the **HACEK** group of bacteria (***H**aemophilus, **A**ggregatibacter, **C**ardiobacterium, **E**ikenella, **K**ingella*).

There are many **symptoms and signs** of endocarditis, although all may not be present in each patient. A common mnemonic is endocarditis **FROM JANE** (because **Janeway** lesions can be present in endocarditis!):

- **F**ever: **Most common symptom,** caused by an immune response to infection of valve.
- **R**oth spots (Fig. 8.36A): Caused by immune complex deposition in the **retina (Roth = retina),** producing inflammation and **white exudate** formation with **hemorrhages,** visible on funduscopic examination.
- **O**sler nodes (Fig. 8.36B): **Painful,** violaceous nodules on the extremities caused by immune complex deposition (**O**sler nodes are painful, **O**uch!).
- **M**urmur: New heart murmur caused by infection and vegetation of the valve.
- **J**aneway lesion: **Nontender,** small hemorrhagic lesions often found on the extremities; can be differentiated from Osler nodes because Janeway lesions are nontender.
- **A**nemia: Anemia of chronic disease secondary to chronic inflammation.
- **N**ailbed (splinter) hemorrhages (Fig. 8.36C): Linear reddish-brown lesions that look like splinters found under the nailbed.
- **E**mboli: Small pieces of the vegetation on the valve can break off, leading to pulmonary emboli (if the right side of the heart is affected) or strokes and peripheral organ infarction (if the left side of the heart is affected).

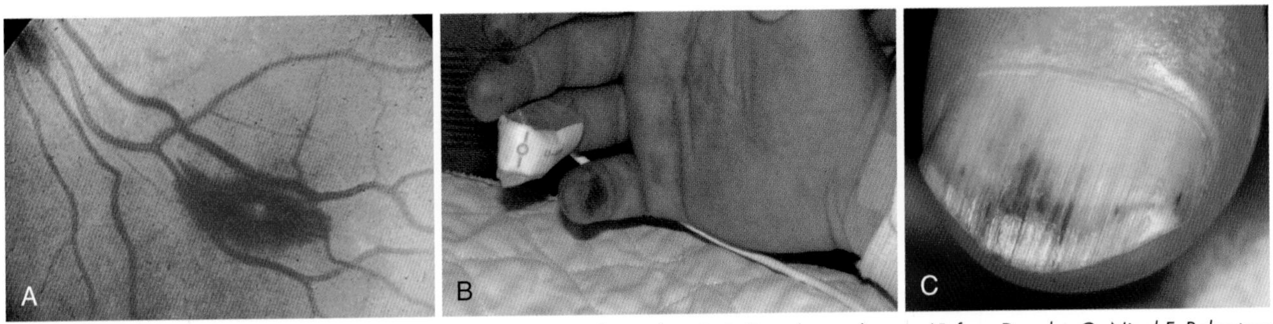

FIG. 8.36 Clinical findings in endocarditis. **A,** Roth spots. **B,** Osler nodes. **C,** Splinter hemorrhages. *(**A** from Douglas G, Nicol F, Robertson C. MacLeod's Clinical Examination. 11th ed. Philadelphia: Elsevier; 2005. **B** from Goldman L, Ausiello D. Cecil's Textbook of Medicine. 23rd ed. Philadelphia: Elsevier; 2008. **C** from Swartz M. Textbook of Physical Diagnosis: History and Examination. 5th ed. Philadelphia: Saunders; 2006:147.)*

Diagnosis is by history and physical examination, **echocardiography** to visualize the vegetation or valvular abnormality, and **blood cultures** to isolate the organism. Treatment is **antibiotics,** usually for at least a month!

Pericardial Disease

Pericarditis is the most common disease of the pericardium, characterized by inflammation that can be caused by a wide variety of agents. It can be either **infectious** (more common) or **noninfectious.**

- **Infectious: Coxsackie B virus** (most common), tuberculosis, other bacteria.
- **Noninfectious:** Uremia (secondary to renal failure), autoimmune (SLE, Dressler syndrome), nearby inflammation (post-MI, myocarditis), metastatic cancer.

The diagnosis of pericarditis can be made both by history and physical examination but also by an ECG.

- **Findings:** Classically, patients will have **chest pain relieved by sitting forward;** on cardiac auscultation, they may have a **pericardial friction rub** because the inflamed pericardium no longer provides a smooth surface for the heart to beat against.
- **ECG:** Because of diffuse inflammation, the ECG shows **diffuse ST-segment elevation** and **PR-segment depression.** The ST-segment elevation can be differentiated from that of a STEMI because it encompasses the entire heart, whereas an MI affects only sections of the heart supplied by the occluded artery.

Although pericarditis is often self-limited and benign, possible complications include **pericardial effusion** (with possible cardiac tamponade) and **constrictive pericarditis.**

- **Pericardial effusion** (Fig. 8.37): The inflammation can lead to fluid accumulation in the pericardial sac. Because the pericardium is fibrous and does not stretch easily, **acute accumulation of fluid in the pericardium can be dangerous and lead to cardiac tamponade.** Chronic fluid accumulation in the pericardium allows for stretching of the pericardium; therefore, larger volumes can build up without causing tamponade. A **hemorrhagic effusion** most likely is due to **tuberculous or malignant pericarditis.** With a large effusion, **electrical alternans** (see Fig. 8.37B) can occur; the heart is essentially swinging in a large effusion and causes the recordings to alternate depending on whether the heart is moving toward or away from the chest wall.
- **Constrictive pericarditis:** The inflammation can lead to scarring, where the two pericardial layers adhere to each other and fill with fibrous tissue, preventing filling of the heart.
- **Cardiac tamponade** is a life-threatening emergency. The heart **becomes compressed** by fluid in the pericardium, preventing filling of the ventricles and subsequently decreased cardiac output. This can be secondary to an effusion or bleeding caused by trauma (such as a knife through the heart), ventricular wall rupture, or extension of an aortic dissection into the heart (see Fig. 8.37A).
- **Beck's triad** (constellation of three findings in tamponade): **hypotension** from decreased cardiac output, **jugular venous distention** from blood backing up into the veins because the heart cannot fill, and **muffled heart sounds** because the heart is being strangled with fluid.

Cardiac tamponade: heart cannot fill because of pressure exerted by pericardial effusion.
Beck's triad of hypotension, jugular venous distention, muffled heart sounds.

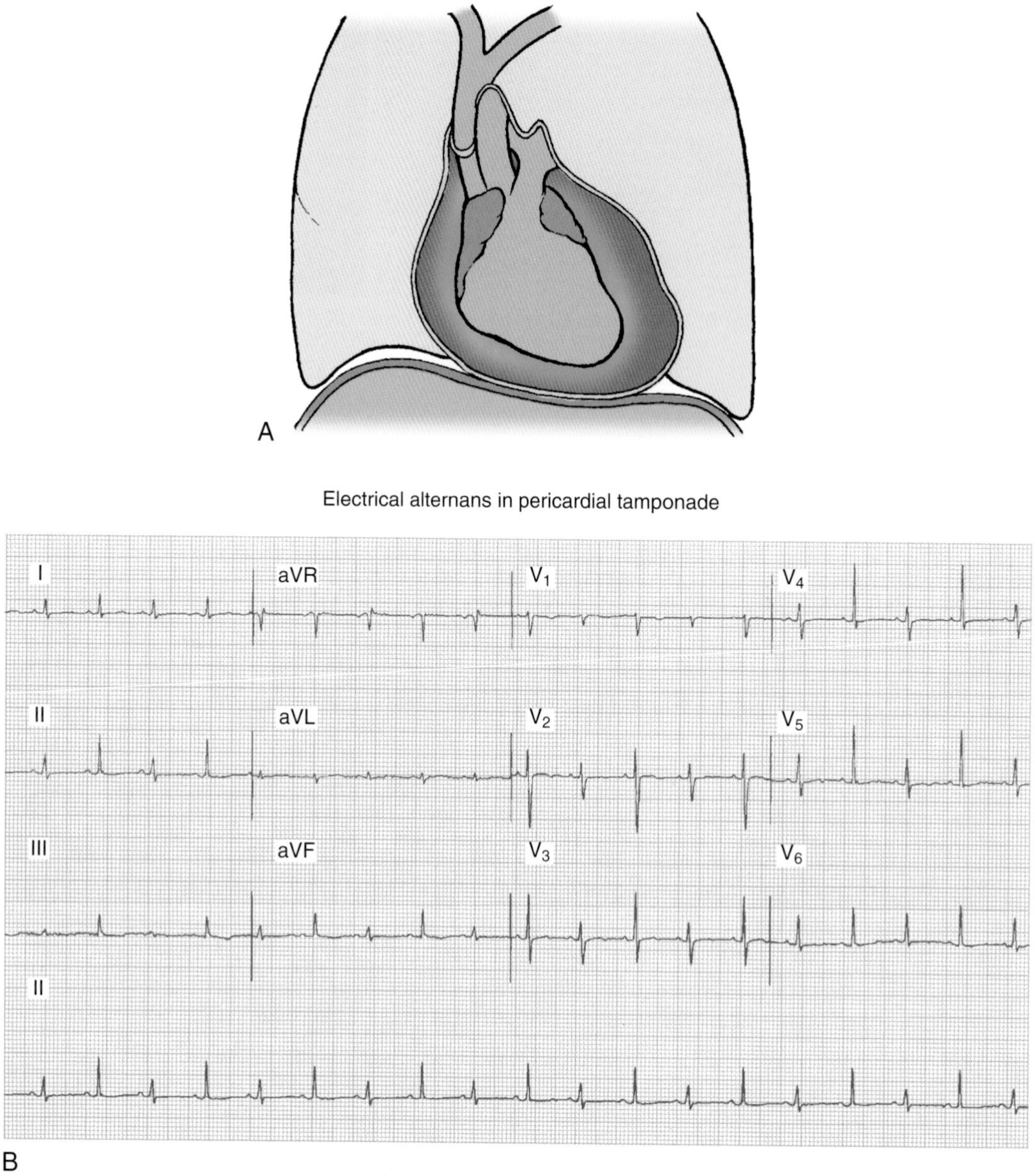

Fig. 8.37 Pericardial effusion. **A,** Image showing significant fluid in the pericardial space. **B,** Electrical alternans, an ECG finding in which a larger effusion causes the heart to "swing" back and forth in the fluid. *(**A** from Dandy DJ, Edwards DJ.* Essential Orthopedics and Trauma. *5th ed. Philadelphia: Elsevier; 2009.* ***B** from Goldberger AL, Goldberger ZD, Shvilkin A.* Clinical Electrocardiography: A Simplified Approach. *8th ed. Philadelphia: Saunders; 2012.)*

- **Pulsus paradoxus** can also be present in tamponade and is an exaggeration of a normal physiologic response. During inspiration, the negative intrathoracic pressure increases venous return to the right side of the heart, filling the right ventricle with more volume. This larger filling of the right ventricle causes the septum between the right and left ventricles to bow toward the left ventricle, reducing left ventricular filling and causing a small decrease in cardiac output and thus blood pressure. In **cardiac tamponade,** because there is so little room in the heart, this effect is exaggerated and the **blood pressure drops by more than 10 mm Hg during inspiration,** called **pulsus paradoxus.**

Treatment of pericarditis involves treating the underlying cause when possible (such as dialysis in uremic pericarditis) as well as using antiinflammatory medications to prevent the inflamed pericardium from developing an effusion or scarring. With tamponade, immediate **pericardiocentesis** (needle drainage of the fluid) is indicated.

Vasculitides

Vasculitis refers to inflammation of the blood vessels, which can be classified as **small vessel vasculitis** (affecting small vessels such as capillaries), **medium vessel vasculitis** (affecting smaller muscular arteries), and **large vessel vasculitis** (affecting the large elastic arteries such as the aorta) (Table 8.3).

Cardiac and Vascular Tumors

Cardiac tumors are uncommon. There are essentially two tumors to remember: (1) **myxomas,** which are found in adults; and (2) **rhabdomyomas,** which are found in children.

- **Myxomas** are almost always found in the left atrium and have the potential to act as a "ball valve" where during diastole, when blood flows from left atrium to left ventricle, the tumor moves with it and blocks flow. This flow obstruction can lead to a transient drop in cardiac output and syncopal

Left atrial myxomas: ball–valve phenomenon cuts off filling of left ventricle, leading to syncope; also can embolize and cause strokes

Table 8.3 Vasculitis Syndromes

DISORDER AND VESSELS AFFECTED	INFORMATION
LARGE VESSEL VASCULITIS	
Takayasu arteritis (pulseless disease) Affects **Aortic arch**	**Affects young Asian women;** called "pulseless disease" because granulomatous damage/narrowing of aortic arch vessels and subclavian artery cause a loss of pulses in upper extremity. Symptoms of **systemic** inflammation occur, such as **fever, weight loss, fatigue, muscle aching.** Skin nodules can also be present. Narrowing of carotid arteries can lead to strokes and visual defects.
Giant cell arteritis (temporal arteritis) Affects **Branches of the carotid arteries** **Superficial temporal artery** **Ophthalmic artery**	**Affects adults** (mostly women) **older than 50 years,** causing inflammation of **branches of the carotid artery.** This leads to **headache,** pain with chewing from stretching of the inflamed artery **(jaw claudication), blindness** from ophthalmic artery involvement, and systemic symptoms such as **fever.** Associated with **elevated ESR,** which is sensitive but not specific. **Half of patients will have polymyalgia rheumatica.** When suspected, **start steroids immediately** and biopsy after— do not wait for biopsy results or blindness may occur!
MEDIUM VESSEL VASCULITIS	
Polyarteritis nodosa Affects **Medium-sized vessels *other than* the pulmonary arteries. (i.e., renal, coronary, arteries to skin, gut)**	**Affects adult men and those with hepatitis B,** causing varied symptoms that depend on which arteries are involved (hence **poly**arteritis—many different arteries affected in different stages): abdominal pain and/or bloody stool (GI arteries), renal failure (renal arteries), skin ulcers (skin arteries), myocardial infarction (coronary arteries). It is important that **the lungs are essentially never affected—important to distinguish this from Wegener granulomatosis. Treat with steroids.**
Granulomatosis with polyangiitis (GPA) (formerly Wegener granulomatosis) Affects **Lung and kidney vessels**	**Affects children and adolescents;** known as a **pulmonary-renal disease** because it primarily affects the lungs and kidneys. This is different from polyarteritis nodosa because the **lung** (both upper airway and lung parenchyma) **is affected in GPA.** Classic findings are **chronic sinusitis with nasal septal perforation** (saddle-nose deformity), hemoptysis from lung involvement, and hematuria from renal involvement. **c-ANCA** is a marker of disease. Treat with cyclophosphamide and steroids. Remember the Cs of GPA: **c-ANCA, corticosteroids, cyclophosphamide.**
Kawasaki disease Affects **Coronary arteries**	**Affects mostly Asian children,** with the potential to cause coronary aneurysms and myocardial infarctions if untreated! Suspect this in **any child with a fever for ≥ 5 days!** Mnemonic **CRASH and burn:** **C**onjunctivitis, **R**ash, **A**denopathy (cervical), **S**trawberry tongue, **H**and or feet changes/swelling/desquamation and **burn** (fever ≥5 days). Treatment is IV immunoglobulin and aspirin (the only time you ever give a child aspirin—remember the association with Reye syndrome!).
Thromboangiitis obliterans (Buerger disease) Affects	**Affects smokers,** causing inflammation and thrombosis of the arteries supplying the hands and feet, leading to claudication, cold sensitivity, ischemic pain, and eventually gangrene with autoamputation of digits. Treatment is **smoking cessation.**
HAND AND FOOT VESSELS	
Raynaud disease Affects **Hand and foot vessels**	Raynaud **disease** is an isolated disease causing inflammation and vasoconstriction in response to cold or stress leading to white digits (lack of blood flow), progressing to blue (cyanosis), and red (reactive hyperemia when blood flow is restored). Treatment is **calcium channel blockers** and **avoiding cold.**

Table 8.3 Vasculitis Syndromes—cont'd

DISORDER AND VESSELS AFFECTED	INFORMATION
Raynaud phenomenon Affects **Hand and foot vessels**	Raynaud **phenomenon** is a phenomenon that **occurs with other autoimmune diseases** such as limited scleroderma (CREST syndrome) and systemic lupus erythematosus. Raynaud phenomenon is usually more severe than Raynaud disease.
SMALL VESSEL VASCULITIS	
Microscopic polyangiitis Affects **Small vessels of skin, lung, kidneys, and other organs**	Presentation can be **similar to Wegener** granulomatosis with lung and kidney involvement, but **there are no granulomas,** unlike in Wegener **granulomatosis.** Small vessel inflammation leads to **palpable purpura**—this is due to inflamed hemorrhagic vessels near the skin. Also associated with ANCA, but **p-ANCA.** Remember the **Ps of microscopic polyangiitis: p-ANCA, palpable purpura.**
Churg-Strauss syndrome Affects **Small vessels of skin, heart, lungs**	**Affects those with allergies/asthma** and is therefore also called **allergic granulomatosis and angiitis.** Can present with any type of organ damage, but with prominent asthma, allergic rhinitis, sinusitis, and potential for peripheral neuropathy. Also associated with **eosinophilia** and **p-ANCA.**
Henoch-Schönlein purpura Affects **Small vessels of skin, kidneys, joints, gut**	**Affects mostly children** (the most common vasculitis of children), **usually after a viral URI** leading to a tetrad of manifestations, including **palpable purpura** on the legs and buttocks from inflamed hemorrhagic vessels, **arthritis** from inflammation of vessels leading to joints, **abdominal pain** and potentially bloody stool from affected gut vessels, and **renal disease** from renal vessel involvement. The inflamed intestines can also lead to **intussusception** because the swelling can act as a lead point to drag itself into the adjacent loop of bowel. **IgA immune complex deposition occurs in capillaries,** accounting for the inflammation.
Cryoglobulinemia Affects **Small vessels of skin, kidneys, gut**	**Affects mostly adults with hepatitis C.** In cryoglobulinemia, there are proteins in the bloodstream that **precipitate in cold** but redissolve with warming. These proteins are usually immunoglobulins and complement proteins, and when deposited in the capillaries, inflammation and vessel damage occur. **C**ryoglobulinemia—**hepatitis C.**

ESR, Erythrocyte sedimentation rate; GI, gastrointestinal; URI, upper respiratory infection.

episodes caused by cerebral hypoperfusion. There is a potential for intravascular tumor embolism (small pieces entering the bloodstream), potentially leading to strokes or other vascular occlusive processes.

- **Rhabdomyomas** are associated tuberous sclerosis and are a tumor of the striated muscle itself. It is benign and may regress.

Vascular tumors include the following:

- **Kaposi sarcoma** is a tumor caused by human herpesvirus 8 (HHV-8); the malignant cells arise from the lymphatic endothelium. Although there are types that do not require an immunocompromised state, the most commonly tested association is with AIDS. The lesions are purple-red macules that subsequently enlarge to papules and nodules and can occur on the skin, intraorally, and in the gastrointestinal tract. AIDS patients who have Kaposi sarcoma often see improvement in these lesions after antiretroviral treatment.
- **Capillary** ("strawberry") **hemangiomas** classically are facial lesions found in infants; they grow rapidly and then slowly fade. Almost all will regress by 9 years of age. No treatment is necessary unless they cause problems such as blockage of nostrils or visual impairment.
- **Angiomyolipomas** are, as the name implies, tumors that include blood vessels (angio-), muscle (-myo-), and fat (-lipo-). Similarly to rhabdomyomas, these tumors are also associated with tuberous sclerosis.
- **Angiosarcomas** are malignant (-sarcoma) neoplasms of endothelial cells and are rare; angiosarcoma of the liver is associated with exposure to vinyl chloride, which is used to make polyvinyl chloride (PVC), the most commonly produced plastic. It is also associated with arsenic and thorium dioxide.

PHARMACOLOGY

Vasopressor agonist activity:
Norepinephrine: α > > β
Epinephrine: β > α, until high doses, when significant α effects occur
Isoproterenol: pure β
Dopamine: D → β → α as dose increases
Phenylephrine: pure α

Vasopressors

Vasopressors (Fig. 8.38) are drugs that work primarily through **increasing systemic vascular resistance** by clamping down blood vessels; they are essentially **"antihypotensive"** agents, most of them **sympathomimetic agents** with α_1 activity. Many of these drugs also have direct **positive inotropic** effects through β_1-receptor agonist activity to increase cardiac output to further correct hypotension. Common vasopressors include **epinephrine, norepinephrine, isoproterenol, and dopamine.** The following section will rely on an understanding of sympathetic adrenergic receptors; please review Chapter 7 if necessary. For the purposes of this section, receptors can be simplified as having α_1-receptor activity, causing increased systemic vascular resistance and therefore increasing blood pressure; β_1-receptor activity, causing increased cardiac output through increased inotropy (contractility) and chronotropy (rate); and β_2-receptor activity, causing vasodilation, decreased systemic vascular resistance, and therefore decreased blood pressure.

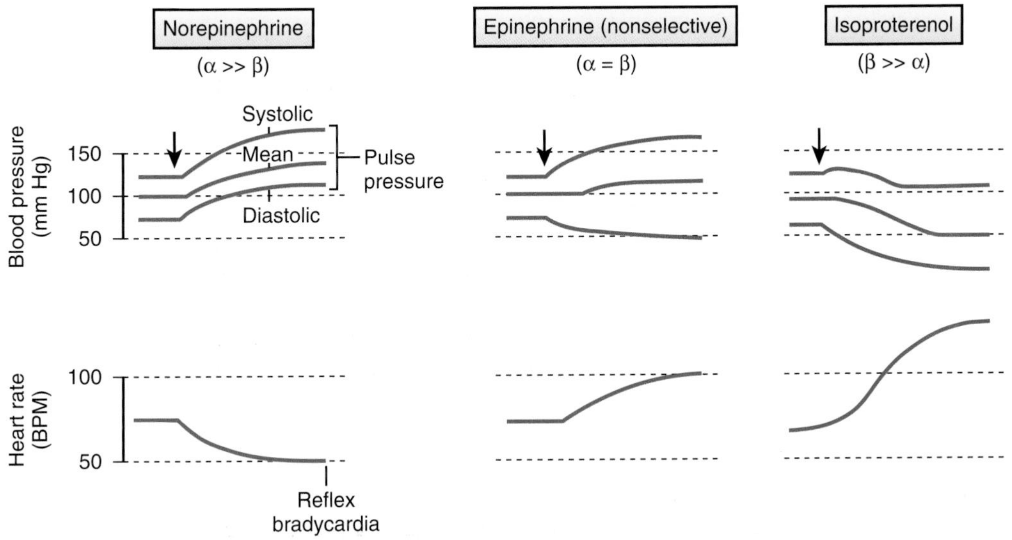

FIG. 8.38 Physiologic effects of vasopressors.

- **Norepinephrine** has predominant **α_1-vasoconstricting effects** but also has β_1 activity. Therefore, when a patient's hypotension is due to vasodilation (such as in septic shock), norepinephrine is the drug of choice because it will increase systemic vascular resistance and increase cardiac output, both contributing to increasing the blood pressure. Because the baroreceptors will see a large increase in blood pressure, vagal tone will be increased, potentially leading to **reflex bradycardia,** especially if the patient is taking a **beta blocker,** which will block the chronotropic effect of norepinephrine's β_1 stimulation.
- **Epinephrine** is an excellent **β_1 and β_2 agonist** (with significant **α activity at higher doses**). Therefore it has effects predominantly on **increasing cardiac output** through β_1 activity but can cause vasodilation as a result of its β_2 activity. The vasodilatory effects can actually cause a **decrease** in blood pressure if the cardiac output increase does not compensate for the vasodilation. The reason for the increased heart rate is twofold: (1) the decreased blood pressure triggers baroreceptor-mediated increases in heart rate, and (2) the direct β_1 receptor has a chronotropic effect. Clinically, epinephrine is used in **anaphylaxis and asthma** for β_2 bronchodilation, but it is also used in **cardiac arrest** because of the cardiac stimulant effect.
- **Isoproterenol** is a pure β agonist (β_1 and β_2) with essentially zero α activity. Therefore it will increase cardiac output but cause vasodilation, potentially dropping blood pressure like epinephrine. However, unlike epinephrine, isoproterenol has no α effect, and therefore the drop in blood pressure with isoproterenol is more profound.
- **Dopamine** is a precursor to norepinephrine and has different effects at different dosages. At **low doses,** dopamine interacts with dopamine receptors, which cause vasodilation in the kidneys and

gut (a clinically insignificant effect); at **medium doses,** it has β_1 activity, increasing cardiac output; at **high doses,** it has significant α_1 activity and acts as a potent vasoconstrictor.

- **Phenylephrine** is a **pure α agonist** and therefore causes significant vasoconstriction and increases blood pressure; the baroreceptors will sense this increase in blood pressure and increase vagal tone to the heart, often leading to **reflex bradycardia.**

ACE inhibitors: can cause cough; are contraindicated in pregnancy (fetal renal agenesis) and bilateral renal artery stenosis

Vasodilators

Vasodilators act to **decrease total peripheral resistance** (when causing smooth muscle relaxation in arterioles) and/or **decrease preload** (when causing venous relaxation). Widely used vasodilator drugs include **ACE inhibitors and angiotensin II receptor blockers (ARBs), nitrates, hydralazine, and calcium channel blockers.**

ACE Inhibitors (-pril drugs—lisinopril, enalapril, captopril):

- **Mechanism of action:** ACE inhibitors work by blocking angiotensin-converting enzyme, preventing the conversion of angiotensin I to angiotensin II and halting the RAA axis (Fig. 8.39). Angiotensin II (AT II) is a potent vasoconstrictor and also causes aldosterone release from the adrenal gland, leading to increased blood pressure and increased sodium reclamation by the kidney. By blocking AT II formation, the vasoconstriction effect is removed and blood pressure falls. In addition, ACE typically also removes bradykinin, a vasodilator, from the bloodstream; increased bradykinin levels cause vasodilation and a further decrease in blood pressure.

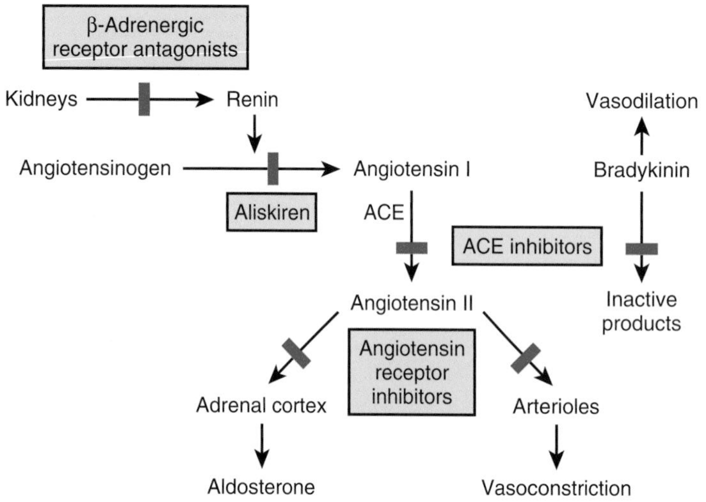

FIG. 8.39 The renin-angiotensin-aldosterone system and the drugs that block various parts of this pathway. *(From Brenner GM, Stevens GW. Pharmacology. 4th ed. Philadelphia: Elsevier; 2012.)*

- **Clinical uses:** ACE inhibitors are typically used in **hypertension** because of the vasodilation effect; in **heart failure** because AT II causes maladaptive remodeling in the failed heart, with ACE inhibition therefore slowing the progression of heart failure; and in **diabetes** because AT II preferentially vasoconstricts the efferent arteriole (the arteriole leaving the glomerulus), and blocking that vasoconstriction decreases glomerular pressure, slowing the progression of kidney damage in diabetes.
- **Side effects:** Increased bradykinin levels cause **cough** in about 20% of patients. Rarely, life-threatening **angioedema** can occur.
- **Contraindications: Bilateral renal artery stenosis** is a contraindication because the kidneys are receiving such small amounts of blood that removing the vasoconstricting effect of AT II on the glomerular arterioles will lead to a large drop in glomerular filtration rate (GFR) and precipitate renal failure. **Pregnancy** is a contraindication because the fetus requires a functioning RAA axis for renal development, and ACE inhibitor use is associated with fetal renal agenesis. **Renal insufficiency** is a contraindication because ACE inhibitors can mildly decrease GFR; those with renal failure cannot afford that drop and can develop **hyperkalemia** from decreased renal potassium excretion.

ARBs (-sartan drugs—losartan, valsartan):

- ARBs are identical to ACE inhibitors except that instead of blocking ACE, they leave the enzyme open and allow AT II to be formed. Instead, ARBs block the AT II receptor directly. This allows bradykinin to be cleared from the bloodstream and therefore does not cause cough as a side effect and is a recommended alternative for patients who develop an ACE inhibitor–associated cough.

Hydralazine:

- **Mechanism of action:** Hydralazine increases cyclic guanosine monophosphate (cGMP) levels, which reduces calcium release from the sarcoplasmic reticulum of smooth muscle, ultimately resulting in smooth muscle relaxation. Therefore hydr**A**lazine acts as an **A**rteriolar **dilator,** reducing blood pressure and afterload by decreasing systemic vascular resistance.
- **Clinical uses:** Used for **severe hypertension** (usually in hospitals, not as home therapy) and often used in **hypertension during pregnancy** because it is not teratogenic (the beta blocker labetalol and the α_2 agonist methyldopa are other pregnancy-safe antihypertensives).
- **Side effects:** Because it is a direct arteriolar dilator, it will lower blood pressure, triggering the baroreceptors to increase sympathetic flow and decrease vagal tone of the heart, leading to **reflex tachycardia.** Cerebral vasodilation is implicated in migraines, so **headache** is also a potential side effect.
- **Contraindications:** Angina and coronary artery disease are contraindications because the reflex tachycardia can **increase myocardial oxygen consumption** and lead to worsening disease.

Nitrates: preload reducers; cause venodilation. Nitric oxide (NO) is produced by endothelial cells but has action on smooth muscle cells.

Nitrates (nitroglycerin, isosorbide dinitrate, isosorbide mononitrate):

- **Mechanism of action:** Nitrates **release nitric oxide (NO),** which activates guanylate cyclase in vascular smooth muscle cells and causes elevated cGMP levels (similar to hydralazine, described previously), causing smooth muscle relaxation (vasodilation). However, **nitrates have greater effect on veins** and therefore cause decreased preload by reducing venous return rather than reducing afterload. This **reduced preload** causes decreased myocardial oxygen consumption, improving ischemia. At higher doses, nitrates act on arterioles as well and reduce afterload. NO is normally produced by the *endothelial cells* of the blood vessel, but the action of NO is on the *smooth muscle cells.*
- **Clinical uses: Angina** is the most common indication.
- **Side effects:** As with hydralazine, if the dose is sufficient to cause arteriolar dilation, reflex tachycardia and headache can occur. In addition, **tolerance** to nitrates occurs quickly, and there must be a daily break from the medication or efficacy will diminish.

Nitroprusside: afterload and preload reduction; can cause cyanide toxicity

Nitroprusside:

- **Mechanism of action:** Nitroprusside has an iron core with **cyanide (CN^-)** and **NO** groups attached. The NO can detach and cause increased cGMP levels similar to hydralazine and nitrates, in this case causing **both arteriolar and venous** dilation and therefore **decreasing preload and afterload.**
- **Clinical uses:** Used in treatment of **malignant hypertension** because it acts quickly (the NO group is readily available) and is easily titrated.
- **Side effects: Cyanide toxicity** can occur with prolonged use because the CN^- groups can detach as well. As with any drug mentioned that decreases afterload, reflex tachycardia can occur as the baroreceptors sense decreased blood pressure and enact compensatory changes. (See the "Toxicology" section of Chapter 7 for discussion of management of cyanide toxicity.)
- **Contraindications:** Relative contraindications include **renal insufficiency** because the metabolites of cyanide (such as thiocyanate) are renally excreted and can build up, as well as **hepatic insufficiency** because the liver can metabolize free cyanide into thiocyanate.

Calcium Channel Blockers (verapamil, nifedipine, amlodipine, diltiazem):

- **Mechanism of action:** Block **L-type calcium channels in cardiac and smooth muscle.** Recall that the L-type calcium channels **mediate phase 2** of the myocyte action potential, which normally allows calcium influx and calcium-induced calcium release to initiate myocyte contraction. Inhibition of these channels results in decreased contractility (inotropy). Vascular smooth muscle also uses L-type calcium channels, and their blockage leads to muscular relaxation and therefore vasodilation. Each calcium channel blocker has a different affinity for either cardiac or vascular smooth muscle:

- Cardiac L-type channels: Verapamil > diltiazem > nifedipine ~ amlodipine (**V**erapamil likes the **V**entricles!).
- Vascular L-type channels: nifedipine ~ amlodipine > diltiazem > verapamil (the exact **opposite** as for L-type channels).

- **Clinical uses:** Because **nifedipine** has vascular preference, it is used to treat **Raynaud** disease to prevent the vasoconstriction of the distal digits. It is used in **hypertension** because it is a vasodilator. **Verapamil** works on the **ventricle** and is therefore used to treat **arrhythmias** and **angina**; it would be a poor choice to use nifedipine for angina because it acts on the blood vessels, causing vasodilation and reflex tachycardia, making angina worse!
- **Side effects: Cardiac** side effects include AV block from decreased L-type calcium channel activity preventing signal transmission and cardiac depression. **Vascular** side effects include **peripheral edema, headache,** and **dizziness.**

Sympatholytics

β-Receptor antagonists (beta blockers) (-lol drugs—β_1 selective: metoprolol, atenolol, esmolol; β nonselective: carvedilol, propranolol, nadolol).

- **Mechanism of action:** β_1-receptor stimulation increases contractility (inotropy), heart rate (chronotropy), and AV conduction, whereas β_2-receptor stimulation dilates the bronchial tree and causes peripheral vasodilation. **β_1 blockade then causes decreased inotropy, heart rate, and AV conduction** and is therefore very useful in a variety of conditions. β_2 blockade is less clinically useful because preventing bronchial dilation is not helpful, although preventing cerebral vasodilation makes β_2 blockade attractive for migraine headache prophylaxis. Therefore most beta blockers in use are **β_1 selective.** Additionally, some beta blockers, such as carvedilol, also have α_1 blocking effects, which is useful in heart failure (decreases afterload).
- **Clinical uses:** Used to treat **hypertension;** used to treat **heart failure** because sympathetic activity on the heart also causes maladaptive remodeling of the failed heart, similar to angiotensin II; used to treat **coronary artery disease** because beta blockade will prevent sympathetic stimulation of the heart, which would increase myocardial oxygen demand.
- **Side effects:** Because beta blockade causes decreased AV conduction, it can precipitate **heart block;** nonselective beta blockers can cause **bronchospasm** because of prevention of β_2-mediated bronchodilation and can also cause **erectile dysfunction** as a result of prevention of β_2-mediated vasodilation. β_1 blockade may also mask the adrenergic symptoms of hypoglycemia. **Overdose can be treated with glucagon,** which directly stimulates myocardial cyclic adenosine monophosphate (cAMP) production; β_1-receptor activation works through the same pathway.
- **Contraindications: Asthma** is a contraindication to the use of nonselective beta blockers.

α_2 Agonists (clonidine, methyldopa):

- **Mechanism of action:** The α_2 receptor acts as **negative feedback** for the sympathetic nervous system. Using an α_2-receptor agonist causes a net decrease in sympathetic outflow.
- **Clinical uses:** Previously used to treat **hypertension** (although **methyldopa** is sometimes still used in the pregnant hypertensive patient); now **clonidine** mostly is used in treatment of opioid withdrawal because sympathetic surges are responsible for some of the side effects.
- **Side effects:** Without sympathetic stimulation, as expected, side effects include **bradycardia, dry mouth (xerostomia), and sedation.** Because it downregulates the sympathetic nervous system, abrupt cessation of α_2 blockers can cause a sympathetic surge and resulting rebound hypertension.

Diuretics

Diuretics (Fig. 8.40) are explained in detail in Chapter 15 but are covered here briefly.

Thiazide diuretics (-thiazide—hydrochlorothiazide, chlorthalidone).

- **Mechanism of action:** Inhibit the sodium chloride cotransporter in the distal convoluted tubule of the nephron, leading to natriuresis (sodium excretion in the urine) and diminished intravascular volume, and thus to decreased blood pressure. Compared with **loop diuretics,** the thiazide diuretics are **longer lasting** but cause **less diuresis.** Thiazide diuretics also **increase calcium resorption** as a

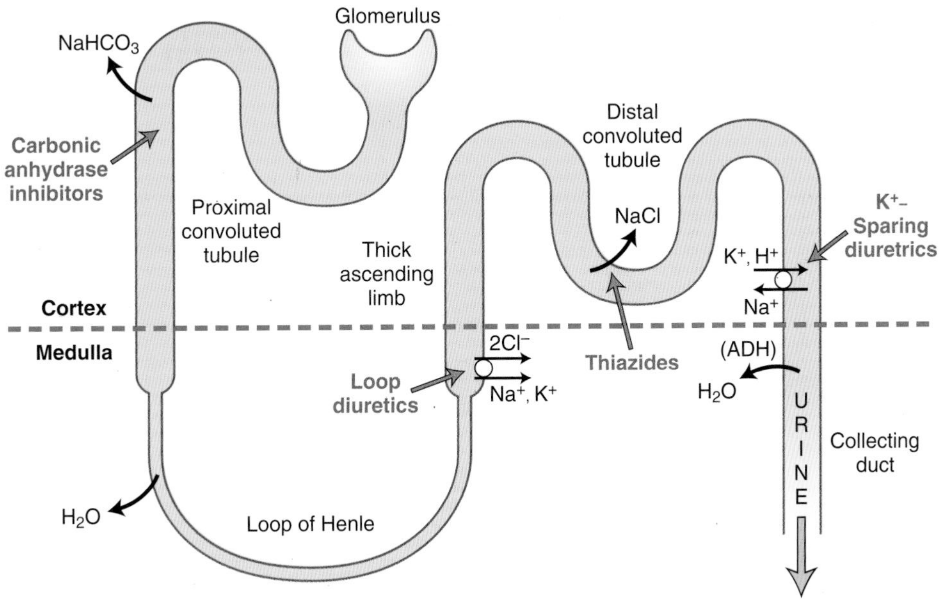

FIG. 8.40 The nephron and sites of action of various diuretics. ADH, Antidiuretic hormone.

result of opening of a voltage-gated calcium channel, leading to decreased calcium excretion in the urine and higher serum levels of calcium.

- **Clinical uses:** Because the thiazide diuretics are longer lasting but less potent, they are useful for the treatment of **hypertension** because rapid diuresis is not necessary. For those with increased calcium in the urine leading to calcium oxalate kidney stones, hydrochlorothiazide can prevent stone formation by increasing calcium resorption.
- **Side effects:** Can cause **hypokalemia** and **metabolic alkalosis** as a result of increased sodium delivery to the distal nephron as well as increased aldosterone secondary to the body's attempt at restoring intravascular volume (mechanism explained in Chapter 15), **hyperuricemia,** and **hypertriglyceridemia.** As mentioned previously, it increases calcium reclamation in the distal nephron and therefore can lead to **hypercalcemia.**
- **Contraindications:** Thiazides are **sulfa drugs** and are contraindicated in sulfa allergy (although this is contentious).

Loop Diuretics (furosemide [Lasix], bumetanide, ethacrynic acid):

- **Mechanism of action:** Inhibits the NaKCC (Na^+, K^+, Cl^-, Cl^-) cotransporter in the thick ascending loop of Henle, leading to significant natriuresis. Loop diuretics can cause **rapid, high-volume diuresis;** in fact, Lasix is so named because it lasts only 6 hours (lasts-six, Lasix)! (Technically, furosemide only lasts 4 hours, but they didn't want to change the brand name.)
- **Clinical uses:** Loop diuretics are used for high-volume diuresis, such as in **pulmonary edema** or decreasing fluid overload in **heart failure.** Because of its calcium-wasting effect, it can be used to treat **hypercalcemia.**
- **Side effects:** As with thiazide diuretics, loop diuretics are **potassium-wasting** diuretics and therefore have the potential to cause **hypokalemia** and **metabolic alkalosis.** Because the resorption of calcium and magnesium requires functional NaKCC cotransporter activity, **hypomagnesemia and hypocalcemia** can occur. Endolymph uses an NaKCC cotransporter as well; blockage can prevent normal electrolyte balance in the ear, causing **ototoxicity.**
- **Contraindications:** Loop diuretics (except for ethacrynic acid) are **sulfa drugs** and are contraindicated in sulfa allergy (although this is contentious).

Potassium-Sparing Diuretics (amiloride, spironolactone, triamterene):

- **Mechanism of action:** Unlike the loop and thiazide diuretics, potassium-sparing diuretics work in mechanisms that **prevent potassium loss in the urine. Amiloride** and triamterene block the sodium channel (ENaC) in the principal cell in the collecting duct, causing natriuresis. Normally,

Table 8.4 Summary Table of Antiarrhythmic Medications

CLASS	MECHANISM OF ACTION	MEDICATIONS, SIDE EFFECTS, CONTRAINDICATIONS
Ia	Blocks fast Na^+ channels (phase 0) Slows conduction velocity Prolongs action potential duration	All: risk for torsades de pointes from prolonging refractory period (QT interval) Procainamide: lupuslike syndrome (rash/arthralgia/fever) Quinidine: "cinchonism"—headaches, tinnitus, altered mental status
Ib	Blocks fast Na^+ channels (phase 0) Slows conduction velocity Binds to ischemic/diseased areas Shortens action potential duration	All: local anesthetic toxicity (CNS symptoms: confusion, seizures)
Ic	Blocks fast Na^+ channels (phase 0) Slows conduction velocity Does not change action potential duration	All: contraindicated in diseased hearts as a result of proarrhythmic effect
II	β-Adrenergic receptor antagonist Decreases sympathetic tone in heart Decreases heart rate Decreases AV nodal conduction	All: beta blocker side effects (heart block from too much AV node depression, impotence, bradycardia, bronchospasm, sedation)
III	Blocks K^+ channels (phase 3) Prolongs action potential Prolongs refractory period *Amiodarone has class I, II, III, IV effects	Amiodarone: check PFTs (pulmonary fibrosis), TFTs (iodine in drug causes thyroid abnormalities), and LFTs (hepatotoxicity) Photosensitivity and blue/gray skin and corneal deposits.
IV	Calcium channel blocker Decreases heart rate Decreases AV nodal conduction	All: edema, heart block, constipation, flushing

CNS, Central nervous system; LFT, liver function test; PFT, pulmonary function test; TFT, thyroid function test.

this sodium channel reclaims sodium at the expense of potassium, and increased sodium delivery here by other diuretics leads to potassium loss. **Spironolactone** causes blockage of the **aldosterone receptor,** preventing upregulation of the activity of the principal cell and leading to decreased sodium reclamation.

- **Clinical uses: Amiloride** is used in the treatment of **heart failure** when hypokalemia is a concern, such as concomitant loop diuretic use. **Spironolactone** is also used in severe **heart failure** as well as in aldosterone-secreting tumors before surgical correction.
- **Side effects: Hyperkalemia** is possible with potassium-sparing diuretics as a result of decreased ability to excrete potassium. **Spironolactone** also blocks the **testosterone receptor,** causing the side effects of androgen antagonism such as gynecomastia (**eplerenone** is an aldosterone receptor antagonist that does not have any antiandrogen effects).

Antiarrhythmics

Various arrhythmias can occur in the heart, most of them causing a fast heart rate (tachyarrhythmia); arrhythmias treatable with **antiarrhythmic** medications include atrial fibrillation and flutter, ventricular tachycardia, and paroxysmal supraventricular tachycardia (PSVT) (Table 8.4). These medications are grouped into **four classes** (I–IV) based on their mechanism of action; class I antiarrhythmics are further classified into Ia, Ib, and Ic.

- **Class I** (Fig. 8.41): All are **fast sodium channel blockers** that affect **phase 0** (depolarization) of the myocyte action potential.
  Class Ia: **D**isopyramide, **Q**uinidine, **P**rocainamide—**D**ouble **Q**uarter **P**ounder.
  Class Ib: **L**idocaine, **M**exiletine, **T**ocainide—**L**ettuce **M**ayo **T**omato.
  Class Ic: **E**ncainide, **Mo**racizine, **F**lecainide, **P**ropafenone—**E**at **Mo**re **F**ries **P**lease.
- Class II: All are beta blockers.
  - **The -lol drugs:** metoprolol, atenolol, carvedilol, esmolol, propranolol.
- **Class III**: All are **potassium channel blockers** that affect **phase 3** (repolarization) of the myocyte action potential.
  - **A**miodarone (has class I–IV activity), **B**retylium, **D**ofetilide, **I**butilide, **S**otalol—**A B**ig **D**og **I**s **S**cary
  - **Sotalol** is "**sota**" (sort of) a beta blocker, except it is a **class III antiarrhythmic.**

There are two Ms in these mnemonics: **Mo**racizine and **Mo**re share the first two letters to differentiate.

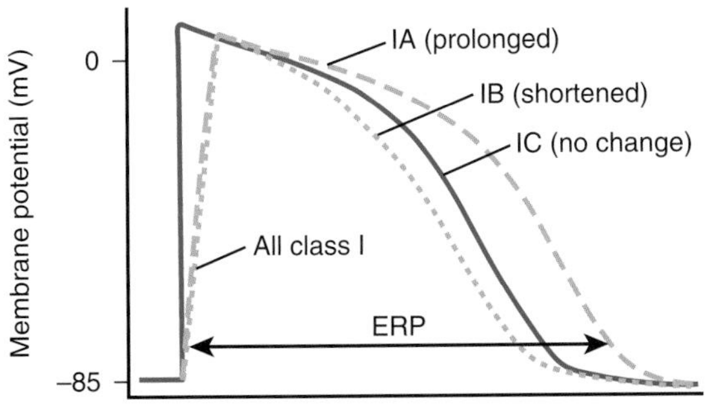

FIG. 8.41 Effects of class I antiarrhythmics on the action potential. ERP, Effective refractory period. *(From Pazdernik T, Kerecsen L. Rapid Review Pharmacology. 3rd ed. Philadelphia: Elsevier; 2010.)*

- **Class IV:** All are L-type calcium channel blockers.
  - Verapamil, diltiazem (nifedipine does not work on myocardial calcium channels enough to classify).

Class I antiarrhythmics are local anesthetics—blocking the Na^+ channels in nerves slows action potentials (APs) in pain fibers, blocking pain; blocking Na^+ channels in cardiac myocytes slows cardiac conduction, blocking some arrhythmias. Therefore all class I medications will slow the initial phase 0 depolarization and slow conduction velocity in the conducting system but are further divided based on whether or not they **P**rolong (class Ia), **S**horten (Ib), or **D**o not change (Ic) the overall action potential duration (and I'll be **PiSseD** if you forget which is which)!

- **Class Ia prolongs AP duration** and therefore also **prolongs the refractory period (QT interval on ECG),** prolonging the time when cells cannot depolarize again. Therefore this can stop arrhythmias that are due to cells depolarizing too frequently such as in **atrial flutter, atrial fibrillation, PSVT, and ventricular tachycardia.** However, because the **QT prolongation** associated with class Ia antiarrhythmics, **there is an increased risk for torsades de pointes.**
- **Class Ib shortens AP duration but preferentially binds to ischemic or abnormal cells** and helps stabilize **ventricular arrhythmias** (ventricular tachycardia) in situations in which the heart is diseased or ischemic **(e.g., post-MI).** Because the **refractory period is not prolonged, torsades de pointes is not a concern.**
- **Class Ic does not change AP duration** but binds to Na^+ channels most avidly out of all class I medications, especially **binding Na^+ channels in the AV node,** and is therefore useful for treatment of **supraventricular tachycardia.** However, class Ic medications are contraindicated in those with diseased hearts because it has been shown to have a **proarrhythmic effect in these patients.**

Class II antiarrhythmics are all **beta blockers** (β-adrenergic antagonists), which help **stop sympathetic activity on the heart.** Recall that the amount of funny sodium channels open (phase 4 of pacemaker cells) depends on sympathetic tone: beta blockade **decreases heart rate** and **decreases AV nodal conduction velocity** (increasing PR interval on ECG). They are useful for treating **PSVT, atrial fibrillation, and atrial flutter** by decreasing the ability to transmit the signal to the ventricles through the AV node.

Class III antiarrhythmics (Fig. 8.42) are **potassium channel blockers;** K^+ channels are responsible for repolarization of the cells (phase 3), with prolongation causing **prolonged action potential duration** and **prolonged refractory period** (QT interval). Again, prolonged QT interval can predispose to **torsades de pointes.** One of the medications in this class, amiodarone, actually has class I, II, III, and IV activity and is therefore helpful for many different tachyarrhythmias—but with many side effects.

Class IV antiarrhythmics (Fig. 8.43) are **L-type calcium channel blockers** that, similar to beta blockers, decrease conduction velocity and heart rate. Also similar to beta blockers, they are used in the treatment of PSVT. Calcium channel blockade slows SA node depolarization, which depends on calcium channels to fully depolarize.

Adenosine: stuns AV node for a very short period to terminate some causes of supraventricular tachycardia

Adenosine

Adenosine is a medication that essentially **stuns the AV node,** causing a **complete (third-degree) heart block** for a **very short duration** (half-life of adenosine is seconds). In any arrhythmia that uses

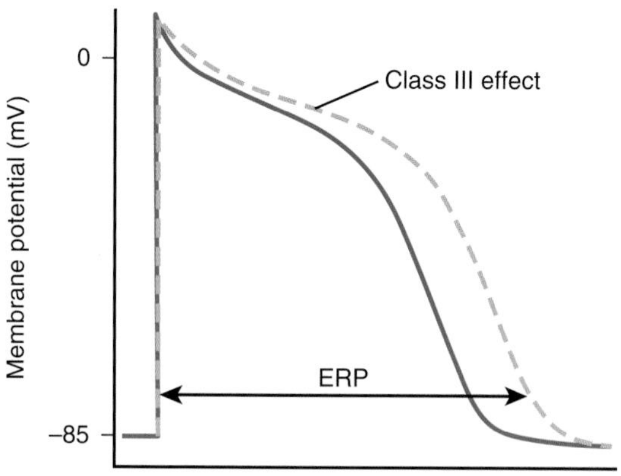

Fig. 8.42 Effects of class III antiarrhythmics on the action potential. ERP, Effective refractory period. *(From Pazdernik T, Kerecsen L. Rapid Review Pharmacology. 3rd ed. Philadelphia: Elsevier; 2010.)*

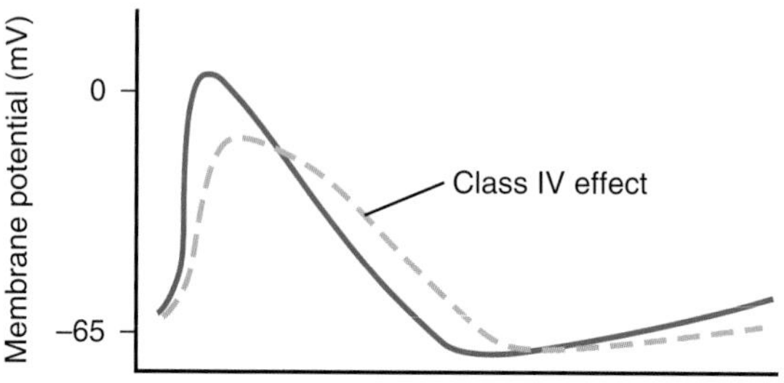

Fig. 8.43 Effects of class IV antiarrhythmics on the action potential of the pacemaker cells. *(From Pazdernik T, Kerecsen L. Rapid Review Pharmacology. 3rd ed. Philadelphia: Elsevier; 2010.)*

the AV node as a focus for reentry, such as AV nodal reentrant tachycardia (AVNRT), the most common supraventricular tachycardia, stunning the AV node causes the reentry circuit to cease and stops the arrhythmia. The underlying conduction abnormality will still be present, however, and therefore the arrhythmia can always return.

- **Mechanism of action:** Adenosine is an endogenous purine nucleoside that acts on **adenosine receptors** that are coupled to inhibitory G-protein–coupled receptors (G_i), inhibiting cAMP formation and subsequently **hyperpolarizing the cell** by promoting K^+ efflux from the cell (remember stage 3 of pacemaker action potentials). This hyperpolarization prevents action potentials for a brief period and effectively stuns the AV node. The hyperpolarization of arterioles of the heart causes transient coronary artery vasodilation as well. Because caffeine binds to the adenosine receptor as well, those who consume caffeine may require higher doses.
- **Clinical uses:** Used in termination of some types of **supraventricular tachycardia.**

Digoxin (Cardiac Glycosides)

Digoxin: blocks Na^+/K^+-ATPase, indirectly increasing Ca^{2+} available to myocytes and leading to increased inotropy

Digoxin is a medication that causes **increased inotropy** by increasing the amount of calcium available to the myocytes for contraction.

- **Mechanism of action** (Fig. 8.44): During myocyte contraction, there are high levels of Na^+ (from depolarization) and Ca^{2+} (for contraction). The Na^+ is normally removed from the cell by the Na^+/K^+-ATPase; some of this can reenter the cell through the Na^+/Ca^{2+} exchanger and help drive Ca^{2+} out of the cell. Digoxin blocks the Na^+/K^+-ATPase by binding to the K^+ site, indirectly shutting down the Na^+/Ca^{2+} exchanger by destroying the sodium gradient that it needs to function. The Ca^{2+} is put back into the sarcoplasmic reticulum instead of being removed from the cell, and subsequently more calcium will be available for contraction (increased inotropy).
- **Clinical uses:** Increases inotropy in **congestive heart failure** (decreases symptoms, but does not improve mortality). Also used for **atrial fibrillation** to slow the ventricular rate. The reason that it is effective in atrial fibrillation is because the increased inotropy from the medication results in **less sympathetic tone** because the contractility is already high. Less sympathetic tone leads to slower AV conduction and therefore slows the ventricular rate in atrial fibrillation.
- **Side effects:** Digoxin toxicity is common, as a result of its **low therapeutic index.** Systemic symptoms include **cholinergic symptoms** such as diarrhea, nausea, and vomiting; **yellow vision** is also

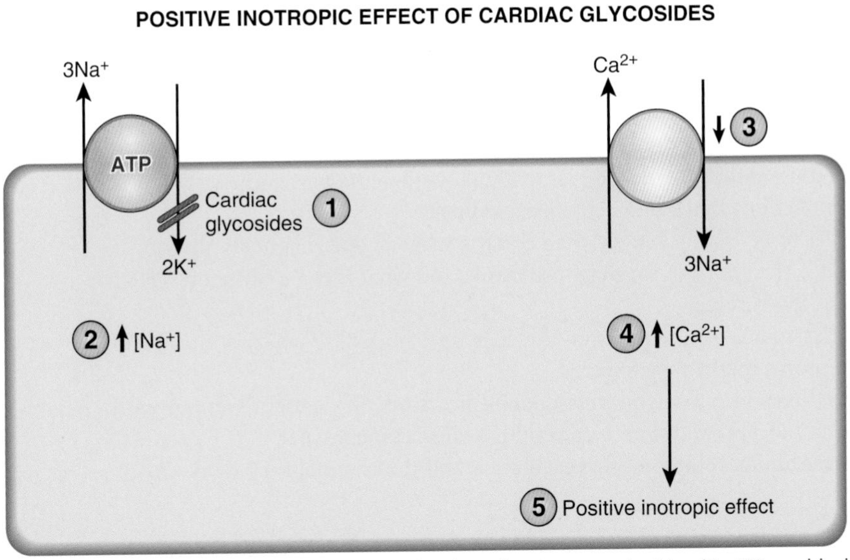

Fig. 8.44 Mechanism of action of digoxin. (1) Digoxin binds to the K^+ site on the Na^+/K^+-ATPase, blocking sodium efflux from the cell; (2) increased intracellular sodium concentration occurs; (3) this decreases the activity of the Ca^{2+}/Na^+ exchanger because the sodium gradient is no longer favorable; (4) increased intracellular calcium occurs, which is reclaimed into the sarcoplasmic reticulum; (5) increased calcium release from the sarcoplasmic reticulum leads to increased actin–myosin interaction and increased contractility. ATP, Adenosine triphosphate. *(From Costanzo LS. Physiology. 4th ed. New York: Elsevier; 2009.)*

possible. Cardiac symptoms include **arrhythmias** and **hyperkalemia.** Digitalis toxicity is treated with **anti-Dig antibody fragments (Fab)** and **correcting potassium** (if it is abnormal).

- **Contraindications:** Because digoxin binds to the K^+ site on the Na^+/K^+-ATPase, **hypokalemia** can result in digitalis toxicity because the K^+ is no longer there to compete for the binding site. Digitalis is renally excreted, and therefore **renal insufficiency** is a relative contraindication.

REVIEW QUESTIONS

(1) Starting from the right atrium, describe the route that a red blood cell takes as it circulates through the body to end up again in the right atrium. Include heart valves, heart chambers, major arteries, capillary beds, and major veins. Assume the red blood cell goes to the kidney (aorta to renal artery) for purposes of this exercise.

(2) Patients with nephrotic syndrome excrete large amounts of protein in the urine (>3.5 g/day). Explain in terms of the Starling forces why these patients develop edema.

(3) What is the mean arterial pressure (MAP) for a patient with a blood pressure of 150/90 mm Hg?

(4) If a patient's heart rate is 80 beats/min, end-diastolic volume (preload) is 120 mL, and end-systolic volume is 60 mL, what is the patient's (a) stroke volume, (b) ejection fraction, and (c) cardiac output?

(5) During hypotension, sympathetic outflow increases α_1-receptor–mediated vasoconstriction at the level of the arterioles to decrease blood flow to organs that are less vital to immediate survival to ensure adequate blood flow to the heart and brain. If the patient's renal arteries constricted to half of their original diameter, what would the resistance be?

(6) What actions occur during each phase of a cardiac myocyte action potential?

(7) Which of the two conditions would lead to increased contractility: (a) increased preload, (b) increased calcium release from the sarcoplasmic reticulum of the myocytes?

(8) For a patient with aortic stenosis, what changes would be seen to the diagrams in (a) Fig. 8.7 and (b) Fig. 8.8?

(9) What type of AV block ("heart block") is described by an ECG that demonstrates randomly dropped beats without progressive PR interval prolongation? Is this particular type of heart block dangerous? If so, why?

(10) During hypotension, are the baroreceptors in the aortic arch and carotid sinus firing more or less often? What net effect does this have on parasympathetic tone and sympathetic tone?
(11) What is the most common cause of right-sided heart failure? What is the pathophysiology for this?
(12) Which cardiomyopathy is classically inherited in an autosomal dominant fashion? What is the physical finding on auscultation, and how does the amount of preload change this finding?
(13) What is the classic presentation and ECG findings in patients with acute pericarditis? What is the most common class of infections that cause acute pericarditis?
(14) In a pediatric patient with a fever lasting longer than 5 days, what is one diagnosis that must always be considered? What is the criterion for diagnosing this, and what is the treatment? What is the feared complication of this disease?
(15) In children with palpable purpura, especially over the legs and buttocks, what is the likely diagnosis? What other symptoms might they have?
(16) What would be the expected response to blood pressure and heart rate if a patient were given a β-adrenergic antagonist (beta blocker) and then received high-dose epinephrine?
(17) Name the classes of antiarrhythmics, some drugs in each class, and the channel they work on.

9 ENDOCRINOLOGY

Ryan A. Pedigo

OVERVIEW OF THE ENDOCRINE SYSTEM

The endocrine system uses hormones to transfer information between different tissues. It is a finely regulated machine that uses feedback loops and sensors to ensure constant homeostasis within the body; the endocrine system plays some form of regulatory role in almost all physiologic processes. It has effects on development, growth, and metabolism and works with almost every organ system, including the nervous and immune systems. In contrast to neurotransmitters, which work in the synapse between the neuron endplate and the receptors they act on, **hormones** are secreted into the circulation and can work on tissues far away from the source of origin.

Hormones

Hormones are secreted by the endocrine glands into the bloodstream. With the exception of the endocrine functions of the reproductive organs, kidneys, and adrenal medulla (see Chapters 16, 15, and 7, respectively), by the end of this chapter the mechanism of action of each of the hormones in Fig. 9.1 will be understood, as well as how they are regulated, what pathologic conditions can occur, and what medications act on these systems.

Regulation

Hormones must be precisely regulated to ensure that homeostasis is maintained. The most common method of hormone regulation is through **negative feedback loops.** Essentially, these loops all function in a similar manner: Some downstream effect or product of the released hormone inhibits further hormone release. That way, when the downstream product or change is made (the goal of the hormone), it will decrease hormone production because the intended goal of the hormone was met. An example of this is parathyroid hormone (PTH): The main stimulus for parathyroid hormone is low ionized calcium levels—when parathyroid hormone has its effects on the body that ultimately increase calcium concentration, that calcium inhibits further PTH secretion because the job of the hormone has been accomplished and further PTH activity would cause hypercalcemia.

A rare method of regulation is the **positive feedback loop,** whereby the end product causes more production of hormone, causing more production of end product, creating a self-promoting loop. This occurs during the menstrual cycle for a brief period to promote ovulation and also occurs during parturition (labor) when oxytocin helps to create uterine contractions; both are covered in Chapter 16.

Types of Hormones

Hormones fall into one of two main types: **peptides/protein hormones** and **steroid hormones.** There are also hormones derived from a single amino acid tyrosine (e.g., the catecholamines, such as epinephrine), covered in Chapters 7 and 8.

- Peptide and protein hormones act on surface receptors of the cells, such as G-protein–coupled receptors (GPCRs) or tyrosine kinases.
- Steroid hormones are lipophilic and can move into the cell, acting on the cytoplasmic and nuclear receptors in the cell to alter gene expression.

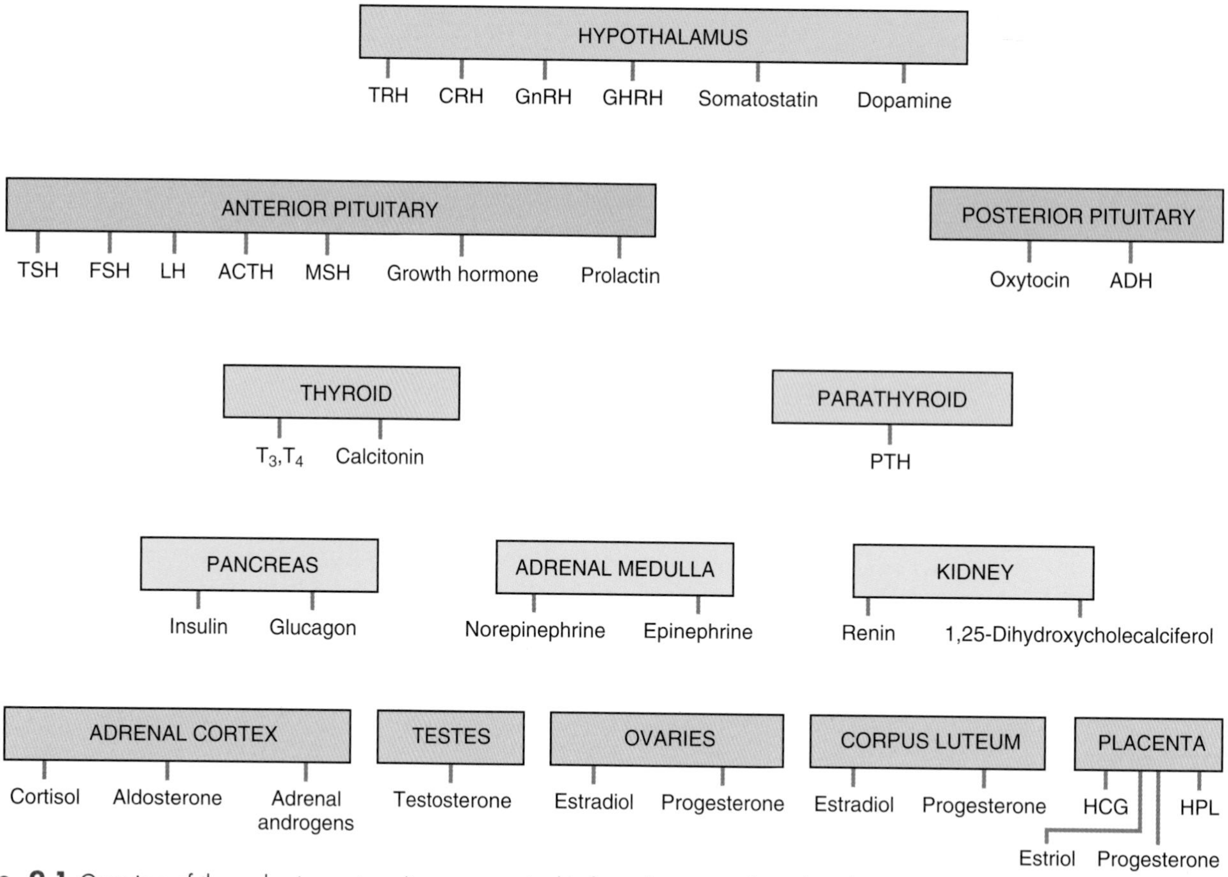

FIG. 9.1 Overview of the endocrine system. Items present in this figure but covered in other chapters include reproductive endocrinology (Chapter 16), renal endocrinology (Chapter 15), and adrenal medulla endocrinology (Chapter 7). ACTH, Adrenocorticotropic hormone; ADH, antidiuretic hormone; CRH, corticotropin-releasing hormone; FSH, follicle-stimulating hormone; GHRH, growth hormone–releasing hormone; GnRH, gonadotropin-releasing hormone; HCG, human chorionic gonadotropin; HPL, human placental lactogen; LH, luteinizing hormone; MSH, melanocyte-stimulating hormone; PTH, parathyroid hormone; TRH, thyroid-releasing hormone; TSH, thyroid-stimulating hormone. (*From Costanzo LS. Physiology. 4th ed. New York: Elsevier; 2009.*)

Terminology of Pathophysiology

Endocrinopathies are generally termed **primary, secondary, or tertiary** (when applicable). The example used for this to demonstrate the terminology is hypothyroidism. Hypothyroidism will be described in detail later, but briefly the hypothalamus generates thyrotropin-releasing hormone (TRH) to stimulate the pituitary to secrete thyroid-stimulating hormone (TSH) to stimulate the thyroid to generate thyroid hormone. When the organ itself fails and causes hypothyroidism, it is termed **primary;** when the stimulus for the organ fails (the pituitary), it is termed **secondary;** when the stimulus for the stimulus for the organ fails (the hypothalamus), it is termed **tertiary** (Fig. 9.2).

- **Primary** dysfunction, such as in primary hypothyroidism, means the **endocrine organ itself** (i.e., the thyroid) is dysfunctional, such as an autoimmune destruction of the thyroid gland.
- **Secondary** dysfunction, such as in secondary hypothyroidism, means the **direct stimulus** for that organ is abnormal (i.e., the pituitary gland failing to produce TSH to stimulate the thyroid; even if the thyroid is functioning normally, it will fail to produce thyroid hormone in the absence of a stimulus); an example would be a tumor destroying the pituitary's function.
- **Tertiary** dysfunction, such as tertiary hypothyroidism, means that the problem is one step further downstream: In the case of tertiary hypothyroidism, it is the hypothalamus failing to secrete TRH, which would normally stimulate the pituitary to secrete TSH to stimulate the thyroid.

Primary dysfunction: problem is with the endocrine organ itself.

Multiple Endocrine Neoplasia Syndromes

The multiple endocrine neoplasia (MEN) syndromes feature **tumors of endocrine organs** and are inherited in an **autosomal dominant** fashion. There are three types: MEN I, IIa, and IIb; each is a

MEN I: the three Ps of pituitary, pancreas, and parathyroid ("pit, panc, and para")

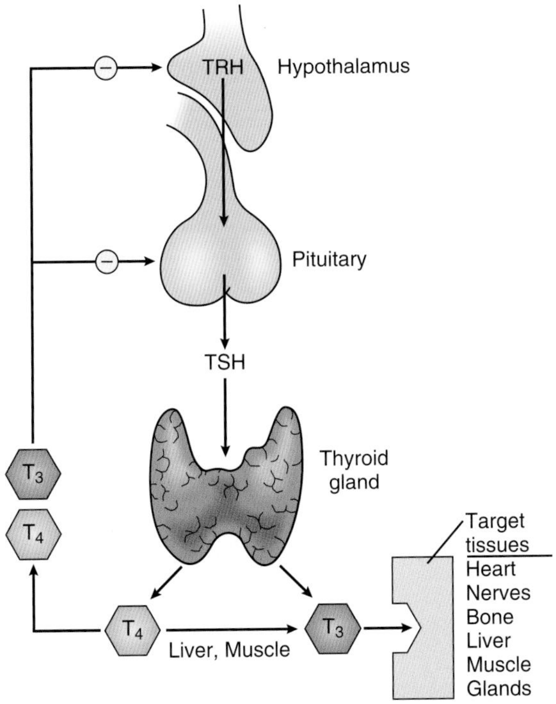

FIG. 9.2 Hypothalamic-pituitary-thyroid axis. Primary hypothyroidism occurs when the endocrine gland itself is the problem; secondary when the stimulus for the gland (the pituitary) is the problem; tertiary when the next stimulus upstream is dysfunctional. Note that there is an exception with tertiary hyperparathyroidism, in which the hyperparathyroidism is due to long-standing hyperplasia of the glands from renal failure and the endocrine gland has lost the ability to respond to calcium levels appropriately. (*From Brenner GM, Stevens GW. Pharmacology. 4th ed. Philadelphia: Elsevier; 2012.*)

TABLE 9.1 Multiple Endocrine Neoplasia (MEN) Syndromes

MEN I: THE THREE Ps, WERMER SYNDROME	MEN IIa: SIPPLE SYNDROME	MEN IIb: WILLIAM SYNDROME
• Pituitary • Pancreas	• Pheochromocytoma • Thyroid (medullary carcinoma)	• Pheochromocytoma • Thyroid (medullary carcinoma)
• Parathyroid	• Parathyroid	• Oral/intestinal ganglioneuromatosis

- **MEN I** (*MEN I* gene): Characterized by the three Ps of pituitary, pancreas, and parathyroid. The **pituitary** lesion is most commonly a prolactin-secreting adenoma. The **pancreatic** lesion is a neuroendocrine tumor such as a gastrinoma (Zollinger-Ellison syndrome). **Hyperparathyroidism** as a result of **hyperplasia** of all four parathyroid glands is the **most common** feature of MEN I.
- **MEN IIa and IIb** (*RET* protooncogene activation mutation): Have two of the three features in common—both can develop pheochromocytomas (catecholamine-secreting tumors of the medulla of the adrenal gland), and both can develop medullary carcinoma of the thyroid. However, the main difference is that those with **MEN IIa** can develop **primary hyperparathyroidism** like those with MEN I, whereas those with **MEN IIb** develop ganglioneuromas of various mucosal sites, such as the mouth and gastrointestinal (GI) tract, and often have a marfanoid habitus.

Remember: There is MEN I, MEN IIa, and MEN IIb. MEN **I** shares **1** condition (parathyroid hyperplasia) with MEN IIa. MEN **IIa** shares **2** conditions (pheochromocytoma and medullary carcinoma of the thyroid) with MEN IIb.

Hypothalamus and Pituitary Gland

Hypothalamus and Pituitary Function Overview

Anterior pituitary hormones (FLAT PeG): FSH, LH, ACTH, TSH, prolactin, GH

The **hypothalamus** is below the thalamus (hence **hypo**thalamus) and is responsible for regulation of numerous aspects of the body (covered in Chapter 13); this chapter will concern itself with the important role the hypothalamus has in **stimulating or inhibiting the pituitary gland** and therefore regulating pituitary gland activity. The pituitary gland has anterior and posterior lobes, which each make a different set of hormones (Table 9.2; Fig. 9.3).

The **anterior pituitary** (previously called the adenohypophysis because *adeno-* refers to "gland") is made up of endocrine glandular cells, which secrete their products into the bloodstream; their

TABLE 9.2 Hormones of the Pituitary Gland

HYPOTHALAMUS	PITUITARY ANTERIOR: "FLAT PEG" MNEMONIC POSTERIOR: ADH AND OXYTOCIN	END ORGAN
Gonadotropin-releasing hormone (GnRH)	Follicle-stimulating hormone (FSH)	Gonads
Gonadotropin-releasing hormone (GnRH)	Luteinizing hormone (LH)	Gonads
Corticotropin-releasing hormone (CRH)	Adrenocorticotropic hormone (ACTH)	Adrenal cortex • Stimulates cortisol (zona fasciculata) and androgen (zona reticularis) secretion
Thyrotropin-releasing hormone (TRH) (dopamine inhibits)	Thyroid-stimulating hormone (TSH) Prolactin Endorphins	Thyroid Breasts
Growth hormone–releasing hormone (GHRH) (somatostatin inhibits)	Growth hormone (GH)	Entire body • Important for growth
	Antidiuretic hormone (posterior pituitary)	Kidneys
	Oxytocin (posterior pituitary)	Uterus, breasts

ADH, Antidiuretic hormone.

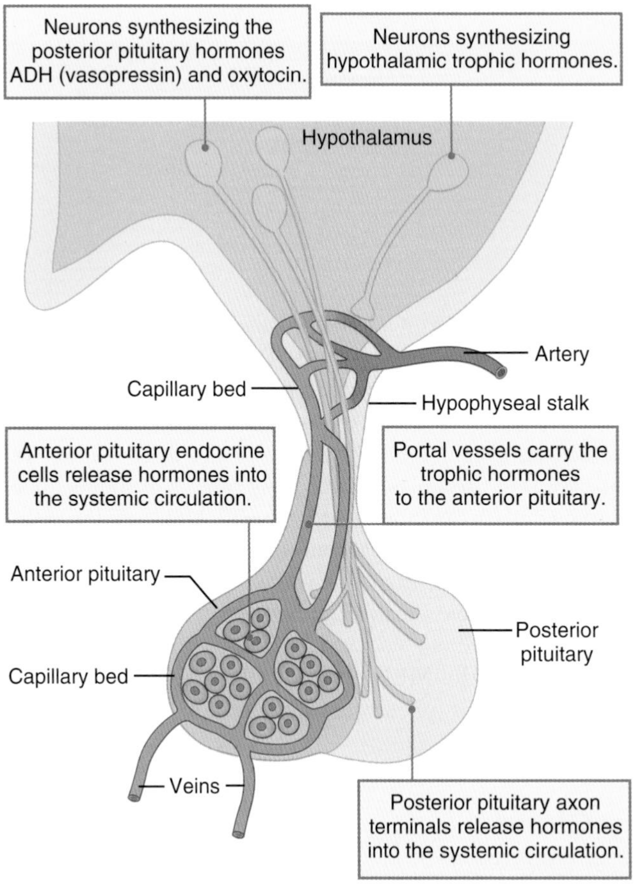

FIG. 9.3 The hypothalamus and pituitary. The anterior pituitary is an endocrine gland; the veins from the hypothalamus directly drain into the anterior pituitary to ensure that the signals from the hypothalamus get there. The posterior pituitary contains the axons of neurons that have their cell bodies in the hypothalamus (supraoptic nuclei and paraventricular nuclei). ADH, Antidiuretic hormone. (*From Carroll RG.* Elsevier's Integrated Physiology. *Philadelphia: Elsevier; 2006.*)

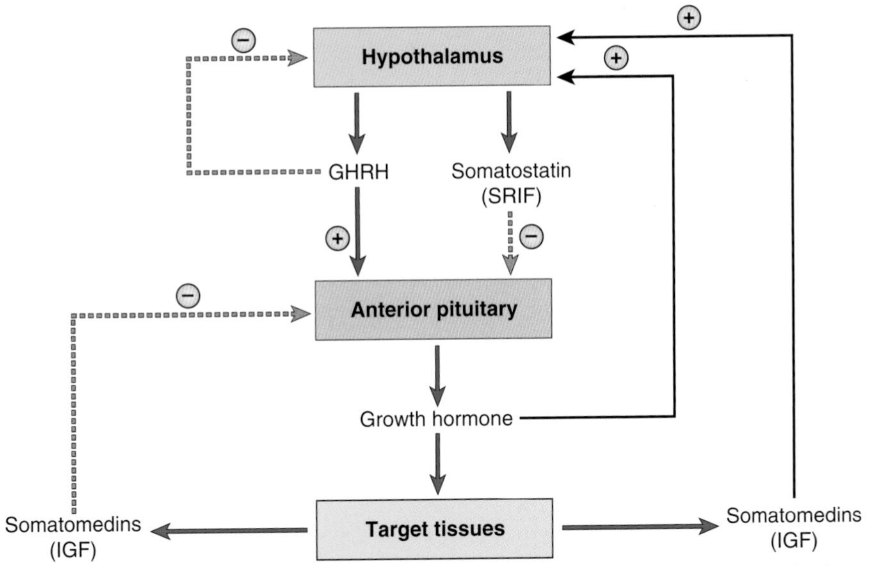

FIG. 9.4 Growth hormone. The stimulus is growth hormone–releasing hormone (GHRH, from the hypothalamus), which is released with starvation and hypoglycemia; the main negative feedback is via the end products (somatomedins), such as insulin-like growth factor 1 (IGF-1). SRIF, somatotropin release-inhibiting factor. (*From Costanzo LS.* Physiology. *4th ed. New York: Elsevier; 2009.*)

hormones can be remembered by the mnemonic **FLAT PeG** (**F**SH [follicle-stimulating hormone], **L**H, [luteinizing hormone], **A**CTH [adrenocorticotropic hormone], **T**SH, **p**rolactin, [**e**ndorphins], **G**H [growth hormone]). Each of these hormones will be covered individually because their function and regulation differ greatly. Because the function of the anterior pituitary is so closely linked with the hypothalamus, the **venous blood from the hypothalamus directly drains into the anterior pituitary** (called the hypothalamic-hypophyseal portal system, similar to the goal of the portal vein draining the intestines into the liver). This close connection ensures that any hormones that the hypothalamus secretes to instruct the anterior pituitary on what to do immediately go in high concentration directly there.

Posterior pituitary hormones: oxytocin and ADH

The **posterior pituitary** (previously called the neurohypophysis) is actually **neural tissue,** with the cell bodies in the hypothalamus and the axons running down into the posterior pituitary. When stimulated, the neurons release their products into the bloodstream, just like a neuron would release its neurotransmitters into a synapse. The posterior pituitary releases **antidiuretic hormone (ADH)** and **oxytocin,** each primarily synthesized by its own set of neuron cell bodies. **ADH** is mainly synthesized by the **supraoptic nuclei,** and **oxytocin** is mainly synthesized by the **paraventricular nuclei,** but both sets of neurons make both hormones to some degree. A helpful way to remember that the paraventricular cells make **oxytocin** is that oxytocin causes contraction of the uterus, just like ventricles of the heart contract (although the paraventricular nuclei are actually named for their location near the third ventricle of the brain). The anatomic structure of the posterior pituitary becomes important in head trauma, where the axons in the pituitary stalk (infundibulum) can become disrupted, causing central diabetes insipidus from the loss of ADH secretion.

Pituitary Hormones Covered Elsewhere

- Follicle-stimulating hormone (FSH), luteinizing hormone (LH), and oxytocin: see Chapter 16.
- **Adrenocorticotropic hormone (ACTH):** see later section, "Adrenal Glands (Cortex and Medulla)"
- **Antidiuretic hormone:** see Chapter 15.

Growth Hormone

Growth hormone, as the name implies, is the main hormone regulating growth; the rapid growth in puberty is a result of increased levels of this hormone (Fig. 9.4). This hormone is secreted in a pulsatile fashion, with **starvation** and **hypoglycemia** acting as two potent stimuli for secretion. **Stimulation** is from the hypothalamus through growth hormone–releasing hormone (**GHRH**) and is **inhibited** by **somatostatin** (which is also secreted by the hypothalamus) and end products such as somatomedins, which are released when growth hormone (GH) has its effect on the end organ on which it is working. The effects of GH are widespread, and after reviewing these effects, the reasons that hypoglycemia and starvation are stimuli for GHRH secretion will become apparent (because initially, starvation and hypoglycemia seem counterintuitive for GH secretion, but GH has a secondary role in maintaining blood sugar levels during periods of starvation and hypoglycemia):

- **Insulin antagonism:** Growth hormone causes insulin resistance with a resultant increase in blood sugar and subsequently increased insulin release by the pancreas. This relative insulin resistance also causes increased lipolysis. Therefore GH simply acts during starvation and hypoglycemia to make blood sugar available to keep the body running (e.g., ensuring that enough blood glucose is available to allow the brain to function because the brain uptakes glucose in an insulin-independent fashion).
- **Increased linear growth:** This is **not** mediated by GH directly but rather because **GH stimulates production of insulin-like growth factor 1** (IGF-1, previously known as somatomedin C) in the liver. IGF-1 acts on osteoblasts and chondrocytes to allow for **long bone growth,** increasing height in those who do not have their growth plates fused yet.
- **Increased synthetic function and organ growth:** Causes increased protein synthesis and growth in nearly all of the body's organs, especially muscle. Coupled with the lipolysis from the insulin resistance, this has the net effect of decreasing fat and increasing lean muscle mass, as well as causing organomegaly.

Growth hormone excess: gigantism if growth plates not fused (accelerated linear growth), acromegaly if they are (no accelerated linear growth)

Just like all hormones, two general pathologic processes can occur: too much hormone or too little hormone.

- **Growth hormone excess:** This can cause one of two conditions—**gigantism** or **acromegaly.** Almost invariably this is due to a GH-secreting pituitary adenoma. Making the distinction between gigantism and acromegaly involves simply finding out the patient's age to determine whether his or her growth plates have likely fused or not. Younger patients who have growth plates that will allow for increased long bone growth (via IGF-1, made in the liver by GH stimulation) will have an extraordinarily tall stature as well as other stigmata of GH excess. Those with fused growth plates will not have increased linear growth but will have all the other problems that come with GH excess, essentially relating to enlarged organs (cardiomyopathy, the most common cause of death); diabetes (from insulin resistance); and classic coarsening of facial features and enlarged hands, head, and feet (probe about hat size changes, ring size changes, and shoe size changes, or ask for an old photo). Diagnosis of this can be made by increased IGF-1 levels as well as **glucose suppression testing**—because hypoglycemia is a stimulus for GH release, giving a glucose load should decrease GH in a normally functioning pituitary gland; failure to do so suggests a GH-secreting tumor in the pituitary. Treatment is surgical removal of the tumor. Nonresectable tumors can be treated with **somatostatin** analogs such as **octreotide,** which will provide negative feedback to attempts to decrease GH levels.
- **Growth hormone deficiency:** Can be caused by many processes. Consider the stimuli and each step of growth hormone activity—problems at any point can cause GH deficiency (e.g., hypothalamus failing to secrete GHRH, pituitary failing to secrete GH, liver failing to produce IGF-1, receptor dysfunction). The symptoms are intuitive: **poor growth** and **delayed puberty.** Treatment is simply giving GH!

Prolactinoma: most common pituitary tumor, may cause bitemporal hemianopsia and decreased GnRH (infertility and loss of libido)

Prolactin

Prolactin, as the name implies, is prolactation. It allows for maternal breast milk production and has a trophic effect on the breast. This hormone normally is only high during pregnancy and lactation but can be increased pathologically with **prolactin-secreting tumors,** with **medications that block dopamine,** or with **hypothyroidism.** The effects of prolactin are twofold:

- **Breast development and support of milk production:** Allows for breastfeeding by promoting mammary duct proliferation and synthesis of milk proteins.
- **Negative feedback on gonadotropin-releasing hormone (GnRH):** Often referred to as "nature's birth control"; in breastfeeding mothers, the persistently high prolactin levels downregulate GnRH to attempt to inhibit ovulation to space out children appropriately.

Although prolactin deficiency can occur from pituitary insufficiency, there are many causes of **hyperprolactinemia,** as alluded to previously. Hyperprolactinemia can lead to **galactorrhea** (milk secretion from the nipples) as well as **infertility** or **loss of libido** as a result of GnRH downregulation.

- **Hypothyroidism:** As can be seen in Fig. 9.5A, TRH from the hypothalamus results in increased prolactin secretion. Those with hypothyroidism have increased TRH to attempt to stimulate the thyroid to increase thyroid hormone output. Treatment is repleting thyroid hormone.
- **Medications that block dopamine:** Dopamine receptor antagonists (classically the antipsychotics, which are D_2-blocking agents) block the dopamine receptors throughout the body, including the anterior pituitary. This shuts off the negative feedback on prolactin secretion, leading to hyperprolactinemia. Treatment is stopping the offending medication if possible.
- **Tumors of the lactotroph cells of the anterior pituitary** (tumors of the cells that make prolactin): Called **prolactinomas** (*white dashed arrow* in Fig. 9.5B), these can cause hyperprolactinemia. **Prolactinoma is the most common pituitary tumor.** Because the pituitary is so close to the optic chiasm (black arrow in Fig. 9.5B), the tumor can press on it, causing bitemporal hemianopsia (see Chapter 13 for visual field defect explanations), which is classic for this tumor if large. Treatment is either surgical removal of the tumor (if large) or giving a **dopamine agonist** such as **bromocriptine** or **cabergoline** to increase negative feedback on the cells to decrease size and output. Serum prolactin levels in prolactinoma are higher than in the other causes, and a serum prolactin level of more than 200 ng/mL is essentially diagnostic of a prolactinoma.

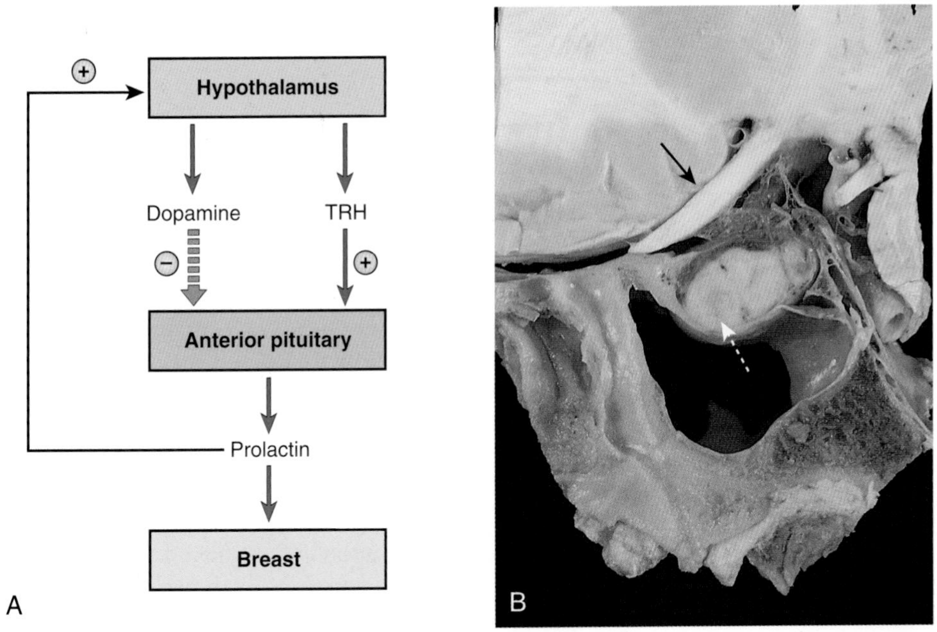

FIG. 9.5 A, Prolactin. The stimulus is thyrotropin-releasing hormone, and the inhibition is via dopamine. Prolactin promotes breast development and milk production and also downregulates gonadotropin-releasing hormone (GnRH) secretion from the hypothalamus. **B,** Prolactinoma, a benign, prolactin-secreting tumor of lactotroph cells in the anterior pituitary. Close proximity to the optic chiasm leads to compressive symptoms such as bitemporal hemianopsia. Increased prolactin secretion can lead to galactorrhea or severely downregulated GnRH secretion, which leads to infertility and/or loss of libido. (**A** *from Costanzo LS.* Physiology. *4th ed. New York: Elsevier; 2009.* **B** *from Burger PC, Scheithauer BW, Vogel KS.* Surgical Pathology of the Nervous System. *4th ed. London: Churchill Livingstone; 2002:444.*)

Causes of Anterior Pituitary Dysfunction

The **anterior pituitary** supplies numerous hormones to the body, and damage to the pituitary (or to the hypothalamus, which sends regulatory signals to the pituitary) can lead to **hypopituitarism.** The main causes of damage to the anterior pituitary gland are **mass effect** (tumors, empty sella syndrome) and **infarction** (Sheehan syndrome, sickle cell anemia).

- **Tumors affecting the pituitary:** Masses can arise from the pituitary, such as **nonfunctioning pituitary adenomas,** which eventually overtake the entirety of the gland, or tumors that exert a mass effect on the pituitary, such as **craniopharyngiomas.** A craniopharyngioma is a remnant of Rathke pouch, which normally is a depression in the roof of the developing mouth that gives rise to the anterior pituitary. Because of mass effect, a craniopharyngioma can press on and destroy the pituitary gland.

- **Empty sella syndrome:** Mainly affects **obese women with hypertension.** This is thought to represent intracranial hypertension. An anatomic defect allows the subarachnoid space to extend into the sella turcica, partially filling it with cerebrospinal fluid (CSF), which then flattens the pituitary gland.
- **Sheehan syndrome** (postpartum necrosis of the pituitary): During pregnancy, the mother's anterior pituitary increases in size significantly as a result of increased hormone requirements. However, the blood supply is not increased to the same degree, leaving the anterior pituitary gland relatively ischemic during this period. If the mother becomes hypotensive, such as from significant hemorrhage during childbirth, the ischemia can progress into pituitary infarction.
- **Sickle cell anemia:** Sickle cell patients often have vasoocclusive crises in which sickled cells cause ischemic injury to the target organ. This can occur in the pituitary and cause dysfunction.

Thyroid Gland

Anatomy, Embryology, and Histology

The **thyroid** gland is located in the **anterior neck,** below and lateral to the thyroid cartilage. It is a **bilobed** gland, connected by the **isthmus** (Fig. 9.6A). This gland was initially an outgrowth near the base of the tongue, migrating down the neck into its current position, and leaving the foramen cecum of the back of the tongue as a remnant. This embryologic movement can malfunction, leading to either a thyroglossal duct cyst or ectopic thyroid tissue.

> Thyroglossal duct cysts: **midline** mass on anterior neck
>
> Branchial cleft cysts: **lateral** mass on anterior neck

- **Thyroglossal duct cyst:** Normally, the thyroglossal duct (the passageway for the thyroid migrating down to its position in the neck) atrophies and closes. Failure of this closure can lead to a cyst, presenting as a midline mass. Because the thyroglossal duct is attached (at the foramen cecum) to the tongue, this cyst will move with tongue movement. The cyst can be asymptomatic (most common) or become infected; rarely, this can cause cancer (thyroglossal duct carcinoma). Because the mass is midline, this can be differentiated from a branchial cleft cyst, which is lateral (see Chapter 4).
- **Ectopic thyroid tissue:** Can present in many forms but simply represents thyroid tissue that did not migrate in a normal fashion. A **lingual thyroid** can occur when the thyroid fails to descend, leading to a mass at the base of the tongue and potentially causing dysphagia (difficulty swallowing).

> C cells: parafollicular cells; create calcitonin; cells that become malignant in medullary thyroid carcinoma (calcitonin used as a tumor marker)

The thyroid is perfused by two major arteries: the **superior thyroid artery** (a branch of the external carotid artery) and the **inferior thyroid artery** (a branch of the thyrocervical trunk, which comes off of the beginning of the subclavian artery; Fig. 9.6B). It is drained by the superior, middle, and inferior thyroid veins.

The histologic image in Fig. 9.7 is of **thyroid tissue.** You should be able to recognize thyroid tissue histologically and understand why it appears the way it does.

- **Follicular epithelial cells:** The rim of cells surrounding the colloid in the center. These are metabolically active cells that pull iodine from the bloodstream (via Na^+/I^- symporters) and begin the synthesis of new thyroid hormone. When the thyroid is stimulated by TSH, these cells take thyroid hormone from the colloid and prepare it for release into the bloodstream. When very active, these cells appear columnar instead of cuboidal.
- **Colloid:** The pink "centers" of the glands contain colloid, which contains formed thyroid hormone and partially formed thyroid hormone attached to a protein called **thyroglobulin.** They will remain stored until the thyroid is stimulated to release hormone.
- **C cells:** Also known as **parafollicular cells** (because they are between the colloid follicles), these are **neural crest** in origin, secreting **calcitonin** to decrease blood calcium level. This also becomes important in **medullary thyroid cancer** (covered later in the section "Pathology"), a cancer of the parafollicular C cells.

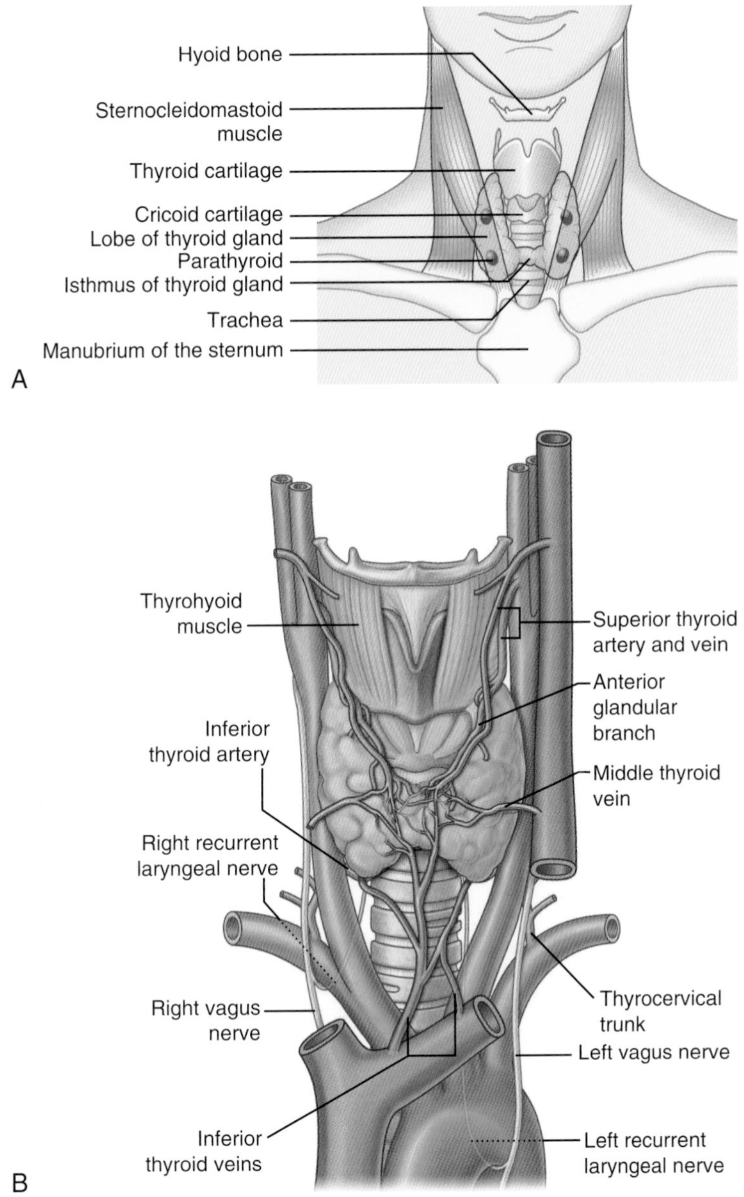

Fig. 9.6 Thyroid anatomy and blood supply. **A,** The thyroid's anatomic position in the neck. **B,** Blood supply of the thyroid with the superior thyroid artery originating from the external carotid artery and the inferior thyroid artery, which is a branch of the thyrocervical trunk (itself the first branch from the subclavian artery). (**A** *from Douglas G, Nicol F, Robertson C.* Macleod's Clinical Examination. *12th ed. Edinburgh: Elsevier; 2009.* **B** *from Drake RL, Vogl AW, Mitchell AWM.* Gray's Anatomy for Students. *2nd ed. Philadelphia: Elsevier; 2009.*)

Thyroid Hormone Physiology

The thyroid gland is responsible for regulation of metabolism and also plays an important role in growth and development—these overarching functions play a role in almost every process in the body; dysfunction therefore leads to widespread symptoms. The thyroid gland generates **thyroid hormone,** both **T_4** (with four iodine molecules attached, inactive) and **T_3** (with three iodine molecules attached, active), into the bloodstream, with T_3 having direct effects on the cells and T_4 being converted to T_3 in the peripheral tissue by **5′-deiodinase enzyme to become active.** The stimulus for thyroid hormone production is **TSH,** produced by the **pituitary.** The pituitary releases TSH when the **hypothalamus** secretes **TRH.** Thyroid hormone has negative feedback on both the hypothalamus (TRH) and the pituitary (TSH), ensuring precise regulation of hormones. Interestingly, **TRH is also a stimulatory signal for prolactin release;** this becomes important in conditions such as primary hypothyroidism,

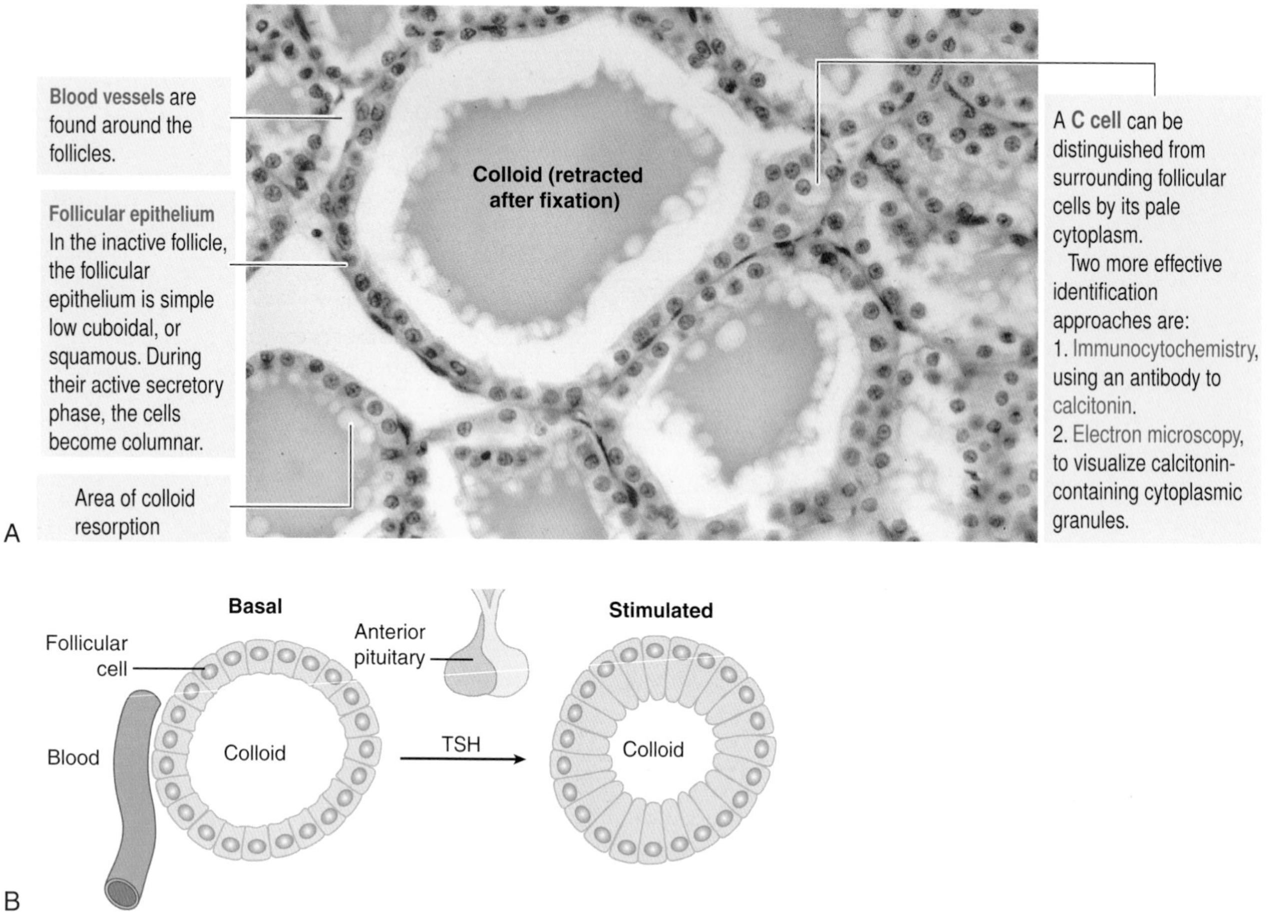
Blood vessels are found around the follicles.
Follicular epithelium In the inactive follicle, the follicular epithelium is simple low cuboidal, or squamous. During their active secretory phase, the cells become columnar.
Area of colloid resorption
A
Colloid (retracted after fixation)
A C cell can be distinguished from surrounding follicular cells by its pale cytoplasm.
Two more effective identification approaches are:
1. Immunocytochemistry, using an antibody to calcitonin.
2. Electron microscopy, to visualize calcitonin-containing cytoplasmic granules.
Basal
Follicular cell
Blood
Colloid
Anterior pituitary
TSH
Stimulated
Colloid
B

FIG. 9.7 Histologic appearance of the thyroid. **A,** Microscopic view of thyroid tissue, demonstrating thyroid follicles filled with colloid. **B,** Illustration of the histologic change in the thyroid follicular epithelium from cuboidal to columnar with increased stimulation from thyroid-stimulating hormone (TSH). (**A** *from Kierszenbaum AL, Tres LL.* Histology and Cell Biology. *3rd ed. St. Louis: Elsevier; 2011.* **B** *from Kester M, Karpa KD, Vrana KE.* Elsevier's Integrated Review Pharmacology. *2nd ed. St. Louis: Elsevier; 2011.*)

in which the hypothalamus generates increased TRH to promote TSH secretion from the pituitary to stimulate the thyroid: This will lead to increased prolactin and even the potential for galactorrhea and infertility. In addition, the **C cells** of the thyroid secrete **calcitonin,** which prevents bone breakdown and stimulates osteoblasts and therefore leads to decreased blood calcium levels (calci**tonin tones down** the calcium level).

Synthesis of thyroid hormone is relatively complex but can be broken down into a few steps (Fig. 9.8):

1. **Iodide (I^-)** is taken into the follicular cells by Na^+/I^- cotransport.
2. This iodide is **oxidized** into iodine (I_2) at the same time as it is moved into the colloid.
3. The I_2 then is attached onto the amino acid tyrosine (termed **organification**) into either **MIT** (monoiodotyrosine, one iodine molecule) or **DIT** (diiodotyrosine, two iodine molecules); these are stored on **thyroglobulin** in the colloid.
4. The MIT and DIT can combine into either T_3 (MIT + DIT, because there are three iodine molecules total), or T_4 (DIT + DIT, because there are four iodine molecules total). More T_4 is generated than T_3.
5. When stimulated (TRH from hypothalamus → TSH from pituitary → TSH stimulation of thyroid), the thyroglobulin with its attached molecules will be endocytosed into the follicular cell, and T_3 and T_4 will be released into the bloodstream. This T_3 and T_4 will then act in a **negative feedback loop** on the pituitary and hypothalamus to decrease thyroid stimulation to ensure the level of thyroid hormone does not become too high.

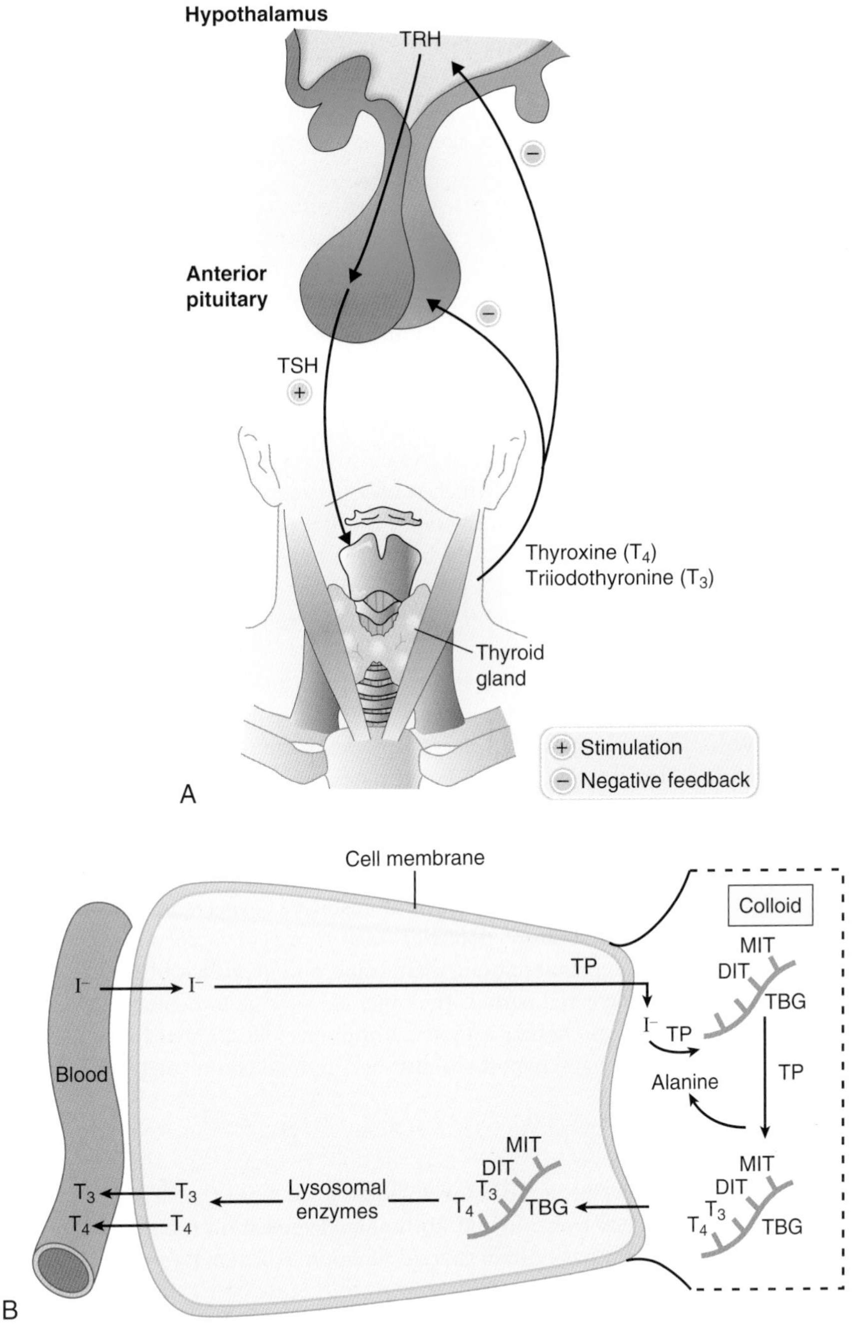

Fig. 9.8 Thyroid hormone synthesis and physiology. **A,** Thyrotropin-releasing hormone (TRH) is secreted by the hypothalamus, triggering the anterior pituitary to release thyroid-stimulating hormone (TSH), which stimulates the thyroid to make and release thyroid hormone (T_3 and T_4). **B,** Thyroid hormone is synthesized in a series of steps (see text for details). TBG, thyroxine-binding globulin; TP, thyroid peroxidase. (**A** *from Damjanov I.* Pathophysiology. *Philadelphia: Elsevier; 2008.* **B** *from Kester M, Karpa KD, Vrana KE.* Elsevier's Integrated Review Pharmacology. *2nd ed. St. Louis: Elsevier; 2011.*)

Wolff-Chaikoff effect: transient **hypothyroidism** after iodine administration

Jod-Basedow phenomenon: transient **hyperthyroidism** after iodine administration

All of the synthetic steps are catalyzed by thyroid peroxidase. Therefore blockage of this enzyme with medications such as **propylthiouracil** or **methimazole** will stop thyroid hormone synthesis, which can be effective in the treatment of **hyper**thyroidism.

Large amounts of iodine administration can have very different effects depending on the initial iodine status of the individual. This can be seen with iatrogenic iodide administration (iodinated contrast material, intravenous or oral iodide administration) or with medications that contain large amounts of iodide (e.g., amiodarone, an antiarrhythmic drug).

- **Wolff-Chaikoff effect:** In a normal individual, giving large amounts of iodine at once will lead to **transient hypothyroidism,** which is counterintuitive. This is because the thyroid has an autoregulatory function; when it sees large amounts of iodide, it shuts down to **prevent massive thyroid hormone generation and release.** Initially it overreacts, leading to transient hypothyroidism before readjusting to normal. This can be a potential therapeutic agent in severe hyperthyroidism to quickly shut down the thyroid.
- **Jod-Basedow phenomenon:** A very different outcome occurs in those with **chronic iodine deficiency.** These individuals have hypothyroidism (iodine deficiency is the most common cause of hypothyroidism in **developing** countries) as a result of lack of iodine available to make thyroid hormone. Therefore their Na^+/I^- cotransporters are heavily upregulated to take up any iodine in the blood, and TSH levels are high to stimulate the thyroid gland to make hormone. When these individuals are given large amounts of iodine, they quickly create large amounts of thyroid hormone from the highly stimulated thyroid, leading to **transient hyperthyroidism** before readjusting.

Once the thyroid hormone (T_3 and T_4) is in the bloodstream, it circulates mostly bound to **thyroxine-binding globulin** (**TBG,** not to be confused with thyroglobulin, which is only present in the thyroid). The rest is bound to albumin or **free in the bloodstream** (only a tiny fraction). This free (unbound) T_3 and T_4 is the thyroid hormone that can have action on the body's cells. It is important to remember that **T_3 essentially has all of the thyroid hormone activity,** and therefore **T_4 must be converted by the tissues to T_3** (by removing one iodine molecule via 5′-deiodinase enzyme) to be active (Fig. 9.9). The effects of thyroid hormone are widespread, including the following:

- **Increasing metabolic rate:** Increases Na^+/K^+-ATPase activity, increasing adenosine triphosphate (ATP) use and therefore increasing metabolic rate.
- **Increasing catecholamine sensitivity:** Increases synthesis of β_1 receptors on cardiac tissue, leading to increased sensitivity of the body to catecholamines, increasing cardiac output (CO) by increasing the heart rate (HR) and stroke volume (SV) (recall that CO = HR × SV). This is to support the increased oxygen requirement by the increased metabolic rate to allow for increased ATP generation.
- **Proper growth and development:** Allows for proper differentiation and maturation of cells; this is why hypothyroidism in the neonate can be so devastating, with symptoms just as expected from before—low metabolic rate leading to low body temperature, poor musculature, excessive sleeping, improper development. Thyroid hormone is also important to brain maturation, and hypothyroidism can lead to irreversible mental retardation in the neonatal period. The other classic clue to neonatal hypothyroidism is a protruding umbilicus (umbilical hernia caused by improper development of anterior abdominal wall). Note that historically, neonatal hypothyroidism was termed cretinism, but the former term is now preferred.

> TSH-secreting tumors essentially do not exist because there is an α subunit and a β subunit generated by different cells. Therefore uncontrolled secretion of one subunit would not be able to generate a functional hormone.

Laboratory Testing

The first study in evaluating thyroid function is checking a **TSH level** (Table 9.3); recall that TSH is produced by the pituitary and has negative feedback from thyroid hormone released from the thyroid. Therefore a normal result ensures that the patient has normal thyroid function. Abnormal results require further workup:

High TSH: Indicates that the pituitary is attempting to stimulate the thyroid to make more thyroid hormone, indicating primary hypothyroidism (such as from autoimmune destruction of the thyroid gland in **Hashimoto thyroiditis**).

- **Low TSH:** Indicates that the pituitary gland is not attempting to stimulate the thyroid to make thyroid hormone, indicating one of two overarching possibilities: (1) the body has too much thyroid hormone (such as in patients taking excess thyroid hormone medication, or in autoimmune stimulation of the thyroid gland as in **Graves disease**), or (2) the problem is upstream of the thyroid—either pituitary dysfunction with failure to secrete TSH or hypothalamic dysfunction in which the pituitary and thyroid may be perfectly fine, but the hypothalamus is not giving the signal through TRH to allow the pituitary to generate TSH to stimulate the thyroid gland.

Because an abnormal TSH usually does not give a single diagnosis, further workup is required, which usually involves getting free T_3 and T_4 levels. **Laboratory tests that quantify total T_3 or T_4 are**

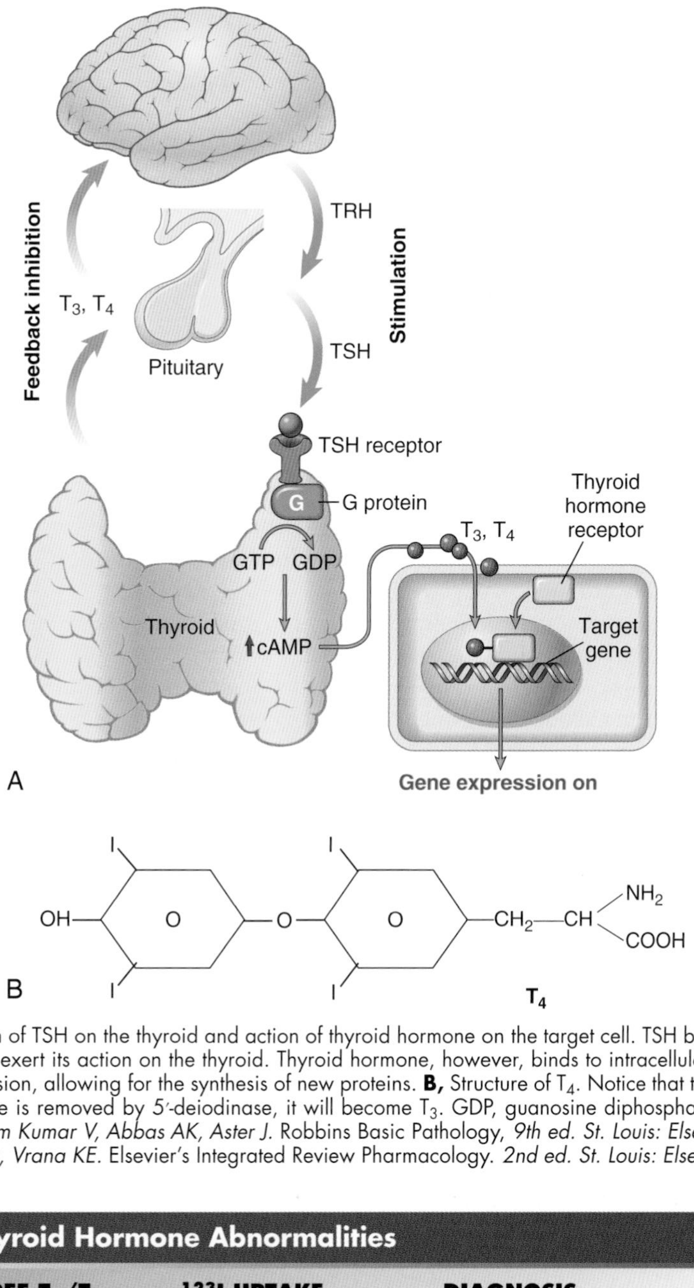

Fig. 9.9 A, Action of TSH on the thyroid and action of thyroid hormone on the target cell. TSH binds to a G-protein–coupled receptor to exert its action on the thyroid. Thyroid hormone, however, binds to intracellular nuclear receptors to alter gene expression, allowing for the synthesis of new proteins. **B,** Structure of T_4. Notice that there are four iodine molecules; when one is removed by 5′-deiodinase, it will become T_3. GDP, guanosine diphosphate; GTP, Guanosine triphosphate. (**A** *from Kumar V, Abbas AK, Aster J.* Robbins Basic Pathology, *9th ed. St. Louis: Elsevier; 2012.* **B** *from Kester M, Karpa KD, Vrana KE.* Elsevier's Integrated Review Pharmacology. *2nd ed. St. Louis: Elsevier; 2011.*)

Table 9.3 Thyroid Hormone Abnormalities

TSH	FREE T_3/T_4	^{123}I UPTAKE	DIAGNOSIS
High	• Low	(unnecessary)	• Primary hypothyroidism
Low	• High	• High, diffuse	• Graves disease
	• High	• High, focal	• Autonomous "hot" nodule(s) producing thyroid hormone
	• High	• Low	• Exogenous thyroid hormone ingestion or initial phase of thyroiditis
	• Low	(unnecessary)	• Secondary or tertiary hypothyroidism

generally less reliable than free levels. Laboratory tests that quantify **free** T_3 and free T_4 are typically most useful. *TBG levels can vary, making total T_3 and T_4 levels unreliable; the free T_3 and T_4 will allow determination of the amount of hormone available to the cells.*

- **Decreased TBG:** Occurs with increased **testosterone** (think that increased testosterone means your body wants to make more muscle, breaking down TBG to make more available protein). Because TBG is made in the liver, **hepatic failure** also causes decreased TBG.

- **Increased TBG:** Occurs with increased **estrogen** (in pregnancy or with oral contraceptive use), which inhibits hepatic breakdown of TBG.

If the cause of hyperthyroidism is not clear, more advanced testing such as radioactive iodine (^{123}I) uptake can occur, which can show whether the thyroid is "hungry" for iodine (actively uptaking iodine to make thyroid hormone, high uptake). (Note that **^{123}I is used for scanning** and diagnostic purposes because it is not toxic to the thyroid, but **^{131}I causes radioactivity** that destroys the thyroid and can be used for therapy of hyperthyroidism—don't mix these up!) This test is helpful when the TSH is low but the free T_3/T_4 is high because iodine uptake scans will show whether the entire thyroid is taking up iodine (diffuse overproduction), if a specific spot in the thyroid is taking up too much iodine (such as small nodules in the thyroid that are autonomously making thyroid hormone independent of stimulation, termed "hot" nodules, which are rarely cancerous), or if none of the iodine is taken up (therefore the thyroid hormone is coming from pills the patient is taking, and not the thyroid).

Pathology

Pathologic conditions of the thyroid are incredibly common; other than malignancies, they can be broken down into two groups: (1) conditions that cause **increased hormone production or secretion,** and (2) conditions that cause **decreased hormone production or secretion.**

Conditions that cause **increased hormone production or secretion** lead to symptoms consistent with thyroid hormone over activity. Any hypermetabolic state characterized by elevated levels of free T_3 and T_4 is known as **thyrotoxicosis.** Because thyroid hormone is involved in metabolic regulation, thyrotoxicosis will lead to increased basal metabolic rate, which will lead to **weight loss** and **heat intolerance** with **diaphoresis** as well as increased catecholamine sensitivity, leading to **tachycardia;** the increased sympathetic drive can even lead to **atrial fibrillation.** Increased stimulation of the gut causes **hyperdefecation,** which is not diarrhea but rather is numerous episodes of defecation from hypermotility.

> Graves disease: the only cause of hyperthyroidism that also causes proptosis (exophthalmos)

Lastly, although it is possible to get **lid lag** (when the patient looks down, the upper eyelid does not move downward quickly) with all forms of hyperthyroidism (because the **superior tarsal muscle** is smooth muscle innervated by the sympathetic nervous system, which is sensitized with thyrotoxicosis), only Graves disease actually causes exophthalmos.

- **Graves disease:** The most common cause of **hyperthyroidism,** in which **B cells produce immunoglobulin G (IgG) autoantibodies** that **stimulate the thyroid's TSH receptors** (making this *a type II hypersensitivity reaction*). There is lymphocytic infiltration of the orbital tissue, and autoantibodies also stimulate fibroblasts to secrete hyaluronic acid (a glycosaminoglycan). These two factors increase the orbital volume, leading to **exophthalmos** (eyes bulging out), which can eventually be so severe as to cause blindness. The increased glycosaminoglycan deposition in the skin also leads to **pretibial myxedema.** It is important to note that these IgG antibodies (like all IgG antibodies) can cross the blood–placenta barrier in pregnant women, leading to potential transient hyperthyroidism in the neonate until they clear the IgG.
- **Toxic multinodular goiter** (Plummer syndrome): The term **goiter** refers to enlargement of the thyroid, and multinodular goiter means that there are many nodules in the thyroid causing this goiter. These diffuse nodules are present throughout the thyroid and are **hyperfunctioning,** working independently of TSH, sometimes because of mutations in the TSH receptor that allow for constitutive activity. Symptoms of hyperthyroidism are present, but there is no exophthalmos and no pretibial myxedema because this is not an autoimmune phenomenon.
- **Exogenous thyroid intake:** Patients taking thyroid hormone in an effort to lose weight will have signs and symptoms of hyperthyroidism. They will also have low TSH and low ^{123}I uptake.
- **Struma ovarii:** A rare syndrome—essentially an ovarian **teratoma** (which can generate many tissue types) that can lead to hyperthyroidism if there is presence of large amounts of thyroid tissue.
- **Early thyroiditis syndromes:** Any time the thyroid is inflamed, it can initially leak a surge of thyroid hormone from the colloid. Afterward, hypothyroidism can occur because the stored hormone has been lost.

Conditions that cause **decreased hormone production or secretion** lead to symptoms that are almost exactly the opposite of hyperthyroidism. The lower metabolic rate leads to **weight gain, cold intolerance, fatigue,** and **dry skin and brittle hair.** Decreased catecholamine sensitivity can lead to **bradycardia.** Decreased gut motility leads to **constipation.** Interestingly, decreased synthesis of low-density lipoprotein (LDL) receptors leads to increased circulating levels of cholesterol, causing hypercholesterolemia. As explained earlier in the section "Thyroid Hormone Physiology," primary hypothyroidism (thyroid gland dysfunction from inflammation or destruction) will lead to increased levels of TRH from the hypothalamus to promote TSH release from the pituitary to stimulate the thyroid gland to make more hormone; this increased TRH can lead to **galactorrhea** as a symptom because TRH is also a stimulus for **prolactin** release. This increase in prolactin may affect gonadotropin function, resulting in decreased libido, infertility, and changes in menstruation.

- **Hashimoto thyroiditis:** The most common cause of **hypothyroidism** in **developed** countries, this is classically seen in **middle-aged women** but can occur in both genders at almost any age. In Hashimoto thyroiditis the body attacks the thyroid directly via $CD8^+$ cytotoxic T cells, leading to cell destruction and release of contents into the bloodstream. These released proteins, such as thyroglobulin and thyroid peroxidase, are usually not present in the bloodstream and are seen as foreign; the B cells then make antithyroglobulin and antithyroid peroxidase antibodies as a response. These antibodies can cause further destruction of the gland. Therefore the damage to the gland is both cell mediated (type IV hypersensitivity) and antibody mediated (type II hypersensitivity). With the initial inflammation of the gland, there can be initial hyperthyroidism because formed hormone leaks from the cell; this is known as Hashitoxicosis.
- **Iodine deficiency:** The most common cause of hypothyroidism and goiter **worldwide**—chronically high TSH levels cause sustained stimulation and growth of the gland (goiter) to attempt to extract any iodine present in the blood.
- **Subacute granulomatous (painful) thyroiditis** (DeQuervain thyroiditis): Often triggered by a **viral infection,** especially **upper respiratory tract infection.** There is either cross-reactivity with a viral antigen or inflammation of the thyroid leading to exposure of a thyroid antigen with subsequent **painful** inflammation of the thyroid. This inflammation can lead to initial hyperthyroidism as preformed hormone is released, but afterward the thyroid can take weeks to return to normal, and hypothyroidism can occur during this time.
- **Subacute lymphocytic (painless) thyroiditis:** A variant of this is the most commonly tested, which is postpartum thyroiditis. This is thought to potentially represent a subset of Hashimoto thyroiditis but is characterized by postpartum hyperthyroidism secondary to follicle rupture with subsequent hypothyroidism. Many of these patients will recover normal thyroid function over weeks to months, but antigen exposure from the follicle rupture may contribute to development of Hashimoto thyroiditis (up to 50% will eventually develop Hashimoto thyroiditis in the future).
- **Riedel thyroiditis:** Very rare disease characterized by ***painless*** **fibrosis** in the thyroid gland and nearby structures in the neck. This can cause **tracheal obstruction** from the **hard, rocklike** fibrous deposition.

Thyroid cancer has four separate types: papillary, follicular, medullary, and anaplastic.

- **Papillary carcinoma** (>85%; Fig. 9.10): The most common thyroid cancer (**p**apillary is **p**opular!), with the major risk factors being exposure to ionizing radiation and family history. Luckily, this usually has an excellent prognosis. Histologically, this is characterized by two items: **Orphan Annie eye nuclei** (Fig. 9.10B), so called because there appears to be nothing inside the nuclei, and (right image) **psammoma bodies,** which are concentrically calcified structures; psammoma is derived from the Greek word *psammos* meaning "sand." Psammoma bodies (Fig. 9.10C) are found in many cancers, but of the thyroid cancers, psammoma bodies are only found in papillary thyroid carcinoma (see Fig. 9.10).
- **Follicular carcinoma** (10%): The second most common thyroid cancer, this occurs in **older women (40–60 years of age),** and the prognosis is directly related to whether metastases are present: When no metastatic disease is present, the prognosis is very good; when metastatic lesions are found, the prognosis is much worse. One unique aspect of this carcinoma is that metastasis occurs by **hematogenous** spread, which is not characteristic of carcinomas (usually carcinomas spread by the lymphatics, and sarcomas spread by hematogenous routes). Histologically, **follicular carcinoma** reveals **colloid follicles** (hence the name), unlike the other carcinomas. This needs to be differentiated

Papillary thyroid carcinoma is **p**opular (most common), has **p**sammoma bodies, and has the best **p**rognosis!

mnemonic
PSa**MM**oma: **P**apillary thyroid cancer, **S**erous cancers of the ovary, **M**eningioma, **M**esothelioma

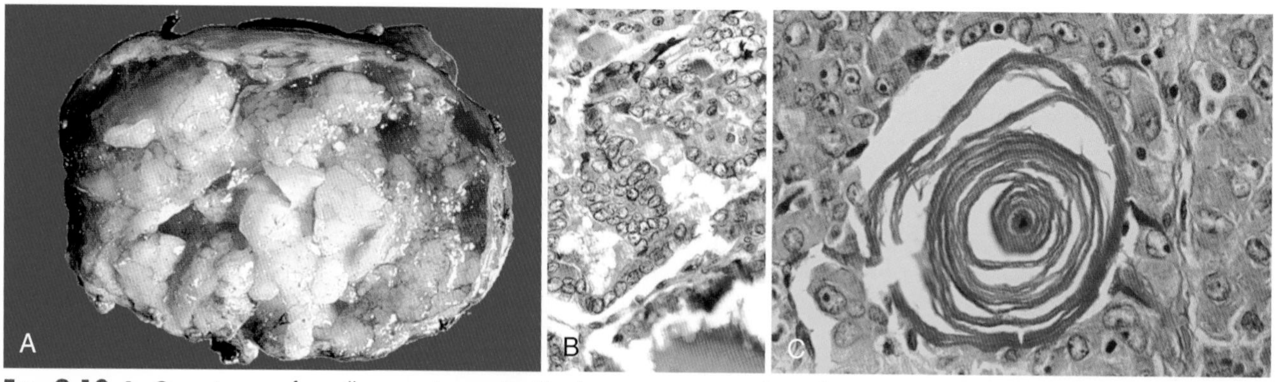

Fig. 9.10 A, Gross image of papillary carcinoma. **B,** Histologic examination of papillary carcinoma, showing classic "Orphan Annie eye" nuclei. **C,** Psammoma bodies, found in papillary thyroid cancer but also in serous cancers of the ovary, meningioma, and mesothelioma. (**A** *and* **B** *from Kumar V, Abbas AK, Fausto N, Aster J.* Robbins & Cotran Pathologic Basis of Disease. *8th ed. New York: Elsevier; 2009.* **C** *from* The AFIP Atlas of Tumor Pathology, *courtesy The Armed Forces Institute of Pathology. Accessed January 10, 2013, from* http://fr.wikipedia.org/wiki/Fichier:Psammoma.jpg.)

from a **follicular adenoma,** which is the most common **benign** tumor and is surrounded by a complete capsule; it is an adenoma (benign) and not a carcinoma (malignant) because the complete encapsulation prevents metastatic spread. It is often hard to differentiate between a follicular carcinoma versus follicular adenoma based just on biopsy unless you see capsular invasion. Thus the only way to definitively tell the two apart is after resection and pathologic evaluation, so all of these are typically removed (Fig. 9.11).

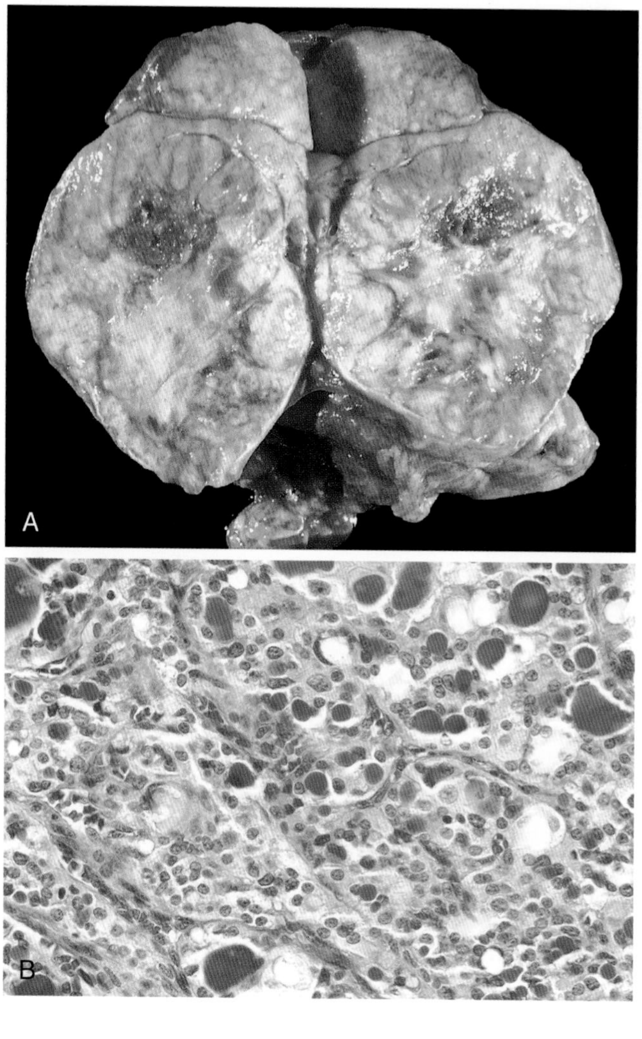

Fig. 9.11 A, Gross image of follicular carcinoma. **B,** Histologic examination of follicular carcinoma, showing some disorganized colloid follicles. (*From Kumar V, Abbas AK, Fausto N, Aster J.* Robbins & Cotran Pathologic Basis of Disease. *8th ed. New York: Elsevier; 2009.*)

- **Medullary carcinoma** (5%; Fig. 9.12): This is a neoplasm of the **parafollicular C cells,** which create calcitonin. This is the type of thyroid cancer **associated with MEN IIa and IIb.** Because they secrete calcitonin, **calcitonin can be used as a tumor marker for recurrence of disease and can be used in immunohistochemical staining of the biopsy to diagnose disease.** The excess secretion of calcitonin builds up and is deposited as **amyloid** in the stroma of the thyroid, which can be seen on histologic examination (Fig. 9.12B). In patients with this rare cancer, checking family history and signs of other MEN IIa and IIb–associated pathology is important (see Fig. 9.12).

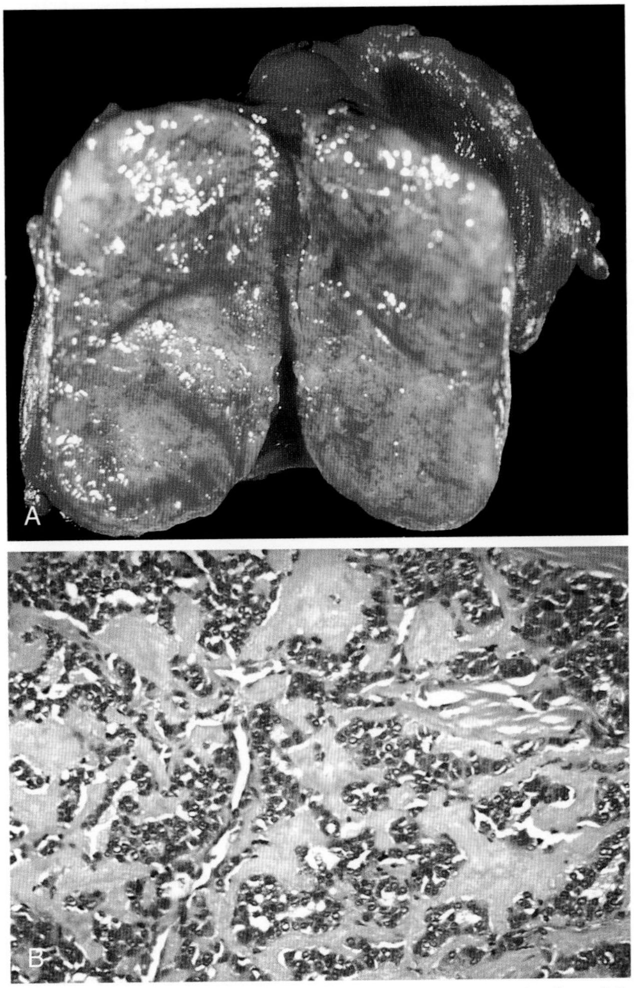

FIG. 9.12 A, Gross image of medullary carcinoma. **B,** Histologic examination of medullary carcinoma, showing amyloid stroma from calcitonin deposition. (*From Kumar V, Abbas AK, Fausto N, Aster J.* Robbins & Cotran Pathologic Basis of Disease. *8th ed. New York: Elsevier; 2009. Courtesy Joseph Corson, MD, Boston, MA.*)

- **Anaplastic carcinoma:** Undifferentiated, rapidly progressive, and almost uniformly fatal, the prognosis for patients with anaplastic carcinoma is often less than 6 months. Some patients will have a history of a prior thyroid cancer.

Pharmacology

The **pharmacology** of the thyroid gland essentially is aimed at either blocking thyroid hormone synthesis and release or providing supplementary thyroid hormone, depending on what needs correcting.

- **Propylthiouracil (PTU) and methimazole:** Inhibit organification of iodide and therefore decrease thyroid hormone synthesis; useful in hyperthyroidism to prevent thyrotoxicosis. Can cause **agranulocytosis** and a skin rash. When taken during pregnancy, methimazole is associated with aplasia cutis congenita (congenital absence of skin, which manifests as a scarlike appearance in a neonate). For this reason, it should be avoided during the first trimester of pregnancy.

- **Levothyroxine** (synthetic T_4) and **triiodothyronine** (also known as liothyronine, synthetic T_3): Replacement thyroid hormones for hypothyroid conditions. T_4 can be converted in the periphery to T_3 and is favored because the half-life of T_4 is considerably longer than that of T_3 (because of greater albumin binding affinity), and therefore blood levels are more stable over time. Toxicity gives symptoms of hyperthyroidism (tachycardia, heat intolerance, tremors).
- **Iodine:** Iodine can be given in thyrotoxicosis to shut down the thyroid through the Wolff-Chaikoff effect. It is important to know that any iodine load can cause this, including unintended administration (such as using iodinated contrast for computed tomography scanning, or the iodine-rich antiarrhythmic drug amiodarone). In addition, ^{123}I is used for diagnostic scanning of the thyroid to visualize uptake. ^{131}I is used in ablation of the thyroid because the thyroid tissue concentrates the iodine and is subsequently destroyed by the ^{131}I radiation.

Adrenal Glands (Cortex and Medulla)

Anatomy, Embryology, and Histology

The **adrenal glands** sit on top of each kidney (superior to the kidney and so also called the **suprarenal glands** by some); therefore like the kidney, the adrenal glands are retroperitoneal. Each adrenal gland has a **cortex** and **medulla,** each with distinctly different functions (Fig. 9.13).

- **Adrenal cortex:** The outer layer of the adrenal gland, consisting of **three layers** (zona glomerulosa, zona fasciculata, and zona reticularis), each of which secretes different steroid hormones because of differences in enzyme activity. Mnemonic: from outside to in, the layers can be remembered by **GFR** (just like the filtration rate of the kidney!)—zona **g**lomerulosa, zona **f**asciculata, zona **r**eticularis.
- **Adrenal medulla:** The inner layer of the adrenal gland, the adrenal medulla is **neuroectodermal** in origin. The medulla is responsible for generation of **epinephrine** and **norepinephrine** to activate the sympathetic nervous system.

It can also be seen in Fig. 9.13 that **because the left kidney is farther away from the inferior vena cava,** the **left** adrenal vein drains into the left **renal** vein, whereas the **right** adrenal vein drains into the **inferior vena cava.** This is the same way that the gonadal (testicular or ovarian) veins drain.

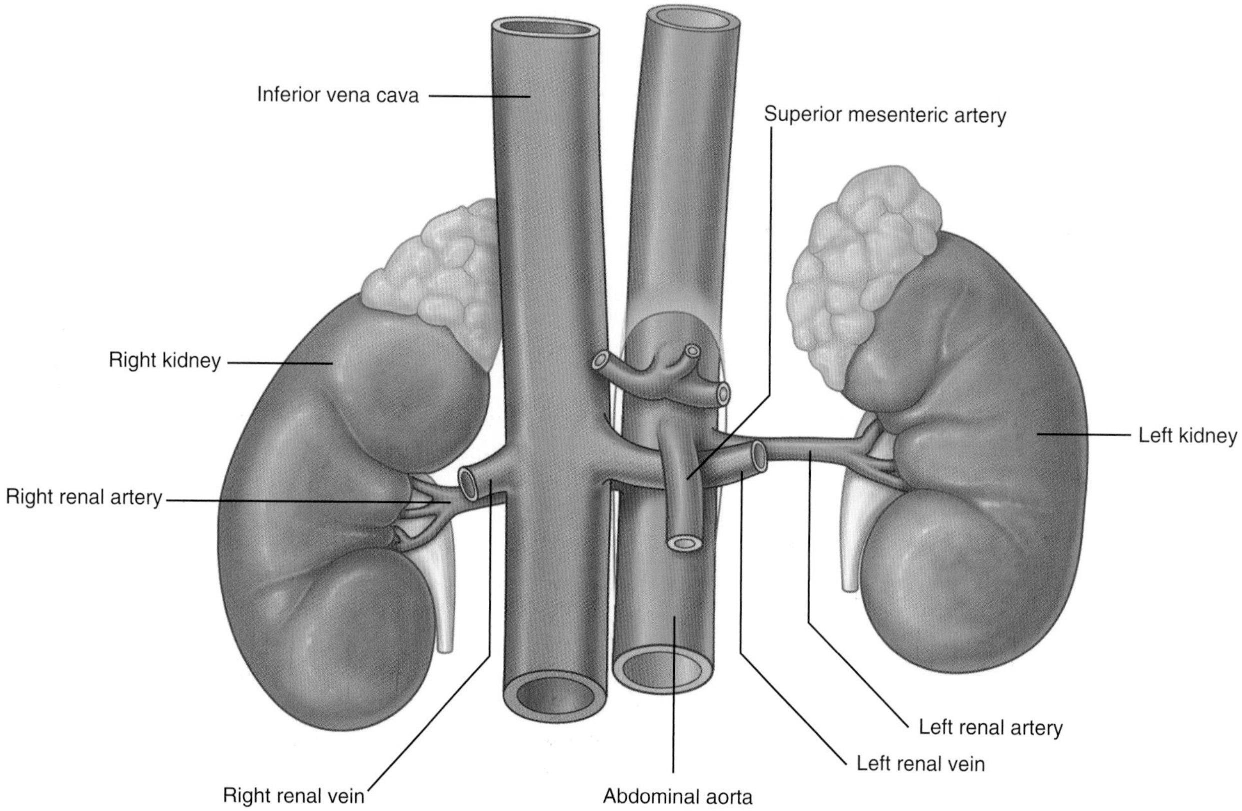

Fig. 9.13 Anatomy of the adrenal glands, demonstrating their location on top of the kidney. (*From Drake RL, Vogl AW, Mitchell AWM. Gray's Anatomy for Students. 2nd ed. Philadelphia: Elsevier; 2009.*)

Adrenal Gland Physiology

The **adrenal cortex,** as mentioned earlier, has three layers, each with different steroid hormone synthetic abilities. The **zona glomerulosa** secretes **mineralocorticoids** such as aldosterone (salt retention); the **zona fasciculata** secretes **glucocorticoids** such as cortisol (blood sugar elevation); and the **zona reticularis** secretes **androgens** (sex steroids). This leads to the mnemonic **the deeper you go, the sweeter it gets** (salt → sugar → sex!) (Fig. 9.14).

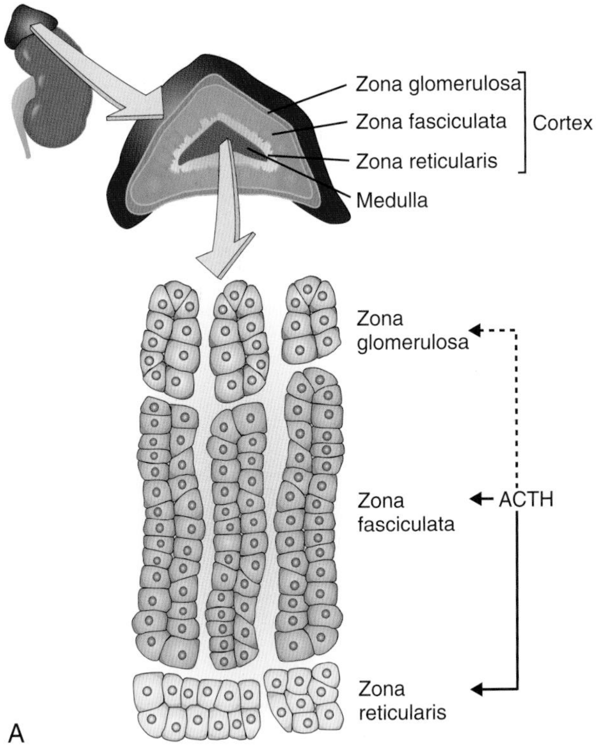

FIG. 9.14 A, Illustration of the zones of the adrenal cortex, including the zona glomerulosa (which makes mineralocorticoids such as aldosterone), zona fasciculata (which makes glucocorticoids such as cortisol), and zona reticularis (which makes androgens such as DHEA sulfate).

Continued

- **Zona glomerulosa:** Responsible for **mineralocorticoid** (aldosterone) secretion—it is the **only** part of the three layers of the adrenal cortex that does not secrete its hormone because of adrenocorticotrophic hormone (ACTH). Instead, as covered in depth in Chapter 15, the trigger for aldosterone release is through the renin-angiotensin-aldosterone axis, with **angiotensin II** causing aldosterone release. The actions of aldosterone are mainly on the **principal cells** of the distal nephron, **increasing sodium reclamation** from the nephron to increase intravascular volume, at the expense of **increasing potassium secretion.** See Chapter 15 for details. It also promotes H^+ secretion through the α-intercalated cells into the lumen of the nephron to promote acid excretion.
- **Zona fasciculata:** Responsible for **glucocorticoid** (cortisol) secretion: The stimulus for its release is ACTH from the pituitary, and it is often a hormone secreted in **response to stress.** There is also a normal daily cortisol spike just before waking in the morning (**diurnal** pattern). **Cortisol** has numerous effects on the body, but the overarching activities of cortisol are a **catabolic** and **diabetogenic** effect, an **antiinflammatory** effect, and causing **catecholamine sensitivity.**
  - **Catabolism:** Provides increased glucose synthesis through gluconeogenesis by breakdown of fat and muscle (catabolism), which is important to maintain blood sugar levels and provide for survival during fasting (ensure a glucose source is available even if no glucose is taken in). In addition, it causes **insulin resistance** (diabetogenic effect) to ensure that glucose is not taken up unnecessarily by cells in times of starvation.

Zona glomerulosa: aldosterone (mineralocorticoids)
Zona fasciculata: cortisol (glucocorticoids)
Zona reticularis: DHEA (androgens)

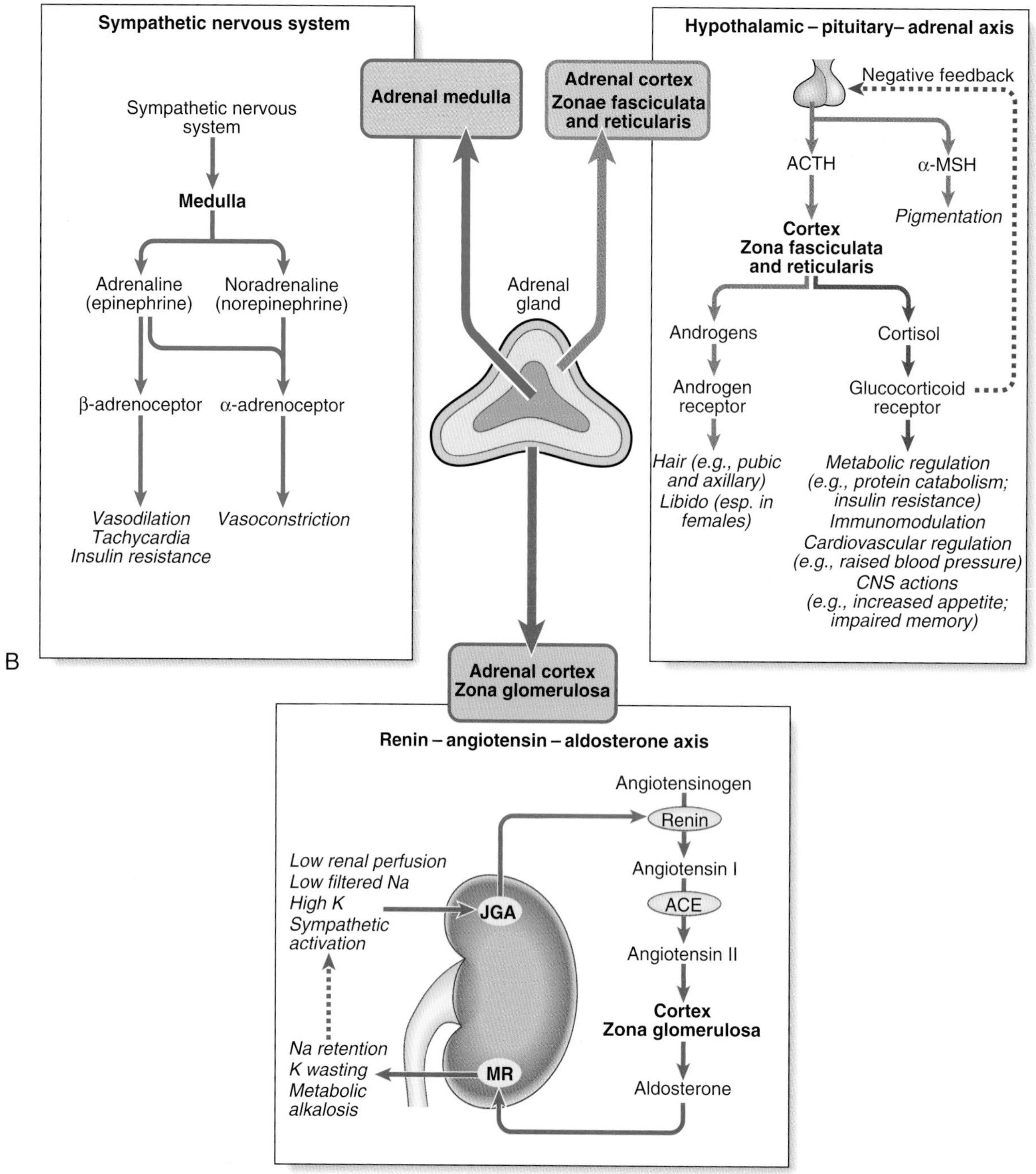

FIG. 9.14, cont'd **B,** Image showing the general mechanism of action of all the products of the adrenal cortex and medulla, as well as the stimulus for their release. ACE, Angiotensin-converting enzyme; JGA, juxtaglomerular apparatus; MR, mineralocorticoid (aldosterone) receptor. (**A** *from Damjanov I.* Pathophysiology. *Philadelphia: Elsevier; 2008.* **B** *from Colledge NR, Walker BR, Ralston SH.* Davidson's Principles and Practice of Medicine. *21st ed. Philadelphia: Elsevier; 2010.*)

- **Inhibition of bone formation:** Decreases **osteoblastic** function and collagen synthesis, leading to cessation of bone formation; this is adaptive in periods of starvation but is the reason that when prescription steroids are used chronically (or another form of hypercortisolism), osteoporosis can develop or worsen.
- **Antiinflammatory:** Increases synthesis of **lipocortin,** which inhibits the normal function of phospholipase A_2 of cleaving arachidonic acid off of lipid membranes to become inflammatory mediators such as prostaglandins and leukotrienes. It also modulates the immune system more directly by preventing T lymphocyte proliferation.

- **Catecholamine sensitivity:** Is said to be **permissive** to catecholamines, meaning that cortisol is required at some level to permit the catecholamines epinephrine and norepinephrine to work effectively by upregulating α_1 receptors, promoting vasoconstriction. This becomes extremely important in the pathology of the adrenal glands because this can lead to blood pressure disturbances when too much or too little cortisol is present.

- **Zona reticularis:** Responsible for **androgen** secretion, most notably **dehydroepiandrosterone (DHEA)** and **androstenedione.** Although this is not important in males (who have testes that are androgen factories), this is the **major androgenic source in females.**

Pathology

Decreased Adrenal Cortex Function: The adrenal cortex can malfunction in a variety of ways, mostly from various causes of **primary adrenal insufficiency** (adrenal gland hypofunction) but also from **pituitary dysfunction** (decreased ACTH) or from **hypothalamic dysfunction** (decreased corticotropin-releasing hormone, or CRH). Because **primary adrenal insufficiency** is the most common, the various causes will be covered in detail; it can be further divided into **acute** and **chronic**.

- **Acute adrenal insufficiency:** Secondary to either (1) **stopping prescribed corticosteroids** without a tapering period, or (2) **bilateral adrenal hemorrhage** (Waterhouse-Friderichsen syndrome). Prolonged (>1 week) use of corticosteroids leads to hypothalamic-pituitary-adrenal axis hypofunction because the exogenous steroids have replaced the need for the adrenal gland to make its own steroids. This can lead to acute adrenal insufficiency and potential hypotension, which is why tapering of steroids is always necessary for longer duration use. **Bilateral adrenal hemorrhage** can occur during sepsis, especially with *Neisseria meningitides* meningococcemia; the endotoxin that it secretes can lead to disseminated intravascular coagulation (DIC) and adrenal hemorrhage, called **Waterhouse-Friderichsen** syndrome. This condition is almost uniformly fatal.
- **Chronic adrenal insufficiency (Addison disease):** This is most commonly **autoimmune** but can be due to **miliary tuberculosis** spreading to the adrenal glands in developing countries with a high prevalence of tuberculosis (TB). Loss of adrenal gland function leads to decreased aldosterone, cortisol, and androgen production. This leads to (1) **hyponatremia** with a **hyperkalemic metabolic acidosis** caused by loss of aldosterone, (2) **hypoglycemia** caused by loss of cortisol, and (3) **hypotension** caused by loss of both aldosterone and cortisol. Because cortisol normally provides negative feedback on the pituitary, loss of cortisol leads to increased ACTH secretion. ACTH has a breakdown product of α-melanocyte–stimulating hormone (α-MSH); this increased melanocyte stimulation leads to **hyperpigmentation** (Fig. 9.15). The last clue to Addison disease is **eosinophilia** as a result of loss of cortisol's immunomodulatory role, which usually also causes apoptosis of eosinophils. Treatment is replacement of both mineralocorticoids and glucocorticoids.

Addison disease: hyperkalemic metabolic acidosis, hyperpigmentation, eosinophilia

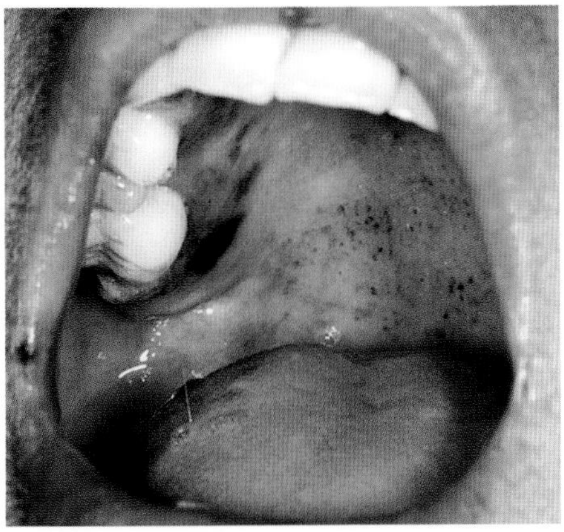

Fig. 9.15 Hyperpigmentation of the buccal mucosa in a patient with Addison disease. This is due to increased ACTH from the pituitary, which subsequently breaks down to α-melanocyte–stimulating hormone (as well as other molecules), stimulating melanocyte production of melanin with resultant hyperpigmentation. (*From Douglas G, Nicol F, Robertson C. Macleod's Clinical Examination. 12th ed. Edinburgh: Elsevier; 2009.*)

Congenital Adrenal Hyperplasia: Like all steroid hormones, the adrenal cortex uses **cholesterol** as a base substrate to generate **aldosterone** (the major mineralocorticoid), **cortisol** (the major glucocorticoid), and the adrenal **androgens** (DHEA and androstenedione). The various modifications require numerous enzymatic steps, but **only the key enzymes shown in** Fig. 9.16 are important to commit to memory because these are the enzymes that can be deficient in various types of **congenital**

adrenal hyperplasia (CAH). With these syndromes, any substrates before the blocked enzyme will build up and take alternative pathways, and of course, substrates after the blocked enzyme will not be used (similar to a roadblock; all the cars take another detour pathway because they need to go somewhere). These disorders are called CAH because the decreased cortisol causes increased ACTH secretion from the pituitary, leading to a tropic effect on the adrenal gland, which causes hyperplasia.

- **21-Hydroxylase deficiency:** The most common cause of CAH. In Fig. 9.16, it can be seen that **both aldosterone and cortisol** require this enzyme; loss of this enzyme therefore leads to **hypoaldosteronemia** and **hypocortisolism,** causing similar symptoms of Addison disease in the neonate (hyperkalemic metabolic acidosis, hypotension). However, with the "roadblock" at the 21-hydroxylase step, the products will instead follow the androgen pathway, and increased androgen levels will occur. Therefore **females** will have **ambiguous genitalia,** and **males** will have **precocious puberty** from the increased male sex steroids.

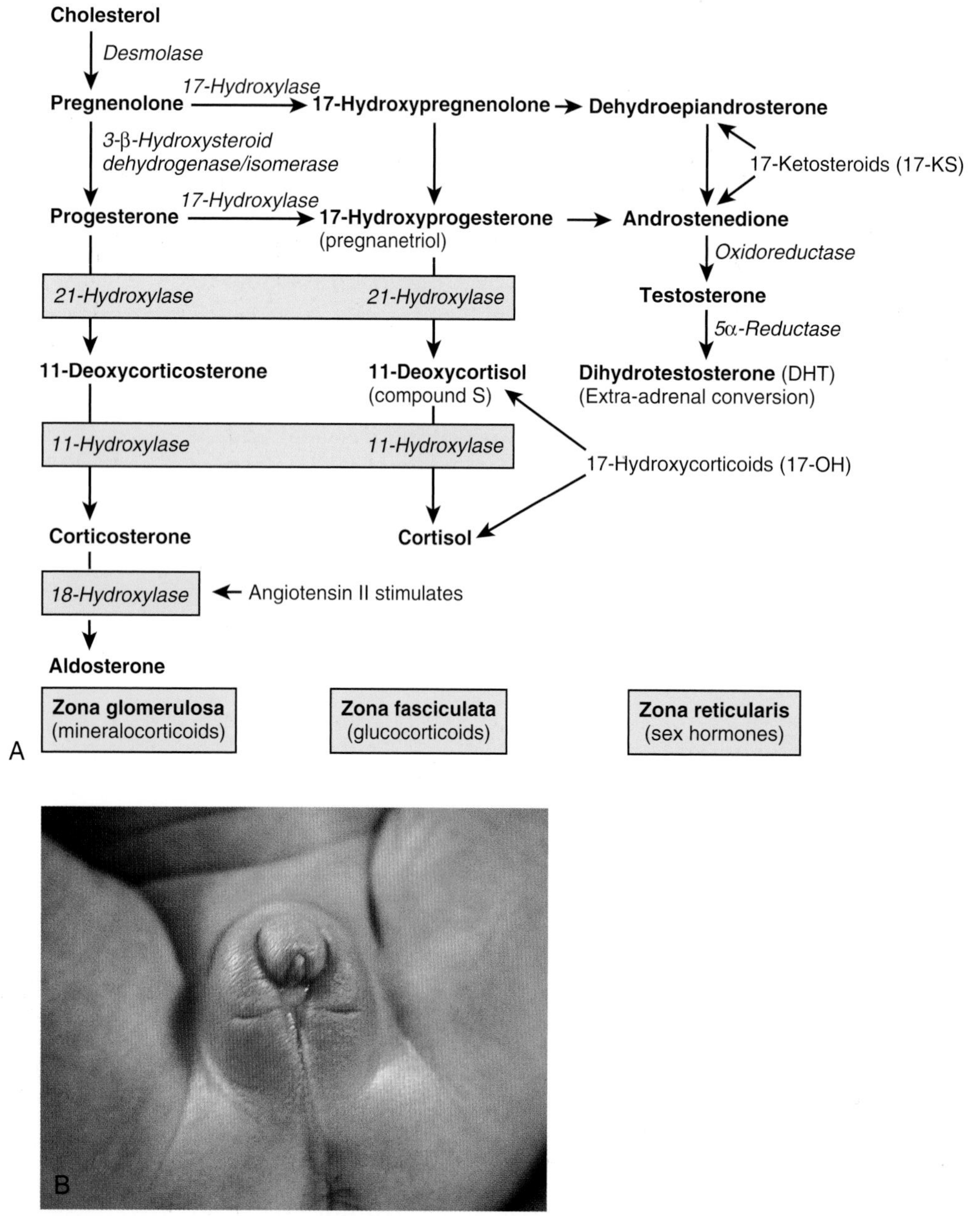

Fig. 9.16 A, Adrenal cortex hormone synthetic pathways, including key enzymes that can be deficient in various forms of congenital adrenal hyperplasia. **B,** Ambiguous genitalia in a female infant with 21-hydroxylase deficiency. (*From Goljan EF. Rapid Review Pathology Revised Reprint. 3rd ed. Philadelphia: Elsevier; 2011. Courtesy Patrick C. Walsh, MD, Johns Hopkins School of Medicine, Baltimore, MD.*)

- **11β-Hydroxylase deficiency:** Also required in the synthesis of both **aldosterone** and **cortisol,** but the main difference here is that 11-deoxycortisol (proximal to the block) will build up. This compound has mineralocorticoid (aldosterone-like) activity. Therefore affected individuals will have the same issue with increased androgens but now will also have stigmata of increased mineralocorticoid activity: hypokalemic metabolic alkalosis and hypertension.
- **17α-Hydroxylase deficiency:** 17α-Hydroxylase is required to make anything other than aldosterone. Therefore **with this deficiency, only aldosterone can be made.** This leads to predictable results: hypokalemic metabolic alkalosis, hypertension (from hyperaldosteronism), and decreased androgens and cortisol.

Increased Aldosterone Secretion: Increased aldosterone secretion can occur from increased production of any part of the renin-angiotensin-aldosterone axis and generally includes juxtaglomerular (JG) cell tumors (secreting renin), renal artery stenosis (causing kidney JG cells to sense less perfusion and increase renin), or aldosterone-secreting tumors.

- **Primary hyperaldosteronism** (Fig. 9.17) (Conn syndrome): Caused by an aldosterone-secreting adenoma in the zona glomerulosa of the adrenal gland cortex, leading to findings of increased aldosterone activity: a **hypokalemic metabolic alkalosis** and potentially **hypertension.** The potassium derangements often lead to weakness. Alkalosis can lead to tetany (calcium normally is bound to albumin; with alkalosis, less H^+ is bound to albumin and can therefore accept more Ca^{2+}, leading to a decreased ionized calcium level and tetany). The main distinguishing factor of primary versus secondary hyperaldosteronism is that in primary hyperaldosteronism, the aldosterone is being secreted **independent of renin** and therefore **renin levels will be low.**

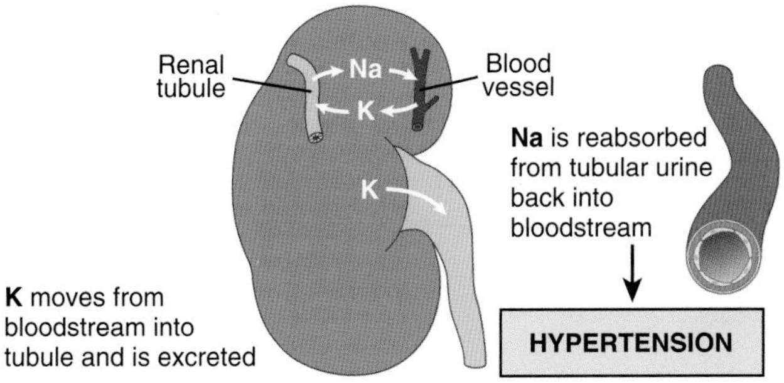

Fig. 9.17 Diagram depicting the action of aldosterone on the kidney, with hyperaldosteronism causing increased potassium and acid (H^+) excretion, sodium retention, and resulting hypertension. (*From Kumar V, Abbas AK, Fausto N, Aster J.* Robbins & Cotran Pathologic Basis of Disease. *8th ed. New York: Elsevier; 2009.*)

- **Secondary hyperaldosteronism:** Can be caused by renal artery stenosis (kidney thinking it is hypoperfused) or a JG cell tumor, or even simply by having actual hypoperfusion (such as in congestive heart failure). Symptoms can be similar, but **renin levels will be high** in all these conditions.
- Treatment involves addressing the underlying cause, but as a temporizing measure, **spironolactone,** an aldosterone-receptor antagonist and K^+-sparing diuretic, can be given to block the effects of the excess aldosterone on the kidney.

Cushing syndrome: buffalo hump, truncal obesity, hemorrhagic purple-red striae, moon facies

Increased Cortisol Secretion: Increased cortisol secretion can occur from increased amounts of anything along the hypothalamic-pituitary-adrenal axis (CRH from hypothalamus, ACTH from pituitary or ectopic site, adrenal gland tumor producing cortisol). The findings in hypercortisolism (Fig. 9.18) (Cushing syndrome) can be striking: Cortisol causes **fat and protein catabolism,** leading to wasted extremities, but the increased insulin causes upregulation of lipoprotein lipase, promoting central fat deposition (so-called **truncal obesity**). The decreased collagen synthesis leads to **hemorrhagic purple-red striae** in the abdomen when the skin stretches because it cannot accommodate the increased truncal fat. Other findings include **moon facies** (fat deposition in the facial area), a **buffalo hump** (dorsocervical [upper back] fat deposition), and even electrolyte derangements seen in hyperaldosteronism. With very high levels, cortisol can attach to the mineralocorticoid receptor and

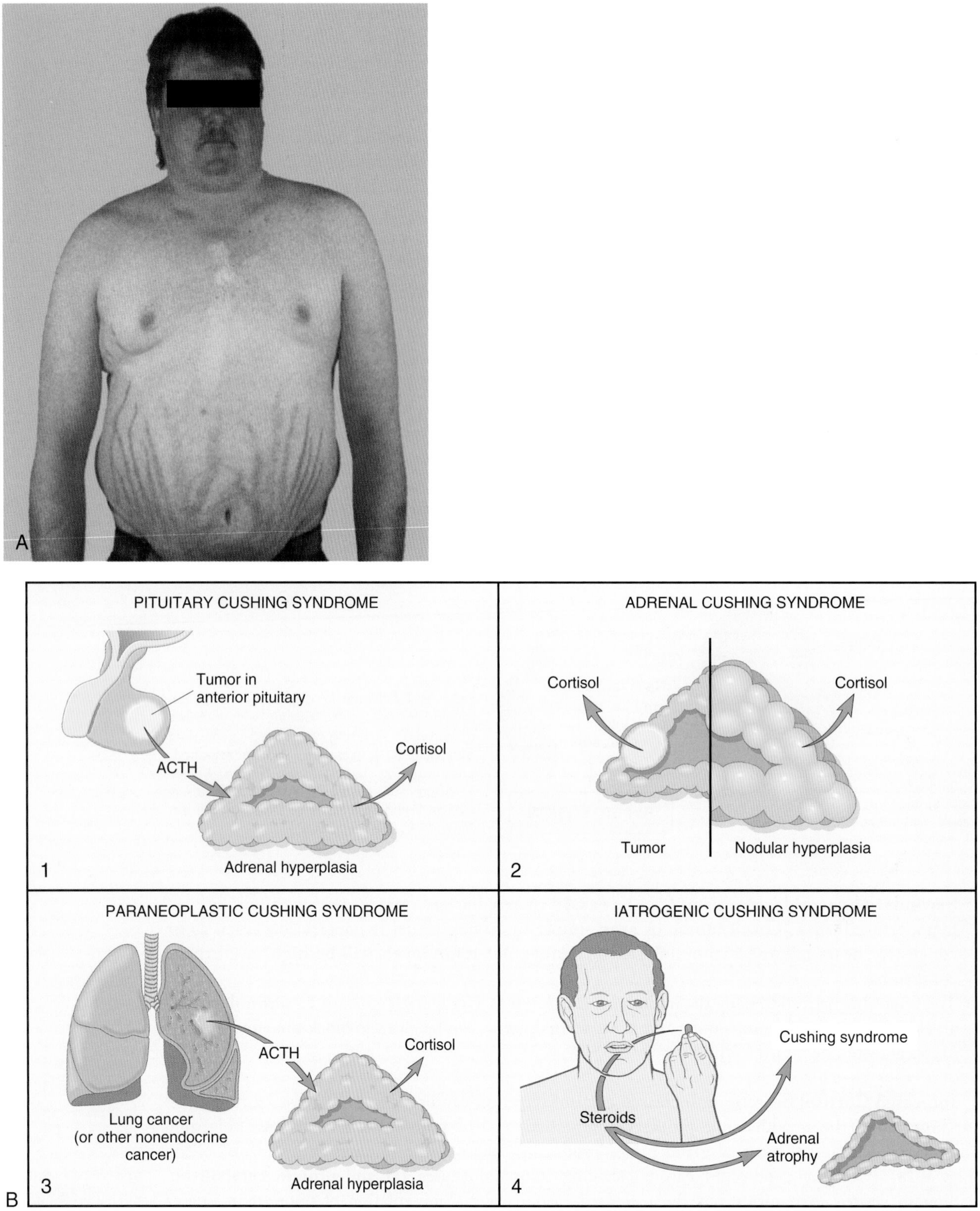

FIG. 9.18 **A,** Purple-red striae, centripetal obesity, and moon facies in a patient with hypercortisolism. **B,** The different forms of hypercortisolism. (1) An ACTH-secreting tumor from the pituitary causing overproduction of cortisol (Cushing disease). (2) Primary cortisol-secreting tumor of the adrenal gland causing overproduction of cortisol. (3) Tumor outside of the pituitary causing ACTH secretion and overproduction of cortisol. (4) Iatrogenic hypercortisolism from long-term prescription corticosteroid use. (**A** *from Lloyd RV, Douglas BR, Young WF.* Atlas of Nontumor Pathology: Endocrine Diseases. *Washington, DC: American Registry of Pathology; 2002.* **B** *adapted from Kumar V, Abbas AK, Aster J.* Robbins Basic Pathology, *9th ed. St. Louis: Elsevier; 2012.*)

have aldosterone-like activity. It is important to first elicit the history from the patient: Iatrogenic hypercortisolism can occur in patients taking chronic glucocorticoid therapy (such as patients with autoimmune diseases or transplants).

- **Adrenal Cushing syndrome:** Excess cortisol is being produced because of an **adrenal gland tumor,** causing high cortisol levels. In this case the **ACTH level will be low** because the tumor will be providing large amounts of cortisol and therefore large amounts of negative feedback on the pituitary.
- **Pituitary Cushing syndrome** (Cushing disease): Only an ACTH-secreting tumor is termed Cushing disease, yet any condition that causes hypercortisolism is referred to as Cushing syndrome. An ACTH-secreting tumor in the pituitary is the most common cause of hypercortisolism after an iatrogenic cause is ruled out. Because the tumor secretes ACTH, it will lead to **high levels of both ACTH and cortisol.**
- **Ectopic (paraneoplastic) Cushing syndrome:** Most often seen in **small cell carcinoma of the lung** (which can also secrete ADH), this will lead to **high levels of both ACTH and cortisol.**

Both pituitary and ectopic Cushing syndrome cause increased ACTH and cortisol, so there must be a way to distinguish the two. The answer is a **dexamethasone suppression test.** In this test, a low dose of dexamethasone (a cortisol analog) is given, and a high dose of dexamethasone is given to **see if negative feedback** is still active to some extent. In the low-dose case, neither pituitary nor ectopic Cushing syndrome will cause a decrease in cortisol production. However, the **high-dose** test can differentiate the two—the **pituitary** still has some negative feedback ability (because it is used to having negative feedback) and will cause **cortisol suppression with high-dose dexamethasone.** Because the ectopic ACTH-secreting tumor does not have a negative feedback loop, it has no suppression with either low or high dose.

Increased Catecholamine Secretion: Increased catecholamine secretion can occur from **tumors of the adrenal medulla** or the **sympathetic nervous chain.** This can be caused by a **pheochromocytoma, paraganglioma,** or **neuroblastoma,** depending on the age of the patient.

- **Pheochromocytoma** (Fig. 9.19): Occurs in **adults** and is a neoplasm of the **chromaffin cells,** which secrete catecholamines such as epinephrine and norepinephrine. Although these are mostly **benign** (meaning they cannot metastasize), they cause the **five Ps of hyperadrenergic states**: **pressure** (hypertension), **pain** (headache), **perspiration** (sweating is sympathetic cholinergic), **palpitations** (tachycardia from β_1-receptor activation on the heart), and **pallor** (from α_1 vasoconstriction). These

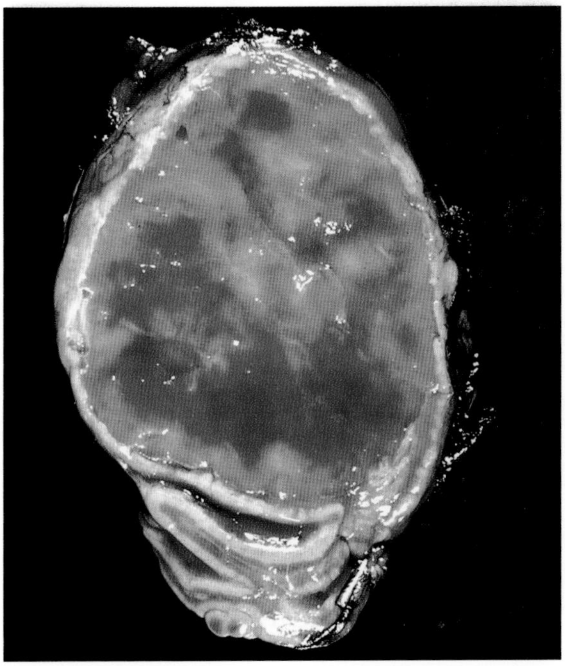

FIG. 9.19 Gross image of a pheochromocytoma, a tumor of the chromaffin cells of the adrenal medulla. *(From Kumar V, Abbas AK, Fausto N, Aster J. Robbins & Cotran Pathologic Basis of Disease. 8th ed. New York: Elsevier; 2009. Courtesy Jerrold R. Turner, MD, PhD, University of Chicago Hospitals, Chicago, IL.)*

symptoms are not constant but rather **occur sporadically.** There is also the **rule of 10%** (which is not quite accurate, but easy to remember):
- 10% are malignant
- 10% are bilateral
- 10% are extraadrenal in the sympathetic chain (paraganglioma)
- 10% are in children
- 10% (actually 30%) are familial (neurofibromatosis, MEN IIa/IIb, von Hippel–Lindau)
- 10% calcify
- … and of course, you're 10 times more likely to see this on an examination than in real life

❍ Diagnosis is by measuring 24-hour urine excretion of catecholamines and total metanephrines (metabolites of catecholamines). Treatment is surgery, but medical interventions to block the excess sympathetic outflow are also required before removal. The medications **phenoxybenzamine** (an **irreversible** α_1 antagonist; **important that it is irreversible because the high levels of catecholamines can outcompete a reversible agent**) and a beta blocker are commonly given.

❍ **Neuroblastoma** (Fig. 9.20) occurs in children and is the fourth most common childhood cancer (after acute lymphocytic leukemia, lymphoma, and medulloblastoma, making it the most common solid extracranial tumor). This is associated with *N-MYC* amplification and can commonly metastasize to **liver, skin, and bones.** Young children (<1 year of age) have a good prognosis, with the tumor often spontaneously disappearing; older children have a very poor prognosis. Histologically, this is a "small cell" tumor (see Fig. 9.20) with **Homer-Wright rosettes;** a rosette is a rose-shaped decoration,

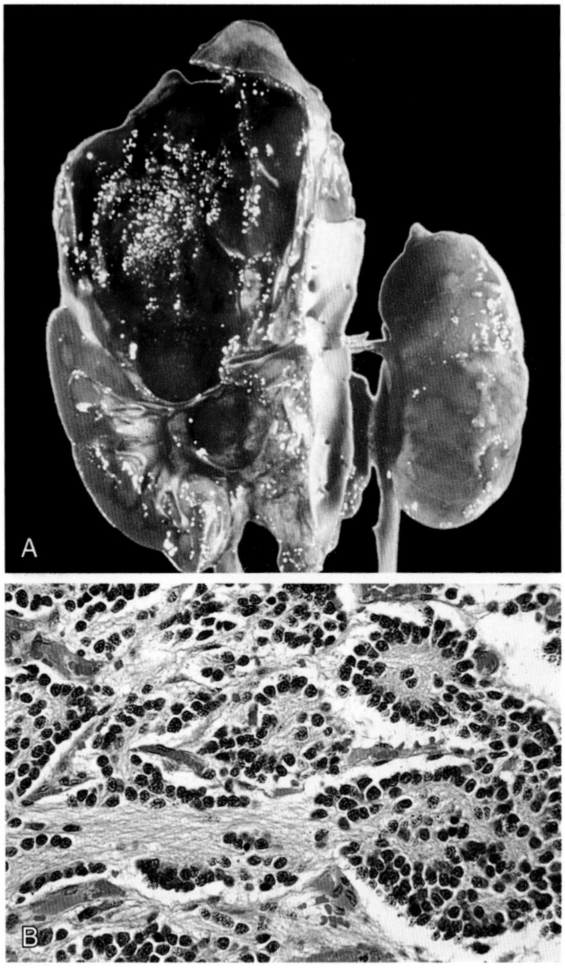

Fig. 9.20 A, Gross image of neuroblastoma. **B,** Histologic examination of neuroblastoma including Homer-Wright rosettes where cells come together like a cluster of roses. (*From Kumar V, Abbas AK, Fausto N, Aster J.* Robbins & Cotran Pathologic Basis of Disease. *8th ed. New York: Elsevier; 2009. Courtesy Arthur Weinberg, MD, University of Texas Southwestern Medical School, Dallas, TX.*)

meaning that all the cells come together in grouped clusters like a bunch of roses. Neuroblastoma may be first suspected by finding an abdominal mass on physical examination. Diagnosis can be confirmed by urinary **homovanillic acid (HVA) levels** (a breakdown product of dopamine). Treatment is surgery.

Endocrine Pancreas

Anatomy, Embryology, and Histology

The **pancreas** is a dual-function organ, having both **endocrine** (hormone release into the blood) and **exocrine** (excreting contents such as enzymes into the pancreatic duct and then the duodenum) functions. The **exocrine** function of the pancreas is covered in Chapter 10, but the endocrine function will be covered here.

The pancreas lies **deep** (posterior) to the stomach and is a **retroperitoneal** organ except for part of the tail of the pancreas (Fig. 9.21). The **ductal system** is important to the exocrine function of the pancreas, but because endocrine hormones are put into the blood and not into ducts, they do not play a role in the endocrine function of the pancreas.

Embryologically, the pancreas is made up of **dorsal** and **ventral** buds that came from the **foregut** (Fig. 9.22). These can fuse abnormally and lead to an **annular pancreas** (see Fig. 9.22) that encircles the duodenum. This can lead to **duodenal stenosis** if the annular pancreas is causing compression.

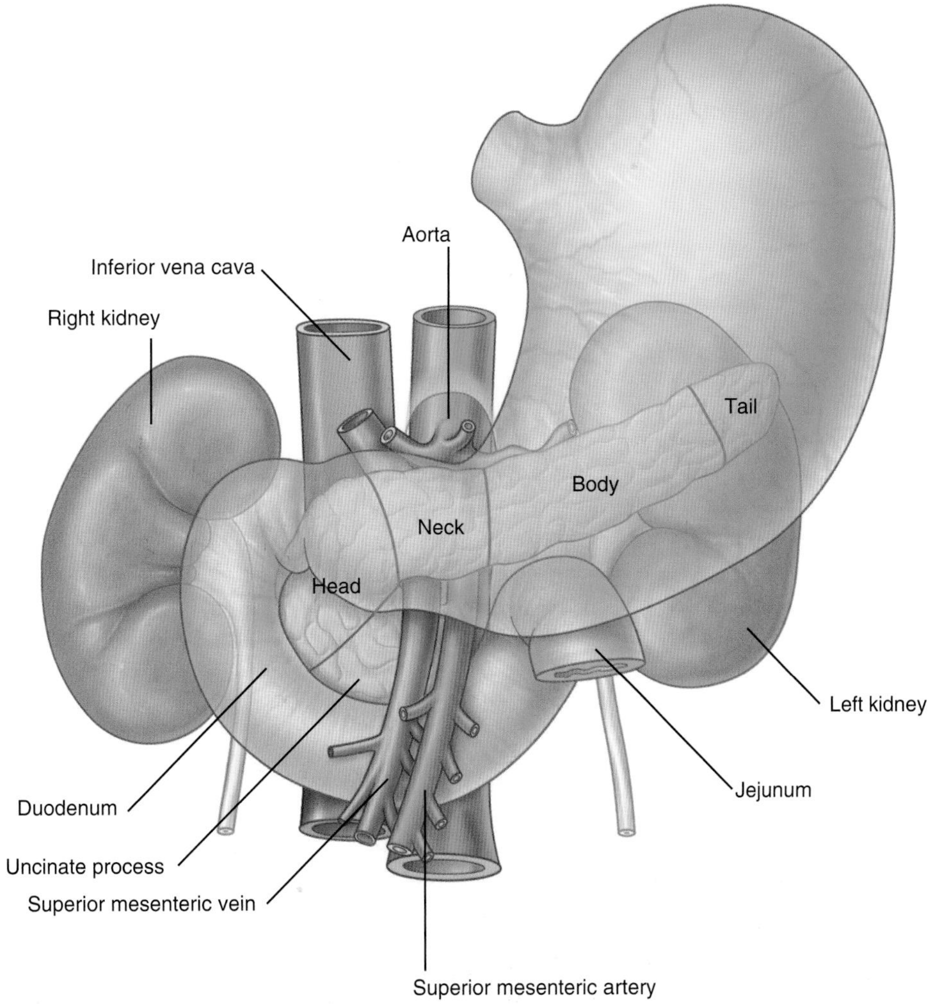

FIG. 9.21 Position of the pancreas as it lies in the abdomen (deep to the stomach). (*From Drake RL, Vogl AW, Mitchell AWM. Gray's Anatomy for Students. 2nd ed. Philadelphia: Elsevier; 2009.*)

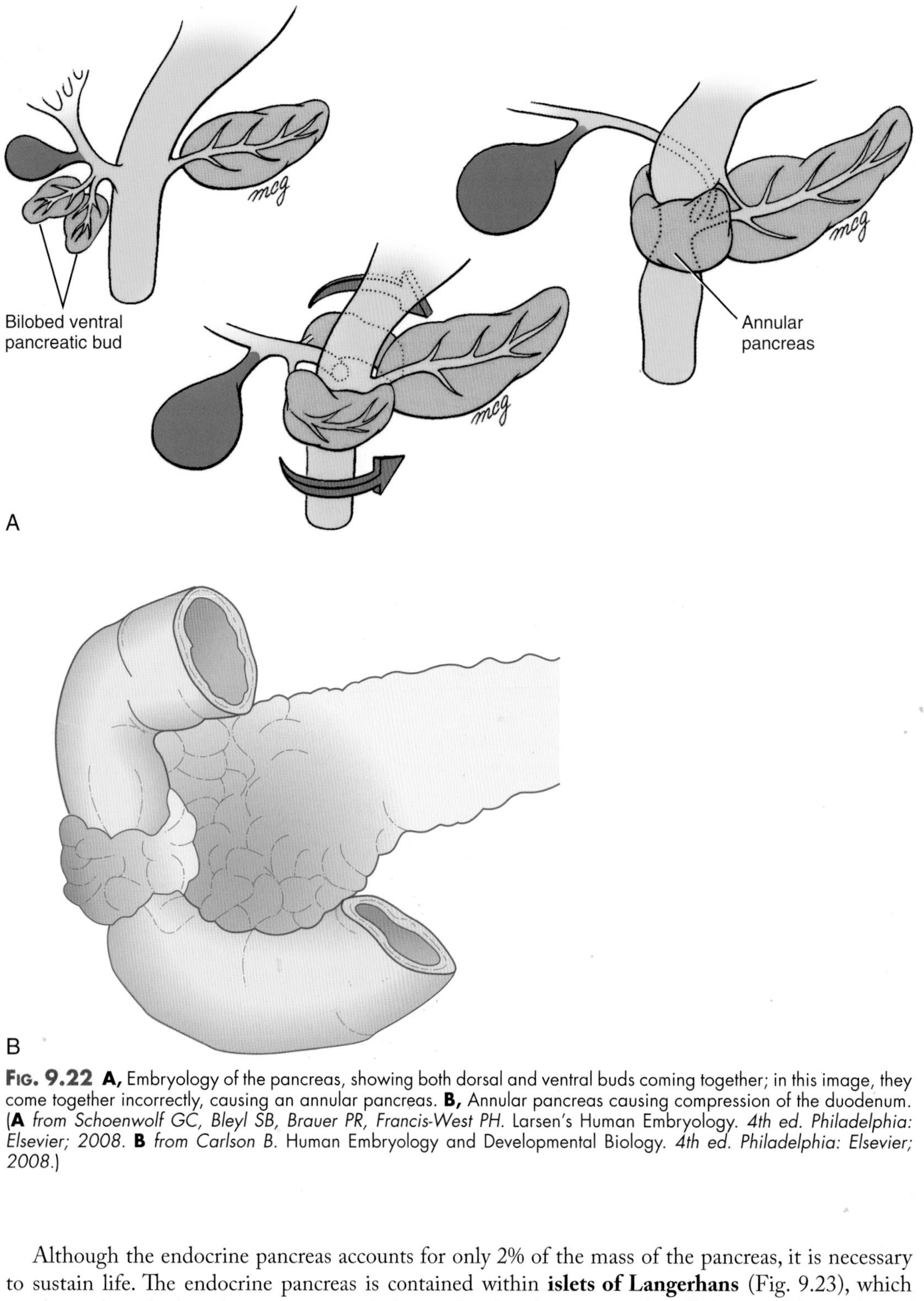

Fig. 9.22 A, Embryology of the pancreas, showing both dorsal and ventral buds coming together; in this image, they come together incorrectly, causing an annular pancreas. **B,** Annular pancreas causing compression of the duodenum. (**A** *from Schoenwolf GC, Bleyl SB, Brauer PR, Francis-West PH.* Larsen's Human Embryology. *4th ed. Philadelphia: Elsevier; 2008.* **B** *from Carlson B.* Human Embryology and Developmental Biology. *4th ed. Philadelphia: Elsevier; 2008.*)

Although the endocrine pancreas accounts for only 2% of the mass of the pancreas, it is necessary to sustain life. The endocrine pancreas is contained within **islets of Langerhans** (Fig. 9.23), which can be seen in the histologic image as a lighter-colored and more scantly cellular area. These islets of Langerhans have alpha (α), beta (β), and delta (δ) cells, which are the main cells that secrete glucagon, insulin, and somatostatin/gastrin, respectively. The **alpha** cells, which secrete **glucagon,** are on the outside (**alpha = away** from center). The **beta** cells, which secrete **insulin,** are toward the center. The delta cells are interspersed among the alpha and beta cells.

Endocrine Pancreas Physiology

Insulin (from the Beta Cells of the Islets of Langerhans): Insulin plays a key role in the regulation of blood glucose levels. Although there are many stimuli for its release, the most important is **elevated**

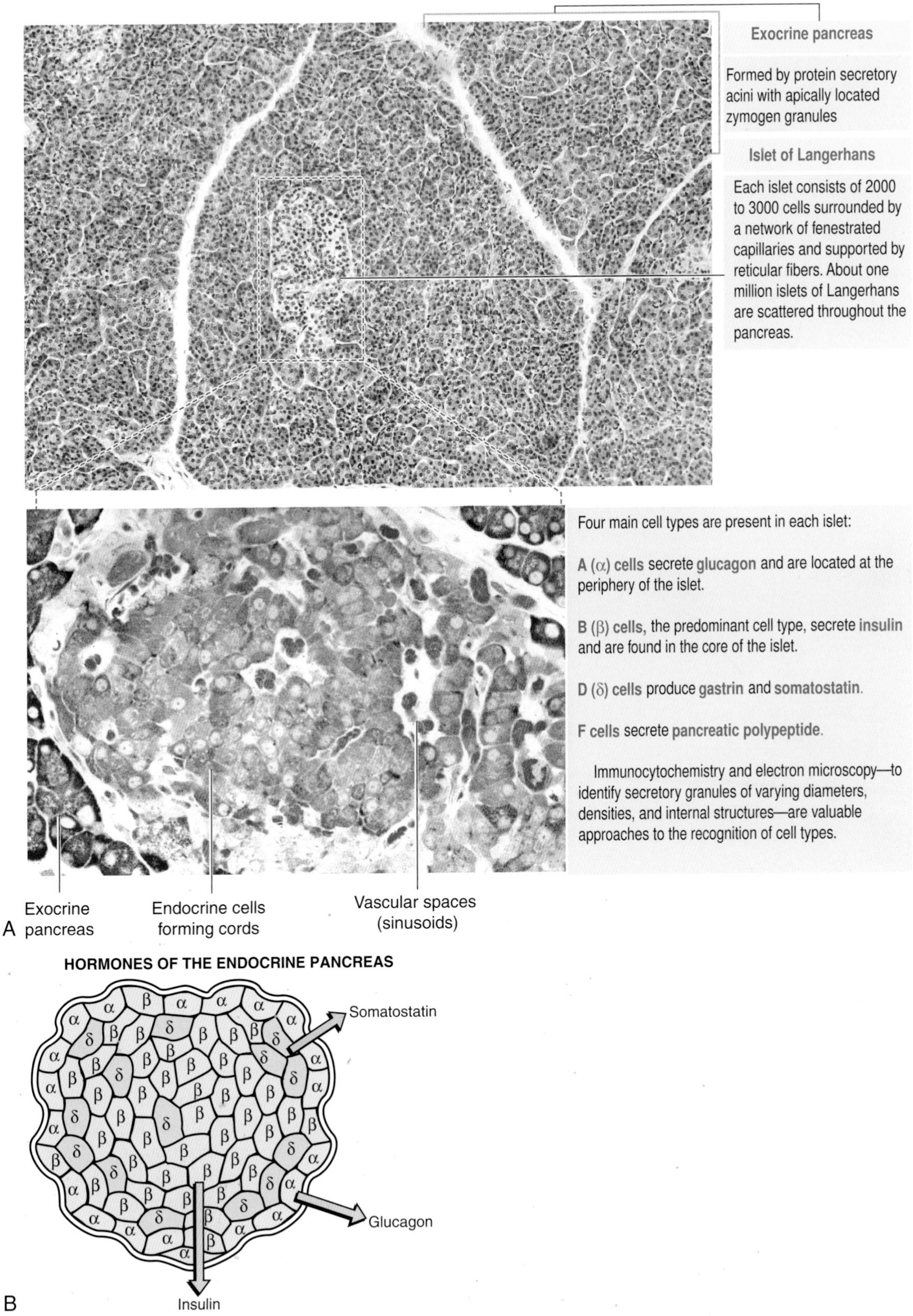
Exocrine pancreas
Formed by protein secretory acini with apically located zymogen granules
Islet of Langerhans
Each islet consists of 2000 to 3000 cells surrounded by a network of fenestrated capillaries and supported by reticular fibers. About one million islets of Langerhans are scattered throughout the pancreas.
Four main cell types are present in each islet:
A (α) cells secrete glucagon and are located at the periphery of the islet.
B (β) cells, the predominant cell type, secrete insulin and are found in the core of the islet.
D (δ) cells produce gastrin and somatostatin.
F cells secrete pancreatic polypeptide.
Immunocytochemistry and electron microscopy—to identify secretory granules of varying diameters, densities, and internal structures—are valuable approaches to the recognition of cell types.
Exocrine pancreas
Endocrine cells forming cords
Vascular spaces (sinusoids)
A
HORMONES OF THE ENDOCRINE PANCREAS
Somatostatin
Glucagon
Insulin
B

FIG. 9.23 A, Histologic examination of the pancreas, with zoom view of an islet of Langerhans, demonstrating the different cell types and their distribution throughout the islet. **B,** Animated representation of the islet of Langerhans, demonstrating the peripheral alpha cells (glucagon), the central beta cells (insulin), and the randomly dispersed delta cells (somatostatin, gastrin). (**A** *from Kierszenbaum AL, Tres LL.* Histology and Cell Biology. *3rd ed. St. Louis: Elsevier; 2011.* **B** *from Costanzo LS.* Physiology. *4th ed. New York: Elsevier; 2009.*)

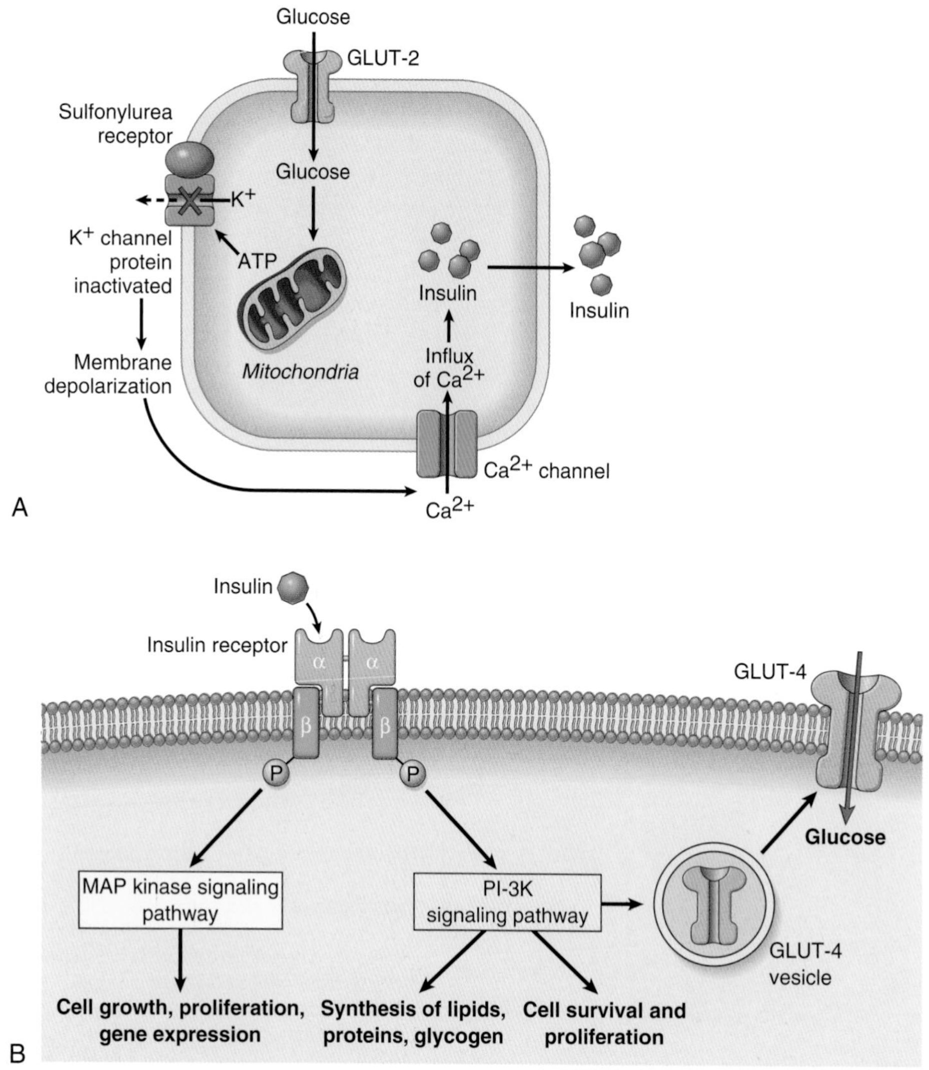

Fig. 9.24 A, Illustration of an insulin-secreting beta cell in the islets of Langerhans, showing the mechanism of insulin secretion. Glucose moves into the cell via GLUT-2. It is then metabolized into ATP, which closes the K^+ channel, stopping the tonic hyperpolarization of the cell. This relative depolarization triggers calcium influx into the cell via a voltage-gated Ca^{2+} channel, and insulin is then released. **B,** Action of insulin on target cells, causing cell growth, anabolic effects, and GLUT-4 glucose channel fusion into the membrane to enhance glucose uptake into insulin-dependent cells. (*From Kumar V, Fausto N, Abbas AK.* Robbins & Cotran Pathologic Basis of Disease. *7th ed. Philadelphia: WB Saunders; 2004.*)

glucose in the blood (hyperglycemia), such as after a meal. Insulin is released from the beta cell of the islet of Langerhans in response to elevated blood glucose by the following steps: (1) glucose goes into the beta cell via **GLUT-2** glucose transporters; (2) glucose is metabolized into ATP; (3) this ATP **closes** the potassium channel that previously was hyperpolarizing the cell, leading to depolarization of the cell; (4) this depolarization triggers a calcium channel to open, facilitating calcium influx into the cell; and (5) the calcium influx into the cell triggers release of preformed insulin into the bloodstream (Fig. 9.24A). In this preformed insulin-containing granule is also a cleavage byproduct of proinsulin called **C-peptide** (connecting peptide)—this will become important in pathology because **C-peptide is present with endogenous insulin but is not present in commercially available injectable insulin;** C-peptide levels in blood can determine whether the insulin is coming from the body or from a needle.

The mechanism of action of the beta cell also becomes important with **sulfonylurea** medications, which attach to the sulfonylurea receptor on the potassium channel. Triggering the sulfonylurea receptor closes the potassium channel (much like ATP did), leading to depolarization and calcium influx, to trigger insulin release from beta cells. **Diazoxide,** on the other hand, keeps this channel open and prevents insulin release and can be used in the treatment of **insulinoma** (described later).

The insulin, now released into the bloodstream, acts on its insulin receptor, starting a cascade mediated by **MAP kinase** and **PI-3 K** (Fig. 9.24B). All these physiologic effects are what would be expected when a lot of sugar is available for the body to use. Insulin is the "hormone of **plenty**" and has an overall anabolic effect. The tissues most dependent on insulin for glucose uptake are **skeletal muscle** and **adipose tissue (GLUT-4).** Some parts of the body, such as the brain and red blood cells, use a different glucose channel (GLUT-1) that is not insulin dependent because these always need glucose regardless of availability (red blood cells do not have nuclei or mitochondria and can only use glucose as a fuel).

- **Fusion of GLUT-4 glucose channels into the cell membrane:** Promotes glucose uptake into cells, reducing serum blood sugar level.
- **Promotes glycogen creation, prevents gluconeogenesis:** This is due to the abundance of sugar with higher insulin levels—promotes storage of sugar as glycogen and prevents gluconeogenesis because there is no need to make glucose if there is adequate glucose available.
- Increases **lipoprotein lipase** activity (which brings fat into cells) and inhibits **hormone-sensitive lipase** activity (which brings fat into the bloodstream). This decreases lipolysis by promoting fat deposition in the adipocytes, making maximum use of the preferred fuel, glucose. Glucagon has the opposite effect on these two hormones.
- **Promotes K^+ uptake into cells** by stimulating the Na^+/K^+-ATPase.

Glucagon (from the alpha cells of the islets of Langerhans): Glucagon (Fig. 9.25) has many effects opposing insulin (the "hormone of **starvation**"). Therefore the major stimulus for glucagon secretion is **hypoglycemia.**

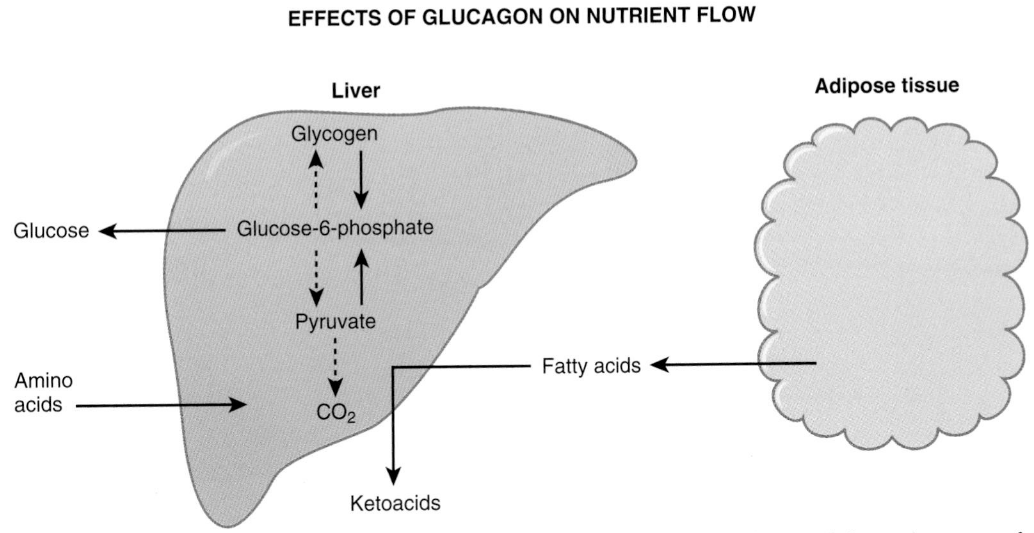

FIG. 9.25 Glucagon is the "hormone of starvation" and acts to promote release of fatty acids from adipocytes to fuel the starving body. It also increases gluconeogenesis and causes breakdown of glycogen to keep blood sugar levels up. *(From Costanzo LS. Physiology. 4th ed. New York: Elsevier; 2009.)*

- Increasing glycogenolysis and gluconeogenesis: Glucagon promotes breakdown of glycogen as well as gluconeogenesis. This is through decreased production of fructose 2,6-bisphosphate, which in turn decreases phosphofructokinase activity. Decreased PFK leads to slowed glucose metabolism, instead favoring gluconeogenesis.
- **Increasing availability of fatty acids:** Glucagon decreases lipoprotein lipase activity (less importing of fat into adipocytes) and increases hormone-sensitive lipase activity (increases exportation of fat from adipocytes into the bloodstream). These are turned into ketoacids after metabolism and account for the ketonuria and ketonemia in starving patients or those who have an absolute insulin deficiency (diabetic ketoacidosis).

Diabetes

Of all functions of the pancreas, the most commonly seen pathologic condition involves disorders of insulin production (type 1 diabetes) and insulin sensitivity (type 2 diabetes) (Fig. 9.26). Both will lead to the cardinal symptoms of **polyuria** (osmotic diuresis) and **polydipsia** (thirst secondary to fluid loss

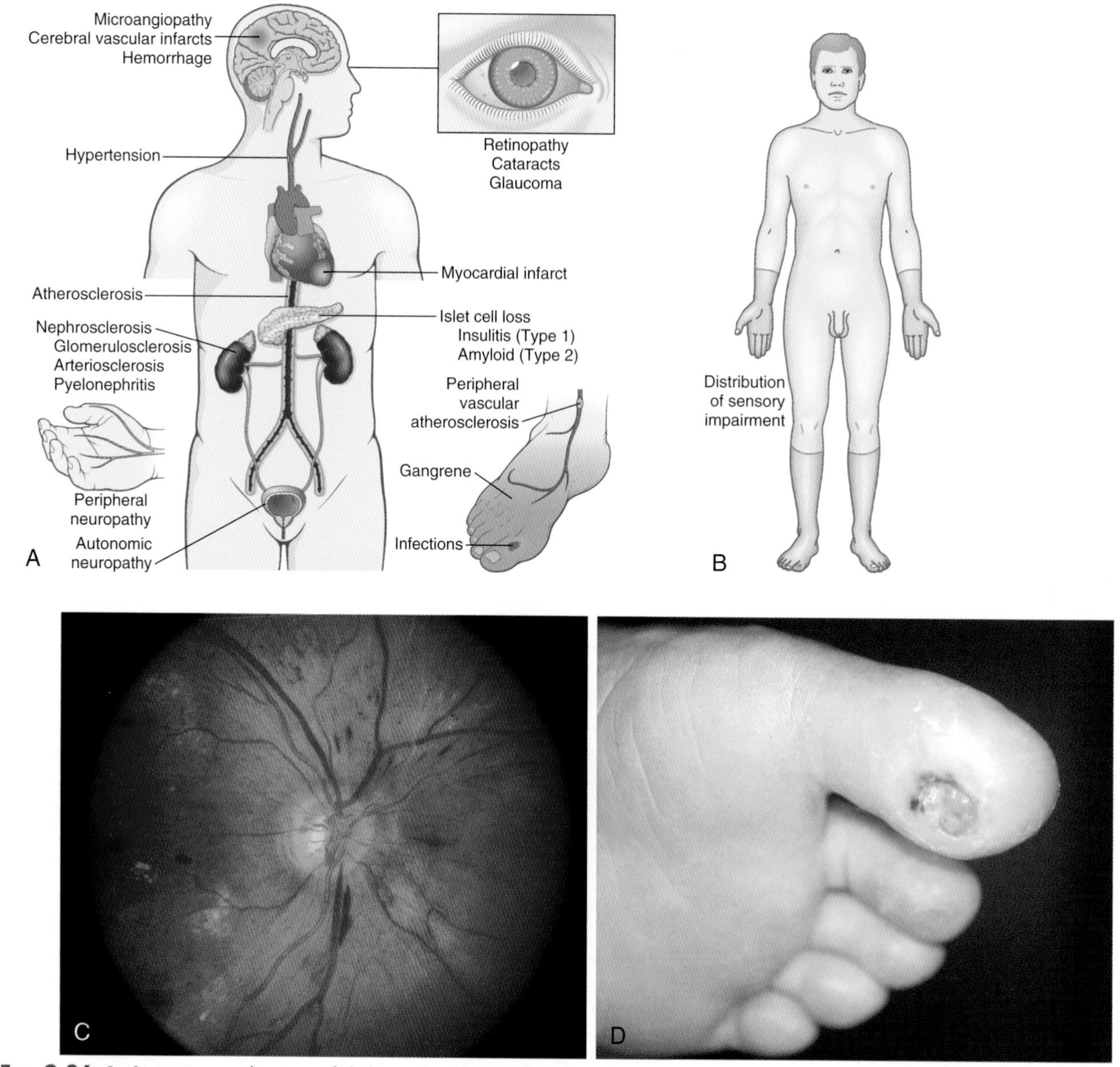

FIG. 9.26 **A,** Systemic complications of diabetes. **B,** Glove-and-stocking distribution of peripheral neuropathy in diabetes. **C,** Diabetic retinopathy. **D,** Foot ulcer as a result of peripheral neuropathy and peripheral vascular disease. (**A** *from Kumar V, Abbas AK, Aster J.* Robbins Basic Pathology. *9th ed. St. Louis: Elsevier; 2012.* **B** *from Douglas G, Nicol F, Robertson C.* Macleod's Clinical Examination. *12th ed. Edinburgh: Elsevier; 2009.* **C** *from Swartz MH.* Textbook of Physical Diagnosis. *4th ed. Philadelphia: Elsevier; 2002.* **D** *from Becker JM, Stucchi AF.* Essentials of Surgery. *Philadelphia: Elsevier; 2006.*)

from osmotic diuresis), but type 2 diabetes is often asymptomatic and incidentally discovered with laboratory screening.

- **Type 1 diabetes mellitus** (10%): Characterized by **autoimmune destruction** of the beta cells of the islets of Langerhans, leading to **absolute insulin deficiency.** Typically affects thin younger people because of lack of insulin to deposit fat into adipose tissue. This is associated with HLA-DR3 and HLA-DR4 in whites, HLA-DR7 in African Americans, and HLA-DR9 in Japanese people. The absolute insulin deficiency can lead to **diabetic ketoacidosis** (DKA), a potentially fatal disease if untreated and often the first manifestation of type 1 diabetes.
- **Type 2 diabetes mellitus** (90%): The most common type of diabetes, characterized by **insulin resistance** secondary to decreased insulin receptor synthesis from increased adiposity. Defects in receptor and signaling pathways also develop, further limiting the effect of insulin in these patients. Initially, patients may be **hyperinsulinemic** as compensation for their decreased insulin sensitivity, but eventually the beta cells fail from the increased demand, and they will have a relative insulin deficiency. The relative insulin

deficiency usually does not lead to ketoacidosis (enough insulin present to prevent widespread lipolysis) but can lead to a **hyperosmolar nonketotic state** (HNS; previously called hyperosmolar hyperglycemic nonketotic coma, HHNKC). HNS is more descriptive because it does not necessarily cause coma. Type 2 diabetes mellitus has a much stronger link to family history than type 1 diabetes mellitus.

Diagnosis of Diabetes

The following are the current criteria used for diagnosis of diabetes. The diagnosis is not met with a single value on a single day; one of the four criteria must be met on **2** separate days.

- Random plasma glucose ≥ 200 mg/dL **with** symptoms of diabetes (polyuria, polydipsia)
- Fasting plasma glucose ≥ 126 mg/dL
- Two-hour plasma glucose level after 75 g of oral glucose administered ≥ 200 mg/dL
- HbA1c ≥ 6.5% (HbA1c is a measure of the level of glycosylation of hemoglobin and is a marker of long-term glucose control over the past few months because red blood cells usually live 120 days)

If there is a suspicion of type 1 diabetes, there are **autoantibodies** that can be tested as well. These include **islet cell autoantibodies, antiinsulin antibodies, and antibodies to glutamic acid decarboxylase** (an enzyme involved in insulin synthesis).

Chronic Effects of Hyperglycemia

There are many problems with long-term hyperglycemia, whether from type 1 or type 2 diabetes. The classic triad of microvascular disease is **retinopathy, neuropathy, and nephropathy**, but there is also macrovascular disease (accelerated atherosclerosis), which leads to increased incidence of strokes and myocardial infarctions. These complications occur through three pathologic processes: **osmotic damage, nonenzymatic glycosylation, and diabetic microangiopathy.**

- **Osmotic damage** (Fig. 9.27A): Glucose can be converted into **sorbitol** by **aldose reductase.** Although some organs have the ability to metabolize sorbitol, the **eye** and the **nerves** do not. This sorbitol gets trapped inside the cell and can cause **osmotic damage** when water rushes into the cell to balance the osmotic forces. This leads to **Schwann cell** damage in neurons and promotes neuropathy through demyelination. In the eye, this can lead to **cataracts** (in the lens) and **retinopathy** (in the retina).
- **Nonenzymatic glycosylation** (Fig. 9.27B): This is when hyperglycemia allows sugar to attach to proteins (without the aid of an enzyme, hence nonenzymatic). This causes dysfunction of the protein; in blood vessels, this leads to increased vessel permeability and predisposes it to atherosclerosis. Not only does this play a role in all three microvascular diseases (retinopathy, neuropathy, and nephropathy) as well as macrovascular disease, but it also gives a way to track glycemic control over the long term, by HbA1c, which is a measure of the glycosylation of hemoglobin. In diabetic patients, the goal is usually an HbA1c of less than 7%.

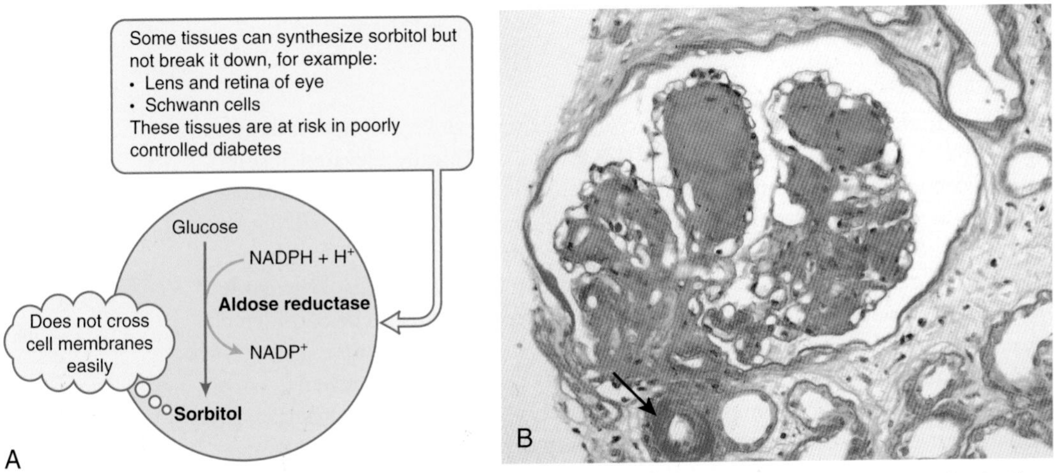

FIG. 9.27 A, Osmotic damage via the aldose reductase pathway. **B,** Diabetic nephropathy with Kimmelstiel-Wilson nodules of type IV collagen, as well as thickening of the arteriole (hyaline arteriolosclerosis) *(arrow)* from nonenzymatic glycosylation. (**A** *from* Clark M. Crash Course: Metabolism and Nutrition. *Philadelphia: Elsevier; 2005.* **B** *from* Kumar P, Clark M. Clinical Medicine. *6th ed. Edinburgh: Elsevier; 2005.*)

- **Diabetic microangiopathy:** With increased blood sugar, the **endothelial cells** that line the blood vessels take in additional glucose. Some of this glucose is made into **glycoproteins,** which are placed on the surface of the endothelial cells and cause **thickening and weakening** of the basement membrane (type IV collagen). This weakening can lead to increased permeability, causing **proteinuria** in the kidney (diabetic glomerulosclerosis with "Kimmelstiel-Wilson nodules," which are actually type IV collagen) and potential for edema and hemorrhage in the retina (diabetic retinopathy). Because there are blood vessels that nourish the nerves (vasa nervorum), damage here can also lead to diabetic neuropathy.

> Diabetic ketoacidosis: absolute insulin deficiency, causing fatty acid breakdown and ketoacid formation, as well as hyperglycemia

Acute Emergencies in Diabetes

As mentioned previously, **type 1 diabetes** predisposes to the potential development of **DKA,** whereas **type 2 diabetes** predisposes to the potential development of **HNS.** These are both acute emergencies that need to be recognized and treated.

- **Diabetic ketoacidosis:** Often seen in patients who are **noncompliant with insulin dosage** when treated for type 1 or because of a secondary illness causing increased stress on the body. This may even be the first manifestation of previously undiagnosed type 1 diabetes mellitus. The **absolute insulin deficiency** leads to **hyperglycemia** from decreased cell uptake of glucose coupled with high levels of gluconeogenesis from high glucagon levels; the hyperglycemia causes subsequent **dehydration** from osmotic diuresis. Despite the abundance of serum glucose, without insulin there is a lack of intracellular glucose. The body shifts toward **lipolysis** (using fat for energy), with **ketoacids** such as acetoacetate and β-hydroxybutyrate being produced as a byproduct of β-oxidation of fatty acids; this is because there is no insulin to inhibit hormone-sensitive lipase or stimulate lipoprotein lipase, which would decrease fat metabolism. Laboratory findings include **hyperkalemic acidosis** with increased anion gap (because of ketones and potentially lactic acidosis if in shock), **hyponatremia** (glucose osmoles draw in water and "dilute" the sodium; this is actually a true hyponatremia and not pseudohyponatremia, but will be corrected with the correction of glucose), and ketonuria and ketonemia. Clinical findings include **Kussmaul respirations** (deep rapid breathing from profound acidosis—respiratory compensation), dehydration with tachycardia (from osmotic diuresis), and a "fruity" odor on the breath from acetone secreted in the saliva. Treatment is fluids and insulin, as well as potassium supplementation. In addition to promoting glucose uptake, insulin upregulates the Na^+/K^+-ATPase, promoting cellular uptake of potassium. Hypokalemia with insulin administration must be carefully monitored in this condition because the patients usually have a global potassium deficit from osmotic diuresis, even if they appear hyperkalemic from the acidosis moving K^+ out of the cells (by H^+/K^+ exchangers).
- **Hyperosmolar nonketotic state (HNS):** Associated with **type 2 diabetes mellitus,** with **severely high blood sugar** (usually > 600 mg/dL) and subsequent hyperosmolarity. This leads to significant dehydration from osmotic diuresis, as well as osmolar shifts, which cause changes in mental status. There is no ketosis because of the presence of insulin, which inhibits lipolysis. This syndrome goes by numerous names, and *hyperosmolar hyperglycemic state (HHS)* and *hyperosmolar nonketotic coma (HONKC)* may also be seen.

Islet Cell Tumors

- **Insulinoma:** A **benign** tumor of the beta cells of the islets of Langerhans, with a strong correlation to MEN I syndrome (pituitary, **pancreas,** parathyroid). This causes chronically elevated insulin levels, leading to **hypoglycemia.** As mentioned before, because this is **endogenous** insulin, there will be high levels of insulin as well as **high levels of C-peptide.** High levels of C-peptide will not be seen with injectable insulin, and therefore the two conditions can be differentiated based on this fact. Treatment is surgery or **streptozocin,** which is a medication that is toxic to beta cells. **Diazoxide** can also help prevent release of insulin and prevent hypoglycemia. Octreotide can also be considered because it will decrease insulin release as well.
- **Glucagonoma:** A **malignant** tumor of the alpha cells of the islets of Langerhans, with **hyperglycemia** from the increased gluconeogenesis and glycogenolysis caused by the glucagon. In addition, there is a characteristic rash called **necrolytic migratory erythema (NME).** Treatment is surgery and **octreotide** (a somatostatin analog), which decreases glucagon production by the malignant tumor.
- **Somatostatinoma:** A **malignant** tumor of the delta cells of the islets of Langerhans. **Somatostatin** inhibits almost every GI-related hormone, including **gastrin, cholecystokinin (CCK),** and **secretin.**

Inhibition of **CCK** causes the gallbladder to fail to contract, leading to cholelithiasis. Inhibition of **secretin** can cause steatorrhea because secretin causes bicarbonate secretion from the pancreas, allowing lipases to work—lack of this can cause the digestive enzymes to be ineffective, leading to malabsorption and steatorrhea.

- **VIPoma:** A **malignant** tumor causing release of vasoactive intestinal peptide. This peptide in high amounts causes what is called **pancreatic cholera,** a cholera-like syndrome characterized by diffuse diarrhea with dehydration, hypokalemic acidosis (GI loss of potassium and bicarbonate), and widespread vasodilation (hence **vasoactive**).
- **Zollinger-Ellison syndrome** (gastrinoma): A **malignant** tumor that secretes **gastrin,** leading to increased acid production with **widespread gastroduodenal ulcers.** The increased acid **denatures** digestive enzymes, leading to malabsorption and diarrhea. Any time multiple or refractory duodenal ulcers are present, you should have a high suspicion for this syndrome. The diagnosis is also suggested by **elevated gastrin levels** (but proton pump inhibitor medication will also cause elevated gastrin as a reflex from the decreased stomach acidity).

Pharmacology of Diabetes Mellitus

Insulin: For those with type 1 diabetes, insulin injections are required to sustain life. For those with type 2 diabetes, insulin may be required because there is progressive beta cell failure over time and subsequent insulin deficiency. Insulin is also the most common medication used to treat pregnant women with gestational diabetes because insulin does not cross the blood–placenta barrier. Insulin is injected subcutaneously or through an insulin pump. Because insulin promotes fatty acid uptake into adipocytes, local **lipodystrophy** can occur. The most common side effect of insulin injections is **hypoglycemia,** especially if a patient forgets to take a meal after dose administration.

- **Rapid-acting insulin preparations:** Insulin aspart, insulin lispro, insulin glulisine
- **Short-acting insulin preparations:** Regular insulin
- **Intermediate-acting insulin preparations:** NPH insulin
- **Long-acting insulin preparations**: Insulin glargine, insulin detemir, insulin degludec

Sulfonylurea Drugs—Glyburide, Glipizide, Glimepiride. Sulfonylurea drugs act to **increase the body's pancreatic production of insulin**. Recall that normally glucose enters the beta cell and is metabolized to ATP. ATP then **closes** a potassium channel that was previously hyperpolarizing the cell (see Fig. 9.24A). This depolarization leads to calcium influx and insulin release. The same potassium channel has a **sulfonylurea receptor** that sulfonylurea can bind to and close the channel independent of ATP, leading to insulin release. Of course, this will only work if there are functional beta cells in the pancreas available to secrete insulin (will not work in type 1 diabetes). The most common side effect of sulfonylurea drugs is **hypoglycemia.**

Biguanides—Metformin: Metformin has numerous actions to reduce hyperglycemia by **decreasing hepatic gluconeogenesis** and acts as an **insulin-sensitizing agent** by promoting glucose uptake in the body's cells. Because this medication prevents hyperglycemia rather than causing hypoglycemia, it is said to be **euglycemic** in that it cannot be a cause of hypoglycemia. Also, because there is no direct action of metformin on the pancreas, this can be used in patients without beta cell function to help lower injected insulin requirements. The most serious side effect is **lactic acidosis**—lactate uptake in the liver is decreased with metformin because lactate is changed into glucose through gluconeogenesis (a process that metformin inhibits). Although this is inconsequential in healthy individuals because the excess lactate can be cleared by the kidneys, patients with renal failure (decreased lactate clearance) or respiratory disease causing relative hypoxia (leading to increased lactate through anaerobic metabolism) can develop lactic acidosis.

Thiazolidinediones—Pioglitazone (-Glitazone Drugs): These medications are **insulin sensitizers** and bind to a nuclear receptor called the peroxisome proliferator-activated receptor gamma receptor **(PPAR-γ).** Activation of PPAR-γ leads to increased synthesis of GLUT-4 glucose channels and other genes involved in insulin sensitivity. Side effects include **water retention,** leading to edema, weight gain, and potentially heart failure from fluid overload. Older preparations of thiazolidinediones caused hepatotoxicity—this has **not** been found in newer preparations (but may be found on an examination regardless).

Incretin Mimetics (-Tides: Exenatide, Liraglutide) and DPP-4 Inhibitors (-Gliptins: Sitagliptin, Linagliptin, Saxagliptin): The **incretin** pathway (Fig. 9.28) is activated when nutrients reach the intestine and act to stimulate insulin release before the glucose actually makes it to the bloodstream to better regulate sugar. These receptors are found in the intestines, so intravenous nutrition will not activate

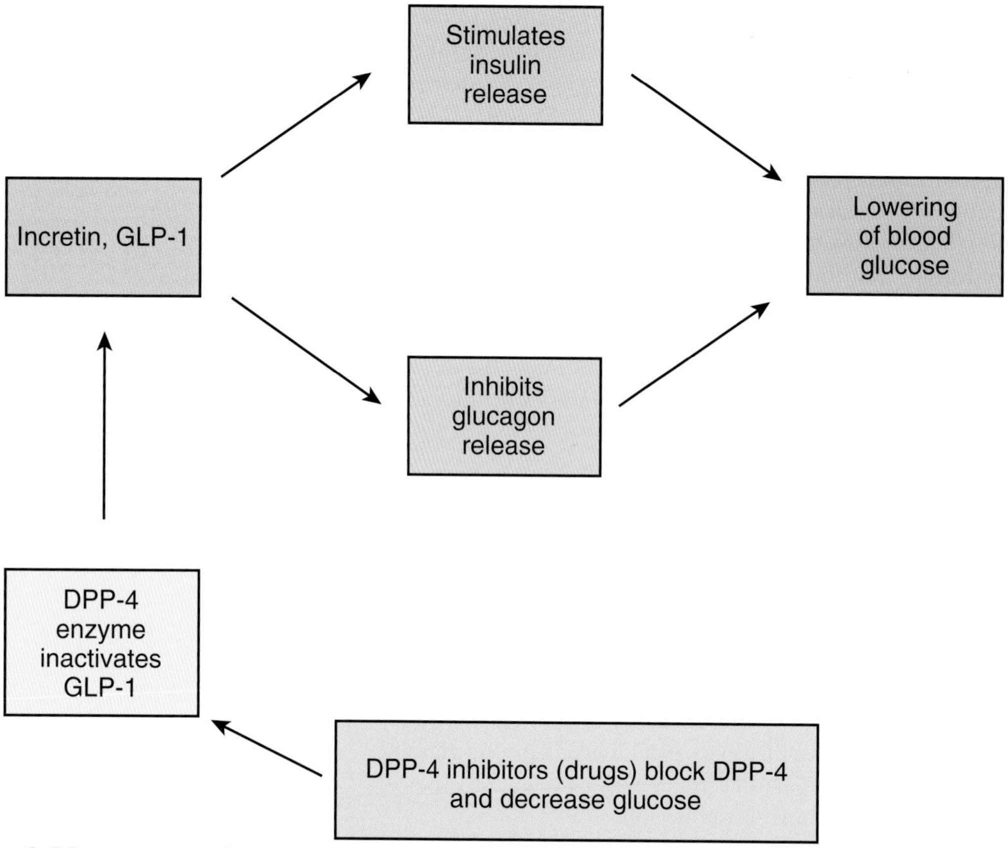

Fig. 9.28 The incretin pathway and the drugs that act on it. (*Drawn in Inkscape by Ilmari Karonen based on w:Image: Incretins and DPP 4 inhibitors.jpg from* http://casesblog.blogspot.com/2006/11/dpp-4-inhibitors-for-treatment-of.html *[uploaded by author]. Accessed January 10, 2013, from* http://en.wikipedia.org/wiki/File:Incretins_and_DPP_4_inhibitors.svg.)

this pathway. **DPP-4 inhibitors such as sitagliptin** prevent breakdown of incretins, whereas incretin analogs such as **exenatide** mimic the incretin GLP-1 and activate the pathway directly. As an interesting aside, exenatide is derived from Gila monster saliva and can potentially cause nausea and **pancreatitis.**

α-Glucosidase Inhibitors—Acarbose, Miglitol: Acarbose inhibits the intestinal brush border α-glucosidase, an enzyme necessary for digestion of carbohydrates, leading to decreased blood sugar by decreased absorption. However, this leftover osmotic agent causes **osmotic diarrhea** and **flatulence** (from bacterial metabolism of carbohydrates, which forms H_2 and CO_2 gas). Because this enzyme breaks down branches of carbohydrates, monosaccharides will still be absorbed normally. Anyone who is lactose intolerant and cannot break down and absorb lactose knows that the osmotic diarrhea and flatulence from bacterial breakdown of the disaccharides is unpleasant; because of these side effects, this medication is rarely used.

Sodium-Glucose Cotransporter 2 (SGLT-2) Inhibitors—Canagliflozin (-Gliflozin Drugs): These drugs block reabsorption of glucose in the proximal nephron, leading to glucosuria. The main side effects of this are those attributable to glucosuria such as dehydration, yeast infections, and urinary tract infections (because yeast and bacteria have more glucose to proliferate). However, the most worrisome side effect is euglycemic diabetic ketoacidosis. If a patient has absolute insulin deficiency and is taking this drug, he or she can develop DKA with a relatively normal blood sugar because the excess glucose is being excreted in the urine but the patient still will have ketoacidosis.

Parathyroid Glands

Anatomy, Embryology, and Histology

The four **parathyroid glands** are the key mediators of calcium and phosphate homeostasis and therefore play an important role in bone growth and development. As the name implies, they are

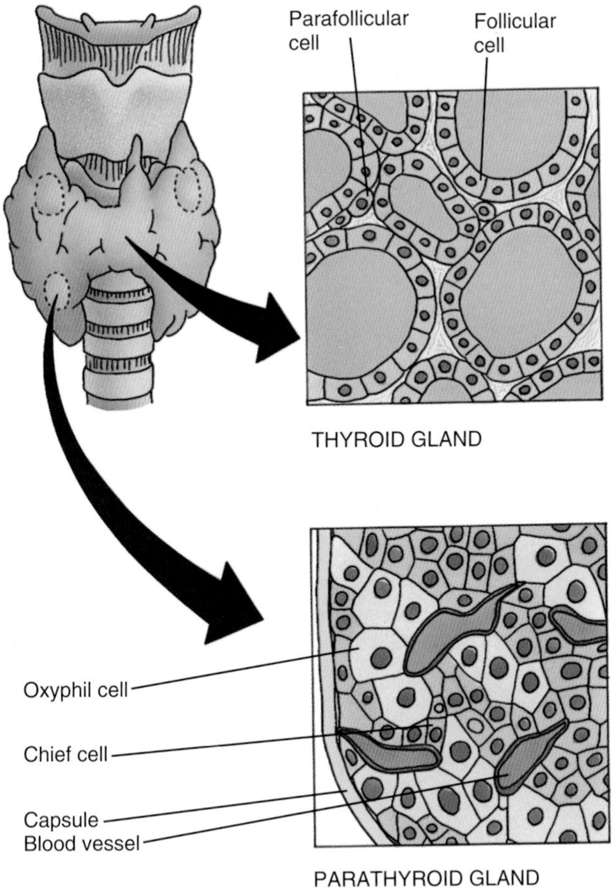

FIG. 9.29 Anatomy of the parathyroid glands and illustrations of their histologic appearance. (*From Gartner LP, Hiatt JL. Color Textbook of Histology. 3rd ed. Philadelphia: Saunders; 2007:313.*)

near the thyroid (usually on the posterior aspect, or inside the thyroid parenchyma; Fig. 9.29). The two **superior** parathyroid glands arise from the **fourth pharyngeal pouch;** the two **inferior** parathyroid glands arise from the **third pharyngeal pouch** (counterintuitive because they swap places!). The embryologic development of these two pouches can fail to develop properly in **DiGeorge syndrome.**

- **DiGeorge syndrome:** Failure of the third and fourth pharyngeal pouches to develop (see Chapter 4). The mnemonic to remember the associated defects is **CATCH-22**—**C**ardiac abnormalities (especially tetralogy of Fallot), **A**bnormal facies, **T**hymic aplasia, **C**left palate, and **H**ypoparathyroidism with hypocalcemia caused by failure of parathyroid development; this disease is a deletion on chromosome **22.**

The **histology** of the gland shows two distinct cell morphologies: **chief cells** and **oxyphil cells.** The chief cells are small, round, eosinophilic cells that **create parathyroid hormone,** which is stored until stimulated for release (the **C**hief cells have a role in **C**alcium). The role of oxyphil cells is unknown.

Overview of Calcium Homeostasis

Calcium (and phosphorus) homeostasis (Table 9.4; Fig. 9.30) are maintained by **hormones** (parathyroid hormone, calcitonin, vitamin D) and the **organs** that react to these hormones (bones, kidneys, and intestines). These hormones mainly regulate the way that each of these organs handles calcium; for example, bone can be deposited or reabsorbed, the intestines can absorb more or less dietary calcium, and the kidneys can reabsorb more or less calcium from the tubules. The major player in calcium homeostasis is **parathyroid hormone,** secreted in response to **low serum ionized calcium** (*ionized*

Table 9.4 Hormones of Calcium Homeostasis

HORMONE	STIMULUS	CALCIUM EFFECTS	PHOSPHATE EFFECTS
PTH	↓ Ionized calcium level	Increases calcium ↑ Renal reabsorption ↑ Bone resorption (although initially it is bone building because PTH receptors are on the osteoblast)	Decreases phosphate ↓ Renal reabsorption (causing phosphaturia)
1,25(OH)-vitamin D (calcitriol)	↑ 1α-Hydroxylase activity (increased PTH, ↓ ionized calcium/phosphorus)	Increases calcium ↑ Renal reabsorption ↑ Intestinal reabsorption	Increases phosphate ↑ Renal reabsorption ↑ Intestinal reabsorption
Calcitonin	↑ Ionized calcium level	Decreases calcium ↓ Bone resorption	

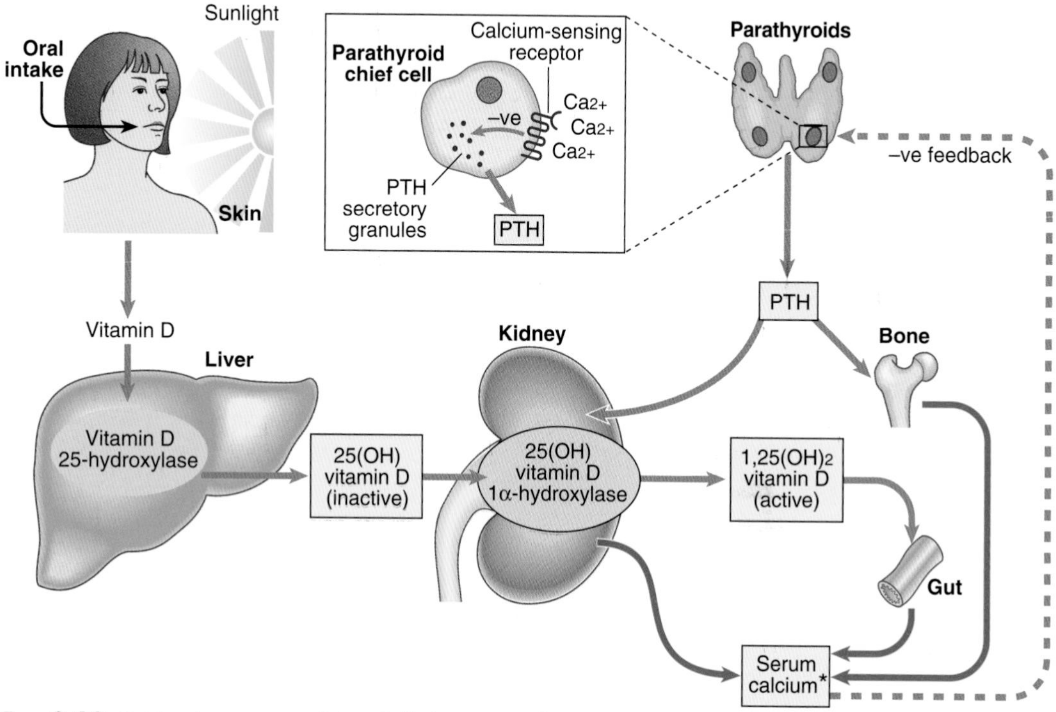

Fig. 9.30 Calcium homeostasis. (*From Colledge NR, Walker BR, Ralston SH.* Davidson's Principles and Practice of Medicine. *21st ed. Philadelphia: Elsevier; 2010.*)

describes free calcium as ions, rather than bound to albumin or other proteins). Follow Fig. 9.30 with the explanation here:

1. The **parathyroid gland** senses **decreased** ionized calcium and **secretes parathyroid hormone (PTH).** Parathyroid hormone has direct actions on the **bones** and **kidneys.**
2. **PTH** activity has three effects on the **kidneys:** (1) PTH **increases expression** of **1α-hydroxylase** in the proximal tubule of the nephron, which will convert vitamin D into its active form; (2) PTH **inhibits** phosphate reabsorption (inhibits Na^+-phosphate cotransporter) also in the proximal tubule causing **phosphaturia** (this is because if both calcium and phosphate were increased in blood, they would precipitate); (3) PTH **increases calcium reabsorption** in the distal convoluted tubule to increase serum calcium levels. As an aside, **PTH** works through the G_s-signaling pathway, which generates increased cyclic adenosine monophosphate (cAMP) as a signaling molecule—the actions on the renal tubular cells cause increased cAMP production, leading to **increased urinary cAMP.**
3. **PTH** activity directly stimulates the **osteoblasts.** This may be counterintuitive when thinking about osteoblasts, which form bone by depositing calcium. The reason for this apparent paradox is that the **osteoblasts in turn signal osteoclasts through RANKL** to reabsorb bone and therefore increase serum calcium. This initial stimulation of osteoblasts, however, is why small bursts of PTH can be used clinically to just stimulate osteoblasts and treat osteoporosis.

4. **Vitamin D,** in its active form (1,25[OH]-vitamin D, "calcitriol"), has its main effect on the **intestines,** increasing synthesis of a calcium-binding protein (calbindin D-28 K) to promote **increased absorption of dietary calcium.** Calcitriol also increases dietary absorption of **phosphate.** Vitamin D also has effects on the **kidneys** (increasing both calcium and phosphate reabsorption) and on **bone** to stimulate resorption of old bone and mineralization of new bone (bone remodeling). The net effect of vitamin D is increasing calcium and phosphate levels through the kidneys, gut, and bone (and subsequently promoting bone remodeling).

Vitamin D can be obtained through **dietary sources** or formed in the skin through **sunlight** (major source). This inactive vitamin D then goes to the liver and, through hepatic 25-hydroxylase, becomes 25(OH)-vitamin D, which is still inactive. It is not until the renal activity of 1α-hydroxylase turns it into 1,25(OH)-vitamin D, or calcitriol, that it is active. Therefore hepatic dysfunction (lack of sufficient 25-hydroxylase activity) or renal dysfunction (lack of sufficient 1α-hydroxylase activity) can lead to a functional vitamin D deficiency.

Calcitonin is also involved in calcium homeostasis but plays a very minor role. **Calcitonin tones down calcium** (lowers serum calcium) by **inhibiting bone resorption** (inhibiting osteoclast activity). Calcitonin is secreted by the parafollicular **C** cells.

Laboratory Testing and Pitfalls

Understanding the laboratory testing necessary to diagnose disorders of calcium and phosphate homeostasis is important. First, it is important to ensure that the calcium level is truly accurate: changes in **albumin** and changes in **acid-base status** can alter total and ionized calcium levels, respectively. Total calcium measures the amount of calcium in the blood; free calcium only takes into account the free (ionized) calcium that is active.

- **Hypoalbuminemia:** Because calcium is attached to albumin, lower albumin levels can lead to a decreased calcium level (1 g/dL of albumin binds 0.8 mg/dL of calcium at physiologic pH). Therefore in the asymptomatic patient, **hypoalbuminemia** is the most common cause of low calcium on a laboratory test. However, this **will not change the ionized** calcium level. The ionized (free, unbound) calcium has not changed, so the patient will not have symptoms related to abnormal calcium levels.
- **Acid-Base Disturbances:** Albumin is a large, negatively charged protein. These negatively charged sites can bind H^+ or Ca^{2+}. In **acidemia,** in which there is excess H^+, the H^+ will take up most of those sites, displacing calcium and leading to **increased ionized calcium** levels because the calcium will have nowhere to bind. Conversely, in alkalemia, in which there are fewer H^+, there are more open sites on albumin for Ca^{2+} to bind, and therefore proportionally more calcium will bind to albumin, leading to **decreased ionized calcium.** Because in both these cases the calcium is just being moved between the bound and unbound state and is not being gained or lost from the body, the **total calcium does not change** in acid-base disturbances. However, the ionized calcium has changed, so the patient may have symptoms related to abnormal ionized calcium levels (Fig. 9.31).

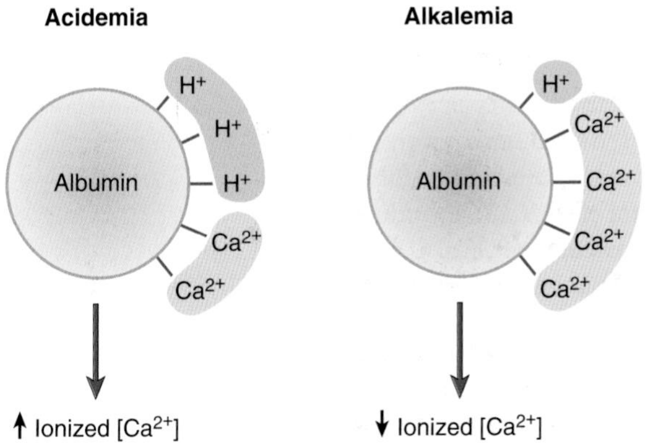

FIG. 9.31 Acidemia and alkalemia and the effect on ionized calcium (no change in total calcium). (*From Costanzo LS.* Physiology. *4th ed. New York: Elsevier; 2009.*)

The etiology of the calcium disturbance can be further elucidated by the use of additional laboratory testing, depending on the pathology. In the next section, each pathologic cause of altered calcium or phosphate levels will be addressed as well as the diagnosis and treatment. It is also important to note that for these disturbances, as well as for endocrine disturbances in general, "normal ranges" for hormones must be taken in their appropriate context. For instance, a normal calcium level is 8.5 to 10 mg/dL and a normal PTH level is 10 to 60 pg/mL. However, if a patient's calcium is 11 mg/dL (high) and PTH level is 50 pg/mL ("normal" range), it is abnormal because **in the context of hypercalcemia,** the normal-range PTH level is much too high; it should be **less than 10 pg/mL** because there should be negative feedback on the parathyroid glands if they are functioning normally. It is important to keep this in mind to prevent being misled.

A. **Primary hypoparathyroidism:** Calcium is low and the parathyroid gland is not attempting to fix it (low PTH).
B. **Hypoalbuminemia:** Decreased albumin leads to decreased total calcium but ionized (free) calcium is normal, and therefore PTH is normal range.
C. **Secondary hyperparathyroidism:** High PTH is unable to correct calcium; this can be seen in renal failure because vitamin D cannot be made to help correct Ca^{2+}. Note that this could also represent pseudohypoparathyroidism, described later.
D. **Respiratory alkalosis:** Total calcium is normal, but alkalosis causes increased binding of calcium to albumin, leading to decreased ionized calcium and subsequent increased PTH level to increase ionized calcium.
E. **Primary hyperparathyroidism:** High calcium, yet PTH is still high.
F. **Hypercalcemia of malignancy:** High calcium, PTH low because parathyroid hormone–related peptide (PTHrP) is being created instead (or direct osteolytic bone metastases).

Refer to Fig. 9.32 when revisiting each pathologic disease to understand why the laboratory values are as described previously.

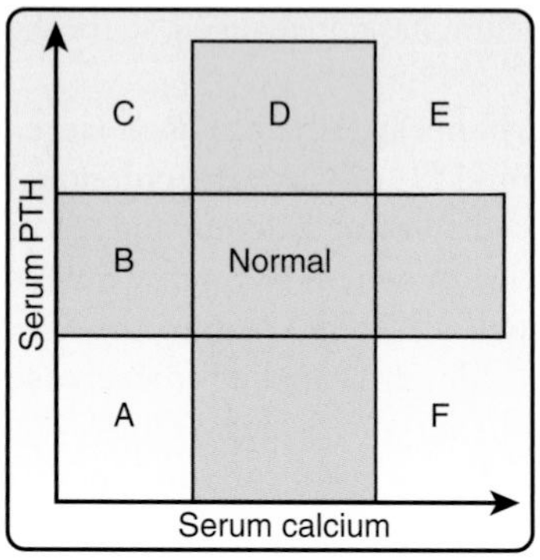

FIG. 9.32 Schematic showing serum calcium and serum PTH; normal is shown by the box in the center. *A* represents primary hypoparathyroidism, *B* represents hypoalbuminemia, *C* represents secondary hyperparathyroidism, *D* represents respiratory alkalosis, *E* represents primary hyperparathyroidism, and *F* represents hypercalcemia of malignancy. (*From Goljan EF.* Rapid Review Pathology Revised Reprint. *3rd ed. Philadelphia: Elsevier; 2011.*)

Pathology Causing Increased Calcium Levels

Hypercalcemia: usually hyperparathyroidism or malignancy

When **hypercalcemia** occurs, the typical symptoms are remembered by "stones, bone, groans, and psychiatric overtones."

Stones: Calcium-containing renal stones are the most common manifestation of hypercalcemia because the increased calcium in the urine promotes stone formation. Gallstones can also occur.

Bones: Depending on the cause of the hypercalcemia, different bone manifestations can occur. In **hyperparathyroidism** the elevated PTH levels cause hypercalcemia (Fig. 9.33), and the effects of sustained high PTH levels on the osteoblasts (which signal the osteoclasts) lead to a syndrome called **osteitis fibrosa cystica,** in which **cystic** and **hemorrhagic** bone lesions develop from high osteoclastic activity and **subperiosteal resorption** of bone, especially in the fingers. High PTH levels also cause osteoporosis for similar reasons. Lastly, there can be a **"salt-and-pepper"** appearance of the skull (Fig. 9.33B) from diffuse osteoclastic activity in the skull.

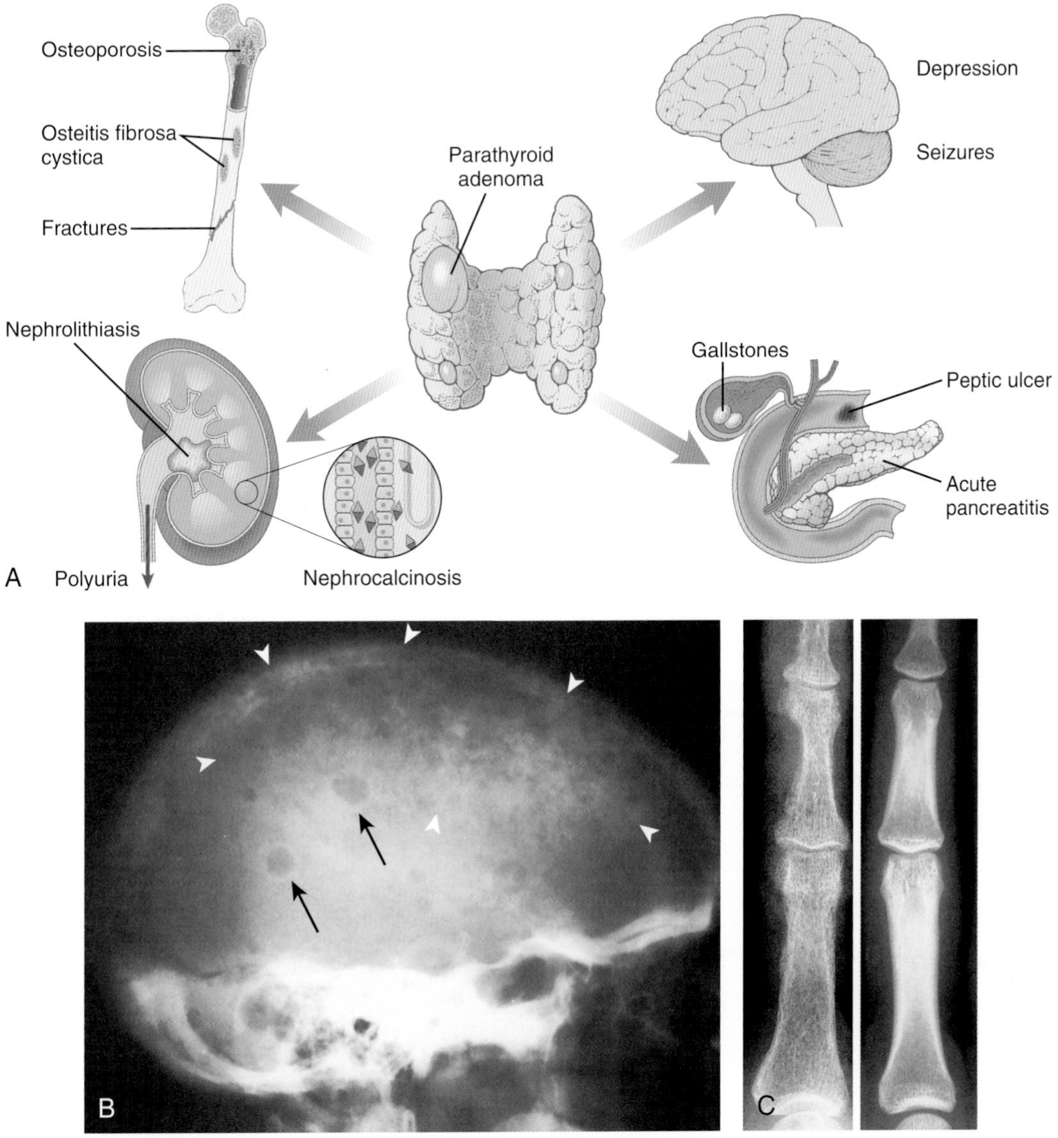

FIG. 9.33 A, Effects of hyperparathyroidism with hypercalcemia. **B,** Salt-and-pepper skull from hyperparathyroidism. **C,** Comparative radiographs of fingers (left finger, hyperparathyroidism; right finger, normal). (**A** *from Kumar V, Cotran RS, Robbins SL.* Robbins Basic Pathology. *7th ed. Philadelphia: Elsevier; 2002.* **B** *from Weissman BN.* Imaging of Arthritis and Metabolic Bone Disease. *Philadelphia: Elsevier; 2009.* **C** *from Underwood JCE, Cross SS.* General and Systematic Pathology. *5th ed. Edinburgh: Elsevier; 2009.*)

Groans: The groans are from **GI** problems such as **abdominal pain, nausea, and vomiting.** This is because **hypercalcemia** is a cause of pancreatitis (from enzyme activation), and calcium also causes increased gastrin production and subsequent acid secretion in the stomach, potentially leading to **peptic ulcer disease.**

Psychiatric overtones: Common, but can have varied findings, ranging from depression and anxiety to psychosis and coma.

The differential diagnosis list for increased calcium levels is long and can be remembered by the mnemonic **CHIMPANZEES.** However, it is worth noting that **primary hyperparathyroidism** and **malignancies** account for almost all causes (>90%) of hypercalcemia and should come to mind first.

- ❍ **C**alcium ingestion (milk-alkali syndrome)
- ❍ **H**yperparathyroidism (most common cause in absence of malignancy)
- ❍ **I**atrogenic

- Multiple myeloma (from bone breakdown)
- Paget disease
- Addison disease (as a result of volume contraction causing increased reabsorption of fluid and electrolytes, including calcium, from the proximal tubule of the nephron)
- Neoplasms (either those secreting PTHrP or from bone metastases)
- Zollinger-Ellison syndrome
- Excessive vitamin D intake or vitamin A intake
- Excessive thyroid hormone (hyperthyroidism causes increased bone turnover)
- Sarcoidosis (or other granulomatous disease, as a result of increased macrophage activity; macrophages have 1α-hydroxylase activity, which leads to hypercalcemia secondary to increased 1,25-vitamin D levels)

Because the two main causes of hypercalcemia are **hyperparathyroidism** and **malignancy,** they will be covered in additional detail.

Hyperparathyroidism (Fig. 9.34) can be **primary** (gland hyperfunction), **secondary** (as a result of hypovitaminosis D or renal failure), or **tertiary** (prolonged secondary hyperparathyroidism causes the glands to become autonomous). **Primary** hyperparathyroidism usually is due to **a single hyperfunctioning adenoma** (80%) but can also be due to diffuse hyperplasia of all four glands (20%). Recall that primary hyperparathyroidism is associated with MEN I and IIa.

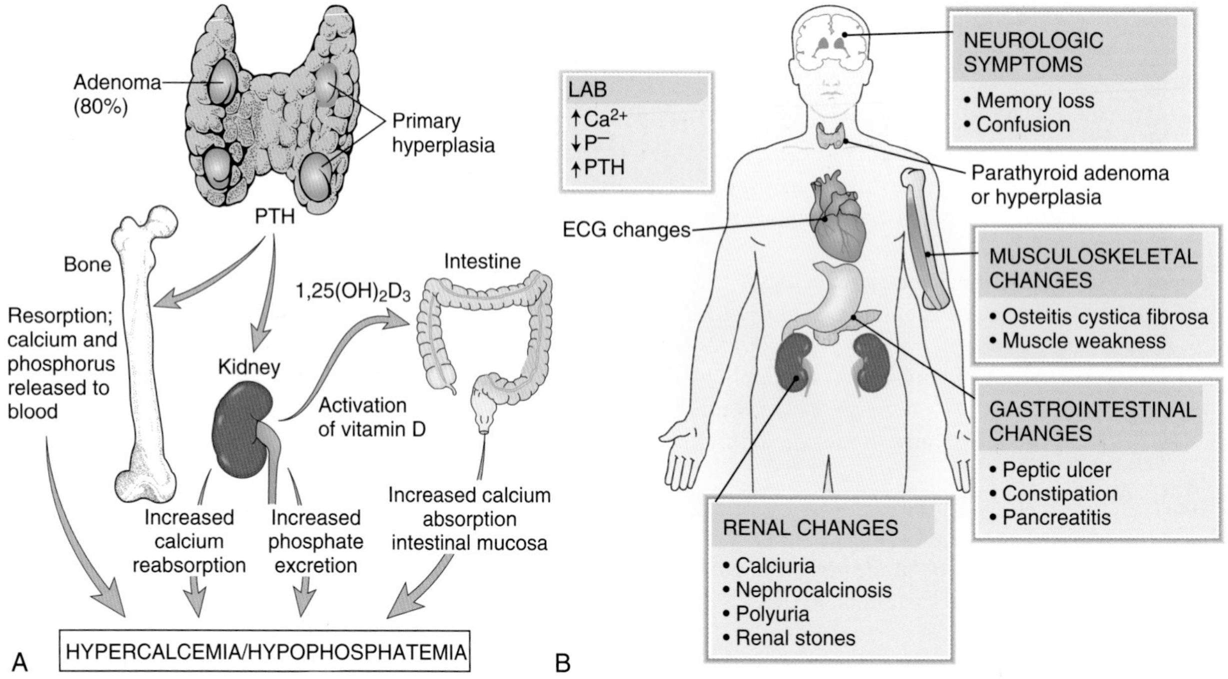

Fig. 9.34 Hyperparathyroidism and the effects downstream of increased PTH and increased calcium. (A) The direct effects of PTH on each organ system. (B) The effects of excessive PTH resulting in hypercalcemia and hypophosphatemia (*From Damjanov I.* Pathophysiology. *Philadelphia: Elsevier; 2008.*)

- **Laboratory diagnosis of primary hyperparathyroidism: Hypercalcemia** in the setting of **normal to high PTH** is diagnostic of hyperparathyroidism as a result of inappropriate secretion of PTH despite high calcium levels.
- **Imaging diagnosis of primary hyperparathyroidism:** A technetium-99m-sestamibi radionuclide scan can indicate whether or not there is a single hyperfunctioning adenoma, which takes up the radiotracer more avidly than the other normal parathyroid glands. In either case (hyperplasia or adenoma) the treatment is surgical.
- **Secondary hyperparathyroidism:** Caused by hypovitaminosis D, either because of dietary deficiency or secondary to renal failure. Because active 1,25(OH)-vitamin D is essential to the

ability of the body to increase calcium levels from inability of conversion of 25(OH)-vitamin D to 1,25(OH)-vitamin D, PTH will have sustained release because of lack of negative feedback from calcium levels. Therefore the laboratory studies will show **high PTH** with **low calcium and high phosphorous.**

- **Tertiary hyperparathyroidism:** With prolonged secondary hyperparathyroidism, the parathyroid glands become autonomous. Even if the underlying cause is fixed (i.e., renal transplantation), PTH will remain high. Sustained high PTH has caused these hyperfunctioning parathyroid glands to lose their negative feedback.
- **Hypercalcemia of malignancy:** Can occur in two settings: (1) a paraneoplastic syndrome from PTHrP secreted by the cancerous cells, and (2) direct bone destruction from metastases leading to increased calcium levels. The best way to distinguish between these two entities is a **PTHrP level.** With hypercalcemia of malignancy caused by PTHrP secretion, the PTH will be low, the PTHrP will be high, and the calcium will be high. The classic cause of this is **squamous cell carcinoma of the lung.** In addition, diffuse lytic metastases to bone can cause destruction, leading to high calcium but low PTH and PTHrP levels.

Hypocalcemia: may just be decreased total calcium but normal ionized calcium—first correct for albumin!

Treatment of any form of hypercalcemia is correction of the underlying cause. However, acute treatment is aimed at (1) diluting the calcium, (2) increasing urinary excretion of calcium, and (3) protecting bone.

- Dilution of the serum calcium occurs from large amounts of intravenous hydration.
- Intravenous furosemide (Lasix) causes calcium to be excreted in the urine (see Chapter 15 for mechanism).
- Bisphosphonates deposit in the bone and prevent osteoclastic release of calcium by preventing breakdown of bone.

Pathologic Causes of Decreased Calcium Levels

Again, when dealing with a low serum calcium level, it is most important to **first correct the calcium for hypoalbuminemia, if present.** This is easily the most common cause of hypocalcemia in an asymptomatic patient. However, a patient who truly has hypocalcemia will often display some of the following symptoms:

- **Tetany:** The decreased calcium level causes hyperexcitability of the muscles; this can be assessed clinically by **Trousseau sign of latent tetany** and **Chvostek sign.** Trousseau sign involves inducing **carpal (or pedal) spasm** by inflating a blood pressure cuff on the arm (or leg) above the patient's systolic pressure. This action allows the limb to develop a mild acidosis, and the subsequent hyperexcitable neurons will fire and trigger muscle contraction. Chvostek sign is tapping on the inferior portion of the zygoma, in the area of the facial nerve, which will subsequently cause facial twitching.
- **Arrhythmias** can occur because hypocalcemia leads to **QT prolongation** of the electrocardiogram, increasing the susceptibility to **torsades de pointes,** which occurs when a premature beat attempts to fire during the repolarization of the heart (termed an *R-on-T phenomenon* because the QRS complex represents ventricular depolarization, which is abnormally occurring during the repolarization of the heart).

The main cause of hypocalcemia is **hypoparathyroidism.** Other causes include **DiGeorge syndrome** (covered earlier in the section "Anatomy, Embryology, and Histology") and **pseudohypoparathyroidism.** Pseudohypoparathyroidism has many subtypes, the most commonly tested being Albright hereditary osteodystrophy (pseudohypoparathyroidism type Ia). This is an autosomal dominant genetic condition in which the G_s subunit of the PTH receptor is broken, leading to ineffective action of PTH on the kidney.

- **Hypoparathyroidism:** Can be caused **iatrogenically** by previous neck surgery, but the most common nonsurgical cause is **autoimmune.** This is characterized by **low PTH levels** in the face of low calcium. Treatment is supplementation with calcium and active vitamin D.
- **Pseudohypoparathyroidism:** There is a dysfunctional PTH receptor on the kidney, but the parathyroid gland itself functions normally. Therefore there will be low calcium (as though the patient had hypoparathyroidism, hence the name **pseudo**hypoparathyroidism), but the **PTH will be high** because the gland is attempting to correct the calcium level. One classic sign of

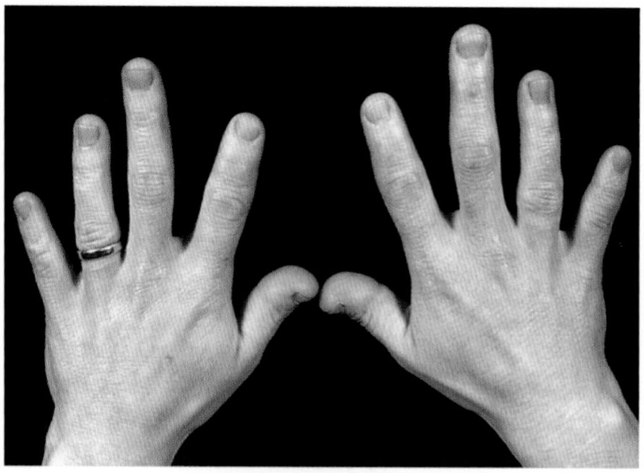

FIG. 9.35 Pseudohypoparathyroidism showing classic "knuckle-knuckle-dimple-dimple" sign. (*From Swash M, Glynn M, Hutchison R.* Hutchison's Clinical Methods. *22nd ed. Edinburgh: Elsevier; 2007.*)

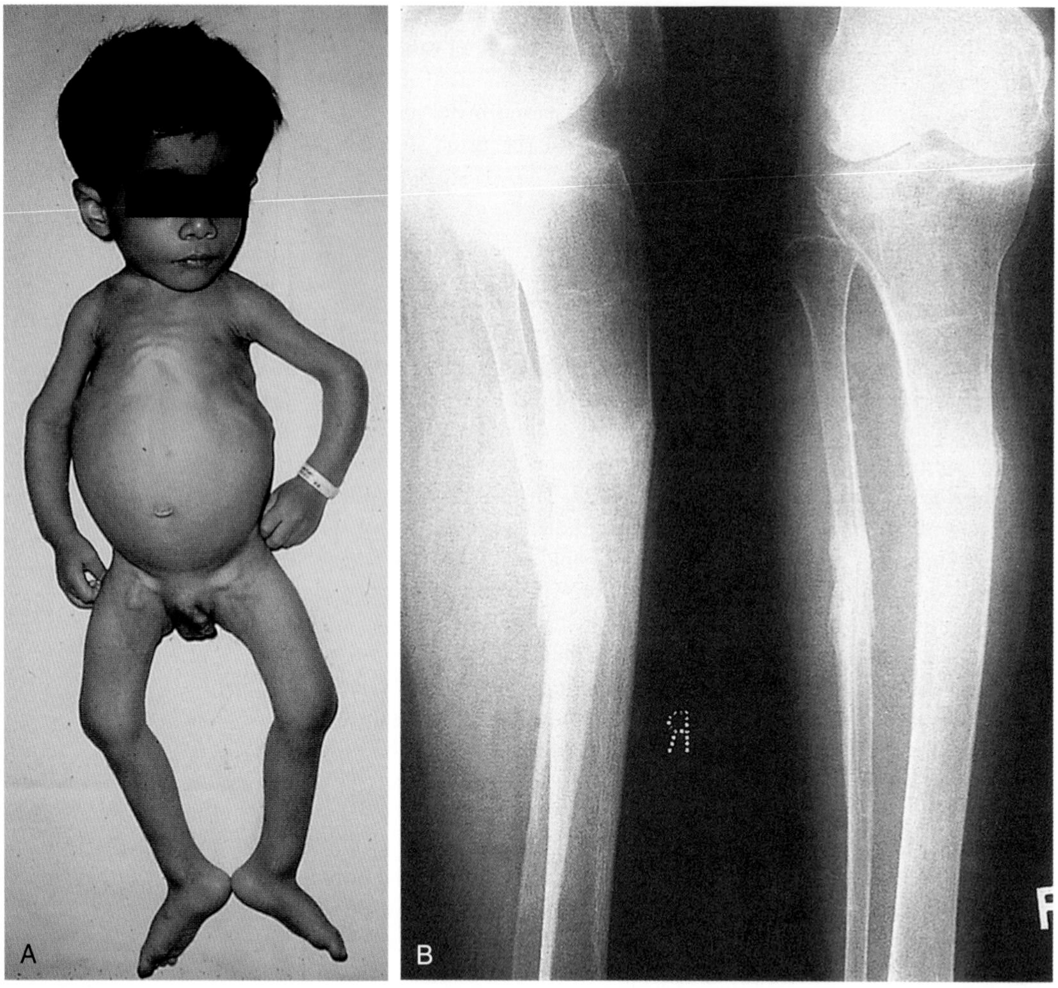

FIG. 9.36 A, Bow legs (genu varum) in a patient with rickets. **B,** Osteomalacia in an adult, showing pathologic fractures. (**A** *from Lissauer T, Clayden G.* Illustrated Textbook of Pediatrics. *3rd ed. Edinburgh: Elsevier; 2007.* **B** *from Dandy DJ, Edwards DJ.* Essential Orthopedics and Trauma. *5th ed. Philadelphia: Elsevier; 2009.*)

pseudohypoparathyroidism is the *knuckle-knuckle-dimple-dimple sign* produced by shortening of the fourth and fifth metacarpals (Fig. 9.35). This is in contrast to Turner syndrome, in which there is a *knuckle-knuckle-dimple-knuckle sign.*

- **Hypovitaminosis D:** Lack of vitamin D leads to two different conditions, depending on whether the patient is a child or an adult. In children, it leads to **rickets** (Fig. 9.36), which causes **insufficient**

bone mineralization for the growing bones, leading to skeletal deformities, especially genu varum (bowing of the femurs). In adults, lack of vitamin D leads to **ineffective mineralization of new bone,** so bone remodeling does not occur properly. This causes osteoporosis and weakening of the bones.

REVIEW QUESTIONS

(1) A patient is found to have hypercalcemia and an elevated PTH. A diagnosis of primary hyperparathyroidism is made. The patient states that he has a family history of primary hyperparathyroidism, and his brothers also have had pituitary tumors. What genetic disease is he likely to have?
(2) What conditions are shared by patients with MEN IIa and MEN IIb? What is the distinguishing condition between them?
(3) A new hormone is discovered and found to be a steroid hormone. Where in the target cell is the receptor likely to be found?
(4) Which causes of hyperprolactinemia relate to: (a) increased pituitary stimulation for prolactin release, (b) decreased negative feedback, and (c) increased primary production of prolactin?
(5) What are the hormones of the anterior pituitary, and briefly what is their overarching function in the body?
(6) An infant is found to have a neck mass. If it were a thyroglossal duct cyst, would it be more likely to be found midline or lateral on the anterior neck? Why?
(7) True or false: Thyroglobulin is normally found in the bloodstream.
(8) If a combination of hyperthyroidism and proptosis is found, what is the most likely diagnosis? What is the pathophysiology of the hyperthyroidism and of the proptosis?
(9) What is the most common form of thyroid cancer? What are some histologic findings?
(10) From outside to inside, what are the layers of the adrenal cortex, and what hormones do they produce?
(11) Why do patients with Addison disease have hyperpigmentation? What would their potassium level likely be and why?
(12) Why is phenoxybenzamine used in treatment of pheochromocytoma? Why would phentolamine not be an acceptable substitute?
(13) Describe the process in which elevated blood glucose levels cause pancreatic insulin release. Bonus: Describe how the incretin pathway enhances this.
(14) Why do patients with absolute insulin deficiency develop diabetic ketoacidosis?
(15) Why do patients with absolute insulin deficiency have hyperkalemia? Give two reasons.
(16) What is the most likely diagnosis if: (a) both the calcium and PTH are high; (b) the calcium is high and the PTH is low, but the PTHrP is high; and (c) both the calcium and PTH are low?
(17) How does hypoalbuminemia change the total calcium and ionized calcium? What about acid-base disturbances?

10 GASTROENTEROLOGY

Thomas E. Blair

ANATOMY

Abdominal Wall: A surgeon cutting through the lateral abdominal wall would cut through anatomic structures in the following order: skin → superficial fascia (Camper and Scarpa fascia) → external oblique → internal oblique → transversus abdominis → transversalis fascia → extraperitoneal fascia → parietal peritoneum (Fig. 10.1).

Camper fascia is the fatty (subcutaneous tissue) layer of the superficial fascia directly under the skin.

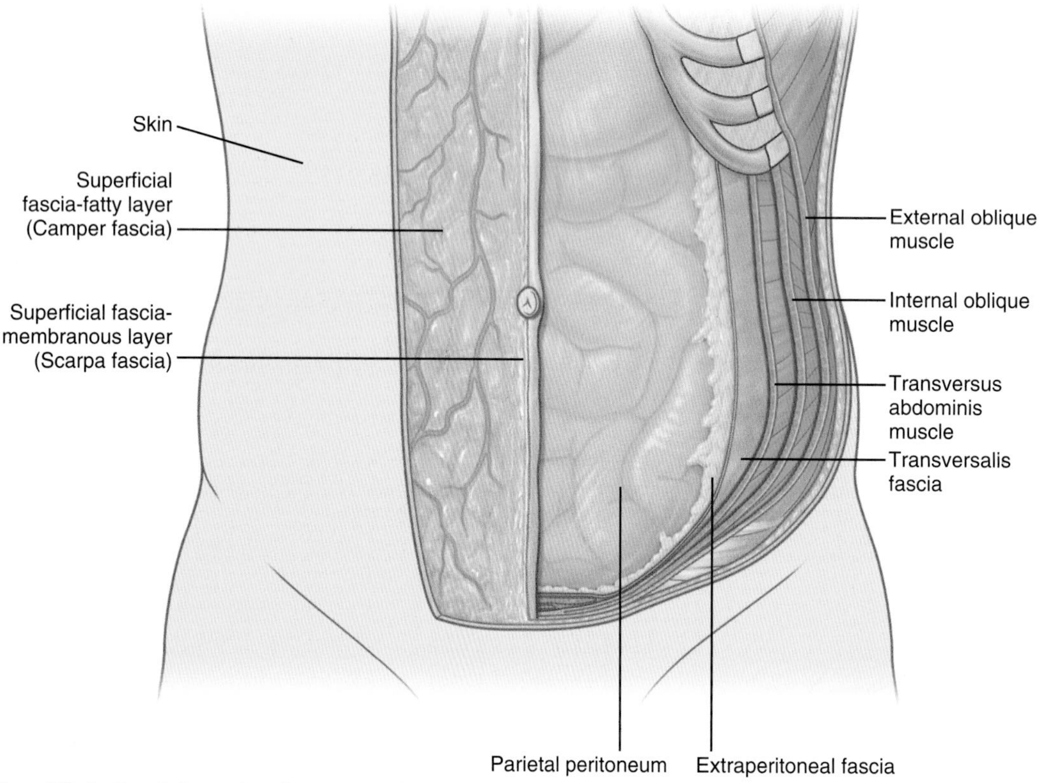

Fig. 10.1 The abdominal wall. (*From Drake RL, Vogl AW, Mitchell AWM.* Gray's Anatomy for Students. *2nd ed. Philadelphia: Elsevier; 2009.*)

The linea alba is the aponeuroses of the rectus sheaths.

A midline incision would cut through the skin → Camper fascia → Scarpa fascia → linea alba (aponeuroses of rectus sheaths) → transversalis fascia → extraperitoneal fascia → parietal peritoneum.

Gastrointestinal Tract: The upper gastrointestinal (GI) tract begins at the mouth and extends to the **ligament of Treitz** (actually not a ligament at all, but the suspensory muscle of the duodenum, which participates in GI motility). The lower GI tract includes everything distal to this point.

The ligament of Treitz separates the lower from the upper GI tract.

Of note, an **upper GI bleed** is a bleed proximal to the ligament of Treitz. It will usually present with hematemesis or melena (although it may present as hematochezia if very brisk). A lower GI bleed is distal to the ligament of Treitz and will usually present as hematochezia, although blood tends to be darker the more proximal the origin of the bleed. Overall, two-thirds of all GI bleeds are from an upper GI source.

Embryologic Divisions: The GI tract can also be divided embryologically into the foregut, midgut, and hindgut, which correspond best with the adult vascular supply. The **foregut consists of the pharynx to the first half of the duodenum** as well as the esophagus, stomach, liver, gallbladder, and pancreas. The vascular supply of the foregut comes from the **celiac trunk** (which gives rise to the **left gastric, common hepatic,** and **splenic arteries**; Figs. 10.2 and 10.3). Parasympathetic innervation comes from the **vagus nerve,** and sympathetic innervation comes from the **thoracic splanchnic nerves (T5–T11).**

The **midgut** includes the distal duodenum, jejunum, ileum, and proximal two-thirds of the transverse colon. The midgut is supplied by the **superior mesenteric artery** and, like the foregut, is innervated by the **vagus nerve and thoracic splanchnics (T11–T12).**

The **hindgut** consists of the distal transverse colon, descending colon, sigmoid colon, and rectum. It is supplied by the **inferior mesenteric artery** and has parasympathetic innervation by the **pelvic splanchnics (S2–S4)** and **sympathetic innervation from the lumbar splanchnics (L1–L2).**

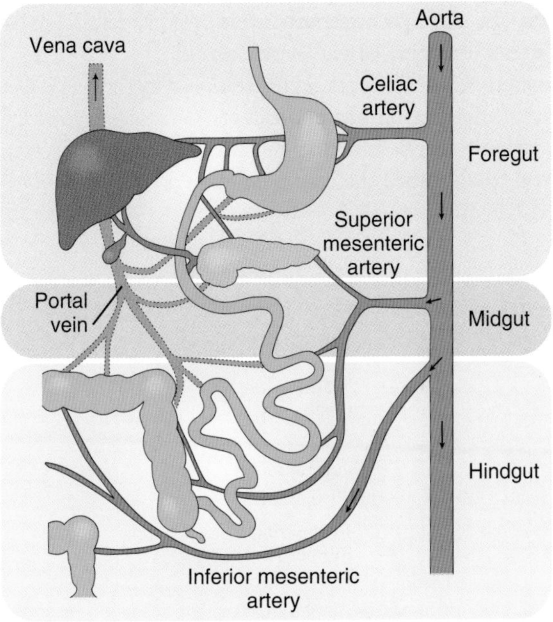

Fig. 10.2 Embryologic divisions of the GI tract. (*From Brown T. Rapid Review Physiology. 2nd ed. Philadelphia: Elsevier; 2011.*)

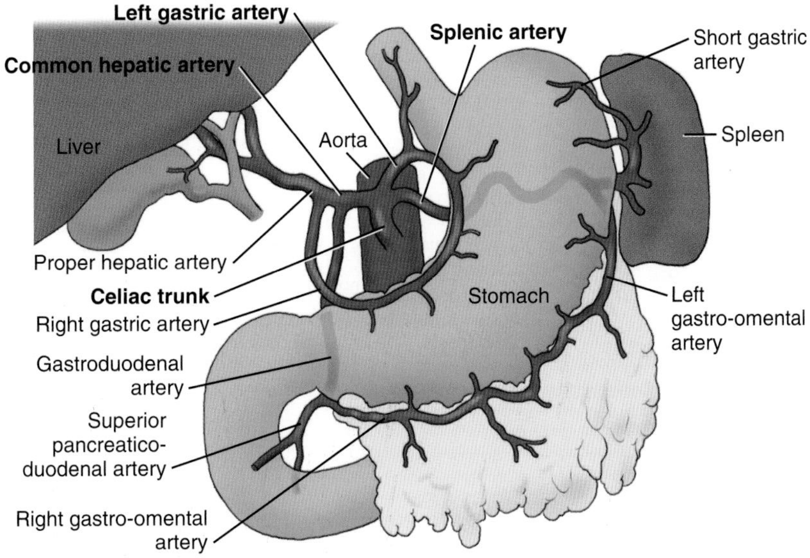

Fig. 10.3 Branches of the celiac trunk. (*From Morton DA, Albertine KH, Peterson KD. Gray's Dissection Guide for Human Anatomy. 2nd ed. Philadelphia: Elsevier; 2006.*)

The splenic flexure is considered a **watershed** area because it is perfused by the most distal branches of the superior mesenteric artery and inferior mesenteric artery. In times of hypoperfusion (e.g., septic shock) this area is the most susceptible to ischemia.

The entire GI tract has **venous drainage** that passes through the liver via the portal circulation, which allows the liver to participate in digestion. Clinically, portal drainage to the liver is relevant for first-pass metabolism of medications and explains why GI cancers tend to metastasize to the liver. The liver is so vascular that it is the most common organ to have metastases from other malignancies. Don't be fooled—a malignancy found in the liver is more likely to be of metastatic than primarily hepatic origin, especially if there are multiple lesions.

Retroperitoneum: The peritoneum is a membranous tissue that lines the abdominal viscera **(visceral peritoneum)** and abdominal wall **(parietal peritoneum).** Several abdominal structures, however, are situated behind the peritoneum (at least in part) and are thus retroperitoneal. These can be remembered with the mnemonic **SAD-PUCKER—S**uprarenal glands (adrenals), **A**orta and inferior vena cava (IVC), **D**uodenum (second through fourth parts), **P**ancreas, **U**reters, **C**olon (ascending and descending), **K**idney, **E**sophagus, and **R**ectum.

Portal Triad: The triad of hepatic artery, portal vein, and bile duct. Portal triads form the six points of a hexagon that make up the liver lobule (Fig. 10.4).

Hepatic Vasculature: Nutrient-rich blood from the GI tract enters the liver via the portal vein, whereas oxygen-rich blood enters the liver via the common hepatic artery (see Fig. 10.4). The blood passes through sinusoids lined by the basolateral surface of a single-layered sheets of hepatocytes (the apical surface faces bile canaliculi). The sinusoids are fenestrated, allowing easy transfer of the products of digestion into hepatocytes. The sinusoids drain into central veins, which empty into the hepatic veins and finally to the IVC. Note that blood drains **away** from the portal triad toward the central vein, whereas bile flows in the opposite direction **toward** the portal triad and bile ducts.

The portal system is responsible for the first-pass effect of medications.

In the portal triad, blood drains toward the central veins. Bile drains toward the bile ducts.

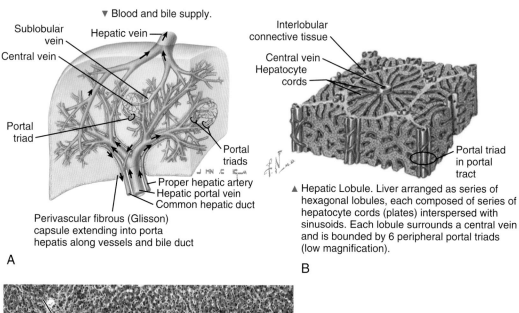

▼ Blood and bile supply.

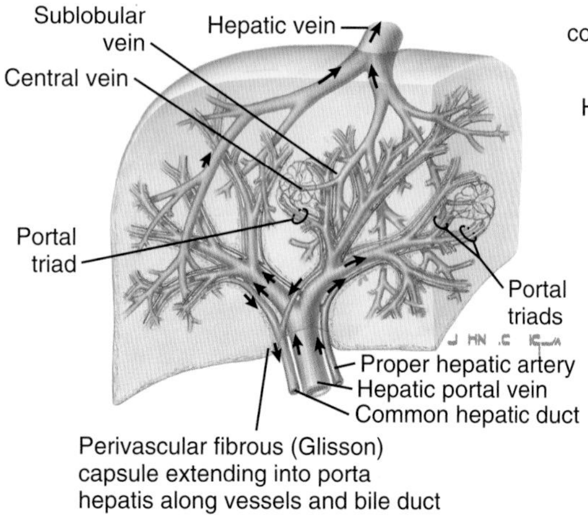

A

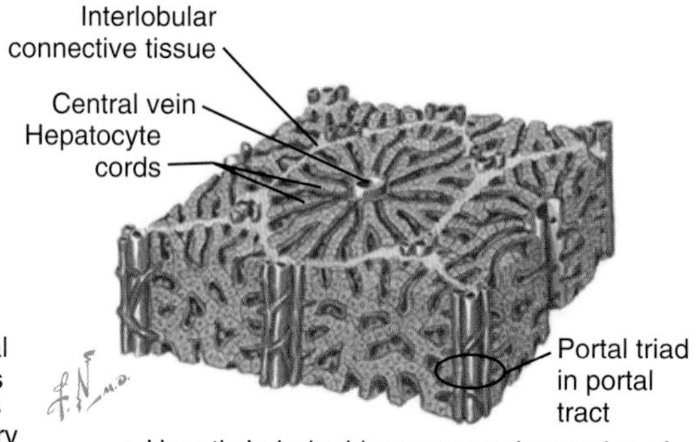

▲ Hepatic Lobule. Liver arranged as series of hexagonal lobules, each composed of series of hepatocyte cords (plates) interspersed with sinusoids. Each lobule surrounds a central vein and is bounded by 6 peripheral portal triads (low magnification).

B

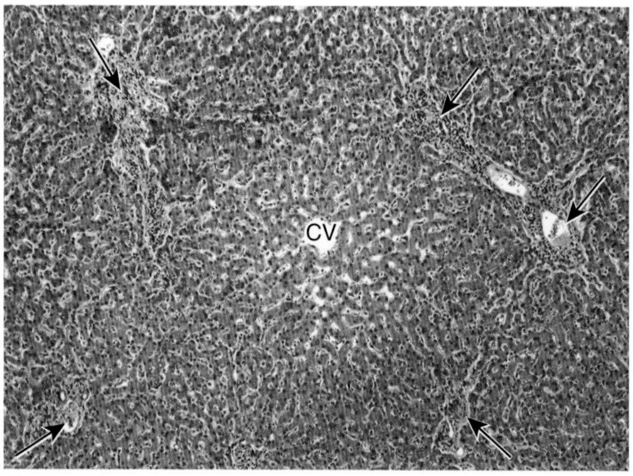

◀ Light micrograph (LM) of a hepatic lobule. It is polyhedral and has a central vein (CV) as its morphologic axis, with plates of hepatocytes radiating from the vein. Its boundaries are marked by portal areas (arrows) at its corners, various amounts of connective tissue, and portal triads. The lobule shows an interlocking mosaic pattern with other lobules. 75×. H&E.

C

Fig. 10.4 **A,** Hepatic vasculature. **B,** The portal triad and the hepatic lobule. **C,** Histologic view of the portal triad and hepatic lobule. 75xH&E, Hematoxylin and eosin. (*From Ovalle WK, Nahirney PC.* Netter's Essential Histology. *Philadelphia: Elsevier; 2007.*)

Biliary Tree and Bile Formation: Bile is created by the hepatocytic breakdown of cholesterol (the primary method of eliminating cholesterol from the body). Bile is secreted from the apical surface of hepatocytes and travels via bile canaliculi into bile ductules. Bile ductules lead to the **left and right hepatic ducts,** which combine to form the **common hepatic duct.** The **cystic duct exits the gallbladder** and joins the common hepatic duct to form the **common bile duct** (CBD). The CBD and pancreatic duct empty into the second part of the duodenum via the **ampulla of Vater, which leads to the major duodenal papilla.** The **sphincter of Oddi** controls the flow of bile and pancreatic enzymes into the duodenum (Fig. 10.5).

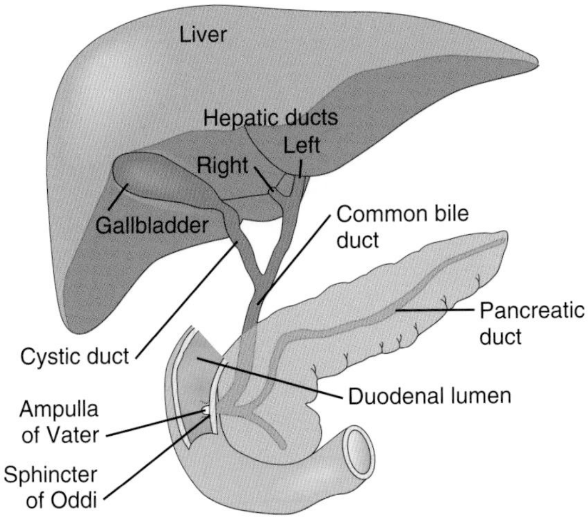

FIG. 10.5 Anatomy of the biliary tree. (*From Brown T. Rapid Review Physiology. 2nd ed. Philadelphia: Elsevier; 2011.*)

When reviewing the biliary pathology section later, consider the clinical importance of each step in the flow of bile. For example, primary biliary cholangitis (PBC) is caused by the destruction of canaliculi, and primary sclerosing cholangitis (PSC) is caused by the destruction of the intra- and extrahepatic bile ducts. Cholecystitis usually results from obstruction of the gallbladder neck or cystic duct. *Choledocholithiasis* refers to a gallstone lodged in the common bile duct. Cholangitis is usually caused by obstruction of the common bile duct (by choledocholithiasis or other means). Obstruction of the pancreatic duct is one cause of pancreatitis.

- Of clinical importance, the liver uses cholesterol to produce bile acids. Statins are a class of medications that interfere with hepatic synthesis of cholesterol by inhibiting **HMG-CoA reductase** (3-hydroxy-3-methyl-glutaryl-CoA reductase). The conversion of **HMG-CoA to mevalonic acid** is the first committed step in the hepatic synthesis of cholesterol (Fig. 10.6). Inhibition of this step causes hepatocytes to absorb cholesterol from the circulation by increasing hepatocyte low-density lipoprotein (LDL) receptors. Decreased synthesis of cholesterol and increased hepatic uptake of serum cholesterol leads to a reduction of serum LDL.

Statins block HMG-CoA reductase and prevent the hepatic synthesis of cholesterol.

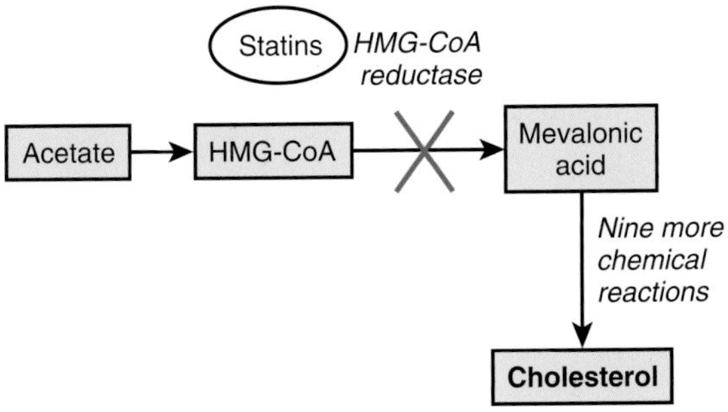

FIG. 10.6 Statins interfere with the hepatic synthesis of cholesterol. (*From Kester M, Karpa KD, Quraishi S, Vrana KE. Elsevier's Integrated Pharmacology. Philadelphia: Elsevier; 2007.*)

Digestive Tract Anatomy

The gut wall is composed of mucosa, submucosa, muscularis propria, and serosa (Fig. 10.7).

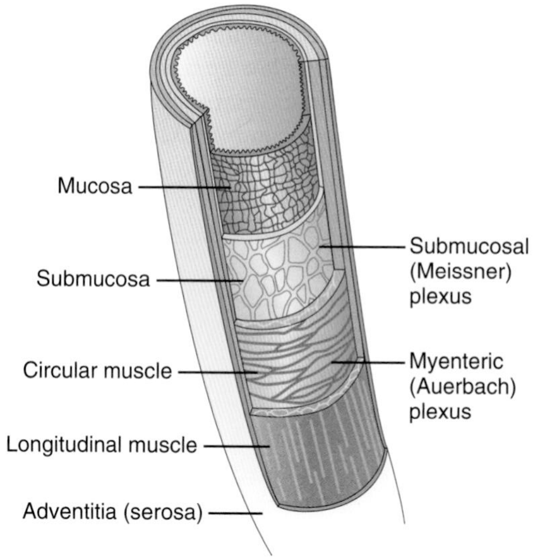

Fig. 10.7 Layers of the gut wall. (*From Brown T.* Rapid Review Physiology. *2nd ed. Philadelphia: Elsevier; 2011.*)

Mucosa: The innermost layer of the GI tract. It consists of the epithelial layer, lamina propria, and muscularis mucosa. Invaginations (e.g., villi at the small intestine) increase the surface area of the **epithelial layer,** which is involved primarily in absorption and secretion. The **lamina propria** contains supportive structures, and the **muscularis mucosa** shapes the underlying epithelium.

Submucosa: Connective tissue that supports the mucosa. Notably, it contains the **submucosal plexus** (Meissner plexus), which innervates the muscularis mucosa and aids in GI motility.

Muscularis propria: Consists of an inner circular muscle and outer longitudinal muscle, which act together to perform **peristalsis.** The **myenteric plexus** (Auerbach plexus) innervates these muscles.

Serosa: Supportive tissue that contains vasculature and lymphatics.

PHYSIOLOGY

Gastric Histology

Fig. 10.8 shows the histologic and anatomic regions of the stomach.

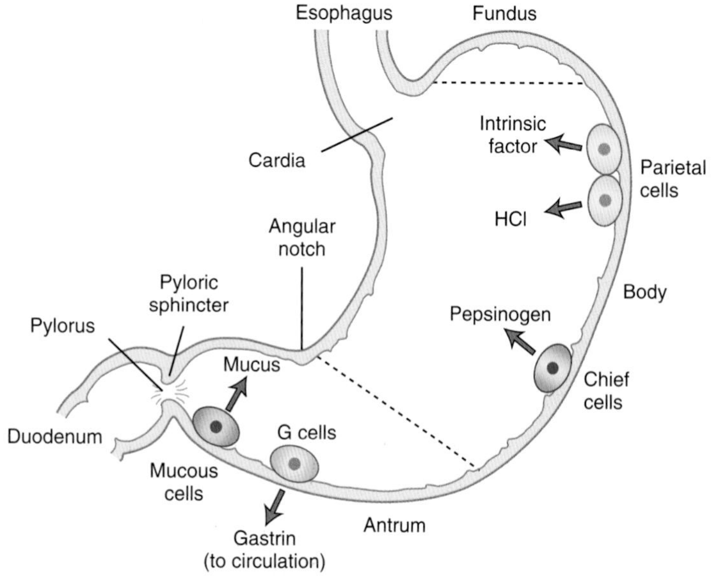

Cell Type	Location	Secretion
Parietal cells	Body	HCl Intrinsic factor
Chief cells	Body	Pepsinogen
G cells	Antrum	Gastrin
Mucous cells	Antrum	Mucus Pepsinogen

Fig. 10.8 Histologic and anatomic regions of the stomach. HCl, Hydrochloric acid. (*From Costanzo LS.* Physiology. *4th ed. New York: Elsevier; 2009.*)

Parietal Cells: Located in the body and fundus of the stomach. These secrete $\mathbf{H^+}$ ions via H^+/K^+-ATPase to lower gastric pH and also secrete **intrinsic factor,** which binds to vitamin B_{12} and facilitates vitamin B_{12} absorption in the terminal ileum. The H^+/K^+-ATPase on parietal cells is the target of proton pump inhibitors (PPIs).

Chief Cells: Secrete pepsinogen (proenzyme for protein digestion active only when the pH is <6). Chief cells also secrete gastric lipase, which plays a small role in lipid digestion.

G Cells: Located in the antrum. These cells secrete gastrin to increase gastric motility and stimulate parietal cells secretion of H^+.

Mucous Cells: Located in the cardia and antrum of the stomach. They secrete mucus (containing HCO_3^-) for epithelial protection.

Parietal cells create the low **pH** of the stomach using a H^+/K^+-ATPase.

Histology of the Intestine

Villi: Fingerlike projections into the intestinal lumen, which increase the surface area for digestion.

Intestinal Crypts: Lying between villi, crypts contain stem cells that replace sloughed enterocytes and secrete digestive enzymes.

Enterocytes: Intestinal columnar epithelial cells. Their apical surface contains a brush border of microvilli, which greatly increases the intestinal surface area and participates in the digestion and absorption of nutrients.

Enteroendocrine Cells: Specialized cells located in the gastrointestinal tract and pancreas involved in the secretion of gastrointestinal hormones (see later) and peptides essential for gastrointestinal regulation and function.

Goblet Cells: These cells lie on intestinal villi and produce a protective and lubricating mucus. The more distal in the small intestine, the more goblet cells are present.

Paneth Cells: Located in intestinal crypts below stem cells, these cells exocytose enzymes that destroy GI microorganisms and participate in the innate immunity of the small intestine.

Duodenal (Brunner) Glands: Submucosal glands of the upper duodenum that secrete bicarbonate and pepsinogen to neutralize gastric acid and facilitate digestion, respectively.

Peyer Patches: Lymph nodules in the lamina propria and submucosa of the ileum. This histologic feature helps **distinguish ileum from jejunum.** They participate in the adaptive immune function of the gut. It is logical that these lymphoid follicles are in the ileum because it is closest to the bacteria-rich colon. Clinically, hypertrophy of Peyer patches has been associated with intussusception (see later).

Colonocytes: Simple columnar epithelial cells of the colon specialized in absorbing water. These are the precursor cells for colon cancer.

Gastrin prepares for the gastric phase of digestion, whereas secretin prepares for the intestinal phase. Somatostatin is inhibitory.

Gastrointestinal Hormones

Gastrin: Prepares for the gastric phase of digestion (Table 10.1). Secreted by antral G cells, gastrin increases gastric motility and parietal cell activity (secretion of intrinsic factor and H^+ ions). Serum levels will be extremely high in patients with a gastrinoma (Zollinger-Ellison syndrome) or if the patient is on a PPI, which raises gastric pH and initiates a feedback loop.

Cholecystokinin (CCK): Greek for "gallbladder move." CCK stimulates gallbladder contraction, relaxation of the sphincter of Oddi, and pancreatic enzyme secretion. Release is stimulated by fatty acids in the GI tract. CCK is secreted by I cells of the duodenum and jejunum. Clinically this hormone is responsible for pain after fatty meals if cholelithiasis is present because it causes the gallbladder to contract against a blocked cystic duct (biliary colic).

Secretin: Prepares for the intestinal phase of digestion by stimulating **secretions** from the pancreas and gallbladder while inhibiting gastric secretions including gastrin and gastric H^+. Like CCK, it is secreted in the duodenum (by S cells). Unlike CCK, secretin tends to stimulate pancreatic bicarbonate secretion, whereas CCK stimulates pancreatic enzyme secretion.

Somatostatin: Acts as the "brakes" of the GI and endocrine systems. Somatostatin decreases the secretion of gastric acid, GI motility, and gallbladder motility. Hormonally, it inhibits insulin, glucagon, thyroid-stimulating hormone, and growth hormone release. It also is a splanchnic vasoconstrictor. **D** cells in the duodenum and pancreas control its secretion.

Glucose-Dependent Insulinotropic Peptide (GIP): As the name suggests, this hormone, GIP, increases pancreatic beta cell release of insulin in response to an oral glucose load. Clinically this means

Table 10.1 Gastrointestinal Hormones

HORMONE	SITE OF SECRETION	STIMULI FOR SECRETION	ACTIONS	COMMENT
Gastrin	Antral G cells	Amino acids, peptides Stomach distention	↑ Parietal cell action ↑ Motility	Elevated in gastrinoma and patients on PPIs. Prepares for gastric phase
Cholecystokinin (CCK)	I cells of duodenum and jejunum	Fatty acids	↑ Gallbladder contraction Relax sphincter of Oddi ↑ Pancreatic enzyme secretion	Worsens pain of cholelithiasis
Secretin	S cells of duodenum	H^+ and fatty acids in duodenum	↑ Pancreatic bicarbonate secretion ↑ Bile secretion ↓Gastrin ↓Gastric H^+ secretion	Prepares for intestinal phase of digestion
Somatostatin	Pancreatic delta cells	Meals (fat, protein, and carbohydrates)	↓GI secretion ↓GI hormones ↓GI motility ↓GH, TSH Splanchnic vasoconstrictor	Brakes of the GI and endocrine systems Octreotide—synthetic somatostatin
Glucose-dependent insulinotropic peptide (GIP)	K cells of duodenum and jejunum	Oral glucose	↑ Insulin release	Oral glucose used faster than IV glucose
Vasoactive intestinal peptide (VIP)	GI mucosal neurons	Vagal parasympathetics	↑ Intestinal and pancreatic secretion of fluids and electrolytes	VIPomas cause profuse watery diarrhea, facial flushing MEN I association
Motilin	Duodenum	Fasting	↑ Migrating myoelectric complexes	So-called housekeeper of gut Causes borborygmi
Ghrelin	P/D1 cells of the fundus	Fasting	Acts on hypothalamus to stimulate hunger	Increased in Prader-Willi syndrome Decreased after Roux-en-Y
Leptin	Adipose tissue	Increased with adipose tissue stores (no short- term increase during feeding)	Acts on hypothalamus to inhibit hunger	Obesity may be related to leptin resistance

GH, growth hormone; MEN, multiple endocrine neoplasia; PPI, proton pump inhibitor; TSH, thyroid-stimulating hormone.

that insulin levels rise more rapidly after an oral glucose load compared with an intravenous glucose load. **K** cells of the small intestine secrete GIP.

Vasoactive Intestinal Peptide (VIP): VIP is released from neurons within the GI mucosa. It increases the intestinal and pancreatic secretion of fluids and electrolytes. It also causes relaxation of smooth muscle. Clinically a VIPoma (often of the pancreas) causes profuse watery diarrhea and facial flushing secondary to fluid secretion and vasodilation, respectively. VIPomas are associated with multiple endocrine neoplasia type I (MEN I syndrome; see Chapter 9).

Motilin: During periods of fasting, the upper duodenum secretes motilin to initiate migrating myoelectric complexes, improving peristalsis. The resulting muscular contractions push indigestible substances (e.g., fiber) through the digestive tract. Motilin functions as a sort of housekeeper of the gut by making room for subsequent meals. Clinically this hormone is responsible for the rumbling sounds (borborygmi) created by the GI tract when fasting.

Ghrelin: During periods of fasting, P/D1 cells of the fundus secrete ghrelin. Ghrelin is thought to act predominantly on the hypothalamus, and it contributes to the sensation of hunger. Not surprisingly, it is found at elevated levels before meals and is decreased after feeding. Clinically, high levels of ghrelin contribute to the insatiable appetite of patients with Prader-Willi syndrome (partial deletion of chromosome 15). Conversely, bariatric surgeries that remove the fundus or exclude it from digestion (e.g., Roux-en-Y surgery) lead to lower levels of circulating ghrelin and contribute to weight loss.

Mnemonic: When hungry, your stomach **growls** because of **ghrelin.**

Leptin: The counterpart of ghrelin, leptin acts on the hypothalamus to inhibit hunger. It is produced in adipose tissue.

Saliva

The parotid, submandibular, and sublingual glands secrete saliva. Saliva provides mechanical lubrication to facilitate swallowing of food boluses. Furthermore, it contains α-amylase and lingual lipase, which initiate digestion of carbohydrates and lipids, respectively. Saliva also contains HCO_3^-, which helps neutralize refluxed gastric contents and inhibits bacterial growth within the mouth. Clinically, patients with Sjögren syndrome produce less saliva and as a result are prone to dental caries. They may also suffer complications of gastroesophageal reflux disease because of decreased salivary buffering activity. Saliva production is stimulated by both **parasympathetic and sympathetic** activity, although the parasympathetic system is dominant. Increased salivation is a symptom of excessive cholinergic activity or acetylcholinesterase inhibition.

DIGESTION AND ABSORPTION

Digestion is the process whereby ingested food is broken down into constituent parts capable of being absorbed. The mechanical activity of chewing and movement of food boluses through the GI tract contribute to the process of digestion, but the major activity takes place at the molecular level.

Carbohydrates: Consist of polysaccharides, disaccharides (including lactose and sucrose), and monosaccharides **(glucose, galactose, and fructose).** Only monosaccharides are capable of being absorbed by the small intestine. Carbohydrate digestion begins with α-amylase in the saliva, which is quickly inactivated in the acidic gastric environment. Once in the duodenum, however, pancreatic amylase continues the process and catalyzes the glycosidic bonds (specifically $\alpha[1-4]$ linkages) in carbohydrates to break down polysaccharides into disaccharides. Intestinal brush border enzymes (lactase, sucrase, and maltase) finish the conversion of disaccharides into monosaccharides. Glucose and galactose are absorbed in the small intestine via secondary active transport (Na^+ cotransport, SGLT-1), whereas fructose is absorbed down its concentration gradient using a transport protein (facilitated diffusion, GLUT-5). All three monosaccharides are absorbed by GLUT-2.

Of clinical importance, lactose intolerance is a disaccharidase deficiency caused by a relative lack of brush border lactase. Undigested lactose remains in the intestinal lumen, resulting in osmotic diarrhea along with symptoms of cramping and bloating because of fermentation by colonic bacteria. An analogous osmotic diarrhea may occur in patients ingesting large amounts of sorbitol (a sweetener often found in sugar-free gum or candy). This monosaccharide is very slowly absorbed and in excess can cause an osmotic diarrhea by drawing water into the lumen.

> Lactose intolerance is a disaccharidase deficiency that causes an osmotic diarrhea.

Dietary lipids: Consist of **cholesterol, triglycerides,** and **phospholipids.** Digestion begins with lingual lipase and gastric lipase hydrolyzing triglycerides into free fatty acids and glycerol. This phase is only responsible, however, for a small fraction of lipid digestion. Once in the duodenum, bile salts emulsify the lipids into **micelles,** hydrophobic products of lipid digestion surrounded by the amphiphilic bile salts. This structure greatly increases their surface area for digestion by pancreatic lipase. When micelles approach the brush border, their lipid contents are absorbed into enterocytes and repackaged as chylomicrons. Chylomicrons then distribute lipids to the rest of the body. Bile salts, on the other hand, remain in the intestinal lumen until they are resorbed in the ileum and recycled via the enterohepatic circulation.

Protein: Protein digestion begins in the stomach with **chief cell** secretion of **pepsinogen,** which is converted to **pepsin** in the acidic environment. Pepsin initiates protein digestion by hydrolyzing internal peptide bonds. However, pancreatic HCO_3^- inactivates pepsin in the duodenum and pancreatic **trypsinogen** takes over. This enzyme is converted to its active form **(trypsin)** by the action of brush border enterokinases. Trypsin not only hydrolyzes peptide bonds but also catalyzes other pancreatic proteases to become active. The end result is protein breakdown into tripeptides and amino acids, which are absorbed via Na^+ or H^+ cotransporters. Clinically, protein malnutrition contributes to poor wound healing. **Kwashiorkor** refers to severe protein-energy malnutrition despite sufficient caloric intake. The lack of protein causes decreased osmotic pressure in blood vessels, resulting in generalized edema (called **anasarca**). Kwashiorkor can be distinguished from **marasmus** (starvation resulting from inadequate intake of all nutrients), a condition characterized by more severe muscle wasting and emaciation without associated edema (Fig. 10.9).

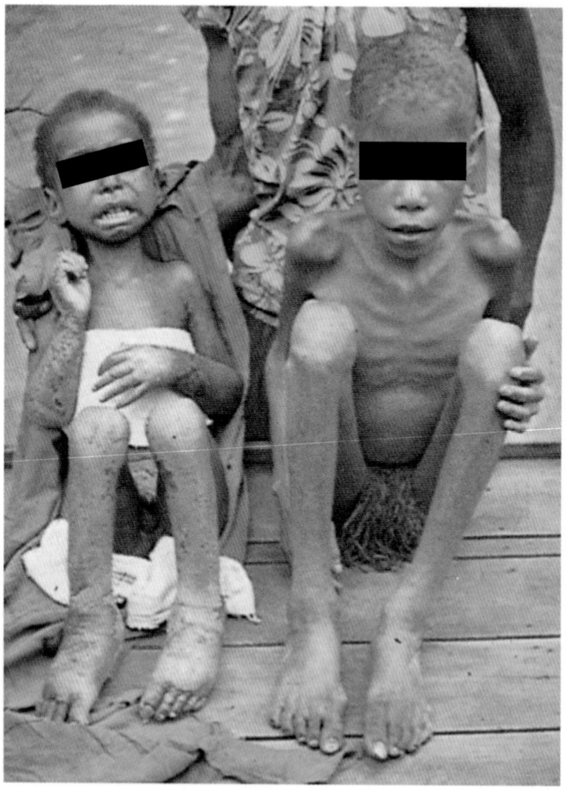

Fig. 10.9 *Left,* Boy with pitting edema of kwashiorkor. *Right,* Boy with emaciation from marasmus. (*From Forbes C, Jackson W.* Color Atlas and Text of Clinical Medicine. *2nd ed. St. Louis, Mosby; 2003:343.*)

PATHOLOGY

Esophageal Pathology

Gastroesophageal Reflux Disease (GERD): GERD is inappropriate relaxation of the lower esophageal sphincter (LES) allowing retrograde flow of gastric contents into the esophagus, causing burning retrosternal pain (especially after meals or when laying flat). It also may present as hoarseness, sour taste in the mouth (water brash), worsening asthma, or chronic cough. Diagnosis is made clinically, but attention must be paid to red flag symptoms such as dysphagia (difficulty swallowing), odynophagia (painful swallowing), and weight loss. If these symptoms are present, additional testing (endoscopy, barium swallow) should be performed to rule out complications such as esophagitis, stenosis, stricture, esophageal mucosal webs, Barrett esophagus, and adenocarcinoma. Treatment of GERD involves diet modification (avoidance of caffeine, alcohol, and spicy foods), H2 blockers, or PPIs. Nissen fundoplication, a surgical procedure in which the gastric fundus is wrapped around the lower esophagus to increase pressure at the lower esophageal sphincter, can be performed in refractory cases.

- **Esophageal stricture:** Chronic gastric acid exposure results in scarring of the esophagus, eventually narrowing the lumen. Dysphagia is the predominant symptom because food has difficulty passing the stricture. Strictures are also a complication of chemical esophagitis from acid or alkali ingestion.
- **Barrett esophagus:** Chronic gastric acid exposure causes intestinal (columnar) metaplasia in place of the normal stratified squamous epithelium at the distal esophagus. This histologic finding predisposes patients to adenocarcinoma. Of note, gastric metaplasia may also occur but is not associated with adenocarcinoma.

Intestinal metaplasia of the esophagus is a risk for cancer. Gastric metaplasia is not.

Hiatal Hernias: A **sliding hiatal hernia** occurs when the gastroesophageal junction (GEJ) herniates through the esophageal hiatus (Fig. 10.10B). The diaphragm is no longer able to contribute to the GEJ pressure gradient, thereby predisposing the patient to GERD; most hiatal hernias, however, are asymptomatic. A **paraesophageal hiatal hernia** occurs when the gastric fundus herniates through the esophageal hiatus (Fig. 10.10C). Because the GEJ is not affected, this anatomic arrangement does not lead to GERD but does put patients at risk for incarceration and strangulation of the fundus. Fortunately, paraesophageal hernias are much less common than the more benign sliding hernias.

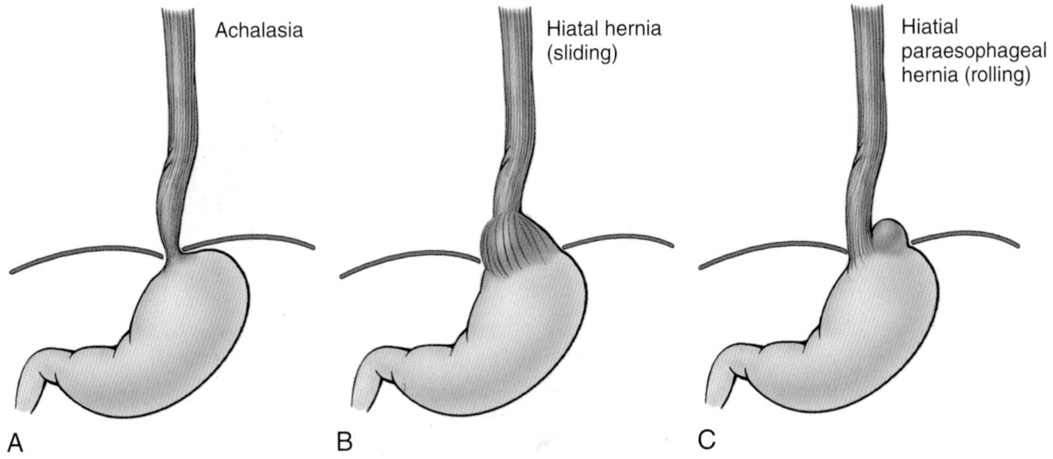

FIG. 10.10 **A,** Achalasia. **B,** Sliding hiatal hernia. **C,** Paraesophageal hiatal hernia. (*From Kumar V, Abbas AK, Fausto N, Mitchell R.* Robbins Basic Pathology. *8th ed. Philadelphia: Elsevier; 2007.*)

Achalasia: A dysfunction of the esophageal myenteric plexus causing increased LES tone and impaired esophageal peristalsis. The failure of LES relaxation leads to food accumulation proximal to the lesion and subsequent dilation of the esophagus. This combination of pathologic conditions results in the bird's beak appearance of achalasia on a barium swallow study (Figs. 10-10A and 10-11). Symptoms include dysphagia, odynophagia, halitosis (bad breath), and regurgitation. Although usually

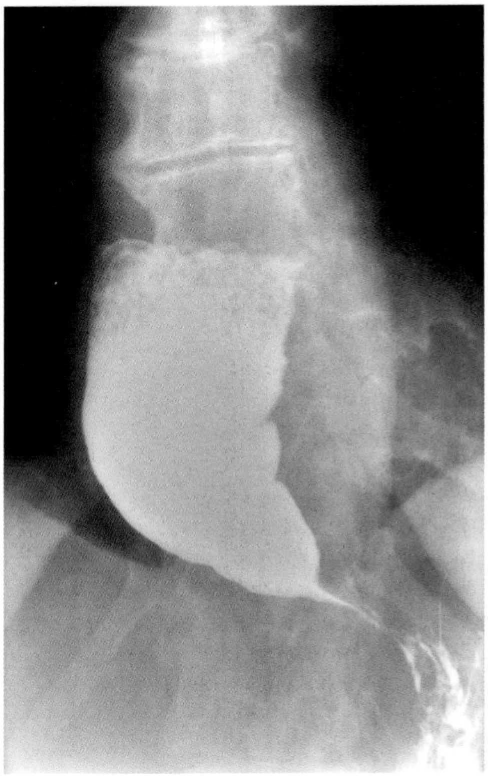

FIG. 10.11 Radiograph of barium swallow demonstrating bird's beak appearance of achalasia. (*From Townsend CM, Beauchamp RD, Evers MB, Mattox K.* Sabiston Textbook of Surgery. *17th ed. Philadelphia: WB Saunders; 2004.*)

idiopathic, Chagas disease, caused by *Trypanosoma cruzi,* causes damage to the myenteric plexus resulting in achalasia. *T. cruzi* can also causes megacolon by the same mechanism (destruction of the colonic myenteric plexus). Endoscopic pneumatic dilation of the LES is a common treatment modality for achalasia. Botulinum toxin can also be injected into the LES to induce relaxation.

Mallory-Weiss Tear: Partial-thickness esophageal laceration caused by forceful retching (e.g., after alcohol consumption, bulimia, food poisoning), which presents as painful, blood-streaked emesis. No treatment is necessary in most cases. This is differentiated from Boerhaave syndrome, which is a serious full-thickness defect in the esophagus that often leads to pneumomediastinum.

Esophageal Perforation: Often caused by forceful vomiting (Boerhaave syndrome) or instrumentation (endoscopy). This life-threatening condition presents as severe chest pain and painful swallowing. Physical examination may reveal crepitus from subcutaneous air (subcutaneous emphysema), and chest x-ray examination may reveal a widened mediastinum or air in the mediastinum (pneumomediastinum). A pleural effusion may also be present because of irritation from the luminal contents. Diagnosis is made with water-soluble contrast esophagraphy. Barium contrast, which will damage and inflame thoracic structures outside the GI tract, should be avoided. Computed tomography (CT) may also be confirmatory.

Esophagitis: Inflammation of the esophageal mucosa. It is most often caused by GERD where acid reflux overwhelms the protective ability of the submucosal glands' mucin and bicarbonate secretions. Pill esophagitis is caused by certain medications becoming lodged in the esophagus (e.g., antibiotics, nonsteroidal antiinflammatory drugs [NSAIDs], bisphosphonates, iron, and potassium chloride). In patients with AIDS or immunosuppression, consider infectious causes such as cytomegalovirus, *Candida,* or herpes simplex virus. Chemical esophagitis occurs after accidental or intentional ingestion of caustic materials such as household cleaners leading to coagulation necrosis (acids) or more severe liquefactive necrosis (alkalis). In all cases endoscopy is diagnostic.

Eosinophilic Esophagitis: Eosinophilic inflammation of the esophagus associated with other atopic conditions (food allergies, asthma, dermatitis, etc.). Symptoms are similar to GERD and include dysphagia and pain, although patients will not respond to antacids. Treatment is with allergen avoidance and steroids.

Zenker Diverticulum: Esophageal diverticulum above the esophageal sphincter at Killian triangle, the region between the cricopharyngeus and the lower inferior constrictor muscles. During swallowing it may trap food causing regurgitation, dysphagia, and halitosis (from trapped rotting food; Fig. 10.12).

Plummer-Vinson Syndrome: Iron deficiency anemia leading to formation of esophageal webs (causing dysphagia) and glossitis (smooth, shiny, inflamed tongue; Fig. 10.13). It is unclear exactly

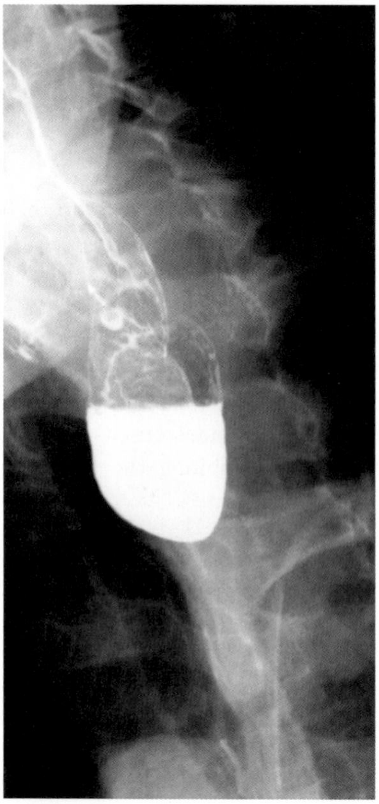

FIG. 10.12 Barium swallow demonstrating Zenker diverticulum. (*From McNally P. GI/Liver Secrets. 3rd ed. Philadelphia: Elsevier; 2009.*)

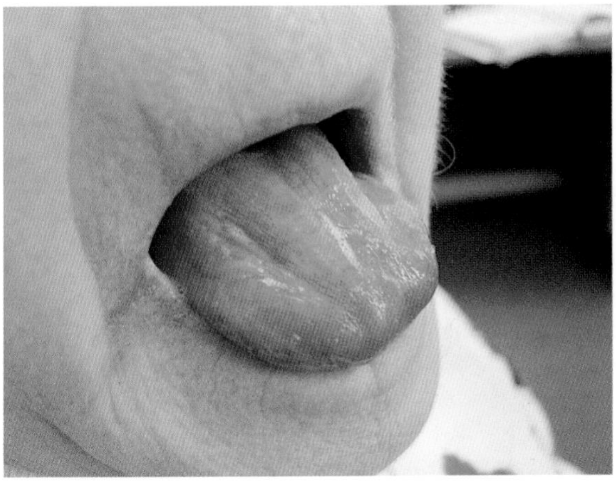

FIG. 10.13 Glossitis. (*From Douglas G, Nicol F, Robertson C. Macleod's Clinical Examination. 11th ed. Philadelphia: Elsevier; 2005.*)

why iron deficiency produces this condition in some patients, but most symptoms respond to iron supplementation. Esophageal webs can also be treated endoscopically.

Esophageal Carcinoma: Presents as progressive dysphagia and odynophagia beginning with bulky foods (e.g., steak), but progressing to liquids. These symptoms contribute to weight loss. It is diagnosed by endoscopy.

- **Squamous cell carcinoma:** More likely secondary to tobacco and alcohol use. Involves the upper two-thirds of the esophagus.
- **Adenocarcinoma:** Often secondary to Barrett esophagus from GERD. Involves the lower third of the esophagus.

Gastric and Duodenal Pathology

Gastritis: Gastric inflammation and associated mucosal injury found on biopsy. However, overall *gastritis* is a term that is not well defined and has several classification systems. A distinction is often made between acute and chronic gastritis. Histopathologically, acute gastritis is neutrophil predominant, whereas chronic gastritis demonstrates a mixture of mononuclear cells. Causes of gastritis include *Helicobacter pylori* infection, alcohol, NSAIDs, and autoimmune conditions.

Of note, **pernicious anemia** is characterized by antiintrinsic factor antibodies and antiparietal cell antibodies. The result is a chronic atrophic gastritis and loss of intrinsic factor, leading to vitamin B_{12} (cobalamin) deficiency and megaloblastic anemia.

Pernicious anemia: Parietal cell loss causes loss of intrinsic factor and therefore inability to absorb vitamin B_{12}, resulting in megaloblastic anemia.

Peptic Ulcer Disease: Erosions of gastric mucosa associated with gnawing, aching, burning epigastric abdominal pain. Ulcers are most commonly caused by *H. pylori* infection or heavy NSAID use. Physiologic stress can also contribute to ulcer formation.

- ***H. pylori:*** Patients with active *H. pylori* infection will have positive stool antigen and urease breath test. The urease breath test involves a patient consuming radiolabeled urea. In the presence of urease from *H. pylori,* the urea will be broken down into CO_2 and ammonia. The radiolabeled CO_2 can then be detected on exhalation. Physiologically, *H. pylori* uses urease to neutralize gastric acid with ammonia and create a more hospitable environment. *H. pylori* serum serology studies indicate only that infection was present at one time but are often used in diagnosis in the appropriate clinical setting (i.e., classic symptoms). Endoscopy, however, remains the gold standard.
- **NSAIDs:** Cause ulcers by inhibiting the production of protective prostaglandins. In general, NSAIDs inhibit cyclooxygenase-1 (COX-1) and COX-2. Because COX-1 is more responsible for the production of protective prostaglandin E2 (PGE_2) in the stomach, selective **COX-2 inhibitors** such as celecoxib are somewhat less likely to contribute to gastritis or ulcer formation.
- **Physiologic stress:** Patients who are critically ill from any cause (trauma, infection, surgery, etc.) may develop gastric ulcers that are caused by inadequate tissue perfusion as a result of splanchnic vasoconstriction and/or systemic hypotension.
  - **Curling ulcers:** Stress ulcers associated with severe trauma/burns caused by systemic hypovolemia, hypotension, and hypoperfusion.

- **Cushing ulcers:** Stress ulcers associated with brain lesions. Elevated intracranial pressure, from tumors or traumatic bleeding, increases vagal stimulation of gastric parietal cells and H^+ secretion.

Complications of peptic ulcers include perforation and bleeding. Malignancies also tend to ulcerate, so one should biopsy ulcers during endoscopy to rule out cancer.

- **Perforation:** Perforation of an abdominal viscus (e.g., perforated peptic ulcers) classically presents as acute-onset abdominal pain and peritonitis. An upright radiograph may reveal free air under the diaphragm (pneumoperitoneum; Fig. 10.14). Emergent surgical consultation is essential.
- **Bleeding ulcer:** If the ulcer overlies a vein or artery (e.g., gastroduodenal or gastric artery), brisk bleeding may occur. Patients with bleeding ulcers most often present with melena, although brisk or large-volume bleeding can result in hematemesis and even hematochezia.

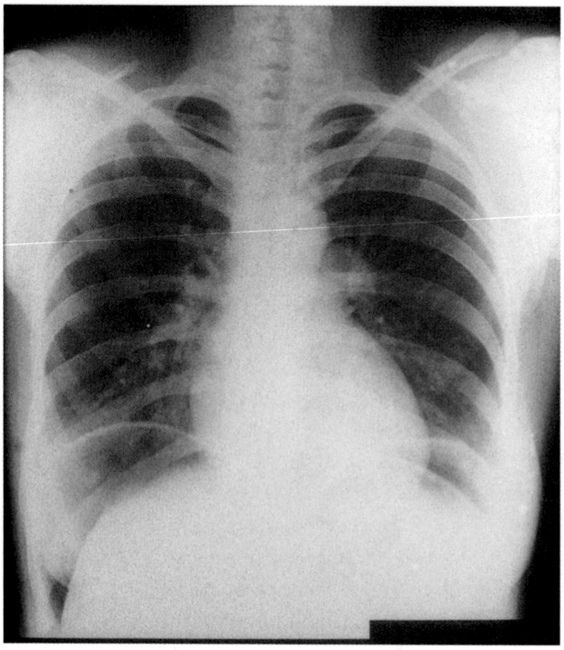

FIG. 10.14 Perforated viscus causing air under the diaphragm on chest radiograph. (*From Lim EKS.* Medicine and Surgery. *Philadelphia: Elsevier; 2007.*)

Zollinger-Ellison Syndrome (ZES): A **gastrinoma** (gastrin-secreting tumor) of the pancreas or small intestine leads to **marked hyperplasia of parietal cells** causing increased H^+ secretion. Symptoms include diarrhea and **multiple recurrent or refractory duodenal ulcers.** Testing reveals **markedly elevated gastrin levels** and a **positive secretin test** (gastrin levels stay elevated even after secretin infusion) ZES should be considered in patients with recurrent or refractory ulcers and in patients with **MEN I syndrome.**

Carcinoid Syndrome: A rare syndrome caused by the release of hormones and products (serotonin, histamine, and others) by neuroendocrine (carcinoid) tumors, most of which originate in the small intestine. Classically the syndrome results in diffuse cutaneous flushing, diarrhea, and right-sided valvular pathologic conditions. Symptoms tend to emerge in the setting of metastatic disease because the first-pass effect of the liver metabolizes serotonin to 5-hydroxyindoleacetic acid (5-HIAA), preventing systemic signs of the disease. Diagnosis can be made with 24-hour collection of urinary 5-HIAA. Must be differentiated from a VIPoma, which also presents with diarrhea and flushing.

Ménétrier Disease (Hypoproteinemic Hypertrophic Gastropathy): Increased levels of transforming growth factor α (TGF-α) cause extreme hypertrophy of gastric rugae. Symptoms include pain, weight loss, and **protein-losing gastroenteropathy** (increased gastric mucosal permeability leads to protein [albumin] loss and subsequent edema from loss of osmotic pressure). Biopsy is diagnostic and reveals mucous cell hyperplasia and gland atrophy.

Because gastric cancers tend to ulcerate, gastric ulcers should be biopsied to exclude cancer.

For a patient with obstruction and previous surgery, think adhesions.

Gastric Cancer: Often presents as weight loss, abdominal pain, and early satiety. Diagnosis is made by endoscopy with biopsy. Gastric cancer is usually **adenocarcinoma (90%).** Risk factors include eating smoked foods and chronic gastritis. *H. pylori* infection is associated with both intestinal type and diffuse type adenocarcinomas as well as mucosa-associated lymphoid tissue (MALT) lymphoma. Common metastatic sites include the **Virchow node** (left supraclavicular lymph node), **Sister Mary Joseph nodule** (periumbilical lymph node), and **Krukenberg tumor** (metastatic growth in the ovary). Because gastric cancer tends to ulcerate, gastric ulcers should be biopsied to exclude malignancy.

- **Intestinal type:** Well-differentiated adenocarcinomas. Risk factors include eating smoked foods, chronic gastritis, and ***H. pylori*** **infection.** Because these cancer cells **produce intercellular adhesion molecules** (E-cadherin), they maintain a glandular structure and the tumors can form ulcerating bulky masses.
- **Diffuse type:** Poorly differentiated adenocarcinoma. They lack **Lacks intracellular adhesion molecules** and therefore spread diffusely along the gastric wall and thicken it. **Linitis plastica** (leather bottle stomach) refers to severe thickening and rigidity of the stomach. The lack of distensibility causes early satiety and vomiting after eating. Biopsy reveals characteristic **signet ring cells,** in which mucin has pushed the nucleus to the periphery, giving the cells the appearance of signet rings (Fig. 10.15).

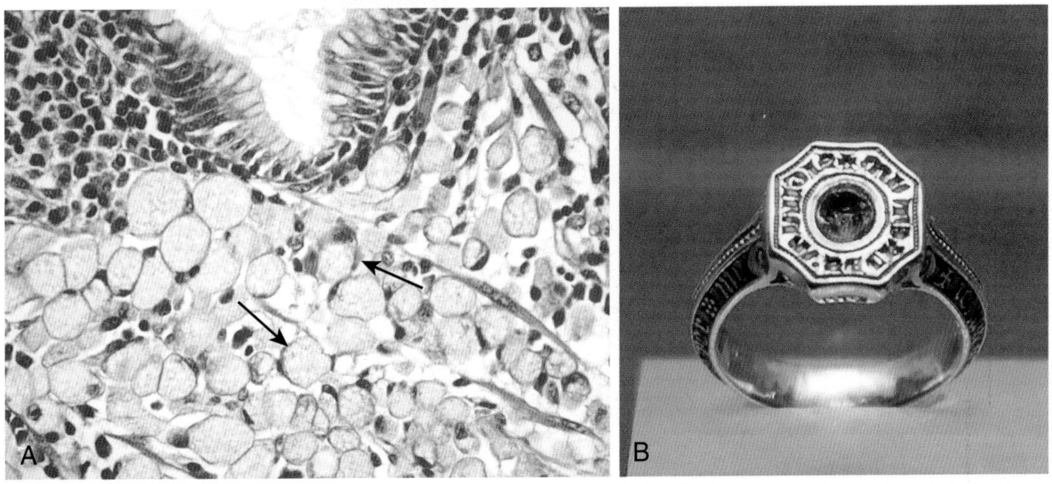

Fig. 10.15 A, Signet ring cell adenocarcinoma. **B,** Signet ring of the Black Prince (1330-1376). (**A** *from Kumar V, Fausto N, Abbas A: Robbins & Cotran Pathologic Basis of Disease. 7th ed. Philadelphia: Saunders; 2004:825;* **B** *from the Department of Decorative Arts, Louvre Museum, Paris.*)

- Gastric **MALT lymphoma:** Highly associated with *H. pylori* and responds very well to eradication, perhaps making it the only cancer that can be cured with antibiotics.
- **GI stromal tumors (GIST):** Arise from interstitial cells of Cajal (the pacemaker cells of gut motility). A gain of function mutation in the *KIT* gene causes a constitutively active tyrosine kinase receptor. In addition to surgical resection, GISTs can be targeted with the **tyrosine kinase inhibitor imatinib.**

Small Bowel and Colon

Small Bowel Obstruction (Fig. 10.16): Presents as colicky abdominal pain, distention, vomiting, and obstipation (inability to pass stool or gas). The pain is colicky because pain is felt specifically when peristalsis causes contraction against the obstruction. An upright abdominal x-ray examination usually reveals dilated loops of bowel, often with multiple air fluid levels (Fig. 10.17). All patients should be made NPO (nothing by mouth) and given intravenous (IV) fluids and medications to control pain and nausea. A nasogastric tube can decompress the bowel.

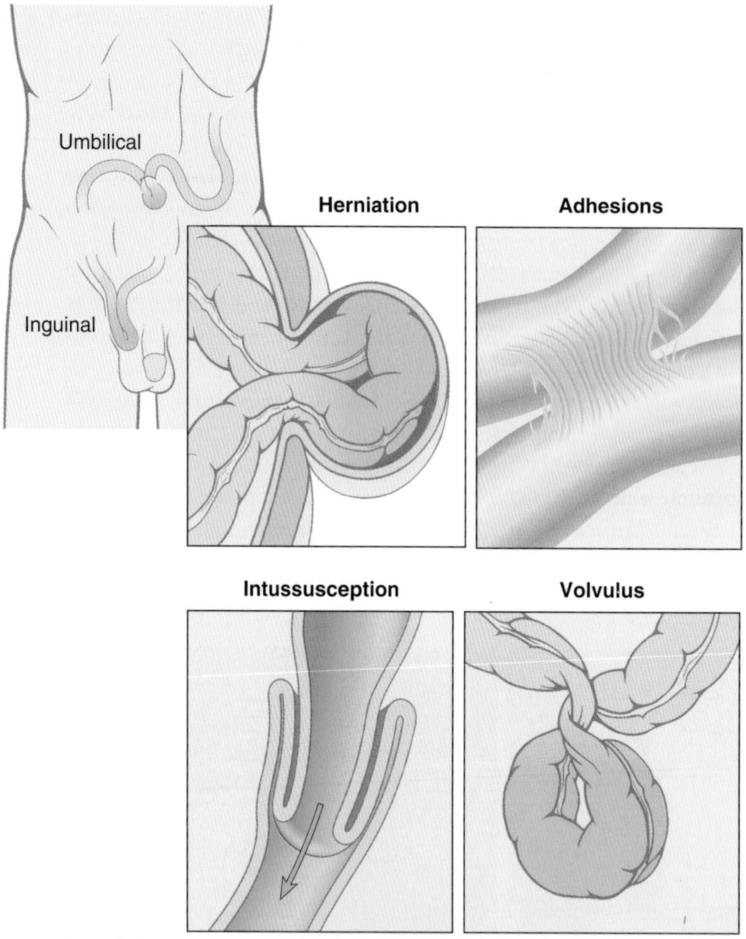

Fig. 10.16 Causes of small bowel obstruction. (*From Kumar V, Abbas AK, Fausto N, Mitchell R.* Robbins Basic Pathology. *8th ed. Philadelphia: Elsevier; 2007.*)

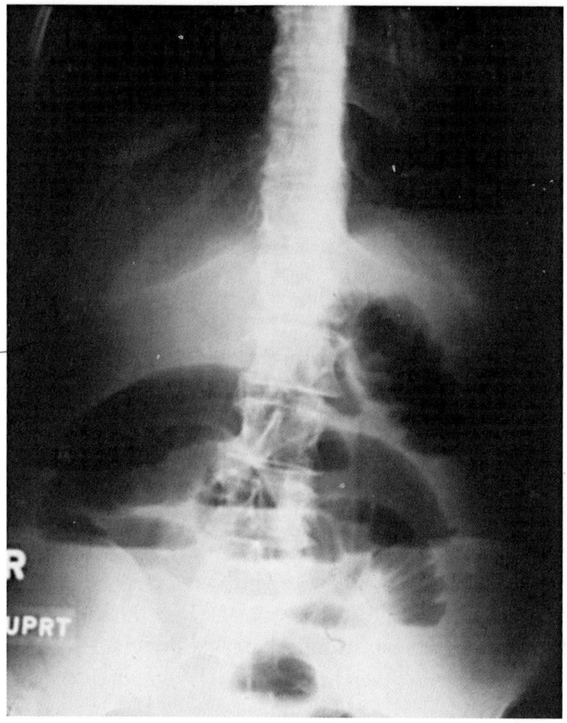

Fig. 10.17 Radiograph of dilated loops of bowel caused by a small bowel obstruction. (*From Lawlor MW.* Rapid Review USMLE Step 2. *Philadelphia: Elsevier; 2006.*)

- **Adhesions:** The most likely cause of obstruction in patients with previous abdominal surgery. Treated with surgical lysis of adhesions in severe cases. Incomplete bowel obstruction may respond to bowel rest (keeping the patient NPO) and nasogastric (NG) tube decompression.
- **Hernia incarceration:** Most common cause of obstruction in adults without history of abdominal surgery (see later).
- **Intussusception:** One piece of small bowel (intussusceptum) telescopes into an adjacent section (intussuscipiens). Most common cause of intestinal obstruction in young children and almost exclusively found in children 6 months to 6 years of age. Two-thirds of cases occur in children younger than 1 year. It occurs commonly after viral illnesses because of lymphatic hypertrophy at the lead point. When it occurs in adults, the lead point is more likely to be a polyp or tumor. Patients present with severe, colicky abdominal pain. Small children often present with alternating periods of crying and lethargy, and parents may describe their child drawing their legs up during painful episodes. Hematochezia is an inconsistent symptom, although many patients will have hemoccult-positive stool, and the classic **"currant jelly stool"** (actually dead mucosa that has sloughed off of ischemic bowel) is an extremely late finding. Physical examination may reveal a palpable, **sausage-shaped** abdominal mass. Ultrasonography, which is currently the first-line diagnostic test in most centers, shows a **bull's-eye lesion** demonstrating one region of bowel surrounding another. Diagnosis and treatment can be accomplished via an air- or contrast-based enema.
- **Volvulus:** Twisting of a loop of bowel around its mesentery, which leads to physical obstruction of the bowel lumen and **ischemia** of the bowel from interruption of the vascular supply. Symptoms include abdominal pain, distention, obstipation, and vomiting. Sigmoid volvulus most often occurs in debilitated older patients who have distended sigmoid colons from chronic constipation. Cecal volvulus most often occurs in middle-aged adults because of increased mobility of the right colon. Midgut volvulus occurs in the first months of life and is caused by congenital malrotation of the gut.

Typically, a sausage-shaped abdominal mass is palpated during intussusception.

Mesenteric Ischemia: Occlusion of the celiac artery, superior mesenteric artery, or inferior mesenteric artery leading to bowel ischemia and infarction. The splenic flexure and rectosigmoid colon are at particular risk because they are watershed bowel segments at the end of their respective arterial supplies.

- **Acute mesenteric ischemia:** Acute arterial occlusion leads to acute-onset severe abdominal pain, **pain out of proportion to the abdominal examination,** and bloody diarrhea from transmural infarction. Occlusion may be from cardiac embolization (e.g., in patients with atrial fibrillation) or may occur from atherosclerotic disease or hypercoagulable states.
- **Chronic mesenteric ischemia:** Progressive atherosclerosis leads to bowel hypoperfusion. Symptoms include **intestinal angina** (abdominal pain that occurs with eating) and associated weight loss. Because this progresses gradually there is growth of collateral blood supply, which may partially compensate.

Angiodysplasia: Abnormal tortuous blood vessels that are susceptible to bleeding. Vessels may bleed slowly, causing minimal or chronic blood loss, or may rupture causing acute or severe GI bleeding with hematochezia (bloody diarrhea). Predisposing conditions include end-stage renal disease, von Willebrand disease, and aortic stenosis.

Celiac Disease (Gluten-Sensitive Enteropathy): A hypersensitivity to wheat—more specifically, sensitivity to the glycoprotein **gliadin** found in gluten. Antigliadin antibodies target gliadin and create a local inflammatory reaction that damages the GI mucosa. Patients present with abdominal pain, vomiting, and diarrhea associated with ingestion of gluten. Laboratory tests often reveal **antitissue transglutaminase antibody and antiendomysial antibody** and may also be consistent with iron deficiency anemia (microcytic) or folate deficiency (macrocytic anemia) because mucosal damage can lead to malabsorption of these micronutrients. It is associated with HLA-DQ8 and HLA-DQ2. Intestinal biopsy reveals increased intraepithelial lymphocytes, **villous atrophy,** and **crypt hyperplasia** (Fig. 10.18). Treatment involves a strict gluten-free diet, which can often lead to resolution of symptoms. Of note, **dermatitis herpetiformis** is a commonly tested dermatologic manifestation of celiac disease characterized by papulovesicular (herpetic appearing) skin lesions, especially on the elbows and other extensor surfaces (Fig. 10.19).

Dermatitis herpetiformis is a commonly tested physical examination finding of celiac disease.

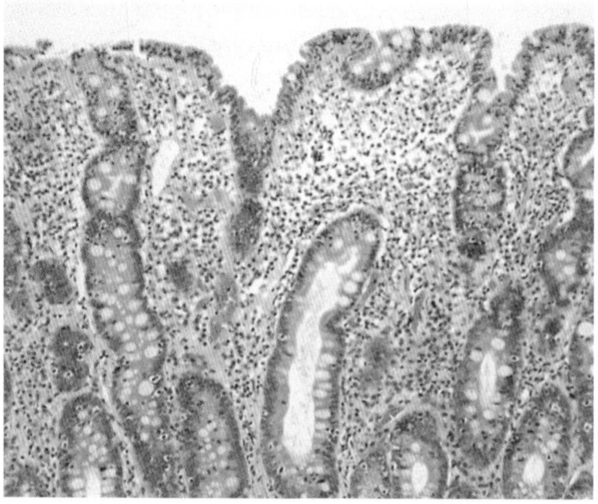

FIG. 10.18 Atrophic villi of celiac disease. (*From Damjanov I, Linder J: Pathology: A Color Atlas. St. Louis: Mosby; 2000:128.*)

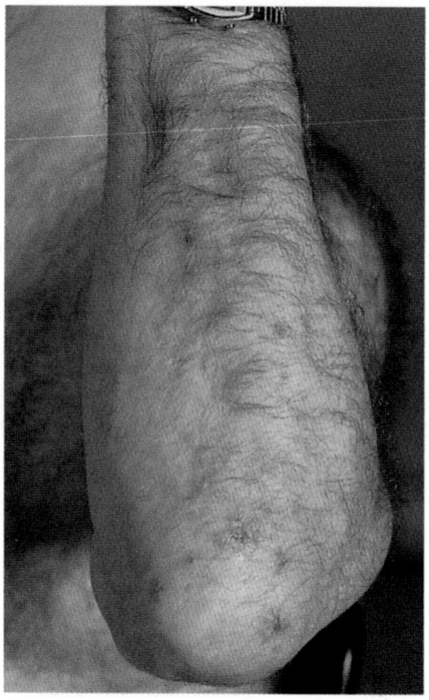

FIG. 10.19 Dermatitis herpetiformis. (*From Savin JAA, Hunter JAA, Hepburn NC: Diagnosis in Color: Skin Signs in Clinical Medicine. London: Mosby-Wolfe; 1997:92.*)

Tropical Sprue: Clinically and histologically indistinguishable from celiac disease, tropical sprue is thought to be caused by an infectious source, although the organism is not known. It is distinguished from celiac because it is found predominantly in the tropics and does not respond to a gluten-free diet. Antibiotics (either tetracycline or doxycycline) are the treatment of choice.

Whipple Disease: Symptoms are similar to tropical sprue and celiac disease; however, biopsy reveals **foamy macrophages** (lipid loaded) that are **periodic acid–Schiff (PAS)–positive**. These bacteria-laden macrophages accumulate in the GI lymphatic system, which impairs drainage and leads to diarrhea and malabsorption. It may spread to other organs, causing joint pain, heart failure, or dementia depending on where it spreads. The intracellular gram-positive bacilli *Tropheryma whipplei* is the causative organism. Treatment is with long-term antibiotics.

Appendicitis: The underlying cause is appendiceal obstruction. Obstruction is often from a fecalith in adults. In children, lymphoid hyperplasia, especially after a viral illness, is commonly the inciting event. Acute appendicitis presents as acute onset of ill-defined periumbilical pain that migrates to the right lower quadrant and then becomes sharply defined. This migration occurs because the inflammation is sensed initially by the poorly defined visceral receptors of the appendix, which synapse in the spinal cord at the same level as the periumbilical region of the anterior abdominal wall. Once the inflammation spreads to the parietal peritoneum, however, the more distinguishing parietal receptors accurately localize the pain to the right lower quadrant. Signs and symptoms of appendicitis include fever, vomiting, and tenderness at **McBurney point** (the location on the abdominal wall one-third the distance between the anterior superior iliac spine and the umbilicus). Patients may also have a positive **psoas** or **obturator signs** (pain with hip flexion or internal rotation, respectively). Bloodwork is of limited use in aiding diagnosis because of poor sensitivity and specificity for the disease but may reveal leukocytosis (a normal white blood cell count does not exclude the diagnosis). CT scanning is usually highly accurate in making the diagnosis, but ultrasound is a reasonable initial diagnostic modality when limiting radiation exposure is a high priority (e.g., in children). Ultrasound can also help distinguish appendicitis from pelvic pathologic conditions, such as an ectopic pregnancy or ovarian torsion. Treatment is with appendectomy and antibiotics. Complications include perforation, which may lead to peritonitis and/or abscess formation. Clinical pearl: *Yersinia enterocolitis* infection and subsequent invasion into the Peyer patches can cause a condition closely resembling appendicitis, called pseudoappendicitis. During laparoscopy, lymphadenopathy and inflammation of the terminal ileum and appendix can be seen.

Appendicitis occurs because of obstruction, often from a fecalith in adults or lymphoid hyperplasia in children.

Irritable Bowel Syndrome (IBS): IBS is abdominal discomfort associated with constipation or diarrhea, often alternating, in the absence of other organic GI pathologic conditions. Mucus may also be found in the stool. Diagnosis is based on the presence of two of three of the following clinical criteria, known as the Rome criteria:

1. Symptoms relieved with defecation
2. Association with a change in stool frequency
3. Association with a change in stool appearance

Inflammatory Bowel Disease

Inflammatory bowel disease is an autoimmune disease of the gastrointestinal tract caused by the interaction between genetics, intestinal microbes, and the immune system. It is divided into ulcerative colitis and Crohn disease.

Ulcerative Colitis (UC): UC is an autoimmune inflammatory condition of the colon. Patients present with relapsing episodes of bloody diarrhea, mucus-covered stools, and cramping. Colonoscopy reveals inflammation that begins in the rectum and spreads continuously as far as the cecum. **Pseudopolyps,** which are areas of normal mucosa that appear polypoid compared with surrounding ulcerated or friable mucosa, may be seen on colonoscopy. Barium enema may reveal absence of haustral markings, known as a lead pipe colon (Fig. 10.20). Histologic examination

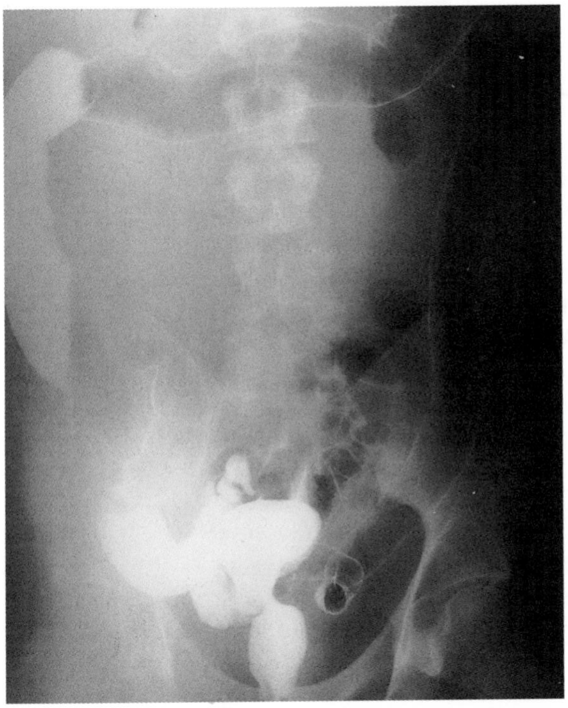

FIG. 10.20 Barium enema study revealing lead pipe colon of chronic ulcerative colitis. (*From Collins P, Lombard M, Horton-Szar D. Collins* Crash Course: Gastroenterology. *3rd ed. Philadelphia: Elsevier; 2008.*)

demonstrates inflammation and ulceration of the mucosa and submucosa as well as crypt abscesses. Unlike in Crohn disease, ulcerations do not involve the full thickness of the bowel and there is no granuloma formation. **Extraintestinal** manifestations of the disease include primary sclerosing cholangitis, polyarthritis, uveitis, pyoderma gangrenosum, and erythema nodosum. Patients with UC are at increased risk for colon cancer and should be screened with colonoscopy starting 8 years after diagnosis. Treatment involves **5-ASA** compounds (e.g., sulf**asa**lazine), steroids, and biologics, including infliximab. Colectomy with ileoanal anastomosis is usually curative for colitis but does not treat extraintestinal manifestations.

UC — PSC

Crohn Disease: An autoimmune inflammatory condition of the entire GI tract but most commonly affecting the ileocecal region. Patients may present with abdominal pain, nausea, vomiting, and diarrhea (often with passage of blood and mucus). Colonoscopy reveals skip lesions—ulcers that may be present anywhere from mouth to rectum. Histologic examination reveals **transmural (full-thickness)** inflammation and may include noncaseating **granulomas.** Complications include **abscesses, strictures, fistulas, and fissures.**

Crohn disease's damage to the ileum (or surgical treatment with resection of the ileum) may cause a deficiency in vitamin B_{12} and bile salts, which are absorbed in the ileum. A relative lack of bile salts can also lead to impaired absorption of fat-soluble vitamins (A, D, E, and K). Also, the presence of bile salts in the colon is cathartic and may worsen diarrhea. Therefore cholestyramine (a bile acid–binding resin) can be used to bind bile salts and prevent their cathartic effect. **Extraintestinal manifestations are similar to UC;** however, primary sclerosing cholangitis is comparatively rare. The risk of colon cancer is elevated in Crohn disease, although less so than in UC. Treatment is similar to UC, but surgery is not curative and recurrent bowel resection may lead to short bowel syndrome—malabsorption and steatorrhea caused by decreased intestinal length. Both UC and Crohn disease are associated with the HLA-B27 major histocompatibility complex (Table 10.2).

Extraintestinal manifestations of irritable bowel disease include polyarthritis, uveitis, pyoderma gangrenosum, and erythema nodosum.

TABLE 10.2 Comparison of Crohn Disease and Ulcerative Colitis

FEATURE	CROHN DISEASE	ULCERATIVE COLITIS
Most common distribution	Ileocecal region	Rectum to cecum
Entire GI tract involvement?	Yes	No
Spread	Skip lesions	Continuous
Biopsy findings	Crypt abscesses Transmural inflammation Noncaseating granulomas	Crypt abscesses Partial-thickness inflammation No granulomas
Cancer risk	+	+++
PSC risk	+	+++
Colectomy curative?	No (symptoms often recur)	Yes (of GI symptoms only)
HLA-B27 association	Yes	Yes
Other	Abscesses, strictures, fistulas, fissures are complications	Lead pipe colon seen on barium enema; pseudopolyps seen on endoscopy

Colonic Polyps: A colonic polyp is a protrusion of mucosal tissue into the colonic lumen. Polyps can be divided into multiple groups by histology and malignant potential:

- **Hyperplastic polyps:** Colonic epithelial proliferation leads to a "piling up" effect of cells. **No malignant potential.**
- **Hamartomatous polyps:** When occurring spontaneously these do not have malignant potential; however, when occurring as part of **juvenile polyposis syndrome** or **Peutz-Jeghers syndrome** there is significant malignant potential.
- **Adenomas:** The most common neoplastic polyp and the precursor lesion to colonic adenocarcinoma. Histologically they display epithelial **dysplasia.** A polyp's risk of malignancy is related to its size, degree of dysplasia, and architecture. From greatest to least risk of malignancy: villous > tubulovillous > tubular histology (Fig. 10.21).

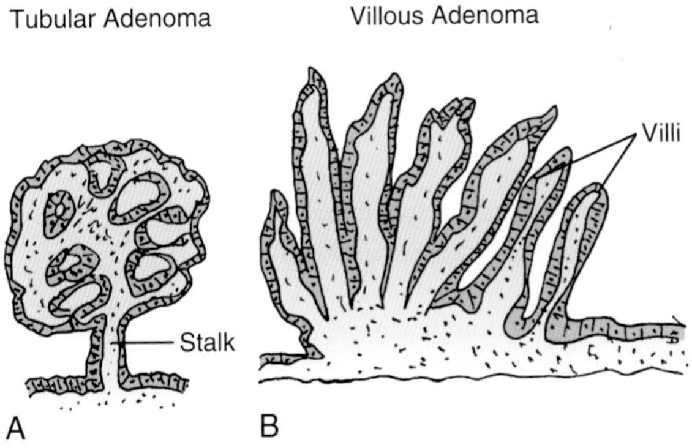

Fig. 10.21 A, Tubular adenoma. **B,** Villous adenoma. (*From Damjanov I. Pathology Secrets. 3rd ed. Philadelphia: Elsevier; 2008.*)

Colon Cancer: Colon cancer is the third leading cause of cancer death in North America. Most are caused by adenocarcinomas. Current guidelines recommend screening for colon cancer every 10 years starting at age 50. In patients with a family history of colon cancer, screening should begin 10 years before the age at which the youngest affected first-degree relative was diagnosed. Patients may be asymptomatic, with cancer found on screening colonoscopy. Patients may also present with hematochezia, obstruction, or small-caliber stools. In general, left-sided cancers tend to obstruct because the colonic lumen is narrower and stool is more solid. Right-sided cancers, on the other hand, tend to bleed. Bleeding may be occult, however, so GI malignancy should be considered in patients with **iron deficiency anemia** or positive fecal occult blood tests.

The liver is the most common site of metastatic disease because of portal drainage; however, perianal lesions drain through the caval system and are thus less likely to metabolize to the liver.

Lynch Syndrome: Also called hereditary nonpolyposis colorectal cancer (HNPCC). Caused by autosomal dominant mutations leading to **defective DNA mismatch repair** and subsequent **microsatellite instability,** leading to increased risk of colon, endometrial, and ovarian cancers. In Lynch syndrome, colon cancer may occur without being preceded by a polyp. It is the most common form of syndromic colon cancer.

Peutz-Jeghers Syndrome: Autosomal dominant condition caused by a tumor suppressor gene mutation. It leads to a syndrome of multiple hamartomatous GI polyps, **mucocutaneous hyperpigmentation,** and high risk of GI (colon, gastric, small intestine) and genitourinary cancers.

Juvenile Polyposis Syndrome: Autosomal dominant condition leading to multiple hamartomatous polyps presenting in children young than 5 years old. These polyps are mostly located in the rectum, and complications include bleeding, obstruction, and intussusception. Approximately 50% of patients will develop adenocarcinoma.

Familial Adenomatous Polyposis (FAP): FAP is caused by the autosomal dominant mutation of adenomatous polyposis coli (APC) gene. The *APC* gene mutation leads to hundreds of polyps in the colon and throughout the GI tract, with the lifetime risk of malignancy approaching 100% without treatment. Treated with prophylactic colectomy.

- Turcot syndrome: Mutation of a DNA mismatch repair gene leading to polyposis and the presence of central nervous system (CNS) tumors, especially medulloblastoma. Essentially, FAP plus medulloblastoma.
- Gardner syndrome: Essentially, FAP plus osteomas.

Diarrhea

Osmotic: Occurs when water is drawn into the bowel because of an increase in luminal osmoles. Osmotic laxatives such as magnesium hydroxide (milk of magnesia) act in this manner. In lactose intolerance (disaccharidase deficiency), lactose is the offending osmole. Sorbitol is poorly absorbed and may cause osmotic diarrhea in patients consuming a lot of low-calorie sweetener (e.g., sugar-free gum). Osmotic diarrhea resolves with fasting or withdrawal of the offending agent.

Secretory: An increase in intestinal secretion of ions and water, causing extremely watery stools. Most notably, *Vibrio cholerae* produces the cholera toxin, which irreversibly activates the enterocyte's Gs subunit. Gs then stimulates cyclic adenosine monophosphate (cAMP)–mediated secretion of ions and water, causing so-called **rice water diarrhea.** It does not improve with fasting.

Cholera toxin activates the Gs subunit, creating a watery, secretory diarrhea.

Exudative: Diarrhea with the presence of blood or pus in the stool is considered exudative. It may be secondary to inflammatory bowel disease (IBD) or infectious in origin. *Shigella* and *Salmonella* spp., enterohemorrhagic *Escherichia coli,* and *Entamoeba histolytica* are the common culprit pathogens. It does not improve with fasting.

Deranged Motility: Anything that reduces gut transit time may lead to an increase in the frequency of loose stools. Surgical resection, carcinoid syndrome, hyperthyroidism, and IBS all cause diarrhea partially through decreasing transit time. GI irritants (e.g., blood) also have decreased transit time and can increase the frequency of stools.

Diverticular Disease: An outpouching of mucosa and submucosa through the muscularis propria that is covered by the serosa (technically pseudodiverticula or "false" diverticula, because they do not contain all layers of the wall; Fig. 10.22). These outpouchings are extremely common and generally asymptomatic. They tend to occur in the sigmoid colon, in which luminal pressure is the highest, and specifically around the vasa recta, where the penetrating blood vessel creates a local area of weakness. Anything that increases colonic pressure is a risk factor, including low-fiber diets, obesity, and straining with defecation.

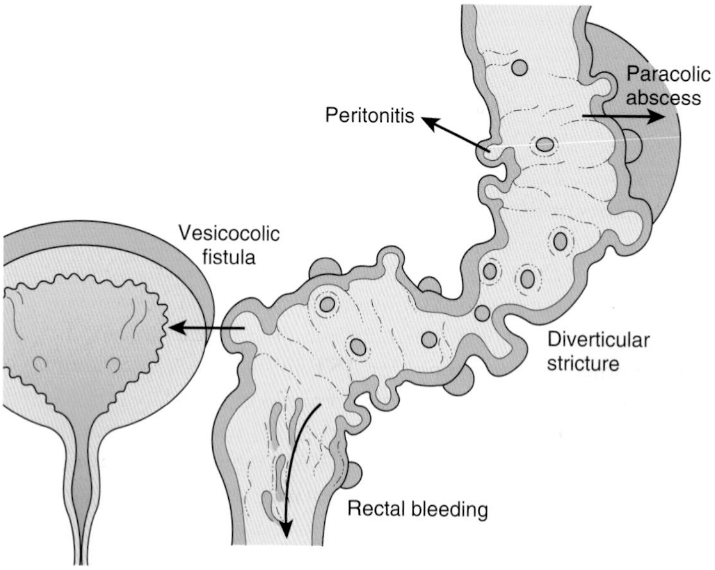

Fig. 10.22 Diverticular disease and its complications. (*From Kontoyannis A, Sweetland H.* Crash Course: Surgery E-Book. *3rd ed. Philadelphia: Elsevier; 2008.*)

Diverticulitis: Occurs when there is a microperforation of a diverticulum leading to inflammation and focal necrosis. Clinically, patients tend to present with more than 24 hours **of left lower quadrant abdominal pain** and tenderness and sometimes low-grade fever, nausea, and vomiting. Because diverticulitis tends to recur, many patients will report similar previous episodes. The history and physical examination alone may be enough to diagnose a recurrence of diverticulitis. Colonoscopy is contraindicated during active inflammation, but CT is diagnostic and will reveal complications. Although the omentum tends to wall off the inflammatory process, complications include peritonitis, secondary perforation, abscess formation, fistulas, and strictures. Uncomplicated diverticulitis can be treated with antibiotics directed against colonic flora, predominantly gram-negative rods and anaerobes. The combination of ciprofloxacin and metronidazole is commonly used.

Diverticula tend to occur around the vasa recta and are thus at risk for bleeding.

Bleeding Diverticulosis: Diverticula tend to occur around the vasa recta, where the penetrating blood vessels create local weakness. The associated vasa recta are then only protected by the overlying mucosa and are at risk for bleeding, even from trivial intraluminal trauma. Bleeding can be profound and presents as hematochezia. Diagnosis and treatment can be achieved via colonoscopy.

Most colonic diverticula are asymptomatic and require no treatment.

Anal fissure

A painful tear in the rectal mucosa below the dentate line. It presents as anal or rectal pain that is exquisitely tender with defecation or digital rectal examination. The fissure may be visible on physical examination or may be associated with a sentinel tag (a perianal skin tag at the site of the fissure). Treatment is with stool softeners, sitz baths, high-fiber diet, and topical anesthetics such as lidocaine.

Hemorrhoids

These are dilated hemorrhoidal veins in the submucosal layer of the rectum. Hemorrhoids are present in approximately 25% of adults. Constipation contributes to their formation. Improvement may be seen with a high-fiber diet and stool softeners, which can reduce straining during defecation. Hemorrhoids may bleed, but rarely is bleeding severe. Most often a small amount of bright red blood is noted on toilet paper with wiping or streaked along the side of a normal stool.

Do not confuse hemorrhoids with perianal skin tags that may represent the sentinel tag of an anal fissure.

Internal Hemorrhoids: Located above the **dentate** (pectinate) line, internal hemorrhoids cause bleeding from the superior hemorrhoidal veins. Because innervation is visceral, internal hemorrhoids are **painless.** They may, however, prolapse and become palpable. Treatment is with band ligation.

External Hemorrhoids: Located below the pectinate line, external hemorrhoids arise from dilation of the inferior hemorrhoidal veins and are covered with squamous epithelium. Because the innervation is somatic, they may be pruritic or **painful,** especially if thrombosed.

Laboratory Tests

Laboratory tests of the liver can be divided into three groups: (1) hepatocyte cytosolic enzymes, (2) biliary analysis, and (3) hepatic synthetic function. Although somewhat of an oversimplification, collectively these tests are referred to as "liver function tests."

Hepatocyte Cystolic Enzymes:

- **Aspartate aminotransferase and alanine aminotransferase:** Aspartate aminotransferase (AST) and alanine aminotransferase (ALT) are hepatocyte cytosolic enzymes important in amino acid metabolism. Clinically they are markers of hepatocyte damage because they are "leaked" into the serum when hepatocytes are injured. The normal reference range for AST and ALT is 5 to 40 U/L. Levels tend to be extremely high (>1000 U/L) in acute viral hepatitis, acetaminophen or other toxin poisoning, and shock liver and more modestly elevated (>100 U/L) in chronic forms of hepatitis. The ratio of ALT to AST can also be useful in diagnosing the cause of liver inflammation. Whenever liver inflammation is present, the rise in ALT tends to be greater than the rise in AST. In alcoholic hepatitis, however, AST is twice as elevated as ALT (think AST—**S**mirnoff vodka). Importantly, the degree of enzymatic elevation does not necessarily correlate with the severity of liver failure. A patient with end-stage liver disease, for example, may only have a slight elevation of AST and ALT levels because most of the liver has already been destroyed. A patient with hepatitis A, on the other hand, may have AST and ALT values >1000 U/L but maintain a fully functional liver after recovery.

Biliary Analysis:

- **Bilirubin:** In the spleen, heme released from senescent red blood cells is broken down to unconjugated bilirubin. The insoluble, inexcretable, unconjugated form travels to the liver bound to albumin, where it is conjugated with glucuronic acid to form conjugated (direct) bilirubin. This form is then excreted from the body in the bile. In the gut, bacteria convert conjugated bilirubin to urobilinogen, part of which is excreted in the feces as stercobilin; the rest is resorbed and excreted again in bile or secreted in the urine as urobilin. Conditions that limit the metabolic function of the liver (e.g., cirrhosis) cause elevations in the unconjugated bilirubin level. Furthermore, an increase in the production of bilirubin (e.g., intravascular or extravascular hemolysis) will also elevate unconjugated bilirubin. On the other hand, a patient with a cholestatic process such as choledocholithiasis will be able to conjugate bilirubin but will be unable to excrete it, resulting in a rise in conjugated bilirubin levels.

Interestingly, hemoglobin is a colorful molecule and, along with its breakdown products, is responsible for the red color of blood, yellow color of urine (urobilin), brown color of feces (stercobilin), and yellow discoloration of jaundice (bilirubin). A patient with a cholestatic process (e.g., choledocholithiasis, cholangiocarcinoma) will be unable to excrete bilirubin into the feces and will have clay-colored (acholic) stools. A patient who cannot conjugate bilirubin will also subsequently lack urobilin so, although the patient may be jaundiced from unconjugated bilirubin, the urine will not appear more yellow because unconjugated bilirubin will not pass through the glomerular basement membrane because it is bound to albumin.

Unconjugated bilirubin does not pass the glomerular basement membrane.

- **Alkaline phosphatase (AP):** AP is a ubiquitous enzyme that, as the name suggests, removes phosphates most efficiently in alkaline environments. This enzyme is particularly concentrated in the biliary tree, bone, and placenta. The AP level is often elevated in cholestatic syndromes and in bile duct obstruction (e.g., cholangitis).
- **γ-Glutamyltransferase:** Another enzyme of amino acid metabolism that is elevated in diseases of the biliary tree. The γ-glutamyltransferase (GGT) level is elevated along with AP but is more specific to biliary disease (e.g., will not be increased in bone disease). It is also raised with alcohol ingestion.

AP is also concentrated in the bone and placenta, not just the biliary tree.

Hepatic Synthetic Function:

- **Prothrombin time and international normalized ratio:** Because the liver makes most clotting factors, an elevation of the prothrombin time (PT) and international normalized ratio (INR) suggests impaired hepatic synthetic function such as in cirrhosis.
- **Albumin:** Albumin is an ubiquitous protein that is made in the liver and is thus a true marker of hepatic synthetic function. It is very important in that it serves to carry factors and molecules (e.g., unconjugated bilirubin, calcium, and many others) throughout the body, as well as provide oncotic pressure to the intravascular fluids. However, albumin can be lowered in nonhepatic pathologic conditions, including nephrotic syndrome and malnutrition. Additionally, albumin is an acute phase reactant and its serum concentration decreases with systemic inflammation.

Hepatic Pathology

Viral Hepatitis: See Chapter 5, Microbiology.

Nonalcoholic Fatty Liver Disease: A spectrum of liver disease that closely resembles alcoholic liver disease but is associated with metabolic syndrome (diabetes, obesity, dyslipidemia, and hypertension). Nonalcoholic steatosis is an early finding with elevation of AST and ALT levels and a hypoechoic (fatty) liver on imaging with no apparent cause except for obesity and/or metabolic syndrome. Treatment involves diet, exercise, and management of metabolic comorbidities, such as diabetes.

Nonalcoholic steatohepatitis (NASH) is nonalcoholic steatosis plus biopsy-proven histologic evidence of inflammation. If untreated, cirrhosis may develop.

Alcoholic Hepatitis: Chronic alcohol consumption leading to fatty infiltration, similar to nonalcoholic steatosis. Eventually transaminase levels will rise secondary to hepatocyte damage. The **AST-to-ALT ratio** may be more than 2:1. **Mallory bodies** (eosinophilic keratin filament inclusion bodies) may be present on biopsy. These are more commonly found in alcoholic hepatitis than in NASH.

Hemochromatosis: Autosomal recessive disorder of the HFE gene (acronym for **h**igh **Fe^{2+}**) leading to dysregulated overabsorption of iron and excessive hemosiderin accumulation, causing free radical damage. Patients present with cirrhosis, bronzed skin, diabetes (pancreatic infiltration), and cardiomyopathy. Diagnosis is suspected with high serum iron and ferritin levels and confirmed with genetic testing. Liver biopsy with Prussian blue staining reveals hemosiderin deposits. Treatment is aimed at normalizing iron stores via repeated phlebotomy. Secondary hemochromatosis is caused by excessive iron intake, usually after repeated red blood cell transfusions, such as for β-thalassemia.

Wilson Disease: Autosomal recessive disorder of Wilson disease protein, an ATPase responsible for transporting copper into bile and important in the formation of ceruloplasmin (the transport protein for copper). The inability to excrete copper leads to an increase in the free serum copper level, although the total serum copper may be high, low, or normal, given the relative lack of ceruloplasmin to transport copper. Consequently, copper accumulates in the liver **(cirrhosis)**, brain (**cognitive deterioration** and **parkinsonism**), and cornea **(Kayser-Fleischer rings).** Diagnosis is based on a decrease in levels of serum ceruloplasmin, an elevation in urinary copper levels, and copper deposits seen on liver biopsy. Treatment involves chelation with **D-penicillamine.**

Wilson disease will cause a decrease in the serum ceruloplasmin level and an increase in the level of urinary copper.

α_1-Antitrypsin Deficiency: Autosomal recessive defect of α_1-antitrypsin (A1AT), a protein that inactivates proteases and protects tissues from their enzymatic destruction. A1AT deficiency leads to early emphysema (see Chapter 17) and accumulation of A1AT in the hepatocyte endoplasmic reticulum, leading to cirrhosis. In a nonsmoker with early-onset emphysema, A1AT deficiency should be considered as the cause of the cirrhosis. Histologic examination reveals PAS-positive granules. It should be noted that null homozygotes (those whose mutation prevents synthesis) do not develop liver pathologic conditions. Liver pathologic conditions are only seen in patients with mutations that cause polymerization of the mutation A1AT protein within hepatocytes, which is most commonly in patients homozygous with the Z allele.

Think of A1AT in early-onset emphysema with cirrhosis.

Cirrhosis: The final common pathway of liver disease and a pathologic diagnosis based on the presence of regenerative nodules surrounded by fibrosis (Fig. 10.23). Sequelae of cirrhosis are secondary to **impaired metabolic function of the liver** and **portal hypertension.**

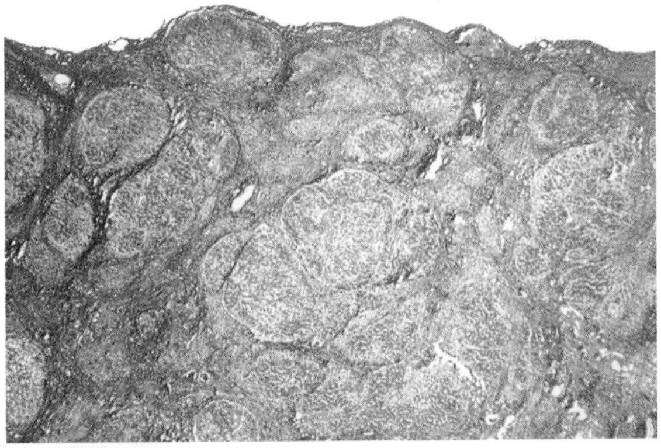

FIG. 10.23 Cirrhosis—regenerative nodules surrounded by fibrotic tissue *(blue)*. *(From Kumar V, Abbas AK, Fausto N, Mitchell R.* Robbins Basic Pathology. *8th ed. Philadelphia: Elsevier; 2007.)*

Impaired metabolic function leads to impaired hepatic breakdown of estrogen, causing **gynecomastia, testicular atrophy, palmar erythema, and spider angioma** (via weakening of vascular walls and localized vasodilation). Impaired synthesis of clotting factors causes a coagulopathy reflected by an elevation of PT/INR values (and later partial thromboplastin time). Finally, **hepatic encephalopathy** may occur, leading to altered mental status and asterixis (flapping tremor of negative myoclonus). Although the mechanism of hepatic encephalopathy is not entirely clear, it is associated with an elevated serum ammonia level (Fig. 10.24). Portal hypertension occurs because the fibrosed liver cannot handle as much blood flow through the portal circulation, leading to complications such as varices and ascites.

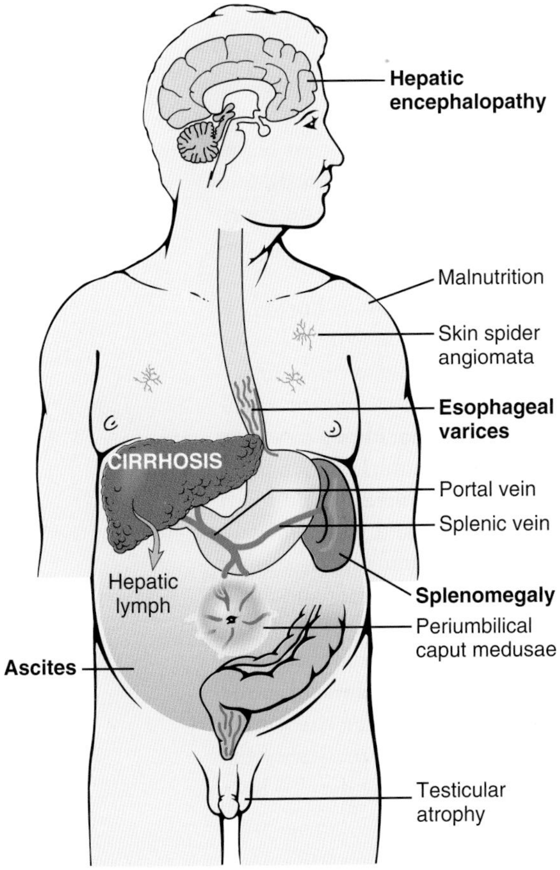

FIG. 10.24 Sequelae of portal hypertension. *(From Kumar V, Abbas AK, Fausto N, Aster J.* Robbins & Cotran Pathologic Basis of Disease. *8th ed. New York: Elsevier; 2009.)*

Portal Hypertension: Defined as a pressure gradient greater than 10 mm Hg between the portal vein (entering the liver) and hepatic veins (leaving the liver). The hypertension is usually intrahepatic (sinusoidal) secondary to cirrhosis (as described earlier). Rarely, however, it may be posthepatic secondary to **hepatic vein thrombosis** (Budd-Chiari syndrome) or prehepatic secondary to portal vein thrombosis. The sequelae of portal hypertension are outlined here.

- **Portosystemic shunting:** As portal pressure rises, more blood is shunted through collateral vessels into the caval system. This results in a dilation of systemic venous collaterals.
  - **Caput medusae:** Dilation of periumbilical veins and abdominal wall veins causing the appearance of the head (caput) of Medusa on the abdominal wall.
  - **Hemorrhoids:** Dilation of veins near the rectum, specifically between the superior rectal and middle/inferior rectal veins.
  - **Esophageal varices:** This is the most clinically important example of portosystemic shunting. Varices are present in 30% to 60% of cirrhotics. Dilated periesophageal veins (fed from collaterals from the left gastric vein) often begin as asymptomatic but may spontaneously rupture, leading to massive upper GI bleeding. A GI bleed in a cirrhotic patient should be considered variceal until proven otherwise, although other causes are possible. Prophylaxis may be accomplished with nonselective beta blockers (e.g., propranolol) or endoscopic banding of varices. Management of acute bleeds involves resuscitation (with IV fluids and blood transfusion as needed) and IV octreotide (a synthetic somatostatin and splanchnic vasoconstrictor that mitigates bleeding). Broad-spectrum antibiotics (e.g., ceftriaxone) are used prophylactically to prevent bacteremia and spontaneous bacterial peritonitis caused by esophageal flora. Endoscopic banding should be attempted emergently.
- **Splenomegaly:** Enlarged spleen secondary to collateral flow via the splenic vein.
- **Ascites:** Portal hypertension causes increased portal hydrostatic pressure. This, combined with decreased osmotic pressure from impaired albumin production, leads to fluid collection in the peritoneal cavity. This process can also lead to generalized edema (anasarca).
- **Hepatorenal syndrome:** Splanchnic vasodilation leading to poor renal perfusion. Hepatorenal syndrome is a late sequela with very poor prognosis.

Triad of Budd-Chiari: abdominal pain, ascites, and hepatomegaly

Budd-Chiari syndrome (hepatic vein thrombosis) is often idiopathic but is associated with hypercoagulable states, especially **polycythemia vera.** It presents with the classic triad of **abdominal pain, ascites, and hepatomegaly.** To remember how to distinguish Budd-Chiari from Arnold-Chiari (a neurologic malformation), think **B**udd for **b**lockage of the hepatic vein.

Hemangiomas are the most common hepatic neoplasms. Do not biopsy them.

Hepatic Neoplasms

Cavernous Hemangioma: Most common benign hepatic tumor caused by a proliferation of blood vessels. It is often asymptomatic and incidentally discovered but may cause abdominal pain. Rarely, hemangiomas will rupture, causing massive blood loss. There is an uncertain link between hemangiomas and hormone use, and some physicians recommend avoiding hormonal contraception if hemangiomas are present. Lesions **should not be biopsied** because this might precipitate bleeding.

Hepatocellular Adenoma: Benign hepatic neoplasm highly associated with the use of **hormonal contraception.** These tumors tend to be avascular and will not bleed if biopsied. Resection of these lesions is the norm to avoid rare complications such as rupture or transformation to hepatocellular carcinoma.

Hepatocellular Carcinoma (Hepatoma, HCC): Most common primary hepatic malignancy and most often secondary to cirrhosis (e.g., viral, alcoholic). Of note, HCC may develop in patients with hepatitis B before cirrhosis occurs, although **this is not the case in hepatitis C.** Overall, however, there is a stronger association between hepatitis C and HCC. Aflatoxin (found in mold contaminated food) is a well-known and often tested carcinogen. Symptoms include jaundice, ascites, and hepatomegaly, but patients with cirrhosis should be monitored because early HCC may be asymptomatic. The tumor marker for HCC is **α-fetoprotein** (AFP), but diagnosis should be confirmed with imaging and often biopsy.

Of note, AFP acts as the fetal form of albumin. Its level is elevated in primary HCC and metastatic disease to the liver and in yolk sac tumors. In neural tube defects, the AFP level is also elevated in the mother's blood because the fetal skin is not fully intact and AFP leaks into the mother's circulation. In Down syndrome, the levels in the mother's blood are decreased, presumably because the size of the fetus and yolk sac are decreased.

It is important to remember that secondary hepatic malignancies are more common than primary hepatic malignancies because of the dual blood supply of the liver and portal drainage.

Cholangiocarcinoma: The second most common primary malignancy of the liver that arises from bile ducts. These tumors may be asymptomatic or may present with biliary obstruction, jaundice, cholangitis, or abdominal pain.

Disorders of Bilirubin Metabolism

Gilbert Syndrome: Common and benign cause of jaundice caused by reduced activity of glucuronyltransferase, the enzyme responsible for the conjugation of bilirubin. Without conjugation, the bilirubin remains insoluble and incapable of being excreted in bile. Those affected may have mild jaundice, especially in times of stress or dehydration, or an **increase in the indirect bilirubin** level found incidentally on laboratory studies. There are no sequelae, and treatment is unnecessary.

conjugation

Crigler-Najjar Syndrome: Rare autosomal recessive condition leading to near-total absence of functional glucuronyltransferase and inability to conjugate (and therefore excrete) bilirubin. Type 1 is most severe and leads to **kernicterus** and early death if aggressive phototherapy and/or plasmapheresis are not initiated. Type 2 is a significant but incomplete absence of glucuronyltransferase, and survival to adulthood is the norm. Laboratory tests reveal **elevated indirect bilirubin** levels.

Dubin-Johnson Syndrome: Rare autosomal recessive condition characterized by inability to excrete conjugated bilirubin into the bile. Characteristically the liver will be black in these patients because of pigment deposition in lysosomes. Most patients are asymptomatic or have only mild jaundice. They rarely require treatment. **Rotor syndrome** is even milder, and the patient's liver does not turn black.

Pigment stones are seen in conditions of high red blood cell turnover, such as sickle cell anemia.

excretion

Autoimmune Disorders

Primary biliary cholangitis (PBC), previously known as primary biliary cirrhosis, is an autoimmune disease caused by the lymphocytic destruction of bile canaliculi and small intrahepatic bile ducts. It is more common in women and is associated with positive antimitochondrial antibody serology. Symptoms begin as fatigue and pruritus and progress to cirrhosis and portal hypertension. Disease progression is slow over the course of decades, however, and many cases are discovered on incidental laboratory finding of elevated alkaline phosphatase or GGT before becoming symptomatic. It is associated with other autoimmune conditions such as Sjögren syndrome, CREST syndrome, and autoimmune thyroiditis.

Primary sclerosing cholangitis (PSC) is caused by destruction farther down the biliary tree of intra- and extrahepatic bile ducts. Preserved sections become dilated, which leads to a beading appearance on imaging with endoscopic retrograde cholangiopancreatography (ERCP) or magnetic resonance cholangiopancreatography (MRCP). Serologic testing may reveal p-ANCA positivity and biopsy reveals the onion skin scar pattern of circumferential bile duct fibrosis. Ulcerative colitis is also present 70% of the time. Like PBC, PSC is often discovered incidentally (especially when people with UC are screened). Symptoms begin as fatigue and pruritus and then progress over years to cirrhosis. Patients are also predisposed to cholangitis, pancreatitis, and cholangiocarcinoma.

GALLBLADDER AND PANCREAS

Gallstones: Risk factors for cholesterol stones include the four Fs—**fat, female, forty,** and **fertile.** These factors combine to create a high-cholesterol, low gallbladder motility environment. Progesterone specifically inhibits gallbladder motility in an analogous manner to its inhibition of uterine smooth muscle contraction during pregnancy. Pigment stones are composed of bilirubin precipitate and are found secondary to high red blood cell (RBC) turnover. For example, a patient with sickle cell anemia and right upper quadrant (RUQ) pain may have symptomatic pigment stone cholelithiasis. In general, stones are best diagnosed with ultrasound because they have a different density from that of the surrounding structures (Fig. 10.25). Although pigment stones are generally radiopaque, conventional radiographs are less helpful because the much more common cholesterol stones are generally radiolucent.

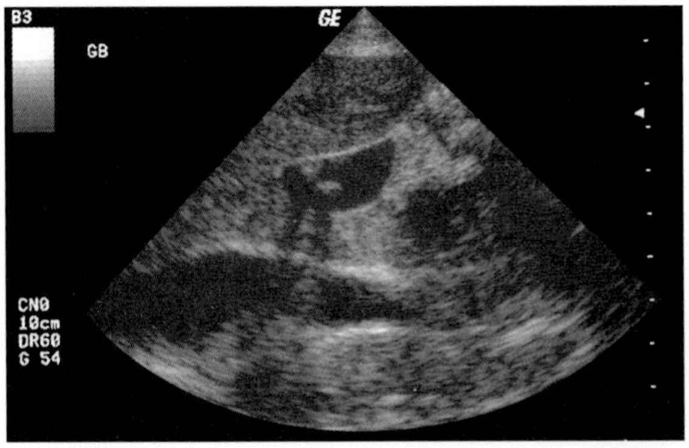

Fig. 10.25 Ultrasound of cholelithiasis—an echogenic gallstone demonstrating acoustic shadowing. (*From Markovchick VJ, Pons PT.* Emergency Medicine Secrets. *4th ed. Philadelphia: Elsevier; 2009.*)

Asymptomatic gallstones found on ultrasound require no treatment. Elective surgery is generally recommended for symptomatic cholelithiasis, whereas cholecystitis, inflammation of the gallbladder and surrounding tissues from an impacted stone, requires antibiotics and urgent surgical attention. Stone impaction within the common bile duct (choledocholithiasis) can lead to cholangitis (ascending infection of the biliary tree). These patients often require endoscopic stone removal via ERCP as well as IV antibiotics.

Symptomatic Cholelithiasis (Biliary Colic): Gallstones, when symptomatic, cause colicky RUQ pain after fatty meals when the gallbladder contracts against a stone lodged in the cystic duct under the stimulation of CCK. Murphy's sign will not be present.

Cholecystitis: An inflammatory process in the gallbladder often secondary to stasis from a stone in the gallbladder neck or cystic duct or (less likely) biliary sludging. Secondary infection often occurs, especially with *Escherichia coli, Enterococcus,* or *Klebsiella.* Clinically acute cholecystitis presents as constant or worsening RUQ pain, fever, and positive Murphy sign. Laboratory testing may reveal leukocytosis, elevated liver enzymes, and elevated alkaline phosphatase Repeated bouts of acute cholecystitis that go untreated may lead to **chronic cholecystitis.** Chronic cholecystitis can lead to calcium deposition, which makes the gallbladder radiopaque and is called a **porcelain gallbladder.** Porcelain gallbladder may predispose patients to adenocarcinoma and so is treated with prophylactic cholecystectomy.

Cholangitis: Bacterial infection of the biliary tree that causes a clinically severe presentation of **fever, RUQ pain, and jaundice** (Charcot triad). It may progress to include **hypotension** and **altered mental status** (Reynolds pentad). Expect elevation in AST, ALT, conjugated bilirubin, and alkaline phosphatase levels. Elevated amylase and lipase levels suggest associated pancreatitis. In this context, abdominal ultrasound revealing gallstones is highly suggestive of cholangitis. Endoscopic retrograde cholangiopancreatography (ERCP) would be diagnostic and therapeutic.

Acute Pancreatitis: Symptoms of epigastric abdominal pain radiating to the back, with elevated amylase and lipase levels (lipase is more specific). Usually caused by gallstones present in the ampulla causing reflux of pancreatic enzymes, leading to autodigestion and inflammation of the pancreas. Alcohol use is also a common cause. Other causes include hypertriglyceridemia (>1000 mg/dL), hypercalcemia, trauma, mumps virus, and medications (especially antiretrovirals and diuretics). An interesting but rare cause of pancreatitis is a scorpion sting. Presentation ranges from mild pain to life-threatening inflammation with multisystem organ failure.

- **Necrotizing pancreatitis** is a particularly severe form of pancreatitis characterized by hemorrhage into pancreatic tissue with associated necrosis of acinar, ductal, and islet tissue.
- **Pancreatic pseudocysts** are a potential complication of acute pancreatitis. Necrotic pancreatic debris becomes surrounded by fibrous tissue. They are termed "pseudo" cysts because they are walled off by fibrous tissue rather than an epithelial cell layer. Pseudocysts may be asymptomatic, but they also may compress local structures or even become infected later on.

Chronic Pancreatitis: Patients may present with exocrine insufficiency (malabsorption) or endocrine insufficiency (diabetes); pain may or may not be a feature. Malabsorption often leads to a deficiency of fat-soluble vitamins (A, D, E, and K). Amylase and lipase levels are often normal. Chronic pancreatitis usually is the result of alcoholism, because ethanol can alter zymogen activation. It may also be a complication of cystic fibrosis caused by thickened pancreatic secretions. Of note, chronic pancreatitis is *not* a complication of gallstones. Abdominal radiography may reveal calcification of the pancreas (Fig. 10.26).

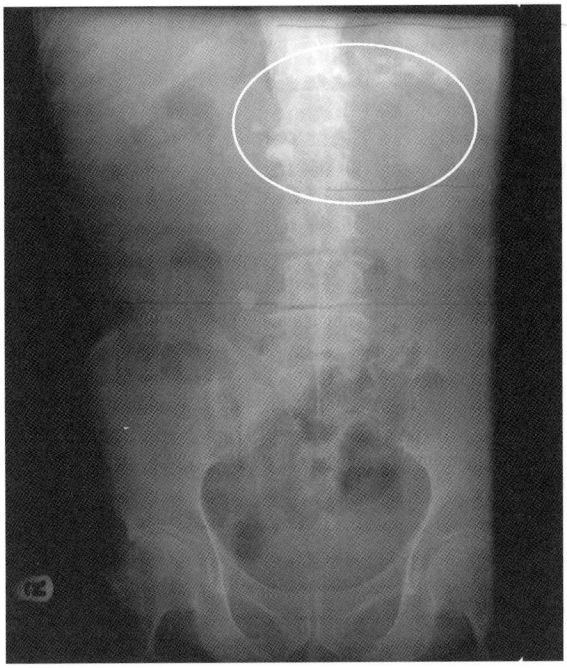

Fig. 10.26 Radiograph showing calcifications of chronic pancreatitis. (*From Lim EKS.* Medicine and Surgery. *Philadelphia: Elsevier; 2007.*)

In an alcoholic suffering from intractable steatorrhea (oily, fat-containing stool), consider chronic pancreatitis. A lack of pancreatic enzymes, including lipase, and subsequent impaired digestion contribute to this malabsorptive syndrome.

Alcohol causes chronic pancreatitis; gallstones do not.

Alcohol causes chronic pancreatitis; gallstones do not.

Pancreatic Adenocarcinoma: Patients often present with **painless jaundice,** weight loss, early satiety, and/or abdominal pain radiating to the back. Physical examination may reveal a palpable gallbladder (Courvoisier sign) or abdominal mass. Laboratory testing shows elevated bilirubin and alkaline phosphatase levels, but only if the tumor obstructs the biliary tree. These findings can be summarized as an obstructive process leading to failure of excretion of bile and bilirubin. Cancer antigen (CA) 19-9 (and to a lesser extent carcinoembryonic antigen [CEA]) are tumor markers than can be used to track response to therapy but are not sensitive or specific enough to be used in screening. Diagnosis requires imaging (often CT) and may be confirmed with biopsy (often performed endoscopically). Pancreatic cancer has a poor prognosis because it often presents late (early stages are asymptomatic) and it responds poorly to chemotherapy. A pancreaticoduodenectomy (Whipple procedure) is potentially curable if the entire mass is resected; however, metastases, especially to the liver, are often already present at the time of diagnosis. Masses in the head of the pancreas have a better prognosis because they are more likely to obstruct early and therefore can be detected early. **Trousseau sign of malignancy (migratory thrombophlebitis)** is recurrent blood clots in multiple superficial veins that occur because of the overall hypercoagulable state of malignancy. It may occur in many malignancies but is particularly associated with pancreatic adenocarcinoma.

Always consider pancreatic cancer in a patient with painless jaundice.

Hernias

A hernia is the protrusion of a peritoneal sac through a musculoaponeurotic barrier, usually a fascial defect. Inguinal hernias are common examples and often present as palpable swellings within defined regions. They may or may not be painful and may or may not be able to be reduced (pushed back into place); however, almost all hernias should be repaired because of the risk of strangulation (compromised blood supply leads to ischemia and infarction).

Inguinal Triangle (Hesselbach Triangle): The anatomic region bounded by the inguinal ligament, inferior epigastric artery, and edge of the rectus abdominis muscle. Inguinal hernias within this region are considered "direct hernias."

Direct Inguinal Hernia: A protrusion of bowel or omentum **medial** to the **inferior epigastric artery** (Fig. 10.27A). The parietal peritoneum forms the hernia sac for direct hernias. **Direct** hernias proceed **directly** through the abdominal musculature and do not pass through the inguinal canal. For this reason, they rarely are found in the scrotum. They are most common in men because of weakening of the abdominal wall.

Indirect Inguinal Hernia: A protrusion of bowel or omentum through the internal inguinal ring, the inguinal canal, and the external inguinal ring (Fig. 10.27B). The hernia sac is formed by the processus vaginalis within the scrotum. Indirect inguinal hernias are more common in infants and children because of the congenital persistence of the processus vaginalis. They occur **lateral** to the **inferior epigastric artery.** Note that **in**direct hernias pass through the **in**ternal ring, **in**to the scrotum, and are common in **in**fancy.

Femoral Hernia: A protrusion of bowel or omentum **inferior to the inguinal ligament** through the **femoral canal** (Fig. 10.27C). **Fem**oral hernias are more common in **fem**ales secondary to the wider structure of the bony pelvis.

Femoral hernias are inferior to the inguinal ligament and are more common in females.

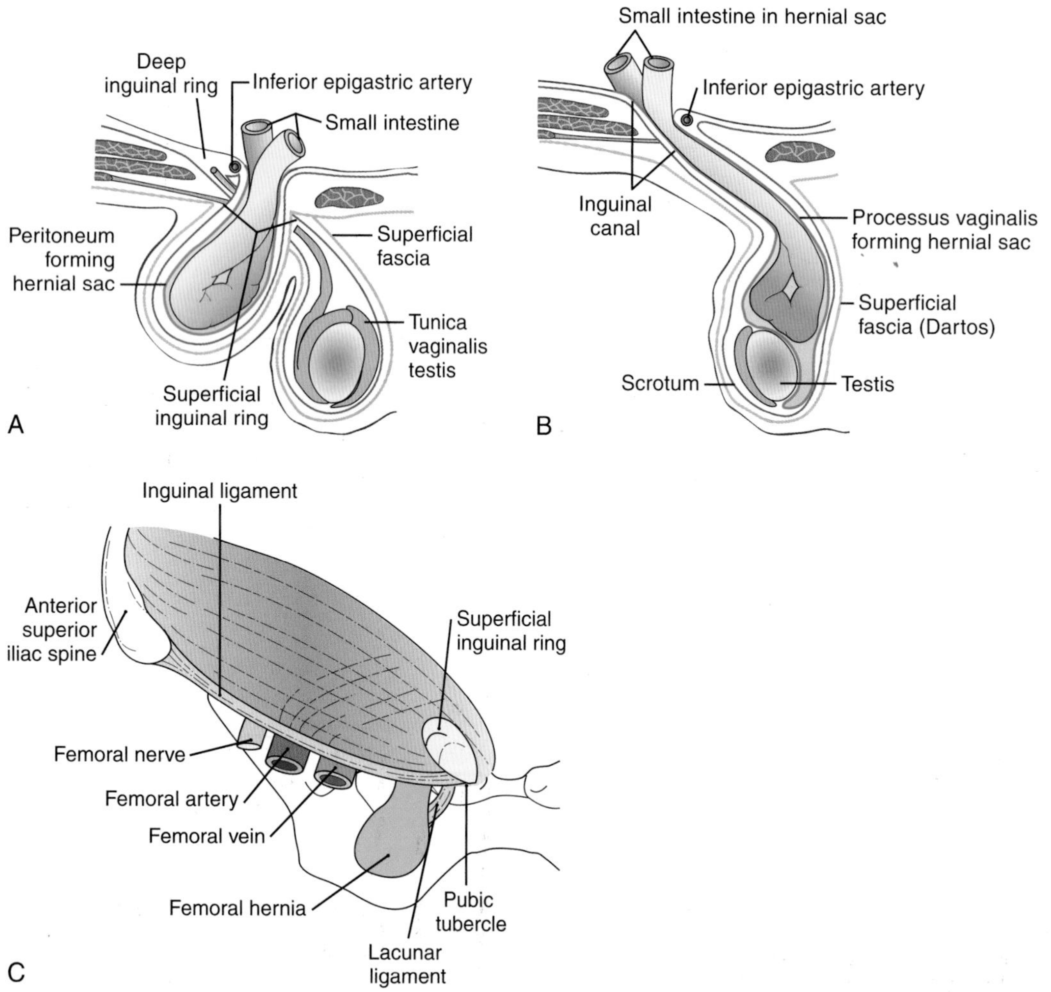

Fig. 10.27 A, Direct inguinal hernia passing medial to the inferior epigastric artery and not entering the scrotum **B,** Indirect inguinal hernia passing lateral to the inferior epigastric artery and into the scrotum. **C,** Femoral hernia passing inferior to the inguinal ligament. (**A, B** *from Moore NA, Roy WA.* Rapid Review Gross and Developmental Anatomy. *3rd ed. Philadelphia: Elsevier; 2010;* **C** *from Kontoyannis A, Sweetland H.* Crash Course: Surgery E-Book. *3rd ed. Philadelphia: Elsevier; 2008.*)

PEDIATRIC GASTROENTEROLOGY AND HEPATOLOGY

Tracheoesophageal Fistula: Congenital abnormal connection between the esophagus and trachea, most often an atresia of the upper esophagus and fistula between the lower esophagus and trachea (Fig. 10.28). It often presents at birth with copious salivation, **choking, and cyanosis** with feeding. There is also an inability to pass a nasogastric tube. It is one of the VACTERL anomalies (see Chapter 4). The presence of congenital gastrointestinal atresia should prompt evaluation for other congenital anomalies.

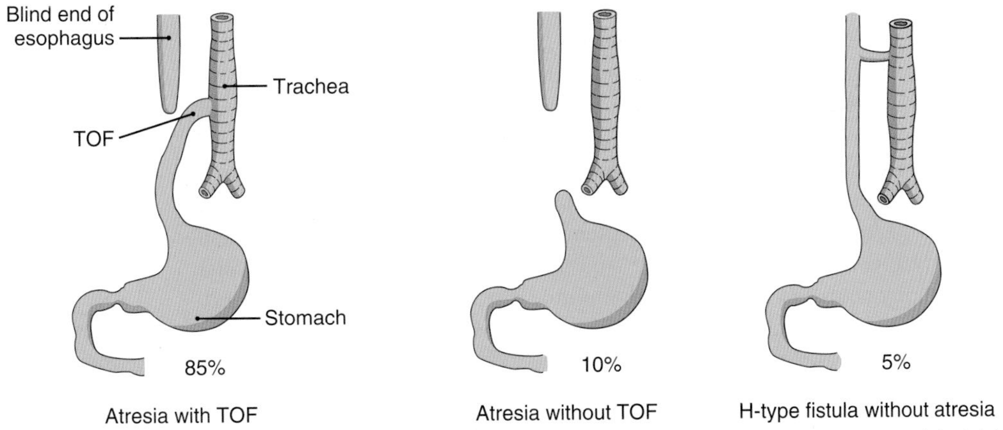

Fig. 10.28 Tracheoesophageal fistula (TOF). (*From Birnkrant J, Alario AJ.* Crash Course: Pediatrics. *Philadelphia: Elsevier; 2007.*)

Pyloric Stenosis: Hypertrophy of the muscularis propria in the pylorus leads to narrowing and lengthening of the canal and inability to pass gastric contents to the small intestine. The underlying etiology is not known, though there is a genetic component, and it is more common in firstborn boys. It presents around the **fourth week of life** as **projectile nonbilious** vomiting after feeds associated with a **voracious appetite.** A right upper quadrant abdominal mass **(palpable olive)** may be felt on physical examination. Diagnosis is accomplished with ultrasound or barium radiography. Surgery is the definitive treatment.

Duodenal Atresia: Congenital intestinal obstruction caused by failure to canalize the duodenum. It presents as **bilious vomiting** in the first days of life, earlier than pyloric stenosis. Abdominal radiography reveals the **double-bubble sign,** two air-filled spaces representing the stomach and duodenum (Fig. 10.29). Duodenal atresia is present in approximately 2.5% of neonates with Down syndrome.

Vomitus in pyloric stenosis is nonbilious. It is bilious in duodenal atresia.

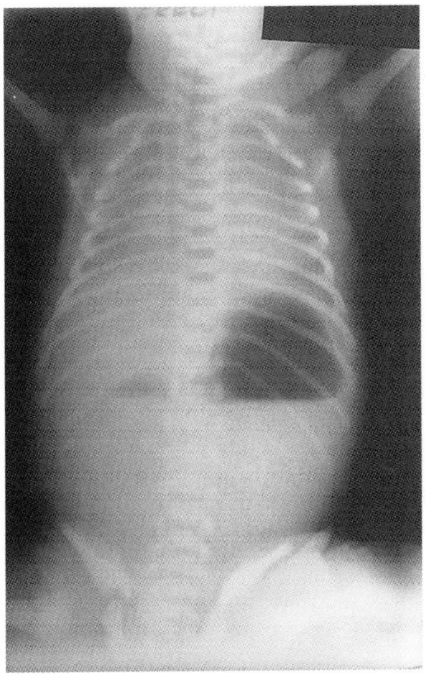

Fig. 10.29 Radiograph of double-bubble sign of duodenal atresia. (*From Lissauer T, Clayden G.* Illustrated Textbook of Pediatrics. *4th ed. Edinburgh: Elsevier; 2011.*)

Meconium Ileus: Presents as failure to pass meconium and almost **pathognomonic of cystic fibrosis.** Abnormal GI secretions cause thickened meconium that can obstruct the lumen of the small bowel. Ileus is actually a misnomer because this is a mechanical obstruction, not a motility disorder.

Congenital Aganglionic Megacolon (Hirschsprung Disease): Presents as failure to pass meconium. This condition is caused by a failure of embryologic **neural crest cell** migration, leading to the absence of the **submucosal and myenteric plexus** in a segment of distal colon. Because there is no functional peristalsis, an obstruction occurs. A digital rectal examination may temporarily dilate the affected section, leading to a large, forceful bowel movement (squirt sign). A barium enema will display a narrowing at the affected site and dilation of proximal segments to compensate for the inability to move stool forward (a massively dilated proximal segment is called "megacolon"). Biopsy is diagnostic and reveals an absence of ganglion cells. Surgery is usually curative.

Imperforate Anus: Congenital anal atresia often presents as failure to pass meconium and absence of an anus on physical examination. Dilation of the colon will also be present. It is associated with Down syndrome and is one of the VACTERL anomalies.

Intestinal Atresia: The most commonly occurring (and tested) forms of intestinal atresia are reviewed earlier and include esophageal atresia (with fistula), duodenal atresia, and imperforate anus. Atresia may also occur at any other location along the GI tract and will usually present with symptoms of bowel obstruction.

Necrotizing Enterocolitis: A condition of premature and low-birth-weight infants in which colonic bacteria take advantage of a neonate's relatively weak immune system to invade the bowel wall. The bacterial invasion leads to pneumatosis intestinalis (air in the bowel wall) and bowel necrosis.

Neonatal Hyperbilirubinemia:

- **Physiologic jaundice:** Unconjugated hyperbilirubinemia caused by the neonatal liver's inability to compensate fully for the rapid turnover of red blood cells during the transition from fetal hemoglobin to adult hemoglobin. Jaundice usually occurs after 24 to 48 hours and improves or resolves after 1 to 2 weeks. **Kernicterus** is a potential complication of all neonatal hyperbilirubinemia and occurs when bilirubin is deposited in the brain, leading to mental disability. If bilirubin levels are concerning, phototherapy can be performed; this converts bilirubin to a water-soluble form that can be excreted without the need for conjugation.
- **Nonphysiologic jaundice:** The most severe form of neonatal jaundice is **hemolytic disease of the newborn.** It occurs when a sensitized Rh-negative mother gives birth to an Rh-positive fetus. These neonates will have an unconjugated hyperbilirubinemia immediately after birth and will have a positive direct Coombs test. Traumatic injuries during birth may also result in hematoma formation and red blood cell breakdown, leading to jaundice. Neonatal jaundice may also indicate enzymatic deficiencies such as those in Gilbert, Crigler-Najjar, Rotor, or Dubin-Johnson syndrome. **Biliary atresia** is one of the most common and severe forms of nonphysiologic jaundice. It is caused by postpartum inflammation of the extrahepatic biliary tree leading to fibrosis and obstruction. The underlying cause is not clear. The condition presents with jaundice, acholic stools, and hyperbilirubinemia in the first 3 months of life. It then progresses to cirrhosis. Definitive treatment is with surgical intervention (Kasai procedure), and many patients require liver transplantation.

> Reye syndrome presents as liver failure and encephalopathy after ingestion of acetylsalicylic acid.

Reye Syndrome: Thought to be secondary to **aspirin** use in children with viral illnesses, this condition leads to mitochondrial dysfunction. Although many systems are affected, liver failure and encephalopathy are the most distinguishing features. Therefore aspirin is generally contraindicated in children. One exception to this rule is for Kawasaki disease (Chapter 8).

Meckel Diverticulum: A true diverticulum (includes all layers of the GI gut wall) caused by a remnant of the vitelline duct (embryologic connection to yolk sac). It is commonly remembered by the **rule of 2**: found in 2% of the population, usually occurs within 2 feet of the ileocecal valve, 2 inches in length, containing two types of ectopic tissue (gastric and pancreatic), and with 2% of those affected becoming symptomatic, usually before 2 years of age. It often presents as a sudden onset of painless melena or hematochezia discovered in the diaper of an otherwise healthy and happy baby. Less commonly, the presence of gastric mucosa may cause intestinal ulcerations that mimic acute appendicitis (as a result of secretion of acid). A technetium scan is used for diagnosis because it detects the ectopic gastric mucosa. Treatment is surgical removal.

Annular Pancreas: Embryologic abnormality in which a bifid ventral pancreatic bud grows around the duodenum. If symptomatic, it can lead to obstruction of the duodenum and projectile vomiting within the first few days of life. This is in contrast to another congenital abnormality, pancreas divisum, where the embryologic dorsal and ventral buds fail to fuse, leading to two pancreatic ducts. May be associated with pancreatitis.

Babies with Meckel diverticulum appear well but often have copious blood in their stool.

PHARMACOLOGY

Antiemetics

Ondansetron

Ondansetron is a serotonin 5-HT3 antagonist. This drug is generally well tolerated with few complications; however, QT prolongation is a potential side effect.

Metoclopramide

Metoclopramide's antiemetic property is from its effects as a **dopamine antagonist,** but its **muscarinic activity** increases upper GI motility. This is why it is also used as a prokinetic agent in conditions such as diabetic gastroparesis. Metoclopramide has an overlapping mechanism of action with antipsychotics, so extrapyramidal side effects (e.g., dystonia, parkinsonism, irreversible tardive dyskinesia) may occur. Metoclopramide should be avoided in patients with suspected small bowel obstruction because the prokinetic activity may actually worsen the symptoms or precipitate perforation. Should also be avoided in patients with Parkinson disease.

Look out for dystonic reactions in patients on metoclopramide.

Antacids

Proton Pump Inhibitors

Proton pump inhibitors directly inhibit H^+-K^+-ATPase on gastric parietal cells, thereby lowering gastric H^+ secretion and raising pH (Fig. 10.30). Medications end in the suffix "-prazole" (e.g., omeprazole, pantoprazole). Note that a higher gastric pH will cause increased gastrin release via a feedback loop. Long-term use has been associated with pneumonia and enteric (including *C. difficile*) infections.

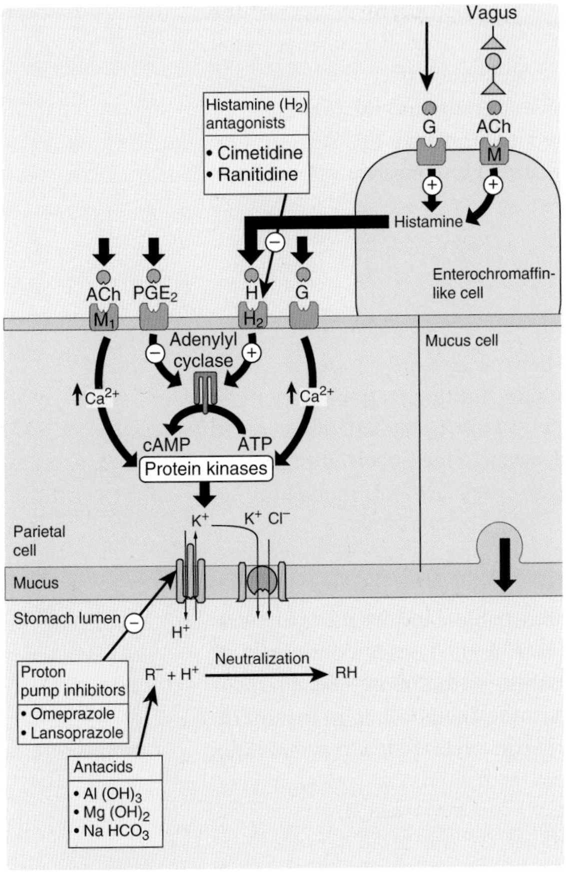

FIG. 10.30 Pharmacologic and physiologic effects on acid secretion by gastric parietal cell. *(From Barnes DW. Crash Course: Pharmacology. Philadelphia: Elsevier; 2006.)*

Histamine-2 Blockers

Histamine-2 (H2) blockers antagonize H2 receptors on parietal cells, causing decreased cAMP activation of H^+,K^+-ATPase (see Fig. 10.30). Medications end in the suffix "-tidine" (e.g., cimetidine, ranitidine, famotidine). Of note, cimetidine inhibits multiple cytochrome P-450 enzymes, leading to elevated levels of interacting medications. Other noninteracting H2 blockers are generally preferred.

H2 blockers decrease cAMP activation in parietal cells.

Weak Bases

Weak bases neutralize gastric hydrochloric acid. Examples include sodium bicarbonate, calcium carbonate, and aluminum hydroxide. They provide symptomatic relief of mild GERD.

Cytoprotective Agents

Bismuth Sucralfate

Bismuth sucralfate binds the ulcer base, protecting it against the acidic environment and digestive enzymes.

Misoprostol

Misoprostol is a prostaglandin E1 analog that promotes gastric secretion of mucus, bicarbonate, and gastrin. It is used to prevent NSAID-induced ulcers. Because misoprostol is a prostaglandin E_1 analog, it is also used as a cervical ripening agent for induction of labor. It can also be used to maintain patent ductus arteriosus in congenital heart anomalies by the same mechanism of action.

Inflammatory Bowel Disease Management

Sulfasalazine

Sulfasalazine is a precursor to the NSAID 5-aminosalicylic acid (5-ASA). This compound is used in the treatment of IBD because it is not converted to its active form until reaching the ileum. Its adverse effects on the gastric mucosa are thus avoided. Furthermore, it is poorly absorbed in the small bowel, so it can reach sufficiently high concentrations to be locally antiinflammatory without causing systemic side effects.

Others

Glucocorticoids may be needed to manage IBD. If still unresponsive, immunomodulators such as 6-mercaptopurine, azathioprine, and methotrexate should be considered (see Chapter 11). Anti–tumor necrosis factor (TNF) biologic therapy such as adalimumab and infliximab is generally reserved for refractory cases (see Chapter 12).

Other Agents

Statins

Statins are HMG-CoA reductase inhibitors, which interfere with hepatic cholesterol synthesis by inhibiting the transformation of HMG-CoA into mevalonic acid, the rate-limiting step in cholesterol synthesis. To have sufficient cholesterol to produce bile acids, hepatocytes must upregulate cholesterol receptors. Increased LDL receptors lead to a decrease in serum LDL levels. Side effects are rare but include hepatotoxicity and myositis, so ALT, AST, and creatine kinase levels are monitored during treatment.

Statins prevent HMG-CoA conversion to mevalonic acid.

Cholestyramine

Cholestyramine is a bile acid–binding resin that renders bile salts unabsorbable. Initially this drug was used to lower cholesterol by increasing the loss of bile salts, thereby increasing the hepatic conversion of cholesterol to bile salts. Currently cholestyramine is generally used for those with disease of the terminal ileum (e.g., Crohn disease). Bile salts that are not absorbed in the terminal ileum act as an irritant in the colon. Cholestyramine binds these irritants and prevents their cathartic effect. Side effects include GI upset and cholesterol gallstones. Because cholestyramine interferes with lipid absorption, it may interfere with the absorption of fat-soluble vitamins and medications.

Loperamide

Loperamide decreases GI motility via **opioid** receptor–induced cholinergic inhibition of the enteric nervous system. Like all opioids, loperamide is an agonist at the opioid receptor. It does not cross the blood–brain barrier, however, so it does not have analgesic properties.

Octreotide

Octreotide is a synthetic somatostatin used in the treatment of esophageal varices because of its effects as a splanchnic vasoconstrictor. Additionally, because of its inhibitory effects on the endocrine system, it is used in the treatment of VIPoma, gastrinoma, glucagonoma, carcinoid syndrome, and acromegaly.

Orlistat

Orlistat is a pancreatic lipase inhibitor that prevents the digestion of triglycerides into free fatty acids. It is used in the treatment of obesity. Because triglycerides are no longer digested or absorbed, they are excreted in the feces. This may cause the predictable side effect of steatorrhea when large quantities of fat are consumed.

Octreotide is a synthetic somatostatin and splanchnic vasoconstrictor.

REVIEW QUESTIONS

(1) If you were to perform a midline incision for an exploratory laparotomy, which layers of the abdominal wall would you cut through?
(2) Which anatomic structures contribute to peristalsis?
(3) After ingesting a steak, what glycoprotein binds vitamin B_{12} (cobalamin)? What type of cell secretes this compound, and where are they both absorbed?
(4) Can you describe the life cycle of a bile salt?
(5) Which enzyme is responsible for fat digestion at each level of the GI tract?
(6) What is the pathologic mechanism of achalasia caused by *Trypanosoma cruzi*?
(7) A 23-year-old woman presents with acute onset of severe chest pain. On physical examination, you note calluses of her knuckles, poor dentition, and swelling of her parotid glands. Laboratory tests reveal hypochloremic metabolic alkalosis. What diagnostic tests should you consider?
(8) A patient with chronic gnawing epigastric pain develops sudden-onset, severe, diffuse abdominal pain. What might be seen on a chest radiograph?
(9) A patient with long-standing abdominal pain and diarrhea presents with erythematous vesicles and papules on his elbows. How would you confirm the diagnosis and what is the best management option?
(10) A 35-year-old woman presents with approximately 2 years of abdominal cramping, which is only relieved with passage of loose stool. She often has several loose bowel movements a day, which occasionally are covered in mucus. Extensive evaluation with laboratory and endoscopic studies are unremarkable. What is the most likely diagnosis?
(11) A patient presents with acute-onset RUQ pain, fever, and jaundice. Laboratory tests reveal elevated AST, ALT, AP, and total bilirubin levels. What is in your differential diagnosis, and how can you determine the cause?
(12) A patient with hereditary spherocytosis has RUQ pain. What should be high on your differential?
(13) A patient with no history of alcohol use and no gallstones develops acute epigastric abdominal pain that radiates to his back. He has a strong family history of cardiac death before age 40. On physical examination, he has yellow papules over his body. What is the likely cause of his symptoms, and what laboratory test would be specific in diagnosing the cause?
(14) A longtime alcoholic presents with gynecomastia, spider angiomata, and nontender swelling of his abdomen and scrotum. Physical examination is notable for a positive fluid wave. What is the pathogenesis of the abdominal swelling?
(15) What is the differential diagnosis for a newborn who fails to pass meconium, and what are the distinguishing features of the top items on your differential?
(16) What is the differential diagnosis for severe vomiting in the neonatal period, and what are the key features of the top items on your differential?

(17) A 2-month-old infant boy presents to the emergency department after his mother discovers a diaper full of bright red blood. The baby is otherwise healthy and is in no distress. What is the pathophysiology of this process?
(18) A patient with GERD is prescribed ranitidine. What is this drug's mechanism of action?
(19) A patient with Crohn disease decides to self-medicate with ibuprofen instead of sulfasalazine. What is the likely result?
(20) A 62-year-old man with chronic lower back pain complains of constipation. His doctor recently prescribed him a new pain medication. What is causing his symptoms?

11 HEMATOLOGY AND ONCOLOGY

Manuel Celedon

Hematology is the study of the physiology and pathology of blood and blood-forming organs. The pluripotent hematopoietic stem cell (HSC) is the precursor to all cells in blood and also gives rise to cells of the lymphoid system. As a result, lymph nodes and lymph tissue are included in the study of hematology. The organs associated with hematology are usually defined by the sites in which pathologic conditions can arise; these include the bone marrow, lymph nodes, and intravascular compartment. The intravascular compartment is where blood cells circulate and includes the endothelial cell lining of blood vessels as well as the proteins in the blood plasma.

ANATOMY

Blood

Blood is a specialized connective tissue composed of red blood cells (RBCs), white blood cells (WBCs), and platelets suspended in plasma.

Blood Cells: Blood cells include three major types: (1) erythrocytes (RBCs), (2) leukocytes (WBCs), and (3) platelets. About 45% of the total blood volume is made up of blood cells.

Plasma: The straw-colored liquid that suspends the blood cells in whole blood. **Blood plasma** is obtained by centrifugation of whole blood and is the acellular liquid that remains after the blood cells are removed. **Plasma contains clotting factors (unlike serum)** and other components, such as dissolved proteins and electrolytes. Blood plasma makes up the other 55% of total blood volume. **Pl**asma is serum **plu**s clotting factors.

Serum: This is blood plasma without clotting factors. As noted, the HSC is the precursor to cells in the blood and lymphoid system. The HSC has the ability to differentiate into one of two cells, the common myeloid progenitor (CMP) cell or the common lymphoid progenitor (CLP) cell (Fig. 11.1). The myeloid system originates from CMP cells which can give rise to RBCs, WBCs, and platelets. The cells of myeloid lineage arise in the bone marrow. CLP cells generate both T and B lymphocytes through a process called lymphopoiesis.

The Myeloid Lineage

Erythrocytes (RBCs) are specialized **biconcave anucleate cells that carry oxygen** to and carbon dioxide from tissues via the hemoglobin protein. To maximize gas exchange (O_2 and CO_2), RBCs have a large surface area–to–volume ratio. Also, in an effort to increase their oxygen-carrying capacity, as RBCs mature, they lose most of their cell contents (including their nucleus and other organelles, such as ribosomes and mitochondria) and replace them with hemoglobin. As a result of the loss of their mitochondria, they can only use glucose as a source of energy and obtain adenosine triphosphate (ATP) mostly via glycolysis (<10% of ATP comes from hexose monophosphate shunt). As the RBC ages, it loses its energy-producing capabilities, causing its cell membrane to stiffen. These "stiff" old RBCs are at increased risk of getting caught up in the splenic circulation and being removed by splenic macrophages. **The RBC life span is about 120 days.**

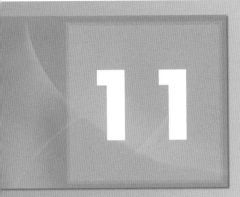

Fetal erythropoiesis, or RBC production, occurs in different places (with some overlap) throughout the lifespan of the fetus. It begins in the **yolk sac** (3-8 weeks), then the **liver** (6 weeks–birth), followed by the **spleen** (10-28 weeks) and **bone marrow** (18 weeks–adulthood). This is popularly summarized through the mnemonic **Y**oung **L**iver **S**ynthesized **B**lood.

Reticulocyte: An **immature RBC** that has expelled most of its cellular content but still **contains a reticular (meshlike) network of ribosomal RNA.** Reticulocytes account for less than 2% of RBCs in the peripheral blood; this percentage is reflected in the reticulocyte count.

Key Definitions

- **Erythrocytosis** or **polycythemia** is an increase in the number of RBCs.
- **Anisocytosis** refers to red blood cells of varying **s**izes.
- **Poikilocytosis** refers to red blood cells of varying sha**pe**s.

Neutrophils **L**ike **M**aking **E**verything **B**etter! WBC differential from highest percentage to lowest: **N**eutrophils **L**ymphocytes **M**onocytes **E**osinophils **B**asophils

Leukocytes

Leukocytes (WBCs) are the blood cells that help the body fight infections or mount inflammatory responses. The normal count ranges from 4,000 to 10,000 cells/μL. Leukocytes can be divided into five subtypes, referred to as the WBC differential (in order, from highest percentage to lowest): **n**eutrophils, **l**ymphocytes, **m**onocytes, **e**osinophils, **b**asophils (see mnemonic in the accompanying box).

Neutrophils: Also referred to as polymorphonuclear neutrophils (PMNs) or segmented neutrophils because they contain a nucleus with multiple segments (see Fig. 11.1). Neutrophils account for 50% to 80% of the total WBC count. These cells are an essential part of the innate immune system. **Neutrophils are typically the first responders in the acute phase of inflammation and are the predominant cells in pus.** They act to phagocytize (engulf) and digest bacteria, cellular debris, and dead tissue. In the circulation, half are marginated (or adherent to the endothelial cells of blood vessels) and the other half are in the peripheral circulation. They exit the circulation via chemotactic stimuli in a process called diapedesis. Neutrophils can be divided into three morphologic groups:

- **Nonsegmented** (band) neutrophils are **immature** neutrophils that can be seen in acute infections or inflammation. The bone marrow is sending out everything it has to fight an infection, even if the cells are not fully mature.
- **Segmented** mature or morphologically appropriate neutrophils with three to five nuclear lobes.

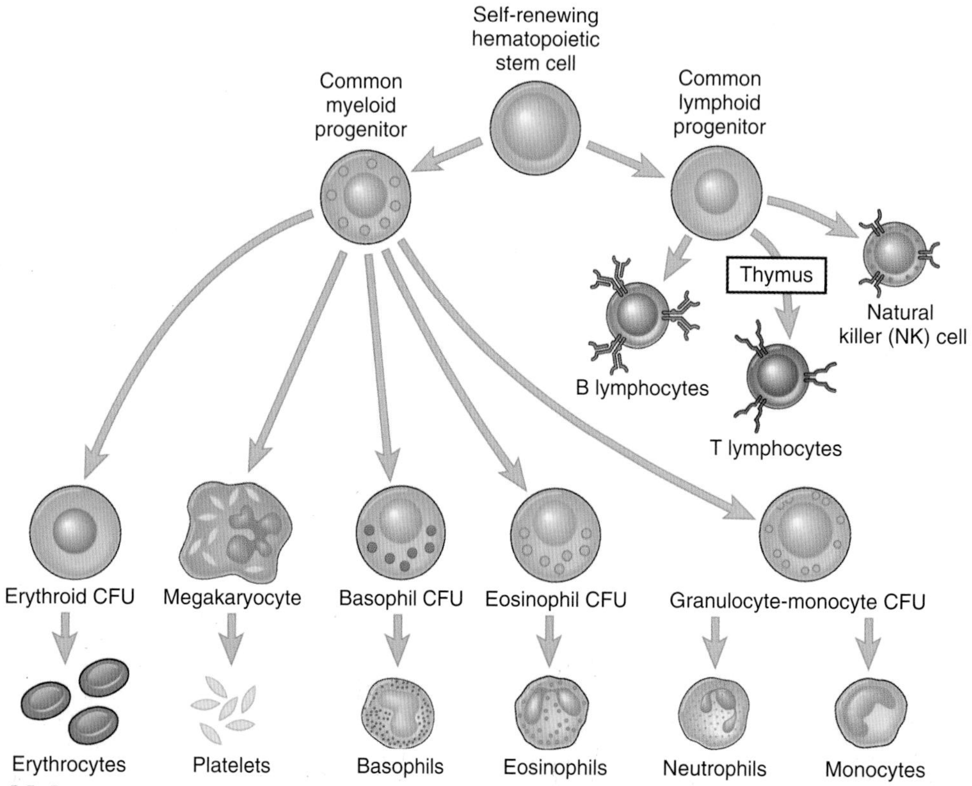

FIG. 11.1 Erythropoiesis and the differentiation of the self-renewing hematopoietic stem cell into a common myeloid progenitor cell, which can make erythrocytes, platelets, basophils, eosinophils, neutrophils, and monocytes, or a common lymphoid progenitor cell, which can make B and T lymphocytes and natural killer cells. CFU, Colony-forming unit. (From Abbas AK. Cellular and Molecular Immunology Updated Edition. *6th ed. New York: Elsevier; 2009.*)

- **Hypersegmented** neutrophils usually have more than five lobes and are associated with vitamin B_{12} or folate deficiencies.

Mnemonic for the causes of eosinophilia: **NAACP**
Neoplasia
Asthma
Allergies
Collagen vascular disease
Parasites

Monocytes are large mononuclear cells that are easily recognizable by their kidney-shaped nucleus and account for 2% to 10% of all WBCs. Monocytes become macrophages when they leave the bloodstream and enter into tissue. **They form part of the mononuclear phagocyte system and act to clean up circulating debris, microorganisms, senescent RBCs, and damaged cells.** Macrophages survive in tissues for up to 80 days and are named by their tissue or origin (e.g., Kupffer cells in the liver, alveolar macrophages in lungs, oligodendrocytes or glial cells in brain). Monocytes and macrophages function as antigen-presenting cells by phagocytosing pathogens and displaying proteins from them on their cell surface (via major histocompatibility complex [MHC] class II) for recognition by lymphocytes.

Eosinophils are cells with bilobed nuclei and have prominent eosinophilic (reddish-orange) granules (see Fig. 11.1). They account for 1% to 6% of WBCs. **They contain proteins, such as major basic protein (MBP), in their granules that are released (degranulated) in response to immune stimulus by foreign proteins.** MBP is important in defending against helminthic and protozoan infections. Eosinophils are increased in invasive parasitic infections, allergic processes, and neoplasms.

Basophils also have bilobed nuclei but have granules that stain **b**lue (**b**asic stain; basophilic granules). They account for less than 1% of WBCs. **They are most commonly involved in inflammatory reactions that cause allergic symptoms.** They express immunoglobulin E (IgE) receptors that release histamine, heparin, prostaglandins, leukotrienes, and other vasoactive amines when stimulated. Basophils are very similar to mast cells, but basophils exist in the blood whereas mast cells exist in the tissue. Mast cells are involved in type I hypersensitivity reactions and mediate allergic reactions via the release of histamine. Basophil levels are often elevated in patients with myeloproliferative disorders such as chronic myelogenous leukemia.

Platelets or thrombocytes are anucleate cell fragments that play a central role in hemostasis (blood coagulation). They are derived from the cytoplasm of megakaryocytes in the bone marrow. The life span of platelets is about 7 to 10 days, with the first 2 days of life spent in the spleen. This becomes important in congestive or inflammatory disorders that can lead to the entrapment of platelets in an enlarged spleen. The normal platelet count ranges from 150,000 to 400,000/mm^3.

The Lymphoid Lineage

Lymphocytes are also leukocytes (as are all white blood cells), but these originate from CLP cells in the bone marrow and are therefore of lymphoid, rather than myeloid, lineage. They are small round cells with a small amount of cytoplasm and densely staining nuclei (Fig. 11.2). They normally account for 25% to 33% of WBCs. There are four types of lymphocytes: T cells, B cells, plasma cells, and natural killer (NK) cells.

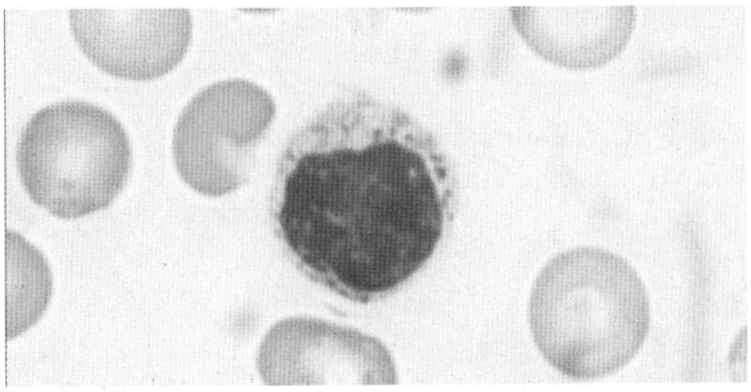

FIG. 11.2 A lymphocyte, showing the characteristic large densely staining nucleus. (*From Stevens A, Lowe JS.* Human Histology. *3rd ed. Philadelphia: Elsevier; 2004.*)

MHC × CD = 8
MHC I × CD8 = 8
MHC II × CD4 = 8

T lymphocytes are **primarily responsible for mediating the cellular immune response.** They are made in the bone marrow and later migrate to the thymus, where they begin to mature. Once they mature, they leave the thymus and reside in the lymphoid tissues. T cells can be distinguished from other lymphocytes by the presence of a T-cell receptor. They differentiate into helper T cells, cytotoxic T cells, and suppressor T cells.

Helper T cells or CD4 T cells help other WBCs complete their immunologic tasks (e.g., maturation of B cells into plasma cells, activation of macrophages or cytotoxic T cells). They express CD4 and recognize their targets by binding MHC II. MHC II is expressed on the surface of antigen presenting cells (see Chapter 6 for a discussion of MHC).

Cytotoxic T cells or CD8 T cells help eliminate tumor cells and cells infected by viruses. They express CD8 and recognize their targets by binding MHC I. MHC I is expressed on the surface of almost every cell in the body except anucleate cells such as platelets and red blood cells.

B lymphocytes are part of the humoral immune system. Their **primary functions are to create antibodies against antigens, act as APCs, and develop into memory cells for future immune response.** They are made in the **b**one marrow, partly mature in the bone marrow, and later migrate to lymphoid tissues. Large quantities of B cells reside in the follicles of lymph nodes and white pulp of the spleen. The terminal differentiation of a B cell happens in the peripheral lymph tissues, such as lymph nodes, when they encounter antigens. Once they encounter an antigen, B cells differentiate into plasma cells that can produce antibodies.

NK cells are a part of the innate immune system and are a type of cytotoxic lymphocyte. They play a large role in the destruction of cells infected by viruses and neoplasms. They work by releasing proteins (perforin and granzyme) that induce programmed cell death (apoptosis).

PHYSIOLOGY

Blood Groups: ABO and Rh Systems

Blood grouping is based on the following: (1) the presence of surface antigen(s) on RBCs; (2) the presence of plasma antibodies (Ab) against antigen(s) that are not present on host RBCs; and (3) the presence or absence of Rh factor.

The **ABO system** is an excellent example of codominant expression of alleles of a gene (Table 11.1), meaning that the contributions of both alleles are visible in the phenotype. If a person has inherited the IA and IB alleles, they will have the AB blood group phenotype and produce both A-type and B-type antigens on the RBC cell surface. **Your body always produces antibodies (Ab) against antigens not present on your RBC cell surface.**

A group: Produces A antigen on RBC surface and anti-B Ab in circulation.

B group: Produces B antigen on RBC surface and anti-A Ab in circulation.

AB group: Produces A and B antigen on RBC surface and no Abs. These patients can receive blood transfusion from all blood types because no Abs against RBC cell surface antigens are produced (universal recipient).

O group: Produces no antigens on RBC surface and anti-A and anti-B Abs. These patients can donate blood to all blood types because their RBCs lack antigen on the cell surface (universal donor).

IgM antibodies do not cross the placenta. They do not interact with the fetal circulation.

IgG antibodies do cross the placenta and can be transferred into the fetal circulation.

The **Rh system** is based on the presence or absence of the five most important antigens—D, C, c, E and e—on the RBC cell surface. However, the most clinically important antigen is the **D antigen** (it is the most immunogenic). Strictly speaking, when a person is said to be **Rh-positive,** that person **produces the D antigen.** Unlike the ABO system, Rh antibodies are only made if an Rh-negative person is exposed to Rh-positive blood. At baseline, **Rh-negative** people **do not produce the D antigen** on their RBC cell surface and do not produce anti-Rh Abs.

At baseline, Rh-negative people do not produce the D antigen on their RBC cell surface and do not produce anti-Rh Abs. Rh-negative individuals can become sensitized (i.e., produce anti-Rh Abs) during a blood transfusion from Rh-positive blood.

Another example of acquiring anti-Rh Abs is during pregnancy. An Rh-negative mother carrying an Rh-positive fetus will be exposed to Rh-positive blood if there is significant fetomaternal hemorrhage (e.g. during a miscarriage or antepartum bleeding), or during delivery. In instances of fetomaternal

TABLE 11.1 Phenotype (Expressed) and Genotype (Genetic Makeup) for Red Blood Cell Surface Proteins

PHENOTYPE	GENOTYPE
A	AA or AO
B	BB or BO
AB	AB
O	OO

hemorrhage Rh immunoglobulin (RhoGAM) is given to Rh-negative mothers. Rh-negative mothers also receive RhoGAM at 28 weeks of pregnancy and within 72 hours after delivery.

Hemostasis: The Coagulation Cascade

Hemostasis is the cessation of blood flow through a blood vessel or body tissue and is the physiologic end point after injury to a vessel wall or tissue. Normally, the endothelial cells of intact vessels prevent hemostasis by continually secreting anticoagulants and inhibitors of platelet aggregation. When injury to the vessel wall occurs, the endothelial cells cease to produce these inhibitors and instead release procoagulation factors (von Willebrand factor and tissue thromboplastin) that initiate hemostasis. Normally, hemostasis and thrombosis result from a careful interplay between protein and cell components. The first component (protein) involves a group of proteins that specialize in **coagulation** (clot formation), **fibrinolysis** (clot dissolution), and **anticoagulation** (regulation of clot formation). The three protein components work to balance each other and localize hemostasis to the site of injury. The second component (cellular) involves platelets, endothelial cells (cells lining the blood vessel wall), neutrophils, and monocytes.

The initial part of hemostasis involves the following: (1) the formation of a platelet plug, followed by (2) blood coagulation and (3) growth of fibrous tissue into the clot to repair the site of injury. A **platelet plug** (Fig. 11.3) begins to form on vessel injury and acts as a temporizing measure to repair injury to blood vessels. This process happens in three steps—**adhesion, aggregation, and platelet swelling.**

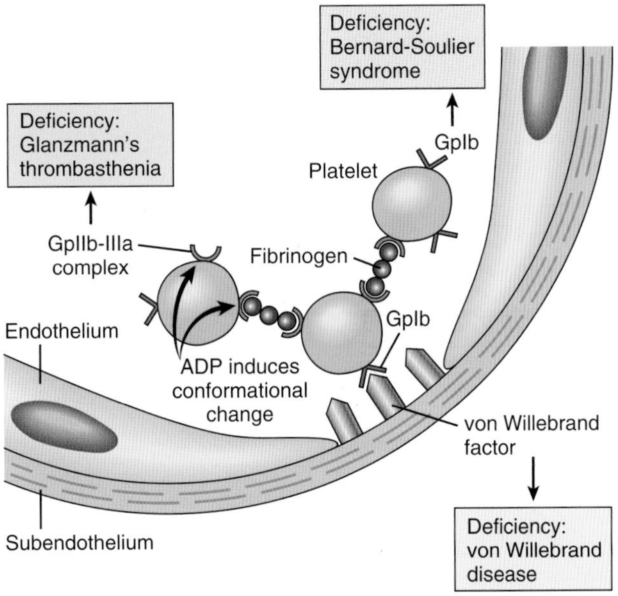

Fig. 11.3 Platelet adhesion and aggregation. von Willebrand factor is the bridge that allows the platelet glycoprotein Ib (GpIb) receptor to adhere to the subendothelium of the damaged blood vessel. To allow platelets to bind to other platelets, fibrinogen is the bridging molecule and uses the platelet GpIIb-IIIa receptor. Also shown are deficiency states causing improper platelet adhesion and/or aggregation. ADP, adenosine diphosphate. (*From Kumar V, Abbas AK, Fausto N, Aster J.* Robbins & Cotran Pathologic Basis of Disease. *8th ed. New York: Elsevier; 2009.*)

Adhesion

This occurs when injury to the blood vessel wall exposes subendothelial collagen. **von Willebrand factor (vWF)** is released and binds to the **glycoprotein Ib (GpIb)** receptor on the platelet surface. At the site of injury, vWF is released from the endothelium and from the platelet, helping to form additional links between the platelets and exposed collagen fibrils. **vWF** also circulates in the plasma bound to factor VIII, acting as a stabilizer for **factor VIII.** Therefore **vWF deficiency also causes decreased factor VIII levels.**

Aggregation

Aggregation involves a complex balance between factors that favor aggregation versus those that prevent aggregation. Undamaged endothelium secretes inhibiting factors (e.g., prostacyclin) that prevent aggregation. Increased turbulence at a site of damaged endothelium promotes aggregation. Activated platelets release adenosine diphosphate (ADP), thromboxane A_2 (TXA_2), vWF, calcium, serotonin, and other factors, which in turn help activate additional platelets and promote aggregation. ADP interacts with the ADP receptor on the platelet surface and initiates a cascade that promotes the insertion of **glycoprotein IIb/IIIa** (GpIIb/GpIIIa) receptors on the platelet surface. The GpIIb/GpIIIa receptor, a **calcium-dependent receptor,** on the platelet surface binds fibrinogen and helps cross-link adjacent platelets, an important final step in primary hemostasis.

Platelet Swelling

Platelet swelling occurs as soon as platelets attach to the injured surface. Activated platelets undergo a conformational change of shape from spherical to stellate (star shaped). These changes help make them stickier by increasing the surface area for fibrinogen to cross-link adjacent platelets via the GpIIb/GpIIIa receptor. The end result is a large accumulation of platelets and **formation of a platelet plug (primary hemostasis)** over the site of injury. This plug is strong enough to stop bleeding until the final product of coagulation cascade, fibrin, helps **stabilize the platelet plug** via the formation of fibrin mesh **(secondary hemostasis).**

The coagulation cascade (Fig. 11.4) is initiated when there is trauma to blood vessels or tissues or if circulating blood comes into contact with subendothelial collagen. There are two basic pathways, both involving plasma clotting proteins—the **extrinsic pathway** and the **intrinsic pathway.** Both these pathways culminate in the activation of **prothrombin** (factor II) to **thrombin** (factor IIa) and **fibrinogen** to **fibrin**.

Extrinsic pathway factor: VII

Intrinsic pathway factors: VIII, IX, XI, XII

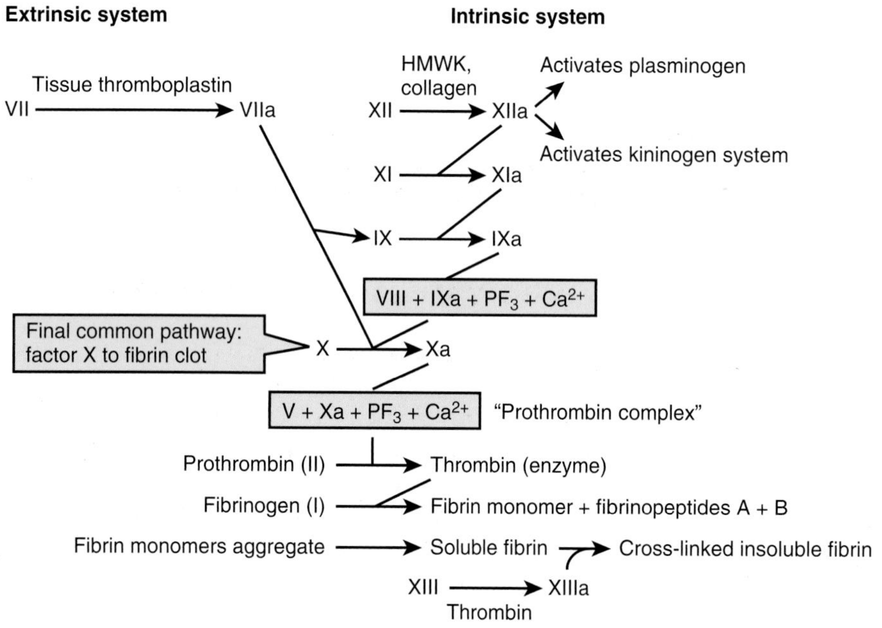

FIG. 11.4 The intrinsic and extrinsic coagulation cascade. The *a* next to the factor name refers to the activated form of that clotting factor. Ca, Calcium; HMWK, high-molecular-weight kininogen; PF, platelet factor. (*From Goljan EF.* Rapid Review Pathology Revised Reprint. *3rd ed. Philadelphia: Elsevier; 2011.*)

The **extrinsic or tissue factor (TF) pathway** begins with trauma to the endothelium of the blood vessel and is the most prominent pathway involved in the clotting cascade. After damage to blood vessels, two initiators of clotting are released, **TF** (factor III) and tissue phospholipids. **Factor VII** (FVII), a plasma-clotting factor in the circulation, comes into **contact with** the exposed **TF** and **forms an activated complex** (TF-FVIIa). FVII is one of the vitamin K–dependent clotting factors and requires calcium to form a complex with TF. The **TF-FVII complex,** along with tissue phospholipids and calcium, then **acts on factor X** to **form activated factor X** (FXa). The activation of FX to FXa is the point at which the extrinsic and intrinsic pathways converge into the common pathway. **FXa,** along with tissue phospholipids, calcium, and **factor V** (which acts as a cofactor to FXa), form a complex that **activates prothrombin** (factor II) to **thrombin** (factor IIa).

1-degree hemostasis = platelet plug formation

2-degree hemostasis = coagulation factors, fibrin strands → strengthen plug

The intrinsic, or contact activation pathway, is initiated on the activation of factor XII (Hageman factor) to factor XIIa (FXIIa). It is known as the contact system because it was discovered that FXII can autoactivate when it comes into contact with a negatively charged surface, such as a glass tube or exposed collagen from a damaged blood vessel. The activation of FXII is also facilitated by circulating high-molecular-weight kininogen (HMWK) in this setting. FXIIa simultaneously activates coagulation and anticoagulation cascades. The coagulation cascade works by amplification and the creation of large amounts of thrombin; activation of the anticoagulation cascade helps localize the thrombin production. The clotting cascade is continued by FXIIa's activation of **factor XI** to **factor XIa** (FXIa), which in turn activates **factor IX (Christmas factor)** to **factor IXa (FIXa).** FIXa forms a four-component complex with **factor VIII** (FVIII), platelet phospholipids, and calcium. This four-component complex merges into the first step of the final common pathway by activating FX to FXa. FXa, along with tissue phospholipids, calcium, and factor V, forms a complex that activates prothrombin to thrombin.

The anticoagulation cascade is initiated by FXIIa via the activation of **plasminogen** and of the **kininogen system:**

- Plasminogen is activated by **tissue plasminogen activator (tPA)** and produces **plasmin,** an enzyme that works to cleave the fibrin meshwork. This cleavage produces fibrin(ogen) degradation products (FDPs) and insoluble fibrin monomers called D-dimers.
- The kininogen system produces **kallikrein** and bradykinin. Kallikrein activates the fibrinolytic system and promotes the activation of plasminogen into plasmin, whereas bradykinin acts as part of the body's inflammatory response to increase vasodilation, vessel permeability, and pain.

Coagulation Cascade: Key Points

Prothrombin (factor II) is a vitamin K–dependent plasma protein that is produced in the liver. In the liver, epoxide reductase converts vitamin K to activated vitamin K, which acts as a cofactor for the vitamin K–dependent coagulation proteins.

The **vitamin K–dependent coagulation proteins** include factors II, VII, IX, and X, protein C, and protein S. **Warfarin** inhibits the vitamin K epoxide reductase enzyme and blocks production of these cofactors.

All vitamin K–dependent proteins require **calcium** as a cofactor.

Vitamin K deficiency leads to decreased production of factors II, VII, IX, and X, protein C, and protein S. Neonates require supplemental vitamin K at birth because their bowel lacks the bacteria that produce vitamin K.

The main actions of **thrombin** (Fig. 11.5) include the following:

- Converting fibrinogen to fibrin
- Activating factor VIII (required for intrinsic pathway) and factor V
- Activating factor XIII (fibrin stabilizing factor)

Factors that are consumed in a clot are factors I, II, V, and VIII. People will be deficient in these factors if they are constantly activating the coagulation cascade (e.g., sepsis).

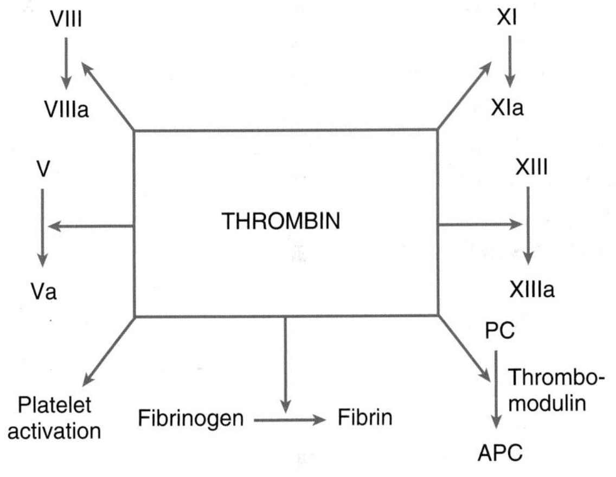

Fig. 11.5 Main actions of thrombin (factor IIa). PC, Protein C. (*From Hudnall SD.* Hematology. *Philadelphia: Elsevier; 2011.*)

Factors that enhance formation of a thrombus in vessels include the following:

- TF (factor III) is a noncirculating protein that is released from injured tissue and initiates the extrinsic pathway by activating factor VII.
- **vWF acts as the "glue" that allows platelets to adhere to exposed collagen on injured endothelium** (platelets bind vWF via GpIb receptors on their surface). It is made by endothelial cells and is also carried within platelets in their α granules.
- **TXA_2** is made within platelets; when it is released, it **acts as a vasoconstrictor** and **enhancer of platelet aggregation by improving fibrinogen attachment to its receptor on the platelet.**

Platelet and Coagulation Tests

The **ristocetin cofactor assay** helps evaluate the function of vWF by promoting platelet agglutination. Platelet agglutination caused by ristocetin (an obsolete antibiotic) can only occur in the presence of functionally normal vWF multimers.

Bleeding time (BT) is used to evaluate the function of platelets. Normal BT is from 2 to 7 minutes. Following are causes of prolonged BT:

- **Aspirin** irreversibly inhibits the platelet cyclooxygenase (COX) enzyme, thereby halting production of TXA_2. Platelet count will remain normal in these patients.
- **Thrombocytopenia** will result in abnormal BT because of the decreased number of platelets in the circulation. An increase in BT will be seen when the platelet count falls below 90,000/mm^3.
- **von Willebrand disease** is an **autosomal dominant** disorder in **which individuals lack vWF** or **have defective vWF protein.** Patients will also have a decrease in FVIII (remember that vWF complexes with FVIII to prevent its degradation), resulting in a combined platelet and coagulation factor disorder. BT and partial thromboplastin time (PTT) will be increased. Patients will also have a correctable abnormal **ristocetin cofactor assay result.** The ristocetin test result will normalize after the addition of normal plasma (which contains normal vWF).
- **Bernard-Soulier syndrome** results when platelets **lack the GpIb receptor** on their cell surface. The GpIb receptor helps bind the platelet to exposed collagen, using vWF as an intermediate; the lack of the receptor results in inappropriate platelet adhesion. This disease is characterized by prolonged BT, thrombocytopenia (because of decreased platelet survival), and increased megakaryocytes. These patients will have an abnormal ristocetin cofactor assay result that is not correctable by the addition of normal plasma; the issue is not with vWF but with abnormal circulating platelets.
- **Glanzmann disease** is an **autosomal recessive disorder in which platelets lack the GpIIb/GpIIIa receptor on their cell surface.** This receptor binds fibrinogen and promotes interplatelet aggregation. BT is significantly prolonged (think of this as a so-called congenital abciximab syndrome).
- **Uremia or renal failure** results in the accumulation of toxic products in the blood that leads to inhibition of platelet phospholipids, thereby producing a platelet aggregation defect. BT prolongation can be reversed with dialysis and desmopressin acetate.

The clinically important **coagulation tests** include PTT and prothrombin time (PT). **PTT** is used to assess the function of the intrinsic pathway and to follow **heparin** therapy. Remember that PTT has an extra T **in**side it and measures the **in**trinsic pathway. A normal PTT ranges from 25 to 40 seconds.

- PTT mainly helps evaluate function of factors VIII, IX, X, XI, and XII.

> H PiTT—heparin therapy followed by PTT (intrinsic pathway)
>
> W PeT—warfarin therapy followed by PT (extrinsic pathway)

PT is used to assess the function of the extrinsic pathway and to follow **warfarin** therapy. A normal PT ranges from 11 to 15 seconds.

- Mainly helps evaluate factor VII function.
- The international normalized ratio **(INR)** is a test that standardizes the PT across different laboratories and allows for its use in following warfarin therapy.

Anticoagulant System

The coagulation cascade is regulated by **two anticoagulant systems** that help **regulate** (by inhibiting) **clot formation.** These systems are the **protein C** and **protein S systems** and the antithrombin **(serine protease inhibitor) system.**

- **Protein C** is a vitamin K–dependent protein that, when activated, will **inactivate** factors Va and VIIIa, thereby **decreasing production of thrombin.** Protein C is activated by thrombomodulin, which is just thrombin bound to an endothelial cell membrane.
- **Protein S** is a vitamin K–dependent protein that works as a cofactor for activated protein C (APC) and helps direct antigen presenting cells to the required site of action.
- **Antithrombin III (ATIII)** is a serine protease inhibitor; therefore, it inhibits all activated serine proteases (basically inhibits all coagulation proteins):
  - Inhibits factors IIa, VIIa, IXa, Xa, XIa, and XIIa and kallikrein.
  - Its **main anticoagulant effect comes from inhibiting factors IIa and Xa.**
  - **Heparin** binds ATIII and greatly increases its anticoagulant activity, by 1000-fold, against factor IIa.

Fibrinolytic System and Tests

Factors that prevent formation of a thrombus (fibrin clot) in vessels include the following:

- **Prostaglandin I_2** (PGI_2), also known as **prostacyclin,** functions as a vasodilator and inhibitor of platelet aggregation. This prostaglandin is constitutionally produced by intact endothelial cells to prevent thrombus formation in vessels.
- Heparin-like molecules act to enhance ATIII activity, thereby inhibiting the function of factors II, IX, X, XI, and XII.
- **tPA** is an enzyme that helps activate plasminogen to plasmin. Plasmin works by degrading coagulation factors and fibrin clots.
- Proteins C and S are vitamin K–dependent factors that work to deactivate coagulation factors V and VIII.

The **fibrinolytic system (which degrades clots)** is initiated by various activators, and all work by converting plasminogen to its active form, plasmin.

- **Plasmin** cleaves the fibrin meshwork created by the coagulation cascade and creates FDPs and **D-dimers.** D-dimers are a type of FDP, so-called because it contains two cross-linked D fragments of fibrinogen. Plasmin also degrades coagulation factors I, V, and VIII.
- Activators of plasminogen include tPA, Hageman factor (factor XIIa), urokinase, and streptokinase.
- An important inhibitor of plasminogen activation is **aminocaproic acids,** used clinically to stop excessive postoperative bleeding or overdoses of tPA and streptokinase.

PATHOLOGY

Anemia

Anemia is defined as a deficiency in the number of RBCs or a below-normal level of hemoglobin (Hb) in the blood. The ability of Hb to bind oxygen by a deformity in the molecule or a decrease in its amount, plays a role in the development of anemia and results in decreased O_2 content in the blood. **General signs and symptoms of anemia include** fatigue, weakness, pallor, malaise, shortness of breath, presyncope or syncope. The anemias are primarily classified by their red cell size (via the mean corpuscular volume [MCV]) and mechanism (e.g., hemorrhage, decreased production, increased destruction). **Anemia is a sign of an underlying disease rather than a specific diagnosis.** See Fig. 11.6 for common causes of anemia and their underlying defect. To initiate appropriate treatment, one must always search for the underlying disease that led to the development of anemia. The complete blood cell count (CBC) and peripheral blood smear (PBS) are important in characterizing the disease processes that lead to anemia.

Laboratory Testing in Anemia

The **CBC** report includes **Hb,** hematocrit **(Hct), MCV, RBC count,** red blood cell distribution width **(RDW),** mean corpuscular hemoglobin concentration **(MCHC),** and mean corpuscular hemoglobin **(MCH).** Some reports will also include the **reticulocyte** count.

- **Hb** is the **most accurate value to screen for and monitor anemia;** it is a direct measure of the concentration of Hb in the blood.

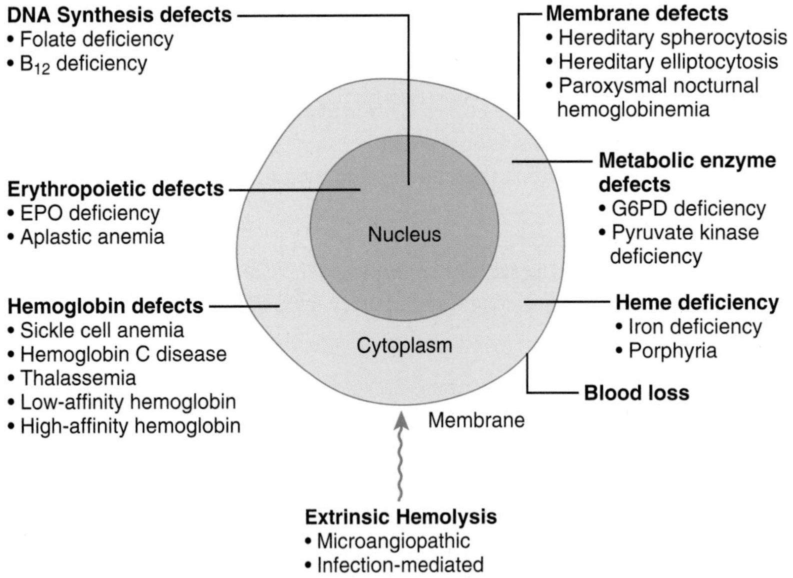

Fig. 11.6 Common causes of anemia and underlying defects. EPO, Erythropoietin; G6PD, glucose-6-phosphate dehydrogenase. (*From Hudnall SD.* Hematology. *Philadelphia: Elsevier; 2011.*)

- **Hct** is a calculated percentage value that represents the volume of RBCs in the blood relative to whole blood.
- **MCV** directly measures the average RBC volume and is obtained by dividing the Hct by the RBC count. It is used to classify anemia. The normal range is 80 to 100 fL, referred to as normocytic. Values lower than normal are referred to as microcytic (small cell); those higher than normal are macrocytic (large cell).
- **RBC count** is a direct measure of the RBCs in the blood (in RBCs per microliter of blood).
- **RBC mass** refers to the total number of RBCs in the body.
- **RDW** is a measure of the variation in width of RBCs. Usually RBCs are a uniform width; however, certain disorders can cause a significant variation in cell size. An **elevated RDW is referred to as anisocytosis.** RDW is most helpful when it is increased.
- **MCHC** is a calculated value determined by dividing the Hb by the Hct. It provides the average concentration of Hb in RBCs. An elevated MCHC, on step 1, usually is a clue for **hereditary spherocytosis.** It may be increased in diseases that result in membrane loss or cellular dehydration. It is decreased in all microcytic anemias.
- **MCH** is a calculated value determined by dividing the Hb by the RBC count. It correlates linearly with the MCV and has little clinical usefulness.

The **reticulocyte count** helps evaluate the bone marrow's response to anemia. It is a valuable test result that helps to determine quickly if anemia is caused by decreased RBC production or decreased survival of RBCs (e.g., hemorrhage, hemolysis). This value is reported as a percentage, with a normal value being lower than 3% when no anemia is present.

- An appropriate bone marrow response to anemia would result in a corrected reticulocyte count greater than 3%. If the bone marrow is not responding appropriately (marrow failure), the corrected reticulocyte count will be less than 3%.
- The value can be incorrectly elevated in anemia; as a result, you must be able to calculate the **corrected reticulocyte count:** Corrected reticulocyte count = (measured Hct/45) × reticulocyte count.
- **Polychromasia** refers to RBCs of multiple colors caused by differing amounts of Hb (Fig. 11.7). If present, you must divide the corrected reticulocyte count by 2 to get an accurate value. **Only do this extra correction if polychromasia is present.**

Hb electrophoresis measures the different types of Hb in the blood and is used in the evaluation of hemoglobinopathies, disorders of Hb structure or synthesis. Using gel electrophoresis, it separates the different types of Hb based on charge (Hb migrates from the negative cathode to the positive anode).

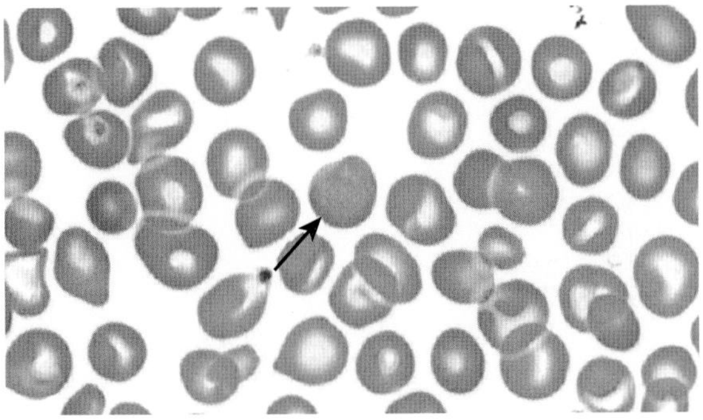

FIG. 11.7 Polychromasia. A reticulocyte *(arrow)* with the characteristic blue discoloration and absence of central pallor; when present, reticulocyte count must be divided by 2. *(From Naeim F. Atlas of Bone Marrow and Blood Pathology. Philadelphia: WB Saunders; 2001.)*

The Hb mutations that lead to the development of various hemoglobinopathies result in a net change in protein charge that is then measured by electrophoresis.

There are several types of Hb:

- **HbA:** Two α- and two β-globin chains; normally 97% of Hb in adults.
- **HbA_2:** Two α- and two δ-globin chains; normally 2% of Hb in adults.
- **HbF:** Two α- and two γ-globin chains; normally 1% of Hb in adults (fetal Hb).
  - HbF has an increased affinity for O_2 and a decreased affinity for 2,3-bisphosphoglyceric acid (2,3-BPG), facilitating oxygen extraction by fetus from maternal hemoglobin.
- **HbS:** Form of Hb found in people with sickle cell disease.
- **HbH:** Four β-globin chains. Seen in α-thalassemia major (three α-gene deletions).
  - **Hb Bart:** Four γ-globin chains (four α-gene deletions); incompatible with life; results in fetal edema and wasting (hydrops fetalis).
  - **HbC:** Abnormal Hb similar to HbS but with a different point mutation leading to the substitution of lysine for glutamic acid at position 6 on the β-globin gene.

> On Step 1, a microcytic anemia with an increased RDW refers to **iron deficiency** anemia.

Haptoglobin is a blood plasma protein that binds free Hb released by RBCs during intravascular hemolysis. It is used to screen for and monitor intravascular hemolytic anemia. Haptoglobin levels drop in intravascular hemolysis. Levels of **haptoglobin will be normal in extravascular hemolysis** because the Hb released by the destruction of RBCs in the spleen (reticuloendothelial system) is not exposed to the circulation and cannot bind haptoglobin (Fig. 11.8).

Approach to Anemia

See Fig. 11.9 for a depiction of a typical approach to anemia.

1. Determine whether patient is anemic by looking at the **Hb.**
2. Classify the anemia as microcytic, normocytic, or macrocytic by looking at the **MCV.**
3. Determine whether the bone marrow is compensating appropriately by looking at the **reticulocyte count** (use correction formulas if necessary).

Microcytic Anemias

Microcytic anemias (MCV < 80 fL) are usually a result of a disorder in the synthesis of Hb. They are further subdivided into those that are acquired and those that are inherited. Acquired microcytic anemias primarily include iron deficiency anemia (IDA), anemia of chronic disease (ACD), and sideroblastic anemia (acquired). Inherited microcytic anemias primarily include thalassemia (α and β) and X-linked inherited sideroblastic anemia.

Acquired Microcytic Anemias:

Iron Metabolism and Iron Deficiency Anemias: Iron is an essential component for the production of the heme in Hb.

Ferritin, an iron-binding protein, is the major storage form of iron. The primary site of storage is in bone marrow macrophages. Circulating serum levels of ferritin correlate with body stores of iron; therefore, **a decreased serum ferritin level is diagnostic** of IDA. Increased levels of ferritin are seen in iron overload disease (hemochromatosis) and ACD.

Hemosiderin is the insoluble degradation product of ferritin (increased deposits of hemosiderin are seen in iron overload diseases).

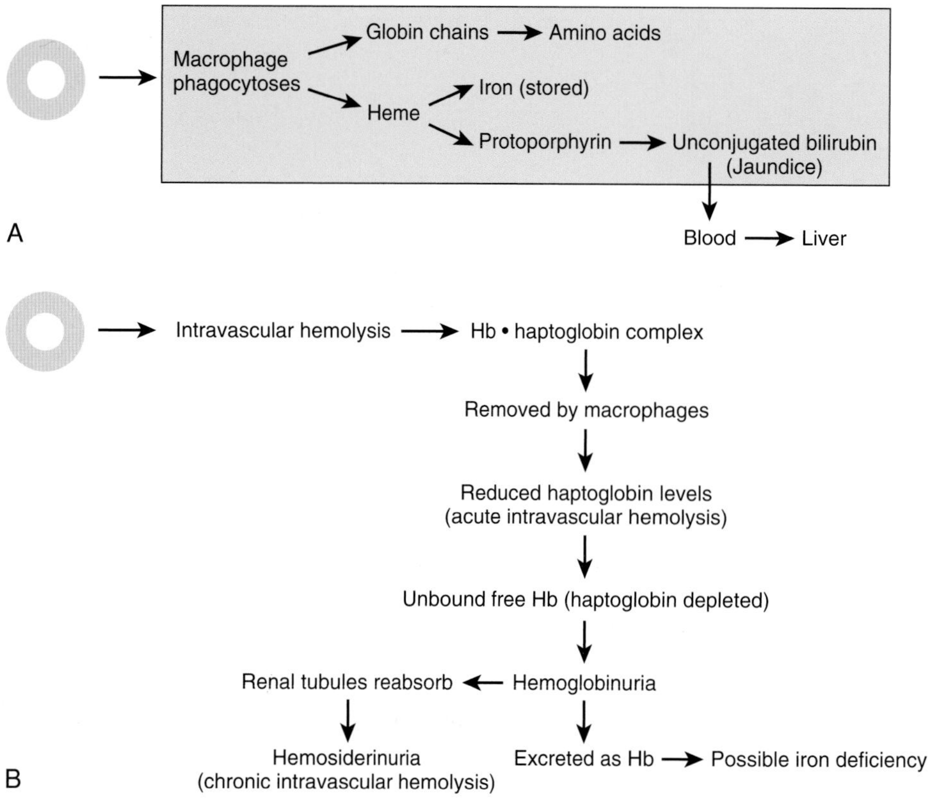

FIG. 11.8 A, Extravascular hemolysis. **B,** Intravascular hemolysis. (*From Goljan EF.* Rapid Review Pathology Revised Reprint. *3rd ed. Philadelphia: Elsevier; 2011.*)

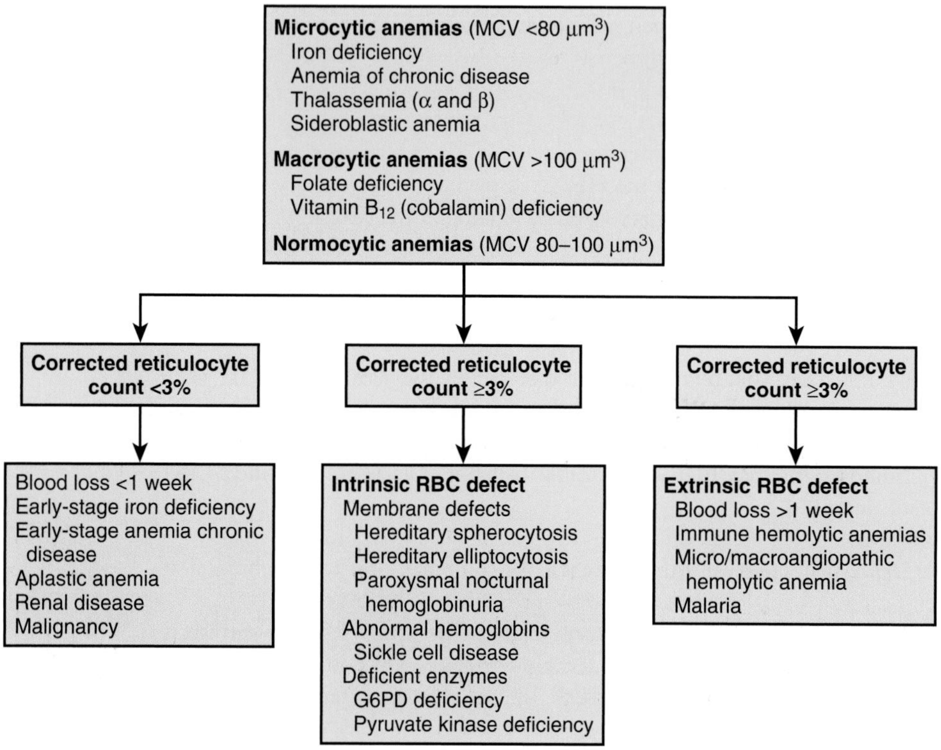

FIG. 11.9 Approach to the patient with anemia. G6PD, Glucose-6-phosphate dehydrogenase. (*From Goljan EF.* Star Series: Pathology. *Philadelphia: WB Saunders; 1998.*)

Transferrin is an iron-binding protein, synthesized in the liver, that carries iron in the blood and is measured when looking at blood iron levels. Transferrin has the capacity to bind up to 300 µg/dL of iron; this value is known as the total iron-binding capacity (TIBC).

Normally, only 33% of transferrin is saturated (referred to as iron saturation percentage). **Transferrin synthesis is inversely related to ferritin stores in macrophages.** When ferritin stores are decreased, the liver synthesizes more transferrin. Conversely, when ferritin stores are high, the liver decreases the production of transferrin. The levels of transferrin, and as a result TIBC, change, depending on several factors:

- Increases in TIBC are seen in iron deficiency, pregnancy, and those on estrogen therapy.
- Decreases in TIBC are seen in inflammation, malignancy, liver disease, and nephrotic syndrome (liver disease and nephrotic syndrome result in decreased protein production and loss of protein in urine, respectively).
- **Ferroportin** is a transmembrane protein that serves as the major regulator of iron transport into and out of a cell. This transport protein is **inhibited by hepcidin,** leading to retention of iron inside cells.

Transferrin synthesis is inversely related to ferritin stores in macrophages.

The average American absorbs 1 to 2 mg of iron/day through the duodenum into the plasma, where it is bound to transferrin. **There are two forms of iron that can be absorbed, heme and non-heme iron.** Meat contains iron in **heme,** or reduced form (ferrous, Fe^{2+}), and is directly resorbed in the duodenum. Plants contain iron in **nonheme** or oxidized form (ferric, Fe^{3+}) and cannot be directly resorbed in the duodenum without first being reduced to Fe^{2+}. Gastric acid plays an important role in releasing the iron from heme and nonheme products; therefore, the absence of stomach acid (achlorhydria) decreases the amount of iron available for reabsorption. Vitamin C (ascorbic acid) is also important in iron reabsorption because it acts to reduce nonabsorbable Fe^{3+} to absorbable Fe^{2+}.

Iron deficiency anemia (IDA) is the most common anemia and can arise from increased iron requirements or inadequate iron supply. Certain physiologic states **can increase iron requirements,** such as growth, pregnancy, or lactation. Other pathologic states **can increase iron requirements,** mainly those involving blood loss (e.g., gastritis, menorrhagia, peptic ulcer disease, Meckel diverticulum, colon cancer, or other malignancy).

- IDA in an adult is caused by blood loss until proven otherwise. Think of colon cancer in an older person with symptoms of anemia and positive heme occult test result.
- An inadequate iron supply can result from decreased intake of iron in diet or decreased absorption (e.g., celiac sprue, post–gastric surgery).

A decreased serum ferritin level is diagnostic of IDA.

Clinical signs of IDA include the following:

- **Pallor,** fatigue, shortness of breath
- **Glossitis**—inflammation of the tongue
- **Koilonychia**—concave or spoon-shaped nails (Fig. 11.10A)
- **Pica**—obsessive craving for nonnutritional materials (e.g., ice, dirt)

Laboratory evaluation in IDA includes the following:

- **The earliest sign on CBC is an increased RDW** because bone marrow will begin to produce small and pale RBCs. Ultimately, the MCV drops as more microcytic and hypochromic RBCs and fewer normal-sized RBCs are produced (Fig. 11.10B).
- Hb, Hct, and MCV are decreased.
- The **serum iron** and **ferritin** levels will be **decreased,** reflecting the depletion of iron stores. **Iron saturation** will also be **decreased** because less iron is available to bind transferrin.
- **TIBC** will be **increased** because the liver creates more transferrin to help bind any remaining available iron.

Plummer-Vinson syndrome—triad of dysphagia (esophageal webs), glossitis, and IDA. Most common in postmenopausal women.

Treatment for iron deficiency anemia includes the following:

- Treatment of the underlying cause
- Oral iron supplementation
- Supplementation with vitamin C (helps convert nonabsorbable Fe^{3+} to absorbable Fe^{2+}).

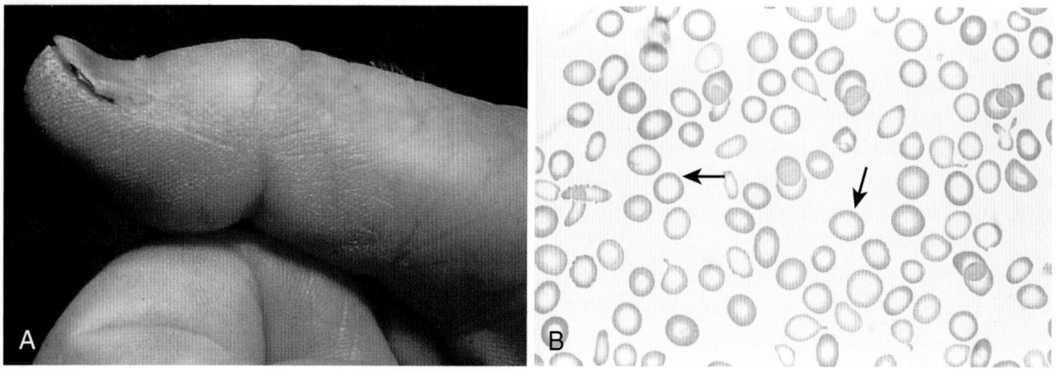

Fig. 11.10 Signs of iron deficiency anemia. **A,** Koilonychia. **B,** Microcytic hypochromic RBCs *(arrows)* on peripheral blood smear. (*From Savin JAA, Hunter JAA, Hepburn NC.* Diagnosis in Color: Skin Signs in Clinical Medicine. *London: Mosby-Wolfe; 1997:118.*)

Anemia of Chronic Disease: ACD is the **most common anemia in hospitalized patients.** Chronic illness leads to continued release of inflammatory cytokines. These inflammatory cytokines, mainly interleukin 6 (IL-6), signal the liver to **increase hepcidin** production, thereby **resulting in increased iron retention by cells.** One hypothesis for this physiologic response, in the short term, is that inflammation acts to help keep iron away from bacterial pathogens in the body, depressing the ability of these pathogens to survive. However, if the inflammation response is prolonged, it results in inadequate levels of iron reaching the bone marrow, leading to decreased production of RBCs. The body cannot distinguish inflammation from infectious versus noninfectious causes, so it responds the same way to both. Although there are other mechanisms that also contribute to the development of anemia during inflammation, this hypothesis acts as an aid in remembering the mechanism of anemia in ACD. Common causes of ACD include the following:

- **Long-term infectious diseases**—osteomyelitis, bacterial endocarditis, and tuberculosis.
- **Chronic noninfectious inflammatory diseases**—rheumatoid arthritis, systemic lupus erythematosus (SLE), ulcerative colitis, and Crohn disease.
- **Neoplasms**—Hodgkin disease, lymphoma, lung and breast carcinoma.

Clinical Signs:

- Pallor and fatigue coupled with signs of a chronic disease listed earlier.

ACD—increased ferritin; decreased iron, and TIBC

Laboratory Evaluation:

- Decreased Hb (rarely < 9 g/dL), Hct, and MCV.
- **Increased ferritin** because iron is being stored inside cells and not released into the circulation. Also, ferritin is an acute-phase reactant (proteins in plasma that increase or decrease in response to inflammatory stimuli).
- **Decreased serum iron, TIBC,** and iron saturation.
- Decreased serum iron because iron is being stored inside cells. Because stores of iron are high in ACD, the liver is not induced to produce transferrin. This results in a low or normal TIBC.

Treatment:

- Treating the underlying condition should resolve the anemia. Administration of erythropoietin may help increase Hb levels in some cases.

Heme Synthesis and Acquired Sideroblastic Anemia: **Sideroblastic anemia results from an inability to form heme molecules in the mitochondria.** The acquired causes of sideroblastic anemia disrupt different steps in heme synthesis, leading to iron deposition inside the mitochondria (forming a ringed sideroblast).

Heme synthesis (Fig. 11.11) mainly occurs in the liver and bone marrow. It is initiated by the synthesis of **δ-aminolevulinic acid (δ-ALA)** from **glycine and succinyl CoA** (obtained from the Krebs cycle) inside the mitochondria. This initial step is the rate-limiting step of heme synthesis and requires the enzyme **δ-ALA synthase** and its cofactor **vitamin B_6,** meaning that all the remaining steps in the pathway depend on the proper functioning of this initial step. This initial **step is regulated** by intracellular **iron levels and** by the concentration of the end product of the whole pathway, **heme (glucose also inhibits this step).** δ-ALA is converted to porphobilinogen by δ-ALA dehydratase and is transported

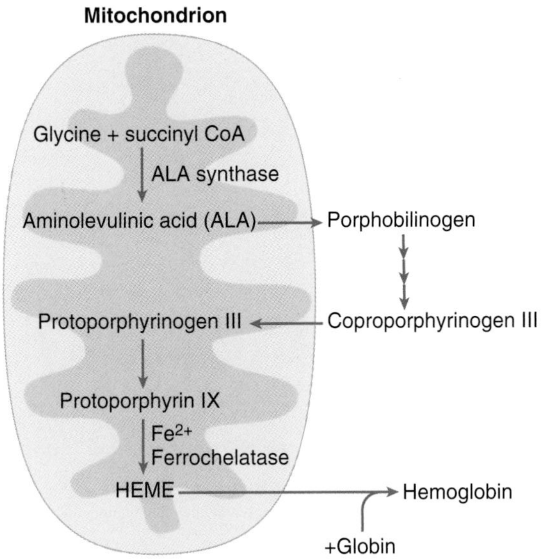

FIG. 11.11 Mitochondrial pathway for heme synthesis. (*From Hudnall SD.* Hematology. *Philadelphia: Elsevier; 2011.*)

out of the mitochondria and into the cytoplasm. In the cytoplasm, **porphobilinogen** is worked on by the enzyme **porphobilinogen deaminase,** the defective enzyme in acute intermittent porphyria, to produce hydroxymethylbilane. Hydroxymethylbilane is then converted to uroporphyrinogen III, and this product is transported back into the mitochondria. **Uroporphyrinogen III** is enzymatically changed to **coproporphyrinogen III by uroporphyrinogen decarboxylase,** the defective enzyme in porphyria cutanea tarda. After a few more enzymatic steps, protoporphyrin is produced inside the mitochondria. The final step involves **incorporating iron** (Fe^{2+}) into **protoporphyrin via ferrochelatase** to produce heme.

In attacks of porphyria, patients are sometimes treated with heme arginate or hematin to inhibit ALA synthase, halting the production of heme and thereby preventing the buildup of toxic intermediates.

Enzyme deficiencies in the early steps of porphyrin synthesis cause neurologic abnormalities without photosensitivity (acute intermittent porphyria). Derangements in the later steps of heme synthesis, after condensation of porphobilinogen (PBG), cause photosensitivity (porphyria cutanea tarda).

Causes of sideroblastic anemia—chronic alcoholism (most common), pyridoxine, lead poisoning

Causes of Sideroblastic Anemia: **Chronic alcoholism** is the most common cause of acquired or secondary sideroblastic anemia. Alcohol damages the mitochondria, which are required for the synthesis of heme.

Vitamin B_6 (pyridoxine) deficiency can lead to sideroblastic anemia. **δ-ALA** synthase requires vitamin B_6 as a cofactor to function properly. Deficiency in this vitamin is commonly seen in patients taking isoniazid (INH) for the treatment of tuberculosis without pyridoxine supplementation. INH binds to pyridoxine, making it unavailable for absorption by the body. Treat with pyridoxine supplementation.

Lead poisoning is the most common cause of acquired sideroblastic anemia in children (≤5 years). Lead **inhibits** two key enzymes in the heme synthesis pathway, **ferrochelatase** and **δ-ALA dehydratase.**

- **Ferrochelatase** is the last enzyme in the heme synthesis pathway; it helps incorporate iron into protoporphyrin to form heme. Because it is inhibited by lead, **iron** and **protoporphyrin build up** in cells.
- **δ-ALA dehydratase** converts δ-ALA to porphobilinogen, one of the early steps of porphyrin synthesis (porphyrins are the intermediates produced during heme synthesis; once iron is incorporated to porphyrins, heme is created). Because it is inhibited by lead, **δ-ALA builds up in cells.**

Clinical Signs Specific to Lead Poisoning:

- Poisoning is usually associated with abdominal, neuromuscular, and neurologic symptoms.
- **Abdominal problems** include **abdominal pain, diarrhea,** anorexia, and weight loss.
- **Neuromuscular symptoms** include peripheral neuropathies, peroneal nerve palsy (foot drop), and radial nerve palsy (wrist drop).
- **δ-ALA,** a neurotoxin, **builds up,** causing neurologic symptoms, headaches, **encephalopathy, learning disabilities, and mental retardation** (in children).
- Lead lines may be seen in the gingivae.

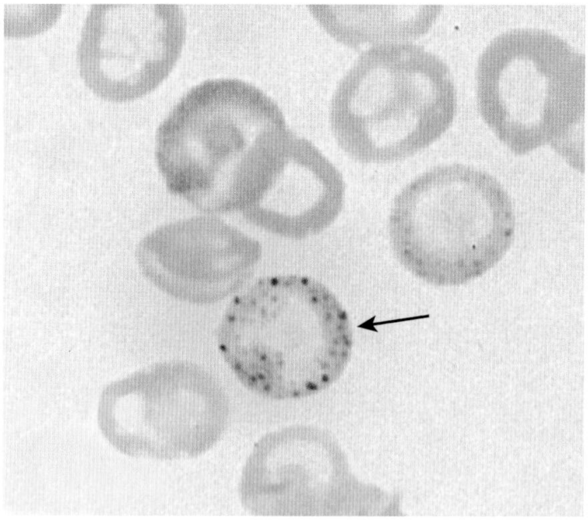

FIG. 11.12 Basophilic stippling *(arrow)* on peripheral smear of patient with lead poisoning. (*From Naeim F.* Atlas of Bone Marrow and Blood Pathology. *Philadelphia: WB Saunders; 2001:27.*)

Laboratory Evaluation Specific to Lead Poisoning:

- **Increased levels of lead** will be found in the urine or whole blood.
- Abdominal radiographs may show **lead chips** (white opacities) in the **intestinal tract.**
- Plain film radiographs of the **epiphysis** will show **lead deposits** (white opacities).
- **Basophilic stippling** is seen on the peripheral smear of patients with lead poisoning. Lead denatures ribonuclease, the enzyme that degrades ribosomes, allowing ribosomes to remain intact inside RBCs (Fig. 11.12).

Treatment Specific to Lead Poisoning: Treatment is chelation with succimer, dimercaprol, or ethylenediaminetetraacetic acid (EDTA).

Laboratory Evaluation of Sideroblastic Anemia:

- Bone marrow aspirate will show **ringed sideroblasts** (Fig. 11.13).
- Hb, Hct, and MCV are decreased.
- **δ-ALA and protoporphyrin are increased.**
- **Serum iron** and **ferritin are increased.**
- **TIBC is decreased** because of high levels of ferritin (and iron).

Inherited Microcytic Anemias:

Thalassemias: Thalassemias are a group of **autosomal recessive** hereditary disorders that arise from a **quantitative defect in the production of Hb (decreased production of normal globin proteins).** They are characterized by an imbalance in globin chain production caused by mutations in the α- or β-globin genes. The production of α- and β-globin chains is a highly regulated pathway that aims to produce equal amounts of both chains. Mutations that lead to a partial or complete inactivation of globin chain synthesis lead to an imbalance in the ratio of α- and β-globin chain production inside RBCs. When the production of one group of globin chains is decreased, the production of another group is increased. The **net production of functional Hb is reduced in thalassemia, but RBC production is usually normal.** As a result, people with thalassemia **develop a microcytosis, with increased RBC count.** The higher number of RBCs compensate for a decrease in the total functional Hb concentration per RBC.

α-Thalassemia: **α-Thalassemia** is more **prevalent** in **South Asian** and **West African** populations. Four genes, two on each copy of chromosome 16, determine the production of α-globin. Because the production of α-globin chains is regulated by four genes, individuals with **one α-gene deletion** are **silent carriers** (no anemia).

α-Thalassemia trait results from the **deletion of two of the four genes** and produces **mild anemia.** This creates a decrease in α-globin and an increase in β-globin (in adults) or γ-globin (in newborns) production. This condition exists in two forms:

1. The cis deletion of both α genes on the same chromosome (–/– α/α) is associated with South Asian populations. They are at increased risk of having offspring with more severe forms of α-thalassemia.
2. The trans deletion of one α gene in each copy of chromosome 16 (α/– α/–) is associated with West African populations.

α-Thalassemia—normal iron studies, normal RDW, increased RBC count, normal Hb electrophoresis

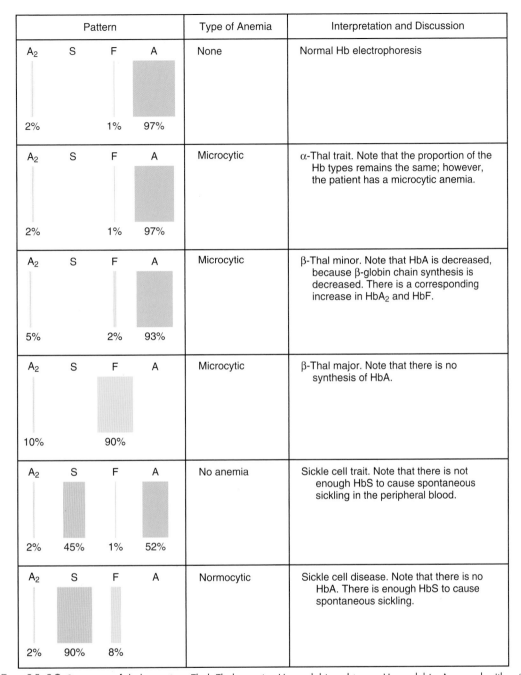

Pattern	Type of Anemia	Interpretation and Discussion
A_2 S F A 2% 1% 97%	None	Normal Hb electrophoresis
A_2 S F A 2% 1% 97%	Microcytic	α-Thal trait. Note that the proportion of the Hb types remains the same; however, the patient has a microcytic anemia.
A_2 S F A 5% 2% 93%	Microcytic	β-Thal minor. Note that HbA is decreased, because β-globin chain synthesis is decreased. There is a corresponding increase in HbA_2 and HbF.
A_2 S F A 10% 90%	Microcytic	β-Thal major. Note that there is no synthesis of HbA.
A_2 S F A 2% 45% 1% 52%	No anemia	Sickle cell trait. Note that there is not enough HbS to cause spontaneous sickling in the peripheral blood.
A_2 S F A 2% 90% 8%	Normocytic	Sickle cell disease. Note that there is no HbA. There is enough HbS to cause spontaneous sickling.

FIG. 11.13 Summary of thalassemias. *Thal,* Thalassemia. Hemoglobin subtypes: Hemoglobin A normal with $\alpha_2\beta_2$ chains, A_2: Hemoglobin A_2, a normal subtype made of $\alpha_2\delta_2$ chains, S: sickle hemoglobin, F: fetal hemoglobin with $\alpha_2\gamma_2$ chains (*From Forbes C, Jackson W.* Color Atlas and Text of Clinical Medicine. *2nd ed. St. Louis: Mosby; 2003:343.*)

Laboratory Findings In α-Thalassemia Trait:

- Decreased Hb, Hct, and MCV
- **Normal iron studies, normal RDW** (differentiates it from IDA), **increased RBC count**
- **Normal Hb electrophoresis** (Fig. 11.14)

Because all the Hb types in the blood require α-globin chains, in α-thalassemia trait you will see an equal decrease in the amount of all of Hb produced but no change in the proportions of each type of Hb (the percentage of each Hb produced stays constant).

Treatment for α-Thalassemia Trait: **There is no treatment.** This disease is often mistakenly diagnosed as IDA and patients are given iron supplementation. **Do not treat with iron because it can cause iron overload.**

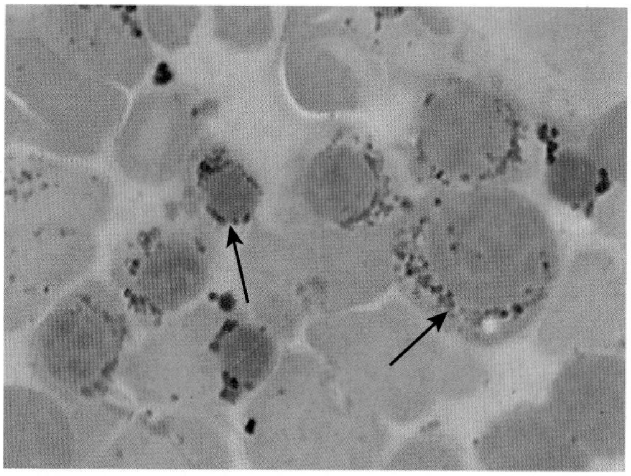

FIG. 11.14 Ringed sideroblasts *(arrows)* in bone marrow aspirate of patient with sideroblastic anemia. *(From Goljan EF, Sloka KI.* Rapid Review Laboratory Testing in Clinical Medicine. *St. Louis: Mosby Elsevier; 2008:159.)*

α-Thalassemia major is a severe form of α-thalassemia that occurs from the deletion of three or four of the four α-globin genes. Anemia can be much more severe than α-thalassemia trait.

Deletion of three α-globin genes results in an excess of free β-globin proteins. These β-globin chains tetramerize, **creating HbH.** These β-tetramers are initially soluble during the production of RBCs in the bone marrow, allowing for proper maturation of RBCs (unlike α-tetramers, which precipitate in RBC precursors). Therefore α-thalassemia is not a disorder of ineffective erythropoiesis. However, with time, the β-tetramers precipitate and form **Heinz bodies** inside the mature RBC. These RBCs with Heinz bodies are destroyed in the spleen, leading to severe hemolytic anemia. As a result, **splenectomy can be an effective treatment for patients with severe HbH disease.**

Four α-globin genes, incompatible with life, form Hb Bart.

Deletion of four α-globin genes is incompatible with life and **results in the formation of Hb Bart.** This disorder is associated with intrauterine fetal death and fetal edema and has potentially fatal complications for the mother if undetected.

β-Thalassemia: **β-Thalassemia** is more prevalent in **Mediterranean populations.** Two genes, one on each copy of chromosome 11, determine the production of β-globin chains. The severity of this disorder depends on the nature of the mutation. All mutations result in decreased or absent production of β-globin chains, leading to an imbalance in the ratio of α- and β-globin production. As a result of the imbalance, there is a decrease or cessation in the production of HbA (requires β-globin chains) and increased aggregation of α-globin chains inside the RBC. In the absence of β-globin, partner α-globin chains will tetramerize and precipitate inside RBC precursors while still in the bone marrow, not allowing RBC maturation. This creates a state of ineffective erythropoiesis and explains why **β-thalassemia is a transfusion-dependent anemia (the body does not produce enough mature RBCs).**

β-Thalassemia trait ($\beta/\beta\beta^+$ or β/β^0) is the milder form of β-thalassemia, in which only **one gene** (heterozygote) **is defective,** resulting in **mild microcytic anemia.** Prevalence is high in the Mediterranean population because of protective effects against *Plasmodium falciparum* malaria.

β-Thalassemia—normal iron, normal RDW, increased RBCs, abnormal Hb electrophoresis

Laboratory Findings in β-Thalassemia Trait:

- Decreased Hb, Hct, and MCV
- **Normal iron studies, normal RDW** (differentiates it from IDA), increased RBC count
- **Hb electrophoresis** (see Fig. 11.4):
  - Mildly decreased HbA levels
  - Mildly increased HbA_2 levels
  - Mildly increased HbF levels

Treatment: Not usually actively treated, given mild symptoms. Monitor frequently for iron overload caused by an increase in intestinal iron absorption seen in all forms of β-thalassemias. **Do not treat with iron!**

β-Thalassemia major (β^0/β^0, β^0/β^+, β^+/β^+), also known as **Cooley anemia,** results from mutations in both β-globin genes. RBCs will have increased amounts of α-globin chains leading to the tetramerization of α-chains, precipitation of tetramers, and destruction of some of the RBC precursors in the bone marrow **(ineffective erythropoiesis).** Because bone marrow production of RBCs is decreased, signs of **extramedullary hematopoiesis** will be seen. RBCs that make it into the circulation are severely distorted in shape and are removed by macrophages in the spleen, leading to **severe hemolytic anemia. Patients will require lifelong transfusions.**

Laboratory and Physical Examination Findings in β-Thalassemia Major:

- Hb, Hct, and MCV are decreased.
- RDW and reticulocytes are increased.
- Patients are at risk of hemosiderosis (iron overload) from constant transfusions.
- Patients will have **high levels of unconjugated bilirubin** and show signs of **jaundice** (from hemolysis).
- **Hb electrophoresis will indicate the following:**
  - Absence of HbA production
  - Significant increase in HbF levels
  - Increased HbA_2 levels
- Splenomegaly may be present.
- Radiographs may show a **crew cut** appearance of the **skull.** You may also see **skeletal deformities** caused by extramedullary hematopoiesis (Fig. 11.15).

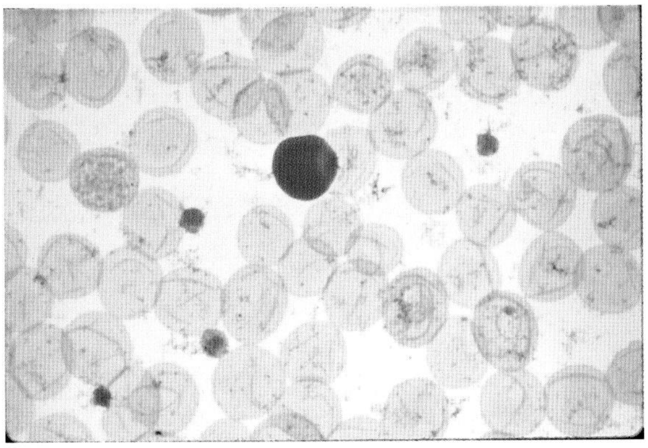

FIG. 11.15 Sickled cells and target cells of sickle cell disease. (*From Hoffbrand AV.* Color Atlas: Clinical Hematology. *3rd ed. St. Louis: Mosby; 2000:103.*)

Treatment:

- Chronic blood transfusions
- Iron chelation treatment to prevent iron overload
- Splenectomy in patients with splenomegaly

Bone marrow transplantation is the only cure. It is indicated only in patients with severe disease.

X-Linked Sideroblastic Anemia: **Inherited sideroblastic anemia** is an X-linked recessive disorder that results in a disruption of heme synthesis similar to that seen in acquired sideroblastic anemia (see earlier). It results from a **defect** in the **δ-ALA synthase gene, producing a defective enzyme.** Laboratory findings will be similar to those seen in acquired sideroblastic anemia (see earlier). This disorder is treated with pyridoxine (vitamin B_6) and, in severe anemia, may require support with blood transfusions.

Normocytic Anemias

Normocytic anemias (MCV = 80 to 100 fL) are the most commonly encountered type of anemia because, in the early stages, almost all anemias are normocytic. Normocytic anemias are the most challenging to diagnose and may reflect an underlying systemic illness or a complex combination of anemias (e.g., a combined folate and iron deficiency). When categorizing normocytic anemias, it is important to determine the response of the bone marrow. These anemias are subdivided into those that have an inappropriate corrected reticulocyte count (<3%) and those with an appropriate corrected reticulocyte count. The **most common** type of **normocytic anemia** is **anemia of chronic disease;** ACD starts off as a normocytic anemia and then develops into a microcytic anemia if the underlying chronic disease persists untreated. **Normocytic anemias with a corrected reticulocyte count** lower than **3%** include early ACD or IDA, acute blood loss, aplastic anemia, chronic kidney disease (CKD), and malignancy. The **normocytic anemias with a corrected reticulocyte count more**

than 3% encompass all the clinically important intrinsic or extrinsic hemolytic anemias, including sickle cell disease, glucose-6-phosphate dehydrogenase (G6PD) deficiency, pyruvate kinase (PK) deficiency, hereditary spherocytosis, hereditary elliptocytosis, paroxysmal nocturnal hemoglobinuria (PNH), HbC disease, immune hemolytic anemias, and microangiopathic and macroangiopathic hemolytic anemias.

Hemolytic anemia is defined by the **premature destruction of circulating RBC**s from numerous inherited or acquired conditions. Causes of hemolysis are traditionally categorized by whether the abnormality is intrinsic or extrinsic to the RBC (intracorpuscular versus extracorpuscular defects) and whether the hemolysis occurs in the vasculature or in the reticuloendothelial macrophages of the liver and spleen (intravascular versus extravascular hemolysis). As a general rule, most inherited conditions leading to hemolytic anemia are due to intrinsic RBC defects, and most immune hemolytic anemias are extravascular.

Intrinsic or **intracorpuscular causes** of hemolytic anemia include issues with the RBC itself, such as the following:

- Defects in hemoglobin structure, function, and production (**sickle cell disease, HbC disease**, and **thalassemia**)
- Defects in red cell metabolism (**G6PD** and **PK deficiency**)
- Defects in RBC cell membrane production (**hereditary spherocytosis,** **hereditary elliptocytosis,** and **paroxysmal nocturnal hemoglobinuria**)

Extrinsic or extracorpuscular defects are those in which external factors in developmentally normal RBCs lead to premature loss of membrane or membrane structural damage. In these cases, RBCs are destroyed as a result of mechanical, immunologic, infectious, metabolic, or oxidant damage (e.g., **autoimmune hemolytic anemia or microangiopathic/macroangiopathic anemia**).

Intravascular hemolysis refers to RBC breakdown that occurs primarily within the blood vessels. This happens when there is significant structural damage to the RBC membrane (e.g., mechanical shearing from prosthetic valve or complement-induced lysis) or when the reticuloendothelial system is overwhelmed. The hallmark of intravascular hemolysis is the **spilling of RBC contents into the bloodstream,** namely the **release of free Hb and lactate dehydrogenase (LDH).** Free Hb then binds to haptoglobin, and the Hb–haptoglobin complex is rapidly removed by the liver, causing a **drop in plasma levels of haptoglobin.** When intravascular hemolysis is severe, circulating haptoglobin is unable to bind all of the free Hb and patients develop dark urine from the spilling of free Hb into the urine (hemoglobinuria). Therefore **intravascular hemolysis** is characterized by **high LDH and low haptoglobin levels.**

Extravascular hemolysis refers to RBC **breakdown that occurs primarily** by the macrophages of the **reticuloendothelial system in the liver, spleen,** lymph nodes, and bone marrow. In this setting RBCs are broken down in a largely contained system, thereby **avoiding direct release of RBC contents into the bloodstream.** Because there is no free Hb floating in the circulation, **haptoglobin levels will not drop** and free Hb does not spill into urine **(no hemoglobinuria).** Severely damaged RBCs that enter the reticuloendothelial system are phagocytosed in their entirety and destroyed within phagosomes of macrophages. Extravascular digestion of RBCs generally occurs in the liver, but in certain circumstances it occurs primarily in the reticuloendothelial system of other organs. For example, the **spleen primarily destroys poorly deformable RBC**s (such as those seen in **sickle cell disease** and **hereditary spherocytosis**) by trapping them in the cords of Billroth.

Normocytic Anemias With Corrected Reticulocyte Count Less Than 3%:

Acute Blood Loss: Acute blood loss occurs in two forms, internal and external bleeding. Internal bleeding can result from blunt trauma (e.g., ruptured spleen) or nontraumatic aneurysm rupture (e.g., stroke, abdominal aortic aneurysm rupture, intestinal bleeding). External bleeding can result from penetrating injury (gunshot wound) or compound bone fractures. **Acute blood loss is the most common cause of hypovolemic shock.** Patients usually present with **sudden** signs of anemia (weakness, fatigue, pallor, dyspnea) and have a history of trauma or bleeding disorders.

> Acute blood loss—Hb and Hct initially normal. After fluid shift, both will decrease.

Laboratory Findings in Acute Blood Loss:

- Hb and Hct are initially normal but decrease as interstitial fluid shifts into the vascular compartment resulting in hemodilution; MCV is normal.
- Reticulocyte will not be increased more than 3% until 1 week after the precipitating event.

Treatment:

- Intravenous fluid replacement
- Blood transfusion (depending on severity)
- Correcting the cause of the hemorrhage

Aplastic Anemia: Aplastic anemia (AA) is a disorder in which the bone marrow does not produce the appropriate amount of new cells to replenish blood cell turnover. It is characterized by **pancytopenia** or **decreased** amounts of all three bloodlines (RBCs, WBCs and platelets) and **decreased** reticulocyte count (reticulocytopenia). Aplastic anemia has many causes and generally results from inhibition, destruction, or a defect in multipotent myeloid stem cells.

Common causes include the following:

- Idiopathic (most common; confers poor prognosis)
  - Normally, the development of myeloid stem cells is suppressed by the immune system. Derangements in the regulation of the immune system, like those seen in autoimmune disorders, are believed to contribute to some idiopathic forms of AA.
- Drugs (**most common known cause; has better prognosis**)—**chloramphenicol**, alkylating agents, antimalarials, sulfonamides
- Exposure to chemical agents—benzene, DDT (insecticide)
- Infection (usually viral)—**parvovirus B19**, Epstein-Barr virus (EBV), HIV, hepatitis C
- Whole-body ionizing radiation

The presentation is often gradual and depends on which blood cell line becomes critically deficient first.

- **Anemia**—decreased RBCs lead to fatigue, malaise, and pallor.
- **Thrombocytopenia**—decreased platelets lead to petechiae (pinpoint red or purple spots on skin), purpura (nonblanching purple spots bigger than petechiae), and mucosal bleeding.
- **Neutropenia**—decreased neutrophils lead to infections.

Aplastic anemia—decreased RBCs, WBCs, and platelets, hypocellular bone marrow and fatty infiltration

Laboratory Findings:

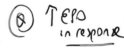

- **Decreased** RBC, WBC, and platelet count
- **Hypocellular bone marrow** and **fatty infiltration** on bone marrow biopsy

Treatment:

- Discontinuation of the offending agent.
- Antibiotics if infection present
- RBC transfusion (if severe anemia)
- Platelet transfusion (if severe thrombocytopenia)
- Immunosuppressive therapy with antithymocyte globulin (ATG) or cyclosporine
- Granulocyte colony-stimulating factor (G-CSF) and granulocyte-macrophage colony-stimulating factor (GM-CSF)
- Allogeneic hematopoietic stem cell transplantation (bone marrow transplant with cells from another individual)

Chronic Kidney Disease: People with CKD experience a normocytic anemia caused by decreased production of erythropoietin (EPO) by the failing kidneys. This EPO deficiency leads to decreased hematopoiesis.

Laboratory Findings:

- Decreased Hb and Hct, normal MCV
- **Burr cells on peripheral smear**
  - Thrombocytopenia; the buildup of toxic metabolites caused by kidney failure results in a functional platelet defect
  - Prolonged bleeding time caused by a reversible platelet aggregation defect (reversible with dialysis)

Malignancy: Malignancy most commonly leads to ACD. Malignancy-related anemia is classified in three main categories:

- RBC losses from the body (e.g., intestinal **blood loss** in colon cancer)
- Increased RBC destruction (e.g., immune **hemolytic anemia** seen in chronic lymphocytic leukemia)

- Decreased red blood cell production (e.g., cancer **metastasis to the bone marrow**)
  - **Myelophthisic anemia** refers to the displacement of normal marrow cells by metastatic cancer cells.

Normocytic Anemias With Corrected Reticulocyte Count More Than 3%:

Sickle cell anemia: Sickle cell disease is an **autosomal recessive disorder** that leads to a structural or **qualitative abnormality** of **Hb** and is associated with hemolysis. It is common in African and African American populations. A **point mutation** in the β-globin gene **substitutes** a **valine** for **glutamic acid** at position 6 (Glu-6-Val) and leads to the production of abnormal **HbS.** The deoxygenated form of HbS can reversibly polymerize with other HbS molecules. The higher concentration of deoxygenated HbS in the RBCs results in a greater rate of polymerization. The polymerization of HbS inside RBCs leads to sickle-shaped cells, which are subject to **destruction by the spleen.** The sickling also **increases** the blood's **viscosity,** leading to **microvascular occlusion.** Sickle cell disorder appears in different forms, each with a differing severity of anemia.

Sickle Cell Trait: These patients are **heterozygous,** having one copy of the HbA and HbS allele. **Genotype is HbSA.** The concentration of deoxygenated HbS in these patients is approximately 40% of total Hb and rarely reaches the threshold concentration necessary to initiate pathologic polymerization of HbS inside RBCs. Instead, these patients benefit from the **protective** effects **against** *P. falciparum* **malaria** that result from this mutation.

Laboratory Findings:

- These patients are **not anemic. Hb, Hct, and MCV are normal.** Peripheral smear is also normal.
- **Hb electrophoresis findings include the following:**
  - Presence of HbS.
  - Decreased HbA levels.
  - HbF and HbA_2 levels do not change.

Sickle Cell Disease: These patients are **homozygous,** having two copies of the HbS allele. **The genotype is HbSS.** The deoxygenated HbS concentration in these patients can rise above the threshold for pathologic polymerization of HbS and results in sickling of RBCs. This polymerization mostly occurs in the **microvascular beds,** in which **acidosis** and **hypoxia** cause Hb to release bound oxygen, increasing the concentration of deoxygenated HbS in RBCs. This polymerization is **reversible** once RBCs are in an environment with higher levels of oxygen (i.e., arteries). Repeated cycles of polymerization and depolymerization result in accumulation of damage to the RBC membrane, which eventually becomes irreversible. The damage to the RBC membrane impairs Na^+/K^+ and water homeostasis, leading to cellular dehydration and increased sickling of RBCs.

Signs and Symptoms of Sickle Cell Disease:

- Periodic episodes of **acute vascular occlusion** called **pain crises** occur beginning at age 1 or 2 years.
- Vascular occlusion can lead to organ dysfunction or failure, causing **bone infarcts, avascular necrosis, acute chest syndrome** (chest pain, shortness of breath [SOB], and pulmonary infiltrates on chest radiograph), **chronic leg ulcers, osteomyelitis (salmonella),** and **stroke.**
- **Dactylitis** (hand-foot syndrome) or swelling of hands and feet can be seen in infants.
- **Recurrent splenic infarction** and **autosplenectomy** occur at a young age. The presence of **Howell-Jolly bodies** on a peripheral smear signifies impaired or absent splenic function. Loss of splenic function makes patients **increasingly susceptible** to infection by **encapsulated bacteria,** and **daily antibiotic prophylaxis** is **required** for the treatment of children.
- **Aplastic crisis** can occur in association with parvovirus B19.
- **Sequestration crisis** results when there is entrapment of sickled RBCs in the spleen, resulting in rapid **splenomegaly.**
- **Renal papillary necrosis** can occur when microinfarcts of the kidney result in microhematuria.

Laboratory Findings:

- Decreased Hb and Hct
- Normal MCV
- Increased reticulocyte count
- **Crescent-shaped RBCs, target cells,** and Howell-Jolly bodies on peripheral smear (see Fig. 11.15)
- **Sickle cell screen** with **sodium metabisulfite**–induced sickling of cells

- **Hb electrophoresis results as follows:**
  - Absence of HbA
  - Increased levels of HbS
  - Increased HbF levels

Plain radiographs of the skull may show a crew cut appearance caused by extramedullary hematopoiesis, as also seen in thalassemias (Fig. 11.16).

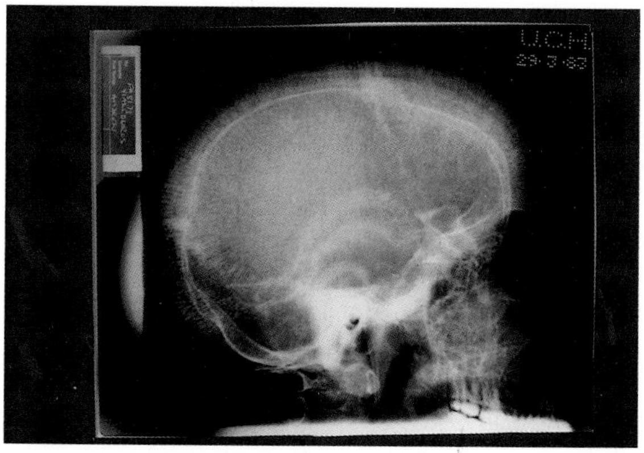

Fig. 11.16 Crew cut appearance of skull radiograph caused by extramedullary hematopoiesis in sickle cell disease and thalassemias. (*From Bouloux P. Self-Assessment Picture Tests: Medicine. Vol 1. London: Mosby-Wolfe; 1997:49.*)

Factors that **increase HbS polymerization and sickling** include any factor that results in the deoxygenation of Hb:
- **Acidosis** results in a right shift of the oxygen-binding curve (OBC) and increased release of oxygen from Hb.
- **Hypoxemia** is defined by decreased levels of arterial Po_2. This results in less oxygen available to bind to Hb.
- **Volume depletion** (dehydrated RBCs) increases the concentration of deoxygenated HbS inside RBCs.
- **Infection** can lead to tissue hypoxemia and acidosis.

Factors That **Prevent or Reverse Sickling** *(and Treatments):*
- Avoidance of hypoxia and dehydration can prevent sickling.
  - **Increased levels of HbF** inhibit HbS polymerization and prevent sickling. **Hydroxyurea** has been shown to increase HbF levels and is used in patients with frequent sickle cell crises. **Newborns are often asymptomatic because of high levels of HbF.**
- Morphine can provide pain relief.
- Exchange transfusion can be used to treat serious forms of vascular occlusion (e.g., acute chest syndrome, stroke, priapism).
- Allogeneic stem cell transplantation is curative in patients with severe clinical disease.
- All patients with sickle cell disease must be up to date on their immunizations (pneumococcal, meningococcal vaccine, Hib, hepatitis B, and influenza vaccines).
- Patients with sickle cell disease should receive folic acid supplementation.

G6PD deficiency: increased stress → oxidation of Hb inside RBCs → Hb molecules precipitate to form Heinz bodies.

G6PD Deficiency: **G6PD,** an **enzyme** that **protects** RBCs from **oxidant stress,** has decreased activity in people with this disorder, leading to increased hemolysis in situations of stress. This enzyme deficiency leads to decreased synthesis of NADPH (a reduced form of nicotinamide adenine dinucleotide phosphate) and glutathione (antioxidants) from the pentose phosphate pathway (Fig. 11.17). Normally, NADPH helps restore glutathione stores so that glutathione can then reduce reactive oxygen species (H_2O_2) to less harmful compounds (H_2O). **Hemolysis** is **mostly intravascular,** but some extravascular hemolysis is also seen. **Increased stress leads to the oxidation of Hb inside RBCs, and Hb molecules precipitate to form Heinz bodies.** Intravascular hemolysis results because Heinz bodies damage the RBC membrane and make RBCs more susceptible to lysis in the circulation. RBCs that do not lyse while in circulation are removed by the spleen, leading to extravascular hemolysis. G6PD deficiency is an **X-linked recessive** disorder common in **black, Middle Eastern,** and **Mediterranean** populations. It is thought to be protective against *P. falciparum* malaria. Hemolysis often results from exposure to oxidative stress, such as the following:
- **Infection** (most common)—acute viral or bacterial infections

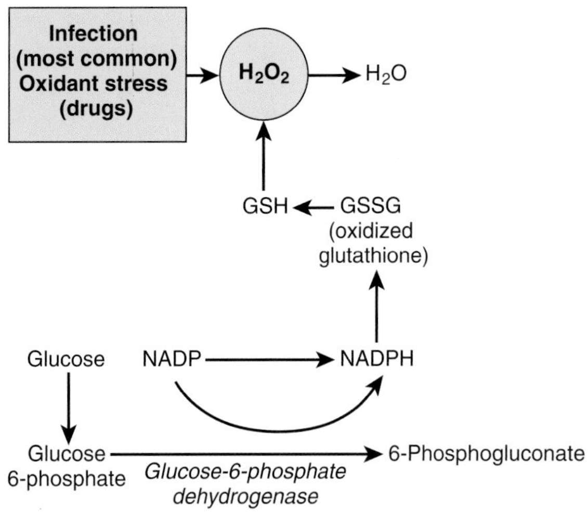

Fig. 11.17 Oxidant stress and G6PD. GSH, reduced glutathione; GSSG, oxidized glutathione. (*From Goljan EF.* Pathology: Saunders Text and Review Series. *Philadelphia: WB Saunders; 1998.*)

- **Drugs—sulfonamides** (trimethoprim-sulfamethoxazole), dapsone, primaquine, chloroquine, nitrofurantoin
- Acidosis (e.g., diabetic ketoacidosis [DKA])
- Fava beans (historically, this condition was called favism)

Signs and Symptoms:

- Most are asymptomatic
- History of neonatal jaundice and cholelithiasis
- Episodic signs of anemia (possibly associated with jaundice and splenomegaly)

Laboratory Findings:

- Decreased Hb and Hct, normal MCV
- **Heinz bodies** and/or **bite cells** on peripheral smear (Fig. 11.18)

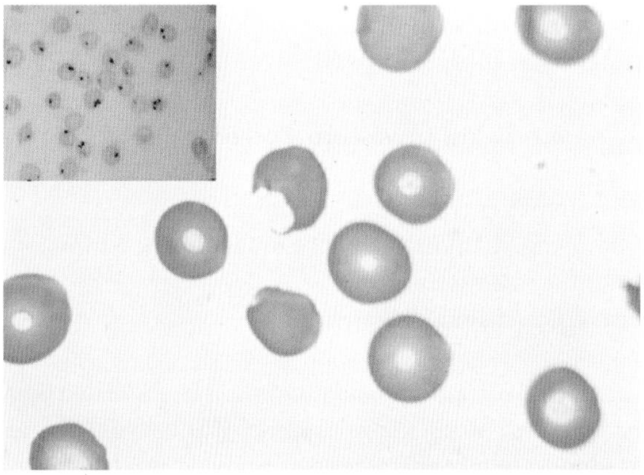

Fig. 11.18 Inset *(upper left)*, RBCs with denatured globin proteins (Heinz bodies) demonstrated by supravital staining. Macrophages will eliminate these inclusions, creating "bite cells." (*From Kumar V, Fausto N, Abbas AK.* Robbins & Cotran Pathologic Basis of Disease. *7th ed. Philadelphia: Saunders; 2004; inset from Wickramasinghe SN, McCullough J.* Blood and Bone Marrow Pathology. *London: Churchill Livingstone; 2003.*)

Measure G6PD enzyme activity after a hemolytic attack. The value will be decreased. It may be falsely elevated or normal in times of hemolysis.

Pyruvate kinase deficiency. PK deficiency is an autosomal recessive disorder that causes chronic lack of ATP in RBCs. PK is an enzyme in the glycolytic pathway that helps synthesize ATP. Because RBCs can only produce ATP via glycolysis, they are dependent on the proper function of the PK enzyme for energy.

The lack of ATP results in accelerated RBC membrane damage and dehydration. It is characterized by chronic extravascular hemolysis with poikilocytosis (RBCs of abnormal shape) and cellular dehydration on blood smear. Patients may present with hemolytic anemia with jaundice since birth.

Laboratory Findings:

- Hb and Hct are decreased; MCV is normal.
- **Echinocytes** are present on peripheral smear (Fig. 11.19).
- **Measure direct PK enzyme activity to diagnose.**

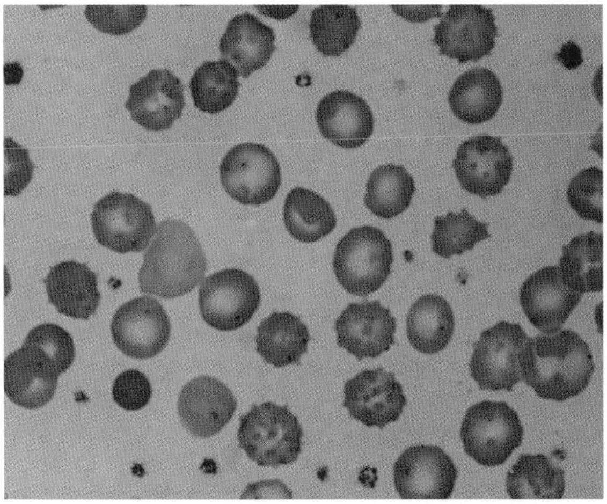

Fig. 11.19 Spiked thorny projections of echinocytes. (*From Wickramasinghe SN, McCullough J.* Blood and Bone Marrow Pathology. *London: Churchill Livingstone; 2003.*)

Treatment: Most patients do not require treatment. Splenectomy may be beneficial in patients with severe disease.

Hereditary spherocytosis (HS): Hereditary spherocytosis (HS) is an **autosomal dominant** hemolytic anemia that results from an abnormality in the RBC membrane. It is characterized by defects in membrane proteins such as **ankyrin (most common), spectrin, or band 3.** RBCs lose their characteristic biconcave shape and instead have a spherical appearance. The spherical shape is less versatile and deformable in circulation, resulting in RBCs becoming trapped and removed in the spleen. Given the inheritance pattern, obtaining a family history aids in the diagnosis.

Signs and Symptoms:

- Patients can be asymptomatic until adulthood.
- **Anemia,** increased unconjugated bilirubin **(jaundice), increased** incidence of **cholelithiasis** (pigment gallstones)

Laboratory Findings:

- Hb and Hct are decreased; MCV is normal.
- **MCHC is increased** (characteristic of this disease on step 1).
- **Osmotic fragility test** will show increased lysis of RBCs in hypotonic solution.
- **Spherocytes** are present on peripheral smear (Fig. 11.20).

Treatment:

- **Splenectomy** (decreases entrapment and destruction of spherocytes in the spleen) is curative but only indicated for patients with severe disease, given the increased risk of infection with encapsulated organisms.
- **Blood transfusion is used in patients with severe disease.**
- Patients must be on folate and iron supplementation given the chronic hemolytic state.

Hereditary Elliptocytosis (HE): HE is an **autosomal dominant** disorder that results from defects in the membrane protein **spectrin** (most common) and **band 4.1.** Signs and symptoms are similar to HS but generally milder (with most patients having no anemia). Peripheral blood smear will show **elliptocytes.** Hemolysis is caused by RBC destruction in the spleen (will result in splenomegaly). **Splenectomy is curative** in symptomatic patients.

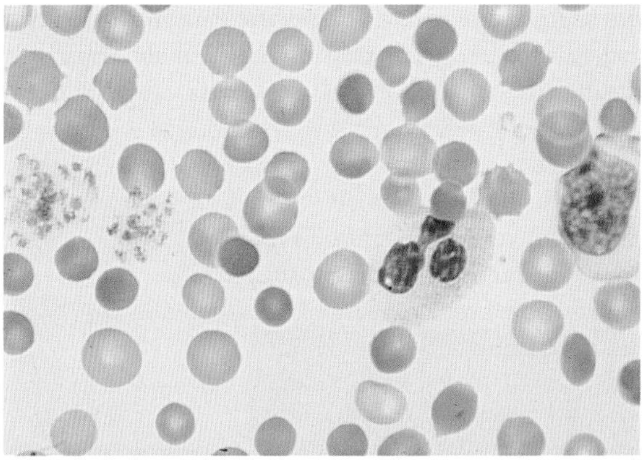

Fig. 11.20 Spherocytes on peripheral smear. (*From Damjanov I, Linder J. Pathology: A Color Atlas. St. Louis: Mosby; 2000:75.*)

Paroxysmal Nocturnal Hemoglobinuria (PNH): PNH results from a rare **acquired** intrinsic defect in the RBC cell membrane that **increases** the **susceptibly** of RBCs to **complement-mediated hemolysis.** Normal RBCs have glycosylphosphatidylinositol **(GPI)** linkage or decay-accelerating factor **(DAF)** proteins on their cell membrane, which act to protect the cell from destruction by the complement system. DAF helps disrupt formation of the membrane attack complex and prevents C9 from binding to the RBCs. Without these protective proteins on their cell surface, RBCs become easy targets for destruction by the complement system, and **intravascular hemolysis** ensues. Complement attachment to RBCs is potentiated in acidotic situations; therefore, there is **increased hemolysis at night** when respiratory acidosis ensues because of the physiologic decrease in respiratory rate while sleeping. PNH **usually occurs in the second decade of life and the incidence increases with age.** Platelets and granulocytes can also be affected by this disease. Patients with this disease are at **increased risk of** developing **aplastic anemia** and **acute leukemia.**

Signs and Symptoms:

- **Hemoglobinuria** (red urine) on awakening

Clinical and Laboratory Findings:

- Triad of Coombs negative hemolytic anemia with pancytopenia and venous thrombosis
- Usually normal MCV but can be microcytic (low MCV) because of long-standing loss of iron in urine (via loss of Hb and hemosiderin in urine)
- Iron deficiency caused by hemoglobinuria and hemosiderinuria
- **Increased incidence of venous thrombosis**
  - The intravascular destruction of platelets results in release of their prothrombotic intracellular granules into the circulation.
- Decreased serum haptoglobin (caused by intravascular hemolysis)
- Low leukocyte alkaline phosphatase (LAP) score

Treatment:

- Correct the anemia and prevent thrombosis.
- **Eculizumab** is a monoclonal antibody that acts as a terminal complement inhibitor.

Hemoglobin C (HbC) Disease: Hemoglobin C disease results from an **autosomal recessive** mutation in β-globin chain **leading to extravascular hemolysis**. An abnormal hemoglobin structure is formed by the substitution of glutamic acid with lysine at position 6 of the β-globin chain (sickle cell is a glutamic acid to valine substitution at the same position). The Hb in **HbC is less soluble than HbA** and **forms hexagonal crystals inside RBCs.** HbC does not polymerize as readily as HbS (sickle cell disease) and will produce less sickling of RBCs. The HbC mutation causes the RBC to lose plasticity, thereby leading to **mild extravascular hemolytic anemia in homozygotes (HbCC). Patients with sickle cell–hemoglobin C (HbSC)** have the gene for HbS inherited from one parent and the gene for HbC from the other parent. HbSC patients will have only a few sickle cells and thereby **have milder disease than HbSS patients.**

Signs and Symptoms:

- Most people have no symptoms.

Clinical and Laboratory Findings:

- Mild extravascular hemolysis in homozygotes or HbCC (people with HbC trait [HbAC] are phenotypically normal)
- **Peripheral smear** with **HbC crystals** seen in RBCs; will also see **target cells**
- Mild splenomegaly
- Mild anemia

Treatment:

- Usually no treatment is needed, but patients may supplement with folate to improve anemia.

Immune Hemolytic Anemias: Immune hemolytic anemias (IHAs) are diseases that develop from antibody or complement binding to antigens on the RBC membrane, leading to hemolysis. IHAs are classified into three groups—**autoimmune** hemolytic anemia (AIHA), **alloimmune** hemolytic anemia, and **drug-induced,** immune-mediated hemolytic anemia.

AIHA results from antibodies directed to an individual's own RBCs, causing them to lyse. These are categorized into **warm antibody** type AIHA and **cold antibody** type AIHA. Almost half of the primary causes of AIHAs are idiopathic. Secondary AIHA can result from underlying diseases or drugs. The presence of antibodies makes these anemias **Coombs test positive** (see later).

Warm antibody type AIHA is the **most common type of AIHA** (70%) and results from the binding of **IgG** to the RBC membrane. This leads to macrophage destruction of RBCs in the spleen (extravascular destruction, more common) or may result in part of the RBC membrane being removed, leading to hemolysis in the circulation (intravascular destruction). The partial removal of the membrane causes RBCs to lose their biconcave form and develop into **spherocytes.** Primary causes of warm-type AIHA are mostly idiopathic. Secondary causes of warm-type AIHA are as follows:

Warm antibody type = IgG
Cold antibody type = IgM

- Lymphoproliferative disorders—chronic lymphocytic leukemia, non-Hodgkin lymphoma
- Connective tissue disorders—systemic lupus erythematosus (most common cause), rheumatoid arthritis
- Medications—methyldopa, penicillin, cephalosporins, quinidine

Signs and Symptoms:

- May present with **jaundice,** cholelithiasis, splenomegaly, or general signs of anemia; may be asymptomatic if hemolysis is well compensated
- May see signs of underlying autoimmune disorder (e.g., rash, fever, lymphadenopathy, renal failure)

Laboratory Findings:

- Decreased Hb and Hct, normal (sometimes high) MCV
- **Spherocytes** on peripheral blood smear
- **Elevated unconjugated bilirubin (extravascular hemolysis)**
- **Decreased haptoglobin, increased urine hemoglobin levels (intravascular hemolysis)**
- **Positive** direct antihuman globulin test (DAT) or direct **Coombs test**
  - Direct Coombs test is when **anti-Ig Ab is added** to the patient's blood, leading to **agglutination of RBCs that already have IgG bound** to them.

Treatment:

- Folic acid supplementation is given because of the high RBC turnover.
- Treat the underlying cause (when secondary).
- When AIHA is not controlled by treating the underlying cause or treating idiopathic warm type AIHA, the following may be used:
  - Corticosteroids (main treatment)
  - RBC transfusion (severe disease)
  - Splenectomy (if the patient fails to respond to steroids)
  - Intravenous immunoglobulin (IVIG)

The most common **cold antibody** type AIHA is **cold agglutinin disease,** accounting for almost 15% of all AIHA. It is a disorder caused by IgM autoantibodies against RBCs that preferentially bind RBCs at low body temperatures. On binding the RBC, the IgM autoantibody will initiate the complement cascade, leading to C3b complement binding the RBC membrane. Once the C3b complement protein is bound to RBC in the circulation, the membrane attack complex is formed, resulting in RBC membrane instability and **intravascular hemolysis** (most common). If RBCs reach the spleen and have IgM bound to them but have not activated the membrane attack complex, they will be removed by splenic macrophages (extravascular hemolysis is less common). Cold antibody type AIHA occurs in chronic and acute forms. The primary causes of cold-type AIHA are mostly idiopathic. Secondary causes of warm-type AIHA are as follows:

- The **chronic form (most common)** is usually seen in older patients with **chronic lymphocytic leukemia,** lymphoma, and Waldenström macroglobulinemia. It is associated with **Raynaud phenomenon** (cold-induced acrocyanosis, blue extremities).
- The **acute form (less common and self-limited)** is usually seen in younger patients and as a rare complication of ***Mycoplasma pneumoniae*** and Epstein-Barr virus infections.

Signs and Symptoms:

- Anemia-related symptoms are usually mild.
- Jaundice and splenomegaly can occur.
- The **major symptom** is **cold-induced acrocyanosis** in which peripheral areas of the body turn blue (fingertips, earlobes, nose).

Laboratory Findings:

- Decreased Hb and Hct, normal MCV
- **RBC agglutination** on peripheral blood smear

Treatment:

- Treat the underlying disease.
- Acute forms are self-limited; supportive measures only are needed.
- **Avoid cold exposure.**
- **Splenectomy** (because mostly intravascular hemolysis) **and steroids are rarely helpful.**

Be aware that **certain drugs** can result in **immune-mediated HA** (drug-induced HA), most commonly by the **hapten mechanism** (Fig. 11.21). A hapten is a small molecule that, when combined with a larger molecule, can elicit the production of an antibody against it. The prototypical drug for this is

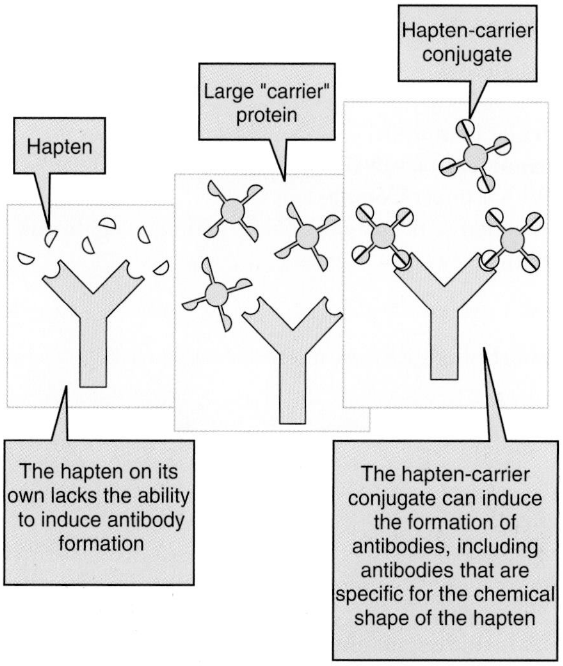

Fig. 11.21 Hapten formation and mechanism for drug-induced hemolytic anemia. (*From Nairn R, Helbert M.* Immunology for Medical Students, *2nd ed. Philadelphia: Elsevier; 2007.*)

penicillin; penicillin will bind with a protein on the RBC surface, leading to the production of antibodies against the penicillin-RBC compound. This results in hemolysis.

Methyldopa and **quinidine** are other medications associated with drug-induced IHA, although they result in hemolysis via a different mechanism than the one described.

Microangiopathic and Macroangiopathic Hemolytic Anemias: **Micro- and macroangiopathic hemolytic anemias** result from mechanical or shear stress destroying the RBC membrane, leading to hemolysis. Microangiopathic hemolytic anemia **(MAHA)** is caused by factors in the small blood vessels that cause them to narrow more than usual. MAHA is usually seen in disseminated intravascular coagulation **(DIC),** thrombotic thrombocytopenic purpura **(TTP),** hemolytic-uremic syndrome **(HUS),** or other disorders that cause increased coagulation, leading to the narrowing of small blood vessels. Macroangiopathic hemolytic anemia results from shear stress caused by turbulent blood flow or occurs in patients with stenosed or prosthetic heart valves.

- General signs and symptoms of anemia will be seen.
- The peripheral blood smear will show **schistocytes,** fragmented pieces of RBCs (Fig. 11.22).

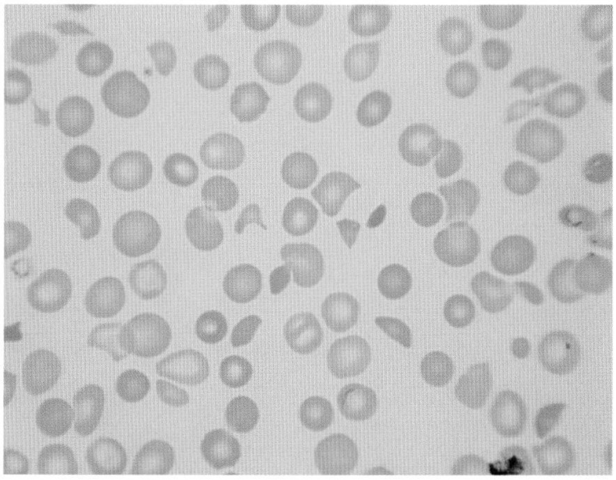

Fig. 11.22 Schistocytes—fragmented RBCs as a result of shear stress. (*From Goldman L, Ausiello D.* Cecil's Textbook of Medicine. *23rd ed. Philadelphia; Saunders Elsevier; 2008:1174.*)

Macrocytic Anemias

Macrocytic anemias (MCV > 100 fL) are divided into megaloblastic and nonmegaloblastic types. **Megaloblastic anemias** are usually related to **disorders of impaired DNA synthesis and have a markedly increased MCV (usually > 110 fL).** The term *megaloblastic* refers to the characteristic morphologic pattern of the hematopoietic cells. **Impairment of DNA synthesis results in arrest of the cell cycle;** blood cells are stuck in the growth phase because they cannot progress to mitosis without new DNA being produced, leading to macrocytosis (large cells). **Megaloblastic cells will have unbalanced cell growth, with dissociation between the maturity of their nucleus and cytoplasm.** The impairment of DNA synthesis causes the **nucleus** of these megaloblastic cells to become **hypersegmented,** a sign of immaturity, whereas the cytoplasm matures normally (Fig. 11.23).

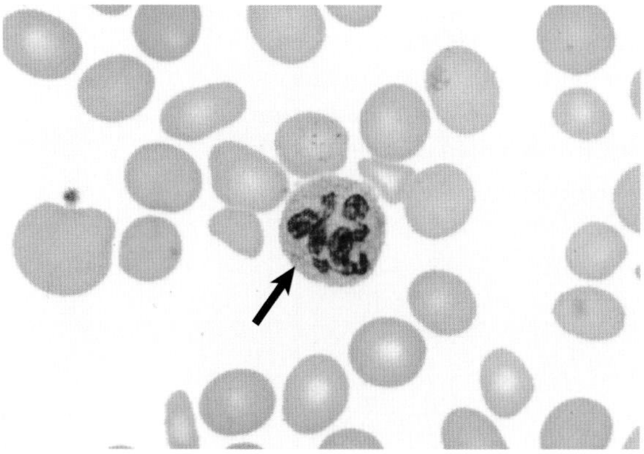

Fig. 11.23 Hypersegmented neutrophil (more than five lobes) seen in vitamin B_{12} or folate deficiency *(solid arrow)*. Macrocytic red blood cell (MCV > 100 fL). (*From Naeim F.* Atlas of Bone Marrow and Blood Pathology. *Philadelphia: WB Saunders; 2001:180.*)

Megaloblastic Anemias: Megaloblastic anemias generally occur as a result of **vitamin B_{12}** (cobalamin) or **folic acid deficiency;** both are coenzymes in DNA synthesis. Another, more rare, form of megaloblastic anemia arises from a defect in uridine monophosphate (UMP) synthase, resulting in the buildup of orotic acid in the urine **(orotic aciduria).**

Megaloblastic anemias = disorders of impaired DNA synthesis and MCV > 110 fL.

Role of Folate and Cobalamin in DNA Synthesis: **Folate** is required for DNA synthesis. It helps in the single-carbon transfer reactions required for nucleic acid synthesis (thymine). In this process, folate needs to be in the form of tetrahydrofolate (THF, or FH_4). To produce THF, folate must first be reduced to dihydrofolate (DHF, or FH_2), which is then further reduced to THF by **dihydrofolate reductase** (inhibited by methotrexate and trimethoprim). Once THF is made, it can participate in single-carbon transfer reactions that result in the conversion of deoxyuridine monophosphate **(dUMP)** to deoxythymidine monophosphate **(dTMP)** by **thymidylate synthase** (inhibited by 5-fluorouracil). **Cobalamin** is required to replenish the supply of THF for use in single-carbon transfer reactions. Cobalamin acts as a carbon acceptor (from methyl-cobalamin) and helps remove a carbon from N-5-methyl-THF (5-MTHF) to regenerate THF. 5-MTHF is the active circulating form of folate in the body. Methylcobalamin then transfers the methyl group to homocysteine to produce methionine (regenerates cobalamin) via methionine synthase (homocysteine methyltransferase). A deficiency in cobalamin or in methionine synthase can result in a methyl trap or folate trap of THF, in which levels of 5-MTHF build up and single-carbon transfer reactions are halted (Fig. 11.24).

dTMP has one more methyl group than dUMP.

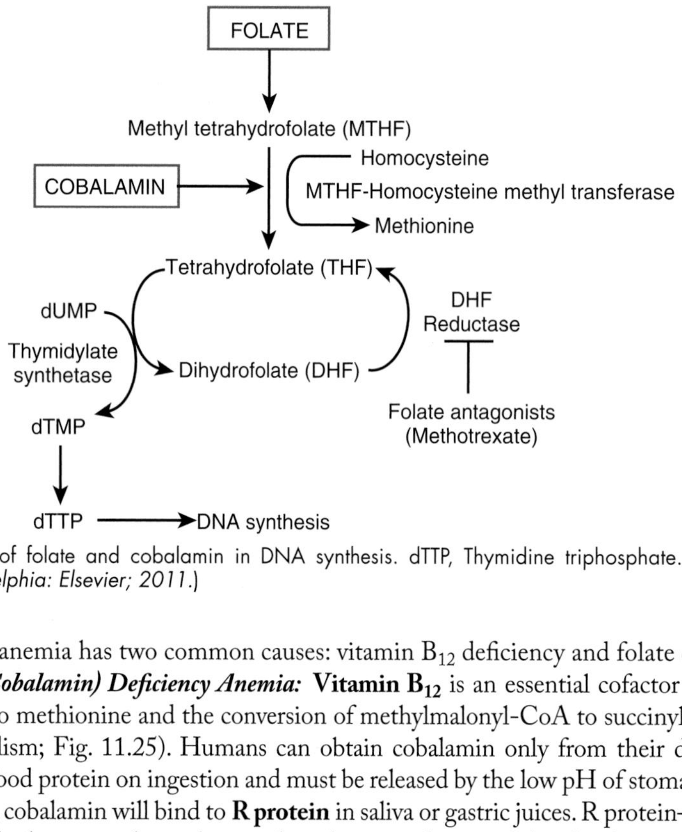

FIG. 11.24 Role of folate and cobalamin in DNA synthesis. dTTP, Thymidine triphosphate. (*From Hudnall SD.* Hematology. *Philadelphia: Elsevier; 2011.*)

Megaloblastic anemia has two common causes: vitamin B_{12} deficiency and folate deficiency.

Vitamin B_{12} (Cobalamin) Deficiency Anemia: **Vitamin B_{12}** is an essential cofactor in the conversion of homocysteine to methionine and the conversion of methylmalonyl-CoA to succinyl-CoA (odd-chain fatty acid metabolism; Fig. 11.25). Humans can obtain cobalamin only from their diet. Cobalamin is usually bound to food protein on ingestion and must be released by the low pH of stomach. Once released from food protein, cobalamin will bind to **R protein** in saliva or gastric juices. R protein–bound cobalamin will travel through the stomach until it reaches the second part of the duodenum, where pancreatic proteases cleave the R protein. The **free cobalamin** will then **bind** to intrinsic factor **(IF).** The **production of IF occurs** in the fundus and cardia of the **stomach parietal cells.** The **IF-cobalamin complex** travels

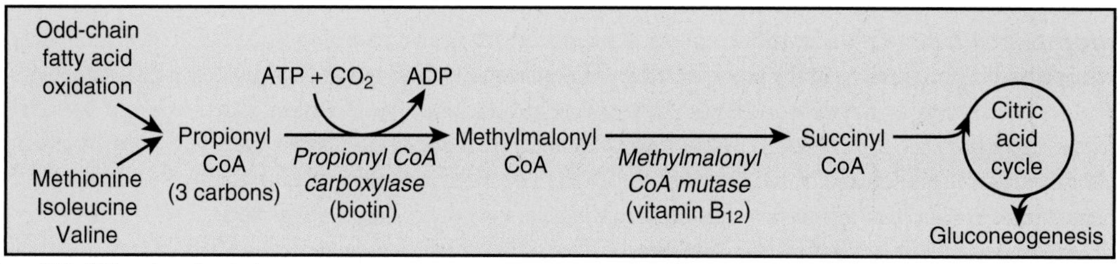

FIG. 11.25 Role of cobalamin in the metabolism of odd-chain fatty acids. (*From Pelley J, Goljan E.* Rapid Review Biochemistry. *2nd ed. Philadelphia: Mosby; 2007:117.*)

through the small intestine until it reaches the IF-cobalamin receptors on the **terminal ileum,** where it is **actively absorbed** into the enterocyte. Cobalamin is stored in the liver, which stores a 3- to 4-year supply.

Deficiency can arise from inadequate intake, impaired absorption, or increased requirement of cobalamin.

- **Inadequate intake**—strict vegetarians are at risk, as are breastfed infants of mothers with subclinical cobalamin deficiency.
- **Impaired absorption**—lack of gastric acid or **achlorhydria** (gastric acid is required to prepare cobalamin for absorption by cleaving R binders), lack of IF, gastric or ileal resection (ileum needed for absorption of cobalamin), Crohn disease or celiac disease in the terminal ileum, *Diphyllobothrium latum* (fish tapeworm), pancreatic insufficiency. **Pernicious anemia** is an autoimmune disorder that results in the destruction of parietal cells in the stomach and lack of IF production. IF is needed by the body to absorb cobalamin.
- **Increased requirements—**such as caused by pregnancy or hyperthyroidism.

Signs and Symptoms of Cobalamin Deficiency:

- **Smooth, beefy, red tongue** (nonhematologic effect of deficiency on epithelial tissues; all body cells rely on DNA synthesis for maintenance and renewal).
- **Peripheral neuropathy—**paresthesias, numbness, absent reflexes (loss of myelin regeneration).
- **Subacute combined degeneration of the spinal cord** is the patchy loss of myelin in the dorsal and lateral columns.
  - Dorsal column dysfunction leads to decreased proprioception and vibratory sensation.
  - Lateral column dysfunction leads to weakness of the legs, arms, and trunk (with tingling).
  - **Dorsal column involvement** leads to loss of vibratory and position senses.
  - **Psychiatric symptoms** include **dementia,** psychosis, and personality change.

Laboratory Findings:

- Hb and Hct are decreased; MCV is increased.
- **Decreased serum cobalamin level is diagnostic** of **deficiency** (this is a reliable measure of total body cobalamin status).
- Peripheral blood smear shows **pancytopenia, oval macrocytosis,** and **hypersegmented neutrophils** (more than five lobes).
- Bone marrow aspirate shows megaloblastic cells.
- **Increased** levels of **homocysteine *and* methylmalonic acid are present. Methylmalonic acid is elevated only in cobalamin deficiency.** The blood levels of both of these will rise before a decline in the total serum cobalamin level is seen.
- **Schilling test** (helps determine the site of the metabolic defect that led to deficiency).
- **Intrinsic factor** and **parietal cell antibody levels** are helpful in diagnosing pernicious anemia.

Treatment: It is important to note that most of the symptoms of cobalamin deficiency are actually folate deficiency symptoms, because all the symptoms are caused by a defect in the nucleic acid synthesis of thymine. If patients with cobalamin deficiency are treated with pharmacologic amounts of folate, almost all the symptoms and hematologic findings will resolve. However, the neuropsychiatric symptoms will not resolve. This is why it is important to differentiate folate from cobalamin deficiency. Intramuscular cobalamin supplementation is commonly used. Oral supplementation is acceptable if the patient does not have pernicious anemia or terminal ileum disease (i.e., patient produces IF and has terminal ileum IF receptors for enteral absorption).

Folate Deficiency Anemia:

Folate Metabolism: Folate is ingested in the form of polyglutamates but can only be absorbed by the body as a monoglutamate. The intestine is lined with an enzyme **(intestinal conjugase)** that helps cleave the polyglutamates to monoglutamate, allowing for its absorption by the jejunum. Anything that disturbs the function of intestinal conjugase (e.g., erosion of intestinal epithelium by Crohn or celiac disease, phenytoin inhibition of the enzyme) results in folate absorption deficiency. Once absorbed, the monoglutamate is converted to the circulating form of folate, 5-MTHF. **Folate** is **stored** in the **liver;** the body normally holds a **3-** or **4-month supply.** This short supply means that **overall, a patient is more likely to have a folate deficiency than cobalamin deficiency.**

Causes of Folate Deficiency: Deficiency arises from inadequate intake, impaired absorption, or increased demand for folate. Some medications result in deficiency.

- **Inadequate intake**—alcoholics are at risk (the absorption of folate is blocked); eating overcooked food can reduce absorption.
- **Impaired absorption**—intestinal malabsorption occurs in patients with celiac or Crohn disease.
- **Increased requirement**—such as occurs in **pregnancy,** lactation, and infancy.
- **Medications**—phenytoin, ethanol, trimethoprim-sulfamethoxazole, sulfasalazine, methotrexate can reduce absorption.

Signs and Symptoms of Folate Deficiency:

- Signs and symptoms are similar to those found in cobalamin deficiency but without the neuropsychiatric manifestations.
- Women with folate deficiency who become pregnant are at increased risk of developing fetal neural tube defects.

Laboratory Findings:

- Hb and Hct are decreased; MCV is increased.
- Peripheral blood smear shows **pancytopenia, oval macrocytosis,** and **hypersegmented neutrophils** (more than five lobes).
- Bone marrow aspirate shows megaloblastic cells.
- **Decreased serum folate levels** are diagnostic of folic acid deficiency. This test can vary depending on recent intake of folate—may show normal folate levels, even if total body levels are low, if the patient recently ate a meal high in folate.
- **The best screening test is measuring RBC folate levels.** This test is not affected by recent intake of folate.
- **Total serum homocysteine levels are elevated with normal methylmalonic acid levels.**

Treatment:

- Oral folic acid treatment is usually sufficient to resolve the deficiency (even in the presence of intestinal malabsorption). Supplementation must be continued until the hematologic findings have resolved.
- Prophylactic folate supplementation should be instituted in **all women thinking about getting pregnant,** pregnant or lactating women, and patients with chronic hemolysis (e.g., sickle cell disease).

Orotic Aciduria: **Orotic aciduria** is an autosomal recessive disorder involving a defect in the de novo pyrimidine pathway enzyme uridine 5′-monophosphate (UMP) synthase. Orotic acid is an intermediate product in the pyrimidine synthesis pathway and is normally converted to UMP. **A deficiency in UMP synthase results in a buildup of orotic acid.** The decreased pyrimidine synthesis results in decreased DNA synthesis and macrocytic RBC membrane formation.

Signs and Symptoms:

- Presents as **failure to thrive and developmental delay** in children, usually in the first year of life.

Laboratory Findings:

- Increased orotic acid crystals in the urine or **orotic aciduria**
- **Megaloblastic anemia** that **does not improve with** administration of **folate** or **B_{12}**
- **No hyperammonemia,** which helps distinguish from ornithine transcarbamylase (OTC) deficiency (OTC deficiency presents with orotic aciduria AND hyperammonemia)

Treatment:

- **Oral uridine** administration (uridine monophosphate)
  - Administration of uridine, which is converted to UMP, will bypass the metabolic block and replenish pyrimidine production.

Nonmegaloblastic Anemia: Nonmegaloblastic anemia is usually caused by **alcohol abuse; the MCV usually ranges from 100 to 110 fL;** there is **no defect in DNA synthesis** and **no megaloblastic cells.** Abstinence from alcohol will reverse the macrocytosis. Other causes of nonmegaloblastic macrocytosis include liver disease, hypothyroidism, Diamond-Blackfan anemia, and spurious myelodysplasia.

Diamond-Blackfan anemia (DBA) is a rare inherited congenital erythroid aplasia that normally presents within the first year of life. It is characterized by a defect leading to a decrease in erythroid progenitor cells in the bone marrow. Features that support a **diagnosis of DBA** include **nonmegaloblastic macrocytosis, elevated fetal Hb** (HbF), and **congenital craniofacial** as well as **upper extremity malformations** (triphalangeal thumbs).

Bleeding and Thrombotic Disorders

Thrombocytopenia is defined as a decrease in the number of circulating platelets in the blood (< 150,000/mm^3). A decrease in the number of circulating platelets results in an increased risk of bleeding events. However, spontaneous bleeding is not usually seen until the count drops below 20,000/mm^3. There are several scenarios that result in thrombocytopenia:

- **Problem of platelet production:** Bone marrow cannot produce platelets to maintain normal basal levels and replenish turnover. Common causes include aplastic anemia, leukemia, and folate or cobalamin deficiency.
- **Problem of platelet destruction:** Bone marrow is producing platelets, but they are being **destroyed** in high numbers by **immune causes** (e.g., autoantibodies against platelet glycoproteins, idiopathic thrombocytopenic purpura [ITP] or drugs) or **nonimmune causes** (e.g., mechanical destruction caused by prosthetic valves, DIC, TTP).
- **Problem of sequestration:** As platelets circulate in the blood, they must pass through the spleen. Normally, up to a third of total body platelets reside in the spleen and the laboratory can only detect platelets that are circulating in the blood. In **patients with splenomegaly,** circulating platelets can get stuck inside the spleen, leading to decreased numbers in the circulation **(platelet sequestration).**
- **Problem of dilution:** This can happen in patients receiving a mass blood transfusion or high volumes of intravenous fluids. Transfused blood often contains no platelets (unless the patient is being transfused with whole blood, which rarely happens), leading to a reduction in the concentration of platelets in the body.

Thrombocytosis is an increase in the circulating platelet level (>400,000/mm^3). The increase in platelets can be primary (e.g., reactive thrombocytosis because of infection) or secondary (e.g., essential thrombocytosis, polycythemia vera):

- **Reactive thrombocytosis** is the body's physiologic response to an injury or inflammation, resulting in a signal for the bone marrow to increase production.
- **Essential thrombocytosis** (ET), or thrombocythemia, is a hematopoietic stem cell disease **(myeloproliferative disorder)** in which there is an increased proliferation of megakaryocytes, leading to increased platelet production (usually > 600,000/mm^3 but > 1,000,000/mm^3 is diagnostic of ET). Most occur as a result of a mutation of the *JAK2* gene. ET is a disorder with an **indolent course** in which **patients often** are **asymptomatic,** with some having **past episodes** of **thrombosis (because of hyperviscosity)** and **hemorrhage (platelets produced are largely nonfunctional).** The **peripheral blood smear** will display very **large platelets** and the **bone marrow biopsy** will reveal hypercellularity, with markedly **increased** numbers of **abnormally large megakaryocytes. Plateletpheresis** is used for the **management of acute events.** Not all patients require **treatment,** but those who do respond well to **hydroxyurea.**

Platelet Abnormalities: All platelet abnormalities present with microhemorrhages, leading to the following:

- Easy bruising or ecchymoses (purpura) and pinpoint hemorrhages (petechiae; Fig. 11.26)

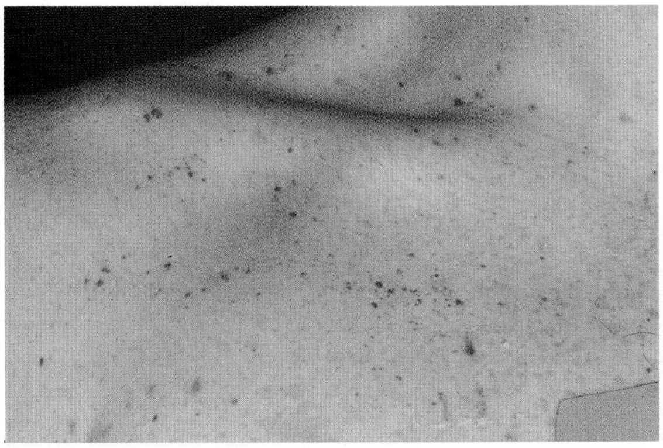

Fig. 11.26 Petechiae seen in a patient with thrombocytopenia. (*From Forbes C, Jackson W. Color Atlas and Text of Clinical Medicine. 2nd ed. St. Louis: Mosby; 2003:343.*)

- Mucosal bleeding, epistaxis
- Menorrhagia, hematuria
- Intracranial or gastrointestinal bleeding

Immune Thrombocytopenic Purpura or Idiopathic Thrombocytopenic Purpura: ITP is commonly an immunologically mediated platelet disorder (some causes are idiopathic) in which the formation of autoantibodies against platelets results in their destruction. There are two types of primary ITP: acute and chronic.

Chronic ITP: This is **an insidious disorder** that involves the formation of IgG **autoantibodies** against platelet membrane **GpIIb/GpIIIa** and megakaryocytes. **Woman are affected more commonly than men** (3:1 female-to-male ratio), and these affected women **tend to be younger than 40 years.** Thrombocytopenia ensues because of the destruction of platelets by splenic macrophages and damage caused to megakaryocytes (less common). Patients typically present with signs of thrombocytopenia, such as petechiae on the skin and mucosa, a history of nose or gum bleeds, hemorrhage in the soft tissues after minor trauma, or menorrhagia. Although the destruction of the platelets is largely occurring in the spleen, **splenomegaly is not usually seen.** The first line of **treatment** is usually **steroids,** but ITP can often be resistant to steroids. In **resistant cases,** the **treatment** is usually **splenectomy** because the spleen is thought to be the site of autoantibody production (and because it is involved in the clearance of antibody-coated platelets). Splenectomy may lead to marked improvement of the disease in up to 80% of patients.

Acute ITP: This is usually a **self-limited** disorder that occurs after a recent viral upper respiratory infection or immunization. Acute ITP is **usually a disorder of children aged 2 to 6 years.** Children will present with **abrupt onset of symptoms of thrombocytopenia** (purpura, epistaxis, petechiae). Like chronic ITP, no lymphadenopathy or splenomegaly develops. **Treatment with steroids** is reserved for severe cases, with very low platelet levels, because it resolves spontaneously in about 2 weeks.

> Chronic ITP—women with thrombocytopenia
>
> Acute ITP—children after upper respiratory infection with thrombocytopenia

Drug-induced Thrombocytopenia: As the name suggests, this disorder develops as an adverse effect of certain medications, namely **heparin,** quinines, and sulfonamide antibiotics.

Heparin-induced Thrombocytopenia (HIT): This can develop in up to 5% of patients who are on heparin therapy. **The thrombocytopenia usually occurs 5 to 14 days after the initiation of heparin treatment. This disorder occurs as a result** of heparin binding to platelet factor 4 (PF4), a normal platelet granule protein and **forming a hapten,** a new molecular structure recognized by the immune system as foreign. The body then makes antibodies against the heparin–PF4 complex (thrombocytopenia develops in 5 or more days because the body first has to make the antibodies), and **these antibodies have the potential to activate platelets.** The activation of platelets by the antibodies results in thrombus (clot) formation and consumption of platelets. Thus paradoxically, **HIT is characterized by excessive thrombi formation, not by excessive bleeding, as is seen in ITP and other thrombocytopenias.** These clots can form in large vessels and lead to life-threatening complications such as a large pulmonary embolism. **Treat by removing the offending agent (heparin).**

Thrombotic Thrombocytopenic Purpura: TTP is a consumptive thrombocytopenia in which there is widespread formation of microthrombi in the small blood vessels throughout the body, leading to decreased platelet levels in the circulation. This disorder is commonly seen in women. TTP occurs because of a deficiency in the ADAMTS-13 enzyme (von Willebrand factor [vWF] metalloprotease), a protease that cleaves multimers of vWF. The ADAMTS-13 enzyme deficiency leads to the accumulation of vWF multimers, creating a prothrombotic environment in which there is increased platelet aggregation, particularly at the arteriole–capillary junction. The thrombus formation is so ubiquitous that it may lead to microangiopathic hemolytic anemia by transforming the previously smooth blood vessel endothelium into a sharp and rough environment for RBCs to circulate through. Similarly to HIT, TTP is a thrombocytopenia that presents with excessive thrombi formation (not bleeding). Patients will present with the clinical pentad of thrombocytopenia, fever, microangiopathic hemolytic anemia, renal failure (microthrombi occlude renal arteries), and transient neurologic deficits. The first-line treatment is plasmapheresis. Patients with disease refractory to plasmapheresis can receive additional immunosuppressive treatment with steroids or vincristine.

> TTP—thrombocytopenia, fever, microangiopathic hemolytic anemia, renal failure, and CNS deficits; more common in adults

> HUS—thrombocytopenia, microangiopathic hemolytic anemia, renal failure; more common in children after GI infection.

Hemolytic Uremic Syndrome: HUS is a disorder similar to TTP that typically occurs in children younger than 10 years after an *Escherichia coli* O157:H7 infection. This strain of *E. coli* produces a Shiga-like toxin that damages the blood vessel endothelium, resulting in increased platelet activation. Patients will present with a similar clinical syndrome as TTP but without the neurologic deficits. The typical triad involves thrombocytopenia, renal failure, and microangiopathic hemolytic anemia.

Both TTP and HUS can be remembered by the mnemonic **FAT RN:** **f**ever, **a**nemia, **t**hrombocytopenia, **r**enal dysfunction, and **n**eurologic symptoms. For the last two words in the mnemonic, remember that in TTP the neurologic symptoms predominate and in HUS the renal dysfunction predominates.

Disseminated Intravascular Coagulation: DIC is a thrombohemorrhagic condition characterized by large amounts of intravascular microthrombi (clots) that consequently deplete platelet (and clotting factor) stores, leading to hemorrhage and thrombocytopenia. DIC happens in two stages, first a prothrombotic and later a prohemorrhagic stage.

Prothrombotic Stage: A systemic inflammatory event occurs (e.g., sepsis) that initiates the clotting cascade throughout the body. The clotting cascade is initiated in a large scale by the release of massive amounts of tissue factor (TF) into the circulation. The clotting cascade works via amplification, so the large amounts of TF released will result in exponentially larger amounts of thrombin (the end result of the clotting cascade) being produced. This abundance of thrombin leads to excessive clotting throughout the body. The formation of these clots leads to the depletion of platelets, fibrin (fibrinogen), and clotting factors (especially II, V, and VIII). The clot formation is so widespread that there is obstruction of blood flow throughout the body, which causes end organ ischemia and damage. Blood vessels are narrowed by the microthrombi, resulting in microangiopathic hemolytic anemia and further intensifying tissue ischemia.

Prohemorrhagic Stage: The body responds to the increase in clot formation by upregulating fibrinolysis. Plasminogen is activated, in the fibrinolytic cascade, in large quantities by tPA and factor XII, forming plasmin. Plasmin degrades the microthrombi by cleaving the cross-linked fibrin proteins, producing fibrin split products (D-dimers). Remember that in the body, coagulation and fibrinolysis occur as delicately balanced processes in which clotting is immediately counteracted by fibrinolysis until homeostasis is reached. In the case of DIC, the body is depleted of its procoagulant abilities and can no longer counteract the massive fibrinolysis that is taking place. This leads to excessive hemorrhaging and shock (caused by hypotension caused by blood loss). Patients will bleed from their mucous membranes, breaks in the skin (petechiae and ecchymoses), or rupture of fragile blood vessels (epistaxis, intracranial hemorrhages).

ITP: ↓ platelets only

TTP and HUS: ↓ platelets + MAHA

DIC: ↓ platelets + MAHA + ↑ PT/PTT

Causes of DIC Include: *the following (mnemonic:* ***STOP Making New Thrombi!****):*

Sepsis (gram-negative), commonly associated with *Neisseria meningitides* and *E. coli* infections
Trauma (severe)
Obstetric complications, such as amniotic fluid embolism, retained fetus, or abruptio placentae.
DIC may occur when amniotic fluid and other fetally derived antigens reach the maternal circulation, leading to a massive inflammatory reaction in the mother.
Pancreatitis
Malignancy
Nephrotic syndrome
Transfusion

Clinical and Laboratory Findings:

- Infarction of any organ, such as the brain, heart, lung, kidneys, adrenals, spleen, liver
- Pulmonary edema caused by increased vascular permeability
- Massive hemorrhaging and shock caused by blood loss (hypotension)
- Mucosal bleeding, petechiae, ecchymoses
- Microangiopathic hemolytic anemia (peripheral blood smear will show schistocytes).
- Increased BT (thrombocytopenia)
- Increased PT and PTT (depletion of clotting factors)
- Decreased fibrinogen level
- Increased levels of D-dimers (fibrin split products)

Treatment:

- Largely supportive, with an emphasis on treating the underlying cause of DIC.

Clotting Factor Deficiencies

Clotting factor deficiencies result in clinical findings similar to the small-vessel bleeds seen in platelet disorders in addition to large-vessel bleeding (hemarthroses or bleeding into the joints, retroperitoneal bleeding, and deep muscular bleeding). These deficiencies lead to decreased production of thrombin and reduced amount of fibrin plug formation at the site of injury. As a result, a weak platelet plug is made, causing delayed and spontaneous bleeding (especially after surgery), with a predisposition for soft tissue and intraarticular bleeding. Clotting factor deficiencies can be hereditary or acquired.

For findings in platelet abnormalities, see "Platelet Abnormalities."

Hemophilia A: Hemophilia A is a **hereditary, X-linked recessive disorder** that results in **decreased production of factor VIII** and is the **most common hemophilia.** The severity of the disease is dictated by the factor VIII activity of the patient, with symptomatic forms having less than 25% activity. These patients **most commonly suffer from acute hemarthrosis** (traumatic or spontaneous), leading to **chronic hemophilic arthropathy** (blood proteases in the synovial space will destroy the joint cartilage). **An increased PTT, normal BT, and normal PT** will be seen. The diagnosis is confirmed by evaluation with a **specific clotting factor assay for factor VIII.** Treatment is with **desmopressin acetate** (increases release of sequestered factor VIII) **in mild cases** or chronic **infusions of recombinant factor VIII in severe cases.**

Hemophilia B: Hemophilia B, also known as Christmas disease, is a **hereditary, X-linked recessive disorder** that results in **decreased production of factor IX** and is **clinically indistinguishable from hemophilia A.** Signs and symptoms are the same as hemophilia A. The diagnosis is made by a **specific clotting factor assay for factor IX.** Mnemonic: Hemophilia is not a **B9** (**b**enign, rhymes with factor **9**) condition.

Vitamin K Deficiency: Clotting factors II, VII, IX, and X and protein C and protein S in the coagulation cascade are vitamin K dependent. Vitamin K (a fat-soluble vitamin) is required for the γ-carboxylation, via epoxide reductase in the liver, that takes place to allow these clotting factors to function properly. In adults, vitamin K deficiency is usually a result of fat malabsorption (from pancreatic insufficiency) or small bowel disease (celiac or Crohn disease). In newborns, deficiency is caused by lack of colonization by vitamin K–producing bacteria (and breast milk does not contain vitamin K). This is why newborns require an intramuscular injection of vitamin K at birth.

Liver Disease: Proper liver function is required for the synthesis and clearance of all coagulation proteins. Patients with liver disease have impaired production of all coagulation factors. Of note, liver disease leads to decreased epoxide reductase activity and subsequent γ-carboxylation of vitamin K–dependent clotting factors. These patients also develop portal hypertension, leading to splenomegaly and platelet sequestration (a double hit). As a result, an increase in PT, PTT, and BT will be seen.

Hereditary Thrombosis Syndromes

Hereditary thrombosis syndromes are autosomal dominant disorders that lead to hypercoagulability. Patients will present with episodes of deep venous thrombosis and pulmonary emboli at a very young age (multiple episodes). These include factor V Leiden, ATIII deficiency, and protein C and protein S deficiencies.

Factor V Leiden: Factor V Leiden is the most common of the hereditary thrombosis syndromes and is characterized by a mutation in the factor V protein that makes it resistant to inactivation by APC. This leads to increased levels of factor Va and increased thrombin formation. Alone, it confers a relatively low risk of thrombosis, but when coupled with other risk factors (e.g., smoking, pregnancy, oral contraceptive pill [OCP] use), it can increase the likelihood of thrombosis.

Protein C and Protein S Deficiency: Normally, APC helps inactivate factors Va and VIIIa, halting clot formation. If there is no APC to inactivate factors Va and VIIIa, thrombin formation will increase, leading to thrombosis. Deficiency in protein C confers a very serious risk of thrombosis; therefore, patients should be started on anticoagulation therapy immediately. Protein C deficiency (a heterozygous defect, because a homozygous abnormality is incompatible with life) is associated with warfarin skin necrosis, a disorder that occurs when patients are started on warfarin therapy. As a result, treat with heparin first and then start low-dose warfarin (slowly titrate up to therapeutic levels) to prevent this complication.

Warfarin skin necrosis or hemorrhagic skin necrosis occurs because **protein C has a shorter half-life (6 hours) than all other vitamin K–dependent clotting factors.** Individuals with protein C deficiency have less than 50% protein C activity. When they are given warfarin (warfarin stops the hepatic production of vitamin K–dependent clotting factors and proteins C and S), their protein C activity drops to 0 within 6 hours. Because the half-life of the other vitamin K–dependent clotting factors is longer than 6 hours, there will be a **window of time during which the individual has no protein C activity (no anticoagulation) while still having vitamin K–dependent clotting factor activity.** Also, during this window of time, the individual will not be able to inactivate factors Va and VIIIa, leading to a so-called double-hit hypercoagulable state, at least until the remaining vitamin K–dependent clotting factors in the circulation degrade, based on their half-lives.

Antithrombin III Deficiency: ATIII is an inhibitor of each of the activated coagulation cascade enzymes, primarily factors IIa and Xa. Heparin enhances the inhibitory ability of ATIII. Individuals with **ATIII deficiency are heterozygous for a mutation that results in reduced ATIII activity.** Persons with this deficiency do not display an increase in PTT after injection with a standard dose of heparin. **Higher doses of heparin are required to reach its anticoagulant effect because not all the circulating ATIII in these individuals is functional.** This is a **severe prothrombotic disorder that requires lifelong anticoagulation therapy.** Treatment is to **give** the patient **higher doses of heparin** to overcome the deficiency and act as a bridge over to warfarin.

Typical age range for leukemias:
ALL, birth to 14 years
AML, 15 to 39 years
CML, 40 to 60 years
CLL, > 60 years

White Blood Cell Neoplastic Proliferation

WBC neoplasms are primarily categorized into **leukemias** and **lymphomas.** Initially they were believed to be separate entities, but the line often blurs between the two.

Leukemias are WBC neoplasms that generally present with widespread malignant involvement of the bone marrow and a large number of tumor cells in the peripheral blood. These cells often infiltrate normal tissues such as the liver, spleen, and lymph nodes. They are subdivided into acute and chronic leukemias. Acute leukemias are characterized by the presence of numerous immature tumor cells (blast cells) in the bone marrow and circulation. Acute leukemias are more aggressive cancers with a short course, usually affecting children or older adults. Chronic leukemias are characterized by the presence of mature tumor cells (or few blast cells) in the bone marrow and circulation. Chronic leukemias have a more indolent course and usually affect adults. The widespread bone marrow infiltration by leukemia often leads to marrow failure, resulting in anemia, thrombocytopenia, and neutropenia (pancytopenia).

Lymphomas are WBC neoplasms that generally proliferate in discrete tissue masses outside the bone marrow and typically present as a solid tumor in the lymph nodes. They are subdivided into Hodgkin lymphoma (presence of Reed-Sternberg cells) and non-Hodgkin lymphoma (lack Reed-Sternberg cells).

Leukemias

Acute Lymphoblastic Leukemia (ALL): ALL is a neoplastic disorder involving immature B or T cells (lymphoblasts). Patients with ALL typically present within days or weeks of onset of symptoms **(acute onset).** The malignant pre-B and pre-T lymphoblasts seen on peripheral smear are morphologically indistinguishable, so the subclassification of ALL is dependent on immunophenotyping. **Most ALLs** (≈ 85%) **are precursor B-cell** (pre–B-cell) **tumors** that typically **manifest in childhood,** with extensive bone marrow and variable peripheral blood involvement. The precursor **T-cell variant occurs in adolescence** and usually **presents with** a **mediastinal mass.** Most cases of ALL occur in those younger than 15 years (mnemonic to remember—ALL is common in children: ALL kids get ALL). The eventual marrow failure that occurs in ALL results in many of the **clinical findings,** such as general weakness and fatigue (anemia), frequent infections (neutropenia), and excessive bruising and bleeding (thrombocytopenia).

Other symptoms result from the voluminous numeric proliferation of the neoplastic pre–B cells or pre–T blast cells (enlarged lymph nodes, hepatomegaly, splenomegaly, bone and joint pain, and altered mental status or headaches [central nervous system (CNS) metastasis]). Testicular enlargement from spread to the testicles may be present in males. Relapses and spread of this disease may occur in the testes and CNS.

Laboratory Findings:

- **Increased WBC count** greater than 100,000 or less than 10,000 cells/mm^3; usually the higher the white count, the worse the prognosis.
- **Low Hb.** Anemia can be normocytic or macrocytic (if the folate level is low).
- **Low platelets** (thrombocytopenia).
- **Peripheral smear with many blast cells.** Lymphoblasts have condensed chromatin, indented nuclei, minimal cytoplasm, and no granules (Fig. 11.27).
- **Bone marrow biopsy** is diagnostic if more than **20% blasts are seen.** Normal marrow cells may be completely replaced by malignant cells.
- **Immunohistochemical testing.** Terminal deoxynucleotidyl transferase **(TdT)** or common acute lymphoblastic leukemia antigen **(CALLA)**–positive findings. TdT is a protein that is a marker for pre–B cells and pre–T cells (sign of immaturity).
- **Cytogenetics.** The most common translocation is t(12;21), and it confers a good prognosis.

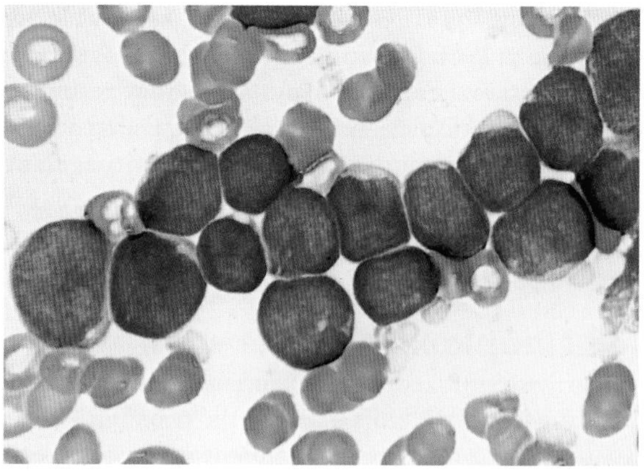

FIG. 11.27 Blast cells of ALL showing condensed chromatin, indented nuclei, minimal cytoplasm, and no granules. (*From Kumar V, Fausto N, Abbas AK. Robbins & Cotran Pathologic Basis of Disease. 7th ed. Philadelphia: Saunders; 2004.*)

Treatment: With aggressive **chemotherapy,** more than 90% of children with ALL achieve complete remission and at least two thirds can be considered cured.

Chronic Lymphocytic Leukemia (CLL) and Small Lymphocytic Lymphoma (SLL): CLL and SLL are disorders of the **malignant proliferation of B cells.** These two diseases are almost indistinguishable and differ only in the degree of peripheral blood lymphocytosis. In CLL, most malignant cells are in the circulation (or marrow), whereas in SLL, they are localized to focal masses (nodal or extranodal). In other words, it is called SLL if cancer is confined to the lymph nodes or CLL if blood cells are found in the peripheral blood. This is the most common type of leukemia and is considered a disease of older adults **(average age of onset, 60 years). Men are more commonly affected** (2:1 male-to-female ratio). The **onset of disease is insidious,** and **individuals are often asymptomatic at presentation** (patients will have an incidentally elevated WBC on routine CBC). **Symptomatic** patients often display the following:

- Painless lymphadenopathy (have a high suspicion in an older man with lymphadenopathy), hepatosplenomegaly (50%-60% of cases), fatigue or weakness (anemia), infection (hypogammaglobulinemia), bleeding (thrombocytopenia) can be present.
- **Anemia** can result from **bone marrow infiltration** of **malignant cells** overwhelming normal hematopoietic cells or, in some cases, the development of a hemolytic anemia.
- **Hypogammaglobulinemia** can result from disruption of normal immune function through uncertain mechanisms and contributes to increased susceptibility to infection.

Laboratory Findings:

- **Increased WBC count** and other CBC findings are similar to what is seen in ALL.
- **Peripheral smear shows few to no blast cells.** The smear contains increased numbers of small round lymphocytes, with scant cytoplasm. These cells are fragile and are often disrupted in the process of making smears, producing so-called **smudge cells** (Fig. 11.28).
- **Bone marrow biopsy** results indicate **less than 10% blast cells.**
- Some patients may have a monoclonal Ig spike.

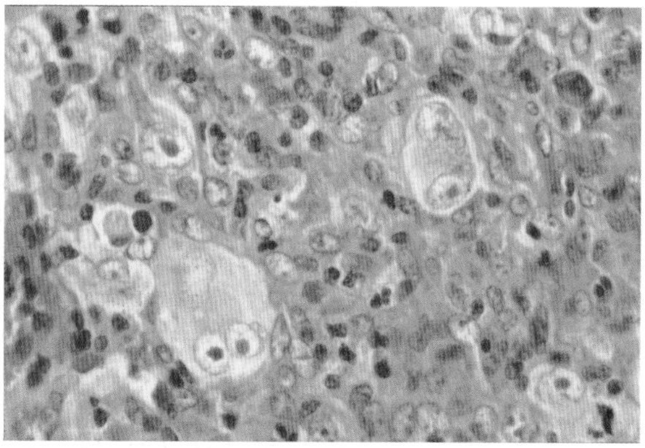

FIG. 11.28 Smudge cells, fragile lymphocytes of CLL disrupted in the preparation of a peripheral smear. (*From Hoffbrand AV. Color Atlas: Clinical Hematology. 3rd ed. St. Louis: Mosby; 2000:179.*)

Immunohistochemical Testing: Tumor cells express B-cell markers CD19 and CD20. **Tumor cells also express CD5 on B cells.** This aids the diagnosis because CD5 is usually only present on normal T cells; CD5 on a B cell identifies it as malignant.

CLL—smudge cells on peripheral smear

Cytogenetics: Unlike most other lymphoid malignancies, chromosomal translocations are rare in CLL and SLL.

Treatment: Because CLL progresses slowly, the goal of treatment is often to control symptoms created by the disease rather than curing it. Average survival is 4 to 6 years, but patients with a minimal initial tumor burden can survive for longer than 10 years.

Acute Myelogenous Leukemia (AML): AML **is a neoplasm of the myeloid line of blood cells** and is the **most common acute leukemia** in **adults.** Because the myeloid cell line produces a variety of cells, AML is a heterogeneous disease, with many subtypes. The median age at diagnosis is 65 years old. Most AMLs are associated with acquired genetic alterations that inhibit terminal myeloid differentiation. As a result, normal marrow elements are replaced by relatively undifferentiated blast cells. The accumulation of these immature neoplastic myeloid precursor blast cells in the marrow suppresses the remaining normal hematopoietic progenitor cells by physical replacement. The eventual failure of normal hematopoiesis results in **anemia, neutropenia,** and **thrombocytopenia,** which cause most of the major clinical complications of AML. As a result, the aim of treatment is to clear the bone marrow of the neoplastic cells, thus permitting normal hematopoiesis. The progression of AML is rapid and can be fatal in weeks to months if left untreated. A common type of AML that is seen and tested on the United States Medical Licensing Examination (USMLE) is acute promyelocytic leukemia (APL, also known as M3 AML under the French American British [FAB] system), which has distinctive histologic characteristics and a different treatment (see later). Although the FAB system has eight different subtypes of AML (M0 through M7), APL (M3) is the most important to recognize because of these differences.

Clinical and Laboratory Findings:

- The **onset** of the disease is **acute,** with most patients presenting within weeks to a few months with symptoms related to anemia **(fatigue),** neutropenia **(fever),** and thrombocytopenia **(spontaneous mucosal and cutaneous bleeding).**
- The **leukemic cells often release procoagulant and fibrinolytic factors,** usually seen in acute promyelocytic leukemia **(APL, M3 AML),** with some **patients presenting with DIC.**
- **Lymphadenopathy** is **rare** in **AML** (helps distinguish it from ALL).
- Some patients present with **swelling of the gums,** usually in **acute monocytic leukemia** (previously M5 AML), from gum tissue infiltration of leukemic cells.
- **A peripheral blood smear** will have increased myeloblast cells. Several types of myeloid blasts are recognized and can be seen in individual patients. **Myeloblasts** have **delicate nuclear chromatin,** two to four nucleoli, **voluminous cytoplasm** compared with lymphoblasts, and peroxidase-positive granules.
- Cells will often contain **Auer rods** (Fig. 11.29), splinter-shaped structures that represent abnormal azurophilic granules (burgundy-colored, peroxidase-positive granules), **especially in APL.** Auer rods are not present in ALL or chronic myelogenous leukemia (CML), helping distinguish these two disorders from AML.
- **Bone marrow biopsy** results will show more than 20% myeloid blast cells.

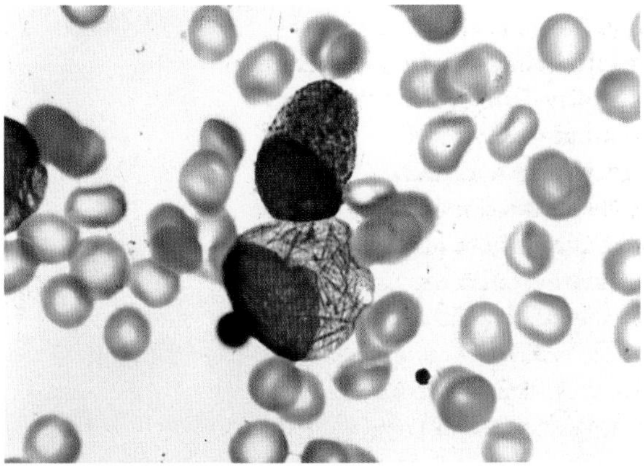

FIG. 11.29 Auer rods in a patient with APL. *(From Damjanov I, Linder J. Pathology: A Color Atlas. St. Louis: Mosby; 2000:79.)*

Immunohistochemical Testing: Because it is often difficult to distinguish myeloblasts morphologically from lymphoblasts in some cases, the diagnosis of AML is typically confirmed by staining cells for myeloid-specific surface markers.

Cytogenetics: The t(15;17) translocation of the retinoic acid receptor α (RARA) to the promyelocytic leukemia protein (PML) is associated with APL, leading to abnormal retinoic acid metabolism, making APL responsive to all-*trans* retinoic acid treatment.

Treatment of APL is with all-*trans* retinoic acid.

Treatment: First-line treatment is chemotherapy, which is divided into two phases, induction and consolidation.

- **Induction therapy** is geared toward **reducing** the **number** of **leukemic** cells to undetectable levels. Cytarabine and daunorubicin are used for induction therapy, with 70% of patients achieving remission with this protocol.
- **Consolidation therapy** is geared toward **eradicating residual disease** and ultimately achieving a cure. Consolidation therapy consists of aggressive chemotherapy with or without radiation.
- **High-dose all-*trans* retinoic acid** is used for patients with APL.

Chronic Myelogenous Leukemia: CML is a leukemia and myeloproliferative disorder that results in the proliferation of **myeloid cells capable of terminal differentiation (mature myeloid cells).** This myeloproliferative disorder is commonly associated with the **BCR-ABL (t[9;22])** translocation, or **Philadelphia chromosome.** The resultant translocation of the *BCR* gene on chromosome 9 to the *ABL* gene on chromosome 22 creates a fusion protein, with constitutively active tyrosine kinase activity. More than 90% of CML cases will display the Philadelphia chromosome on karyotyping. The *BCR-ABL* fusion gene continuously activates a cascade of proteins that control the cell cycle, causing unregulated myeloproliferation. Additionally, the BCR-ABL fusion protein inhibits DNA repair, resulting in genomic instability and increased susceptibility to further genetic mutations. The unregulated proliferation of leukemic cells overcrowds the bone marrow and prevents normal cell production. Normal bone marrow is usually about 50% cellular and 50% fat; the marrows of CML patients are usually 100% cellular, with maturing granulocytic precursors comprising most of the increased cellularity. The onset of **symptoms** is **insidious** and **nonspecific,** with many patients being asymptomatic at diagnosis (incidentally elevated WBCs on routine CBC). Some patients present with **mild anemia** and hypermetabolism (because of increased cell turnover) leading to easy **fatigability**, weakness, **weight loss,** and anorexia.

CML—defined by *BCR-ABL* gene. Treat with Gleevec.

Clinical and Laboratory Findings:

- **Splenomegaly** is common, with some patients presenting with left-sided pain.
- Generalized painless lymphadenopathy can be present.
- Anemia and thrombocytopenia occur in 50% of patients.
- **WBC count is increased (50,000 to 200,000 cells/mm^3).**
- **Thrombocytosis may be seen in up to 50% of patients** with CML (as opposed to most leukemias, which present with thrombocytopenia).
- CML is often suspected on the basis of the CBC, with increased numbers of granulocytes of all types.
- Peripheral smear will show a mix of neutrophils, metamyelocytes, and other mature myelocytes, as well as increased levels of basophils and eosinophils.
- **Elevated levels** of **basophils** and **eosinophils** (along with mature myeloid cells) helps distinguish CML from leukemoid reaction (see later). Another **differentiation** from **leukemoid reaction** is that **CML does not have elevated levels of LAP** (levels are decreased in CML).
- **Definitive diagnosis is made with polymerase chain reaction (PCR) analysis revealing BCR-ABL fusion protein.**
- Very few (<10%) myeloblasts are seen on peripheral smear and bone marrow biopsy.
- **Blast crisis** may occur later in the evolution of CML. These events are characterized by increased number (>20%) of myeloblasts or lymphoblasts in the blood or marrow. These blasts will not contain Auer rods, helping distinguish a CML blast crisis from AML. Blast crisis behaves like an acute leukemia.
- Bone marrow biopsy results will be hypercellular, but diagnosis is mainly made by PCR assay.

Cytogenetics:

- 90% of patients will have t(9;22) translocation.

Treatment:
- **Imatinib mesylate (Gleevec)** is the first-line treatment. It **is a tyrosine kinase inhibitor** and helps halt the progression of CML in most patients, allowing for regrowth of normal marrow. Overall survival 5-year rate is 90% in patients on imatinib.
- The natural history of CML is one of slow progression, and even without treatment, a median survival of 3 years can be expected. After a variable period averaging 3 years, approximately 50% of patients enter an accelerated phase, during which there is increasing anemia and thrombocytopenia and sometimes voluminous peripheral blood basophilia or a blast crisis. Eventually patients exhibit increasing episodes of an accelerated phase, or blast crises.
- Allogeneic bone marrow transplantation.

Leukemoid Reaction: Leukemoid reaction is defined as an exaggerated response to stress or infection that leads to a markedly elevated WBC count (as opposed to a primary blood malignancy, such as leukemia). The white count is typically elevated to more than 50,000 cells/mm^3, with a significant increase in neutrophils, lymphocytes, and/or eosinophils. Leukemoid reactions with neutrophil precursors (i.e., band forms) are the most common. The term *increased white count with left shift* is often used to describe an elevated WBC count with a predominant increase in neutrophil precursors or band forms (usually a sign of infection). It is important to differentiate this from acute and chronic leukemias. In leukemoid reactions, **a mix of mature myelocytes, metamyelocytes, promyelocytes,** and **myeloblasts** are seen **in the peripheral blood** smear. This is different than in **acute leukemia,** in which a predominance of **immature** myeloid cells is seen. The blood smears in CML and leukemoid reaction are similar, with a few exceptions:
- In a **leukemoid reaction,** the LAP level is **elevated** because the leukocytes are functioning normally (malignant cells have lost the ability to produce LAP).
- CML more commonly has **basophilia** and **eosinophilia** in the peripheral smear (along with an increase in other mature myeloid cells).
- CML will be Philadelphia chromosome positive.

Hairy Cell Leukemia (HCL): HCL is a **rare B-cell neoplasm** that predominantly **affects middle-aged white men** (4.1 male-to-female ratio). Its name derives from the morphologic appearance of the leukemic cells, which have fine, hairlike cytoplasmic projections (Fig. 11.30). **The bone marrow is always involved** in this disease, leading to marrow failure and **pancytopenia** (anemia, thrombocytopenia, neutropenia). The spleen is another common site of proliferation, with almost **90% of patients presenting with splenomegaly** (sometimes the only clinical finding). Interestingly, **this is the only leukemia that presents without lymphadenopathy.** Examination of the **bone marrow** will demonstrate **diffuse proliferation of tumor cells that stain positive for tartrate-resistant acid phosphatase (TRAP), which clinches the diagnosis.** Not all patients require treatment (usually reserved for highly symptomatic disease); treatment success does not depend on treating the disease at an early stage. **HCL** is very responsive to purine analog treatment (cladribine and pentostatin).

TRAP-positive stain is diagnostic of HCL.

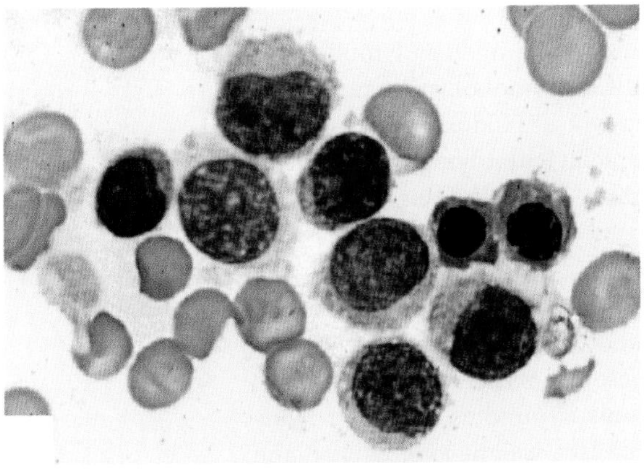

FIG. 11.30 Fine, hairlike cytoplasmic projections of hairy cell leukemia. (*From Naeim F.* Atlas of Bone Marrow and Blood Pathology. *Philadelphia: WB Saunders; 2001.*)

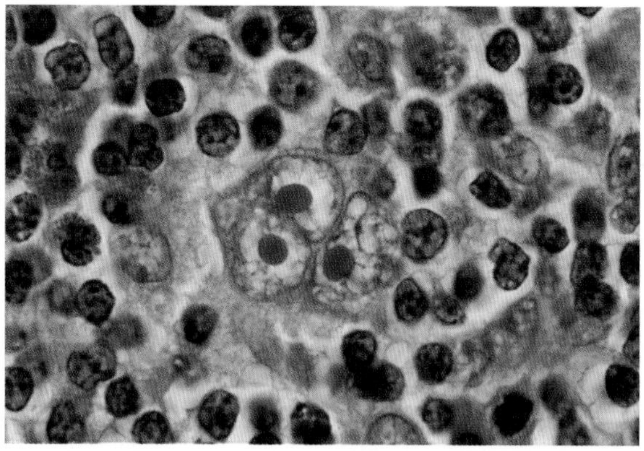

Fig. 11.31 Reed-Sternberg cell—multinucleated giant cell, with two mirror image nuclei (owl's eyes), each with an eosinophilic nucleolus. These are characteristic of Hodgkin lymphoma. (*From Damjanov I, Linder J. Anderson's Pathology. 10th ed. St. Louis: Mosby; 1996:1145.*)

Lymphomas

Hodgkin Lymphoma (HL): HL is a distinct type of lymphoma characterized by the **orderly spread of Hodgkin cells from lymph node (LN) group to LN group** and the presence of **Reed-Sternberg** cells (RSCs). These features help differentiate it from non-Hodgkin lymphoma (NHL), a group of disorders that spread in a less predictable manner and do not have Reed-Sternberg cells. The **RSC** is a **multinucleated giant cell,** usually with two mirror image nuclei **(owl's eyes)**, each with an eosinophilic nucleolus (Fig. 11.31). These cells are usually **transformed** germinal center **B cells** and have a **CD30⁺** and **CD15⁺** immunophenotype. RSCs release factors that recruit reactive lymphocytes, histiocytes, granulocytes (eosinophils), and plasma cells, which make up most of the cellularity of the tumors. RSCs can also take a variety of forms and help in the diagnosis of HL. There are **four major subtypes of HL** based on RSC morphology and the characteristics of the cell infiltrate seen in the lymph nodes (cell composition surrounding the RSC):

- **Nodular sclerosing** is the **most common** subtype, named for the prominent collagen fibrosis (sclerosis) surrounding the scattered (few) RSCs and lacunar cells (a variant RSC seen in this subtype). It occurs more commonly in women. Mediastinal lymph nodes are usually involved, and it is usually EBV negative. Patients commonly present at stage I or II. Nodular sclerosing HL has a good prognosis.
- **Mixed cellularity** is the **second most common** subtype and is named for the prominence of **numerous RSCs admixed with numerous inflammatory cells** (lymphocytes, histiocytes, eosinophils, and plasma cells) without surrounding sclerosis. This subtype may display the mononuclear variant RSC and is usually seen in men older than 50 years. This type is commonly associated with EBV infection. It presents with increased eosinophils, histiocytes, and plasma cells.
- **Lymphocyte-depleted** is a **rare** subtype named for the **presence of numerous RSCs,** with few surrounding inflammatory cells (few lymphocytes, histiocytes, eosinophils, plasma cells). Most cases that used to be diagnosed under this subtype have now been recategorized as a variant of nodular sclerosis HL or as variants of diffuse large cell NHL. This subtype also occurs in men older than 50 years or in HIV-positive individuals. It is the most aggressive form of HL, and patients often present with disseminated disease. **This has the worst prognosis of all of the HL subtypes.**
- **Lymphocyte-predominant** is a **rare** subtype that is often confused with nodular lymphocyte–predominant B cell NHL because it is **difficult to find typical RSCs.** Lymphohistiocytic variant RSC (popcorn cells) may be seen. As a result, it is not considered a typical Hodgkin lymphoma. It usually presents in **young men with asymptomatic cervical or supraclavicular lymphadenopathy.** The immunophenotype is usually negative for CD20⁺, CD15⁻, CD30⁻, and EBV. This subtype **has the most favorable prognosis.**

HL characteristics:
- RSCs present
- Orderly spread from LN to LN group
- Constitutional B symptoms (advanced disease)
- Splenomegaly rare

The **most common sign** of HL is **painless cervical or supraclavicular lymphadenopathy** (mediastinal lymph nodes may also be affected and are seen on a chest radiograph). HL rarely affects the Waldeyer ring (tonsils and adenoids) or mesenteric nodes, whereas these lymph nodes are more often affected in NHLs. HL patients **present with constitutional B symptoms,** symptoms that affect many different organ systems in the body, such as low-grade fever, night sweats, weight loss, fatigue, and malaise. Constitutional symptoms are usually a marker for advanced disease (stages III and IV), with earlier stages often being asymptomatic. **Gross splenomegaly is rare in HL** and more commonly occurs in NHL. Half of patients with HL are associated with an EBV infection, but the precise contribution of EBV remains unknown. HL is more commonly seen in whites than blacks. The **age distribution is bimodal,** affecting the young (20s) and older (>50s), with average age at diagnosis being 32 years old. **All subtypes,** except nodular sclerosing, **affect men more commonly than women.** HL **is diagnosed based on lymph node biopsy** and the following: (1) the presence of the diagnostic RSCs or (2) the presence of a variant RSC with a background of reactive inflammatory cells (lymphocytes, histiocytes, eosinophils, plasma cells).

Types of HL:
- Nodular sclerosing (most common)
- Mixed cellularity
- Lymphocyte depleted
- Lymphocyte predominant

Clinical and Laboratory Findings:
- Normocytic anemia
- Painless enlargement of single groups of contiguous lymph nodes (usually above the diaphragm)

Treatment:
- The clinical stage of HL is more important for prognosis than subtype of HL.
- Standard of treatment is the ABVD chemotherapy regimen for 6 to 8 months:
  - **A:** **A**driamycin (doxorubicin)
  - **B:** **B**leomycin
  - **V:** **V**inblastine
  - **D:** **D**acarbazine

NHL characteristics:
- No RSCs
- Multiple peripheral LN involved (no orderly spread of disease)
- Extranodal involvement
- Constitutional symptoms less common
- Splenomegaly more likely

Non-Hodgkin Lymphoma (NHL): NHL is a broad category of **B-cell (occasionally T-cell) blood cancers** that include all lymphomas except for Hodgkin lymphomas. NHL is classified into different categories based on the normal cell type that most resembles the tumor. For example, a lymphoma composed of cells that resemble cells of the normal mantle zone of the lymphoid follicle is called Mantle cell lymphoma. There are three large groups of NHL—B-cell, T-cell, and NK-cell lymphomas (B- and T-cell tumors will be discussed in detail; NK-cell tumors are rarely tested on Step 1):
- **B-cell tumors**—SLL (see earlier, "Leukemias"), follicular lymphoma, diffuse large B-cell lymphoma, Mantle cell lymphoma, Burkitt lymphoma, extranodal marginal zone B-cell lymphoma or mucosa-associated lymphoid tissue (MALT) lymphoma
- **T-cell tumors**—adult T-cell lymphoma, mycosis fungoides (Sezary syndrome)
- **NK-cell tumors**—extranodal NK-cell lymphoma, blastic NK-cell lymphoma

NHLs account for almost 60% of adult (mostly B-cell type) and childhood (mostly T-cell or Burkitt) lymphomas. They are often associated with immune suppression (e.g., HIV, chronic steroid therapy). NHLs are distinguished from HL by the fact that they do not produce Reed-Sternberg cells, lymphadenopathy **usually presents in multiple groups of peripheral lymph nodes,** and there may be **extranodal tumor involvement.** Also unlike HL, **NHLs do not spread in a contiguous manner.** Patients are **less likely to develop constitutional B symptoms** on presentation. Common risk factors associated with the development of NHL include the following:
- EBV infection (also a risk factor in Hodgkin lymphoma)
- Human T-cell leukemia virus type 1 (HTLV-1; adult T-cell lymphoma, leukemia)
- Hepatitis C infection
- *Helicobacter pylori* (MALT lymphoma)
- Immune suppression (AIDS)
- Prior high-dose radiation therapy (treatment of HL often risk factor for developing NHL)

B-cell Lymphomas:

Follicular Lymphoma (FL): This is one of the **most common** (almost 45% of adult lymphomas) adult forms of **NHL** in the United States. FL cells **closely resemble the normal germinal center B cells** of the lymphoid follicle (the tumor actually forms follicles, like normal tissue). As a result, it can be confused microscopically with physiologically reactive follicular hyperplasia, except that the follicles in FL do not generally respect the normal anatomic architecture of the lymph node, and **nodal architecture is effaced by nodular expansion** (Fig. 11.32). Microscopically, you will see a predominantly nodular or nodular and diffuse growth pattern in the involved lymph node.

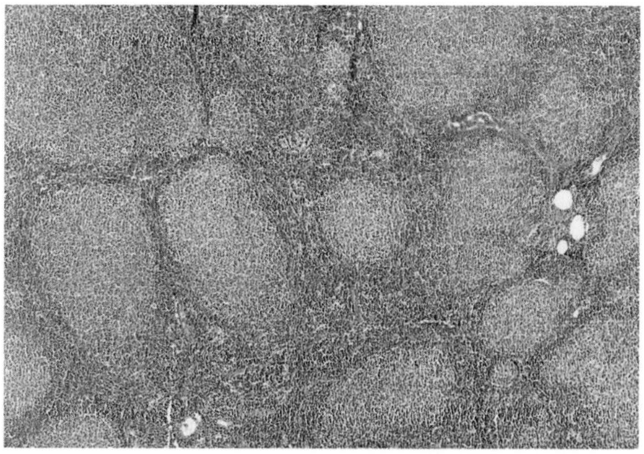

Fig. 11.32 Follicles effacing lymph node architecture in follicular lymphoma. (*From Goljan EF. Rapid Review Pathology Revised Reprint. 3rd ed. Philadelphia: Elsevier; 2011.*)

Nodules vary in size and contain two principle cell types, predominantly small lymphocytes with cleaved nuclei **(centrocytes)** along with variable numbers of larger cells with vesicular chromatin and prominent nucleoli **(centroblasts).** A key hallmark of classic FL is a **t(14;18) translocation** that fuses the IgH locus (chromosome 14) onto the BCL-2 locus (chromosome 18), leading to **increased *BCL-2* expression (an antiapoptosis gene)** and inhibition of cell apoptosis. Histologic transformation may occur in 30% to 50% of FLs, most often to diffuse large B-cell lymphoma. Patients will usually **present during middle age,** with **men and women affected equally**. FL usually follows an **indolent waxing and waning course.** Patients **typically present with painless, generalized lymphadenopathy.**

Treatment:

- This disease is **incurable** and treatment is variable depending on age, stage, and prognostic scores. Survival is also variable, with median survival from 7 to 9 years.
- Asymptomatic patients may benefit from a watchful waiting approach.
- Because this disease is not improved by aggressive therapy, the usual clinical approach is to **palliate patients with low-dose chemotherapy or radiation when they become symptomatic.**

Diffuse Large B-cell Lymphoma (DLBCL): DLBCLs are another **common** (40%-50% of adult lymphomas) **adult form of NHL.** This is a **very aggressive tumor that is rapidly fatal if left untreated.** It is the most commonly encountered (80%) subtype of the diffuse large-cell lymphoma group (diffuse large T-cell lymphomas make up the other 20%). They resemble the large lymphocytes that usually reside in normal follicles and are **derived from germinal centers.** DLBCLs rarely display a follicular pattern **(they lack follicular architecture),** helping differentiate them from normal germinal centers. They obtain their name from the fact that lymphomas that do not form follicles are referred to as diffuse lymphomas. Microscopically, you will note **sheets of large cells** with **prominent nucleoli** that can take **many forms** (may be two or three nucleoli located peripherally to the nuclear membrane or may be single and centrally placed). Their molecular profile is heterogeneous and does not have a defining translocation or mutation (although 10%-20% will exhibit the t(14;18) translocation seen in FLs. Remember that some FLs may transform into DLBCLs. The chromosome abnormalities that may be observed include anomalies in the *BCL-2, BCL-6,* or *MYC* genes (some have a combination of one to three of these anomalies). **The median age at diagnosis is 60 to 70 years** but has a wide age range (up to 5% of all childhood lymphomas). Like many NHLs, there is a **slight male predisposition.**

Clinical and Laboratory Findings:

- May **present with a rapidly enlarging, often symptomatic, mass at a single nodal** or **extranodal site.** Extranodal disease may arise within the gastrointestinal (GI) tract, skin, bone, brain, and other sites (can arise at almost any site). There may be primary or secondary involvement of the liver and spleen in the form of large destructive masses.
- Bone marrow involvement happens late in disease.
- **Immunophenotype:** These mature B-cell tumors express B-cell markers CD19 and CD20.
- Diagnosed via mass or nodal biopsy.

Treatment:

- The standard of treatment is **CHOP.** The expanded **CHOP-R** protocol may confer improved survival:
  - **C:** **C**ytoxan (cyclophosphamide)
  - **H:** **H**ydroxydaunorubicin (doxorubicin)
  - **O:** **O**ncovin (vincristine)
  - **P:** **P**rednisone
  - **R:** **R**ituxan (rituximab)
- Complete remission can be achieved in 60% to 80% of patients, and about 50% remain disease-free for several years.

Mantle Cell Lymphoma (MCL): MCL is an **extremely rare form of NHL** composed of cancerous cells that **resemble mantle zone B lymphocytes** (cells present at the perimeter of the germinal center) in the normal lymphoid follicle. Microscopically, MCL is normally diffuse but sometimes tumor cells may be seen surrounding benign germinal centers. The proliferation consists of a homogenous population of small lymphocytes, with round to occasionally deeply clefted (cleaved) nuclear contours. **The presence of cells with cleaved nuclei gives it some similarity to FL, but MCL is distinguished by the lack of centroblasts.** MCLs can also be confused with CLL and SLL because they share some immunophenotypic features—namely, the presence of CD5 on the malignant B-cell surface. **MCL is usually $CD23^-$ and does not usually present with proliferation centers** (helping distinguish it from CLL and SLL). It is important to distinguish MCL from CLL and SLL because although both are incurable diseases, **MCL is clinically more aggressive. It is associated with the t(11;14) translocation** involving the fusion of the IgH locus (chromosome 14) to the cyclin D1 (or bcl-1) locus on chromosome 11. This translocation is detected in up to 70% of cases and leads to **increased expression of cyclin D1** (promotes progression of the G1 to the S phase in the cell cycle and basically leads to increased proliferation of cells). It usually presents in older **men (≥60 years old).** Patients are typically male (**4:1 male-to-female predominance)** and present with advanced disease in their 60s. Almost half of patients have some combination of symptoms of fever, night sweats, or weight loss.

Clinical and Laboratory Findings:

- Lymphadenopathy and splenomegaly that are usually painless can be present.
- Patients are highly likely to have GI, liver, or bone marrow involvement at presentation.
- Immunophenotype is $CD5^+$, $CD23^-$, with increased expression of cyclin D1.

Treatment:

- Chemotherapy, usually CHOP-R, is a common treatment. There is no proven standard chemotherapeutic treatment regimen.
- MCL is an aggressive lymphoma with median survival rate from 3 to 4 years. Most patients eventually succumb to organ dysfunction caused by tumor infiltration.

Burkitt Lymphoma: Burkitt lymphoma is a **neoplasm of mature B-cell origin** that occurs in three main variants— endemic, sporadic, and immunodeficiency associated. These variants can be differentiated only on clinical presentation; they are histologically and immunophenotypically identical.

- The **endemic variant** arises in **equatorial Africa** and characteristically **involves the lymph nodes of the head and neck** (jaw bone marrow involvement). It **is the most common childhood neoplasm** of the region and is linked to infection with EBV. It is believed that many of the children that present with the disease are also chronically infected with malaria, decreasing their ability to fight the EBV infection.
- The **sporadic** or nonendemic variant is found outside of Africa. It is histologically similar to the endemic variant and is also associated with EBV infection. This variant is more commonly seen in the United States and occurs in the lymphoid tissue of the distal small bowel (jaw marrow is less commonly involved). It accounts for 30% to 50% of childhood lymphomas.
- The **immunodeficiency-associated** variant, as its name implies, is associated with states of immune suppression. It can be an AIDS-defining manifestation (in HIV-positive individuals) or can present in the setting of patients taking immunosuppressive medications.

Burkitt lymphoma does not usually form follicles and is believed to originate from the germinal center. **Microscopically** it appears as sheets of lymph cells, with a very high mitotic index and apoptosis. These lymphoid cells are interspersed with reactive macrophages (histiocytes) containing dead tumor cells and debris, giving it the **characteristic starry sky appearance** (the stars are the reactive macrophages and the night is represented by sheets of malignant cells; Fig. 11.33). **All forms are associated with the t(8;14) translocation,** which results in **fusion of the *c-myc* oncogene** (chromosome 8) onto the heavy-chain Ig gene (chromosome 14). This very aggressive disorder presents largely in children or young adults.

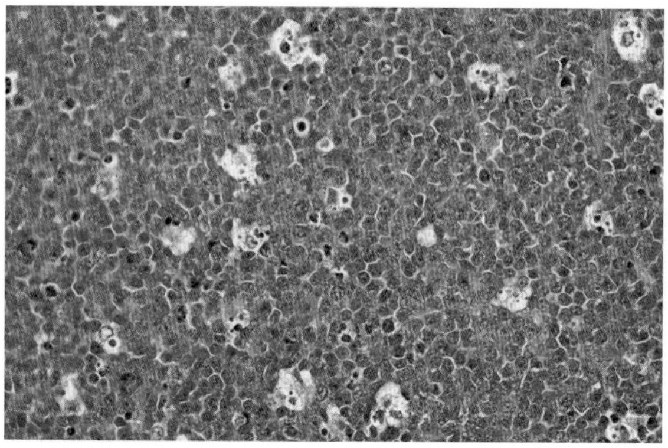

FIG. 11.33 Burkitt lymphoma with characteristic starry sky appearance. The "stars" represent the reactive macrophages and the "sky" represents sheets of malignant cells. (*From Rosai J, Ackerman LV. Surgical Pathology. 9th ed. St. Louis: Mosby; 2004:1955.*)

Clinical and Laboratory Findings:

- Endemic variant usually presents with a mass involving the mandible (may also involve the kidneys, ovaries, and adrenals).
- Sporadic variant usually presents with an abdominal mass involving the ileocecum and peritoneum.

Treatment:

- Responds to short-term, high-dose chemotherapy, with younger patients having better outcomes than older adults.

MALT Lymphoma: MALT lymphoma is a **low-grade tumor of B-cell origin** (a subtype of marginal zone lymphomas). Lymphoid tissue is present throughout the gastrointestinal tract and is referred to as MALT. It most commonly presents with involvement of the **stomach, small and large bowels,** and salivary glands. In the stomach and small bowel, this disorder **is associated with *H. pylori*** infection (gastritis, peptic ulcer disease [PUD]). Antibiotic **treatment against *H. pylori* can lead to regression of disease** in the stomach.

Primary Central Nervous System Lymphoma (PCNSL): Primary central nervous system lymphoma is a rare variant of extranodal NHL that **appears mostly in immunocompromised patients** (typically from AIDS but also seen in those iatrogenically immunosuppressed). It is also referred to as microglioma or primary brain lymphoma and it usually involves the brain, leptomeninges, eyes, or spinal cord without evidence of systemic disease. In immunocompromised patients the **prognosis is usually poor,** and it does not have a predilection for any particular age group. PCNSL can affect immunocompetent patients, usually appearing in older patients, with a median age at diagnosis in the fifth decade. Presenting signs and symptoms may vary, usually depending on the site of involvement. PCNSL usually **presents with seizure,** headache (increased intracranial pressure), **altered mental status, progressive dementia,** or memory loss. **PCNSL is considered an AIDS-defining lesion.**

T-cell Lymphomas:

Adult T-cell Lymphoma or Leukemia (ATL): ATL is a rare neoplasm of mature T cells associated with HTLV-1 infection. This disorder is seen more commonly in areas in which HTLV-1 is endemic, such as southern Japan, the Caribbean, South America, and Africa. It is a very aggressive type of NHL without a characteristic histologic finding other than a diffuse pattern of malignant mature T cells. ATL often has a leukemic phase (will see malignant cells in the circulation). ATL is an adult disease and typically presents with skin lesions and lytic bone lesions (resulting in hypercalcemia). The malignant T cells are CD4 positive and TdT negative (usually TdT negativity indicates that it is a mature lymphocyte).

Clinical and Laboratory Findings:

- Generalized lymphadenopathy and hepatosplenomegaly
- **Skin infiltration**
- Elevated WBC count in leukemic phase
- **Hypercalcemia** (because of release of osteoclast-activating factor by tumor cells, leading to lytic bone lesions)
- **Immunophenotype**—CD4 positive and TdT negative

Treatment:

- **There is no established standard of treatment.** Usually patients treated with zidovudine (to fight off virus) or chemotherapy (CHOP) to fight off proliferation of cancer cells.
- Mean survival is 1 year after diagnosis.

Mycosis Fungoides and Sezary Syndrome: Mycosis fungoides is a **neoplasm of peripheral CD4 helper T cells** and is the **most common form of cutaneous T-cell lymphoma.** It is **characterized by skin involvement** in the form of rashlike patches or nodules. Initially, it is difficult to diagnose because the rashlike patches resemble those of eczema or psoriasis; however, skin biopsy aids in the diagnosis. Mycosis fungoides **occurs in adults** and has an **indolent progression,** with **most patients presenting with disease localized to the skin** (but may progress internally over time if untreated). **Treatment** is **variable** but includes sunlight, UV light, topical steroids, and systemic chemotherapy. The disease is incurable but, with successful treatment, can remit to an indefinite nonprogressing state.

Sezary syndrome is a condition in which the skin involvement presents as generalized exfoliative lesions (particularly on the face), resulting in **leonine facies.** These patients will also have a leukemic phase, with the presence of **Sezary cells.**

Histiocyte Disorders

Langerhans Cell Histiocytosis (LCH) and Histiocytosis X

LCH is **a rare disorder** characterized by the **proliferation of specialized histiocytes (monocytes).** In LCH, the proliferating cell is the dendritic (or Langerhans) cell, which derives from monocyte lineage. In the past, these disorders were referred to as histiocytosis X and were subdivided into three categories—**Letterer-Siwe syndrome, Hand-Schuller-Christian disease,** and **eosinophilic granuloma.**

Letterer-Siwe Disease: This occurs **most commonly before 2 years of age**. It is characterized by the development of **cutaneous lesions resembling a seborrheic eruption** (usually the trunk and scalp), caused by infiltrates of Langerhans cells over the affected areas. Most of those affected have concurrent bone marrow failure, hepatosplenomegaly, lymphadenopathy, and destructive osteolytic bone lesions. The course of untreated disease is rapidly fatal, and treatment is with intensive chemotherapy. It has a 5-year survival rate of 50%.

Eosinophilic Granuloma: This is considered a benign histiocytosis that usually occurs in adolescents and young adults. It results from erosive accumulations of unifocal or multifocal Langerhans cells within the medullary cavities of bones (or in the lungs). The lesions can be asymptomatic or can cause pain and pathologic fractures. This is an indolent disorder that can heal spontaneously or be cured by local excision or irradiation.

Hand-Schuller-Christian Disease (Multifocal LCH): This usually affects young children. The classic Hand-Schuller-Christian triad includes calvarial bone defects (lytic lesions in the skull), diabetes insipidus, and exophthalmos (infiltration of orbit by tumor cells). Patients may present with fever and eruptions on the scalp and ear canals. They also display multiple erosive bony masses that sometimes expand into adjacent soft tissue. In about half of patients, involvement of the posterior pituitary stalk of the hypothalamus leads to diabetes insipidus. Many patients experience spontaneous regression; others can be treated successfully with chemotherapy.

These three conditions are now considered different expressions of the same basic disorder, but the USMLE Step 1 may still test on the historic names. **The tumor cells express S-100 and CD1a.** Microscopically, the presence of **Birbeck granules in the cytoplasm is characteristic. Birbeck granules** have a **tennis racket appearance** of rodlike tubular structures with a dilated terminal end (Fig. 11.34).

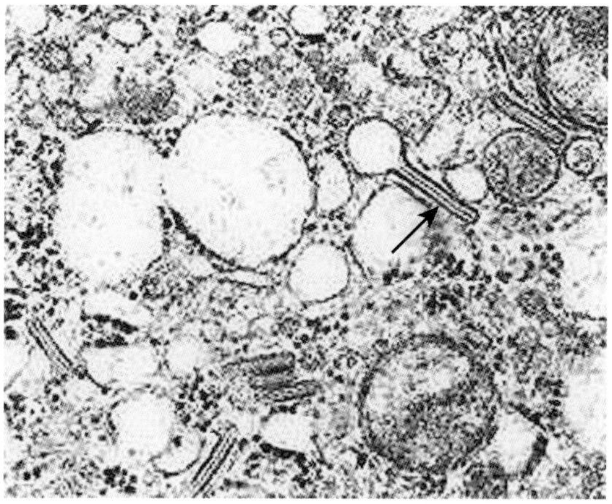

FIG. 11.34 Birbeck granules demonstrating the classic tennis racket appearance of rodlike tubular structures with a dilated terminal end. High-powered electron micrograph. (*From Goljan EF.* Rapid Review Pathology Revised Reprint. *3rd ed. Philadelphia: Elsevier; 2011.*)

Plasma Cell Disorders

Plasma cell disorders involve the **malignant transformation of terminally differentiated B cells** (plasma cells), resulting in unregulated proliferation of plasma cells in the bone marrow and monoclonal secretion of immunoglobulins (also called paraproteins) in the circulation. The increase in monoclonal immunoglobulins is detected as a monoclonal spike referred to as the **M component** (Fig. 11.35). The physiologic balance between the production of light and heavy chains is disturbed. Heavy chains are not produced in high enough quantities to couple with the light chains, which are produced in high volume by the cancer, leading to increased amounts of free light chains in the circulation (called **Bence Jones proteins**) and their excretion in the urine.

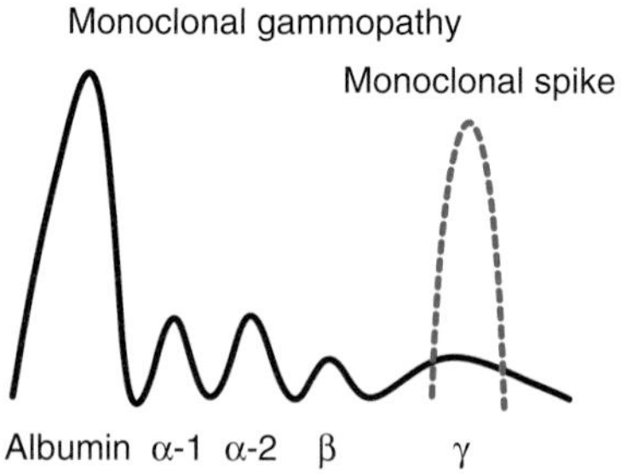

FIG. 11.35 Monoclonal spike (M component) of plasma protein electrophoresis secondary to a plasma cell disorder. (*From Goljan EF, Sloka KI.* Rapid Review Laboratory Testing in Clinical Medicine. *St. Louis: Mosby Elsevier; 2008:284.*)

Multiple Myeloma (MM)

MM is a monoclonal **plasma cell cancer** that arises in the bone marrow, interfering with the production of normal blood cells. The **unregulated proliferation of plasma cells** results in the **production of large amounts of monoclonal immunoglobulins,** mostly IgG. This is a disorder of older patients, with a **peak incidence at 50 to 60 years of age** (incidence increases with age). MM is **more common in African Americans than in whites (2:1 ratio)**. Many organ systems may be affected by the disorder, and presentation is variable. The production of cytokines, such as IL-1 or osteoclast-activating factor, by the malignant plasma cells and the deposition of monoclonal antibodies in organs produce most of the localized damage (osteoporosis and organ damage, respectively). It is helpful to use the **mnemonic CRAB** to remember the **common tetrad of findings in MM:**

- **C:** **C**alcium (elevated)
- **R:** **R**enal failure
- **A:** **A**nemia
- **B:** **B**one lesions (bone pain)

Signs and Symptoms:

- **Bone pain, lytic bone lesions, and hypercalcemia.** The **bone pain arises from the accumulation of plasma cells in local areas,** usually involving the pelvis (low back pain), ribs, clavicles, and femurs. The increased levels of osteoclast-activating factor produced by the plasma cells results in **bone breakdown and release of calcium into the circulation** (hypercalcemia). The **bone lesions** usually occur in the ribs, skull, and pelvis. They are best seen on radiographs and **have a punched-out appearance.** The bone lesions may present with pathologic fractures (ribs).

- **Renal failure.** Renal failure (with or without proteinuria) develops through a variety of different mechanisms including the following:
  - **Hypercalcemia.** Hypercalcemia leads to **increased deposition of calcium phosphate in normal tissue** (called metastatic calcification), resulting in calcification of renal tubules and collecting ducts.
  - **Production of Bence Jones (BJ) proteins.** The **excretion of BJ proteins is directly toxic to the kidneys,** damaging the renal epithelium and producing an intratubular giant cell reaction (further damaging the kidneys). Tubular casts of BJ proteins and giant cells are seen.
  - **Primary amyloidosis.** The increased levels of circulating light-chain proteins may result in their deposition in the kidney and subsequent conversion to amyloid.
  - **Infiltration of malignant plasma cells in kidneys (rare).** Infiltration of renal parenchyma by myeloma cells disrupts normal renal cell function, similarly to how they disrupt normal hematopoietic cell function in the bone marrow.
- **Anemia.** The anemia seen in MM is **normocytic** and happens as a result of infiltration (and replacement) of normal bone marrow cells with tumor cells. Also contributing to the inhibition of hematopoiesis is the increased cytokine production by the tumor cells, creating an environment of inflammation similar to that seen in anemia of chronic disease.
- **Recurrent infections.** The **unregulated production of monoclonal immunoglobulin leads to** increased blood immunoglobulin levels. However, these monoclonal antibodies cannot be used to fight off infection because they are not directed to a specific infectious pathogen. The increased production of Ig by the malignant plasma cells leads to decreased production of normal Ig by normal plasma cells, creating **a relative immunodeficiency state.** As a result, patients are commonly at **increased risk of developing pneumonia and pyelonephritis** (increased susceptibility to *Streptococcus pneumoniae, Staphylococcus aureus, E. coli,* and other gram-negative rods).
- **Neurologic symptoms.** The resultant **hypercalcemia leads to many of the neurologic findings in MM** (e.g., weakness, confusion, fatigue). Hyperviscosity syndrome can result from the increased levels of Ig protein in the circulation, leading to headaches, visual changes, and congestive heart failure. Cord compression can occur because of the extension of tumor cells from vertebral bodies to the spinal cord, resulting in radicular pain and loss of bowel or bladder control. Peripheral neuropathies (carpal tunnel syndrome) may result from amyloid deposition in peripheral nerves.

C: Calcium (elevated)
R: Renal failure
A: Anemia
B: Bone lesions (bone pain)

Diagnostic Criteria: **Symptomatic myeloma:** Bone marrow (or other tissue) biopsy result with more than 10% clonal plasma cells is diagnostic (Fig. 11.36); there is typically no evidence of end organ damage caused by tumor cells.

PCT: Sun-induced blistering, accumulation of iron and uroporphyrin

AIP: No sun-induced blistering, accumulation of ALA and porphobilinogen

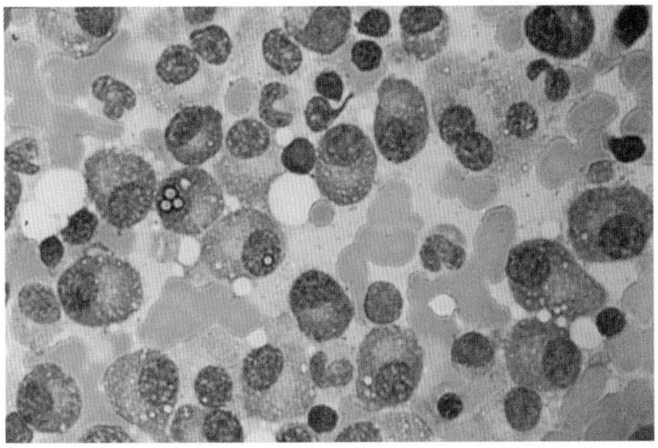

FIG. 11.36 Malignant egg-shaped plasma cells of multiple myeloma demonstrating eccentric nuclei. (*From Goldman L, Ausiello D. Cecil's Textbook of Medicine. 23rd ed. Philadelphia: Saunders Elsevier; 2008:1430.*)

Monoclonal Gammopathy of Undetermined Significance (MGUS):
- Bone marrow (or other tissue) biopsy with < 10% clonal plasma cells
- Increased serum monoclonal protein levels
- No evidence of end organ damage caused by tumor cells

Laboratory Findings:
- Bone marrow biopsy demonstrating more than 10% clonal plasma cells. Tumor cells have a characteristic fried egg appearance.
- Peripheral blood smear showing RBCs stacked like poker chips (rouleaux formation)
- Serum protein electrophoresis (SPEP) demonstrating increased monoclonal Ig spike (usually IgG, M component)

- 24-hour urine protein showing increased light-chain (BJ) proteins
- Increased erythrocyte sedimentation rate (ESR)—plasma cells release inflammatory cytokines
- Hypercalcemia, anemia, increased creatinine level

In the process of diagnosis, you must do a complete skeletal survey to evaluate for lytic ('punched-out') lesions.

Treatment:

- This is an **incurable disease** and treatment is aimed toward therapy that will decrease the proliferation of malignant plasma cells (signs and symptoms caused by proliferation of tumor cells).
- **High-dose chemotherapy** is administered with addition of bisphosphonates to prevent pathologic fractures.
- **Autologous stem cell transplantation (ASCL)**—the transplantation of one's own normal stem cells into the bone marrow—can be considered.
- With treatment, median survival is 3 to 4 years (6-month survival without treatment).

Waldenström Macroglobulinemia (Lymphoplasmacytic Lymphoma)

Waldenström macroglobulinemia (WM) is a **disorder of neoplastic lymphoplasmacytoid B cells secreting IgM monoclonal proteins.** Plasmacytoid lymphocytes are cells between B lymphocytes and plasma cells on the maturity level spectrum. **It is a disorder seen in older men** (>50 years). The main **risk factor for developing this disease is a history of MGUS.** The clinical presentation is related to bone marrow infiltration, visceral organ infiltration, and effects of the increased IgM levels.

Bone marrow infiltration results in marrow failure, leading to anemia, thrombocytopenia (bleeding), and neutropenia (infection). It **does not result in lytic bone lesions** (this tumor cell does not secrete cytokines because it has not yet matured into a plasma cell). **Visceral organ infiltration** results in **lymphadenopathy, hepatosplenomegaly,** and cutaneous lesions (all three not present in MM). The **IgM immunoglobulin is a very large pentamer** molecule; high levels of this protein thickens the blood **(hyperviscosity syndrome).** Hyperviscosity syndrome may lead to the development of stroke, myocardial infarction (MI), priapism, or visual impairment. **IgM cold antibody autoimmune hemolytic anemia** is sometimes seen.

Clinical and Laboratory Findings:

- Bone marrow findings are similar to MM.
- Biopsy results of enlarged lymph nodes demonstrate proliferation of lymphoplasmacytoid cells.
- Serum protein electrophoresis will show a clonal IgM spike.
- Bone lesions and renal failure are uncommon in WM. Fewer than 10% of cases will have BJ proteinuria. Initial 24-hour urine collection is usually not required if there are no signs of renal insufficiency. Skeletal survey is not usually required if the patient does not report bone pain.
- Obtain cryoglobulins and cold agglutinin levels in patients with symptoms of hemolytic anemia.

Treatment:

- Similar to MM; treatment aims at reducing the tumor cell burden and focuses on treating the symptoms.
- **Chemotherapy** is similar to that used for CLL; bone marrow transplantation is not part of therapy.
- Frequent **plasmapheresis** is required for removal of IgM, helping resolve symptoms of hyperviscosity and hemolytic anemia.
- Median survival with treatment is 4 years.

Monoclonal Gammopathy of Undetermined Significance

MGUS is the most **common monoclonal gammopathy** and, like MM, it **occurs in older adults.** This is a **diagnosis of exclusion** after MM and WM have been ruled out. **Patients will often present asymptomatically,** with increased serum protein levels (small IgM spike). **Bone marrow evaluation will reveal fewer than 10% clonal plasma cells and BJ proteins will not be seen in the urine.** In general, this is a benign condition, and most patients do not require treatment. However, these patients are **at increased risk for developing WM or MM.** It is important to follow these patients closely with regular serum protein levels, skeletal surveys, and 24-hour urinalysis for BJ proteins.

Myeloproliferative Disorders

Myoproliferative disorders (MPDs) are a group of neoplastic disorders that involve the proliferation of myeloid stem cells. This category of neoplasms includes polycythemia vera, essential thrombocythemia (see earlier, "Bleeding and Thrombotic Disorders"), CML (see earlier, "Leukemias"), and myeloid metaplasia with myelofibrosis. With the exception of CML, these disorders are associated with a mutation in the *JAK2* gene and can be treated with hydroxyurea.

Polycythemia Vera

Polycythemia vera (PV) is a myeloproliferative disorder that leads to the unregulated production, by myeloid stem cells, of increased levels of RBCs (may also produce WBCs and platelets). The term *polycythemia* refers to a state of increased Hb and Hct values above the normal range. **PV is a true polycythemia,** and the first step in its diagnosis is to distinguish it from a **relative polycythemia (e.g., one caused by plasma volume contraction)** or a secondary true polycythemia. True polycythemias are categorized into primary and secondary polycythemias. In **primary polycythemia,** the production of RBCs results from an **EPO-independent pathway,** as in PV. In **secondary polycythemia,** the increased production of RBCs results from the **excess secretion of EPO** that is physiologically appropriate or pathologic.

In **relative polycythemia,** the most common polycythemia, a loss in plasma volume (dehydration) results in hemoconcentration of the blood. In other words, the amount of solute (RBCs and other blood products suspended in the plasma) stays the same while the amount of solution (plasma volume in which blood products are suspended) is decreased, leading to a higher concentration of solute (not an absolute increase in RBC amount). **RBC mass is used to distinguish relative from true polycythemias;** RBC mass is always elevated in true polycythemias.

Relative Polycythemia Laboratory Findings:

- Normal oxygen saturation (Sa_{O_2}), so no physiologic stimulus for EPO release (normal EPO)
- Increased RBC count (concentration of RBCs has increased)
  - Remember, the RBC count is a measure of the concentration of RBCs in the blood (number of RBCs per microliter of blood).
- Normal RBC mass (amount of RBCs has not changed because there is no EPO stimulus to create more RBCs)
  - Remember, RBC mass is a measure of the number of RBCs in the blood.
- Decreased plasma volume

Tissue hypoxia of any cause (e.g., high altitude, pulmonary disorders, decreased Hb oxygen-carrying capacity) results in increased EPO secretion and leads to **physiologically appropriate secondary polycythemia.** The body is attempting to overcome the hypoxic state by upregulating the production of Hb (and RBCs), thereby increasing the oxygen-carrying capacity of the blood.

Physiologically Appropriate Secondary Polycythemia Laboratory Findings:

- **Decreased oxygen saturation (Sa_{O_2})** acts as a stimulus for EPO release.
- **RBC count, RBC mass, and EPO** will be **increased.** EPO causes the bone marrow to increase the production of RBCs, resulting in an increase in the RBC count and RBC mass.
- **Plasma volume** will be **normal** (the amount of solute has increased by bone marrow production of RBCs, not the amount of solution).
- Certain **cancers** (e.g., renal cell carcinoma, hepatocellular carcinoma) **secrete EPO** in an autonomous fashion and **lead to physiologically inappropriate (pathologic) secondary polycythemia.**

Pathologic Secondary Polycythemia Laboratory Findings:

- Oxygen saturation (Sa_{O_2}) is normal, so there is no physiologic stimulus for EPO release. However, ectopic release of EPO from tumor cells results in increased EPO levels.
- RBC count and mass are increased.
- Plasma volume will be normal.

Polycythemia vera, similarly to the other MPDs, is **associated with a mutation in the *JAK2* kinase gene.** PV is an **insidious disorder** that is **usually diagnosed in older adults (>60 years)** but can occur in any age group. PV patients may enter a spent phase many years after diagnosis (develop anemia and have fibrotic bone marrow). Most **symptoms of PV are caused by the hyperviscosity of**

the blood (from increased RBCs) and its effects on organs, such as headaches, vertigo, mental status and visual changes (congestion of retinal vein), and **splenomegaly** (from congestion or extramedullary hematopoiesis).

As a result, **individuals will be at increased risk of thrombotic events** causing significant morbidity and mortality, such as cerebrovascular accidents (strokes), MIs, deep venous thrombosis, **splenic infarction,** and Budd-Chiari syndrome (hepatic vein thrombosis).

A subset of patients may be **largely asymptomatic,** not displaying symptoms of hyperviscosity or thrombotic events. In these patients, the **only presenting symptom may be pruritus after a warm bath** (caused by abnormal histamine release by mast cells).

Clinical and Laboratory Findings:

- Hepatosplenomegaly may be present.
- **Left upper quadrant pain** can be present (from splenomegaly or splenic infarct).
- A **ruddy complexion** and **conjunctival plethora** can be noted from congestion of blood vessels.
- **Peptic ulcer disease** may be present (unclear cause, possibly increased histamine release seen in this disorder).
- **Gouty arthritis** is a result of increased cell turnover caused by cancer.
- **RBC count and mass are increased.**
- **EPO is decreased** (remember, PV is an EPO-independent polycythemia). The EPO is low because the body's physiologic response to abnormally high RBC levels is to decrease the production of RBCs by decreasing its secretion of EPO.
- **Leukocytosis** or **thrombocytosis** may be seen in some patients. Bone marrow aspirate may show hyperplasia of all three myeloid cell lines.
- Patients in the spent phase will have a fibrotic bone marrow.
- **Differentiate from CML by absence of Philadelphia chromosome** and increased LAP score (LAP is decreased in CML).

Treatment:

- **Fatal if left untreated (1- to 3-year survival).**
- **With treatment, expected survival can be more than 10 years.**
- Nonmyelosuppressive agents include the following:
  - Periodic phlebotomy to keep Hct less than 45%. Treatment is effective, but chronic phlebotomy may result in IDA and reactive thrombocytosis (patients will have increased risk of thrombotic events in first few years of this therapy).
- Myelosuppressive agents, such as **hydroxyurea** (with reduced rate of periodic phlebotomy) and **interferon-α (IFN-α),** may also be used.

Myeloid Metaplasia with Myelofibrosis

Myeloid metaplasia with myelofibrosis (MMM) is a **myeloproliferative disorder caused by neoplastic changes in the myeloid stem cells that lead to the pathologic proliferation of fibroblasts, causing marrow fibrosis.** Neoplastic cells produce ineffective RBCs, WBCs, and platelets. The findings in MMM are similar to those in the spent phase of PV, in which there is a replacement of marrow with collagen fibrosis. MMM is also associated with a mutation of the *JAK2* gene (chromosome 9). *Myeloid metaplasia* is another term for extramedullary hematopoiesis. Hematopoiesis can occur in almost every tissue in the body. **In MMM, the main site of extramedullary hematopoiesis is the spleen, which is enlarged in more than 90% of patients.** The myelofibrosis develops early in this disease because of the increased release of platelet-derived growth factor and transforming growth factor β (TGF-β) by the neoplastic megakaryocytes. These growth factors promote the growth of nonneoplastic fibroblasts, leading to increased production of collagen and fibrosis in the marrow. MMM occurs primarily in **individuals older than 60 years.** The **typical presentation is one of marrow failure** (anemia, thrombocytopenia, neutropenia), with **left upper quadrant pain** (splenomegaly and resultant splenic infarction). Constitutional symptoms are also common, such as weight loss, low-grade fever, night sweats, and fatigue.

Clinical and Laboratory Findings:

- **Widespread extramedullary hematopoiesis may be present.**
  - **Splenomegaly (left upper quadrant pain) may lead to splenic infarction.**
  - Hepatomegaly results from increased splenic hematopoiesis, which increases portal blood flow and leads to portal hypertension and hepatomegaly.

- **Hematopoiesis** of serosal surfaces **can lead to large pleural or pericardial effusions.**
- Initially the bone marrow is hypercellular, but early in the disease progression it becomes **hypocellular and fibrotic,** with increased collagen and reticulin fibers (Fig. 11.37).

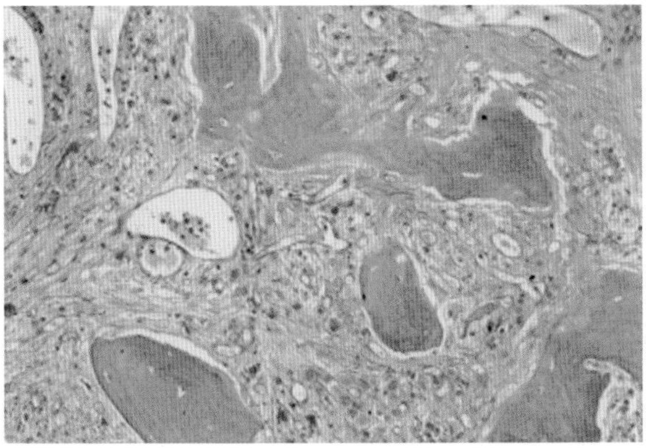

Fig. 11.37 Hypocellular, fibrotic bone marrow biopsy from a patient with myeloid metaplasia with myelofibrosis. (*From Goldman L, Ausiello D.* Cecil's Textbook of Medicine. *23rd ed. Philadelphia: Saunders Elsevier; 2008:1125.*)

- **Leukoerythroblastosis** (or myelophthisis) on peripheral blood smear. This is defined as the presence of immature granulocytic precursors and nucleated RBCs found on the smear. The **RBCs will have a characteristic teardrop shape (called dacrocytes,** from RBCs being squeezed out of fibrotic marrow).
- **Normocytic anemia** (from leukoerythroblastosis) may occur.
- WBC and platelet count is variable. **Platelets are abnormally large.**

Treatment:

- Splenectomy if complications develop from massive splenomegaly
- **Hydroxyurea**
- Interferon-α

Disorders of Heme Production

The production of heme is a highly regulated biochemical process; a defect in any step results in the accumulation of pathway intermediates. The accumulation of certain heme intermediates can be toxic, leading to the development of a disorder called porphyria. See "Heme Synthesis and Acquired Sideroblastic Anemia" section for heme synthesis pathway.

Porphyria Cutanea Tarda

Porphyria cutanea tarda (PCT) is a genetic or acquired disorder of heme production and the most common porphyria. PCT develops from decreased activity of the enzyme in the fifth step of heme synthesis, uroporphyrinogen decarboxylase (UROD). This deficiency leads to the accumulation of heme pathway intermediates such as uroporphyrin and iron. The pathology of this disease is directly associated with the buildup of uroporphyrin and iron. PCT is characterized by sun-induced blistering and erosion of the skin caused by accumulation of uroporphyrin deposits in the skin. Patients also may develop hyperpigmentation, hypertrichosis (increased hair growth, mainly on face), and skin fragility. The accumulation of iron results in siderosis (iron overload) primarily affecting the liver, resulting in hepatic inflammation and cirrhosis. Inherited causes of PCT are mostly sporadic mutations (80%) in the UROD gene, and the remaining 20% of cases of PCT are inherited in an autosomal dominant manner. It is unclear how PCT is acquired, but several risk factors have been observed that cause and exacerbate the disease. These included hepatitis C virus (HCV) infection, alcohol abuse, excess iron, estrogens, and exposure to chlorinated cyclic hydrocarbons. Diagnosis is made by measuring urine uroporphyrin (increased). Treatment is aimed at eliminating exposure to precipitants, decreasing iron levels, and increasing the excretion rate of porphyrins by the liver.

Patients are instructed to **avoid alcohol** consumption, **iron** supplementation, **sunlight** exposure, intake of **estrogens**, and exposure to chlorinated cyclic hydrocarbons. Excess iron is managed by **routine phlebotomy. Low-dose antimalarials** (chloroquine or hydroxychloroquine) help increase the removal of porphyrins from the liver by increasing their rate of excretion. Patients with HCV should have their infection controlled with antiviral medication for proper control of PCT.

Acute Intermittent Porphyria

Acute intermittent porphyria (AIP) is a rare **autosomal dominant disorder of heme production.** Individuals with AIP are deficient in porphobilinogen deaminase (or uroporphyrinogen synthase, an enzyme in the heme synthesis pathway), resulting in the **accumulation of upstream intermediates** inside the cytosol—namely, **PBG and δ-ALA.** Buildup of these two intermediates is toxic to cells and can also cause degeneration of myelin. The symptoms of AIP are variable, with **severe poorly localized abdominal pain being the most common.** The symptoms **can be categorized by the 5 Ps of AIP:**

- **P**ainful abdomen (often confused for acute abdomen, leading to a belly full of scars)
- **P**ort wine–colored urine (urine is colorless initially, but exposure to light causes PBG in urine to oxidize and gives urine its color).
- **P**eripheral neuropathy (patchy numbness and paresthesias)
- **P**sychological disturbances (anxiety, confusion, psychosis, dementia)
- **P**recipitated by drugs (drugs that enhance cytochrome P-450 activity, sulfa drugs, barbiturates, some antipsychotics, alcohol)

A feature that distinguishes AIP from other porphyrias is that it has **no sun-induced blistering of the skin or rashes. Diagnosis** is obtained by observing the **presence of increased urinary excretion of PBG and genetic testing** (can also measure porphobilinogen deaminase activity but this is less helpful in diagnosis). **Treatment** is aimed at decreasing factors that precipitate attacks (discontinue any offending drugs) and at halting the endogenous heme production pathway.

Endogenous heme production can be decreased by inhibiting ALA synthase (the rate-limiting step in heme synthesis). **ALA synthase is inhibited by heme,** the end product of heme synthesis (feedback inhibition), **and by glucose.** Patients should **receive a high-carbohydrate (glucose) infusion during acute attacks** and **hematin or heme arginate to help resolve severe attacks** (both are hemelike substances).

PHARMACOLOGIC TREATMENT

Anticoagulants

Heparin

Heparin is a glycosaminoglycan, administered parenterally (intravenously or subcutaneously), that binds ATIII with high affinity. This fast-acting anticoagulant (onset of action is seconds) works by inducing a conformational change in ATIII that results in a 1000-fold increase in its protease activity. **Clinically** it is used as prophylaxis as well as treatment of venous thrombosis and pulmonary embolism. Heparin also is used as adjuvant therapy for unstable angina, MI, and stroke. Heparin can be safely administered for anticoagulation during pregnancy because it does not cross the placenta. **Side effects** include bleeding, and HIT. Clinical effects are reversed by protamine sulfate and are followed by measuring the PTT. **Contraindications** include active bleeding, bleeding disorders, history of HIT, and aortic dissection.

Direct Thrombin Inhibitors (Lepirudin/Bivalirudin and Dabigatran)

A **direct thrombin inhibitor** (DTI), as the name implies, acts by directly inhibiting circulating and clot-bound thrombin (also known as factor IIa) and provides ATIII-independent anticoagulation. **Lepirudin** and **bivalirudin** are hirudin analogs that differ from **dabigatran** in how they bind to inactivate the thrombin enzyme as well as route of administration (dabigatran is given orally). **Clinically** it is used as an alternative anticoagulant (administered intravenously [IV]) for patients with a history of HIT or heparin allergy. **Side effects** include bleeding. No therapeutic drug monitoring is widely available for DTIs. Theoretically may use the thrombin clotting time to monitor, but it is not generally used in clinical practice. **Contraindications** are similar to those of heparin.

Direct Factor Xa Inhibitors (apiXaban and rivaroXaban): Direct factor Xa inhibitors are another class of ATIII-independent anticoagulants that act to directly inhibit circulating and clot-bound factor Xa. Currently these medications are only available clinically in oral formulations and are used as an alternatives to warfarin or heparin. **Clinically** they are used for stroke prevention in atrial fibrillation as well as pulmonary embolism (PE) or deep vein thrombosis treatment and prophylaxis. They have a rapid onset and offset of action, which reduces the need for "bridging." Additionally, they do not require frequent monitoring or redosing because they have few drug interactions and no food interactions (relative to warfarin). **Side effects** include bleeding. **Contraindicated** in severe renal impairment.

Warfarin (Coumadin)

Warfarin is an oral anticoagulant that inhibits the normal production of vitamin K–dependent clotting factors in the liver. It functions by inhibiting epoxide reductase, the enzyme that helps regenerate vitamin K from its epoxide form to its reduced (active) form. Warfarin basically induces a functional vitamin K deficiency state in the body. Clotting factors II, VII, IX, and X and proteins C and S depend on vitamin K as a cofactor for their complete synthesis. **Clinically** it is used for the treatment and prophylaxis of venous thrombosis and pulmonary embolism. Additional uses include anticoagulation therapy for atrial fibrillation and patients with mechanical heart valves. **Side effects** include bleeding. Clinical effects are monitored by following the PT and INR. Effects are reversed immediately with administration of fresh-frozen plasma and, within a few hours, with vitamin K infusion. **Contraindications** include history of bleeding disorders and active pregnancy (warfarin crosses the placenta and is teratogenic).

Antiplatelet Agents

Aspirin

Aspirin is the prototypical nonsteroidal antiinflammatory drug (NSAID). The mechanism of action of NSAIDs involves the inhibition of cyclooxygenase (COX-1 and COX-2) enzymes, thereby preventing the conversion of arachidonic acid to prostaglandins or TXA_2. Aspirin differs from other NSAIDs in that it irreversibly inhibits COX enzymes. The inhibition of prostaglandin synthesis results in its antiinflammatory and analgesic (decrease in prostaglandin E_2) actions. The inhibition of TXA_2 production leads to decreased platelet aggregation, producing an anticoagulant effect. **Clinically** it is used as an antipyretic, analgesic, antiinflammatory, and anticoagulant (antiplatelet) drug. **Side effects** include gastric ulcers and bleeding, central effects (hyperventilation, tinnitus), and Reye syndrome. Clinical effects are monitored by measuring the BT (will be increased). **Contraindicated** in children and adolescents because it can lead to Reye syndrome.

Thienopyridine Derivatives (Clopidogrel and Ticlopidine)

Clopidogrel and ticlopidine are thienopyridine-derived antiplatelet medications that act via a mechanism other than that of aspirin. Clopidogrel works by irreversibly inhibiting the binding of ADP to its receptor on platelets, thereby reducing platelet aggregation. **Clinically** it is often used in conjunction with aspirin to decrease ischemic events in patients with a previous history of stroke, coronary artery disease, and peripheral arterial disease. It is also used to reduce thrombosis after cardiac stent placement or in patients who cannot tolerate aspirin therapy. **Side effects** include bleeding, severe neutropenia, TTP, rashes, and dyspepsia (ticlopidine is associated with a worse side effect profile than clopidogrel). **Contraindicated** in patients with active bleeding.

Abciximab

Abciximab is a monoclonal antibody that works as a platelet aggregation inhibitor by binding the GpIIb/GpIIIa receptor on activated platelets. This blockade prevents platelets from sticking together and inhibits thrombus formation. **Clinically** it is used as an anticoagulant in acute coronary syndrome and also to prevent restenosis after coronary angioplasty. **Side effects** include bleeding (GI bleed) and thrombocytopenia. **Contraindicated** in patients with active bleeding, recent GI bleed (within 6 weeks), or thrombocytopenia. (also eptifabatide, tirofiban)

Phosphodiesterase III inhibitors (Cilostazol, Dipyrimadole)

Phosphodiesterase III (PDE3) inhibitors stop clot formation by blocking the enzymes that normally inactivate cyclic AMP (cAMP), leading to increased levels of cAMP in platelets. As you may remember, cAMP is an important mediator of platelet activity and increased levels lead to inhibition of platelet aggregation. These medications also act as direct arterial vasodilators by inhibiting the cellular reuptake of adenosine, leading to increased levels of extracellular adenosine. Increased adenosine levels then act as a local vasodilator. **Clinical uses** include angina prophylaxis, intermittent claudication, prevention of stroke or transient ischemic attack (when combined with aspirin). **Side effects** are related to its function as a vasodilator, including headache, nausea, hypotension, palpitations (arrhythmias), GI upset, and thrombocytopenia. **Contraindications** include heart failure (especially New York Heart Association [NYHA] class III and IV failure), tachycardia, and hypovolemia.

Thrombolytics

Alteplase (tPA), Reteplase (rPA), Tenecteplase (TNKase), Streptokinase: Thrombolytics are medications that help dissolve blood clots by a process referred to as thrombolysis. These agents catalyze the formation of endogenous plasmin (the protease that removes clots or thrombi) **from plasminogen.** Plasmin cleaves fibrin as well as thrombin clots. You will see **elevation of PT and PTT,** without any change in platelet count. **Clinically** this class of medications are used for treatment of MI, ischemic stroke, or massive PE. **Side effects** include bleeding, specifically hemorrhagic stroke. **Contraindicated** in patients with a history of hemorrhagic stroke, known intracranial malignancy, known cerebral vascular lesion (arteriovenous malformation), recent ischemic stroke (within last 3 months), known bleeding disorder or active bleeding, suspected aortic dissection, or significant closed head/facial trauma (within 3 months). Relative contraindications include severe hypertension, recent major surgery, or pregnancy.

Antineoplastics

Antimetabolites

Methotrexate (MTX): Methotrexate is an antimetabolite medication that is an analog of folic acid. Folic acid is required to carry out one-carbon transfer reactions in various synthetic pathways, specifically the synthesis of purine nucleotides (thymidylate) and some amino acids (serine and methionine). Methotrexate inhibits dihydrofolate reductase (DHFR) and prevents the regeneration of folate for continued use in DNA synthesis. This antifolate agent is not selective for tumor DHFR versus normal DHFR; therefore, it can affect the DNA synthesis and cell growth of normal and tumor cells. However, it does have a greater toxic effect in the DNA synthesis (S phase) of cells that are rapidly dividing. **Clinically** it is used as an antineoplastic agent used with other chemotherapeutic agents to treat leukemias, NHL, and other malignancies. It is also used as an immunosuppressant in the treatment of rheumatoid arthritis. Methotrexate is used in the medical management of ectopic pregnancy. **Side effects** commonly include bone marrow suppression, liver damage, and neurotoxicity. Toxic effects can be diminished with the administration of leucovorin (folinic acid), which is taken up in disproportionate amounts by normal cells (versus tumor cells).

5-Fluorouracil (5-FU): 5-FU is a pyrimidine analog that acts during the S phase of the cell cycle. Similarly to MTX (they work synergistically by inhibiting different enzymes in the DNA synthesis pathway), 5-FU halts DNA and protein synthesis. 5-FU is an antimetabolite that irreversibly inhibits thymidylate synthase, thereby blocking the synthesis of thymidine. It is enzymatically converted to its active form, 5-fluorodeoxyuridine (5-FdUMP), which in turn inhibits thymidylate synthase and halts DNA synthesis. This leads to an imbalance in cell development and thymineless death of the cell. Thymineless death occurs when bacterial, yeast, or human cells are deprived of thymidine triphosphate (dTTP), an essential precursor for DNA synthesis, thereby initiating irreversible cell death. **Clinically** it is used in the treatment of colon cancer and superficial tumors (basal cell carcinoma). **Side effects** include myelosuppression, GI mucositis, and photosensitivity. Side effects cannot be reversed by leucovorin.

Azathioprine and 6-Mercaptopurine (6-MP): Azathioprine is a prodrug that is nonenzymatically cleaved to create 6-MP. 6-MP (analog of adenine) is an antimetabolite that works by inhibiting many enzymes involved in de novo purine synthesis (S phase). This immunosuppressive medication must first be converted by hypoxanthine-guanine phosphoribosyltransferase (HGPRT) to exert its clinical effects. **Clinically** these medications are used for the treatment of leukemias and lymphomas. They are also immunosuppressants used to treat certain autoimmune disorders, including rheumatoid arthritis, SLE, and inflammatory bowel disease. **Side effects** include bone marrow suppression, GI mucositis, and liver damage. 6-MP is metabolized by xanthine oxidase and may result in increased toxicity in patients taking allopurinol.

6-Thioguanine (6-TG): 6-TG is a guanine analog antimetabolite that works similarly to 6-MP. It blocks the synthesis of guanine nucleotides and results in the arrest of DNA and RNA synthesis (S phase). Unlike 6-MP, it is metabolized by thiopurine methyltransferase and is safe to give with allopurinol. **Clinically** it is used in the treatment of acute leukemias and chronic myeloid leukemia. **Side effects** are similar to 6-MP except that it can be given with allopurinol.

Cytarabine: Cytarabine is an S phase–specific antimetabolite (analog of deoxycytidine, a deoxyribonucleoside resembles cytidine, with one oxygen atom removed) that blocks DNA synthesis by incorporating itself into the internucleotide linkages in DNA. **Clinically** it is used in the treatment of acute leukemias (AML, ALL) and in lymphomas (induction therapy). **Side effects** include bone marrow suppression and GI mucositis.

Cladribine (2-CDA): Cladribine is a synthetic purine analog that is used in the treatment of hairy cell leukemia. It is an immunosuppressant that inhibits DNA processing by cells. It is an adenosine deaminase inhibitor. **Clinically** used for treatment of hairy cell leukemia. **Side effects** include bone marrow suppression, neurotoxicity, and renal toxicity.

Antitumor Antibiotics

Dactinomycin

Dactinomycin (actinomycin D) is an antibiotic used as a chemotherapy medication, which disrupts the cell cycle by inhibiting transcription. It works by binding double-stranded DNA and blocking elongation of the chain by RNA polymerase. **Clinically** it is used to treat Wilms tumor in children (may be curative if combined with surgery and radiation), rhabdomyosarcoma, Ewing sarcoma, and choriocarcinoma. **Side effects** include bone marrow suppression and GI mucositis.

Doxorubicin

Doxorubicin (Adriamycin), an antibiotic, is the A part of the ABVD chemotherapeutic regimen. It works by intercalating within DNA to disrupt replication and transcription. Doxorubicin inserts itself into DNA, leading to breaks in the chain. **Clinically** it is used in the treatment of multiple myeloma, leukemias, HL, sarcomas, and solid tumors (breast, ovary, bladder, and lung). **Side effects** include significant cardiotoxicity (leading to dilated cardiomyopathy), bone marrow suppression, and alopecia.

Bleomycin

Bleomycin is a G2 phase–specific drug and is the B part of the ABVD chemotherapeutic regimen. This agent is a mixture of glycoproteins that produce free radicals on binding DNA. The free radicals create breaks in DNA, which accumulate and lead to cell death. **Clinically** it is used in the treatment of HL, testicular carcinoma, and squamous cell carcinomas. **Side effects** include skin changes (hyperpigmentation, ulcers, alopecia) and life-threatening pulmonary fibrosis (pulmonary function must be monitored). It produces minimal bone marrow suppression.

Alkylating Agents

Cyclophosphamide and Ifosfamide

Cyclophosphamide is an alkylating mustard agent. Like other alkylating agents, it exerts its effects by alkylating DNA (lethal to cells) and is most toxic to rapidly dividing cells. It is the most commonly used alkylating agent. Cyclophosphamide is unique in that it can be administered orally. Both cyclophosphamide and ifosfamide require activation by the liver's P-450 system to function properly. **Clinically** it is used to treat NHL, breast carcinoma, and ovarian carcinomas. It also acts as an immunosuppressant. **Side effects** include hemorrhagic cystitis, leading to bladder fibrosis (this side effect is decreased by aggressive hydration and administration of mesna) and myelosuppression.

Nitrosoureas

Nitrosoureas (e.g., carmustine, lomustine, semustine, streptozocin) are DNA alkylating agents used in chemotherapy. Nitrosoureas are a subgroup of medications that work by alkylating the cross-link strands of DNA to create breaks and inhibit its replication (also leading to inhibition of RNA and protein synthesis). These medications must be metabolized into their active products. Carmustine (BCNU) and lomustine (CCNU) are two closely related nitrosoureas that are highly lipophilic and readily cross the blood–brain barrier, so they are used in the treatment of many brain tumors. **Side effects** include myelosuppression, renal toxicity, and pulmonary fibrosis (after prolonged use).

Busulfan

Busulfan is an alkyl sulfonate that acts as a nonspecific alkylating agent. It acts similarly to other alkylating agents and forms reactive intermediates that alkylate DNA bases (mostly purines) leading to cross-linking of bases, abnormalities in base pairing, and DNA strand breakage. **Clinically** it was used as the main treatment for CML until imatinib (the gold standard treatment for CML) was discovered, although it continues to play a role in the treatment of CML. Busulfan is also used in bone marrow transplantation (kills bone marrow cells in preparation for the procedure). **Side effects** include pulmonary fibrosis (main side effect) and hyperpigmentation.

Microtubule Inhibitors

Vincristine and Vinblastine

Vincristine (Oncovin) is a vinca alkaloid used as the O part of the MOPP chemotherapeutic regimen. Vincristine is an M phase inhibitor of the cell cycle and works by binding to tubulin, thereby preventing polymerization of microtubules and spindle formation. Inhibition of microtubule formation leads to arrest of the cell cycle (at metaphase) and stops mitosis. Vinblastine is a similar medication that is the V part of the ABVD chemotherapeutic regimen. **Clinically** it is used in the treatment of HL, leukemias, Wilms tumor, and choriocarcinomas. **Side effects** include peripheral neuropathy and constipation. Vincristine causes minimal myelosuppression. Vinblastine, on the other hand, produces significant myelosuppression.

Paclitaxel

Paclitaxel (Taxol) is the first of the taxane family of chemotherapeutic agents. It is an M phase agent that prevents the breakdown of the mitotic spindle and inhibits completion of anaphase. Paclitaxel, a derivative from the yew tree, acts by binding tubulin and promoting polymerization and stabilization of microtubules (unlike the vinca alkaloids, which inhibit polymerization). The microtubules created are highly stable but dysfunctional, leading to mitotic arrest and cell death. **Clinically** it is used against ovarian carcinomas, breast cancer, squamous cancers of the head and neck, and other cancers. **Side effects** include serious hypersensitivity reactions (e.g., dyspnea, urticaria, hypotension), peripheral neuropathy, and bone marrow suppression.

Topoisomerase inhibitors

Podophyllotoxins (Etoposide and Teniposide)

Etoposide and teniposide are podophyllotoxin-derived chemotherapeutic medications. Members of the podophyllotoxin drug class are G2 phase specific and act by inhibiting topoisomerase II. They form a three-part complex with DNA and topoisomerase II, leading to the inhibition of topoisomerase II and an accumulation of breaks in the DNA (topoisomerase II normally reseals double-stranded DNA breaks). The accumulation of breaks leads to degradation of DNA and cell death. Clinically etoposide and teniposide are used to treat lung and prostate carcinomas (small cell carcinomas), testicular cancers, lymphoma (ALL), and AML. **Side effects** include bone marrow suppression and possible high rate of secondary leukemias (in children treated with etoposide) with characteristic 11q23 translocation due to DNA breaks induced by medication.

Teniposide also inhibits topoisomerase II and is mainly used in the treatment of ALL. Side effects include severe myelosuppression, gastrointestinal toxicity, hypersensitivity reactions, and alopecia.

Camptothecan Analogs (Irinotecan and Topotecan): Irinotecan and topotecan are camptothecan derivatives that act as topoisomerase I inhibitors. Topoisomerase I is an enzyme that changes DNA structure by facilitating the relaxation of DNA supercoiling during the process of replication and transcription. **Clinical uses** include colon cancer (Irinotecan), ovarian cancer, and small cell lung cancer. **Side effects** include diarrhea and severe bone marrow suppression.

Steroid Hormones and Their Antagonists

Prednisone

Prednisone is a strong synthetic glucocorticoid that is the last P in the MOPP regimen. It has many actions on the body. Prednisone must be metabolized to prednisolone (active form), after which it binds a cytosolic receptor and is transported into the nucleus, activating specific corticosteroid response genes. Prednisone acts as an antiinflammatory and immunosuppressant agent by blocking proliferation of activated T cells and inhibits production of inflammatory mediators (also inhibits antibody production). It may trigger apoptosis of immune cells, especially lymphocytes. Prednisone also produces neutrophilia (without bandemia) via demargination of neutrophils in the circulation. It helps maintain blood glucose levels by increasing gluconeogenesis; it increases muscle catabolism and increases lipolysis. It also acts as a weak mineralocorticoid. **Clinically** it is used in the treatment of autoimmune diseases such as rheumatoid arthritis and asthma but is also used in leukemias (CLL) and HLs. **Side effects** include hypercortisolism (Cushing syndrome), hyperglycemia, an increased risk of infections, osteoporosis, muscle wasting, skin thinning, fat deposition, and psychosis.

Tamoxifen and Raloxifene

Tamoxifen is a selective estrogen receptor modulator (SERM) that acts primarily as an antiestrogen but has weak estrogenic activity. It competes with estrogen for the estrogen receptor (tamoxifen is not effective in premenopausal women because they produce enough estrogen to "out-compete" tamoxifen for the estrogen receptor) and creates a nonproductive complex with its receptor, failing to induce estrogen-responsive genes and RNA synthesis. This results in suppression of growth in estrogen-responsive tissues. As a result of its partial estrogen agonist activity, tamoxifen reduces the severity of osteoporosis in postmenopausal women, but it can stimulate endometrial growth and increases the risk of endometrial cancer. It also increases high-density lipoprotein (HDL) levels, protecting against atherosclerosis and cardiovascular disease. Raloxifene (endometrial estrogen antagonist), a drug similar to tamoxifen, does not stimulate endometrial growth and therefore does not increase the risk of endometrial cancer. It also protects against osteoporosis. **Clinically** it is used in the treatment of estrogen receptor–positive breast cancer and to prevent osteoporosis in postmenopausal women. **Side effects** include nausea, vomiting, hot flashes, and increased risk of endometrial cancer (tamoxifen only).

Other Agents

Cisplatin and Carboplatin

Cisplatin is a platinum-containing compound that is a member of the platinum coordination complex class of anticancer medications. Cisplatin acts similarly to the alkylating agents; it enters the cell and creates interstrand and intrastrand DNA crosslinks. These crosslinks result in DNA instability and cell death. **Clinically** it is used in the treatment of testicular and lung carcinomas. **Side effects** include significant nephrotoxicity, ototoxicity (cranial nerve [CN] VIII damage), and mild myelosuppression. Carboplatin is a similar agent, with less toxicity but greater bone marrow suppression.

Hydroxyurea

Hydroxyurea is an S phase–specific medication that inhibits DNA synthesis by blocking ribonucleotide reductase, stopping the conversion of ribonucleotides to deoxyribonucleotides. Hydroxyurea also acts by increasing the circulating levels of fetal hemoglobin. **Clinically** it is used in the management of sickle cell anemia and various myeloid cancers (CML). **Side effects** include bone marrow suppression, nausea, vomiting, and diarrhea (at high doses).

Trastuzumab

Trastuzumab (Herceptin) is a monoclonal antibody that binds and inhibits the Erb-B2/HER-2 receptor (a family of tyrosine kinases) expressed in some breast cancers. The HER-2 pathway promotes cell survival, growth, and division. **Clinically** it is used in the treatment of metastatic breast cancer. **Side effects** include cardiomyopathy.

Imatinib

Imatinib (Gleevec) is a monoclonal antibody that acts by binding and inhibiting the tyrosine kinase produced by the *ABL* and *C-KIT* genes (there are a large number of tyrosine kinase enzymes in the body). The Philadelphia chromosome in CML is produced by a fusion of the *BCR-ABL* genes creating a constitutively active tyrosine kinase. The *C-KIT* gene also produces a tyrosine kinase whose active site can be inhibited by imatinib. Gastrointestinal stromal tumors often arise from mutations in the *C-KIT* gene. **Clinically** it is used as the first-line treatment for CML. It is also used to treat gastrointestinal stromal tumors. **Side effects** include weight gain (most common), edema, bone marrow suppression, and possibly congestive heart failure (CHF).

Rituximab

Rituximab is an anti-CD20 monoclonal antibody that is **used clinically** to treat malignancies (NHL, CLL) and autoimmune diseases (rheumatoid arthritis, ITP). Many B-cell neoplasms are $CD20^+$; however, CD20 is also found on normal B cells and rituximab will destroy both. **Side effects** include fatal infusion reaction (deaths within 24 hours of infusion), reactivation of hepatitis B and other viral infections (JC virus infection leading to PML), mucocutaneous reactions, and diarrhea.

Erlotinib

Erlotinib (Tarceva) is a reversible epidermal growth factor receptor (EGFR) tyrosine kinase inhibitor **used clinically** to treat non–small cell lung cancer. Its main **side effect** is a rash that resembles acne and primarily involves the face as well as neck.

Bevacizumab (Avastin)

Bevacizumab is a medication that inhibits angiogenesis (growth of new blood vessels). It is a monoclonal antibody against vascular endothelial growth factor A (VEGF-A). VEGF-A is a chemical signaler that promotes angiogenesis. **Clinical uses** include many solid tumors such as colon cancer, renal cancer, ovarian cancer, lung cancer, and glioblastoma multiforme. **Side effects** include GI perforations, impaired wound healing (because it blocks growth of new blood vessels), and hemorrhage.

Vemurafenib

Vemurafenib is a B-Raf enzyme inhibitor that is **used clinically** for the treatment of advanced melanoma. Most common **side effects** include arthralgia and rash.

Cetuximab

Cetuximab is an EGFR inhibitor **used clinically** to treat metastatic colon cancer (KRAS wild-type), non–small cell lung cancer, as well as head and neck cancer. Most common **side effect** is acnelike rash.

REVIEW QUESTIONS

(1) What cells would you expect to be elevated in neoplastic disorders of myeloid progenitor cells?
(2) What cells would you expect to be elevated in neoplastic disorders of lymphoid progenitor cells?
(3) What will cause an increase in eosinophils in the blood?
(4) For what would you expect a patient with neutropenia (decreased blood levels of neutrophils) to be at increased risk?
(5) A 24-year-old primigravida at 10 weeks' gestation is brought to the emergency department (ED) because of vaginal bleeding. The patient is diagnosed with an incomplete abortion. She is treated with dilation and curettage (D&C) and all the products of conception are removed. Her blood type is AB Rh-negative. What is the most appropriate next step in management?
(6) A deficiency in proteins C and S would lead to what clinical disorder?
(7) An individual presents to your clinic complaining of recurrent bouts of epistaxis and easy bruising. He was told by another physician that he had "a problem with a platelet receptor or protein in his blood." His BT is prolonged, platelet count is low, and ristocetin assay is abnormal. He was transfused with normal plasma, and the ristocetin assay result remained abnormal. What is his most likely diagnosis?
(8) A 60-year-old man presents with fever, night sweats, weight loss, and hemoptysis. On evaluation he is found to have tuberculosis. He is started on one medication for 6 months. At his 6-month follow-up, his CBC shows a microcytic anemia and peripheral blood smear shows ringed sideroblasts. He also has symptoms of peripheral neuropathy. What other laboratory findings do you expect?

(9) A 75-year-old man with no medical history presents for an annual checkup. He reports some increased dyspnea on exertion, along with an overall feeling of fatigue for the past few months. Physical examination is negative except for a heme occult–positive stool test. What is the most likely reason for his symptoms and what would his peripheral blood smear show?

(10) What four disorders cause microcytic, hypochromic anemia?

(11) A 24-year-old African man comes to your office as a new patient. He recently moved from Africa and, when asked about medical history, he says he has a problem with his blood. He reports frequent pain and mentions that his family members have similar blood problems. On examination, his sclera are icteric. What type of hematologic disorder should you suspect in this patient?

(12) An otherwise healthy Kenyan man is prescribed trimethoprim-sulfamethoxazole for an infection. He presents to the ED with new onset of fatigue, jaundice, and confusion. What is his clinical diagnosis and what may you expect on a peripheral blood smear?

(13) List the disease associated with each of the following peripheral smear findings: (1) bite cell, (2) elliptocyte, (3) schistocyte (helmet cell), (4) spherocyte, (5) Heinz body, (6) Howell-Jolly body, (7) target cell, (8) acanthocyte (spur cell), and (9) teardrop cell.

(14) What is the mechanism that results in the formation of hypersegmented neutrophils in megaloblastic anemia?

(15) A person with suspected megaloblastic anemia is treated with folate supplementation. After a few months of treatment, the anemia symptoms resolve but the patient's psychiatric symptoms do not. What went wrong?

(16) List the expected BT, PT, PTT, and platelet findings in each of the following bleeding disorders: (1) vWD disease; (2) ITP, TTP, HUS; (3) DIC; (4) hemophilia A; (5) NSAID use; (6) warfarin or heparin. (Answers in the following table.)

CONDITION	BT	PT	PTT	PLATELET COUNT
vWD disease				
ITP, TTP, HUS				
DIC				
Hemophilia A				
NSAIDs				
Warfarin or heparin				
Vitamin K deficiency				
Bernard-Soulier syndrome				
Glanzmann disease				

(17) What differentiates TTP from HUS?

(18) List the seven causes of DIC.

(19) What are the typical age ranges for ALL, AML, CML, and CLL?

(20) A 3-year-old presents with a 1-week history of fever, pallor, headaches, and bone tenderness. On examination, he has a fever, hepatosplenomegaly (HSM), and generalized lymphadenopathy. Peripheral smear reveals an absolute lymphocytosis with abundant TdT-positive lymphoblasts. What is the diagnosis?

(21) A 60-year-old man has complained of fatigue and anorexia for 6 months. On examination, he has generalized lymphadenopathy and hepatosplenomegaly. His white count is 250,000, Hb is 9.0, and direct Coombs test is positive. His peripheral blood smear shows numerous small round lymphocytes and smudge cells. What is the diagnosis?

(22) A 35-year-old man presents with fever and an abdominal mass. He reports weight loss and night sweats over the past 6 weeks. On examination, he has enlarged abdominal lymph nodes. A lymph node biopsy demonstrates a starry sky appearance. What is the diagnosis, and which virus is most likely associated with the condition?

(23) A patient presents with cervical lymphadenopathy. You perform a lymph node biopsy and see a nodular lymphoma with follicle formation. What is the most likely diagnosis and with what translocation is this disorder associated?

(24) A 40-year-old woman presents with 2 months of fever, night sweats, and weight loss. On examination, you notice cervical lymphadenopathy and hepatosplenomegaly. Her CBC reveals leukocytosis, and a chest radiograph demonstrates bilateral hilar lymphadenopathy. The nodal biopsy reveals the presence of a few RSCs, with surrounding fibrosis. What is the most likely diagnosis?

(25) A 60-year-old African American man presents with constipation and generalized bone pain. The examination is unremarkable, but the patient is found to be hypercalcemic, and his skull radiograph shows lytic lesions. What is the diagnosis and what other abnormalities are to be expected?

(26) A 64-year-old woman is seen in your clinic to follow up on test results for anemia. She was found to have anemia of chronic disease. As part of the testing, she was found to have elevated serum protein levels. Her serum protein electrophoresis showed a singular protein spike and bone marrow biopsy specimen with 5% plasma cells. What do you tell this patient about her disease?

(27) What is the best way to differentiate PV from CML?

(28) A 62-year-old woman complains of headaches, vertigo, and pruritus after showering. On examination, she has a ruddy complexion, mild hypertension, and splenomegaly. What is the diagnosis? List the expected RBC mass, RBC count, and EPO level.

(29) A 17-year-old woman is admitted to the psychiatric ward because she reports that everyone is trying to kill her. Four days after her admission, she develops severe abdominal pain, fever, and vomiting. A nurse tells you that she noticed her urine turns red when left standing. What is the diagnosis?

12 MUSCULOSKELETAL/ RHEUMATOLOGY

Thomas E. Blair

ANATOMY AND PHYSIOLOGY

Bone: Bone formation begins with **osteoblasts producing osteoid,** which is composed primarily of type I collagen. The osteoid matrix acts as a scaffold onto which minerals from the blood deposit to form hydroxyapatite crystals and eventually rigid bone. **Osteoclasts** migrate from the bone marrow and are responsible for bone **remodeling.** Remodeling functions to repair bony microdamage and maintain calcium homeostasis. Remodeling is under hormonal control, so when calcium is high, calcitonin is released to inhibit osteoclast function directly. When calcium is low, parathyroid hormone (PTH) is released, which induces osteoblasts to activate osteoclasts. Osteoclasts then resorb bone and release calcium into the circulation. Osteoblasts will eventually produce more osteoid to replace the resorbed bone.

Osteoblasts produce osteoid, a collagen scaffold for hydroxyapatite deposition.

Mnemonic: Osteo**B**lasts **B**uild bone. Osteo**C**lasts **C**onsume bone. Calci**tonin** **"tones** down" calcium.

Long Bone: Weight-bearing bones, such as the tibia and femur, are important for skeletal mobility. These bones grow via endochondral ossification (cartilage-dependent growth) at the epiphyseal plate (growth plate). Long bones are divided into the epiphysis, epiphyseal plate, metaphysis, and diaphysis (Fig. 12.1).

Flat Bone: These bones provide broad, flat surfaces for muscle attachment or protection. Examples include the pelvis and skull. Growth is through intramembranous ossification (cartilage-independent growth).

Cartilage: Produced by chondrocytes and composed primarily of type 2 collagen, ground substance, and elastin. **Hyaline** cartilage provides a compressible, low-friction, high-strength material ideal for cushioning joints. **Elastic** cartilage contains relatively more elastin and forms structures such as the pinna of the ear and epiglottis. Because cartilage is avascular, chondrocytes must rely on diffusion to obtain nutrients. Cartilage has only a minimal capacity for regeneration because of the low numbers of highly specialized chondrocytes.

Ligament: Fibrous connective tissue composed of collagen that connects bone to bone.

Fascia: Fibrous connective tissue composed of collagen that connects muscle to muscle.

Tendon: Fibrous connective tissue composed of collagen that connects muscle to bone. The points at which tendons insert into bone are called **entheses.**

Skeletal Muscle: Voluntarily controlled muscle tissue innervated by the somatic nervous system. Individual muscles are composed of bundles of fascicles, which are composed of bundles of muscle fibers. The muscle fibers are the "muscle cells" referred to as myocytes. At the subcellular level, muscle fibers contain bundles of myofibrils (Fig. 12.2). Each myofibril consists of proteins (e.g., actin, myosin) that form thick and thin filaments that repeat along the myofibril. These repeating units are called **sarcomeres.**

Sarcomere: This basic contractile unit of muscle is composed of actin and myosin (Fig. 12.3). The A band contains thick myosin filaments. The M line bisects the center of the A band and contains proteins that link the myosin filaments together. The I bands fall on either side of the A band and contain thin actin filaments. Contraction occurs when the actin and myosin fibers overlap in the presence of Ca^{2+} and ATP, allowing cross-bridge cycling.

The sarcomere is the basic contractile unit of muscle.

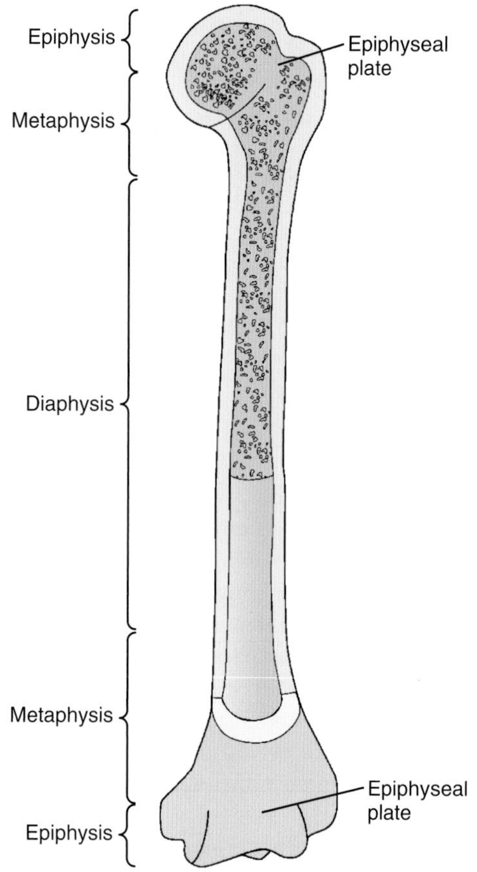

FIG. 12.1 A long bone can be divided into the epiphysis, epiphyseal plate, metaphysis, and diaphysis. (*From Rakel RE, Rakel DP.* Textbook of Family Medicine. *8th ed. Philadelphia: Elsevier; 2011.*)

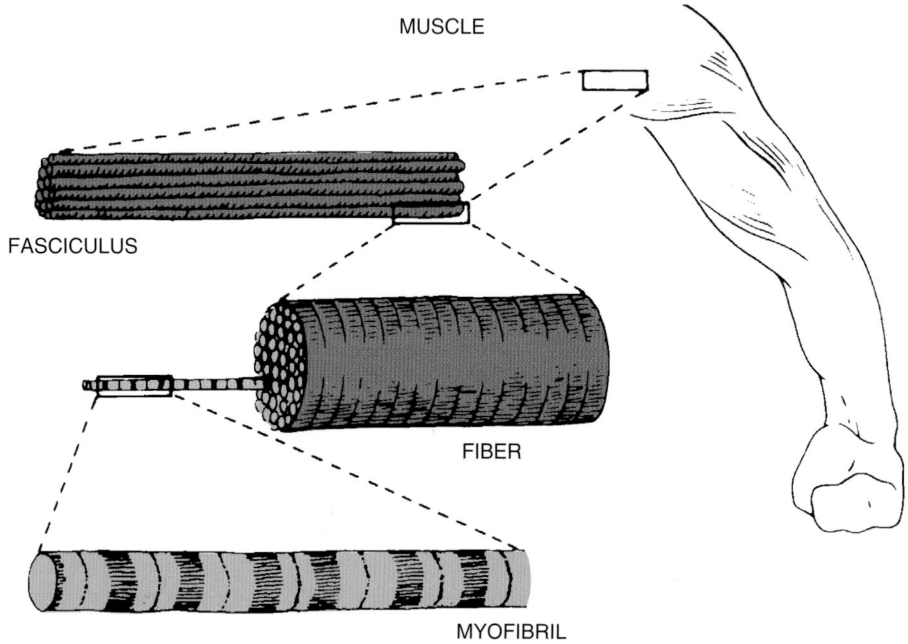

FIG. 12.2 Constitutive parts of skeletal muscle. (*From Berne MN, Levy BA, Koeppen BM, Stanton RM.* Physiology. *Philadelphia: Elsevier; 2003.*)

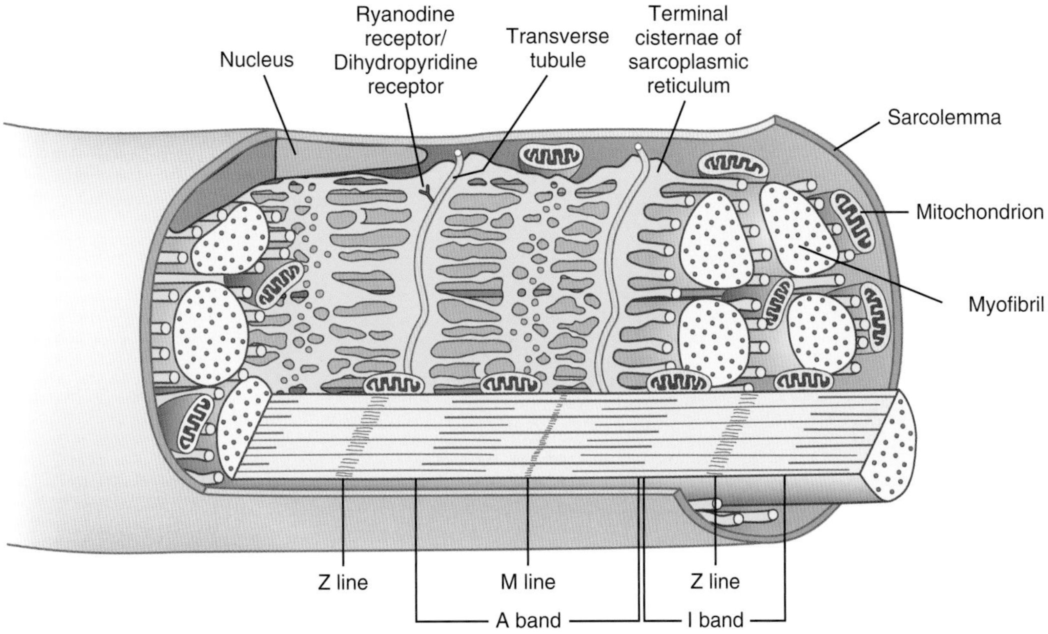

FIG. 12.3 Sarcomere, the basic contractile unit of muscle composed of actin and myosin. (*From Gartner LP, Hiatt JL.* Color Textbook of Histology. *3rd ed. Philadelphia: Saunders; 2007.*)

Type 1 Fibers: Slow twitch muscle is **red** because of its dense concentration of capillaries, mitochondria, and myoglobin. These fibers specialize in the **aerobic metabolism** needed for sustained muscle contractions.

Type 2 Fibers: Fast twitch muscle is **white** because of relatively sparse mitochondria and myoglobin. These fibers specialize in **anaerobic bursts** of activity for fast, forceful muscle contractions.

Type 1 muscle: Slow, red, aerobic, sustained

Type 2 muscle: Fast, white, anaerobic, bursts

Skeletal Muscle Contraction:

- Action potentials release acetylcholine from the presynaptic neuron into the neuromuscular junction.
- **Nicotinic acetylcholine** receptors open ligand-gated ion channels, allowing Na^+ to rush in and generate a depolarizing endplate potential.
- Transverse tubules (T-tubules), which form invaginations in the sarcolemmal (muscle cell) membrane, carry the depolarizations deep into the myofibers to cause a conformational change of the voltage-sensitive **dihydropyridine receptors.** Dihydropyridine receptors are in the sarcolemmal membrane, but thanks to the T-tubules, are positioned next to the sarcoplasmic reticulum (SR).
- The dihydropyridine receptor's conformational change opens the **ryanodine receptor** on the sarcoplasmic reticulum (SR) and allows the large Ca2+ stores of the SR to diffuse into the cytoplasm.
- Calcium binds **troponin C**, causing a conformational change of tropomyosin and exposing the myosin-binding site of actin.
- Myosin heads can now form cross bridges with actin to allow cross-bridge cycling (Fig. 12.4).
- As long as Ca^{2+} is bound to troponin and ATP is present, cross-bridge cycling will continue. Once the Ca^{2+} ATPase sequesters Ca^{2+} back in the SR, there is no longer sufficient Ca^{2+} to bind troponin C. Tropomyosin then returns to its resting position, blocking the formation of actin-myosin cross-bridges, and resulting in muscle relaxation. If, on the other hand, Ca^{2+} remains present and ATP is absent, the muscle will enter a state of rigor (prolonged contraction).

T-tubules transmit depolarization to dihydropyridine receptors on the sarcolemmal membrane. This stimulates ryanodine receptors to release Ca^{2+} from the SR.

Smooth Muscle: Nonstriated muscle under involuntary control of the autonomic nervous system. Smooth muscle provides vascular tone within blood vessels and is the contractile force for involuntary movements throughout the body including the gastrointestinal, genitourinary, and respiratory tracts.

Smooth Muscle Contraction (Fig. 12.5):

- Action potentials depolarize smooth muscles, which open voltage-sensitive Ca^{2+} channels in the sarcolemma.
- Ca^{2+} flows into the cell down its concentration gradient and binds **calmodulin.**
- The Ca^{2+}calmodulin complex activates **myosin light-chain kinase (MLCK).**
- Activated MLCK phosphorylates myosin light-chains and increases their ATPase activity. Increased ATPase activity promotes cross-bridge cycling.

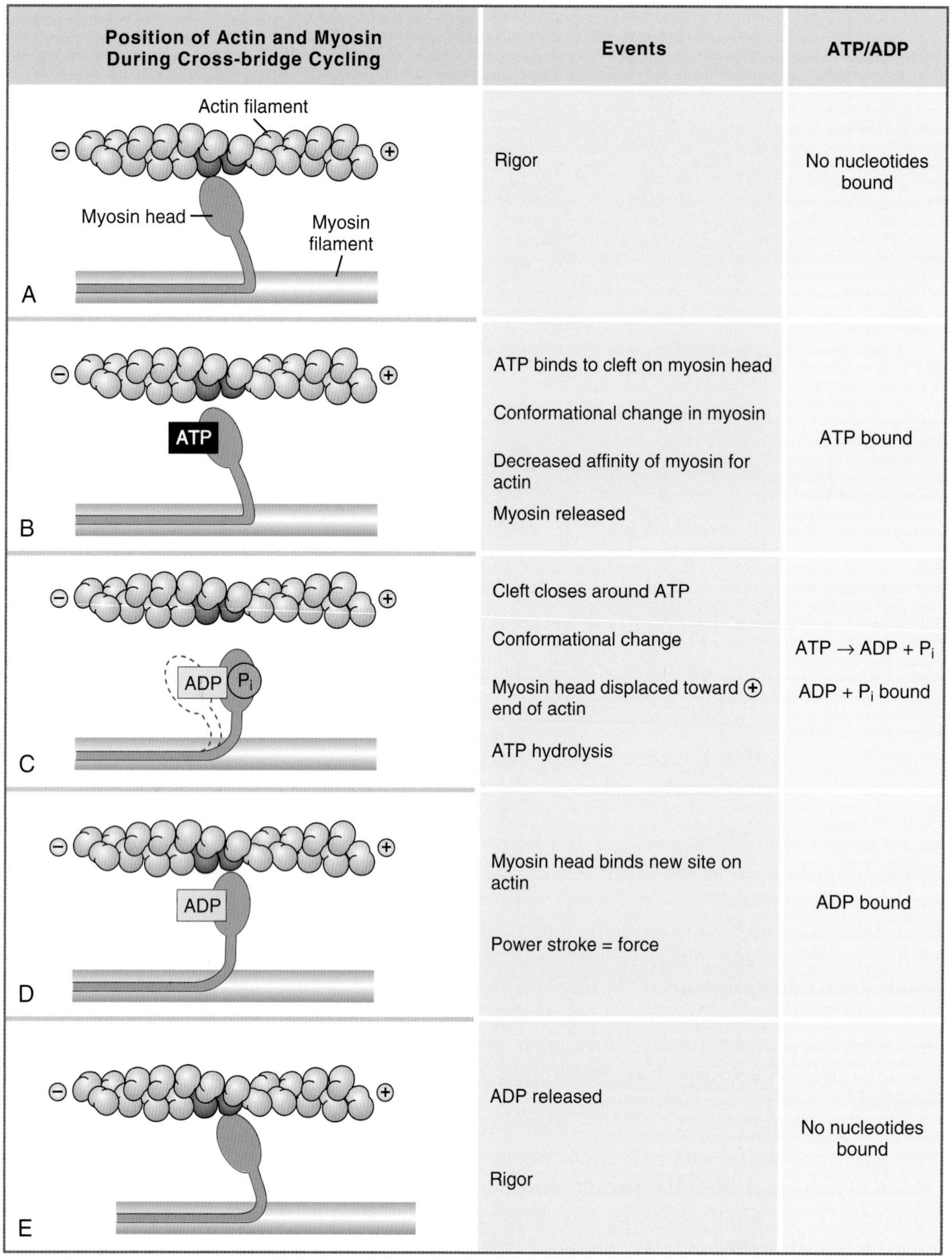
Position of Actin and Myosin During Cross-bridge Cycling
Events
ATP/ADP
Actin filament
Myosin head
Myosin filament
A
Rigor
No nucleotides bound
ATP
B
ATP binds to cleft on myosin head
Conformational change in myosin
Decreased affinity of myosin for actin
Myosin released
ATP bound
ADP
Pi
C
Cleft closes around ATP
Conformational change
Myosin head displaced toward ⊕ end of actin
ATP hydrolysis
ATP → ADP + Pi
ADP + Pi bound
ADP
D
Myosin head binds new site on actin
Power stroke = force
ADP bound
E
ADP released
Rigor
No nucleotides bound

Fig. 12.4 Cross-bridge cycling and muscle contraction of skeletal and cardiac muscle. (*From Costanzo LS.* Physiology. *4th ed. New York: Elsevier; 2009.*)

- **Myosin light-chain phosphatase** eventually inhibits contraction by dephosphorylating myosin-light chains.
- Individual smooth muscle cells are connected via **gap junctions.** This means one neuron can stimulate one smooth muscle cell, but an entire group of cells will depolarize and contract together.

Cardiac Muscle: Provides the contractile force of the myocardium and is composed of cardiac myocytes. Cardiac muscle has some properties of striated muscle and some of smooth muscle. Like skeletal muscle, cardiac muscle is striated, with sarcomeres of actin and myosin. Contraction is very similar to skeltal muscle contraction; Na^+ influx induces depolarizations, which spread down T-tubules. Unlike skeletal muscle, however, depolarization of cardiac myocytes triggers extracellular calcium to flow

The Ca^{2+} calmodulin complex activates MLCK, which phosphorlyates myosin light chains, thus increasing their ATPase activity.

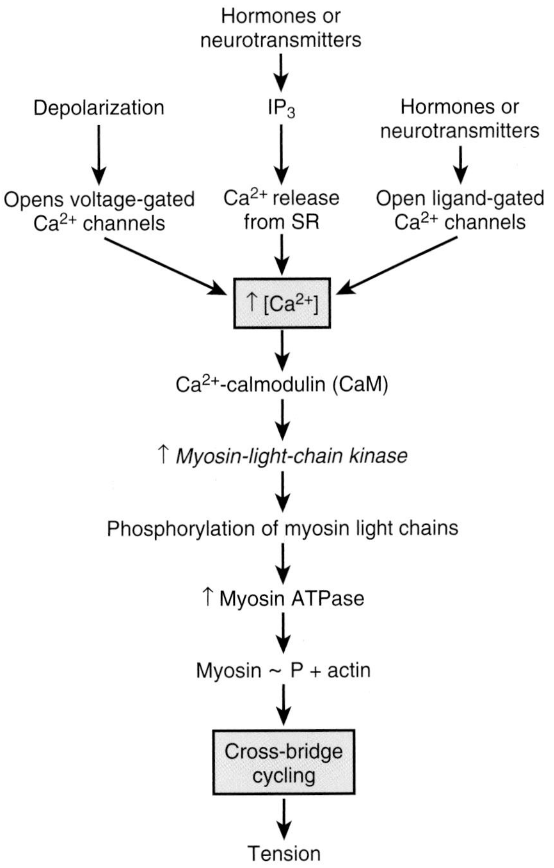

FIG. 12.5 Smooth muscle contraction. (*From Costanzo LS.* Physiology. *4th ed. New York: Elsevier; 2009.*)

inward through L-type calcium channels, which triggers ryanodine receptors to release Ca^{2+} from the SR (**calcium-induced calcium release** rather than dihydropyridine receptor–induced calcium release).

Cardiac muscle is like smooth muscle in that it is under involuntary control, and cells are linked together via gap junctions, which allow coordinated contraction.

Of note, cardiac muscle contains a unique type of troponin that functions in a similar manner to skeletal muscle troponin. This protein is leaked during cardiac myocyte damage, and measurement of troponin is very sensitive for detecting myocardial infarction.

> Cardiac myocyte contraction relies on Ca^{2+}-induced Ca^{2+} release.

> Troponin is a sensitive marker for myocardial infarction.

Upper Extremity Anatomy

Brachial Plexus: Bundle of nerve fibers responsible for sensory and motor innervation to the upper extremity. For the purposes of Step 1, it is valuable to know all **r**oots, **t**runks, **d**ivisions, **c**ords, **b**ranches, and associated lesions (Figs. 12.6 and 12.7). The muscular and sensory innervation of nerves should also be memorized (Table 12.1).

Mnemonic: **R**eal **T**exans **D**rink **C**old **B**eer.

Axillary Nerve: Composed of nerve roots C5-C6, the axillary nerve provides sensory innervation from the shoulder (over the deltoid muscle). It innervates the deltoids and teres minor (shoulder abduction). Injury is usually from a proximal arm injury (e.g., proximal humeral fracture, anterior shoulder dislocation).

Long Thoracic Nerve: Composed of nerve roots C5-C7, the long thoracic nerve innervates the serratus anterior muscle, which pulls the scapula forward with relation to the thorax. Damage causes winged scapula (Fig. 12.8). Injury may occur from a stab wound or surgical procedure.

Musculocutaneous Nerve: Composed of nerve roots C5-C7, the musculocutaneous nerve innervates the biceps brachii and brachialis muscle, which are responsible for elbow flexion and supination. Injury may occur because of forced stretching between the shoulder and head, damaging the upper trunk.

Median Nerve: Composed of nerve roots C8-T1, the median nerve provides sensory innervation from the palmar surface of the hand and the first 3½ digits (Fig. 12.8). It innervates

> The median nerve innervates all forearm flexors except flexor carpi ulnaris (ulnar nerve).

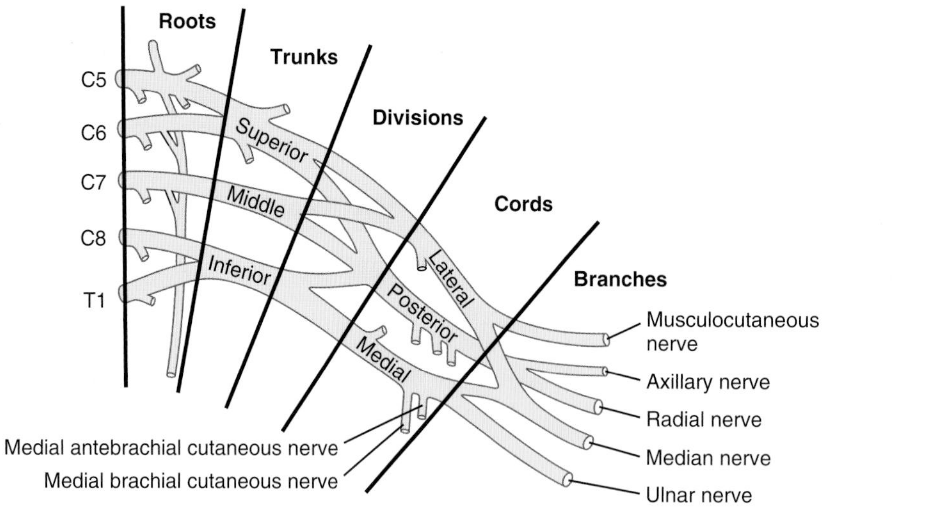

FIG. 12.6 Roots, trunks, divisions, cords, and nerves of the brachial plexus. (*From Miller RD:* Miller's Anethesia. *6th ed. Philadelphia: Churchill Livingstone; 2005.*)

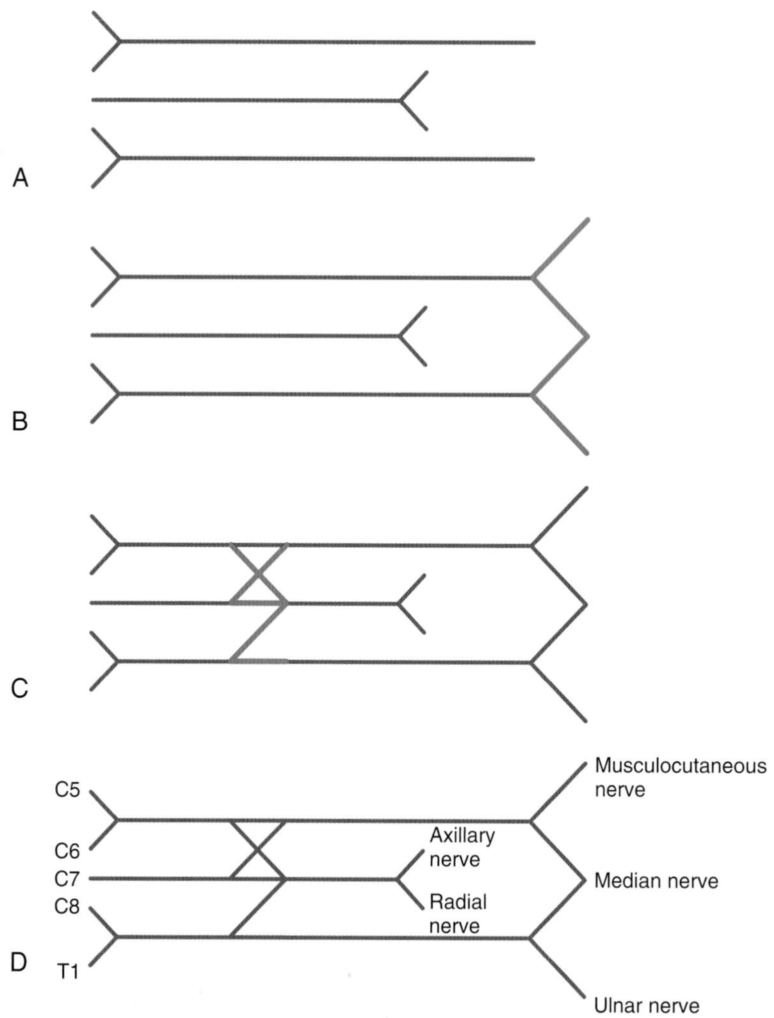

FIG. 12.7 Tips for memorizing the brachial plexus anatomy. **A,** Draw two headless arrows to the right and one headless arrow to the left. **B,** Draw a "W" on the right. **C,** Draw an "X" above and a "Z" below. **D,** Label C5-T1 and the major nerves.

TABLE 12.1 Upper Extremity Nerves and Their Corresponding Injuries

NERVE INJURY	NERVE ROOTS	CAUSE	SENSORY LOSS	MOTOR LOSS	COMMENT
Upper brachial plexus	C5-C6	Shoulder dystocia		Deltoid, infraspinatus, biceps brachii	**Erb palsy** (waiter's tip)—inability to abduct shoulder, externally rotate, or supinate arm
Axillary	C5-C6	Proximal humeral fracture; shoulder dislocation	Shoulder(over deltoid muscle)	Deltoid, teres minor	Inability to abduct shoulder
Long thoracic	C5-C7	Knife, surgical injury		Serratus anterior	**Winged scapula—** inability to hold scapula against rib cage
Musculocutaneous	C5-C7	Upper trunk injury		Biceps brachii, brachialis	Inability to flex or supinate arm
Radial nerve	C5-T1	Midshaft humeral fracture; axillary compression	Dorsum of hand (except fifth and lateral fourth digit)	Triceps brachii, extensor carpi radialis	**Wrist drop—** inability to extend wrist
Median	C8-T1	Distal humeral fracture; carpal tunnel syndrome	Palmar surface of hand; first, second, and third digits	Forearm flexors, opponens pollicis, lateral lumbricals	**Ape hand—** nonopposable thumb **Bottle sign—** inability to flex second and third digits, causing inability to hold a bottle
Ulnar	C8-T1	Distal humeral fracture; wrist (hamate) fracture	Fifth digit; lateral fourth digit	Wrist-finger flexors, intrinsic muscles of the hand	**Ulnar claw (Pope's blessing)—** flexion of fourth and fifth digits
Lower brachial plexus	C8-T1	Traction on raised arm (e.g., during birth or falling from a tree)		Finger extensors, lumbricals	**Klumpke palsy—** total clawing of hand

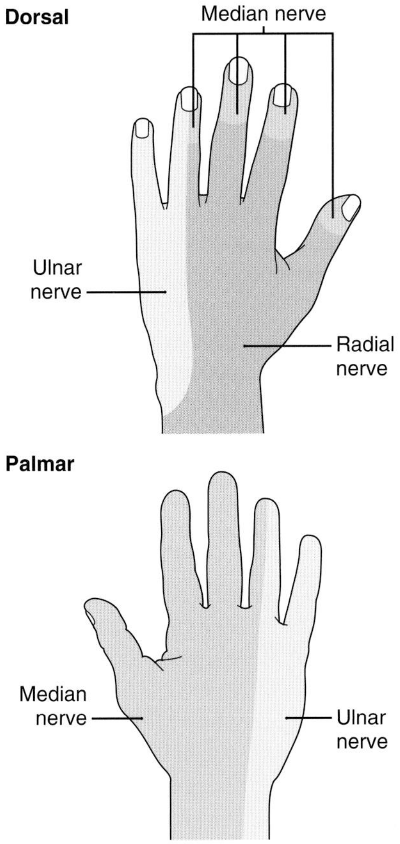

FIG. 12.8 Sensory innervation to the hand. Consider tracing this image on your hand while you study. (*From Marsland D, Kapoor S.* Crash Course: Rheumatology and Orthopaedics, *2nd ed. Philadelphia: Elsevier; 2008.*)

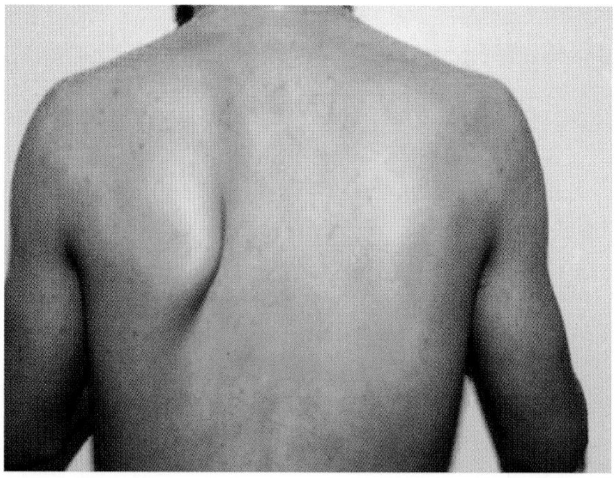

Fig. 12.9 Winged scapula from damage to the long thoracic nerve. (*From Douglas G, Nicol F, Robertson C. Macleod's Clinical Examination. 11th ed. Philadelphia: Elsevier; 2005.*)

all the forearm flexors except the flexor carpi ulnaris (ulnar nerve). It is also responsible for flexion of the lateral digits (lateral lumbricals) and opposition of the thumb (opponens pollicis) muscle. Proximal injury causes inability to oppose the thumb, so-called ape hand. Distal injury causes the bottle sign (inability to flex second and third digits, resulting in inability to hold a bottle). Damage may be caused by fracture of the distal humerus proximally or compression from carpal tunnel syndrome more distally.

Ulnar Nerve: Composed of nerve roots C8-T1, the ulnar nerve provides sensory innervation from the fifth digit and lateral fourth digit (Fig. 12.8). It innervates some of the wrist and finger flexors and the intrinsic muscles of the hand. Injury may be caused by fracture of the distal humerus, wrist (hamate) fracture, or compression of the cubital tunnel.

Radial Nerve: Composed of nerve roots C5-T1, the radial nerve provides sensory innervation from the dorsum of the hand, except the fifth and lateral fourth digits (Fig. 12.8). It is responsible for **extension** of the elbow (triceps brachii), wrist (extensor carpi radialis), and fingers. For this reason it is called the "great extensor" of the arm. Damage causes wrist drop. Injury may occur because of a midshaft humeral fracture or axillary compression (e.g., poorly fitted crutches or drooping one's arm over the edge of a bar ["Saturday night palsy"]).

The radial nerve is known as the "great extensor" of the arm.

Brachial Plexus Syndromes

Winged Scapula: Damage to the long thoracic nerve (C5-C7) causes paralysis of the serratus anterior muscles and a winged scapula because of inability to hold the scapula against the rib cage (Fig. 12.9). This injury is more pronounced when the patient faces a wall and presses the hands against the wall.

Erb Palsy (Waiter's Tip): Damage to the upper brachial plexus roots causes weakness of abduction from deltoid paralysis (C5), weakness of external rotation from infraspinatus paralysis (C5), and loss of flexion from biceps paralysis (C6). The internal muscles of the hand are unaffected. Think of it as damage to the roots supplying the axillary and musculocutaneous nerves. The result is an arm that hangs limply by the side in extension and internal rotation (Fig. 12.10). Injury is usually caused by shoulder dystocia, in which the infant's shoulder cannot pass the maternal pubic symphysis during birth. The result is traction on the shoulder, which damages the upper brachial plexus roots.

Erb palsy is often a result of shoulder dystocia causing upper brachial plexus damage.

Klumpke Palsy: Injury to the lower roots of the brachial plexus (C8-T1) causes total clawing of the hand because of paralysis of the lumbricals and finger extensors (Fig. 12.11). Injury occurs when the raised arm is forcibly pulled upward, as may occur during birth or, for example, if a patient catches himself or herself by a branch while falling from a tree.

Klumpke palsy causes total clawing of the hand because of lower brachial plexus injury.

Thoracic Outlet Syndrome: Compression of the brachial plexus above the first rib, causing numbness and weakness of the affected arm, especially after protracted usage or reaching overhead (common in weight lifters). On physical examination, the patient's radial pulse may disappear on tilting the head toward the unaffected side (Adson sign) because of compression of the subclavian artery at the thoracic outlet.

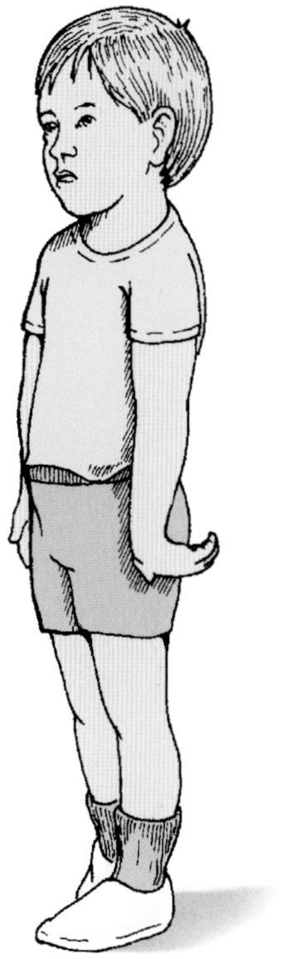

Fig. 12.10 Erb palsy (waiter's tip) from damage to roots C5–C6 of the brachial plexus. (*From Dandy DJ, Edwards DJ.* Essential Orthopaedics and Trauma, *5th ed. Philadelphia: Elsevier; 2009.*)

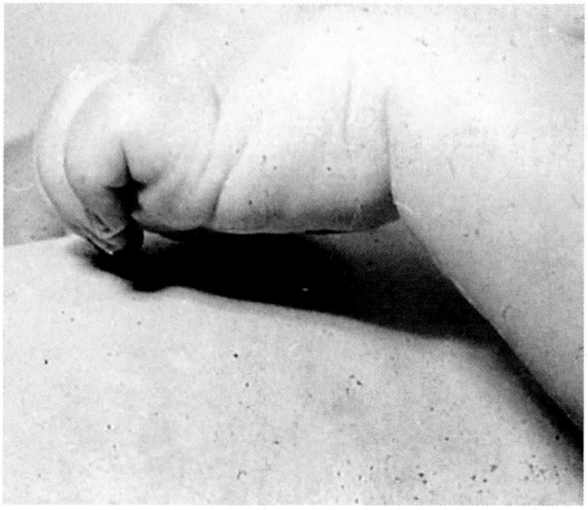

Fig. 12.11 Klumpke palsy, total clawing of the hand caused by trauma to the lower brachial plexus. (*From Pope BA, Painter MJ.* Neurologic sequelae of birth, *2008 http://www.glowm.com/ section_view/ item/198/recordset/18975/value/198.*)

Peripheral Nerve Lesions of the Upper Extremity

See Table 12.1.

Ulnar Claw (Pope's Blessing): Damage to the ulnar nerve at the medial epicondyle or wrist, causing lumbrical weakness and flexion (clawing) of fourth and fifth digits.

Wrist Drop: Compression of the radial nerve results in unilateral wrist drop because the radial nerve innervates the finger and wrist extensors. Compression may be in the axilla because of the use of crutches or at the midshaft of the humerus because of a fracture. Lead poisoning can lead to wrist drop through its effect on the radial nerve. Wrist drop also classically occurs when a patient becomes drunk and falls asleep with his or her arm draped over the bar. This compresses the radial in the axilla and is called Saturday night palsy.

Radial nerve injury causes wrist drop.

Ape Hand (Nonopposable Thumb): Median nerve injury, causing weakness of the opponens pollicis muscle and inability to abduct or oppose the thumb.

Bottle Sign: Distal median nerve injury causes weakness of the lateral lumbricals and inability to flex the second and third digits. Patients are therefore unable to hold a bottle.

Carpal Tunnel Syndrome: The carpal tunnel is a narrow tunnel of the anterior wrist. The carpal bones form the floor, and the flexor retinaculum (transverse carpal ligament) forms the roof. The tunnel contains nine flexor tendons and the **median nerve** (Fig. 12.12). Compression of the median nerve causes pain and numbness in the lateral palmar surface of the hand. Chronic compression may also cause weakness of palmar abduction and thenar atrophy. Patients may have a positive Tinel sign (paresthesia with percussion of carpal tunnel) or Phalen maneuver (paresthesia with forced wrist flexion). Conservative treatment is a night splint. Medical treatment involves steroid injections. Surgical treatment, which is definitive, occurs when the flexor retinaculum is released. Anything that compresses the median nerve may cause this syndrome, including myxedema from hypothyroidism, fluid compression within the carpal tunnel (during pregnancy), compression from synovitis secondary to constant wrist flexion (during sleep or while typing), or inflammation (rheumatoid arthritis).

The carpel tunnel contains the median nerve. Compression causes lateral palmar numbness.

Ulnar Tunnel Syndrome (Guyon's Canal Syndrome): Compression of the radial nerve at the wrist causes paresthesias of the medial surface of the hand (ring and little finger). Clasically occurs in cyclists due to compression of the ulnar tunnel against the bicycle handlebars.

Lower Extremity Anatomy

Lumbosacral Plexus: Unlike the brachial plexus, it is probably not high yield to memorize the lumbosacral plexus in detail. The muscular and sensory innervation of major nerves should be known, however (Table 12.2).

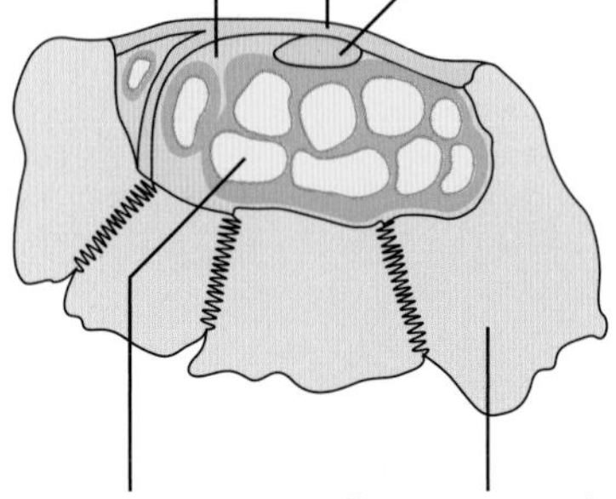

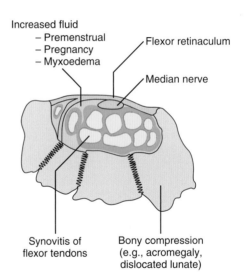

Fig. 12.12 Anatomy of the carpal tunnel and pathophysiology of carpal tunnel syndrome. (*From Douglas G, Nicol F, Robertson C. Macleod's Clinical Examination. 11th ed. Philadelphia: Elsevier; 2005.*)

Table 12.2 Lower Extremity Nerves and Their Corresponding Injuries

NERVE INJURY	SENSORY LOSS	MOTOR LOSS	COMMENT
Femoral	Anterior thigh, medial leg	Iliacus, anterior compartment of thigh	Inability to flex thigh or extend the leg
Obturator	Medial thigh	Medial compartment of thigh	Inability to adduct hips
Fibular branch of sciatic	Anterior shin, dorsum of foot	Anterior compartment of leg	**Foot drop**—inability to dorsiflex foot or toes
Tibial branch of sciatic	Sole of foot	Hamstrings, soleus, gastrocnemius	Inability to flex knee, foot, or toes
Superior gluteal		Gluteus medius, gluteus minimus, tensor fasciae latae	**Trendelenburg sign**— hip dropping on the contralateral side when standing on the affected leg
Inferior gluteal		Gluteus maximus	

Femoral Nerve: Composed of nerve roots L2-L4, the femoral nerve provides sensory innervation to the anterior thigh and medial leg. It innervates the iliacus and all the muscles of the anterior compartment of the thigh (quadriceps and sartorius). It is therefore responsible for thigh flexion and leg extension (the motion of a high kick). Injury may occur because of fracture of the pelvis.

Obturator: From the Latin "to close." Composed of nerve roots L2-L4, the obturator nerve provides sensory innervation from the medial thigh. It also innervates the muscles of the medial compartment of the thigh (gracilis, adductors, and obturator externus). It allows for hip adduction (i.e., closing the thighs).

The obturator nerve is responsible for closing the thighs (adduction).

Sciatic Nerve:

Fibular (Peroneal) Branch: Composed of nerve roots L4-S2, the fibular nerve provides sensory innervation to the anterior shin and dorsum of the foot. It innervates the anterior compartment of the leg and is responsible for foot and toe dorsiflexion. Injury causes **foot drop.**

Fibular nerve damage causes foot drop. Superior gluteal damage causes Trendelenburg gait.

Tibial Branch: Composed of nerve roots L4-S3, the tibial nerve provides sensory innervation to the sole of the foot. It innervates the hamstrings, soleus, and gastrocnemius muscles and allows for knee, foot, and toe flexion.

Superior Gluteal: Composed of nerve roots L4-S1, the superior gluteal nerve innervates the gluteus medius, gluteus minimus, and tensor fasciae latae muscles (thigh abduction). Injury causes inability to abduct the thigh while walking, which can cause Trendelenburg gait.

Inferior Gluteal: Composed of nerve roots L5-S2, the inferior gluteal nerve innervates the gluteus maximus muscle (hip extension).

Peripheral Nerve Lesions of the Lower Extremity

See Table 12.2.

Foot Drop: Compression of the common fibular (peroneal) nerve at the head of the fibula causes weakness of the anterior tibialis muscle and inability to dorsiflex the foot. Patients may present with a **steppage gait,** where they lift the affected thigh high enough to prevent their toes from dragging on the ground. Nerve compression is most frequently caused by simply crossing the legs in a way that causes pressure on the fibular head. Fibular head and neck fractures are also occasionally implicated. Sensory loss may be concurrent and occurs in the anterolateral shin and dorsum of the foot (superficial peroneal nerve distribution).

Prolonged crossing of the legs can cause foot drop.

Trendelenburg Gait: Injury to the superior gluteal nerve causes weakness of the gluteal muscles and inability to abduct the hip. On examination, positive Trendelenburg sign is hip dropping on the contralateral side to the affected lesion when standing on ipsilateral leg (i.e., if the right superior gluteal nerve is damaged, then standing on the right leg will result in left hip drop; Trendelenburg sign; Fig. 12.13). When walking, they will compensate by leaning their trunk over the affected side (i.e., if the right superior gluteal nerve is damaged the patient will lean their trunk to the right when walking; Trendelenburg gait).

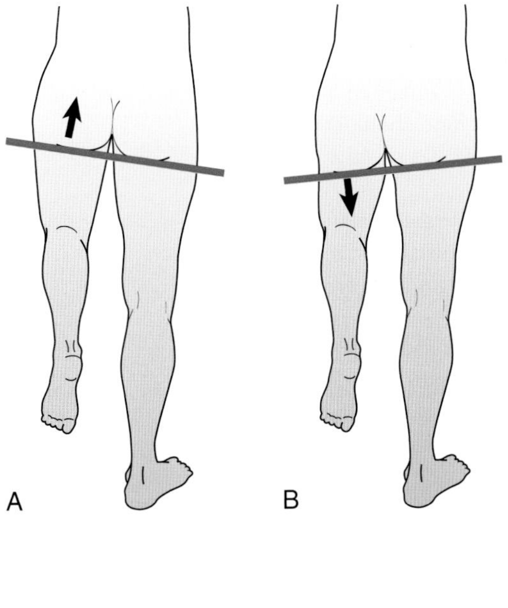

Fig. 12.13 Injury to the superior gluteal nerve results in drooping of the affected buttock on raising the affected leg (Trendelenburg sign). **A,** Normal physical examination. **B,** Trendelenburg sign. (*From Moore NA, Roy WA. Rapid Review Gross and Developmental Anatomy. 3rd ed. Philadelphia: Elsevier; 2010.*)

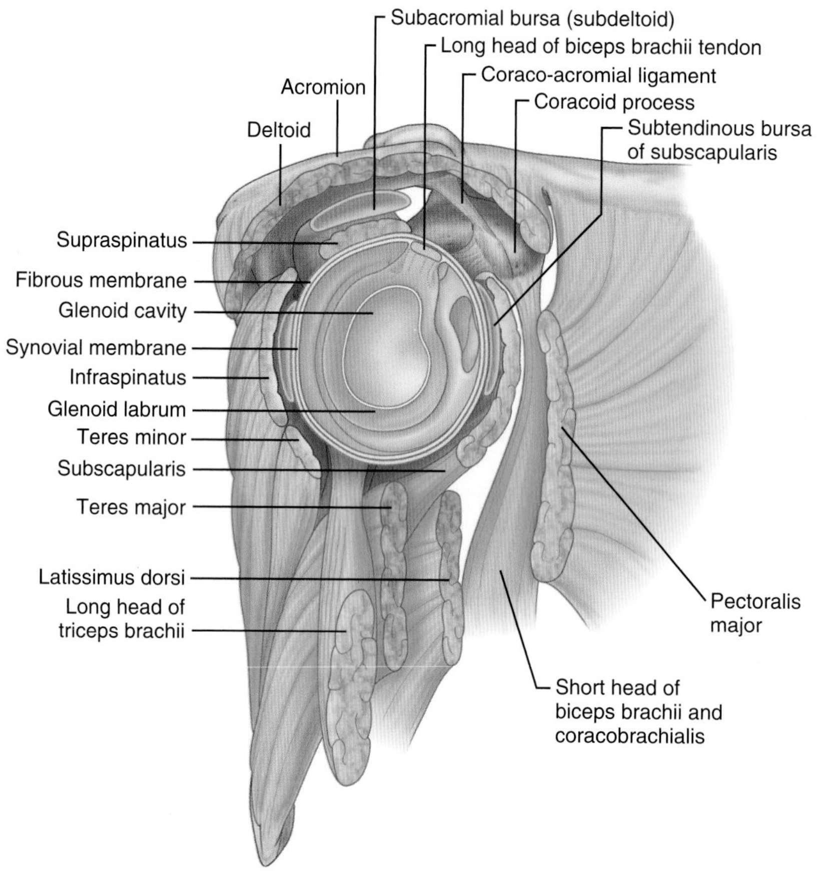

Fig. 12.14 Muscles of the rotator cuff. *(From Drake RL, Vogl AW, Mitchell AWM. Gray's Anatomy for Students. 2nd ed. Philadelphia: Elsevier; 2009.)*

Joints

Shoulder: The shoulder is formed mostly by the humeral head as it sits in the glenoid fossa. The rotator cuff is a group of four tendons that support the glenohumeral joint.

The muscles involved can be remembered by the mnemonic: **SItS**—**S**upraspinatus (abduction), **I**nfraspinatus (external rotation), **t**eres minor (abduction), and **S**ubscapularis (internal rotation; Fig. 12.14).

Rotator Cuff Tear: Most frequently affects the supraspinatus and may be detected by a positive **drop arm** test (inability to keep arm abducted below 90 degrees).

Rotator cuff: Supraspinatus, infraspinatus, teres minor, subscapularis

Impingement Syndrome: Occurs when the supraspinatus tendon becomes inflamed as it passes between the acromion process and the head of the humerus. Symptoms include shoulder pain and weakness, especially with overhead movements. Physical examination may reveal a positive Neer's or Hawkin's test.

Knee: The ligamentous structures of the knee add stability to the joint. Extracapsular ligaments include the lateral and medial collateral ligaments, which resist valgus and varus forces, respectively. The patellar ligament connects the patella to the tibial tuberosity. Intracapsular ligaments are described later (Fig. 12.15).

Anterior Cruciate Ligament (ACL) Tear: The ACL originates on the posterior surface of the femur and travels to the anterior surface of the tibia. It functions to prevent anterior translation of the tibia in relation to the femur. Injury often occurs secondary to forced hyperextension or noncontact injury during pivoting (e.g., while skiing). Patients will report an immediate "pop" sensation and inability to bear weight, followed by swelling of the affected knee (secondary to hemarthrosis). Physical examination will reveal joint instability, with a positive anterior drawer and Lachman test (forced anterior translation

ACL tears present with a popping sensation, inability to bear weight, and hemarthrosis.

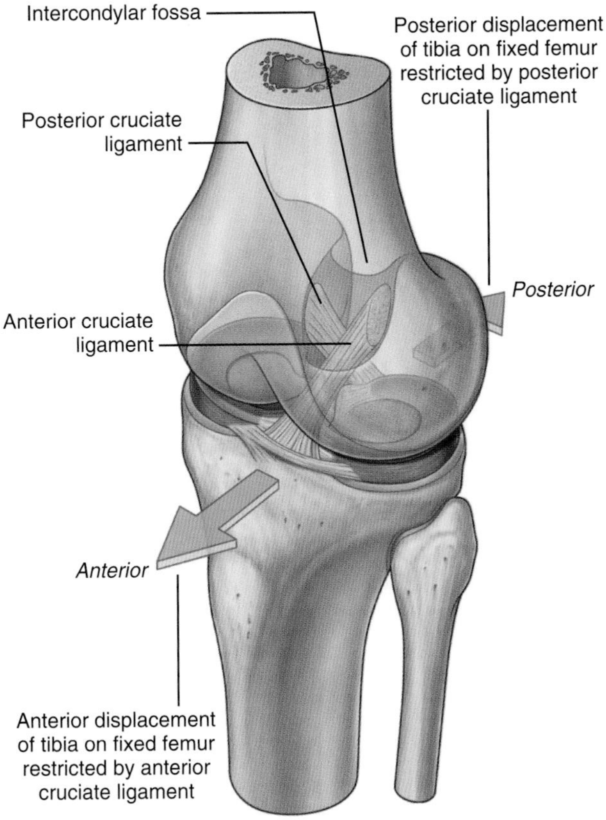

FIG. 12.15 Ligaments of the knee. (*From Drake RL, Vogl AW, Mitchell AWM.* Gray's Anatomy for Students. *2nd ed. Philadelphia: Elsevier; 2009.*)

of the tibia on the femur). X-rays are nondiagnostic, but magnetic resonance imaging (MRI) will reliably reveal a tear. Treatment may be conservative or surgical.

Posterior Cruciate Ligament (PCL) Tear: The PCL originates on the anterior surface of the femur and travels to the posterior surface of the tibia. It functions to prevent posterior translation of the tibia in relation to the femur. Physical examination will reveal a positive posterior drawer test (forced posterior translation of the tibia on the femur) and posterior sag test (posterior translation of the tibia on the femur due to gravity).

Medial and Lateral Menisci Tear: These C-shaped fibrocartilage rings provide structural support to the knee and reduce friction within the joint. Physical examination of meniscal tear may reveal decreased range of motion and joint line tenderness.

Unhappy Triad: Refers to simultaneous injury of the ACL, medial collateral ligament, and either the medial or the lateral meniscus, which may occur with lateral impact to the knee when the foot is planted on the ground.

Ankle Sprains: Ankle sprains are most common after "rolling" the ankle (forced ankle inversion). The weakest ligament, the **anterior talofibular ligament,** is the most frequently involved. Medial ankle sprains are quite rare (forced ankle eversion) because of the strength of the medial deltoid ligament. This is intuitive by simply noting the ease of ankle inversion compared with the difficulty of ankle eversion.

The anterior talofibular ligament is the most likely ligament sprained after "rolling" the ankle.

PATHOLOGY

Neuromuscular Junction Disorders

Myasthenia Gravis (MG): Autoimmune condition in which antibodies attack postsynaptic nicotinic acetylcholine receptors at the neuromuscular junction (NMJ). The result is muscle weakness and easy fatigability that worsens throughout the day and with repetitive movement. Muscles of the face are particularly affected, and patients often present with ptosis or difficulty keeping their eyes open by the

Think myasthenia gravis in a patient with ptosis at the end of the day.

end of the day. Myasthenic crisis occurs when weakness significantly affects the muscles of respiration. Diagnosis of myasthenia gravis can be suggested by the ice pack test. Because NMJ transmission is more efficient at lower temperatures, an ice pack applied to the eyes improves ptosis. Injection of edrophonium, a short-acting acetylcholine esterase inhibitor, also improves ptosis by increasing acetylcholine at the NMJ. This is rarely used as a diagnostic tool anymore, however, since the surge of acetylcholine can also cause bradycardia and bronchospasm. It is still tested on Step 1 though because it addresses the underlying pathophysiology of MG. Diagnostic laboratory tests reveal the presence of **anti–acetylcholine receptor antibodies.** The **thymus** is often the culprit in the production of these antibodies. Computed tomography (CT) or MRI of the chest should be performed to investigate for thymoma. A therapeutic thymectomy may halt progression of the disease. Additionally, **acetylcholine esterase inhibitors** (e.g., pyridostigmine) provide symptomatic improvement by increasing the concentration of acetylcholine at the NMJ. Finally, immunosuppressants may decrease the autoimmune response.

> Pyridostigmine, an AchE inhibitor, can treat MG and LEMS.

Lambert-Eaton Myasthenic Syndrome (LEMS): Autoimmune condition in which antibodies attack **presynaptic voltage-gated calcium channels** at the NMJ, thereby decreasing release of acetylcholine. Unlike MG, symptoms are less likely to involve facial muscles and more likely to involve proximal muscles. Proximal muscle weakness presents as difficulty climbing stairs or rising from a chair. Unlike MG, symptoms will improve with repetitive movements (Lambert sign). LEMS is a paraneoplastic syndrome highly associated with **small cell lung carcinoma.** Treatment with pyridostigmine and immunosuppressants is similar to MG. Treatment should also be aimed at any underlying malignancy.

> MG worsens with repetitive movements; LEMS improves.

Muscular Dystrophy

Duchenne Muscular Dystrophy: X-linked recessive mutation of the **dystrophin** gene. Dystrophin connects the myocyte cytoskeleton to the surrounding extracellular matrix. Because dystrophin is the **longest human gene,** it is susceptible to spontaneous mutations. Without functional dystrophin, myocytes undergo damage and cell death. The result is progressive muscular weakness and atrophy, usually beginning before age 5 years. Patients are usually wheelchair-bound by age 12. The hips, pelvis, and thighs are affected first. Patients may present with **pseudohypertrophy** of calf muscles (calf enlargement caused by muscle tissue being replaced by fat and fibrous tissue) and **Gower sign** (patients rise to stand upright by walking their hands up their legs). Patients usually die in their 20s because of cardiac and diaphragmatic involvement. Elevated serum creatine kinase levels and characteristic findings on muscle biopsy are diagnostic.

> Dystrophin is the longest human gene and thus more subject to mutation.

Becker Muscular Dystrophy: Milder form of muscular dystrophy caused by dysfunctional, but not absent, dystrophin protein. Also inherited in an X-linked recessive pattern. Onset is later, and patients may survive to adulthood.

Mechanical Injuries

Sprain: Ligamentous injury as a result of forceful stretching, especially of the ankle, knee, and wrist. In severe forms, ligamentous rupture may occur producing a popping sound. Physical examination may reveal joint instability, ecchymoses, and effusion.

Strain: Muscle injury as a result of forceful stretching; colloquially known as a pulled muscle.

Shoulder Dislocations: In general, there is a tradeoff between range of motion around a joint and stability of that joint. It is not surprising then that the shoulder is the most commonly dislocated joint because of the phenomenal range of motion and relative instability of the glenohumeral joint. **Anterior dislocation** accounts for **95% of cases.** It is caused by pressure to the abducted, externally rotated, extended arm, as may occur during a fall on an outstretched hand. Anterior shoulder dislocations can potentially damage the axillary nerve. Posterior dislocations only account for about 5% of shoulder dislocations and are caused by violent contractions as in seizures or electrocutions. An incredibly rare cause of shoulder dislocation (but sometimes tested) is luxation erecta, which is an inferior shoulder dislocation. This results in the patient's arm being stuck in the raised position, as if raising their hand to ask a question.

> Assume anterior shoulder dislocation on Step 1 except after seizures or electrocutions.

Hip Dislocation: Rare because of the relative stability of the femoral head within the acetabulum. **Posterior hip dislocation accounts for 90% of all cases.** They are often caused by car accidents, in which the knee is forced against the dashboard, pushing the femoral head posteriorly against the acetabulum.

Epicondylitis: Repetitive use injury causing tendon damage leading to pain and tenderness of the lateral epicondyle **(tennis elbow)** or medial epicondyle **(golfer elbow).**

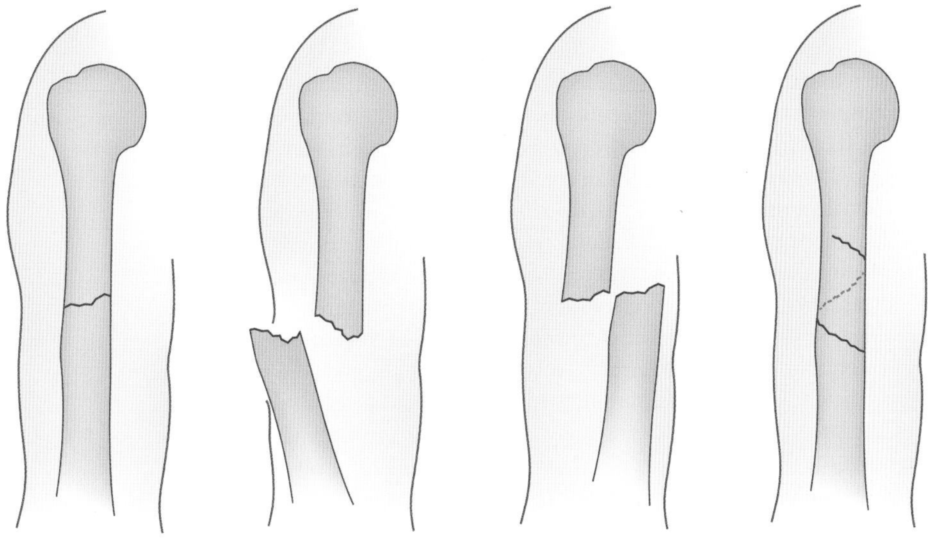

Fig. 12.16 Classification of long-bone fractures. **A,** Closed. **B,** Open. **C,** Displaced. **D,** Spiral.

Fracture: Simply a break in the continuity of bone (Fig. 12.16). There are a number of high-yield facts that can be remembered about fractures. As a general rule, fractures should be reduced to anatomic position and immobilized.

Closed, Simple: Uncomplicated fracture in which the bone does not pierce the overlying skin.

Open, Compound: The bone is exposed to the environment through the wound so is at risk for infection. Procedural washout and antibiotics should be used in the treatment of these fractures.

Displaced: The bone is separated in a nonanatomic position. It must be reduced before healing.

Pathologic: Bones break after trivial trauma. Although osteoporosis often is the pathology underlying these fractures, underlying malignancies or bone cysts should also be considered.

Spiral: When torque is applied as the bone fractures, it may break in a spiral pattern. These are significant because they may indicate child abuse in the appropriate clinical scenario (e.g., fracture from twisting the child's arm or leg). The spiral fracture of the distal tibia **(toddler's fracture)** is less concerning because it may occur with rotational force during normal activity.

> Spiral fractures are concerning for child abuse except the "toddler's fracture"

Stress (Hairline Fracture): Fracture caused by constant or repeated stress instead of acute severe stress. Often of weight-bearing bones, including the tibia and metatarsals. X-ray may not immediately reveal the fracture, so other modalities (e.g., CT) may be necessary. Treatment or immobilization based on clinical suspicion is often reasonable.

Basilar Skull Fracture: Usually secondary to trauma and may present as periorbital ecchymoses (raccoon eyes), mastoid ecchymoses (Battle sign), blood in the middle ear (hemotympanum), cerebrospinal fluid leakage through the ears (otorrhea), or nose (rhinorrhea with salty, metallic taste).

Scaphoid Fracture: Often secondary to a fall on an outstretched hand. Patients will have pain at the anatomic snuffbox, but x-ray is usually unremarkable during the first week. Patients still must be splinted or the proximal scaphoid may undergo avascular necrosis because blood flow to the scaphoid is retrograde, distal to proximal.

Hip Fracture: Proximal femoral fractures notable for the association with osteoporosis and high mortality in older adults.

Nonaccidental Trauma: In children, a handful of fractures are highly suspicious for nonaccidental trauma. These include rib fractures, spiral fractures (other than toddler's fracture), and multiple fractures of different ages. In shaken baby syndrome, subdural hematomas and retinal hemorrhages may also be found. Child services should always be notified.

Complications of Fracture

Fractures that cause reduced mobility may predispose patients to deep vein thromboses and pulmonary emboli. Anticoagulation should be considered in at-risk patients.

In long bone fractures, **fat emboli** can occur if bone marrow leaks into local venules and embolizes to the lung. Patients present with hypoxia, altered mental status, and petechial rash.

Fat embolism: Hypoxia, altered mental status, and petechiae after a long-bone fracture

Tissue swelling or bleeding after a fracture may also increase local pressure because the surrounding fascial compartment may not stretch. **Compartment syndrome** occurs when this increased pressure compromises the vascular supply to the extremity. The forearm and leg are the areas most often affected. Patients will experience severe pain, and examination will reveal a tense, woodlike compartment. Diagnosis can be confirmed by measuring the intracompartmental pressure. Treatment is fasciotomy (surgical incision of the fascia). Mnemonic: History and physical reveals the five **P**s: **P**ain, **P**allor, **P**aresthesias, **P**ulselessness, **P**aralysis.

Osteoarthritis: Degenerative joint disease caused by mechanical wear and tear. Damage manifests as breakdown of cartilage, injury of subchondral bone, and changes to all articular structures. It is the most common type of arthritis. It presents as pain in weight-bearing joints that **worsens with use.** It may also be associated with decreased range of motion, a "cool" (noninflammatory) effusion, crepitus, and bony deformities (e.g., Heberden or Bouchard nodes). The joints most commonly affected are the distal interphalangeal, proximal interphalangeal, knees, hips, toes, and spine. Radiography reveals (1) osteophytes, (2) joint space narrowing, (3) subchondral cysts, and (4) subchondral sclerosis (Fig. 12.17). Treatment involves weight loss (to decrease stress on all joints), nonsteroidal antiinflammatory drugs (NSAIDs), acetaminophen, physical therapy, and/or intraarticular injections of steroids or hyaluronic acid. Surgery may also be indicated.

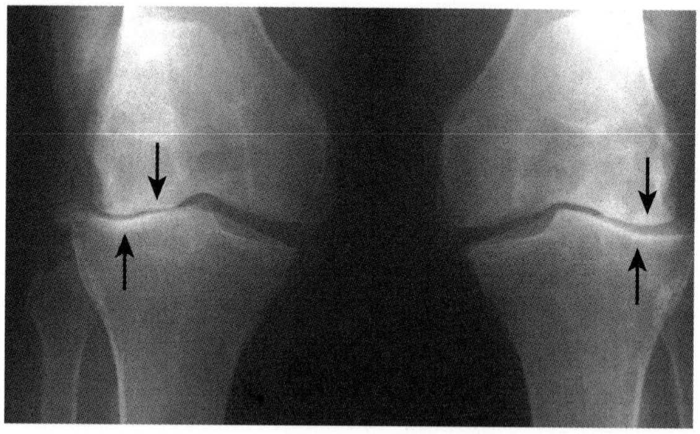

FIG. 12.17 Radiographic image of osteoarthritis with joint space narrowing *(arrows)*, sclerotic bone, osteophytes, and subchondral cysts. (*From Kelly IC, Bickle BE.* Crash Course Imaging. *Philadelphia: Elsevier; 2007.*)

Charcot Joint: Neuropathy, usually secondary to diabetes, reduces pain sensation and proprioception in the affected joint. Without these protective senses, joint destruction can be rapid and profound.

Disease of Bone

Osteomyelitis: Infection of bone caused by (1) direct inoculation (e.g., penetrating trauma), (2) contiguous spread (e.g., cellulitis), or (3) hematogenous spread. Osteomyelitis is diagnosed by plain films or MRI.

Osteomyelitis, temporal arteritis, and polymyalgia rheumatica are the few conditions that elevate ESR > 100 mm/hr.

Of note, it is one of the few conditions that can raise an erythrocyte sedimentation rate (ESR) higher than 100 mm/hr. Overall, *Staphylococcus aureus* is the most common causative organism, but some populations deserve special mention:

- Patients with sickle cell anemia: *Salmonella*
- Diabetic foot infections: *Pseudomonas* or polymicrobial
- Prosthetic joints: *S. aureus* and *S. epidermidis*
- After nail puncture through rubber-soled shoe: *Pseudomonas*

Avascular Necrosis (Osteonecrosis): Bone infarction due to insufficient blood flow which causes pain at the affected site. Fractures are the most obvious cause due to direct vascular trauma. Steroid use and sickle cell crises are other commonly tested causes of avascular necrosis. The femoral head is most commonly affected.

Osteoporosis: Decreased bone density with normal bone architecture. Defined as bone density >2.5 standard deviations below that of a young/healthy reference group. Bone density is measured by dual-energy x-ray absorptiometry (DXA) scan and expressed as a T score. Osteopenia is defined as a T score between −1 and −2.5 and osteoporosis is defined as a T score below −2.5. Patients may be asymptomatic but are prone to fractures.

Of note, vertebral compression fractures may lead to loss of height, kyphosis, and possibly back pain, with or without radiculopathy. Hip fractures are of particular concern because of their high mortality rate. Risk factors include age, smoking, female gender, and glucocorticoid use. Weight-bearing exercise is protective. Treatment may involve adequate intake of calcium and vitamin D. Bisphosphonates inhibit osteoclast resorption of bone and are first-line pharmacotherapy.

Osteomalacia: Adult-onset vitamin D deficiency causing bony pain, "soft bones," and fractures. Low vitamin D leads to decreased serum calcium, which causes elevated PTH. PTH, in turn, raises serum calcium at the expense of mineralized bone. Patients with fractures accompanied by malnutrition, malabsorption, or intestinal bypass should be considered for osteomalacia. Pertinent laboratory values can be deduced: low vitamin D → low calcium → elevated PTH → low phosphate (caused by decreased renal reabsorption).

Rickets: Vitamin D deficiency in childhood, leading to defective mineralization at the growth plate. Compromised bony stability may cause bowing of long bones (genu varum; Fig. 12.18).

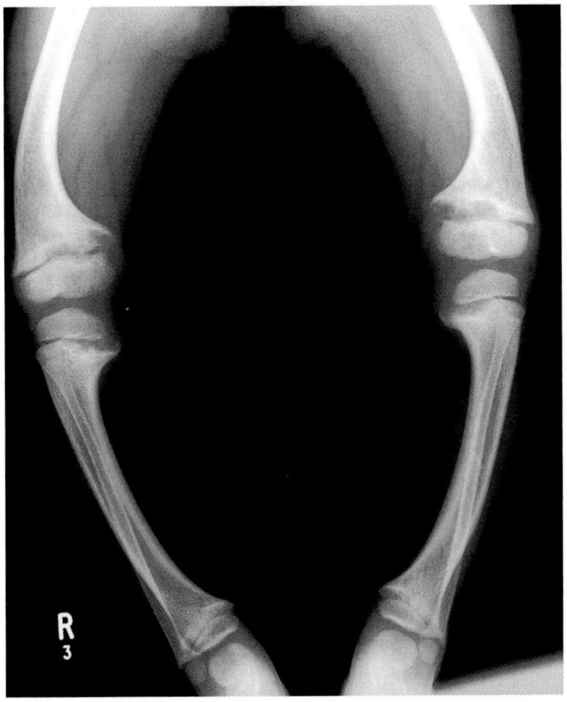

FIG. 12.18 Rickets, bowing of long bone secondary to vitamin D deficiency in childhood. (*From Kelly IC, Bickle BE.* Crash Course Imaging. *Philadelphia: Elsevier; 2007.*)

Osteogenesis Imperfecta (Brittle Bone Disease): Autosomal dominant disorder of type I collagen leading to **blue sclerae** (Fig. 12.19), brittle bones, and hearing loss (ossicle damage). The severity of the disease is highly variable, ranging from being fatal in utero to a mildly increased risk of fractures. Because these patients present with multiple fractures of different ages, your goal on Step 1 may be to distinguish this condition from child abuse (look for blue sclerae as a hint).

Osteogenesis imperfecta causes blue sclerae.

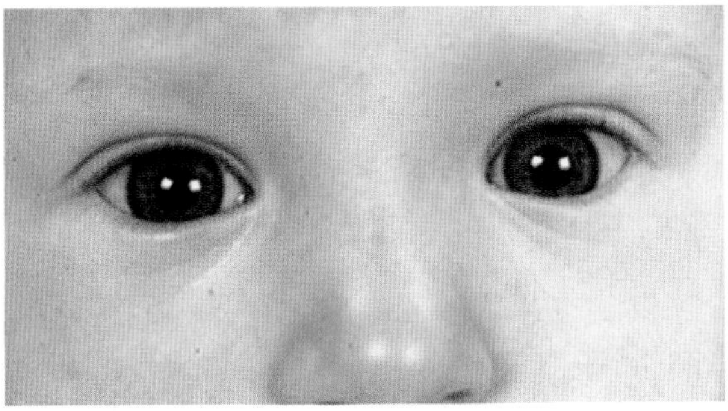

FIG. 12.19 Blue sclerae of a patient with osteogenesis imperfecta. (*From Lissauer T, Clayden G.* Illustrated Textbook of Paediatrics. *4th ed. Edinburgh: Elsevier; 2011.*)

Achondroplasia: Autosomal dominant form of dwarfism caused by mutation of fibroblast growth factor receptor-3 (FGFR3). This receptor becomes constitutively active and results in paradoxical inhibition of longitudinal bone growth (endochondral ossification), making the limbs comparatively shorter than the near- normal skull and trunk. Pituitary dwarfism, by comparison, causes proportional decrease in size caused by lack of growth hormone secretion.

Paget Disease of Bone (Osteitis Deformans): Disorganized bone remodeling from increased osteoclast and osteoblast activity, which results in overgrowth of affected bone. The cause is unknown, with genetics and environment playing a role. Most patients are asymptomatic. They may be diagnosed incidentally based on **elevated alkaline phosphatase** levels and radiographic abnormalities. Levels of serum calcium, phosphorus, and PTH are not affected. Symptoms include pain and deformity of affected bones. Complications include fractures (especially chalkstick fractures), nerve compression (e.g., hearing loss), and high-output heart failure (from increased vascularity of bone). Patients are also at **increased risk for osteosarcoma.** Treatment is with bisphosphonates. Radiography may reveal **cotton wool** appearance of bone (Fig. 12.20).

Paget disease of bone increases the risk of osteosarcoma.

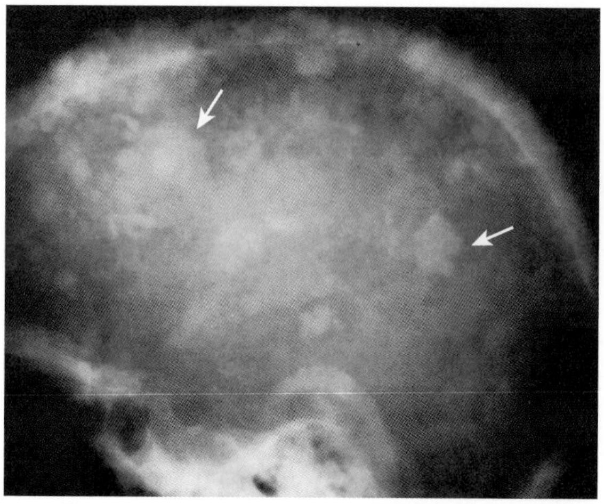

Fig. 12.20 Paget disease of bone. Shown is the cotton wool appearance of bone on a skull radiograph *(arrows)*. (*From Lawlor MW.* Rapid Review USMLE Step 2. *Philadelphia: Elsevier; 2006.*)

Osteopetrosis (Marble Bone Disease): Defective osteoclast resorption of bone secondary to carbonic anhydrase deficiency. Unopposed osteoblast activity leads to thickened, brittle bones that are prone to fracture. Invasion of bone marrow leads to pancytopenia and splenomegaly secondary to extramedullary hematopoiesis.

Osteitis Fibrosa Cystica: Elevated parathyroid hormone overstimulates osteoclasts to resorb bone. Laboratory values can be deduced—primary hyperparathyroidism → elevated PTH → elevated calcium, elevated alkaline phosphatase (from bone resorption), and low phosphate (from renal wasting). Substantial resorption of bone causes cystlike **brown tumors** within the bone, consisting of fibrous tissue and woven bone without matrix.

Polyostotic Fibrous Dysplasia: Problem of osteoblastic maturation, in which fibrous tissue forms instead of medullary bone. The result is painful, swollen bones that are prone to pathologic fractures. The ribs and femur are most commonly affected. These lesions can be confused with the brown tumors of osteitis fibrosa cystica, but the pathophysiology is different.

McCune-Albright Syndrome: Triad of polyostotic fibrous dysplasia, precocious puberty, and unilateral café-au-lait spots.

Rheumatology

Inflammatory Arthritis

Rheumatoid Arthritis (RA): Autoimmune condition causing symmetric joint destruction. It presents as joint pain and stiffness, particularly of the metacarpophalangeal, metatarsophalangeal, proximal interphalangeal, and **wrist joints.** Large joints and the cervical spine may also be involved. Symptoms are worse in the morning and **improve with use.** Decreased range of motion, effusions, and muscle atrophy may be present, along with swan neck deformity, boutonniere deformity, ulnar deviation (Fig. 12.21B), or arthritis mutilans (bag of bones deformity). There is a genetic association with HLA-DR4. Diagnosis is clinical, but **rheumatoid factor** and anti–cyclic citrullinated peptide (CCP) antibody may be helpful. Later in the disease, radiography reveals deformity joint space narrowing and erosions. Treatment is based on DMARDs (disease-modifying antirheumatic drugs), particularly methotrexate. Tumor necrosis factor (TNF) inhibitors are also commonly used. Flares can be treated

RA is more likely to occur in the wrists. Symptoms improve with use.

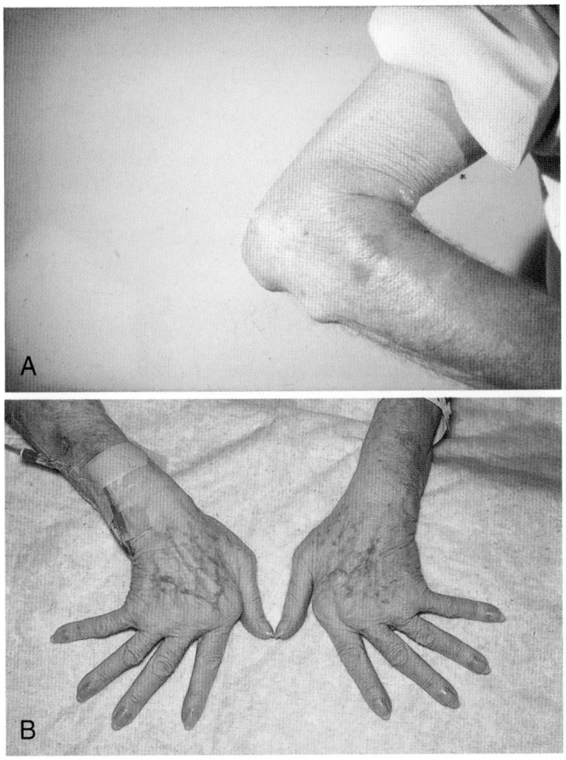

FIG. 12.21 Physical findings of rheumatoid arthritis. **A,** Rheumatoid nodules. **B,** Ulnar deviation. (***A*** *From Talley NJ.* Clinical Examination. *5th ed. Philadelphia: Elsevier; 2005;* ***B*** *from Swartz MH.* Textbook of Physical Diagnosis, History and Examination. *6th ed. Philadelphia: Elsevier; 2009.*)

with NSAIDs and/or steroids. Systemic manifestations include fever, fatigue, anemia of chronic disease, and **rheumatic nodules** (subcutaneous nodules on extensor surfaces; Fig. 12.21A).

Systemic Lupus Erythematosus (SLE): Relapsing and remitting autoimmune disease in which antibodies directly damage tissues (type II hypersensitivity) or form destructive immune complexes (type III hypersensitivity). Patients have a collection of symptoms, which can include arthritis, fevers, malar rash (Fig. 12.22), oral and nasal ulcerations, photosensitivity, pleuritis, pericarditis, seizures, and psychosis. Immune deposits can also cause lupus glomerulonephritis and renal failure. Like many rheumatic conditions, SLE predominantly affects women (90%). African Americans are especially at risk.

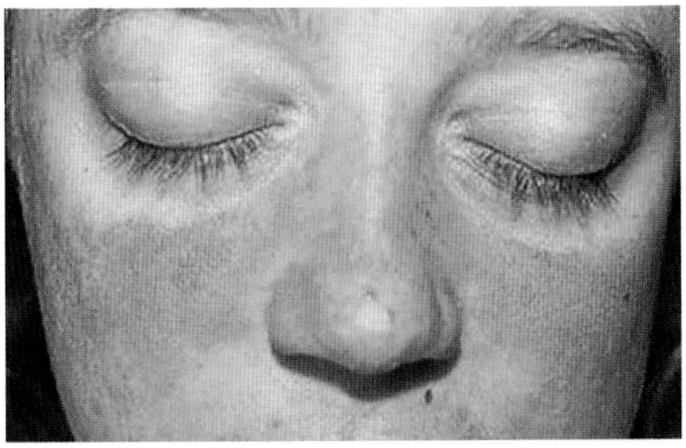

FIG. 12.22 Malar rash of SLE, sparing the nasolabial folds. (*From Lim E, Loke YK, Thompson A.* Medicine and Surgery. *Philadelphia: Elsevier; 2007.*)

Diagnosis is based on a combination of clinical and laboratory findings that can be remembered by the mnemonic **SOAP BRAIN MD:** **S**erositis (pleuritis/pericarditis), **O**ral ulcers, **A**rthritis, **P**hotosensitivity, **B**lood (anemia/leukopenia/thrombocytopenia), **R**enal disorders, positive **A**ntinuclear antibody (ANA), **I**mmunologic phenomena (anti-dsDNA, antiphospholipid, anti-Sm antibodies), **N**eurologic (psychosis or seizures), **M**alar rash ("butterfly rash"), **D**iscoid rash.

SLE causes a false-positive Venereal Disease Research Laboratory test (VDRL) result. Don't assume syphilis.

A negative ANA is very sensitive (rule out) and a positive dsDNA is very specific (rule in) for SLE.

ANA is very sensitive for lupus. Anti-dsDNA is specific.

Drug-Induced Lupus: A mild lupus syndrome with positive ANA and **antihistone** antibody can occur as a result of certain drugs, including hydralazine (antihypertensive) and procainamide (antiarrhythmic).

Sjögren Syndrome: Autoimmune lymphocytic inflammation of joints and exocrine glands causing **arthritis, xerophthalmia** (dry eyes), **xerostomia** (dry mouth), and parotid gland enlargement. Additionally, lack of salivary protection predisposes to dental caries, and chronic inflammation predisposes to lymphoma. Diagnosis of Sjögren Syndrome is supported by the presence of **anti-SSA (Ro), anti-SSB (LA) antibodies,** and rheumatoid factor. On biopsy, lymphocytic salivary gland infiltrate is also suggestive.

Sjögren syndrome: Dry eyes, dry mouth, and arthritis; SSA, SSB, RF+

Scleroderma: Rheumatic condition characterized by dysregulated matrix synthesis causing collagenous deposition in tissues and blood vessels (luminal narrowing). Tissue is damaged directly by matrix deposition and by subsequent inflammation. Skin becomes thickened and taut, causing sclerodactyly and contractures (Fig. 12.23).

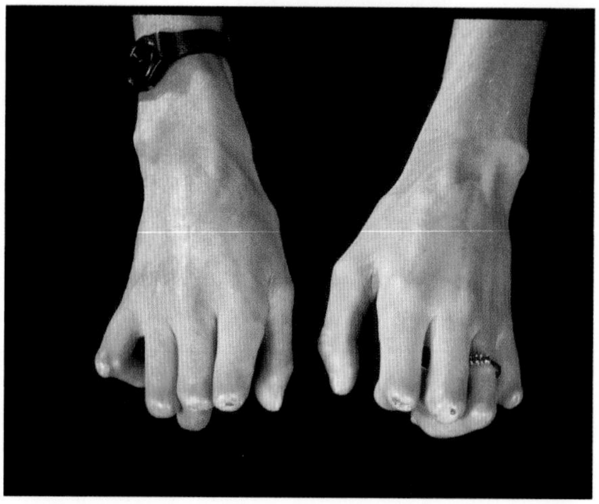

Fig. 12.23 Calcinosis and sclerodactyly of scleroderma. (*From Talley NJ.* Clinical Examination. *5th ed. Philadelphia: Elsevier; 2005.*)

- **Diffuse systemic sclerosis:** Diffuse skin and organ involvement, including skin, kidneys (scleroderma renal crisis), gastrointestinal (GI) tract (dysmotility), and the most severe—lungs (interstitial lung disease). There is an association with **anti-SCL70** antibody.
- **Limited systemic sclerosis (CREST):** Calcinosis (subcutaneous calcium hydroxyapatite deposition), Raynaud phenomenon, Esophageal dysmotility, Sclerodactyly, and Telangiectasias. **Anticentromere** antibody may be present. There is also a risk for pulmonary disease.

Seronegative Spondyloarthropathies

These conditions share common features of **rheumatoid factor negativity,** asymmetry, oligoarticular involvement, and association with the **HLA-B27 allele.** They have common extraarticular manifestations, including uveitis, rashes, and occasional GI symptoms. They are remembered by the acronym **PAIR.**

Psoriatic Arthritis: An inflammatory peripheral arthritis may arise in addition to the skin findings of psoriasis (silver plaques and nail bed pitting). **Distal interphalangeal (DIP) joints** are particularly affected; fingers take on a characteristic **sausage digit** appearance (dactylitis). Radiography reveals a so-called pencil in cup deformity. See Chapter 3 for details on skin manifestations and management.

Sausage digits are characteristic of psoriatic arthritis.

Ankylosing Spondylitis: Greek for "bent spine," this condition begins as sacroiliac joint stiffness and progresses up the spinal column. The pathophysiology involves inflammatory cells causing cartilage destruction and pannus formation, leading to joint space fusion (ankylosis). Uveitis is the most common extraarticular manifestation. Diagnosis is made based on sacroiliac tenderness, lower back pain that is worst in the morning and improves with exercise, and decreased range of motion. Radiology may reveal a "bamboo spine" from ankylosis (Fig. 12.24). Complications may result from fracture of fused spinal segments, which can lead to cord impingement.

Think ankylosing spondylitis in a patient with sacroiliac tenderness.

Inflammatory Bowel Disease (IBD): Of patients with IBD, 2% to 20% may have an inflammatory arthritis in addition to GI symptoms (see Chapter 10).

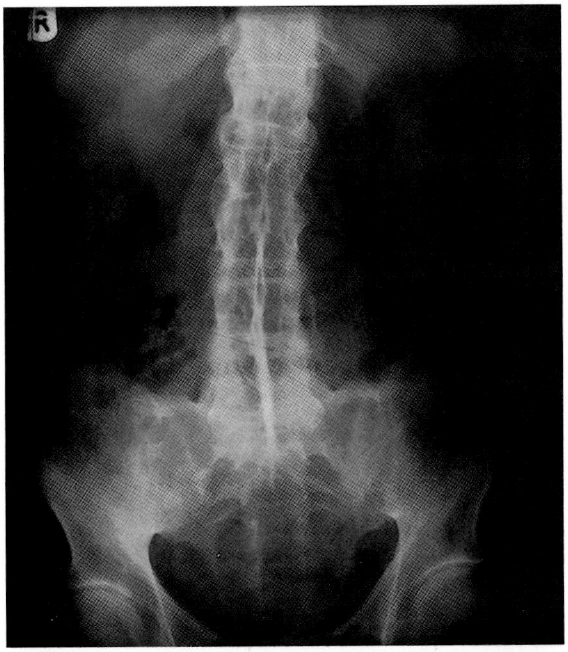

FIG. 12.24 Radiograph demonstrating so-called bamboo spine in a patient with ankylosing spondylitis. (*From Kumar P, Clark M. Clinical Medicine. 5th ed. Philadelphia: Elsevier; 2002.*)

TABLE 12.3 Autoantibodies and Laboratory Findings Associated with Various Rheumatic Conditions

STUDY	CONDITION
Antinuclear antibody (antismith and anti–double-stranded DNA)	Systemic lupus erythematosus (SLE)
Anti–histone antibody	Drug-induced lupus
Anti-**SS**A (Ro)	**S**jögren **S**yndrome, SLE
Anit-**SS**B (La)	**S**jögren **S**yndrome
Anticentromere antibody	CREST syndrome (limited systemic sclerosis)
Scl70	**Scl**eroderma (diffuse systemic sclerosis)
Antitopoisomerase antibody	Scleroderma (diffuse systemic sclerosis)
Anti-Jo antibody	Polymyositis
Voltage-gated calcium channel antibodies	Lambert-Eaton myasthenic syndrome
Anti–acetylcholine receptor antibody	Myasthenia gravis
Anti–cyclic citrullinated peptide (CCP)	Rheumatoid arthritis
Rheumatoid factor	Rheumatoid arthritis, Sjögren syndrome
HLA-DR4	Rheumatoid arthritis
HLA B27	Psoriasis, ankylosing spondylitis, inflammatory bowel disease, rheumatoid arthritis

Reactive Arthritis: Inflammatory arthritis as a reaction to prior infection. Pathogens include *Chlamydia trachomatis* and GI pathogens (*Salmonella, Shigella,* and, *Campylobacter).* Clinically, patients present days to weeks after an instigating infection with the triad of **urethritis, conjunctivitis** (or uveitis), and **arthritis** remembered by the mnemonic—"can't pee, can't see, can't climb a tree."

Table 12.3 reviews the antibodies and laboratory findings associated with these rheumatologic conditions.

Monoarticular Disease

Infectious Arthropathy

Synovial aspiration with >50,000 neutrophils → septic arthritis.

Septic Arthritis (acute): Given the severity of this condition, all arthritides affecting a single joint should be considered septic arthritis until proven otherwise. It is the result of joint space invasion by an infectious organism, with subsequent inflammation. Infection typically spreads hematogenously, but direct inoculation may also occur (e.g., trauma). Septic arthritis presents as a red, swollen, hot joint with loss of motion and inability to bear weight. Fever may also be present. *S. aureus* and streptococcal subspecies are the most common pathogens. A synovial fluid aspiration is always necessary and will reveal more than 50,000 neutrophils. Gram stain or culture may reveal the causative organism. Treatment is with procedural joint washout and IV antibiotics. Failure to treat promptly results in permanent functional impairment and may also lead to sepsis and death.

Disseminated Gonococcus: Gonorrhea may produce a migratory monoarthritis associated with tenosynovitis and dermatitis. Urethritis may also occur. It is less severe but is treated similarly to nongonococcal septic arthritis, including antibiotics and a possible need for joint washout. Do not confuse this with reactive arthritis, which presents with ocular symptoms.

Reactive arthritis: Arthritis, urethritis, **conjunctivitis**

Gonococcus: Arthritis, urethritis, **dermatitis**

Chronic Infectious Arthritis: Disseminated tuberculosis, Lyme disease, and fungal infections may cause chronic monoarticular joint disease. Systemic signs will often point to these infections.

Crystal Arthropathy

Gout: Uric acid crystal (monosodium urate) deposition in joints, causing swelling and **recurrent** bouts of inflammation. The first metatarsophalangeal joint is commonly affected (podagra; Fig. 12.25), but any joint may be involved. Gout is associated with hyperuricemia through decreased renal excretion of uric acid, increased production of uric acid (chemotherapy), or increased ingestion of purines (e.g., red meat, shellfish, wine). Acute changes in uric acid level precipitate flares. Diagnosis is made with needle aspiration of crystals that demonstrate **negatively birefringent,** needle-shaped crystals. Negative birefringent crystals are blue when perpendicular and ye**ll**ow when para**ll**el. Treatment of acute flares involves NSAIDs and colchicine. Long-term management involves dietary modification (decreases purine intake), allopurinol (decreases uric acid production), and probenecid (increases uric acid renal excretion). Thiazide diuretics should be avoided because they decrease excretion of uric acid. Chronic gout may lead to uric acid deposition in tophi and joint destruction.

Gout: Negative birefringent needle-shaped crystals (ye**ll**ow when para**ll**el)

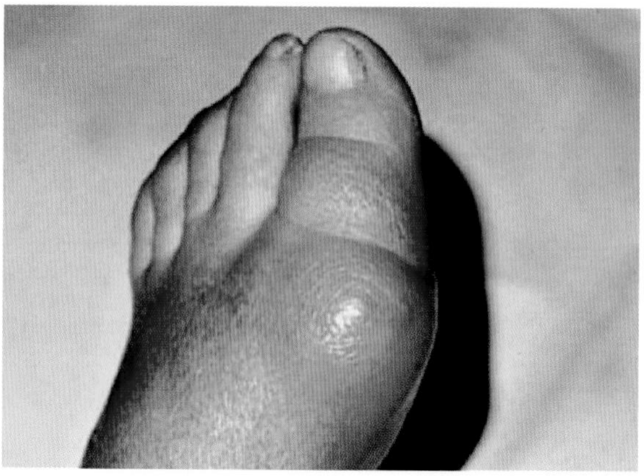

Fig. 12.25 Podagra, painful swelling of the first metatarsophalangeal joint. (*From Luqmani R, Robb J, Porter D.* Textbook of Orthopaedics, Trauma, and Rheumatology. *Philadelphia: Elsevier; 2008.*)

Of note, **Lesch-Nyhan syndrome** is caused by an X-linked recessive mutation of hypoxanthine-guanine phosphoribosyltransferase (**HGPRT**), an enzyme of the purine salvage pathway. Without purine salvage, uric acid builds up in the blood and urine, which presents as **gout, mental retardation, self-mutilation,** and **uric acid crystal** formation in the urine (**orange-colored crystals** found in a baby's diaper).

Lesch-Nyhan syndrome: Orange crystals in diaper, gout, and self-mutilation

Pseudogout: Presentation identical to gout, but caused by deposition of calcium pyrophosphate dihydrate crystals (CPPD). Aspiration reveals **positively birefringent,** rhomboid-shaped crystals.

Positive birefringence refers to crystals appearing yellow when perpendicular and blue when parallel to the plane of light. Think **P**ositive for **P**yrophosphate in **P**seudogout.

Pseudogout: Positive birefringent, rhomboid-shaped crystals

Pediatric Conditions

Transient Synovitis: Joint pain and inflammation (often of the hip) causing limited range of motion. Often occurs after a viral infection. The difficulty of this benign condition is that it may mimic septic arthritis. In transient synovitis, unlike septic arthritis, patients are unlikely to have fever, leukocytosis, or elevated ESR. These patients can be treated with NSAIDs; however, if septic arthritis cannot be ruled out, a joint aspiration should be performed.

Slipped Capital Femoral Epiphysis (SCFE): Typically occurs in obese children between 11 and 15 years of age. Typically presents as hip pain and altered gait secondary to slippage at the epiphyseal plate (growth plate), in which the epiphysis remains in the acetabulum and the metaphysis becomes displaced. On AP and frog-leg lateral x-rays, this appears as a so-called **ice cream scoop** slipping of the cone (Fig. 12.26). Treatment involves surgical stabilization with pinning. If untreated, patients are at risk for avascular necrosis of the femoral head.

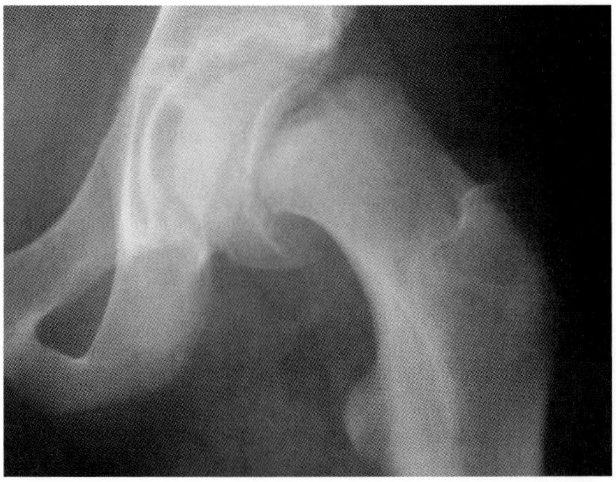

FIG. 12.26 Radiograph demonstrating slipped capital femoral epiphysis. Note the appearance of "ice cream slipping of the cone." (*From South M, Isaacs D, Roberton DM.* Practical Paediatrics. *6th ed. Philadelphia: Elsevier; 2007.*)

Sarcoidosis: Cough, bilateral hilar adenopathy, and elevated ACE. Treat with corticosteroids.

Developmental Dysplasia of the Hip: Congenital instability of the femoral head within the acetabulum leading to hip dislocation (Fig. 12.27). Screening should be performed on physical examination of all neonates and may reveal asymmetry of leg creases. Clicks and clunks on forced adduction or abduction of the hip indicate positive Barlow and Ortolani maneuvers. Risk factors include female gender, family history, and breech presentation. Patients are often managed with a Pavlov harness. If left untreated, patients may slowly develop hip pain, gait abnormalities, or leg length discrepancies.

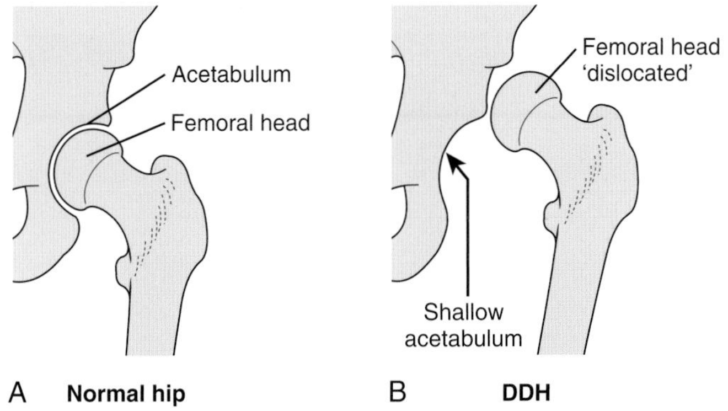

FIG. 12.27 A, Normal hip. **B,** Developmental dysplasia of the hip. The femoral head is easily dislocated from the shallow acetabulum. (*From Marsland D, Kapoor S.* Crash Course: Rheumatology and Orthopaedics. *2nd ed. Philadelphia: Elsevier; 2008.*)

Legg-Calvé-Perthes Disease: Idiopathic avascular necrosis of the femoral head causing hip pain and inability to bear weight. Patients are usually between the ages of 5 and 7 years. Don't forget that hip pain can be referred to the knee or groin in any condition. X-rays may be normal in early disease, so MRI may be indicated.

Osgood-Schlatter Disease: Avulsion of the patellar tendon (Fig. 12.28) causing pain and tenderness at the tibial tuberosity. Avulsion is secondary to repetitive stress on the patellar tendon from sports or exercise. The typical patient is an athletic adolescent boy. Treatment is conservative and braces or casts are rarely required.

Osgood-Schlatter: Tibial tuberosity tenderness in an adolescent boy

Other Conditions

Sarcoidosis: Condition characterized by noncaseating granulomas in various tissues. More common in African American women. Pulmonary sarcoidosis is the most common presentation, which can manifest

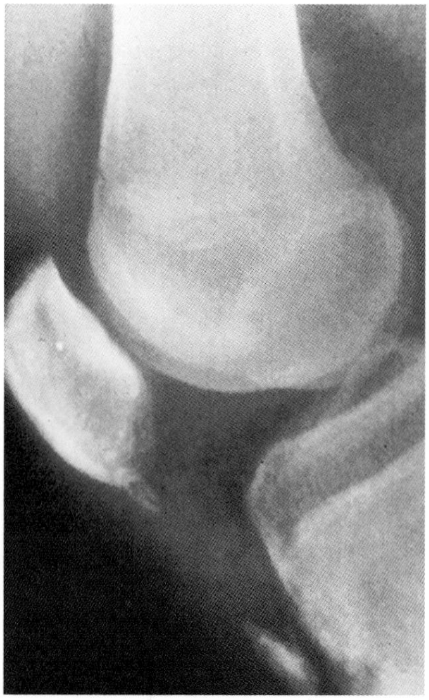

FIG. 12.28 Avulsion of the patellar tendon from the tibial tuberosity in Osgood-Schlatter disease. (*From Scudieri G [ed]:* Sports Medicine: Principles of Primary Care. *St. Louis: Mosby; 1997.*)

clinically as shortness of breath and cough. Patients also frequently present with erythema nodosum. Chest x-ray reveals **bilateral hilar adenopathy** (Fig. 12.29), and labs may reveal elevated serum levels of angiotensin-converting enzyme (ACE), since ACE is produced within the granulomas. Symptoms may remit spontaneously, but severe cases can be treated with corticosteroids. Although almost every organ can be affected in sarcoidosis, the information in this section should suffice for your Step 1 examination.

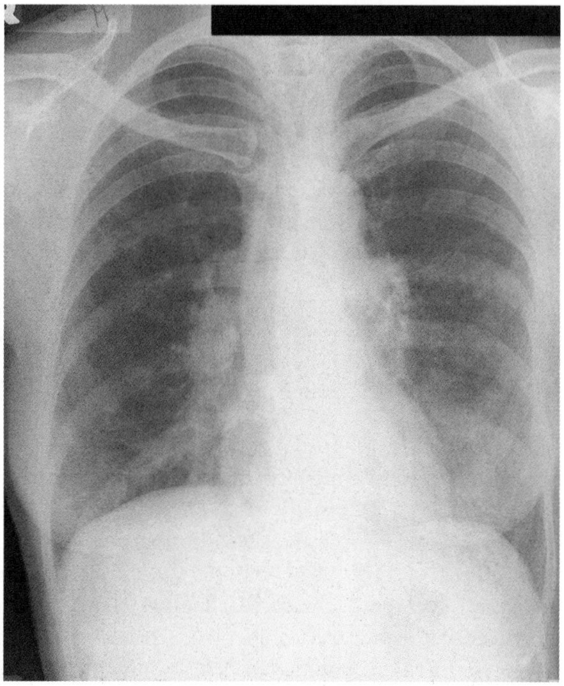

FIG. 12.29 Bilateral hilar lymphadenopathy of sarcoidosis. (*From Kelly B, Bickle IC.* Crash Course Imaging. *Philadelphia: Elsevier; 2007.*)

Polymyalgia Rheumatica (PMR): Autoimmune condition of adults characterized by pain of proximal muscles (hips and shoulders) that is worse in the morning. Pain must also be accompanied by ESR >40 mm/hr and/or elevated C-reactive protein (CRP) level. It is one of the few conditions in which the **ESR may be greater than 100** mm/hr (also consider osteomyelitis and temporal arteritis). Treatment is with prednisone. There is a strong **association with temporal arteritis,** so ocular symptoms and headaches may necessitate temporal artery biopsy.

PMR: Pain and elevated ESR

Polymyositis: Weakness and elevated CK

Polymyositis: Connective tissue disease of muscle characterized by weakness in proximal muscles. Polymyositis may present as difficulty ascending stairs or rising from a chair. Labs reveal an **elevated creatine kinase (CK)** level and positive **anti–Jo** antibody. Muscle biopsy is diagnostic. Treatment is with steroids. There is an association with internal malignancy.

Dermatomyositis: Connective tissue disease similar to polymyositis, but with dermatologic manifestations, including **Gottron papules** (Fig. 12.30A), **heliotrope rash** (Fig. 12.30B), and shawl sign (erythematous rash in the distribution of a shawl; Fig. 12.30C). As in polymyositis, there is an elevated CK level, and muscle biopsy is diagnostic. Compared with polymyositis, there is an even stronger association with internal malignancy.

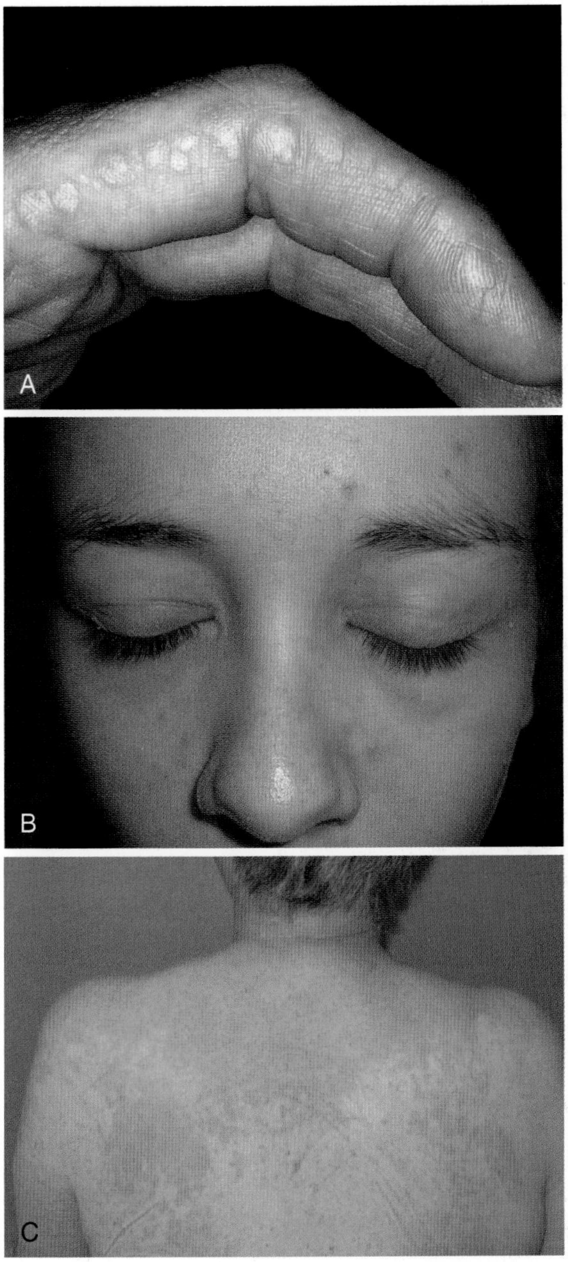

Fig. 12.30 Physical examination findings in a patient with dermatomyositis. **A,** Gottron papules. **B,** Heliotrope rash. **C,** Shawl sign. (***A*** *from Habif TP.* Clinical Dermatology. *5th ed. London: Elsevier; 2009.* ***B*** *from Rakel RE, Rakel DP.* Textbook of Family Medicine. *8th ed. Philadelphia: Elsevier; 2011.* ***C*** *from Hochberg MC, Silman AJ, Smolen JS, et al.* Rheumatology. *5th ed. Philadelphia: Mosby; 2010.*)

Mixed Connective Tissue Disease: Overlap disease that may have features of scleroderma, lupus, RA, and polymyositis, but does not fit specifically into one diagnostic category. Associated with the anti-RNP antibody.

Fibromyalgia: Trigger point tenderness, fatigue, and joint stiffness thought to be caused by abnormal processing of painful signals. On Step 1, look for a patient with persistent pain despite lack of diagnostic findings, except for tenderness over multiple trigger points.

Neoplasms of Bone

Benign

Osteochondroma: Most common benign tumor of bone. Cartilage-forming tumor that presents between 10 and 20 years of age. Described as **mushroom-shaped** because of its cartilage-capped outgrowth on a bony stalk. Most commonly presents in the metaphysis of the distal femur. Malignant transition to chondrosarcoma is rare, and management involves simple excision.

Osteochondroma: Mushroom-shaped

Osteoma: Gardner syndrome association

Osteoblastoma: Aspirin relief, radiolucent nest

Giant cell: Soap bubble

Osteoma: Benign tumor of bone that presents between 10 and 20 years of age. It most frequently protrudes from the skull, and symptoms are related to their interference with surrounding structures. Osteomata are also found in **Gardner syndrome** accompanied by multiple colonic polyps.

Osteoblastoma, Osteoid Osteoma: Originally thought to be variants of the same disease (e.g., that an osteoblastoma was a large osteoid osteoma), but may actually be separate entities. Osteoblastomas have pain that is not relieved by aspirin, whereas osteoid osteomas typically are smaller and the pain can be relieved by aspirin or NSAIDs. Both are benign tumors of bone that presents between 10 and 20 years of age as localized and **severe bony pain** caused by prostaglandin production. Tumors most often occur in the cortex of the tibia or femur. Radiography reveals a central **radiolucent nest** (nidus) representing osteoid, with surrounding reactive sclerotic bone.

Giant Cell Tumor: Benign tumor, which appears histologically as spindle cells with **multinucleated giant cells.** Its most distinguishing feature is a **soap bubble** appearance on radiography, a large lytic (bone-destroying) lesion without calcification.

Malignant

Metastases: The most common malignancy of bone is from metastatic disease, especially of the **b**reast, **l**ung, **t**hyroid, **k**idney and **p**rostate.

Mnemonic: **BLT** with a **K**osher **P**ickle.

Breast, lung, thyroid, and renal cell carcinomas tend to be lytic. **Prostatic metastases are blastic.** In addition, multiple myeloma may present as multiple, punched-out lytic bone lesions characteristic of the condition (Fig. 12.31).

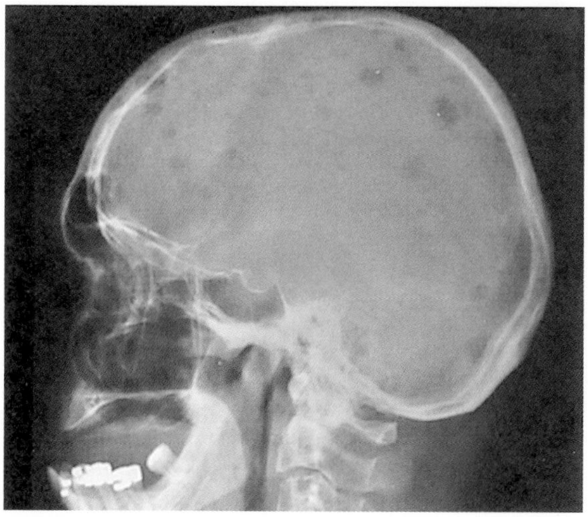

Fig. 12.31 Multiple punched-out lytic bone lesions of multiple myeloma. *(From Lawlor MW. Rapid Review USMLE Step 2. Philadelphia: Elsevier; 2006.)*

Osteosarcoma: Accounts for about 35% of primary bone malignancies. Patients often present **between 10 and 20 years** of age with pain or swelling, especially of the **distal femur**. Note that this occurs around the adolescent growth spurt and most frequently occurs in areas of rapid growth. The tumor is composed of osteocytes surrounded by osteoid. Radiography reveals a characteristic **sunburst pattern** (spiculated calcifications) and **Codman triangle** (raised periosteum in triangular shape) (Fig. 12.32). Because the bone is weak, it may also present as a pathologic fracture. The tumors

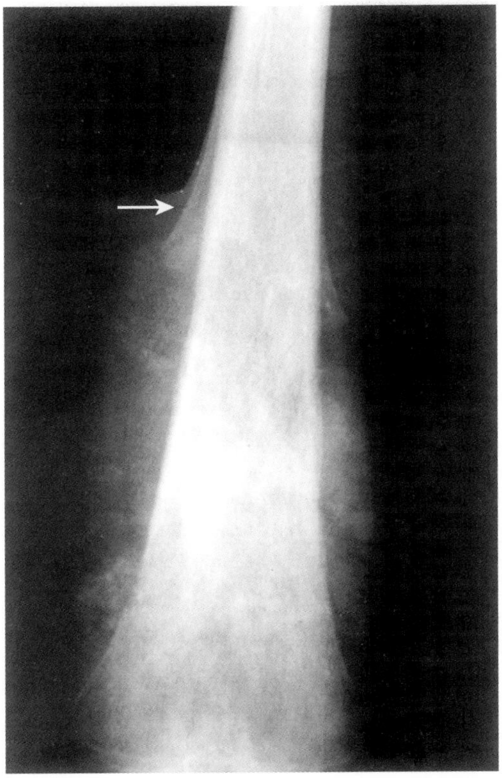

FIG. 12.32 Osteosarcoma of the distal femur with sunburst pattern of spiculated calcifications. Note the *white arrow* pointing to raised periosteum in a triangular shape (Codman triangle). Step 1 may ask that you recognize the diagnosis based solely on a similar image. (*From Kumar V, Abbas AK, Fausto N, Aster J.* Robbins & Cotran Pathologic Basis of Disease. *8th ed. New York: Elsevier; 2009.*)

are fast-growing and have a 60% 5-year survival rate. They frequently metastasize to lung. Paget disease is a risk factor.

Chondrosarcoma: Accounts for about 30% of primary bone malignancies. Slow-growing malignant tumor of cartilage, most frequently occurring in the **proximal femur or pelvis**. Patients are typically males **older than 45 years**. Radiography reveals bony destruction with calcified spots. Histology reveals **gelatinous lobules of cartilage with local necrosis and calcification.**

Ewing Sarcoma: Accounts for about 15% of primary bone tumors. Primitive neuroectodermal malignancy that often presents between 10 and 20 years of age. It manifests with localized pain and swelling, especially of the diaphysis of the femur. It is one of the few bone tumors that is more common in females. It is distinguished radiographically by its periosteal **onion skinning** appearance. Histology reveals anaplastic small blue cells. A combination of surgery, chemotherapy and radiation therapy is often indicated.

Mnemonic: eWings with a side of **onion** rings.

Osteosarcoma: Sunburst, Codman triangle

Chondrosarcoma: Gelatinous lobules

Ewing: Onion skinning

Neoplasms of Soft Tissue

Lipoma: This benign proliferation of mature adipocytes is the most common soft tissue neoplasm. It presents as a soft subcutaneous nodule. Malignant transformation is very rare, so excision is solely for cosmetic purposes.

Liposarcoma: Rare malignant tumor of fat cells.

Rhabdomyoma: Benign tumor of striated muscle. Cardiac rhabdomyomas are associated with **tuberous sclerosis**.

Rhabdomyosarcoma: Rare malignant tumor of striated muscle found in the pediatric population.

PHARMACOLOGY

Nonsteroidal Antiinflammatory Drugs

NSAIDs interfere with the arachidonic acid inflammatory pathway (Fig. 12.33) by nonselectively inhibiting cyclooxygenase-1 and cyclooxygenase-2 (COX-1, COX-2). COX is an enzyme

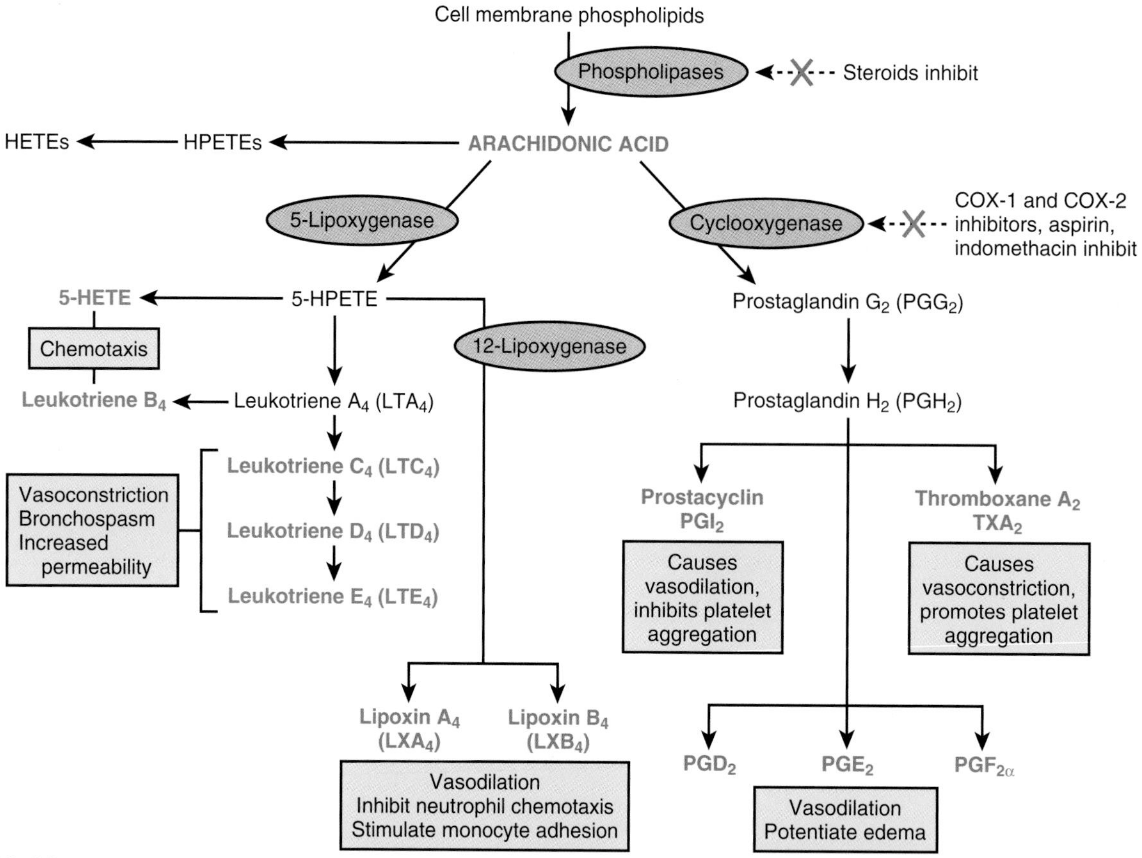

Fig. 12.33 Inflammatory cascade of arachidonic acid. 5-HETE, 5-Hydroxyeicosatetraenoic acid; HETE, hydroxyeicosatetraenoic acid; HPETE, arachidonic acid 5-hydroperoxide (5-hydroperoxy- eicosatetraenoic acid. (*From Kumar V, Cotran RS, Robbins SI.* Basic Pathology. *7th ed. Philadelphia: Elsevier; 2002.*)

that converts arachidonic acid into prostaglandin G_2 (PGI_2), which is eventually converted into the prostanoids (prostaglandins, prostacyclin, and thromboxane [TX]). By inhibiting this pathway, the inflammatory, vasoactive (PGI_2, TXA_2), pyrogenic (PGE_2), and painful effects are also inhibited. NSAIDs include ibuprofen, naproxen, ketorolac, indomethacin, and diclofenac. Side effects include gastritis, **gastric ulcers, and GI bleeds** secondary to inhibition of mucosa-protecting prostaglandins. **Renal failure** may also occur secondary to inhibition of prostaglandins that physiologically vasodilate the glomerular afferent arterial, thereby reducing glomerular perfusion pressure . NSAIDs are contraindicated in pregnancy because they may prematurely close the ductus arteriosus.

Aspirin (ASA): Unique among NSAIDs in that it covalently and **irreversibly binds COX.** It also preferentially inhibits COX-1 over COX-2. Because most cells in the body can simply produce more COX enzymes, the overall effects are similar to those of other NSAIDs (antipyretic, antiinflammatory, and analgesic). Platelets, however, contain no nuclei and are unable to produce more COX. Inhibition therefore limits their ability to form TXA2 to become activated. This antiplatelet effect lasts for the lifetime of a platelet (≈5 to 9 days). ASA is therefore used prophylactically in patients at high risk for thrombotic events and used acutely for the management of myocardial infarction. Toxicity is similar to other NSAIDs, but bleeding is more common. ASA is also contraindicated in children with viral illnesses out of fear of Reye's syndrome (liver failure and encephalopathy).

COX-2 Inhibitors: Although COX-1 is a ubiquitous constitutively expressed enzyme, COX-2 is a facultatively expressed enzyme found in inflammatory cells (COX-1 is maintenance and COX-2 is reactive). COX-2 inhibition theoretically has the antiinflammatory benefits, with less risk of GI side effects from prostaglandin inhibition. COX-2 is also found in vascular endothelium and produces the antithrombotic PGI_2. Selective inhibition may put patients in a prothrombotic state because of unopposed action of the prothrombotic TXA_2.

COX-2 inhibitors: Fewer GI side effects, more cardiovascular complications.

Acetaminophen: Analgesic and antipyretic that functions by inhibiting cyclooxygenase in the **central** nervous system. Its antiinflammatory activity is limited, however, because it is not active peripherally. Acetaminophen overdose is the most common cause of **acute liver failure** because of its toxic metabolite. The antidote is *N*-acetylcysteine (see Chapter 7).

Acetaminophen inhibits COX in the central nervous system but is not peripherally active.

Glucocorticoids

Antiinflammatory steroid hormone that functions by forming a complex with glucocorticoid receptors and activating nuclear transcription of antiinflammatory mediators. Ultimately, they interfere with phospholipase A_2's production of inflammatory cytokines. Glucocorticoids include hydrocortisone, prednisone, prednisolone, and dexamethasone. There are many side effects to steroids, including hyperglycemia, weight gain (moonlike facies, central obesity, buffalo hump, purple striae), osteoporosis, adrenal insufficiency, cataracts, and immunosuppression.

Osteoporosis Medications

Calcium and Vitamin D: Adequate consumption of these compounds may result in positive calcium balance and may slow or reverse bone loss. Supplementation is indicated for those with osteoporosis and inadequate dietary intake. The active form, vitamin D_3 (cholecalciferol), is preferred to its precursor, vitamin D_2. Calcium supplementation may be falling out of favor with some practitioners.

Bisphosphonates: First-line therapy in the treatment of osteoporosis. This class of medications becomes concentrated in bone and ingested by osteoclasts. Bisphosphonates then prevent bone remodeling by inducing osteoclast apoptosis or inhibiting resorption of hydroxyapatite. Medications have the suffix "-dronate" (e.g., alendronate, ibandronate). Bisphosphonates can also be used to prevent the pathologic remodeling of Paget disease. They are known to cause pill esophagitis, so patients should ingest with water and remain upright afterward.

Skeletal Muscle Relaxants

Centrally acting class of medication that reduces muscle tone. These are used in combination with NSAIDs to decrease acute muscle spasm. Examples of this class of medication include baclofen and cyclobenzaprine. Baclofen functions as a gamma-aminobutyric acid B ($GABA_B$) receptor agonist in the central nervous system and acts analogously to benzodiazepines while producing less sedation. The mechanism of action of cyclobenzaprine is less clear. Side effects include sedation and dizziness.

Gout Medications

Colchicine: Used in **acute flares** of gout. It acts by binding tubulin, which **prevents microtubule formation** and therefore neutrophil motility. Its action is thus antiinflammatory. Because microtubules are essential for mitotic spindles, this drug is also considered a mitotic poison. This can lead to side effects such as bone marrow suppression and hair loss. GI upset, however, is more common.

Allopurinol: Used to prevent flares of gout by reducing serum uric acid concentration; not useful in acute flares. Allopurinol is a **xanthine oxidase inhibitor,** which prevents the conversion of hypoxanthine to xanthine and eventually uric acid. Allopurinol is also used prophylactically in patients with lymphoma and leukemia who are undergoing chemotherapy to prevent tumor lysis syndrome. Febuxostat is a newer xanthine oxidase inhibitor that can be used for patients intolerant of allopurinol.

Colchicine: Decrease inflammation

Allopurinol: Decrease urate production

Probenecid: Increase urate excretion

Probenecid: Used to prevent flares of chronic gout by reducing serum uric acid concentration, but not useful in acute flares. It functions by inhibiting the nephron's organic anion transporter, thereby inhibiting the renal reabsorption of uric acid.

Methotrexate: Used in the treatment of malignancies, methotrexate acts as an inhibitor of dihydrofolate reductase. It is also used, however, as a disease-modifying antirheumatic drug. (See Chapter 11 for details.)

TNF Inhibitors: These biologic agents are used in the treatment of autoimmune conditions such as rheumatoid arthritis, ankylosing spondylitis, psoriasis, and Crohn disease. They act by blocking TNF-α, an inflammatory cytokine secreted from monocytes. Side effects are related to impaired immunity; they include opportunistic infections and malignancies.

Etanercept: Functions as a decoy TNF receptor, thereby decreasing the level of circulating functional TNF-α.

Infliximab, Adalimumab: Monoclonal antibodies that directly target TNF-α, thereby decreasing its circulating levels.

❍ The mechanism of action of these biologic agents is hidden in their name. Etaner**cept** is a decoy re**cept**or. Inflixi**mab** and adalimu**mab** are **m**onoclonal **a**nti**b**odies.

Rituximab: Anti-CD20 monoclonal antibody (anti–B cell) used in the treatment of autoimmune conditions, often after an inadequate response to TNF-α inhibitors.

Botulinum Toxin (Botox): Prevents presynaptic release of acetylcholine at the neuromuscular junction. Without acetylcholine to stimulate the endplate, the muscle is paralyzed. Botox is used not only for cosmetic purposes, but also to relieve muscle spasms and dystonias.

Botox interferes with presynaptic Ach release, which causes muscle paralysis.

❍ Botulinum toxin is produced by the gram-positive rod ***Clostridium botulinum.*** Infant botulism occurs when infants ingest the microbe (typically in honey), leading to colonization of the immature GI tract. The subsequent toxin formation leads to **floppy baby syndrome.** The adult GI flora is resistant to *C. botulinum* colonization, but the microbe may colonize wounds or form preformed toxins in home-canned foods (in which anaerobic conditions permit bacterial growth). Foodborne botulism begins with GI upset and proceeds to flaccid paralysis, especially of the cranial nerves.

REVIEW QUESTIONS

(1) A patient has primary hyperparathyroidism from a parathyroid adenoma. What effects will this have on his or her bone?

(2) Using the above information about skeletal muscle contraction, deduce the process of rigor mortis.

(3) A 50-year-old woman presents complaining of weakness that progresses over the course of the day. By evening she can barely keep her eyes open. Which tests might confirm your diagnosis and what medication might improve the patient's symptoms?

(4) A 3-month-old male presents to the emergency department with a midshaft spiral fracture of the tibia. On questioning, his parents state that he rolled off the changing table when the fracture occurred. Is this fracture suspicious for nonaccidental trauma?

(5) A 70-year-old woman presents with long-standing morning pain of her neck, shoulders, and hip associated with an ESR of 105 mm/hr. She presents to the emergency department for severe headache. What is the likely chronic condition and what is the acute complication?

(6) Identify the likely skeletal pathology based on patient characteristics alone. A, Obese 12-year-old boy with hip pain. B, 7-year-old with inability to bear weight. C, Newborn with asymmetric gluteal skin folds.

(7) A 28-year-old African American woman presents with cough, shortness of breath, and painful swollen nodules overlying her shins. Chest x-ray reveals bilateral hilar lymphadenopathy. What is a biopsy of the involved lymph nodes most likely to reveal?

(8) Identify the following neoplasms based on one of their defining features: A, Soap bubble appearance B, Codman triangle C, Mushroom shape D, Onion skinning E, Radiolucent nest.

(9) A 16-year-old male presents with fever and inability to bear weight on his left leg. He has lost all range of motion. What steps should be taken to diagnose this condition.

(10) A 62-year-old man presents to his primary care physician complaining of hearing loss. Further questioning reveals a recent increase in the man's hat size. What studies would confirm the diagnosis, and which medication may prevent progression?

(11) After months on a new medication, a patient presents with purple striae and new-onset diabetes. Which medication was the patient prescribed, and what is its mechanism of action?

(12) An 81-year-old woman with severe osteoarthritis (OA) is found to have creatinine elevated at 4.1 mg/dL on laboratory analysis. What medication might be responsible for this result?

13 NEUROLOGY

Manpreet Singh

ANATOMY AND PHYSIOLOGY

Neurohistology

The nervous system is composed of **two general components, neurons** (nerve cells), which are the functional units involved in nerve transmission (which occurs via a synapse), and **glial cells,** which are the supporting (nonneuronal) cells that serve different functions such as modulating nerve transmissions at the synapse itself or myelinating nerves.

Rough endoplasmic reticulum (RER) and polyribosomes (Nissl bodies) are only found in the cell body and dendrites (not axon).

Neurons: These are the nondividing functional units of the nervous system, which can be classified according to function (motor, sensory, or interneurons). Each neuron is broken into a cell body, receiving dendrites, and a single projecting axon. Of the three components, clumps of rough endoplasmic reticulum (RER) and polyribosomes (referred to as Nissl bodies) are only found in the cell body and dendrites (not axon). The dispersion of these Nissl bodies (which appear dark when using the Nissl stain) is a prominent feature in axonal injury and is appropriately termed *chromatolysis.*

Glial Cells: There are **four central nervous system (CNS)** glial cell types (astrocytes, oligodendrocytes, microglia, and ependymal cells) and **one peripheral nervous system (PNS) glial cell** type (Schwann cells).

Astrocytes: These are the most abundant and largest of the glial subtypes. Although thought of as support, they play a far greater role. Their most notable role is the metabolism and recycling of certain neurotransmitters (glutamate, serotonin, and γ-aminobutyric acid [GABA]). They also buffer the extracellular potassium concentration, respond to injury **(gliosis),** and make up the blood–brain barrier. They contain glial fibrillary acidic protein **(GFAP),** which is a marker used in brain cancers such as astrocytoma and glioblastoma.

One oligodendrocyte myelinates multiple neurons in the CNS. One Schwann cell myelinates one neuron in the PNS.

Oligodendrocytes: These cells **myelinate neurons within the CNS** (one cell myelinates multiple neurons; Fig. 13.1A) and are damaged in disease processes such as multiple sclerosis (MS) and leukodystrophies.

Microglia: These cells arise from monocytes (hematopoietic precursor) and thus are the resident macrophages of the CNS. Their function is to protect the CNS. When the brain is damaged or infected, they become activated and multiply quickly to perform functions such as phagocytosis and presenting antigens. Microglia cells are implicated in neurodegenerative diseases such as Alzheimer disease and Parkinson disease, as well as infections, such as human immunodeficiency virus (HIV) infection, where they form multinucleated giant cells.

Ependymal Cells: These ciliated cells line the cavities of the CNS (ventricular system) in the choroid plexus, where they are involved in the production of cerebrospinal fluid (CSF) and are part of the blood–CSF barrier. They are implicated in disease processes such as ependymomas and syringomyelia.

Schwann Cells: These cells are derived from **neural crest origin** and are similar to oligodendrocytes but instead myelinate neurons of the PNS (one cell myelinates one neuron; Fig. 13.1B). They are implicated in diseases such as Guillain-Barré syndrome (GBS), Charcot-Marie-Tooth disease (CMT), chronic inflammatory demyelinating polyneuropathy (CIDP), schwannomas, and acoustic neuromas (also known as vestibular schwannomas).

Sensory Receptors

Sensory neurons receive signals from external or internal stimuli via numerous sensory receptors. Each type of sensory receptor conveys a unique type of sense such as vibration, pressure, pain, and temperature.

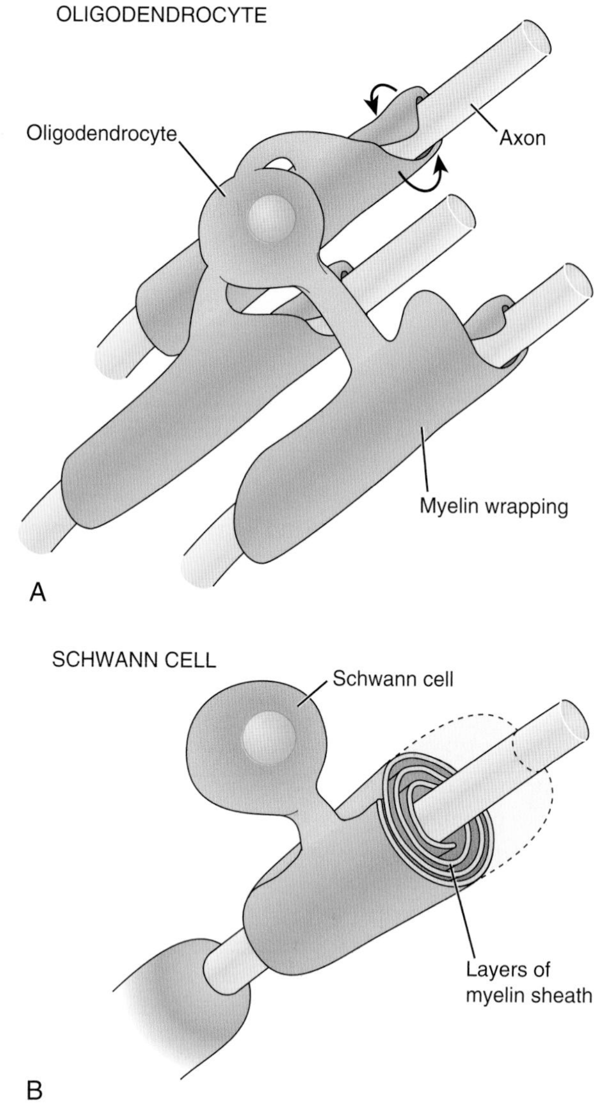

Fig. 13.1 A, One oligodendrocyte myelinates multiple central nervous system (CNS) neurons. **B,** One Schwann cell myelinates only one peripheral nervous system (PNS) neuron. (*From Boron WF, Boulpaep EL. Medical Physiology. 2nd ed. Philadelphia: Elsevier; 2008.*)

In addition to classifying receptors based on the sense they convey, we can also classify them according to location (cutaneous versus muscle), morphology (free, nonencapsulated versus encapsulated), and rate of adaptation to a stimulus (slow-adapting versus fast-adapting). Slow-adapting receptors (e.g., muscle spindles, Merkel disks, Ruffini corpuscles) steadily detect the stimulus and steadily produce a signal over the duration of the stimulus. In contrast, fast-adapting receptors (e.g., Meissner corpuscles, Pacinian corpuscles) quickly generate action potentials that diminish soon after the onset of the stimulus. This gives us a sense of the stimulus duration and intensity. This is why we stop feeling our clothes soon after we have them on.

Slow-adapting receptors: Muscle spindles, Merkel disks, and Ruffini corpuscles

Fast-adapting receptors: Meissner corpuscles and Pacinian corpuscles

Cutaneous Receptors

- **Free nerve endings:** These are nonencapsulated nerve endings, located throughout the epidermis and some viscera. They convey information regarding **pain** and **temperature.** Some of these nerve endings are associated with C fibers, which are slow (unmyelinated), convey warm temperature, and are involved in referred pain. Others are associated with Aδ fibers, which are fast (myelinated), convey cold temperature (see also Krause end bulbs, below), and are involved in localized pain.
- **Merkel disks:** These are nonencapsulated, large, slow-adapting, myelinated fibers located in hair follicles. These convey the senses of position (location) and static touch (e.g., textures).

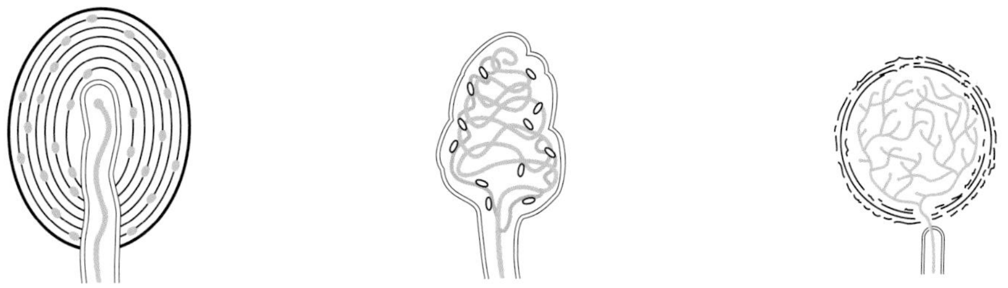

	Pacinian corpuscles	Meissner corpuscles	Krause end bulbs
Location:	Ligaments, joint capsules, serous membranes	Palms, soles, digits	Skin, mucous membranes, conjunctiva
Detects:	Pressure, coarse touch, vibration, tension	Light touch on hairless skin	Cold, mechanical stimulation

Fig. 13.2 *Left,* Pacinian corpuscles are for pressure and vibration. *Middle,* Meissner corpuscles are for light touch. *Right,* Krause end bulbs are for cold (like Santa Claus). (*From Burns R, Cave MD.* Rapid Review Histology and Cell Biology. *2nd ed. Philadelphia: Elsevier; 2007.*)

- **Pacinian corpuscles** (Fig. 13.2, *left*): These are encapsulated, large, fast-adapting myelinated fibers found in the dermis, ligaments and joints. They convey the senses of vibration and deep pressure.
- **Meissner corpuscles** (Fig. 13.2, *middle*): These are encapsulated, large, fast-adapting myelinated fibers found in the epidermis of hairless (glabrous) skin (e.g., fingers and lips). These convey the senses of position (location) and dynamic touch (e.g., light touch).
- **Krause end bulbs** (Fig. 13.2, *right*): These are primarily for the sensation of cold; think **Krause** sounds similar to Santa **Claus,** who is always **cold** in the North Pole.
- **Ruffini corpuscles:** These are encapsulated fibers, which adapt slowly, are found in the dermis and convey the senses of pressure and skin stretch (e.g., joint change).

Muscle Receptors

The main sensory muscle receptors are muscle spindles, which detect change in the length of skeletal muscle fibers and Golgi tendon organs, which are placed at the junction of the tendon and muscle fibers and sense the force of contraction.

Muscle Spindles: The muscle spindles are present in **intrafusal** fibers, which run parallel to the actual contractile muscle fibers (the contractile muscle fibers are also referred to as **extrafusal** fibers). By running in parallel (along with) the contraction of the muscle, intrafusal fibers can detect when the length of the muscle shortens or lengthens. This can be better understood with a clinical example, such as the myotactic reflex, in which hitting the patellar tendon with a reflex hammer causes the knee to jerk (Fig. 13.3). The tendon is stretched with the hammer, pulling on the muscle spindle. This then sends information to the spinal cord, which stimulates the knee extensor muscles to contract (causing the knee to jerk). It also inhibits the knee flexor muscles from contracting. A quick way to remember which nerve roots are tested by which reflexes is simply to count to eight: ankle (S1-2), patellar (L3-4), biceps (C5-6), triceps (C7-8).

Nerve roots of reflexes:
Ankle (S1-2)
Patellar (L3-4)
Biceps (C5-6)
Triceps (C7-8)

Golgi Tendon Organ: Located at the junction of muscle fibers, with its tendons arranged **perpendicular** to extrafusal muscle fibers (Fig. 13.4). This receptor conveys a sense of muscle tension via afferent nerves and provides an autogenic inhibition reflex (also called the inverse myotatic reflex), which causes muscle relaxation before a tendon can be torn. This is why weight lifters may drop a heavy weight before it's too late and why this sensory receptor overrules the muscle spindle.

Neurotransmitters

Neurotransmitters (NTs) are substances found in synaptic vesicles that are secreted into the synaptic cleft from a presynaptic neuron to a postsynaptic neuron. They are classified according to chemical composition and the action elicited, which can be excitatory or inhibitory. See Chapter 7 for details of synaptic transmission and metabolism of many of these neurotransmitters.

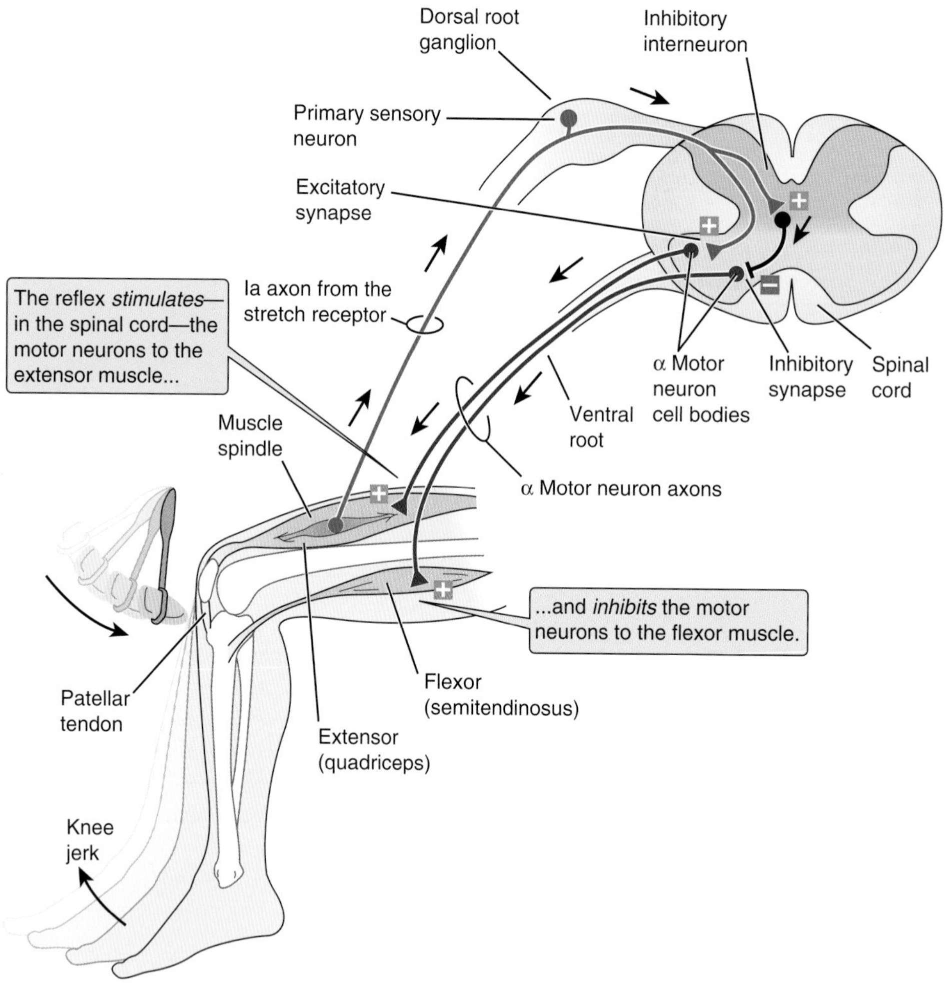

Fig. 13.3 Muscle spindles sense muscle stretch and send a signal to the spinal cord. In the case of the patellar tendon reflex (shown), this causes activation of the extensor muscles and inhibition of the flexor muscles, causing the knee to jerk. (*From Boron WF, Boulpaep EL.* Medical Physiology. *2nd ed. Philadelphia: Elsevier; 2008.*)

Amino Acids

- **Glutamate:** As part of the glutamatergic pathway, glutamate has an excitatory effect, specifically on *N*-methyl-D-aspartate (NMDA) receptors, and is involved in cognition functions (learning and memory) in the hippocampus. In brain injury or disease, such as a stroke or seizure, excitotoxicity from excess glutamate release can lead to neuronal damage and death from the resulting excess calcium influx into the neuron.
- **Gamma-aminobutyric acid (GABA):** This is an inhibitory NT found in the nucleus accumbens and is involved in regulating excitability throughout the nervous system. It is decreased in anxiety and Huntington disease.
- **Glycine:** This is an inhibitory NT used by the Renshaw cells of the spinal cord. Strychnine, which can be fatal to humans, blocks its action.
- **Acetylcholine:** Found in the basal nucleus of Meynert, this NT is involved in functions such as learning, short-term memory, arousal, and reward. In Alzheimer disease, there is a loss of neurons in the nucleus of Meynert and thus the amount of NT released is reduced.
- **Opioid peptides:** Include endorphins, enkephalins, and dynorphins; involved in analgesia.

Monoamines and Catecholamines

Dopamine (DA): This NT is involved in functions such as nausea, reward, cognition, the motor system, and the endocrine system through four discrete pathways:

Nigrostriatal pathway is part of the motor system. It projects from the substantia nigra (in the midbrain) to the striatum; destruction of these neurons can lead to parkinsonism and extrapyramidal symptoms (side effect of antipsychotic drugs).

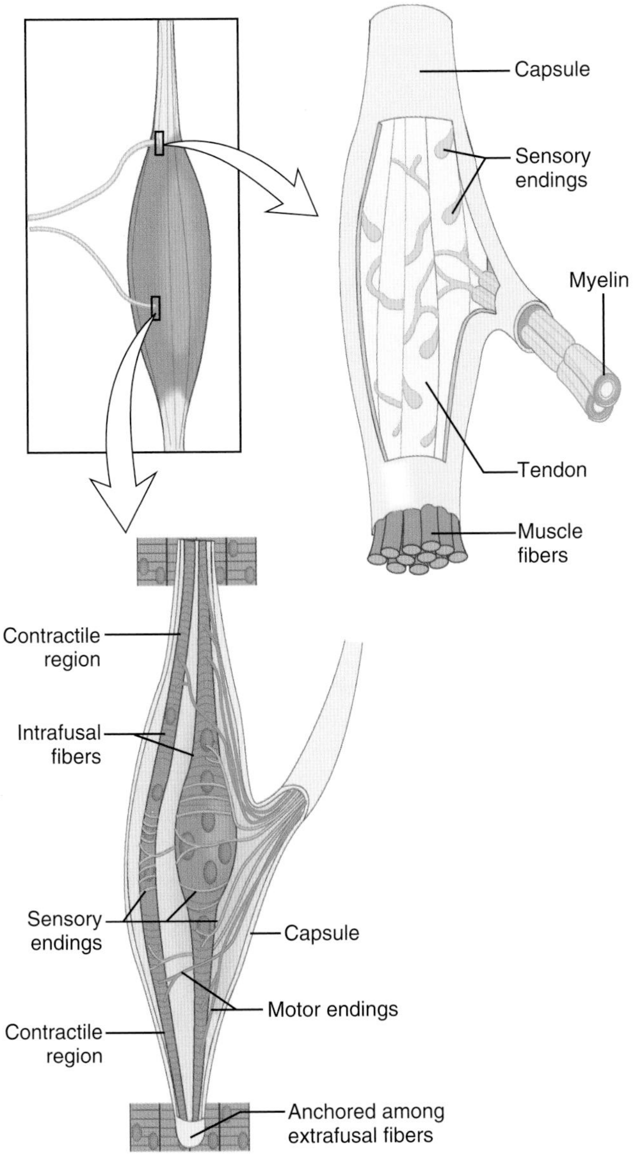

Fig. 13.4 Location and anatomy of Golgi tendon organs *(top right)* and muscle spindles *(bottom)*. The Golgi tendon organs are located at the junction of the muscle and tendon and are perpendicular to the extrafusal (contractile) fibers to be able to sense the force that the contractile fibers are generating. If this force is too high and places the tendon at risk of rupture, it will send inhibitory signals to stop exerting force. The muscle spindles are in parallel with the extrafusal fibers and therefore can sense length. *(From Nolte J.* Elsevier's Integrated Neuroscience. *Philadelphia: Elsevier; 2007.)*

Nigrostriatal DA pathway: Movement and parkinsonism

Mesolimbic DA pathway: Reward and hallucinations

Mesolimbic pathway is found projecting from the ventral tegmentum (in the midbrain) to the nucleus accumbens; this is generally considered the "reward pathway" of the brain. It has also been linked to the positive symptoms of schizophrenia (hallucinations and delusions), which is the target for many antipsychotic drugs

Tuberoinfundibular pathway is found projecting from the arcuate nucleus of the hypothalamus to the portal vessels of the infundibulum; DA in this case inhibits prolactin release in the anterior pituitary. As a result, symptoms such as gynecomastia, galactorrhea, and menstrual dysfunction may result from DA-blocking agents (including antipsychotic medications).

Mesocortical pathway is found projecting from the arcuate nucleus to the frontal lobes; this has been linked to negative symptoms of schizophrenia (causing the characteristic hypoactive, flat affect).

Norepinephrine (NE): Found in the locus ceruleus (found in the pons), lateral tegmental areas, reticular formation, and solitary tracts, this NT is involved in the arousal, reward, and maintenance of mood. In depression, NE is decreased. In states such as mania, anxiety, or stimulant drug use (amphetamines and cocaine), NE is elevated. Of note, in Alzheimer disease, there is substantial loss of the locus ceruleus.

Serotonin (5-HT): Found only in the raphe nucleus of the brainstem, this NT is involved in functions such as mood, sleep, and pain. It is elevated during mania and reduced in depression, anxiety, and insomnia.

5-HT is found in the raphe nucleus of the brainstem.

Others

Adenosine: Generally acts as an inhibitory neurotransmitter. Caffeine acts as a stimulant by antagonizing adenosine receptors. Of note, adenosine is commonly used in the treatment of atrioventricular nodal reentry tachycardia (AVNRT), a specific type of supraventricular tachycardia (SVT), especially in higher doses when it comes to patients drinking caffeine.

Nitric oxide (NO): Formed from the conversion of arginine to citrulline, this NT is involved in memory formation through paracrine signaling. NO has been linked to reperfusion injury when blood flow is reestablished in an ischemic region.

Substance P: Excitatory NT involved in pain transmission.

Cerebral Perfusion Pressure (CPP)

CPP is the tight autoregulation of the net pressure causing brain perfusion. This net pressure, typically defined as CPP, is the difference between mean arterial pressure (MAP) and intracranial pressure (ICP) (that is, CPP = MAP – ICP). With autoregulation between MAP and ICP, CPP is maintained between 50 and 150 mm Hg. However, outside the limits of autoregulation, increased ICP (e.g., in traumatic brain injury from trauma, cerebral edema from stroke or DKA, vasogenic/cytotoxic edema) leads to decreased CPP, which is detrimental. To address this detriment, therapeutic hyperventilation is often used, where decreased pCO_2 results in cerebral vasocontriction and decreased cerebral blood flow. ICP can also be relieved with measures such as administration of hypertonic saline or mannitol, or by dramatic measures such as craniotomy.

ANATOMY

Frontal lobe: Primary motor cortex and Broca's area

Temporal lobe: Primary auditory cortex and Wernicke's area

Parietal lobe: Primary somatosensory cortex

Occipital lobe: Primary visual cortex

Each cerebral hemisphere is divided grossly into four lobes—frontal, parietal, occipital, and temporal (Fig. 13.5A). Each lobe specializes in certain functions (Fig. 13.5B). The **frontal lobe** provides crucial executive functions such as cognition, planning, decision making, error correction, and troubleshooting. The frontal lobe houses the frontal eye fields (which are involved in voluntary eye movements), premotor area (generates execution or plan of movement), and primary motor cortex. The frontal lobe also houses Broca's area in the dominant hemisphere (usually the left hemisphere, regardless of whether or not the person is right- or left-handed), to which the motor aspect of speech production is linked. The function of the **parietal lobe** includes integrating sensory modalities and housing the principal sensory areas. The **temporal lobe** is involved in auditory perception; it is home to the primary auditory cortex. It also houses Wernicke's area (associative auditory cortex) in the dominant hemisphere, in which

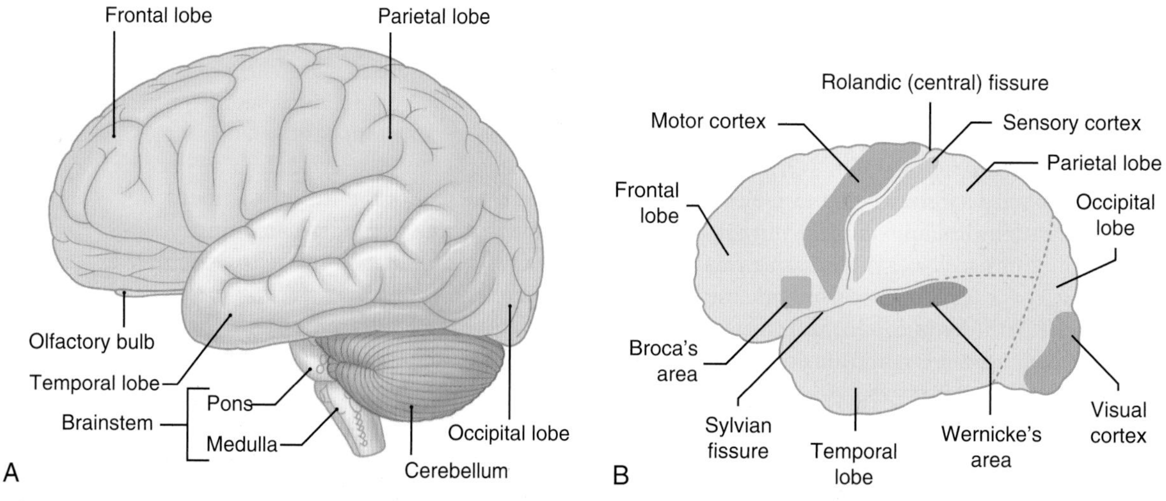

FIG. 13.5 **A,** Gross anatomy of the brain. **B,** Selected areas of importance. (***A*** *from Moses K, Nava P, Banks J, Petersen D.* Atlas of Clinical Gross Anatomy, *2nd ed. St. Louis: Elsevier; 2012;* ***B*** *from Lim EKS.* Medicine and Surgery. *Philadelphia: Elsevier; 2007.*)

written and spoken language is understood. Broca's and Wernicke's areas are interconnected by the arcuate fasciculus, which aids in language processing. The **occipital lobe** is involved in the processing and integration of visual information.

The cortical homunculus is a pictorial representation of the anatomic divisions of the primary motor cortex (frontal lobe) and primary somatosensory cortex (parietal lobe); it shows the portion of the human body involved in sensory and motor function mapped onto the cerebral hemisphere (Fig. 13.6). It is important to note that some regions (e.g., hands, face, lips) are disproportionately larger in comparison to the rest of the body. This is because fine motor control and skills are needed in these particular parts of the body; more neurons need to be devoted to fine motor control of the hand compared with the hip. The homunculus is important in allowing one to localize a lesion based on the specific defects noted on neurologic examination. The middle cerebral artery (MCA) provides circulation to the lateral aspect of the cerebral hemisphere (resulting in neurologic deficits in the face and upper extremities if occlusion occurs), whereas the anterior cerebral artery (ACA) provides circulation to the medial aspect of the cerebral hemisphere (resulting in lower extremity and trunk neurologic deficits if occlusion occurs).

Basal Ganglia

Basal ganglia: Voluntary motor control, procedural learning, eye movement, and cognition

This subcortical structure is a group of nuclei whose main function is to modulate voluntary motor control. The basal ganglia are also involved in procedural learning, eye movement, and cognition. It consists of the following components (Fig. 13.7):

- Striatum, which is subdivided into the caudate (deals with cognition) and putamen (deals with motor control).
- Globus pallidus, which is subdivided into the externa (lateral external segment) and interna (medial internal segment), abbreviated GPe and GPi, respectively. Both segments have inhibitory GABAergic neurons that operate using a disinhibition principle. They are steadily firing at a high rate in the absence of signal, but may pause or reduce the rate in response to an inhibitory (GABA) signal from the striatum. As a result, there is a net reduction of this tonic inhibition on their targets.
- Subthalamic nucleus, which is the only portion of the pathway to produce the excitatory NT glutamate.
- Substantia nigra, which is subdivided into the pars compacta (SNc; DA-producing) and pars reticulata (SNr), which works in unison with the GPi.

The basal ganglia consist of a complex circuit that ultimately aids in communication between the cortex, thalamus, and basal ganglia (see Fig. 13.7). The signal starts at the primary motor cortex (precentral

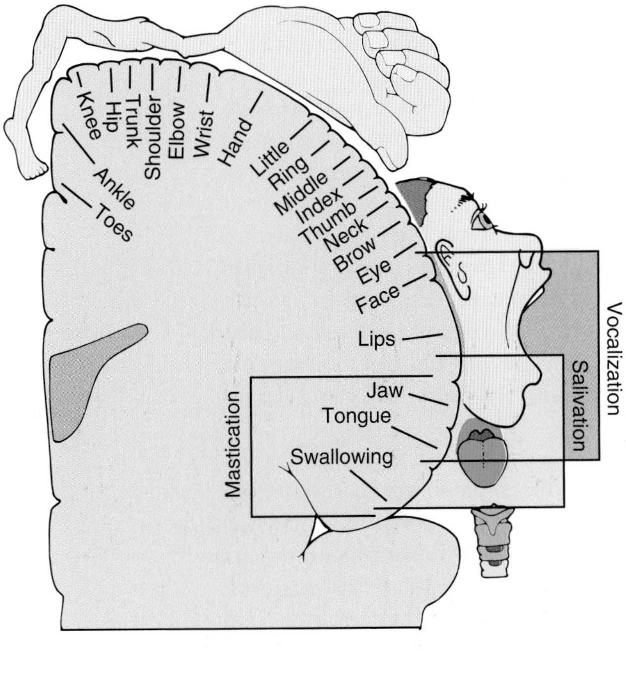

Fig. 13.6 The motor homunculus mapped out onto the cerebral cortex. The medial side is supplied by the anterior cerebral artery, leading to trunk and leg weakness in anterior cerebral artery strokes. The rest is supplied by the middle cerebral artery, leading to arm weakness in middle cerebral artery strokes. (*From Levy MN, Bruce M, Koeppen BM, Stanton BA.* Berne & Levy Principles of Physiology, *4th ed. Philadelphia: Elsevier; 2005.*)

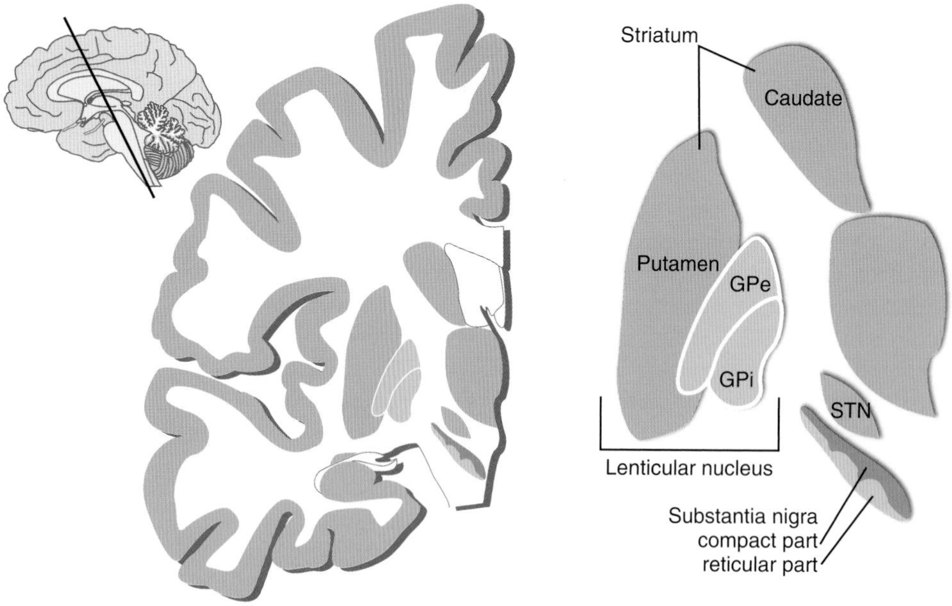

FIG. 13.7 Nomenclature of the basal ganglia. The striatum includes the putamen and caudate nucleus. The lentiform nucleus includes the putamen and globus pallidus. (*From Nolte J.* Essentials of the Human Brain. *Philadelphia: Elsevier; 2009.*)

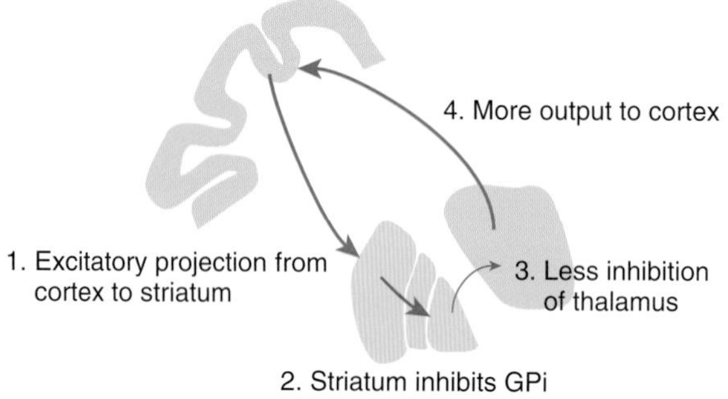

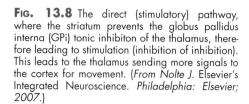

FIG. 13.8 The direct (stimulatory) pathway, where the striatum prevents the globus pallidus interna (GPi) tonic inhibiton of the thalamus, therefore leading to stimulation (inhibition of inhibition). This leads to the thalamus sending more signals to the cortex for movement. (*From Nolte J.* Elsevier's Integrated Neuroscience. *Philadelphia: Elsevier; 2007.*)

gyrus), which projects excitatory (glutaminergic) cortical neurons onto the striatum. From there, the signal can take two different directions, giving rise to two major pathways—the direct excitatory or **in**direct **in**hibitory pathways. These are involved in triggering motion; the direct pathway stimulates it, and the indirect pathway inhibits it.

The direct pathway stimulates motion; the indirect pathway inhibits motion.

Direct (stimulatory) pathway: See Fig. 13.8. Initially, the cortex stimulates the striatum. Through this pathway, the striatum **inhibits the globus pallidus interna (GPi)**. Normally, the GPi tonically inhibits the thalamus, so therefore the direct pathway **inhibits the inhibition of the thalamus.** Therefore this leads to increased thalamic output to the cortex.

Indirect (inhibitory) pathway: Remember that **in**direct **in**hibits. This pathway is more complicated (Fig. 13.9). Again, the cortex stimulates the striatum to cause inhibition. However, here the striatum **inhibits the globus pallidus externa (GPe)** instead. The GPe normally provides inhibition to the subthalamic nucleus (STN); therefore this inhibition of the STN is turned off when the striatum inhibits GPe. The STN is ultimately stimulated to excite the GPi. Recall that the GPi normally inhibits the thalamus, so therefore increased GPi activity leads to increased thalamic inhibition. Thus the thalamus will have less output to the cortex.

In summary, whereas the direct (stimulatory) pathway allows for increased thalamic transmission to the cortex by inhibiting the GPi inhibition of the thalamus, the indirect (inhibitory) pathway leads to increased GPi inhibition of the thalamus and less thalamic transmission to the cortex. The interplay between the excitatory and inhibitory signals is mediated by **dopamine** via the **substantia nigra pars compacta (SNc)**. Dopamine stimulates the direct ("excitatory") pathway upon binding to D_1 receptors, while those binding to D_2 receptors inhibit the indirect (inhibitory) pathway. Pathology with the basal

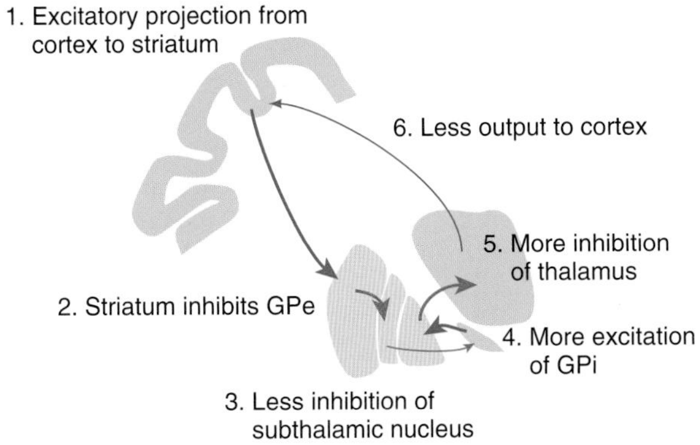

FIG. 13.9 The indirect (inhibitory) pathway starts the same as the direct pathway (cortex excites striatum) but the differences are that the indirect pathway stimulates the GPe first, and there is involvement of the subthalamic nucleus, which has excitatory output to the GPi, ultimately leading to increased thalamic inhibition. (*From Nolte J.* Elsevier's Integrated Neuroscience. *Philadelphia: Elsevier; 2007.*)

ganglia therefore, unsurprisingly, leads to movement disorders such as Wilson's disease, tardive dyskinesia, Parkinson disease, and Huntington disease (see later).

Basal ganglia pathologic conditions: Wilson disease, tardive dyskinesia, Parkinson disease, and Huntington disease

Hypothalamus

The hypothalamus is a major subcortical structure that consists of distinct nuclei that are involved in various functions. Mnemonic: The hypothalamus makes me hungry for **HAM BEETS** (**H**unger, **A**utonomic nervous system, **M**emory, **B**ehavior, **E**ndocrine, **E**motion, **T**emperature, **S**leep-Wake cycle, and **S**exual urges).

Instead of memorizing all the distinct nuclei and their individual functions, a better way to look at the hypothalamus is to break it into two contrasting regions (anterior and posterior) and two contrasting areas (lateral and medial), with distinct functions.

Anterior: Deals with parasympathetics and cooling.
- Destruction leads to hyperthermia (e.g., hypothalamic stroke).

Posterior: Deals with sympathetics and heating (e.g., shivering).
- Destruction leads to a poikilothermic (cold-blooded) individual (**posterior** destruction, **poikilothermic**).
- A functioning posterior hypothalamus keeps your posterior warm, like a functioning heater.

Lateral: Deals with thirst and hunger. Stimulated by grehlin. Inhibited by **l**eptin.
Mnemonic: **Late**ral makes you hungry for a **late** night snack and makes your waist grow laterally.
- Destruction leads to anorexia in adults and failure to thrive (FTT) in infants.

Medial: Deals with satiety. Stimulated by leptin.
- Destruction (e.g., craniopharyngioma) leads to hyperphagia.

The following are distinct nuclei of which you should be aware:
- **Supraoptic nucleus and paraventricular nucleus:** See Chapter 9 for more details. These two nuclei play a significant role in the posterior pituitary's release of antidiuretic hormone (ADH) (supraoptic) and oxytocin (paraventricular).
- **Arcuate nucleus:** This nucleus plays a significant role in releasing hormones from the anterior pituitary.
- **Suprachiasmatic nucleus:** Receives input from the retina via the optic chiasm; this plays a significant role in circadian rhythm. (You need enough sleep via the suprachiasmatic nucleus to be charismatic.)

Thalamus

The thalamus is a subcortical structure that **functions like a switchboard** in relaying sensory information to the cortex. It can be divided into functional nuclei (Fig. 13.10).

Anterior Nuclear Group (A): Relays input from the fornix to the cingulate gyrus as part of the Papez circuit; this plays a role in learning and memory.

Dorsomedial Nucleus (DM): Relays input from the prefrontal cortex and the limbic system; plays a crucial role in memory, attention, planning, organization, and abstract thinking. A lesion of this nucleus is associated with Korsakoff syndrome (see later).

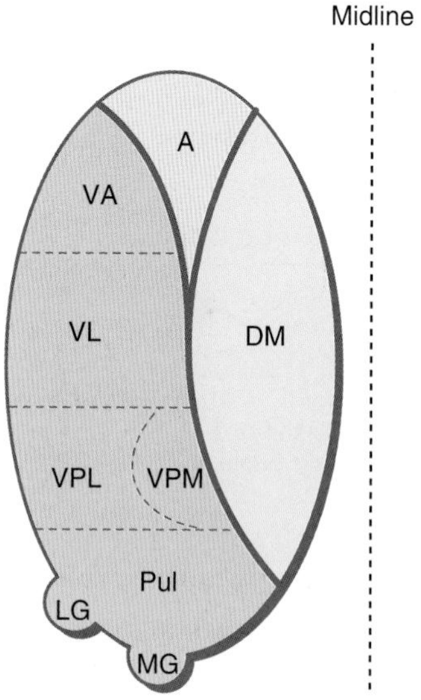

Fig. 13.10 Anatomy of the thalamus. Note that this thalamus has been compressed into one layer; each nucleus is not actually present at each level. A, Anterior nuclear group; DM, dorsomedial nucleus; LG, lateral geniculate nucleus; MG, medical geniculate nucleus; Pul, pulvinar; VA, ventral anterior; VL, ventral lateral; VPL, ventral posterior lateral; VPM, ventral posterior medial. (*From Nolte J.* Essentials of the Human Brain. *Philadelphia: Elsevier; 2009.*)

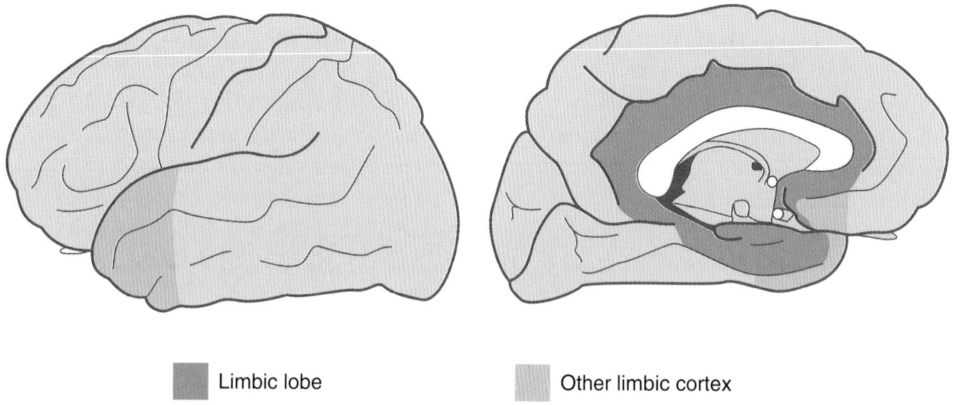

Fig. 13.11 The limbic system. (*From Nolte J.* Essentials of the Human Brain. *Philadelphia: Elsevier; 2009.*)

Ventral Nuclear Group:

- Ventral anterior, lateral nuclei relay **MOTOR** input from basal ganglia and cerebellum to the primary motor and premotor cortex and functions in coordination and planning of movement.
- Ventral posterior medial (VPM), and ventral posterior lateral (VPL) nuclei relay **SENSORY** input from the face (VPM) via the trigeminal nerve (cranial nerve [CN] V) and from the body (VPL) via **dorsal columns** and **spinothalamic tract.**

Medial Geniculate Nucleus (MGN): Relays **auditory** input from the inferior colliculus to the primary auditory cortex. **M**edial for **m**usic.

Lateral Geniculate Nucleus (LGN): Relays **visual** input from the retina to the optic cortex via the optic radiations. **L**ateral for **l**ooking.

Pulvinar: Integration of visual, auditory, and somatosensory input.

Limbic System

The limbic system (Fig. 13.11), which consists of the hippocampus, amygdala, limbic cortex, fornix, and mammillary body, provides myriad functions, such as memory, emotion, award, fear, pleasure, addiction, and olfaction.

Mnemonic for limbic system functions: **Five Fs** = **F**eeding, **F**leeing, **F**ighting, **F**eeling and… **S**ex.

Ventricular System

The ventricular system (Fig. 13.12) is a set of caves connected by tunnels in the brain that is continuous with the central canal of the spinal cord and subarachnoid space. It contains CSF, which functions

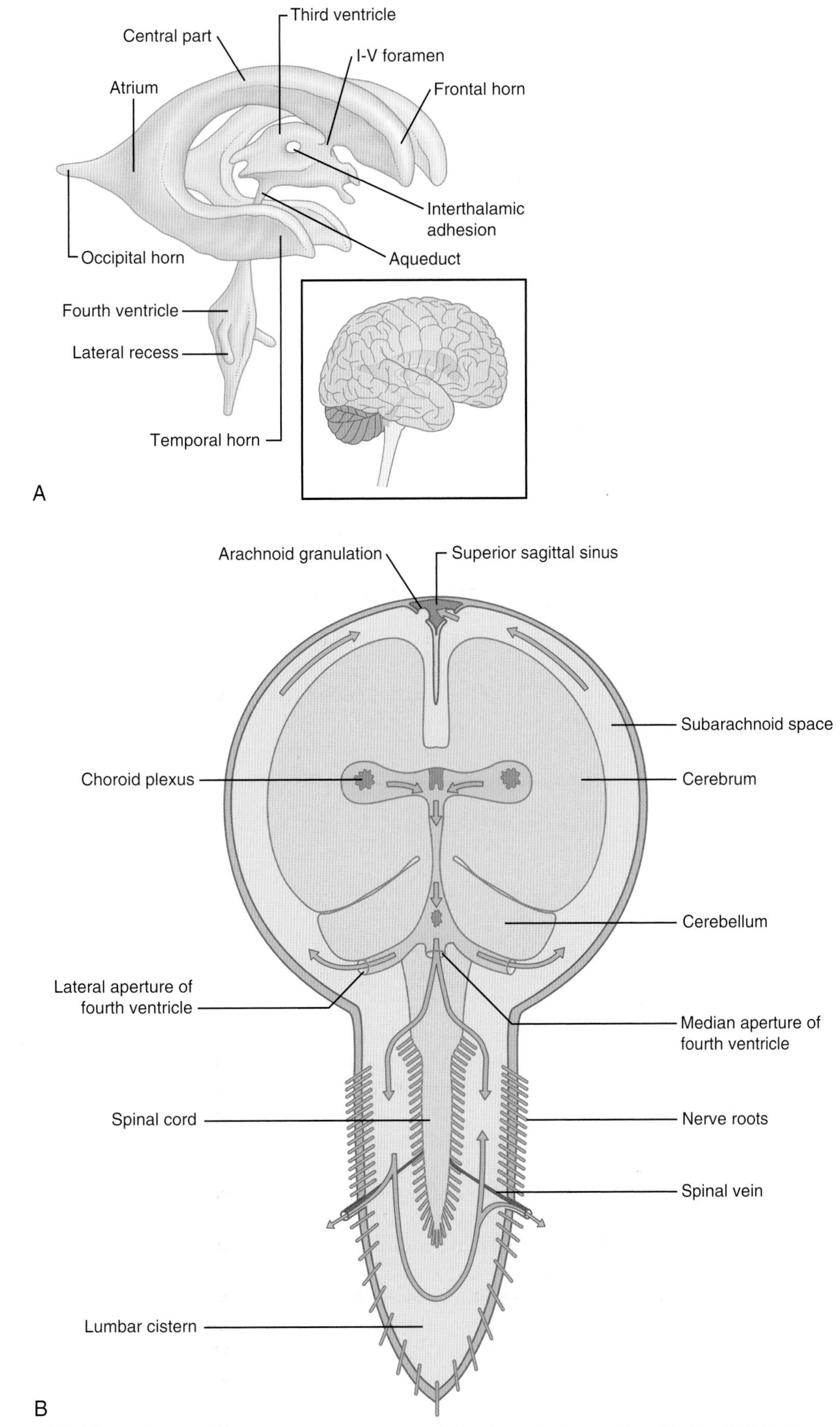

Fig. 13.12 A, The ventricular system. **B,** Its anatomic relationship to the brain. (*From FitzGerald MJT, Gruener G, Mtui E.* Clinical Neuroanatomy and Neuroscience. *6th ed. Philadelphia: Saunders; 2011.*)

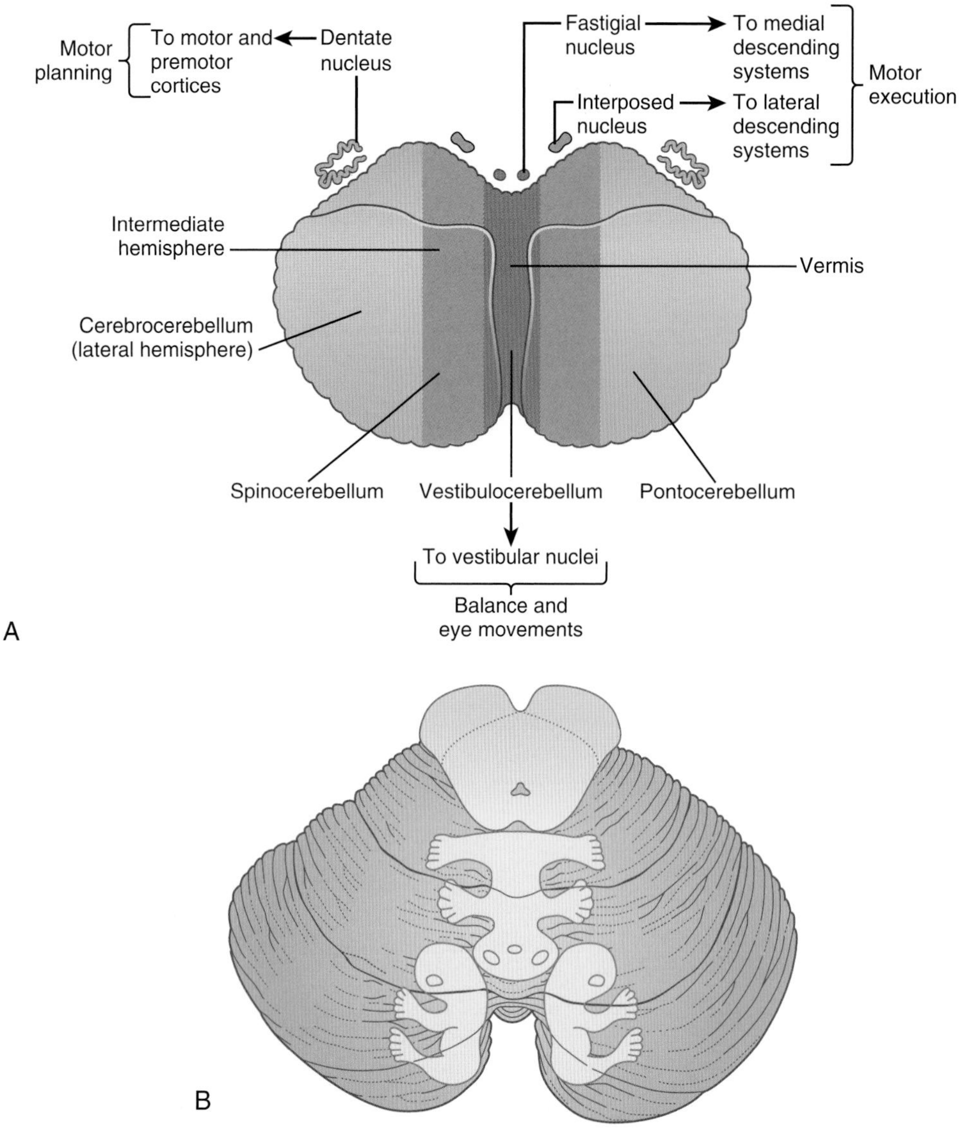

FIG. 13.13 A, Cerebellar anatomy and function. **B,** Cerebellum homunculus. (***A*** *from FitzGerald MJT, Gruener G, Mtui E:* Clinical Neuroanatomy and Neuroscience. *5th ed. Philadelphia: Saunders; 2007;* ***B*** *from FitzGerald MJT, Gruener G, Mtui E.* Clinical Neuroanatomy and Neuroscience. *6th ed. Philadelphia: Saunders; 2011.*)

as a cushion in protecting the brain, providing buoyancy in suspending the brain against gravity and maintaining chemical stability. CSF starts in two lateral ventricles and moves into the third ventricle via the interventricular foramina of Monro and then into the fourth ventricle via the cerebral aqueduct of Sylvius.

From there it can flow into the central canal of the spinal cord or into the cisterns of the subarachnoid space via three small foramina: the **m**edian aperture (foramen of **M**agendie) and the right and left **l**ateral apertures (foramina of **L**uschka). Because the foramen of Magendie is the median aperture, there is only one (but there are two lateral apertures of Luschka). Once the CSF is in the subarachnoid space, it can flow down the spinal cord into the lumbar cistern at the end of the cord around the cauda equina (where lumbar punctures are performed) or flow around the superior sagittal sinus to be resorbed via the arachnoid villi into the venous system. The ventricular system is implicated in pathologies such as hydrocephalus (abnormal enlargement of ventricles), meningitis, ventriculitis, and subarachnoid hemorrhage, which will be discussed in more detail later (see "Pathology").

Obstructing lesions of the ventricular system cause hydrocephalus above the lesion.

Cerebellum

The cerebellum (Fig. 13.13) is a structure located below the cerebral cortex and behind the pons component of the brainstem, where it plays a crucial role in the coordination, accuracy, and timing of our

Lesions of the cerebellum affect the ipsilateral side of the body.

movements. It houses four deep nuclei, which from lateral to medial are the **d**entate, **e**mboliform, **g**lobose, and **f**astigial nuclei.
Mnemonic "**D**on't **E**at **G**reasy **F**oods."

These nuclei receive inhibitory GABAergic input from Purkinje cells and excitatory glutaminergic input from mossy and climbing fibers via the inferior cerebellar peduncle (ipsilateral proprioception input) and medial cerebellar peduncle (contralateral cortical input). Once input is received, modulated output signals are projected from the dentate nuclei by Purkinje fibers via the superior cerebellar peduncle to the contralateral VA and VL nuclei of the thalamus. Because of these connections, it is important to note that a lesion of the cerebellum results in ataxias (incoordination) of the **ipsilateral side of the body**. Based on anatomy, the cerebellum can be subdivided to understand the functional denomination:

1. Lateral cerebellar hemisphere: Dentate nuclei aid in voluntary movement of the extremities as part of the cerebrocerebellum pathway.
2. Midline-medial vermis: Interposed (emboliform and globose) and fastigial nuclei aid in balance and fine-tuning of body and limb movements as part of the spinocerebellum pathway.
3. Flocculonodular lobe: Fastigial nuclei aid in balance and eye movement as part of the vestibulocerebellum pathway using visual and vestibular input from the retina and semicircular canals.

Blood Supply

Cerebral circulation is provided by the left and right **internal carotid arteries** and the left and right **vertebral arteries.** The **anterior** circulation is provided by the **internal carotid** arteries, which branch into the anterior and middle cerebral arteries. The **posterior** circulation is provided by the **vertebral** arteries, which fuse to form the basilar artery (supplies brainstem and cerebellum) which in turn branches into the posterior cerebral arteries. The left and right anterior cerebral arteries are connected by the anterior communicating artery. The internal carotid is interconnected with the posterior circulation via the posterior communicating arteries in the cerebral vault. Together, these connections form the circle of Willis (Fig. 13.14), which allows for collateral (backup) circulation if one of the artery supplies becomes stenosed or occluded. The circle of Willis includes the anterior cerebral artery, anterior communicating artery, internal carotid artery, posterior cerebral artery, and posterior communicating artery.

> Cerebral circulation is provided by the internal carotid arteries and vertebral arteries.

The cerebral circulation is supplied by three main arteries—the anterior, middle, and posterior cerebral arteries. Each artery supplies distinct parts of the cerebral hemisphere (Fig. 13.15). The anterior cerebral artery supplies the anteromedial surfaces, which include the frontal and parietal lobes, anterior portion of the basal ganglia and internal capsule, and medial motor homunculus. The middle cerebral artery supplies the lateral surfaces, which include the anterior and inferior temporal lobes, insular cortices, lateral surfaces of the hemispheres, and deep branches of the basal ganglia. The posterior cerebral artery supplies the posterior and inferior surfaces, which are primarily formed by the occipital lobe.

Venous drainage of the brain includes superficial (superior sagittal sinus) and deep subdivisions (inferior sagittal sinus) that connect at the confluence of sinuses before bifurcating into two transverse sinuses (Fig. 13.16). The transverse sinuses travel laterally and inferiorly in an S-shaped curve that forms the sigmoid sinuses, which go on to form the internal jugular veins.

Brainstem

The brainstem (Fig. 13.17), which consists of the medulla, pons, and midbrain, is a continuous structure adjoining the brain to the spinal cord and has conductive and integrative functions. It includes many of the motor and sensory tracts (corticospinal, spinothalamic, and posterior column) from the spinal cord, as well as motor and sensory innervations from the face via CNs III to XII).

Cranial Nerves

See Table 13.1.

Unlike spinal nerves, which emerge from the spinal cord, CNs emerge directly from the brain (brainstem or cerebrum; see Table 13.1). A good way to remember where each cranial nerves emerge is the "2, 2, 4, 4" rule, where the first two CNs emerge above the brainstem (CNs I, II), the next two emerge in the midbrain (CNs III, IV), the next four in the pons (CNs V, VI, VII, VIII), and the final four in the medulla (CNs IX, X, XI, XII).

> "2, 2, 4, 4 rule":
> CN I, II: Above brainstem
> CN III, IV: Midbrain
> CN V, VI, VII, VIII: Pons
> CN IX, X, XI, XII: Medulla

Mnemonic for the names of each CN: "**O**n **O**ld **O**lympus' **T**owering **T**op, **A** **F**riendly **V**iking **G**rew **V**ines **A**nd **H**ops."

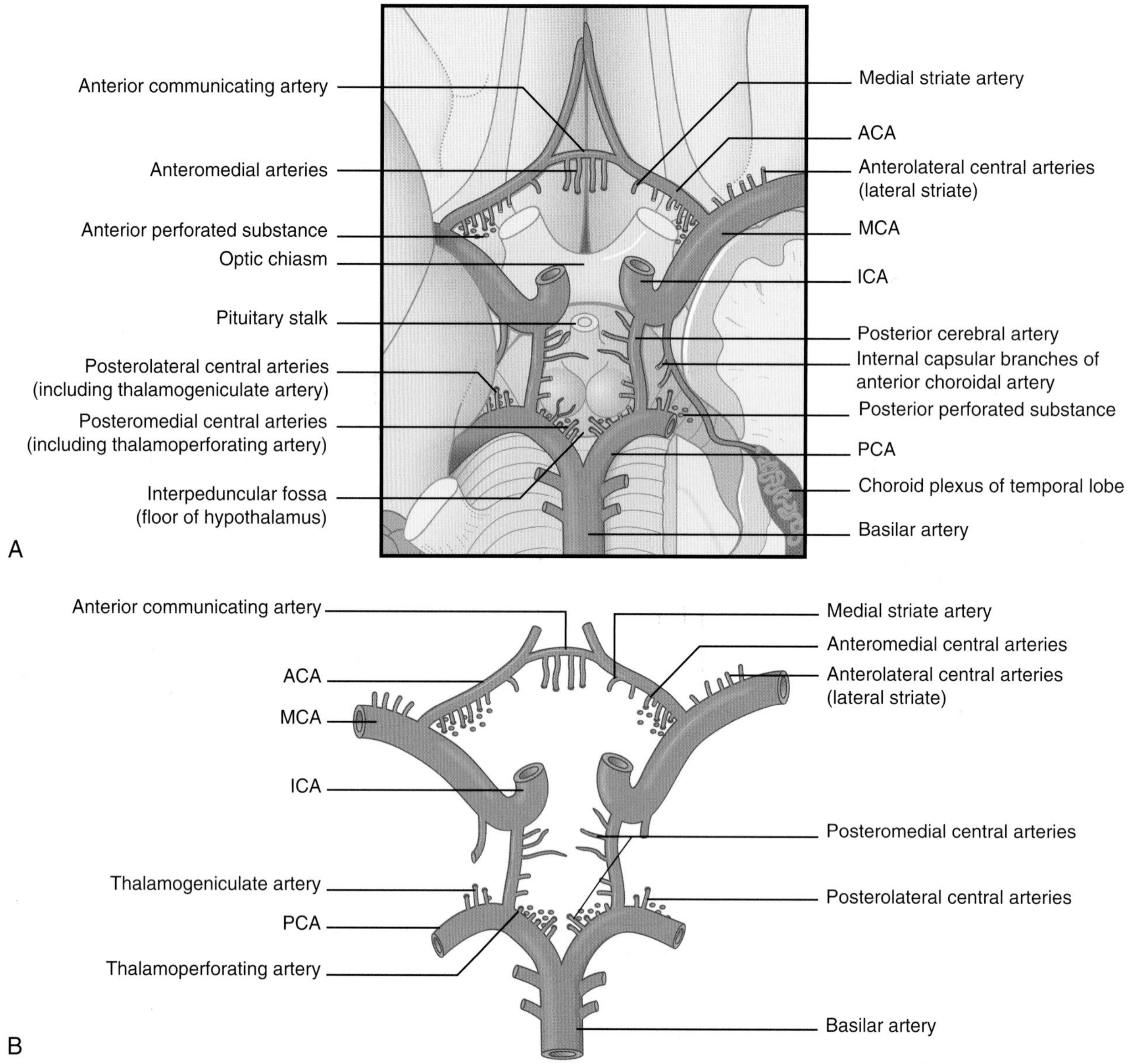

Fig. 13.14 A, The circle of Willis as viewed on the inferior surface of the brain. **B,** The circle of Willis viewed in isolation. ACA, anterior cerebral artery; ICA, internal carotid artery; MCA, middle cerebral artery; PCA, posterior cerebral artery. (*From FitzGerald MJT, Gruener G, Mtui E.* Clinical Neuroanatomy and Neuroscience. *6th ed. Philadelphia: Saunders; 2011.*)

Mnemonic of whether the cranial nerve (listed in order of CNs I through XII) carries **s**ensory signals, **m**otor signals, or **b**oth: "**S**ome **S**ay **M**arry **M**oney, **B**ut **M**y **B**rother **S**ays **B**ig **B**usiness **M**akes **M**oney."

In addition to knowing the name and functions of each CN, it is important to know the pathway they take in the base of the skull (Fig. 13.18). These pathways become important when discussing pathology.

Cribiform Plate: CN I goes through this and can be injured or transected in a trauma (e.g., nasal fracture), which can lead to temporary or permanent anosmia.

> The trigeminal nerve has "**S**tanding **R**oom **O**nly."
> V1: **S**uperior orbital fissure
> V2: Foramen **r**otundum
> V3: Foramen **o**vale

Middle Cranial Fossa

Optic canal: CN II, ophthalmic artery and central retinal vein.

Superior orbital fissure: CN III, IV, V1, VI, ophthalmic vein, and sympathetic fibers. Nerve blocks can be performed here for lacerations in the V1 distribution.

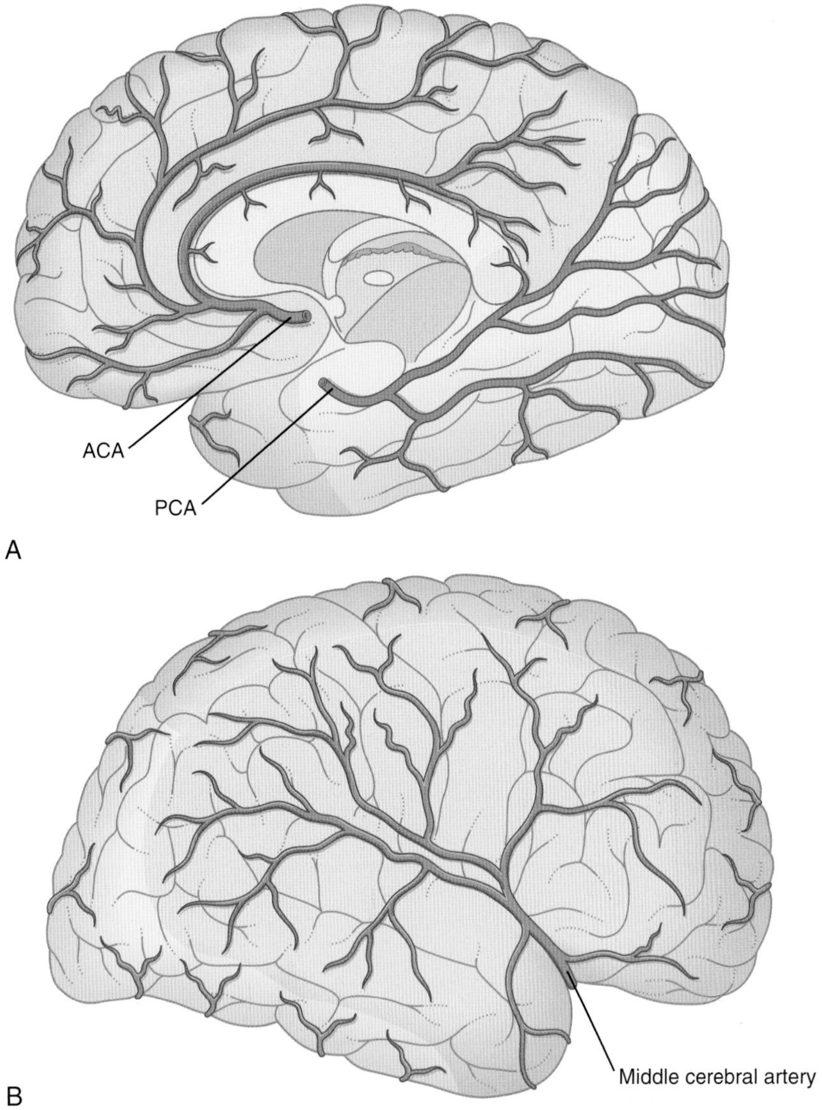

FIG. 13.15 Cerebral circulation with anterior cerebral artery (ACA) territory in blue, middle cerebral artery territory in red, and posterior cerebral artery (PCA) territory in orange. **A,** Medial view. **B,** Lateral view. (*From FitzGerald MJT, Gruener G, Mtui E.* Clinical Neuroanatomy and Neuroscience. *6th ed. Philadelphia: Saunders; 2011.*)

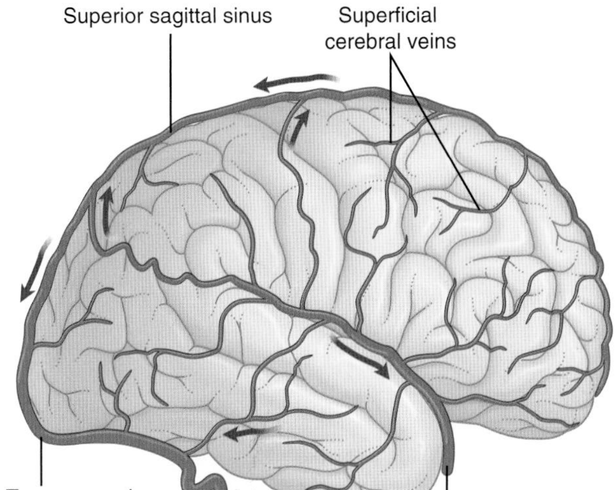

FIG. 13.16 Venous drainage of the brain. (*From FitzGerald MJT, Gruener G, Mtui E.* Clinical Neuroanatomy and Neuroscience. *6th ed. Philadelphia: Saunders; 2011.*)

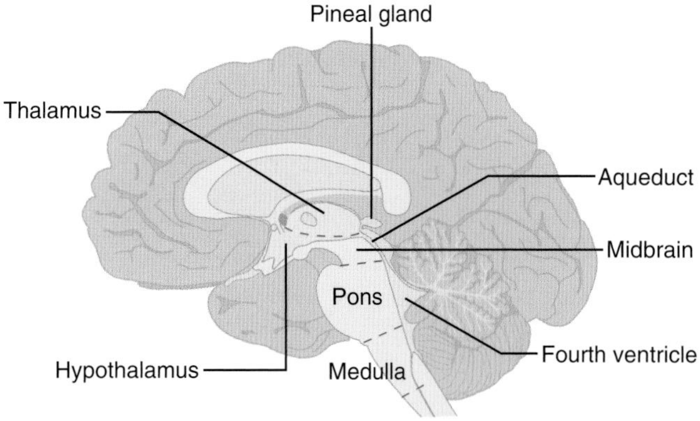

Fig. 13.17 Location of the medulla, pons, and midbrain. (*From Nolte J.* Elsevier's Integrated Neuroscience. *Philadelphia: Elsevier; 2007.*)

Table 13.1 The Cranial Nerves

NERVE NAME	CN	TYPE	FUNCTION
Olfactory	I	Sensory	Transmits sense of smell directly to cortex without thalamic relay
Optic	II	Sensory	Transmits visual signals from retina of the eye to the brain
Oculomotor	III	Motor	Eye movement (innervates the superior rectus, inferior rectus, medial rectus, inferior oblique); pupillary constriction (contains parasympathetics) via sphincter pupillae; eye accommodation via ciliary muscles; eyelid opening (innervates the levator palpebrae)
Trochlear	IV	Motor	Eye movement (innervates the superior oblique)
Trigeminal	V	Both	Motor—mastication (masseter, temporalis, medial pterygoid muscle to close jaw; lateral pterygoid muscle to open the jaw) Sensory—facial sensation via three divisions: ophthalmic (V1), maxillary (V2), and mandibular (V3). V1 is the afferent component of the corneal reflex.
Abducens	VI	Motor	Eye movement (innervates lateral rectus).
Facial	VII	Both	Motor—facial movement for expressions, lacrimation, salivation (except parotid), eyelid closing (orbicularis oculi muscle), sound dampening (stapedius ear muscle), and efferent component of corneal reflex. Sensory—taste (salt and sweet) from anterior two thirds of tongue (chorda tympani).
Vestibulocochlear	VIII	Sensory	Hearing and balance (rotation and gravity).
Glossopharyngeal	IX	Both	Motor—elevates pharynx and larynx via stylopharyngeus muscle, and salivation (parotid only). Sensory—taste from posterior third of tongue (sour and bitter), and monitors carotid body, sinus chemoreceptors and baroreceptors
Vagus	X	Both	Motor—laryngeal and pharyngeal muscles except stylopharyngeus muscle (swallowing, palate elevation, midline uvula, talking, coughing) Sensory—taste from epiglottis, parasympathetic autonomic nervous system fibers to thoracoabdominal viscera up to the splenic flexure, and aortic arch chemoreceptors and baroreceptors
Accessory	XI	Motor	Innervates sternocleidomastoid and trapezius muscles (head turning and shoulder shrug)
Hypoglossal	XII	Motor	Innervates all tongue muscles (end in *-glossus*) except palatoglossus (CN X) in tongue movement (swallowing and speech articulation)

Foramen rotundum: CN V2: Nerve blocks can be performed here for lacerations in the V2 distribution.

Foramen ovale: CN V3: Nerve blocks can be done here for lacerations in the V3 distribution.

The trigeminal nerve (CN V) is packed full of so many branches of nerves that there is **S**tanding **R**oom **O**nly (V1: **s**uperior orbital fissure; V2: foramen **r**otundum; V3: foramen **o**vale).

Foramen spinosum: Middle meningeal artery, a branch of the internal maxillary artery. Trauma to the head can damage this artery and cause an epidural hematoma.

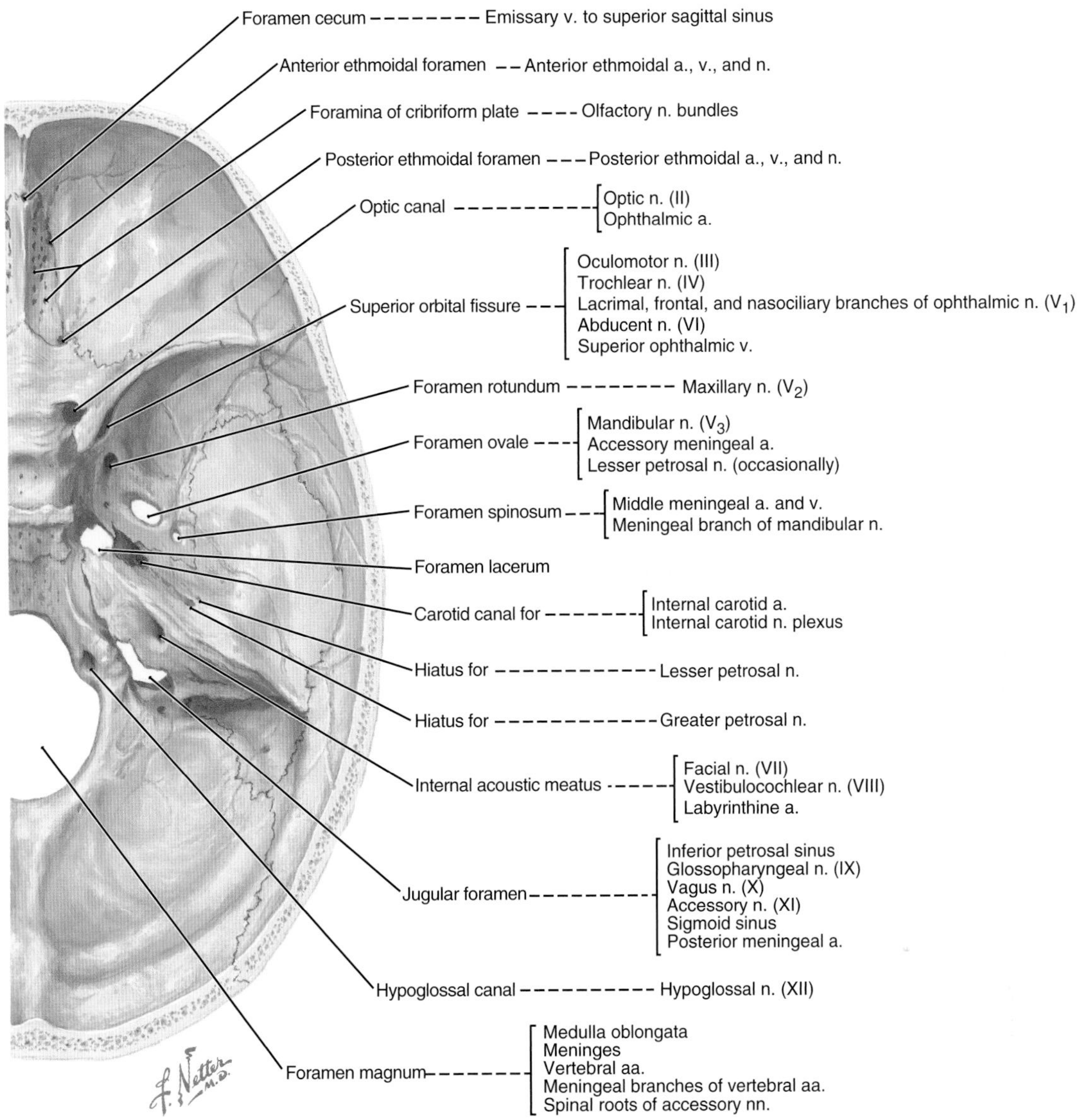

FIG. 13.18 Fossa in the cranium and the structures that pass through it. (*From Hansen J.* Netter's Clinical Anatomy, *2nd ed. Philadelphia: Elsevier; 2009.*)

Posterior Cranial Fossa

Internal auditory meatus: CNs VII, VIII: Schwannomas growing near this cause hearing loss.

Jugular foramen: CNs IX, X, XI, jugular vein: Lemierre's syndrome—thrombophlebitis of the internal jugular vein caused by head and neck infections.

Foramen magnum: CNs XI spinal roots, brainstem and vertebral arteries. Of note, this means that CN XI begins outside the skull, enters the skull through the foramen magnum, and then exits the skull again via the jugular foramen—the only CN to enter and exit the skull.

Hypoglossal canal: CN XII.

Cavernous Sinus

A collection of veins within the skull located lateral to the pituitary gland and superior to the sphenoid sinus (Fig. 13.19). It drains blood from the ophthalmic vein and superficial cortical veins into the internal jugular vein. It is important to know the structures running through this sinus because pathology affecting the cavernous sinus can affect the structures running through it.

One mnemonic for remembering the contents is "O TOM CAT": **O**culomotor nerve (CN III), **T**rochlear nerve (CN IV), **O**phthalmic nerve (CN V1), **M**axillary nerve (CN V2), **C**arotid artery (internal), **A**bducens nerve (CN VI), and **T**rochlear nerve (repeat).

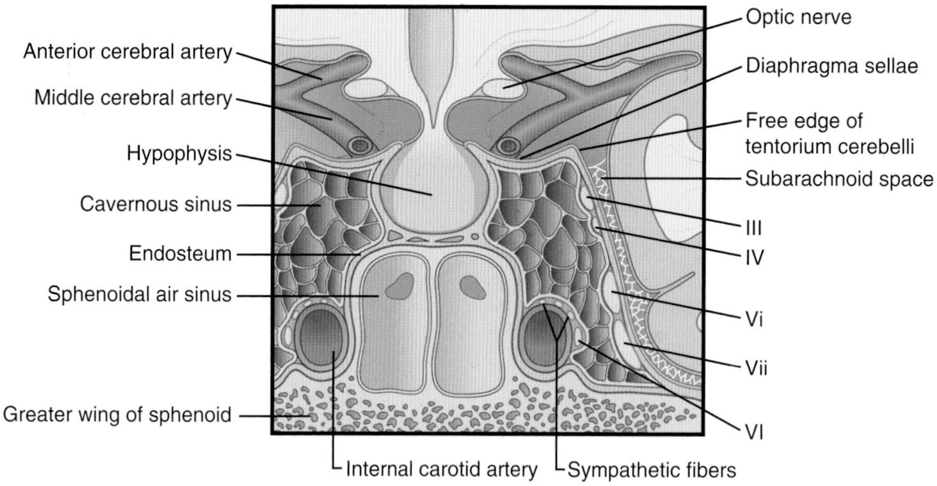

FIG. 13.19 Anatomy of the cavernous sinus. (*From FitzGerald MJT, Gruener G, Mtui E.* Clinical Neuroanatomy and Neuroscience. *6th ed. Philadelphia: Saunders; 2011.*)

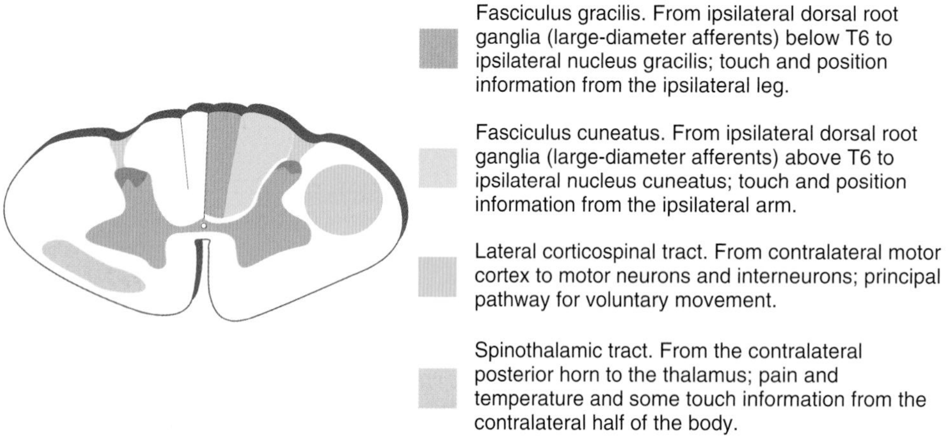
Fasciculus gracilis. From ipsilateral dorsal root ganglia (large-diameter afferents) below T6 to ipsilateral nucleus gracilis; touch and position information from the ipsilateral leg.
Fasciculus cuneatus. From ipsilateral dorsal root ganglia (large-diameter afferents) above T6 to ipsilateral nucleus cuneatus; touch and position information from the ipsilateral arm.
Lateral corticospinal tract. From contralateral motor cortex to motor neurons and interneurons; principal pathway for voluntary movement.
Spinothalamic tract. From the contralateral posterior horn to the thalamus; pain and temperature and some touch information from the contralateral half of the body.

FIG. 13.20 Cross section of the spinal cord. The dorsal columns are composed of the fasciculus gracilis (legs) and fasciculus cuneatus (arms). (*From Nolte J.* Essentials of the Human Brain. *Philadelphia: Elsevier; 2009.*)

When looking at the orientation of these structures, it is important to note that the abducens nerve and carotid artery run through the middle of the sinus, whereas other structures run along the lateral walls:

Mnemonic: CN "six sticks" to the carotid.

All the nerves pass through the superior orbital fissure, with the exception of CN V2 (exits via the foramen rotundum). The most commonly tested pathology of the cavernous sinus is the **cavernous sinus thrombosis,** where a blood clot forms in the cavernous sinus, usually as a result of an infection nearby spreading into the sinus. The classic symptoms include **visual changes, exophthalmos** (from an enlarged cavernous sinus pushing on the eye), **headache**, and **cranial nerve palsies**. The most commonly affected cranial nerve is the **abducens nerve (CN VI)**.

O TOM CAT
Oculomotor nerve (CN III)
Trochlear nerve (CN IV)
Ophthalmic nerve (CN V1)
Maxillary nerve (CN V2)
Carotid artery (internal)
Abducens nerve (CN VI)
Trochlear nerve (repeat)

Spinal Cord

The spinal cord houses the major motor and sensory tracts that interconnect the rest of the body to the brain (Fig. 13.20). It consists of **three major motor and sensory tracts**—dorsal (posterior) columns (Fig. 13.21), lateral corticospinal tracts (Fig. 13.22), and spinothalamic tracts (Fig. 13.23). Each specializes in conducting specific sensory information to the brain. The **dorsal column** provides **ascending** pressure, vibration, touch, and proprioceptive sensory information. The dorsal column is organized such that the axons responsible for touch sensation of the arms are located laterally, while those responsible for the legs are located medially. The lateral group of axons are called the fasciculus cuneatus (conveying sensory information from the upper body and upper extremities via C2-T6), and the medial group of axons are called the fasciculus gracilis (conveying sensory information from the lower body and lower extremities via T7 and below).

Mnemonic: Dancers are **graceful** because they know where their legs are, thanks to the fasciculus **gracilis**.

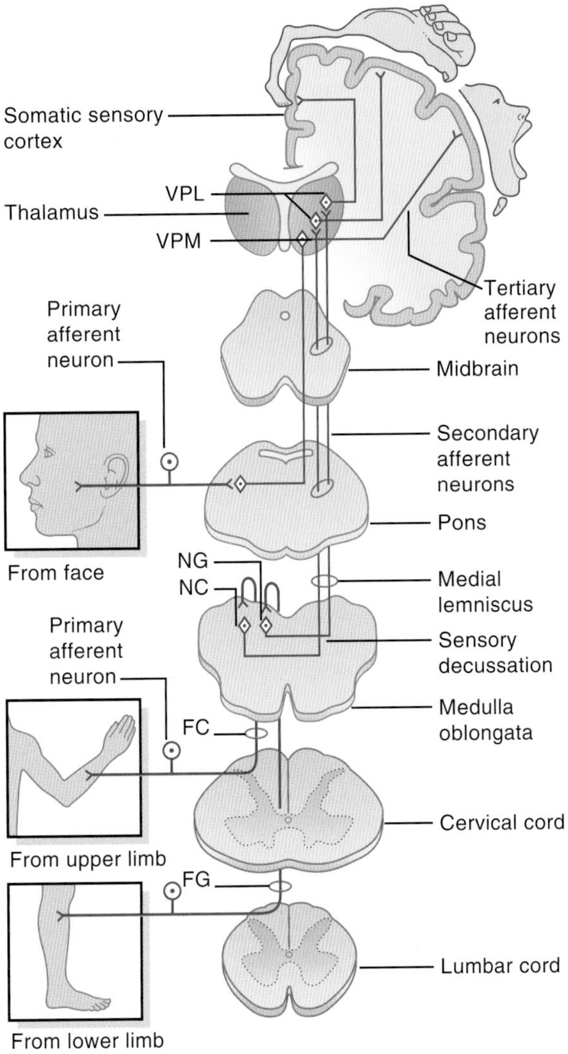

FIG. 13.21 Posterior (dorsal) column, medial lemniscal pathway. As shown, the decussation is in the brainstem; therefore, spinal lesions will cause ipsilateral loss of proprioception and vibratory sensation, whereas cortical lesions will cause contralateral loss. FC, Fasciculus cuneatus; FG, fasciculus gracilis; NC, nucleus cuneatus; NG, nucleus gracilis; VPL, VPM, ventral posterior lateral, ventral posterior medial nuclei of thalamus. (*From FitzGerald MJT, Gruener G, Mtui E.* Clinical Neuroanatomy and Neuroscience. *6th ed. Philadelphia: Saunders; 2011.*)

The **spinothalamic tract** provides **ascending** pain and temperature sensory information. The axons of the spinothalamic tract first ascend (travel rostrally) for a few spinal cord segments before crossing in the spinal cord via the anterior white commissure (anterior and midline in the spinal cord). The **lateral corticospinal tract** provides **descending** voluntary motor information to the contralateral limbs. These latter two tracts are organized as if someone is diving into the spinal cord, where the hands are medial and legs are lateral. The dorsal (posterior) columns and lateral corticospinal tracts cross sides (decussate) in the brainstem, whereas the spinothalamic tracts cross in the spinal cord. This nuance is important when talking about injuries to just half of the spinal cord (Brown-Séquard syndrome; see later).

Spinal nerves are a part of the PNS, where they exit the spinal cord carrying a **mix** of motor, sensory, and autonomic signals. There are 31 pairs of spinal nerves, which include 8 cervical spinal nerve pairs (C1-C8), 12 thoracic pairs, 5 lumbar pairs, 5 sacral pairs, and 1 coccygeal pair. Cervical spinal nerves (C1-7) exit above the corresponding vertebra, whereas the remaining spinal nerves exit below. The clinical significance of these nerves is that each spinal root supplies a specific myotome and dermatome, which can be used to localize lesions depending on the neurologic deficits seen on examination. For example, if vertebral disk herniation occurred at the nerve roots between L5 and S1 (the most common site of disk herniation), this could lead to difficulty with toe walking.

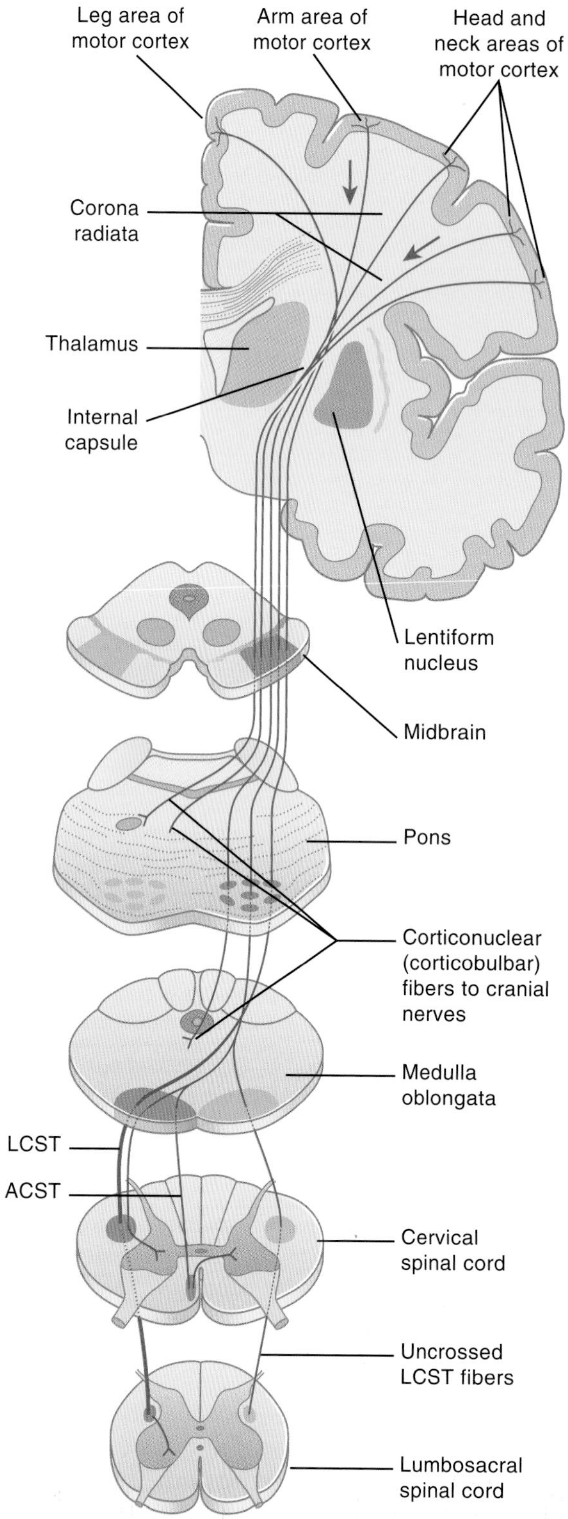

FIG. 13.22 Lateral corticospinal tract pathway. As shown, the decussation is in the brainstem; therefore, spinal lesions will cause ipsilateral paralysis, but lesions above the medulla will cause contralateral paralysis. ACST, anterior corticospinal tract; LCST, lateral corticospinal tract. (*From FitzGerald MJT, Gruener G, Mtui E.* Clinical Neuroanatomy and Neuroscience. *6th ed. Philadelphia: Saunders; 2011.*)

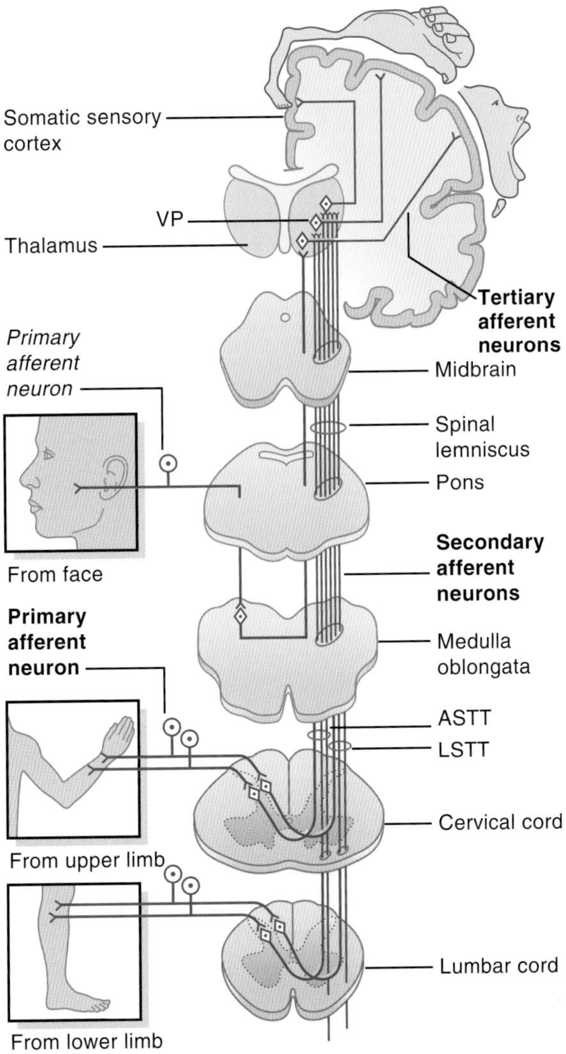

Fig. 13.23 Spinothalamic tract. The decussation of these fibers is different than that of the posterior (dorsal) column, medial lemniscal pathway, and lateral corticospinal tract pathway in that the decussation of the fibers is in the spinal cord itself. This becomes important in conditions such as Brown-Séquard syndrome. ASTT, anterior spinothalamic tract; LSTT, lateral spinothalamic tract; VP, ventral posterior nucleus of thalamus. (*From FitzGerald MJT, Gruener G, Mtui E.* Clinical Neuroanatomy and Neuroscience. *6th ed. Philadelphia: Saunders; 2011.*)

Important **dermatomes** to memorize in localizing lesions (Fig. 13.24) include **T4** (the nipple), **T10** (the umbilicus), **L1** (inguinal ligament), and the various parts of the feet. The medial foot is **L4,** the top of the foot is **L5,** and the lateral foot is **S1.**

Auditory Pathway

The ear is divided into three sections, with each playing a unique role in detecting sound. The external ear acts like a satellite dish to capture pressure waves (sound) and focus them on the eardrums. The air-filled middle ear (Fig. 13.25A) contains three ossicles (malleus, incus, and stapes). These ossicles mechanically convert the low pressure vibrations at the ear drum into amplified high pressure waves to cause fluid (perilymph) movement in the inner ear via the oval window. This fluid movement stimulates hair cells in the inner ear (cochlea), which transforms this mechanical movement into electrical signals in neurons (Fig. 13.25B). The electrical nerve impulses are now transmitted down cochlear fibers to the brain via the vestibulocochlear nerve. Before reaching the thalamus (medial geniculate nucleus [MGN]), and being relayed to the primary auditory cortex on the temporal lobe, they are processed at intermediate stations, such as the cochlear nuclei and superior olivary complex of the brainstem and inferior colliculus of the midbrain.

Before reaching the thalamus (MGN), auditory signals are processed at the cochlear nuclei, superior olivary complex, and inferior colliculus.

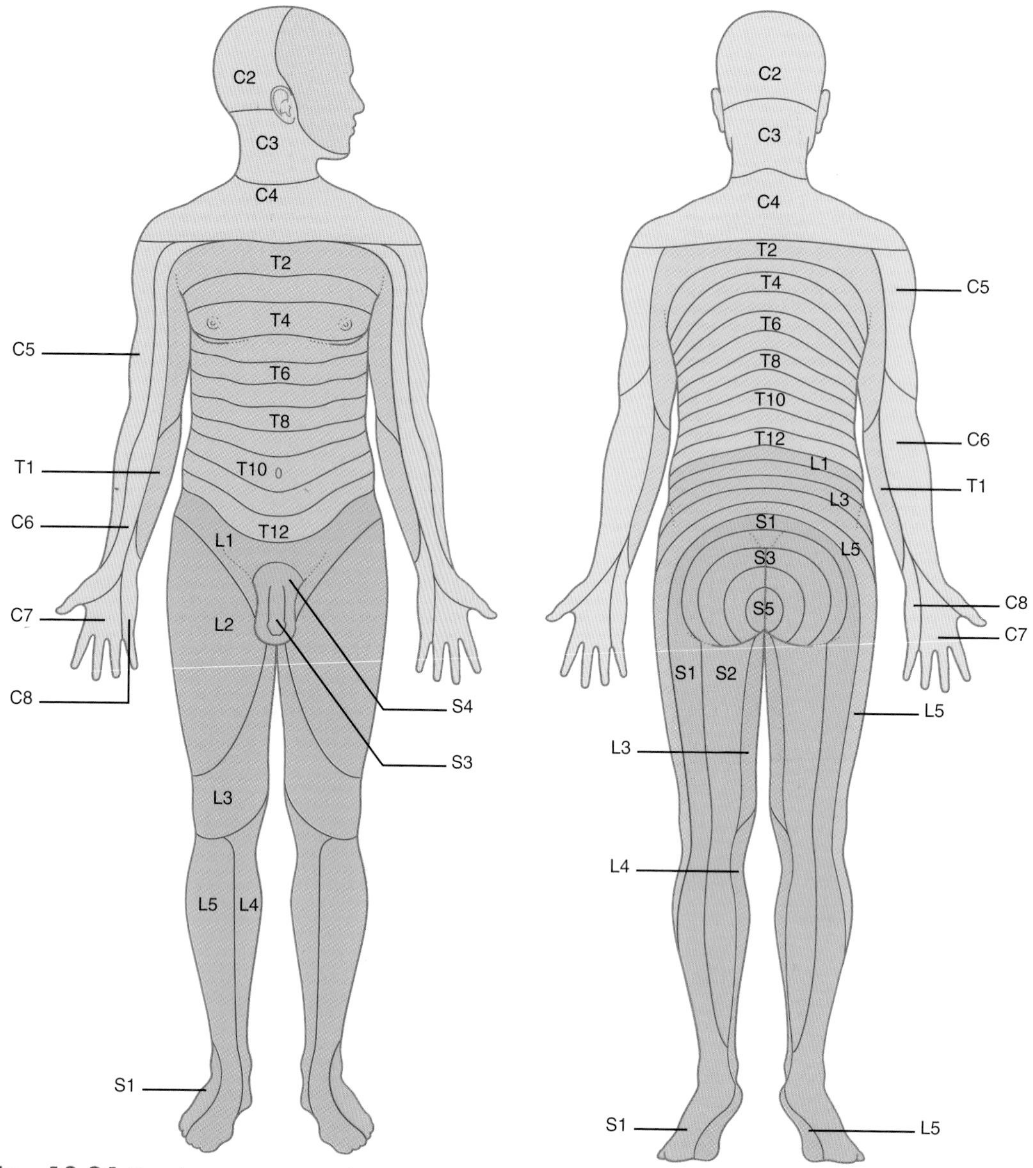

FIG. 13.24 The dermatome map. (*From FitzGerald MJT, Gruener G, Mtui E. Clinical Neuroanatomy and Neuroscience. 6th ed. Philadelphia: Saunders; 2011.*)

Vestibular Pathway

The vestibular system (Fig. 13.26) is another component of the inner ear, which is dedicated to balance. Three canals, oriented perpendicular to each other, provide sensory input for rotary movements, with the horizontal canal detecting horizontal head movement (e.g., spinning), and the superior and posterior canals detecting vertical head movement (e.g., nodding head). Each canal opens into the utricle and has a dilated sac at one end (ampulla), which houses the crista ampullaris (hair cells and supporting cells) in a gelatinous structure (cupula). Each canal is filled with endolymph, which lags behind as the head moves. This lag pushes opposite of the cupula, causing hair cells to bend, and depending on the tilt of the hair cells, excitatory (depolarizing) or inhibitory neural electrical signals are generated.

Visual System

The eye muscles (Fig. 13.27) are innervated by three cranial nerves (CNs III, IV, and VI). A good way to memorize which muscles are innervated by which cranial nerves is to think of the fictional molecule $LR_6SO_4R_3$, where the **L**ateral **R**ectus is innervated by CN **6**, **S**uperior **O**blique is innervated by CN **4**, and the **R**est innervated by CN **3**. Damage to a cranial nerve leads to specific findings when looking at the eye and testing these extraocular muscles (see later, "Eye Pathology").

Extraocular muscle innervation: $LR_6SO_4R_3$

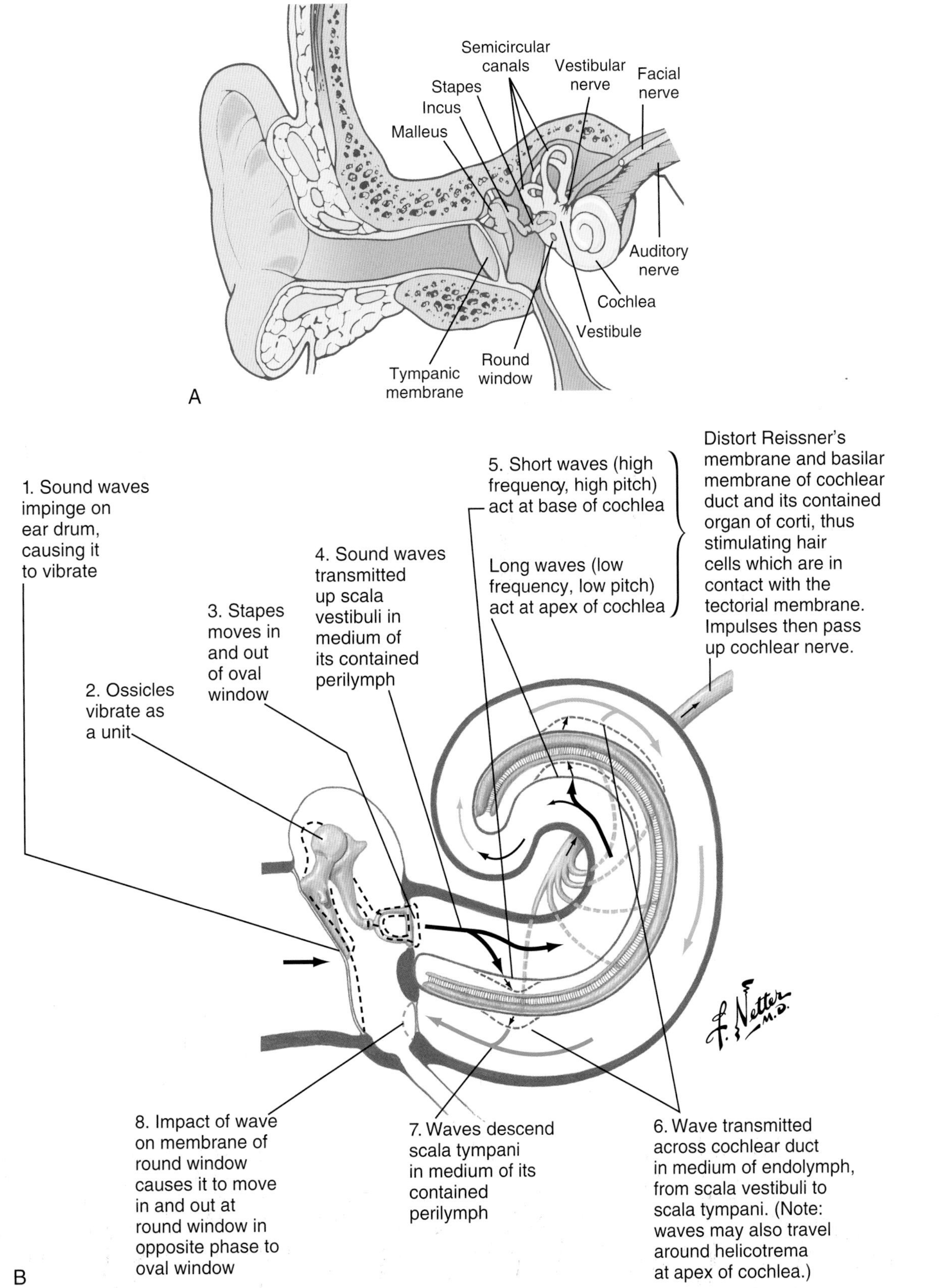
Semicircular canals
Vestibular nerve
Facial nerve
Stapes
Incus
Malleus
Auditory nerve
Cochlea
Vestibule
Round window
Tympanic membrane
A
1. Sound waves impinge on ear drum, causing it to vibrate
2. Ossicles vibrate as a unit
3. Stapes moves in and out of oval window
4. Sound waves transmitted up scala vestibuli in medium of its contained perilymph
5. Short waves (high frequency, high pitch) act at base of cochlea
Long waves (low frequency, low pitch) act at apex of cochlea
Distort Reissner's membrane and basilar membrane of cochlear duct and its contained organ of corti, thus stimulating hair cells which are in contact with the tectorial membrane. Impulses then pass up cochlear nerve.
8. Impact of wave on membrane of round window causes it to move in and out at round window in opposite phase to oval window
7. Waves descend scala tympani in medium of its contained perilymph
6. Wave transmitted across cochlear duct in medium of endolymph, from scala vestibuli to scala tympani. (Note: waves may also travel around helicotrema at apex of cochlea.)
B

Fig. 13.25 A, Auditory anatomy. **B,** The cochlea and the transmission of sound. (**A** *from Levy MN, Bruce M. Koeppen BM, Stanton BA.* Berne & Levy Principles of Physiology, *4th ed. Philadelphia: Elsevier; 2005;* **B** *from Felten DL, Shetty AN.* Netter's Atlas of Neuroscience. *Philadelphia: Elsevier; 2009.*)

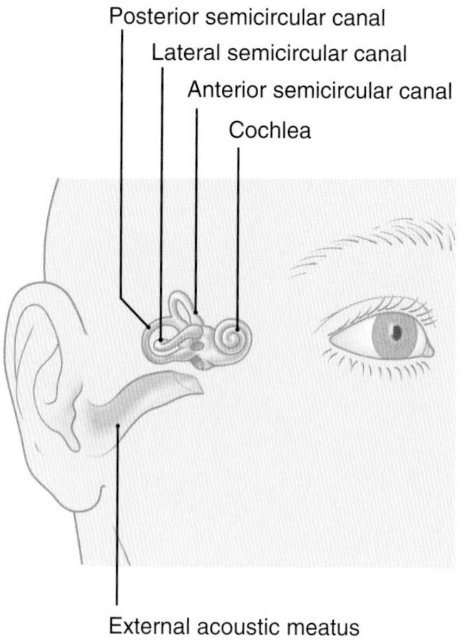

Fig. 13.26 The vestibular system is composed of three semicircular canals. The lateral canal detects horizontal head movements, whereas the superior and posterior canals detect vertical head movements. (*From Moses K, Nava P, Banks J, Petersen D.* Atlas of Clinical Gross Anatomy, *2nd ed. St. Louis: Elsevier; 2012.*)

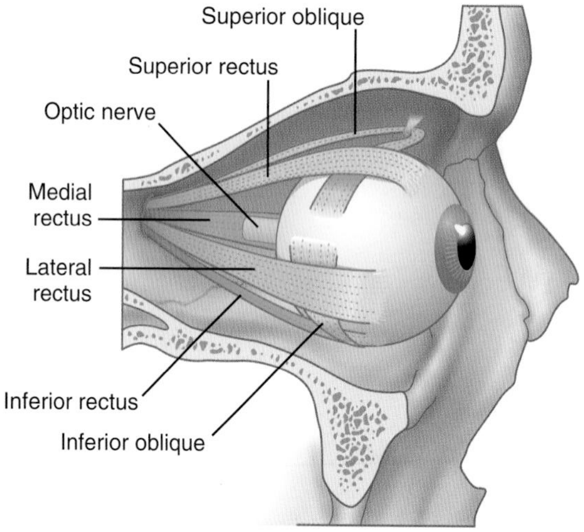

Fig. 13.27 Extraocular muscles. (*From FitzGerald MJT, Gruener G, Mtui E.* Clinical Neuroanatomy and Neuroscience. *6th ed. Philadelphia: Saunders; 2011.*)

The eyes convert light waves into electrochemical signals via the retina. Light is first refracted by the cornea, goes through the pupil (opening that is controlled by the iris), and is further refracted by the lens (whose shape is changed by the ciliary body) to project an inverted image on the retina (Fig. 13.28).

Rods: Contain rhodopsin

Cones: Contain photopsin (opsin + retinal)

The retina consists of layers that house two types of photoreceptor cells, cones (found in high density in the fovea, which is the most sensitive part of the macula; these are responsible for color perception, high visual acuity, and are light-adapted) and rods (found in retinal periphery, responsible for monochromic [black-white], night vision, low visual acuity). It also houses bipolar cells, which are an intermediary in transmitting signal from photoreceptors to ganglion cells. Photoreceptors contain rhodopsin (rods) or photopsin (cones), which are comprised of a large plasma membrane protein (opsin) bound to retinol (a vitamin A derivative), that is very important in the visual phototransduction process (light → electrochemical signal). Retinal exists as cis-retinal, which changes configuration into transretinal on light exposure and leads to activation of transducin (G protein), which activates cyclic guanosine monophosphate (cGMP) phosphodiesterase. This enzyme breaks down cGMP, leading to closure of sodium channels, hyperpolarizing the cell and stopping the release of NTs. These NTs generally inhibit the bipolar cells in the dark, but in the light they allow bipolar cells to transmit the signal to the optic nerve.

The signal is carried from the optic nerve to the optic chiasm, where nasal retinal fibers cross over. Nasal retinal fibers are those fibers on the retina closest to the nose, whereas temporal fibers are those

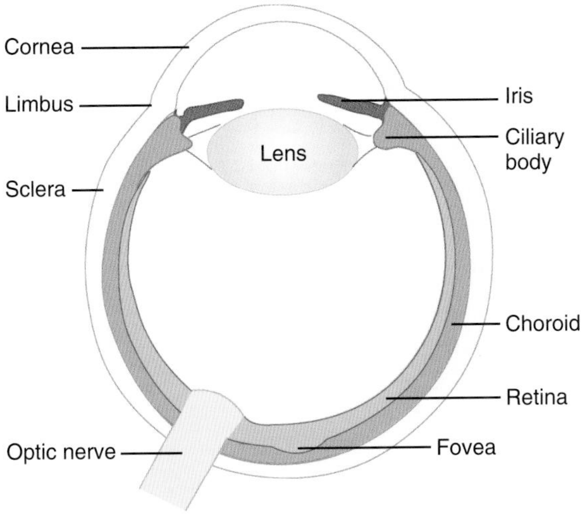

FIG. 13.28 Basic structures in the eye. (*From Telser AG, Young JK, Kate M. Baldwin KM.* Elsevier's Integrated Histology. *Philadelphia: Elsevier; 2007.*)

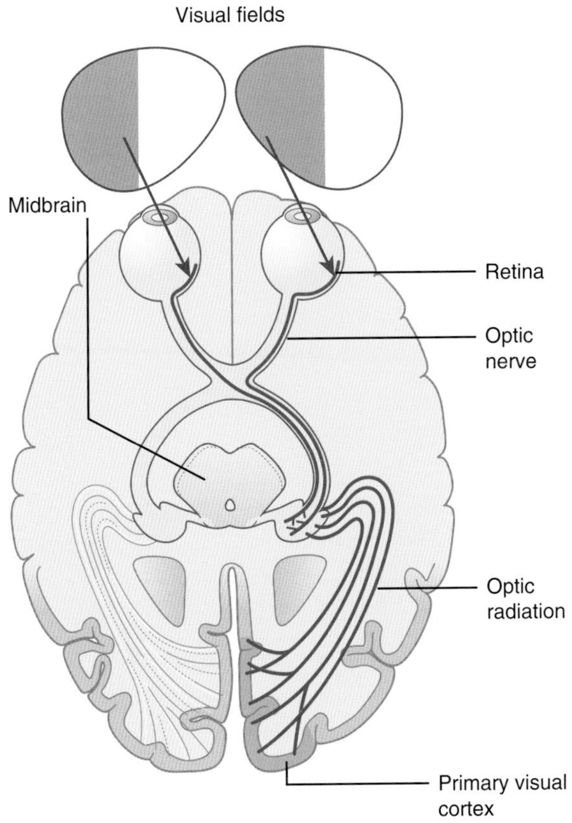

FIG. 13.29 The visual pathway, from the retina to the visual cortex. (*From FitzGerald MJT, Gruener G, Mtui E.* Clinical Neuroanatomy and Neuroscience. *6th ed. Philadelphia: Saunders; 2011.*)

on the lateral retina, closest to the temples. Beyond the optic chiasm, the optic nerve continues as the optic tract, which carries the crossed and uncrossed fibers to the LGN of the thalamus. From the LGN, the signal is carried to the pretectal nucleus of the midbrain (involved in pupillary reflex) and the visual cortex (occipital lobe) by optic radiations (Fig. 13.29). The optic radiations are split into two parts. Fibers from the inferior retina (Meyer's loop) carry information from the superior part of the visual field, passing through the temporal lobe by looping around the temporal horn of the lateral ventricle, and synapsing in the occipital cortex. Fibers from the superior retina (Baum's loop) carry information from the inferior part of the visual field on a shorter pathway (less susceptible to damage) through the parietal lobe. Lesions along these pathways, from the retina to the visual cortex, can lead to various visual field defects (see later, "Eye Pathology").

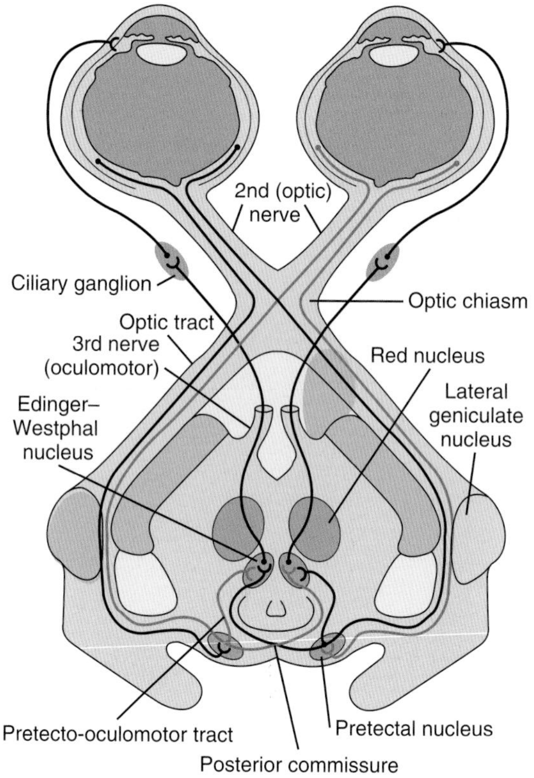

FIG. 13.30 The pupillary light reflex. (*From Liporace J: Crash Course: Neurology. Philadelphia: Mosby; 2006.*)

In the pupillary light reflex (Fig. 13.30), neurons from the pretectal nucleus run to the Edinger-Westphal nucleus, which receives bilateral input from the pretectal nuclei. From here, presynaptic neurons synapse at the ciliary ganglion and postsynaptic neurons innervate the pupillary sphincter muscle (sphincter pupillae), causing pupillary constriction (miosis).

Electroencephalogram (EEG)

Similar to how an electrocardiogram (ECG) records the electrical activity of the heart, an EEG records the electrical activity of the brain. Clinically, neurologists can use the EEG for the diagnoses of epilepsy (ictal discharges), coma, encephalopathies (triphasic waves), and brain death. It is important to keep the following in mind:

Awake:

- Eyes open → beta waves (high frequency, low amplitude).
- Eyes closed → alpha waves.

Sleep: As discussed earlier, the circadian rhythm is oscillated by the suprachiasmatic nucleus in the hypothalamus, which is regulated by one's environment (i.e., light via photosensitive ganglion cells). The pineal gland acts as a transducer upon stimulation by norepinephrine release from the suprachiasmatic nucleus to release melatonin.

As one goes into deeper stages of sleep, these waves slow down.

- Stage 1 → theta waves (presleep, or nodding off with slow eye movement). Also known as relaxed wakefulness.
- Stage 2 → sleep spindles and K complexes (most prominent form with NO eye movement; accounts for ≈50% of sleep during the night).
- Stage 3 → delta waves (this is the stage where sleep walking, bedwetting, parasomnias and night terrors occur).
- Rapid eye movement (REM) → beta waves (EEG looks as if the patient were awake, but muscles are paralyzed. REM sleep is when dreams occur. Disrupted REM sleep is thought to be the cause of sleep paralysis).
  - Disrupted REM sleep associated with alcohol, benzodiazepines and barbiturate use.

PATHOLOGY

Developmental Disorders

Disruption during the development of the nervous system can be disastrous, leading to a variety of conditions listed below.

Neural Tube Defects

Failure of the neural tube to close can lead to a continuum of these defects extending from anencephaly to subtypes of spina bifida (see Chapter 4).

Hydrocephalus

This literally translates to "water in the brain" caused by the excess accumulation of CSF in the ventricular system of the brain from impaired CSF flow (e.g., obstruction), resorption, or excessive production of various causes. Because of the enclosed space of the skull, signs of increased intracranial pressure (ICP) develop, such as headaches, nausea, vomiting, papilledema, sleepiness, coma, and even death caused by herniation. It is important to note that in infants, ICP symptoms present as irritability, poor feeding, muscle hypertonia, hyperreflexia, and a bulging fontanelle. Treatment often includes opening up the ventricles (ventriculostomy) or placement of cerebral shunts. Shunts can bypass outflow obstructions or drain excessive CSF into body cavities, such as the abdominal peritoneal cavity, where it can be resorbed. Based on the underlying mechanism, hydrocephalus can be categorized into communicating and noncommunicating categories. They can be further subdivided into congenital or acquired.

Noncommunicating, Obstructive

There is CSF **outflow obstruction** in the ventricular system.

Congenital: Caused by atresia or webs within the ventricular system (e.g., within the cerebral aqueduct of Sylvius), Arnold-Chiari malformation, or Dandy-Walker syndrome.

- Arnold-Chiari malformation: Malformation of the brain in which there is a downward herniation of the cerebellar tonsils through the foramen magnum. Conditions associated with this malformation include syringomyelia and connective tissue disorders, such as Ehlers-Danlos and Marfan's syndrome.
- Dandy Walker syndrome (DWS): Consists of partial or complete absence of the cerebellar vermis, enlargement of the fourth ventricle, and cyst formation near the internal base of the skull. DWS is associated with corpus callosum absence and karyotype abnormalities.

> Arnold-Chiari malformation: Congenital downward herniation of cerebellar tonsils through the foramen magnum

Acquired:

- Following subarachnoid hemorrhage, causes obstruction within the channels of the ventricular system (e.g., stenosis of aqueduct of Sylvius).
- Underlying brain tumor (e.g., ependymoma, medulloblastoma, colloid cyst) within the ventricular system or one causing external compression of the ventricular system.

Communicating, Nonobstructive

There is **impaired CSF resorption** by arachnoid granulations or villi caused by scarring or fibrosis following infectious, inflammatory, or hemorrhagic events, such as postmeningitis or arachnoid bleeds.

Normal pressure hydrocephalus (NPH): This disease entity is **often misdiagnosed** as Parkinson disease or Alzheimer disease because of the chronic, insidious nature of the symptoms. Because of the chronic dilation of the ventricular system, NPH presents classically with the **triad of urinary incontinence, gait disturbance (ataxia), and dementia** in older adults, despite having normal CSF pressures on lumbar puncture. This constellation of symptoms is often termed ***wet, wobbly, and wacky.*** The gait disturbance is typically an early and prominent feature of NPH and can help distinguish this disease from other forms of dementia, in which gait disturbance may be a late symptom. Treatment is with a ventriculoperitoneal shunt that drains the excess CSF to the abdominal peritoneal cavity. If performed early, shunting can reverse the symptoms.

Hydrocephalus Ex Vacuo: There is a compensatory enlargement of CSF because of **atrophy or loss of brain parenchyma** caused by various diseases, despite no increased CSF pressure (e.g., posttraumatic brain injury) and dementias (e.g., Alzheimer, Pick's, Huntington dementia).

Signs of increased ICP, such as papilledema, can also be confused with another disease process known as idiopathic intracranial hypertension (IIH), formerly known as pseudotumor cerebri. IIH is seen in young obese females, who present with headache, nausea and vomiting. They may also complain of pulsatile tinnitus (described as whooshing or buzzing), diplopia (CN VI palsy), and deteriorating vision, eventually leading to blindness if not treated. The mechanism of this disease process is poorly understood, with speculation that it is caused by increased CSF production or decreased venous drainage from the brain. On funduscopy, these patients have papilledema. Computed tomography (CT) scans will reveal no mass, but sometimes small slitlike ventricles and an empty sella sign can be seen. Diagnosis is usually made by measuring the opening lumbar puncture (LP) pressure, which is greatly elevated.

Think IIH in young obese women with headache and papilledema.

Treatment of this condition starts with drainage of excess CSF by LP; serial LPs may be necessary. Acetazolamide also decreases CSF production. Patients should also discontinue medications that increase ICP, such as high-dose vitamin A derivatives (e.g., isotretinoin for acne), tetracycline, hormonal contraceptives and danazol. Surgery is a last resort, in which a CSF shunt (lumboperitoneal) and optic nerve decompression via fenestration can be performed.

Syringomyelia: Also known as a **syrinx.** A cystic cavity forms within the spinal cord, which expands over time, leading to pain, weakness, and paralysis. Upper extremities are usually affected because of a mass effect on the spinothalamic tracts. The **dorsal column is usually spared** (pressure, vibration, touch and proprioception remain intact). Typically, this disease presents as a **capelike** loss of pain and temperature sensation in the back and arms. A syrinx can be congenital or associated with Arnold-Chiari malformation. It can also be acquired as a complication of trauma, meningitis, or tumor.

Syringomyelia is highly associated with Arnold-Chiari malformation. Look for loss of sensation in a capelike distribution.

Neurocutaneous Syndromes

Also known as phakomatoses, theses syndromes present with lesions on the skin or eye.

Neurofibromatosis (NF):

- NF type 1 autosomal dominant mutation of NF1 on chromosome 17, which is a tumor suppressor that inhibits p21 ras oncoprotein. This mutation leads to uncontrolled cell proliferation. Characteristics include subcutaneous neurofibromas, groin and axillary freckling, café au lait spots (light brown macules), Lisch nodules (iris hamartomas), optic nerve gliomas, and epilepsy.
- NF type 2 (central NF) autosomal dominant mutation of merlin on chromosome 22, which is also a tumor suppressor gene. This leads to **bilateral vestibular schwannomas** (formerly known as acoustic neuromas) that cause sensorineural hearing loss. Schwannomas of other cranial nerves, meningiomas, and ependymomas may also be seen. Think **NF 2: 2-22-2** (NF **2** is chromosome **22** and can cause **2** [bilateral] acoustic neuromas).

NF1: Neurofibromas, axillary freckling, café au lait spots, iris hamartomas, optic gliomas, and epilepsy

NF2: Bilateral acoustic neuromas (schwannomas)

Tuberous Sclerosis: Autosomal dominant mutation of hamartin or tuberin, which are tumor suppressors, leading to a **multisystem disease** that has a **variable penetrance.** Signs include facial angiofibromas (adenoma sebaceum), hypomelanic macules (ash leaf spots), Shagreen patches (a raised or textured skin lesion), cortical tubers, cardiac rhabdomyomas, and renal angiomyolipomas.

Sturge-Weber Syndrome: Occurring sporadically because of embryonal development anomalies (GNAQ mutation), this syndrome presents with seizures at birth and is associated with **port wine stain** of the face ("nevus flammeus" in CN V_1/V_2 distribution [forehead and upper eyelid]), early onset glaucoma, mental retardation, and **ipsilateral leptomeningioma,** which increases contralateral seizure/epilepsy likelihood.

von Hippel-Lindau (VHL) Disease: Autosomal dominant mutation of VHL tumor suppressor gene on chromosome 3 leads to hemangioblastomas (retina, kidney, spine, brainstem, or cerebellum) and angiomatosis (various organs), often associated with renal angioma, renal cell carcinoma, pancreatic cysts, cystadenomas and pheochromocytoma.

Brain Lesions

Understanding anatomy and relating it to the respective function is key in localizing neurologic lesions. Table 13.2 is a list of common pathologic examples that can be encountered.

Aphasia

Aphasia is an impairment of language ability that ranges from not remembering words to being completely unable to speak, read, or write, depending on the area and extent of the dominant side of the brain affected (Table 13.3). It usually follows a stroke, but can develop from conditions such as an infection, tumor, or brain injury. In contrast, dysarthria is the motor inability to speak.

Table 13.2 Brain Lesions and Their Resulting Symptoms

LOCATION	RESULT
Frontal lobe	Lack of executive functions leads to disinhibition and reemergence of primitive reflexes.
Nondominant parietal lobe	Hemispatial neglect (agnosia of the contralateral side of the world)
Dominant parietal lobe	Gerstmann syndrome—agraphia, acalculia, finger agnosia
Amygdala	Klüver–Bucy syndrome—disinhibition, psychic blindness (visual agnosia), hyperorality, hypersexuality
Hippocampus	Unable to form new memories (anterograde amnesia); unable to form new long-term memories if bilateral lesion
Basal ganglia	Motor symptoms, such as tremor, chorea, athetosis
Mammillary bodies	Wernicke-Korsakoff syndrome, which consists of Wernicke encephalopathy (confusion, ophthalmoplegia, ataxia) and Korsakoff psychosis (anterograde and retrograde memory loss, confabulation, personality changes); petechial hemorrhages seen in limbic system on pathology.
Subthalamic nucleus	Contralateral hemiballismus
Cerebellar hemisphere	Ipsilateral deficits, including tremor and limb ataxia
Cerebellar vermis	Dysarthria and truncal ataxia
Frontal eye fields	Eyes deviate toward lesion.
Paramedian pontine reticular formation	Eyes deviate away from lesion.
Superior colliculus	Parinaud syndrome—upward gaze paralysis
Reticular activating system	Reduced level of conscious, leading to difficulty in arousal and wakefulness

Table 13.3 Aphasias

APHASIA TYPE	FLUENCY	COMPREHENSION	NAMING	REPETITION	LESION	PRESENTATION
Broca (motor, expressive)	Nonfluent	Intact	Difficult	Impaired	Inferior, frontal gyrus	Broken speech of Broca aphasia (speaks in short meaningful phrases)
Wernicke (sensory, receptive)	Fluent	Impaired	Difficult	Impaired	Superior, temporal gyrus	Long wordy speech of Wernicke with no meaning
Global	Nonfluent	Impaired	Difficult	Impaired	Both Wernicke and Broca areas	Limited speech and comprehension
Anomic	Fluent	Intact	Difficult	Preserved	Temporal or parietal area	Unable to recall words or names
Conduction	Fluent	Intact	Intact	Impaired	Arcuate fasciculus	Connection between speech comprehension and production area impaired

Vascular Dysfunction

Causes of embolic stroke: Carotid stenosis, atrial fibrillation, endocarditis, PFO (paradoxical emboli)

Similar to a myocardial infarction (MI), a stroke is caused by impeded blood flow leading to specific neurologic deficits, depending on the area of the brain affected. Just as time is muscle in a myocardial infarction, time is brain in a stroke. Irreversible damage develops within a few minutes, so reperfusion with therapies such as tissue plasminogen activator (tPA; see later, "Pharmacology") quickly is important. Strokes can be classified by their etiology, either ischemic or hemorrhagic. Most strokes are ischemic (85%) because of embolic phenomenon from atherosclerotic lesions or atrial fibrillation. Carotid dissection (primary or secondary to aortic dissection), endocarditis, or a patent foramen ovale (allowing a blood clot in the leg that travels from the right atrium to the left atrium, and then to the left ventricle and brain; these are called "paradoxical emboli") also cause ischemic strokes. Approximately 15% of strokes are hemorrhagic, in which intracerebral bleeding results directly from vessel rupture or hemorrhagic conversion from an ischemic stroke because of increased vessel fragility. A CT scan is used to differentiate between ischemic and hemorrhagic stroke initially, followed by magnetic resonance imaging (MRI; diffusion-weighted imaging). Before a stroke, a patient may have experienced a transient ischemic attack (TIA), in which they experience brief neurologic dysfunction that lasts less than 24 hours without acute infarction. For example, some patients experience **amaurosis fugax**, which is a painless transient loss of vision caused by atherosclerotic embolization, usually at the carotid body, to the retinal arteries, while others may

Table 13.4 Brainstem Strokes

OCCLUSION SYNDROME	VASCULATURE AFFECTED	SYMPTOMS
Medial medullary syndrome	Vertebral artery, anterior spinal artery	Contralateral hemiparesis (arm + leg), contralateral decreased proprioception/sensation, ipsilateral tongue (hypoglossal nerve) paralysis; facial sparing
Lateral medullary syndrome (Wallenberg syndrome)	Posterior inferior cerebellar artery (PICA)	Contralateral loss of pain and temperature, ipsilateral facial pain and temperature (sensory signs and symptoms only), vomiting, vertigo, nystagmus (vestibular nuclei), dysphagia, hoarseness (nucleus ambiguous).
Lateral inferior pontine syndrome	Anterior inferior cerebellar artery (AICA)	Ipsilateral facial pain and temperature loss, ipsilateral facial paralysis
Locked-in syndrome	Basilar artery	Anterior pons infarction leads to quadriparesis (face and eyes also), but vertical gaze (CN III), pontine tegmentum, and reticular formation spared (consciousness preserved).
Foville syndrome	Perforating basilar arteries	Contralateral hemiparesis, hemisensory loss, and internuclear ophthalmoplegia (INO); ipsilateral horizontal gaze palsy and facial paralysis
Weber syndrome	Paramedian branches of posterior cerebral artery (PCA)	Contralateral parkinsonism, hemiparesis, lower facial muscle paralysis, and hypoglossal nerve paralysis; ipsilateral CN III palsy.

have aphasia, slurred speech (dysarthria) or confusion. TIAs are usually a harbinger of an impending stroke and usually warrant a workup as an outpatient or inpatient depending on various factors (e.g., $ABCD^2$ score).

Stroke

- **Anterior cerebral artery:** Supplies anteromedial hemispheric surface, where leg-foot motor and sensory areas are affected.
- **Middle cerebral artery:** Supplies lateral hemispheric surface, where face-arm motor and sensory areas are affected. In addition, patients may show aphasias (Broca or Wernicke's aphasia) if the dominant lobe is involved (usually the left).
- **Posterior cerebral artery:** Supplies posterior and inferior hemispheric surface, where homonymous hemianopsia with macular sparing can occur.

Aneurysm: An aneurysm is a balloon-like bulge of a blood vessel that involves all three layers of an artery (intima, media, and adventitia). An aneurysm may rupture, causing subarachnoid hemorrhage.

- **Saccular or Berry aneurysm:** Occurs at bifurcations in the circle of Willis, where rupture leads to hemorrhagic strokes or subarachnoid hemorrhage. Often associated with Marfan's syndrome, Ehler-Danlos syndrome, and adult polycystic kidney disease.
  - Anterior communicating artery: Most common location of aneurysm, where lesions lead to bitemporal hemianopsia
  - Posterior communicating artery: Common site of aneurysm, which can lead to CN III palsy (eyes down and out)
- **Charcot-Bouchard microaneurysm:** Chronic hypertension leads to rupture of small vessels, usually within the basal ganglia, pons and thalamus, which is not typically seen on angiograms.

Venous:

- **Dural sinus thrombosis**: Rare stroke that results from the thrombosis of the dural venous sinus, resulting in strokelike symptoms, headaches, weakness and seizures. A CT scan shows an empty delta sign (contrast enhancement of the sinus wall and periphery of the clot, but not within the clot itself).

Brainstem: Unlike cerebrum strokes, brainstem strokes often involve cranial nerves (Table 13.4). Most notably, brainstem strokes show alternating signs; CN involvement and hemiparesis are on opposite sides.

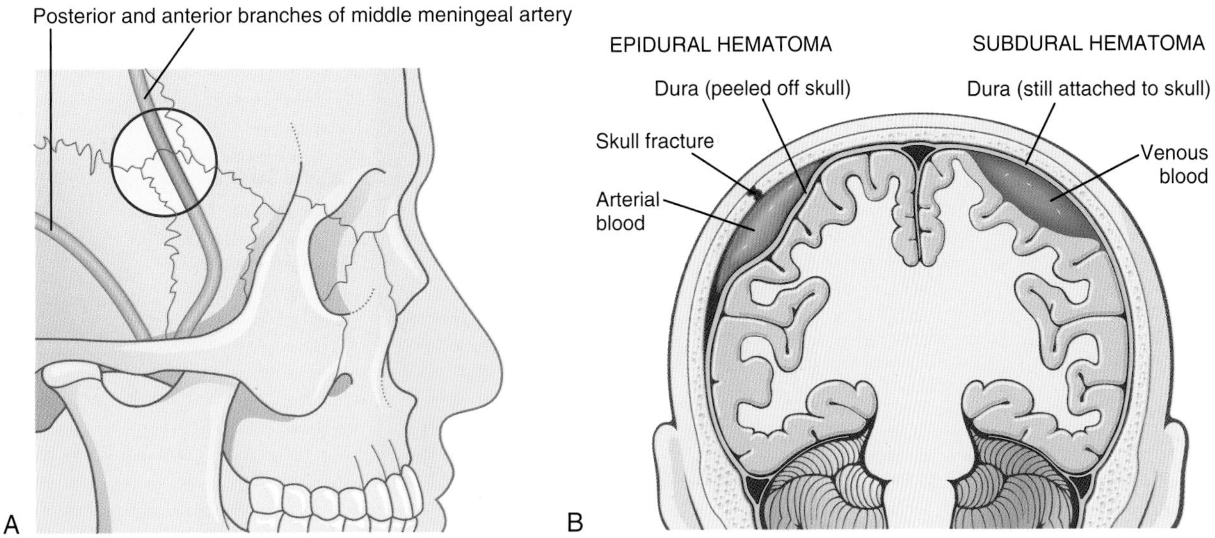

Fig. 13.31 **A,** The middle meningeal artery is injured in epidural hematomas. The blue circle is over the pterion. **B,** Comparison between epidural and subdural hematomas. Note that because the dura is so firmly adherent to the skull at the suture lines, epidural hematomas are not strong enough to peel the dura off the sutures and therefore cannot cross suture lines. However, subdural hematomas are under the dura (hence, subdural) and therefore can cross suture lines. (***A*** *from FitzGerald MJT, Gruener G, Mtui E.* Clinical Neuroanatomy and Neuroscience. *6th ed. Philadelphia: Saunders; 2011;* ***B*** *from Kumar V, Abbas AK, Fausto N, Aster J.* Robbins & Cotran Pathologic Basis of Disease. *8th ed. New York: Elsevier; 2009.*)

Trauma

Traumatic brain injury (TBI) is a major cause of death and disability worldwide, especially for young adults. In TBI, or any situation of altered mental status, a patient's level of consciousness (eye, verbal and motor response) is graded based on the Glasgow Coma Scale (GCS). The scale ranges from 3 to 15 and classifies brain injuries as mild (13 to 15), moderate (9 to 12), or severe (3 to 8). Endotracheal intubation is generally recommended in severe head injury (GCS ≤8).

Classification

Diffuse:

- Diffuse axonal injury is a devastating type of TBI due to shearing forces from a sudden acceleration or deceleration of the head. Diagnosis is usually made via MRI because it is difficult to detect on a CT. Patients generally end up staying in a coma and never regaining consciousness.

Focal:

Epidural hematoma: As a result of temporal bone fracture from trauma at the **pterion** (weakest part of skull; Fig. 13.31A), the **middle meningeal artery** can rupture, leading to a buildup of the blood between the dura mater and skull. Patients generally have a **lucid interval**, but soon rapidly deteriorate because of transtentorial herniation (see later) as a result of expansion of the hematoma under systemic arterial pressure. CT generally shows a **"biconvex" lens** that **does not cross suture lines**, but can cross the falx and tentorium (dural reflections).

> Epidural hematoma CT: "Biconvex" lens that does not cross suture lines

Subdural hematoma (SDH): Bleeding between the dura and arachnoid membrane (Fig. 13.31B) from the rupture of **small bridging veins** as a result of rapid changes in velocity (acceleration or deceleration in whiplash or shaking). It is commonly seen in older adults and alcoholics because of **brain atrophy**, which increases the subdural space and results in a wider distance in which the veins have to travel, making them vulnerable to tear. The same principle applies to children from shaken baby syndrome, who tend to have larger subdural spaces because of their smaller brains. Unlike an epidural hematoma, subdural bleeds are **slow venous bleeds with delayed onset of symptoms**. As pressure (ICP) gradually increases, patients begin to have increasing headache and confusion. CT generally shows blood collecting in a **crescent-shaped** pattern that **crosses suture lines**, but cannot cross the dural reflections.

> Infants, alcoholics, and older adults are all at risk for subdural hematomas.

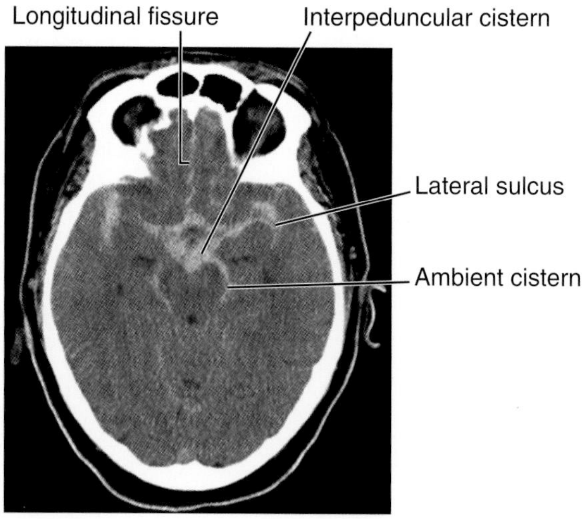

FIG. 13.32 CT scan of subarachnoid hemorrhage showing blood (the more dense white signal) in the areas normally occupied by the cerebrospinal fluid (normally a less dense and more black signal), such as the cisterns shown in the image. This is why a lumbar puncture can be used for diagnosis; the blood is in the CSF itself. (*From Nolte J.* The Human Brain. *6th ed. Philadelphia: Elsevier; 2008.*)

Subarachnoid Hemorrhage (SAH): Bleeding between the arachnoid membrane and pia mater surrounding the brain results from **rupture of a cerebral aneurysm** (especially berry aneurysms in Marfan's syndrome, Ehlers-Danlos syndrome, and polycystic kidney disease) or arteriovenous malformation (AVM), spontaneously or from trauma (Fig. 13.32). Patients generally complain of sudden onset of the **"worst headache of my life"** or may present beforehand with warning leaks as general headaches. Most SAHs are detected on CT after the onset of bleeding, which shows blood in the cisterns and filling of blood along the sulci and fissures. If a CT scan is negative, a lumbar puncture is performed and CSF collected, which may show elevated blood cells equally in all tubes collected, or the CSF may appear yellow **(xanthochromic)** because of the bilirubin (breakdown of heme from red blood cells). Treatment consists of preventing rebleeding (clipping or coiling aneurysms), seizures, vasospasm (treat with calcium channel blocker nimodipine), and hydrocephalus.

Intracerebral Hemorrhage (ICH): This is bleeding within the brain tissue itself that can occur as a result of trauma (e.g., skull fracture, AVM), stroke, bleeding within a tumor, or amyloid angiopathy. ICH risk factors include hypertension, diabetes, menopause, current cigarette smoking, and alcoholism.

Basilar Skull Fracture: Traumatic fracture involving the base of the skull (temporal, occipital, sphenoid and ethmoid bone), leading to damage to the meninges. As a result, there can be CSF rhinorrhea or otorrhea and ecchymosis of the mastoid process of the temporal bone **(Battle sign)** or periorbital ecchymosis (**raccoon eyes**) (Fig. 13.33).

Basilar skull fractures may present with raccoon eyes, Battle sign, and CSF rhinorrhea or otorrhea.

Cerebral Contusion: This is literally a bruise to the brain caused by **multiple microhemorrhages** from small blood vessel leaks. An example is **coup contrecoup** injury, in which the coup injury occurs at the site of impact and the contrecoup injury occurs on the side opposite the impact, where the brain recoils against the skull.

Herniation

This is a serious consequence of very high ICP or mass effect that results from a traumatic brain injury, tumor, or stroke. The skull is a closed cavity that cannot expand to accommodate increasing ICP, so the brain shifts around structures such as the falx cerebri, tentorium cerebelli, and foramen magnum in an attempt to decompress. This places extreme pressure on delicate neural structures, which often leads to coma and death. Herniated patients typically exhibit the following two abnormal postures (Fig. 13.34):

- **Decorticate posturing**: As a result of lesions above the red nucleus in the midbrain, a patient presents with arms flexed and hands clenched and bent inward over chest and the legs extended, with feet inward. The former is caused by red nucleus disinhibition, which favors motor neurons to the flexor muscles of the upper extremities. The latter is caused by lateral corticospinal tract disruption, which normally supplies motor neurons to the flexor muscles of the lower spinal cord.
- **Decerebrate posturing**: This is a more serious lesion involving damage below the red nucleus (usually a brainstem lesion). Patients present rigid with clenched teeth, arched head back, and arms, elbows, and legs extended.

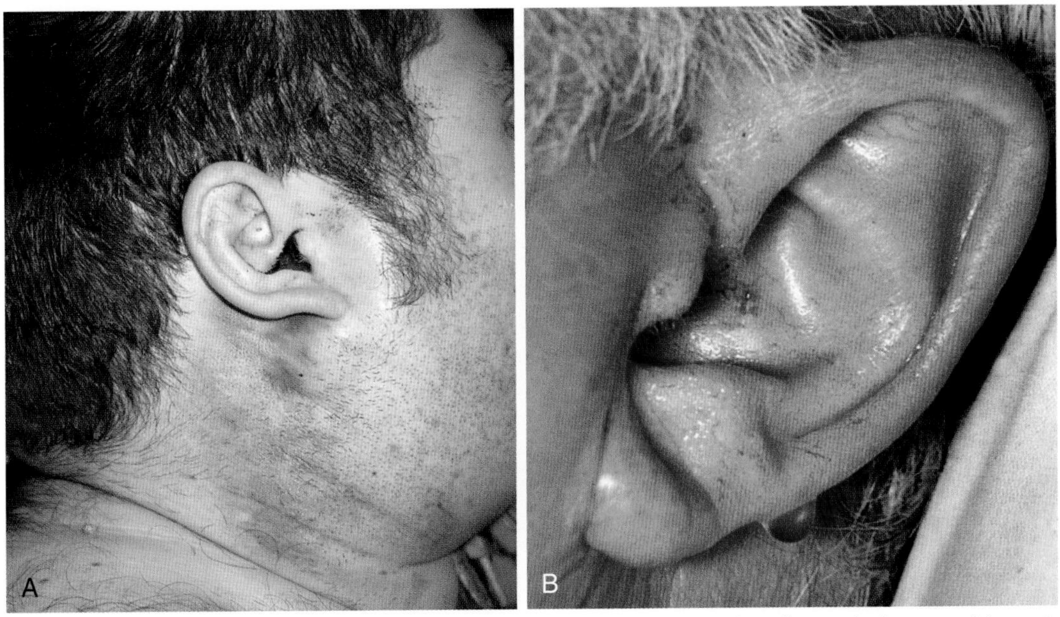

FIG. 13.33 Basilar skull fracture causing Battle sign **(A)** and CSF otorrhea (**B**; literally, CSF leaking out of the ear). (*From Swash M, Glynn M.* Hutchison's Clinical Methods. *22nd ed. Edinburgh: Elsevier; 2007.*)

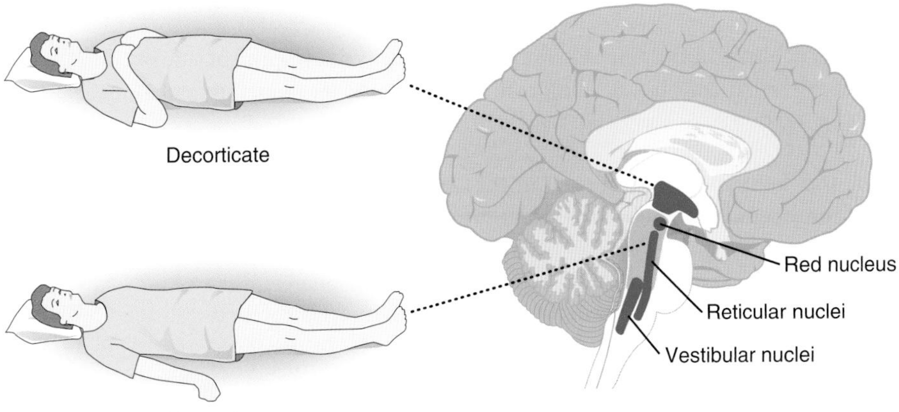

FIG. 13.34 Decorticate posturing (above the red nucleus), and decerebrate posturing (below the red nucleus). The red nucleus sends signals to the upper extremity that favor flexion of the arms; therefore, lesions below the red nucleus will sever these flexor tracts and lead to decerebrate posturing. (*From Weyhenmeyer J, Gallman E:* Rapid Review Neuroscience. *Philadelphia: Mosby; 2007.*)

Herniation (Fig. 13.35) can be categorized into two major classes, **supratentorial** and **infratentorial,** depending on whether the lesion is above or below the tentorium cerebelli, consisting of subtypes according to which direction the brain moves in response to increasing pressure.

Supratentorial

- Uncal: Downward transtentorial herniation of the innermost part of the temporal lobe (uncus) through the tentorium cerebelli (dura that separates the cerebellum from the cerebrum), which can be associated with the following:
- Kernohan's notch: Uncal herniation causes an indentation of the contralateral cerebral peduncle or crus, which contains descending corticospinal fibers, leading to ipsilateral hemiparesis at the side of herniation because it is above the decussation (crossing of the fibers). This is often termed a *false localizing sign* because the herniation creates injury on the opposite side of the brain.
- Compression of the ipsilateral posterior cerebral artery leads to contralateral homonymous hemianopsia.
- "Blown pupil": This is one of the earliest signs of uncal herniation. As the third cranial nerve (CN III) is compressed, parasympathetic neurons surrounding the nerve are affected first, resulting in

Transtentorial herniation can cause compression of sympathetic fibers on CN III, leading to mydriasis ("blown pupil").

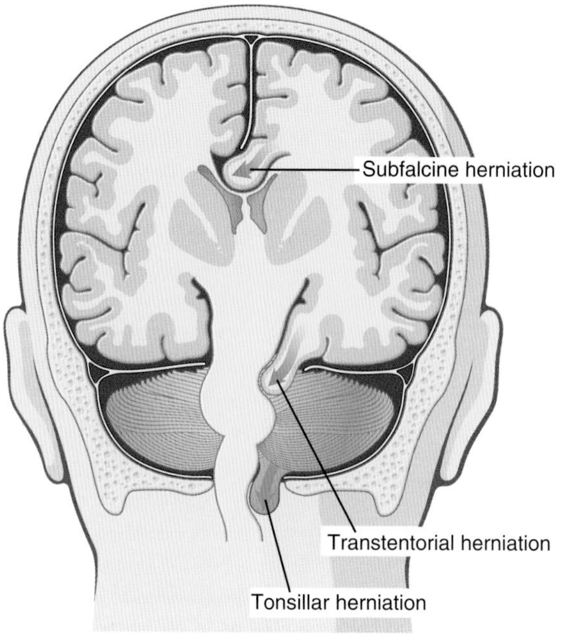

FIG. 13.35 Selected herniation syndromes. Shown are subfalcine herniation under the falx cerebri, uncal transtentoral herniation under the tentorium cerebelli, and tonsillar herniation, in which the cerebellar tonsils move downward through the foramen magnum. (*From Kumar V, Abbas AK, Aster J. Robbins Basic Pathology, 9th ed. St. Louis: Elsevier; 2012.*)

Herniation of the cerebellar tonsils compresses the medullary respiratory center, leading to respiratory arrest.

unopposed sympathetic drive and pupillary dilatation (mydriasis). As compression progresses, the innermost motor part of CN III is affected, leading to ptosis (CN III innervates levator palpebrae) and eye deviation (down and out).

- Duret hemorrhages are parenchymal bleeds in the pons and midbrain caused by tearing and bleeding in the small paramedian arteries of the basilar artery, leading to abnormal posturing, coma (reticular formation), and death.

Downward cerebellar (tonsillar): "Coning" of the cerebellar tonsils downward through the foramen magnum. The cerebellar tonsils can compress the brainstem and cause the medullary respiratory centers to cease to function, leading to apnea or abnormal breathing. As noted, this can also occur in Arnold-Chiari malformation.

Central: Downward transtentorial herniation of both parts of the cerebral hemispheres through a notch in the tentorium cerebelli. Duret hemorrhages can also result from this.

Cingulate (subfalcine): Most common type of herniation, in which the innermost part of the frontal lobe herniates under the falx cerebri (dura that separates the two brain hemispheres). The frontal lobe can then press on the anterior cerebral artery and mimic symptoms of anterior cerebral artery ischemia or stroke.

Transcalvarial: Brain squeezes through a fracture or surgical site (e.g., craniectomy).

Infratentorial: Upward cerebellar: As a result of increasing posterior fossa pressure, the cerebellum can move up.

Spinal Cord

Motor Neuron Signs: Differentiating between upper (descending) and lower motor neurons can assist in localizing the damage/lesion along the motor tracts.

- Upper motor (UMN) signs: Hyperreflexia and increased tone with positive Babinski.
- Lower motor (LMN) signs: Hyporeflexia and decreased tone with atrophy and fasciculations.

UMN signs: ↑ Reflexes, ↑ tone, + Babinski

LMN signs: ↓ Reflexes, ↓tone, + muscle atrophy, + fasciculations

Spinal Cord Lesions

Brown-Séquard Syndrome: Hemisection of the spinal cord leads to the following findings (Fig. 13.36):

- Below lesion level:

Ipsilateral UMN signs (corticospinal tract)

Ipsilateral dorsal column signs (loss of tactile, vibration, and proprioception)

Contralateral spinothalamic signs (pain and temperature loss) that begin a few spinal cord levels below the lesion; recall that the spinothalamic tract travels rostrally for a few segmental levels before crossing in the anterior white commissure of the spinal cord.

Poliomyelitis affects the anterior horn cells causing lower motor neuron signs.

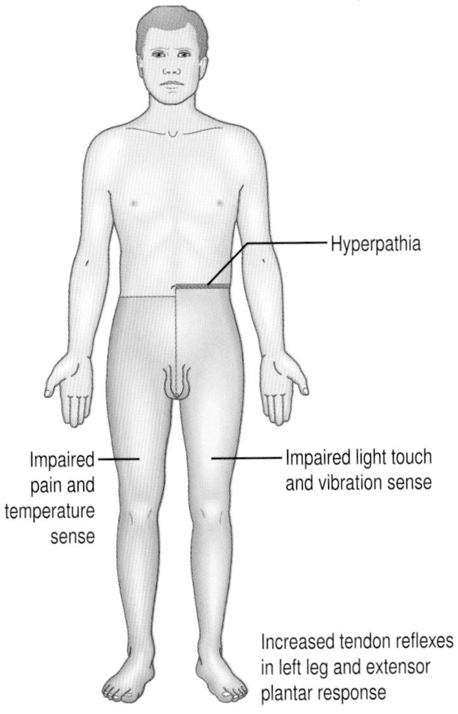

Fig. 13.36 Brown-Séquard syndrome, showing the characteristic ipsilateral loss of vibration and proprioception as well as loss of motor control, with contralateral loss of sensation of pain and temperature. (*From Douglas G, Robertson C.* Macleod's Clinical Examination. *11th ed. Edinburgh: Elsevier; 2005.*)

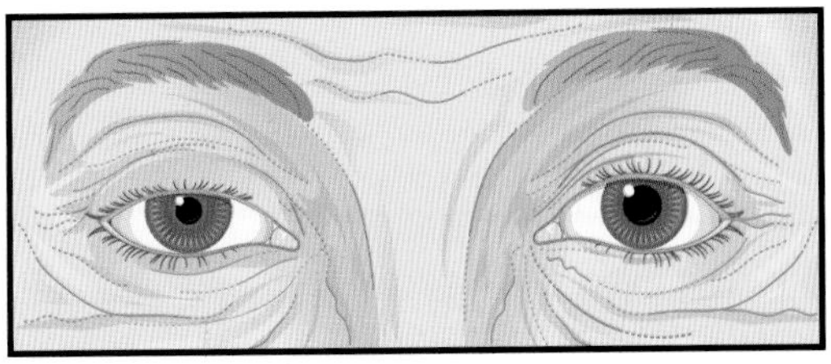

Fig. 13.37 Horner syndrome, with characteristic ptosis and miosis of the (patient's) right eye indicating disruption of ipsilateral sympathetic activity. (*From FitzGerald MJT, Gruener G, Mtui E:* Clinical Neuroanatomy and Neuroscience. *5th ed. Philadelphia: Saunders; 2007.*)

- At the lesion level:
  - Ipsilateral loss of all sensation
  - LMN signs

Poliomyelitis: Spread through the fecal-oral route, the polio virus replicates in the oropharynx and small intestine before spreading hematogenously to the CNS, where it leads to destruction of anterior horn cells and to LMN signs.

Tabes Dorsalis: Degeneration of the **dorsal columns** of the spinal cord as a result of **tertiary syphilis.** Patients can present with a variety of symptoms, such as weakness, paresthesias (shooting, lightning, burning, pricking pain), tabetic gait (high-stepping gait, with foot striking ground), loss of coordination, impaired response to light (Argyll Robertson pupil; see later, "Eye Pathology"), progressive joint degeneration (Charcot joint caused by neuropathic osteoarthropathy—destruction → resorption → deformity → ulceration → infection; can also be caused by diabetes), positive Romberg test (tests proprioceptive sensory loss), absence of deep tendon reflexes (DTRs; Westphal sign), and tabetic ocular crisis (sudden, intense ocular pain with lacrimation and photophobia, known as Pel crisis). Treatment often consists of IV penicillin, with pain control and physical therapy.

Horner's Syndrome: Ipsilateral presentation of facial **r**ubor (flushing), **a**nhidrosis (absence of facial sweating), **m**iosis (pupil constriction), and **p**tosis (superior tarsal muscle) [mnemonic—**RAMP**], which results from lesions of the sympathetic outflow on the affected side (Fig. 13.37). Many diseases can be the cause, including apical lung tumors (e.g., Pancoast tumor), Brown-Séquard syndrome, lateral medullary syndrome, cluster-migraine headache, trauma, thoracic aortic aneurysm, multiple sclerosis,

Table 13.5 Interpreting CSF results

MENINGITIS TYPE	PROTEIN	GLUCOSE	CELLS
Bacterial	↑	↓	PMNs >300/mm^3
Viral	Normal or ↑	Normal	Lymphocytes
Fungal	↑	↓	Lymphocytes <300/mm^3
Tuberculosis	↑	↓	Lymphocytes, PMNs <300/mm^3 ± acid fast bacilli
Malignant	↑	↓	Lymphocytes and malignant cells

PMN, Polymorphonuclear leukocyte.

late-stage syringomyelia, and carotid artery dissection (usually will not exhibit anhidrosis as these sympathetic fibers travel along the external carotid artery).

Infection

Meningitis: This is inflammation of the meninges, which houses CSF; it is the protective membrane surrounding the brain and spinal cord. Patients typically present complaining of headache and neck stiffness associated with fever, altered level of consciousness (e.g., confused and lethargic), photophobia, and phonophobia. In meningococcal meningitis (caused by *Neisseria meningitidis*), a rapidly spreading **petechial rash** (nonblanching) can be seen on the trunk, extremities, mucous membranes, and conjunctiva. On examination, patients generally have **signs of meningismus,** which include **nuchal rigidity** (inability to flex the neck passively), **Kernig knee sign** (knee pain with passive extension), and **Brudzinski neck sign** (neck flexion causes involuntary flexion of the knee and hip). Ultimately, diagnosis is made by lumbar puncture (LP), which can differentiate the various causes of meningitis, ranging from bacterial to aseptic (nonbacterial) causes, such as viral and fungal, by looking at specific factors within the CSF (Table 13.5). CSF can also be sent for more specialized tests to look for certain causes, such as VDRL (syphilis), India ink (*Cryptococcus*), viral polymerase chain reaction (PCR) assay (enterovirus, herpes simplex virus [HSV]), and titers (neurosyphilis, Lyme disease, *Coccidioides*).

Initial treatment should include IV fluid resuscitation if hypotension or shock is present. Because bacterial meningitis can be life-threatening, antibiotics should be immediately started if there is a high clinical suspicion before obtaining blood work, LP, or blood cultures. Adjuvant treatment with corticosteroids should also be given to reduce overall inflammation, leading to reduced mortality, **hearing loss,** and **neurologic sequelae** (e.g., learning and behavioral disabilities). Viral meningitis typically requires supportive therapy alone (e.g., fluids, analgesics) because of the benign course. However, if a patient is relatively young and presents with some behavioral changes or a seizure, suspect HSV, which has a predilection for affecting the temporal lobes. The CSF in HSV encephalitis also typically has an elevated RBC count. In this case the addition of acyclovir is warranted. Despite ideal management of meningitis, complications can arise, such as deafness, epilepsy, seizures, hydrocephalus, disseminated intravascular coagulation (DIC), **Waterhouse-Friderichsen syndrome** (adrenal hemorrhage with hypotension and hyperkalemia), and sepsis, leading to death.

Encephalitis: Encephalitis is an acute inflammation of the brain that presents as fever, headache, confusion, drowsiness, and fatigue, with a viral or bacterial cause. Some common viruses to keep in mind are herpes simplex, rabies virus, poliovirus, and West Nile virus. Some common bacterial causes include syphilis, Lyme disease, and pathogens that cause meningitis.

Abscess: A brain abscess is a collection of infected material formed from distant infectious sources or local spread (e.g., meningitis, mastoiditis, dental abscess, otitis, sinusitis). Patients will have increased ICP and focal neurologic signs caused by this space-occupying lesion. A right to left cardiac shunt is also a risk factor. As a result, a patient will appear very ill, with a fever, headache, and focal neurologic findings. Diagnosis is established by CT, which typically will show a ring-enhancing lesion. LP is contraindicated because of risk of herniation. Treatment ultimately consists of a combination of antibiotics and surgical drainage of the abscess, depending on the location.

In an AIDS patient with deteriorating neurologic status think PML from JC virus.

Viral Infections

West Nile Virus is caused by **Flaviviridae,** usually affecting humans through infected mosquitoes. At first, a patient may be asymptomatic, but can eventually develop a fever and encephalitis.

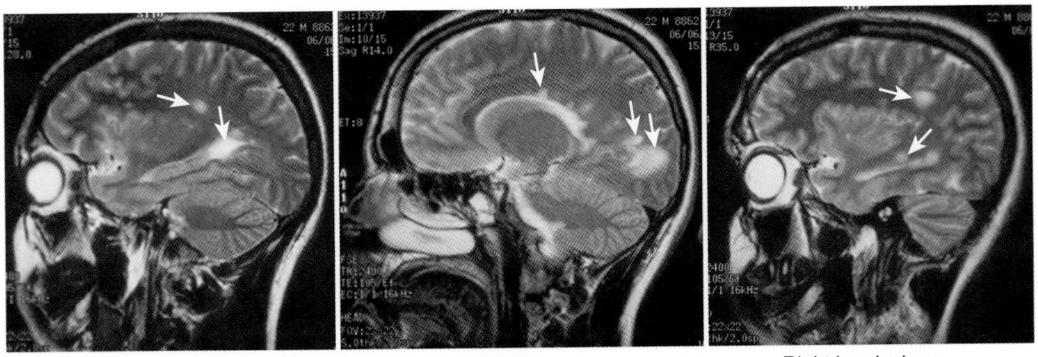

Fig. 13.38 Multiple demyelinating plaques *(arrows)* can be seen on this MRI image of the brain. Note the classic periventricular lesions (Dawson fingers), best seen on the midline image. (*From Weyhenmeyer J, Gallman EA.* Rapid Review Neuroscience. *Philadelphia: Elsevier; 2006.*)

Progressive multifocal leukoencephalopathy (PML) is a disease caused by the **John Cunningham virus (JCV; polyomavirus)** leading to quickly progressing **demyelination of oligodendrocytes.** Normally, JCV is kept under control by the immune system. It causes disease only when the immune system has been severely weakened, especially in AIDS patients, or by immune-modulating therapies (e.g., rituximab, natalizumab).

Parasitic Infections

Toxoplasmosis is a parasitic disease caused by ***Toxoplasma gondii*** that affects humans through **contaminated cat feces or ingestion of meats (pork, lamb, venison)** infested with cysts. The disease spectrum includes encephalitis, chorioretinitis, cutaneous lesions, and congenital lesions.

Taenia solium, also known as **pork tapeworm**, is the most common tapeworm infection of the brain worldwide. It causes **neurocysticercosis,** which is the leading cause of seizures and epilepsy in the developing world. This disease develops from **eating raw or undercooked pork** or from the ingestion of tapeworm eggs via the **fecal-oral route.** The eggs hatch in the intestine and pass through the intestine wall to migrate preferentially toward the brain and muscles, where they form cysts that can remain dormant for years. However, once active, they may cause a local inflammatory reaction causing myalgias or seizures. Treatment with **albendazole** and **steroids** is only warranted if a patient is symptomatic (e.g., having seizures). Otherwise, if one coincidentally finds an asymptomatic patient with neurocysticercosis on CT, no treatment is needed.

Prion: A prion is an **infectious misfolded protein** that accounts for transmissible spongiform encephalopathies, such as bovine **spongiform encephalopathy** (mad cow disease) in cows and **Creutzfeldt-Jakob disease** (CJD), **kuru, fatal familial insomnia,** and **Gerstmann-Straussler-Scheinker (GSS)** syndrome in humans. Prions can arise from sporadic mutation or genetic transmission, or they can be acquired. Once acquired, these misfolded proteins act as a template to induce preexisting, properly folded proteins in neural tissues to convert into misfolded ones (**α helix → β sheets**), which continue the same process in a chain reaction cycle that exponentially grows the population of misfolded proteins. Patients typically present with **rapid neurologic deterioration,** starting with personality and psychiatric changes and ataxia, which leads to dementia and loss of the ability to speak. Findings on examination generally include **myoclonus** (involuntary jerking movements), with EEG showing **periodic sharp wave complexes.** Once acquired, the end result is universally fatal, and patients are generally given supportive and comfort care. Strict sterilization in denaturing the protein's tertiary structure is key in preventing further transmission. The mainstay of sterilization is the combination of heat, pressure, and chemical cleaners.

Demyelinating Diseases

In young women with multiple focal neurologic lesions distributed over time, think MS.

Multiple Sclerosis (MS): MS is an autoimmune disorder of the CNS, mostly affecting women in their 20s and 30s, which eventually leads to **demyelination** (Fig. 13.38) and **inflammation** of the CNS. As the name implies, multiple sclerosed plaques involving the **white matter** of the brain and spinal cord (and including cranial nerves) result from repeated damage and destruction to the **oligodendrocytes** over time. In addition to demyelination, inflammation results from T cell entry into the brain via the blood-brain barrier (BBB), where it recognizes myelin as a foreign molecule and triggers inflammatory cytokines. The BBB is normally not permeable to any type of cell unless the integrity of the tight junctions forming the barrier becomes compromised.

MS can present as a **variety of neurologic symptoms**, such as visual problems (e.g., nystagmus, optic neuritis, diplopia), dysarthria, dysphagia, muscle weakness, spasms, or paralysis, hypoesthesia or paresthesia, or bowel and bladder difficulties (constipation, diarrhea, frequency, retention, incontinence). Sometimes patients may complain of worsening of symptoms when the body becomes overheated (e.g., stepping into a hot tub, during hot weather, or exercise). The increased temperature slows or blocks nerve impulses. In other cases, some complain of electrical shock sensation down the spine (**Lhermitte sign**) or symptoms of trigeminal neuralgia. Typically, a patient presents with **Charcot triad** (**SIN mnemonic**) of **s**canning-telegraphic speech, **i**ntention tremor (**i**ncontinence and **i**nternuclear ophthalmoplegia), and **n**ystagmus. The most common presentation is optic neuritis, where the patient complains of sudden vision loss (partial or complete), blurry or foggy vision, pain with eye movement, and some subtle loss of color vision, especially red.

Because of the wide array of symptoms, MS can be difficult to diagnose. The **McDonald criteria** combine clinical, laboratory and radiologic data. Neuroimaging using MRI with gadolinium contrast is the gold standard, in which **multiple lesions or plaques of demyelination can be seen anywhere from the brain down to the spinal cord.** Lesions around the ventricle-based brain veins are classic (**Dawson fingers**). LP can show signs of chronic inflammation and typically shows increased **oligoclonal IgG bands** on electrophoresis. In addition, there is increased **p100 latency** of nerves when doing visual, auditory, and sensory evoked potentials caused by demyelination. Treatment of an acute attack of MS generally consists of **high doses of IV corticosteroids** for the inflammation and symptomatic treatment of pain, spasticity (e.g., baclofen), and fatigue (e.g., amantadine). Long-term disease-modifying treatments include immunomodulators, such as interferon-β, fingolimod, glatiramer acetate, mitoxantrone, and natalizumab. Deficits suffered during an acute attack may resolve or persist. Ultimately, the overall treatment goal is to prevent the increasing disability that results over time from recurrent episodes of relapsing-remitting MS and prevent development into progressive MS.

Acute Disseminated Encephalomyelitis (ADEM): Similar to MS, ADEM is an autoimmune disease that produces multiple inflammatory lesions in the brain and spinal cord. However, it generally affects children and adolescents after viral, bacterial, or parasitic infection and requires an extended period of time to recover completely

Transverse Myelitis: This demyelinating inflammatory process occurs **across the thickness of the spinal cord** after infection, immunization, or the development of MS. Depending on the level of the spinal cord and the tracts involved, patients present with motor, sensory, and sphincter (bowel, bladder) deficits. Transverse myelitis should be on the differential of acute onset of extremity weakness and numbness. Other conditions on the differential should include Guillain-Barré syndrome, acute spinal cord trauma, compressive spinal cord lesions, and spinal cord infarction.

Central Pontine Myelinolysis (CPM): CPM, also known as osmotic demyelination syndrome, is a complication of **overly rapid correction of severe hyponatremia.** The serum osmolarity is low in hyponatremia; with chronic hyponatremia, the cells make intracellular adaptations to equalize the osmolarity between the serum and inside the cell. However, if the hyponatremia is rapidly corrected (more than 12 mmol/L/day), the serum osmolarity will now be significantly higher than the intracellular osmolarity. This rapidly draws water out of the cell and damages the myelin. Patients generally develop an acute onset of dysphagia, dysarthria, and paralysis. No specific treatment other than supportive care is available once demyelination occurs. Although most patients die, some may live with disability, ranging from mild tremors and ataxia to spastic quadriparesis and locked-in syndrome.

Leukodystrophy: This is a **group of inherited disorders** that leads to **impaired growth and development of the myelin sheath**. Leukodystrophy can be inherited in a recessive, dominant, or X-linked manner (e.g., adrenoleukodystrophy—excessive buildup of long fatty acids in nervous system, testes, and adrenal glands leads to progressive adrenal crisis and coma/death).

GBS: Ascending paralysis caused by autoimmune demyelination, often after *C. jejuni* or cytomegalovirus (CMV) infection

Guillain-Barré Syndrome (GBS): GBS, also known as acute inflammatory demyelinating polyneuropathy, is an autoimmune disorder affecting the PNS. Because of molecular mimicry after infections (often *C. jejuni* or CMV), there is an autoimmune attack on myelin of the peripheral sensory and motor nerves. A patient may present with symmetric ascending weakness starting distally in the hands and feet and migrating toward the trunk. Bulbar cranial nerves can also be affected, leading to facial weakness or paralysis, dysphagia, drooling, and difficulty swallowing and maintaining an open airway. Commonly, respiratory support is needed (e.g., endotracheal intubation) because of impending respiratory failure. Sensory loss is manifested as loss of both proprioception and reflexes, along with bladder dysfunction. Autonomic dysfunction can also be seen in severe cases (e.g., cardiac arrhythmia, fluctuating blood pressure). Suspect GBS if a patient presents with rapid onset of muscle paralysis, areflexia, absence of fever, and a GI or respiratory infection in the past 30 days. Diagnosis is confirmed with LP, which shows CSF with an albuminocytologic dissociation (increased protein without increased cell count), and nerve conduction study (NCS) or EMG showing prolonged distal latencies and conduction slowing. There are two treatment options: (1) plasmapheresis to filter antibodies out of the blood system; and (2) IV immune globulin (IVIG) to neutralize antibodies. Most patients recover weeks to months after onset, but some may have residual disability. Some patients may have one or more relapses of similar symptoms, classifying them as chronic inflammatory demyelinating polyneuropathy (CIDP).

Charcot-Marie-Tooth (CMT) disease: An **incurable, hereditary, sensorimotor neuropathy** that consists of a group of clinical and genetic subtypes, in which there is a defect in the production of neuronal proteins involved in the myelin sheath and axon of **peripheral nerves.** Initially there are intermittent severe painful muscle contractions that are disabling, but over time there is loss of muscle tissue and touch sensation in the extremities. Generally, **high-arched cavus feet** are associated with this disease.

Subacute combined degeneration (Lichtheim disease): As discussed in the spinal cord pathologies, there is **patchy loss of myelin in the dorsal and lateral columns** caused by **vitamin B_{12}** deficiency. Patients typically present with weakness, paresis, numbness, and/or tingling in the legs, arms and trunk. If the B_{12} deficiency is not corrected, damage may be irreversible. If a patient has B_{12} and folic acid deficiencies, the vitamin B_{12} deficiency should be corrected first to avoid precipitating this condition. Administration of nitrous oxide anesthesia has been shown to precipitate this disease in patients with subclinical vitamin B_{12} deficiency, while chronic exposure (recreational abuse) can cause it in people with normal B_{12} levels.

Neurodegenerative Diseases

Alzheimer disease (AD): AD is the **leading cause of dementia,** in which there is **reduced overall synthesis of the neurotransmitter acetylcholine and diffuse cortical atrophy** (especially in the hippocampus) because of the loss of neurons and synapses. Although the exact cause of AD is not known, higher amounts **of extracellular β-amyloid core** (amyloid β [Aβ] protein or senile plaques), and **intracellular abnormally phosphorylated tau protein** (neurofibrillary tangles) are seen on histology.

ApoE4, trisomy 21, and presenilin mutations are all associated with Alzheimer disease.

AD develops sporadically in most cases; 10% of cases are familial and tend to be earlier in onset. Early onset AD is also seen in Down syndrome patients (trisomy 21), who carry an extra copy of the gene for Aβ precursor protein (APP). Early onset AD is also seen in mutations in presenilin-1 and -2 (chromosomes 14 and 1, respectively), which are subcomponents of an enzyme responsible for converting APP to Aβ protein. Late-onset AD is seen in those carrying apolipoprotein E4 (ApoE4), which is an isoform allele of the gene found on chromosome 19. Another isoform, ApoE2, serves a protective role in AD. AD is a **diagnosis of exclusion** that is clinically diagnosed. Short-term memory loss is usually the initial symptom. As the disease progresses, problems with long term memory, executive function, and behaviors develop.

ALS is one of the few conditions with upper *and lower* motor neuron findings.

Amyotrophic lateral sclerosis (ALS; Lou Gehrig's disease): ALS is a **fatal** disorder that affects **both lower motor neurons and upper motor neurons**. The autonomic nervous system and cognition are spared. It is characterized by a rapidly progressive weakness, muscle atrophy and fasciculations (LMN signs), spasticity (UMN sign), dysphagia, dysarthria, and eventually respiratory compromise and death. Although the pathophysiology is not completely understood, it is linked to a mutation in the **superoxide dismutase (SOD)** enzyme, which is an antioxidant that generally neutralizes superoxide, a toxic free radical. Other than symptomatic treatment, **riluzole** is the only treatment known to improve survival by preventing glutamate excitotoxicity indirectly.

Spinal muscle atrophy (SMA): This autosomal recessive disease is caused by a mutation in a gene coding a crucial protein (SMN) for motor neuron survival. As a result, anterior motor neuron death results, leading to diffuse, whole-body atrophy and LMN signs (e.g., fasciculations). SMA can manifest from infants to adults in varying forms of severity. In infants, it is most severe and called **Werdnig-Hoffmann disease,** or **floppy baby syndrome** because of the abnormally low muscle tone observed. In addition to palliative care, no cure exists for SMA, but gene therapy, stem cell therapy, and SMN activation may eventually play a role in treatment.

Movement Disorders

These are neurologic disorders characterized by various abnormal or dysfunctional movements. **Chorea,** for example, is a sudden, jerky, purposeless movement generally seen with lesions to the basal ganglia, which can evolve into **athetosis,** which is a slow, writhing movement, especially of the fingers. In contrast to other movements, **hemiballismus** is a sudden wild flailing of one arm caused by a contralateral subthalamic nucleus lesion. Other movements can include **myoclonus**, and **dystonias**, which are sustained, involuntary muscle contractions.

The nigrostriatal dopaminergic pathway is damaged in Parkinson disease.

Parkinson disease (PD): PD is a degenerative disorder of the CNS in which the dopamine-producing cells of the **substantia nigra** in the midbrain undergo cell death for unknown reasons. It has been postulated that the accumulation of **Lewy bodies** (alpha-synuclein intracellular inclusions) and its progression in location from the brainstem to the cortex plays a role in PD development. Referring back to the basal ganglia section in physiology, keep in mind that dopamine plays a significant role in motor movement modulation. In general, high dopamine levels promote motor activity, whereas low levels, such as those in PD, decrease it. As a result of the loss of dopaminergic neurons, patients develop a collection of **motor symptoms,** known as **parkinsonism**. Classic symptoms include **rigidity** (increased muscle tone often described as "cogwheel"), **bradykinesia-akinesia** (slowness of or no movement), **postural instability** (impaired balance and frequent falls), and **tremor** (pill-rolling tremor at rest only). Other common symptoms include a festinating shuffling gait (short steps) with decreased arm swing and turning en bloc, hypophonia (soft speech), micrographia (small, cramped handwriting), and hypomimia ("masklike" emotionless face). In addition to motor symptoms, patients also develop sleeping difficulties (REM disorders precede motor findings) and neuropsychiatric symptoms affecting mood, cognition, behavior, or thought (e.g., depression, apathy, anxiety). Similar to AD, primary idiopathic PD is diagnosed clinically with a medical history and neurologic examination. When dealing with a patient with parkinsonism, secondary or acquired causes must also be ruled out. Methyl-phenyl-tetrahydropyridine (MPTP), a contaminant in illicit street drugs, can cause selective destruction of dopaminergic neurons, whereas drug-induced parkinsonism can result from antipsychotics (e.g., haloperidol) because of dopamine D_2 receptor blockade (D_2 receptor binding by dopamine normally inhibits the inhibitory pathway thereby increasing movement/motion). **Parkinson plus syndromes** are conditions in which parkinsonism exists with some other dominating feature. For example, **multiple system atrophy (MSA)**, also known as Shy-Drager syndrome, is a combination of parkinsonism, ataxia, and autonomic dysfunction. **Progressive supranuclear palsy (PSP)** is a combination of parkinsonism with predominantly visual symptoms (especially inability to move the eyes vertically), causing early falls (Fig. 13.39).

Huntington disease (HD): An **autosomal dominant** neurodegenerative genetic **trinucleotide repeat disorder.** The Huntington gene on **chromosome 4** contains a sequence of **CAG (glutamine)** that is repeated. This **polyglutamine sequence** normally consists of fewer than 36 repeats in normal individuals; once it is 36 or more repeats, the Huntington protein possesses different characteristics and is considered a mutant form. This mutant form leads to neuronal death via NMDA receptor binding and **glutamate excitotoxicity**. Patients typically present with a **triad of early dementia** (ages, 20s to 50s), **behavioral changes** (e.g., emotional lability, aggression, hypersexuality), and **choreiform movement.** CT scanning of the brain generally shows **atrophy of the striatum,** which consists of the caudate nucleus (cognition) and putamen (motor). Once the disease is suspected, genetic testing is crucial in confirming physical findings, and providing the patient with genetic counseling is crucial. The trinucleotide CAG is unstable during replication (only with paternal spermatogenesis), and its instability increases with the number of repeats present. As a result, **genetic anticipation** is seen—with each successive generation, the numbers of repeats increases, along with the severity and earlier onset of HD. There is no cure for HD, and symptoms are treated as appropriate (Fig. 13.40).

Friedreich ataxia: An **autosomal recessive** inherited disorder in which **trinucleotide repeats (GAA)** lead to decreased transcription of the **frataxin** protein. As a result, **mitochondrial dysfunction** occurs because of free radical damage from cytoplasmic **iron buildup.** Patients present from the age of 5 to 30 years with signs and symptoms such as kyphoscoliosis, ataxia (wide-based gait), dysarthria (slurred speech), nystagmus, and high plantar arches (pes cavus). Patients develop heart disease (e.g., conduction defects, cardiomyopathy) and diabetes. Death is usually secondary to **hypertrophic cardiomyopathy.**

Dementia

Dementia (Table 13.6) is an irreversible global decrease in cognitive ability beyond what is expected with age. It is important to differentiate it from delirium, which is often reversible and waxing and waning. Further differentiation is discussed in Chapter 14. Before making the diagnosis of dementia, other organic causes must be ruled out, such as syphilis, HIV, vitamin B deficiency, Wilson's disease, and hypothyroidism.

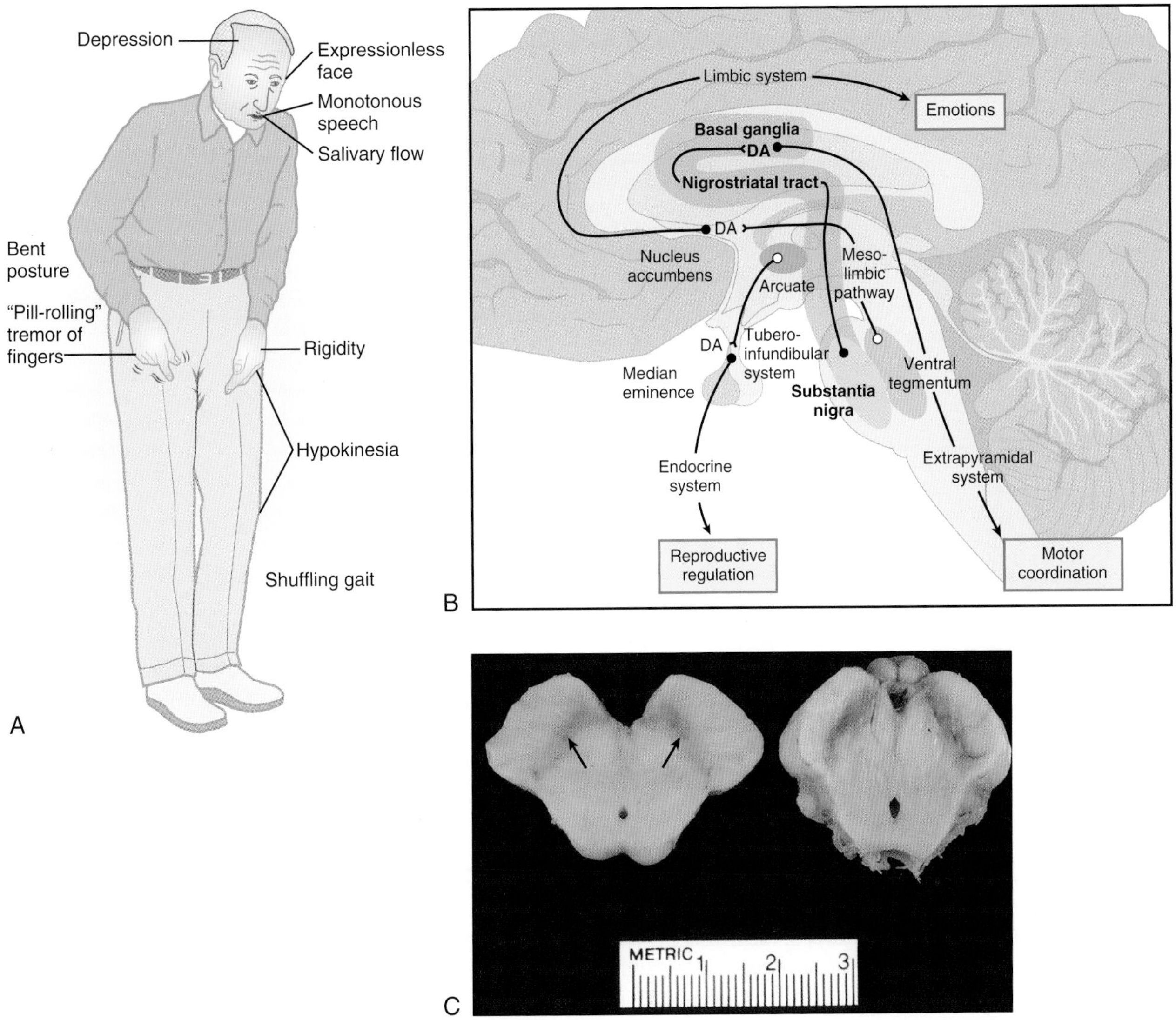

Fig. 13.39 Parkinson disease. **A,** Classic symptoms of Parkinson disease. **B,** Dopaminergic pathways that are altered in Parkinson disease, leading to the symptoms shown in **A**. **C,** Cross section of the midbrain showing the substantia nigra (*arrows,* "black substance"; *left*), with significantly fewer dopaminergic neurons; compare with a normal midbrain and normal substantia nigra *(right)*. *DA,* dopamine. (**A** *from Damjanov I.* Pathophysiology. *Philadelphia: Elsevier; 2008;* **B** *from Kester M, Karpa KD, Quraishi S, Vrana KE.* Elsevier's Integrated Pharmacology. *Philadelphia: Elsevier; 2007;* **C** *from Adkison LR, Brown MD.* Elsevier's Integrated Genetics. *Philadelphia: Elsevier; 2007.*)

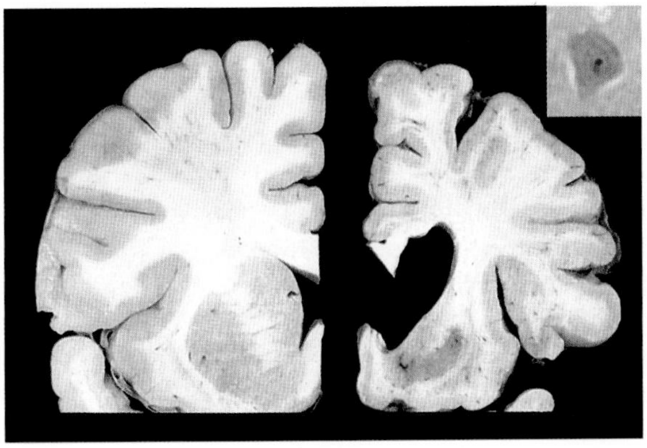

Fig. 13.40 Huntington disease, showing a normal brain with normal striatum *(left)* and the brain of a patient with Huntington disease *(right)*. *Inset,* Histology slide with an intranuclear inclusion that is strongly immunoreactive for ubiquitin (H&E stain, 6.25 micrometers). (*From Kumar V, Abbas AK, Aster J.* Robbins Basic Pathology. *9th ed. St. Louis: Elsevier; 2012.*)

TABLE 13.6 Subtypes of Dementia

DISEASE	HIGH-YIELD FACTS
Alzheimer disease	Most common form of dementia; diffuse cortical atrophy
Pick disease (frontotemporal dementia)	Caused by frontotemporal atrophy; characterized by personality changes (disinhibition, emotional blunting); aphasia is also a common feature
Lewy body dementia	Visual hallucinations are a key feature, but others include parkinsonism and mental status fluctuations. Hallucinations often made worse with anticholinergics.
Vascular dementia	Results from multiple vascular infarcts over time leading to step-wise decline in cognition. Often diagnosed on CT/MRI, which shows multiple cortical/subcortical infarcts.

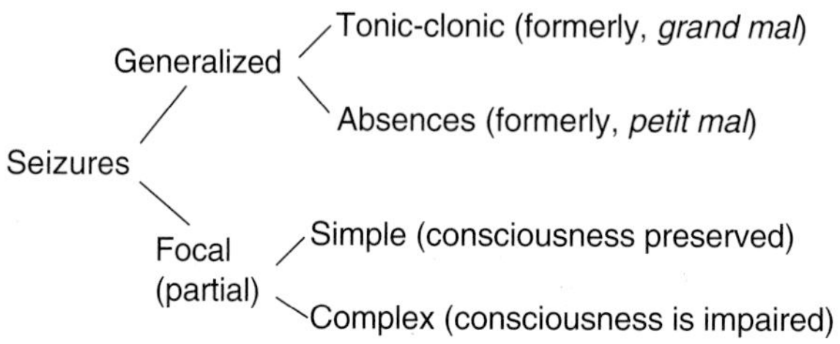

FIG. 13.41 Classification of seizure disorders. (*From FitzGerald MJT, Gruener G, Mtui E. Clinical Neuroanatomy and Neuroscience. 6th ed. Philadelphia: Saunders; 2011.*)

Seizures

A seizure is an episode in which there is an **abnormal excess of synchronous neuronal firing** that leads to **transient symptoms**, such as tonic-clonic movements, behavioral alterations, or sensory alterations (e.g., déjà vu, burning rubber olfactory hallucination). Many conditions can bring about an episode of a seizure, including hypoglycemia, hyponatremia, fever, delirium tremens, infection, stroke, and brain tumors. Epilepsy is a term used specifically to describe recurrent, spontaneous, unprovoked seizures from an underlying alteration of brain function. Epilepsy is a continuum of seizure disorders that differ in terms of clinical presentation, underlying causes, and pathophysiology, which is classified according to site of origin and pattern of spread (see Fig. 13.41).

Partial seizures: Arise in a **localized, focal area** of the brain, but **can spread** to nearby areas that can ultimately become secondarily generalized seizures with diffuse brain involvement. For example, a **Jacksonian seizure** starts in one area of the brain and moves along the motor homunculus. Typically, a "Jacksonian march" starts with tingling in the fingers moving more proximally, leading to arm, head, and eye movements. Sometimes the seizure can cross to the other side of the brain, leading to a secondarily generalized seizure.

- **Focal seizure without impairment of awareness (simple partial):** Seizures present as motor, sensory, autonomic, or psychological symptoms, depending on origin. **Consciousness is not impaired;** however, the seizure can spread, leading to a complex partial seizure or generalized seizure.
- **Focal seizure with impairment of awareness (complex partial):** A seizure preceded by an aura, in which **consciousness is impaired.** Patients may remain motionless or engage in repetitive behaviors, called automatisms (e.g., grimacing, lip smacking). Although it may arise from any lobe of the brain, it most commonly arises from the **mesial temporal lobe.** Occasionally, mesial temporal sclerosis may be seen on imaging, indicating gliosis and atrophy from neuronal loss.

> Do not confuse absence seizures with attention deficit disorder. Treat with ethosuximide.

Generalized seizures: Diffuse brain involvement that impairs consciousness.

- **Absence:** Formerly known as **petit mal seizures,** these are brief seizures of sudden onset and termination, with no postictal confusion. Because this often presents with staring spells in children it may be confused with attention deficit disorder; however, absence seizures may still have automatisms. EEG shows **3-Hz generalized spike and slow wave discharges.** Treatment is mainly with **ethosuximide** or valproic acid.
- **Myoclonic:** Rapid involuntary contraction of muscles described as "jumps." In juvenile myoclonic epilepsy, seizures begin between puberty and adulthood, where seizures affect the neck, shoulders, and upper arms. They generally occur shortly after waking.

- **Tonic-clonic**: This is the **most common form** of epilepsy, formerly known as grand mal seizures. Episodes are divided into **two phases,** the **tonic phase** and **clonic phase.** It first begins with the tonic phase, which will cause the patient to fall down. Muscles suddenly contract, causing the extremities to be rigidly pulled toward or away from the body. Following this, the clonic phase consists of rapid muscle contractions and relaxations, causing convulsions. Clinically, the patient may be rolling on the ground with the extremities violently shaking.
- **Atonic**: Also known as **drop seizures,** in which patients have a brief lapse of muscle tone leading to drop attacks, and they collapse to the ground. These seizures must be differentiated from similar looking attacks that may occur in cataplexy or syncope.

When encountering a patient that presents with seizure-type symptoms, further history and physical examination needs to be done to confirm if it was a seizure, and if so, what the underlying cause may be (epilepsy vs. metabolic vs. tumor vs. infection vs. stroke). In general, the patient's age may shed light on possible causes. For children, it is typically genetic or infectious (febrile), which differs from adults or older patients, in whom tumors and strokes are more common.

Headache (HA)

Primary Headaches

These exist independently from other medical conditions or diseases.

Acute cluster headaches respond well to the inhalation of 100% oxygen.

Tension-type HA: This is the **most common type** of HA, often described as a **bilateral pressure or "bandlike"** pain around the head. Precipitating factors often include stress, sleep deprivation, hunger, and eye strain. Although painful, these HAs are not harmful, and symptoms improve with nonsteroidal antiinflammatory drugs (NSAIDs) or acetaminophen. It is important to note that frequent use of pain medication to relieve tension-type HA can lead to the development of medication overuse HA (rebound HA).

Migraine HA: This typically presents as a **disabling unilateral, pulsating HA associated with autonomic symptoms,** such as nausea, vomiting, phonophobia, and photophobia for 4 to 72 hours (**POUND** mneumonic - **P**ulsatile quality of headache, **O**ne-day duration (actually four to 72 hours), **U**nilateral location, **N**ausea or vomiting, **D**isabling intensity – 4 of 5 symptoms with 92% probability of migraine). An aura generally precedes the HA in a third of sufferers, in which the patient may have transient visual deficits, sensory hallucinations, or even motor and language disturbances. Although the exact cause is highly debated, it is believed to be a neurovascular disorder, in which the brain blood vessels undergo constriction and neurogenic inflammation because of changes in the levels of serotonin, histamine, and substance P.

Cluster HA: Presents rapidly as a severe, excruciating unilateral orbital-supraorbital eye pain associated with autonomic symptoms, such as ptosis, miosis, conjunctival injection, rhinorrhea, lacrimation, facial swelling, flushing, and sweating, lasting 15 minutes to 4 hours or longer. A distinguishing feature is the **regularity** of the attacks (occurring at the same time each day), speculating a connection with circadian rhythm. It is often referred as **"alarm clock HA"** because of the ability to wake a person from sleep with regular timing. Generally, many patients respond to inhalation of **100% oxygen.** It is also more commonly seen in men.

Trigeminal neuralgia: Also known as **tic douloureux.** It presents as episodes of unilateral severe pain described as **stabbing electrical shocks,** burning, crushing, or shooting pain in the distribution of the trigeminal nerve across the face. Although it may occur paroxysmally, with no stimulations, it can be triggered by common activities, such as brushing teeth, shaving, combing hair, eating, or talking. External stimuli, such as the wind or loud noises, may also trigger attacks. Trigeminal neuralgia is usually treated with **carbamazepine,** which prevents depolarization by inhibiting voltage-gated sodium channels, as well as with intravenous phenytoin.

Secondary Headaches

These are headaches caused by an underlying condition.

Think of pseudotumor cerebri in obese women with headache and papilledema.

Subarachnoid hemorrhage (SAH): Presents as a "thunderclap" HA. Typically described as the "worst headache of my life" or "like being kicked in the head." SAH is usually associated with vomiting, neck stiffness, confusion, altered level of consciousness, oculomotor palsy, or seizures. See earlier ("Trauma") for further details.

Table 13.7 Tumors of Adulthood

ADULT TUMORS	DESCRIPTION	KEY HISTOLOGIC FEATURES
Glioblastoma multiforme	Most common primary brain tumor; very aggressive tumor with poor prognosis; called "butterfly glioma" because it can cross corpus callosum	Stains GFAP +; "palisading" pleomorphic tumors with central necrosis, hemorrhage
Meningioma	Resectable tumors because they occur outside hemispheric convexity	Psammoma bodies (laminated calcification), whorled pattern concentrically arranged spindle cells
Schwannoma	Schwann cell origin usually affecting CN VIII (vestibular schwannoma) at cerebellopontine angle	S-100 positive. A cause of sensorineural hearing loss. Treat with resection or stereotactic radiosurgery
Oligodendroglioma	Frontal lobe tumor with chicken wire capillary pattern	"Fried egg" cells; often calcified
Pituitary adenoma	Presents as prolactinoma or bitemporal hemianopsia	Derived from Rathke's pouch

GFAP, Glial fibrillary acidic protein.

Idiopathic intracranial hypertension (IIH): Also known as pseudotumor cerebri, IIH results from increased intracranial pressure, with the absence of tumor or disease. The HA is usually associated with nausea, vomiting, visual changes (double vision and visual loss from long-term untreated papilledema), and pulsatile tinnitus (whooshing sensation or buzzing in ear). See earlier ("Developmental Disorders") for further details.

Meningitis: Always consider this diagnosis when a patient presents with a HA and fever. See earlier ("Infection") for further details.

Giant cell arteritis (GCA): Generally known for affecting the temporal artery in **temporal arteritis,** GCA is a form of **vasculitis** that affects large and medium-sized vessels, such as the aorta. It is named according to the type of inflammatory cells found on biopsy (giant cell from union of several macrophages). Generally affecting women more than men, patients present with symptoms such as HA, jaw-tongue claudication, tinnitus, and visual changes (diplopia or blurred vision). If left untreated, the inflammation can affect the ophthalmic artery, leading to **sudden blindness,** so GCA is considered a medical emergency. On examination, a patient may have prominent temporal arteries, which are exquisitely **tender to palpation**. Definitive diagnosis is made via biopsy, but **elevated inflammatory markers (erythrocyte sedimentation rate [ESR] or C-reactive protein [CRP])** support it. If GCA is suspected based on the history and physical examination, treatment with **high-dose steroids** should be started before biopsy confirmation. It is important to note that GCA is **associated with polymyalgia rheumatica,** which presents as pain and stiffness in the neck, shoulders and hips, and treated similarly.

New onset of headaches in patients > 40 years old is a red flag. Be sure to consider SAH, GCA, and closed-angle glaucoma.

Brain tumors: Similar to IIH, brain tumors can raise ICP to cause a HA. However, depending on the location, surrounding brain structures can be damaged, leading to focal neurologic deficits. This will be discussed in further detail in the brain tumor section (see later).

Closed-angle glaucoma: Raised intraocular pressure leads to a **painful red, middilated eye** causing a HA associated with visual abnormalities, nausea, and vomiting. More details are given later.

Carbon monoxide (CO) poisoning: This colorless, odorless, tasteless, toxic gas is usually emitted from gasoline-powered tools, heaters, furnaces, and cooking equipment. Typically, a **cherry red** patient with altered mental status presents with a history of living in a garage (using a heater). Also consider CO poisoning when several members of a family have simultaneous onset of headaches and nausea. Patients with CO poisoning may have normal oxygen saturation, but CO oximetry is used to determine carboxyhemoglobin levels, which misrepresent oxyhemoglobin. Treatment consists of administration of 100% oxygen via a nonrebreather mask to displace CO from hemoglobin; hyperbaric oxygen therapy is also used in cases of pregnancy, neonates, and certain other circumstances.

Brain Tumors

Primary brain tumors are slow-growing cancers that usually are not noticed until they begin to affect nearby structures. Patients can present with seizures, unrelenting headaches, altered mental status, or dementia. Primary brain tumors rarely metastasize. In general, brain tumors are supratentorial in adults (Table 13.7) and infratentorial in children (Table 13.8).

Table 13.8 Tumors of Childhood

CHILDHOOD TUMORS	DESCRIPTION	KEY HISTOLOGIC FEATURES
Pilocytic (low-grade) astrocytoma	Well-circumscribed cystic-solid tumor found in posterior fossa. Benign, good prognosis	GFAP-positive; Rosenthal fibers (eosinophilic corkscrew fibers)
Medulloblastoma	Solid cerebellar tumor that is highly malignant; form of a primitive neuroectodermal tumor (PNET); seen in Turcot syndrome; presents as obstructive hydrocephalus (fourth ventricle compressed)	Homer Wright rosettes; cells are very radiosensitive, so can be used in therapy
Ependymoma	Ependymal cells typically found in fourth ventricle leading to obstructive hydrocephalus; can seed (metastasize to) the cerebrospinal fluid	Perivascular pseudorosettes; rod-shaped blepharoplasts near nucleus (basal ciliary bodies)
Hemangioblastoma	Cerebellar tumor associated with von Hippel-Lindau syndrome, which can produce EPO (polycythemia vera)	Foamy cells with high vascularity.
Craniopharyngioma	Benign tumor that is calcified and rich in cholesterol; often confused with pituitary adenoma.	Derived from Rathke's pouch remnants

EPO, Erythropoietin; GFAP, glial fibrillary acidic protein.

Table 13.9 Cranial Nerve Lesions

CRANIAL NERVE (CN)	PRESENTATION
Trigeminal (CN V)	Jaw deviates **toward** the side of the lesion because there is an unopposed lateral pterygoid, which receives bilateral cortical input.
Vagus (CN X)	Uvula deviates **away** from the side of the lesion because the affected side has weak muscles compared with the nonaffected side.
Accessory (CN XI)	Weakness on turning head to **contralateral** side of lesion for the sternocleidomastoid muscle (SCM); ipsilateral shoulder droop due to trapezius innervation.
Hypoglossal (CN XII)	Tongue deviates **toward** the side of the lesion ("lick your wounds") because the opposite side overpowers the affected side.

Cranial Nerve Lesions

See Table 13.9 and Fig. 13.42.

Facial nerve paralysis: CN VII lesions most commonly affect the muscles of **facial expression,** but it is important to keep in mind the other functions that may be compromised, such as **lacrimation** (dry eyes), **corneal reflex** (cannot blink), **taste,** and **sound dampening** (hyperacusis). When a facial nerve lesion is suspected, it is very important to classify it as an UMN lesion (usually from stoke) or a LMN lesion (e.g., compression from a parotid tumor). On physical examination, forehead involvement should be assessed by asking the patient to raise the eyebrows. The forehead is spared (e.g., patient can furrow forehead) in UMN lesions because it is innervated by both cerebral hemispheres. The following are some causes of facial nerve paralysis:

- **Supranuclear, nuclear:** Infarcts to internal capsule (lacunar stroke), pons (CN VII nucleus), or face area of motor cortex homunculus.
- **Infranuclear:** Bell's palsy (linked to herpes simplex so treated with steroids and acyclovir), Lyme disease (bilateral facial palsy; associated with cardiovascular arrhythmias in stage 2), GBS (bilateral facial palsy), herpes zoster oticus (Ramsay-Hunt syndrome), AIDS, sarcoidosis (bilateral facial palsy; sign of neurosarcoidosis), tumors (acoustic neuroma, parotid, cholesteatoma), and diabetes mellitus.

UMN facial paralysis: Forehead is spared.

LMN facial paralysis: Forehead is affected.

Mnemonic: My **L**ovely **B**ella **H**as **A**n **STD**: **L**yme disease, **B**ell's palsy, **H**erpes Zoster, **A**IDS, **S**arcoidosis, **T**umors-**T**rauma, **D**iabetes mellitus.

Treatment for the typical Bell's palsy entails protection of the eye from abrasions (eye shield) and dryness (lubrication via artificial tears or ointment), and a course of antiretrovirals (e.g., acyclovir) with possible steroids.

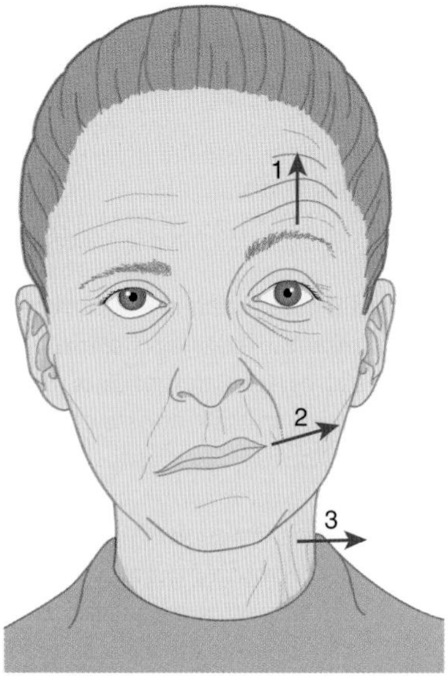

FIG. 13.42 Right facial nerve paralysis. The patient is unable to smile *(arrow 2)* or furrow his brow on the affected side *(arrow 1)*. *(From FitzGerald MJT, Gruener G, Mtui E.* Clinical Neuroanatomy and Neuroscience. *6th ed. Philadelphia: Saunders; 2011.)*

Ear Pathology

Vertigo: An illusion of movement, despite being in a stationary position (sensation that "the room is spinning"). When evaluating a patient with vertigo, it is crucial to categorize vertigo as peripheral or central. Peripheral causes affect the vestibular system in the inner ear. Central causes affect the CNS. Central causes include migraine headaches, lateral medullary syndrome, vertebrobasilar TIA, cerebellar infarction, and multiple sclerosis. Peripheral causes are discussed here.

- **Benign paroxysmal positional vertigo (BPPV):** This is the most common cause of vertigo. It presents as short, intermittent episodes of dizziness provoked by head movements and associated with nausea and nystagmus. BPPV is caused by **calcium crystals (otoliths)** that affect the cupula or cause abnormal endolymph movement. Otoliths are typically found in the utricle, but over time they may migrate into one of the semicircular canals (posterior is most common). BPPV is diagnosed clinically, but can be confirmed by the **Dix-Hallpike** and **roll tests**, which test the posterior and horizontal semicircular canals, respectively. Treatment aims to reposition the otoliths out of the semicircular canals through the **Epley maneuver.** Antivertigo medications that include **antihistamines (meclizine)** and **anticholinergics (scopolamine)** can be given for symptomatic management.
- **Ménière's disease:** Typically, this presents as **vertigo, tinnitus, hearing loss, and fullness or pressure** in one or both ears, but not all patients experience the same symptoms. It is believed to be caused by **excess endolymph** buildup in the inner ear, which over time causes dilation and blockage to cochlear structures. Herpesvirus has also been linked to this disease, and acyclovir can be used as a possible treatment. It is a diagnosis of exclusion; physical examination, brain MRI, and audiometry should be done to rule out other entities such as schwannoma. Treatment aims to reduce further fluid buildup (low-salt diet or diuretics [**acetazolamide**]) and symptomatic control of nausea and vomiting. Surgery is a last resort; destructive (vestibular neurectomy) and nondestructive (shunt) procedures can be done.

Otitis externa pathogens: *Pseudomonas* and *S. aureus*

Otitis media pathogens: *S. pneumoniae, H. influenzae,* and *M. catarrhalis*

- **Vestibular neuritis:** This generally presents after or during a viral syndrome, with a sudden onset of vertigo associated with nystagmus, nausea, vomiting, and gait instability. Unlike labyrinthitis, there are no hearing symptoms. Because of the clinical overlapping picture, it is crucial to differentiate it from acute vascular events, particularly cerebellar strokes. Treatment consists of a short corticosteroid taper.

Infection

Acute otitis externa: A common cause of an earache, or otalgia, this is an inflammation of the outer ear (pinna) and external auditory canal caused by pathogens such as *Pseudomonas aeruginosa* and *Staphylococcus aureus.* Typically, it is known as "swimmer's ear," occurring after swimming, in which the remaining water serves as a moist environment for bacterial growth. It can also be caused by trauma (ear scratching or cotton swabs), occlusive ear devices (ear phones, hearing aids), and dermatologic conditions (psoriasis). In addition to otalgia, swelling can cause conductive hearing loss and, in severe cases, canal obstruction. Treatment consists of thoroughly cleaning the ear canal (remove cerumen) and treating inflammation and infection with topical antibiotics and steroids.

Of note, when dealing with older diabetic individuals or immunocompromised patients, consider malignant (necrotizing) external otitis, which can spread to the skull base and requires emergent ENT evaluation.

Acute otitis media (AOM): Also a common cause of otalgia, this is an inflammation of the middle ear usually caused by pathogens such as ***Streptococcus pneumoniae, Haemophilus influenzae,*** and ***Moraxella catarrhalis.*** The most important factor in the pathogenesis of AOM is eustachian tube dysfunction, which occurs secondary to allergic rhinitis or upper respiratory tract infections. Treatment strategy is controversial, but generally consists of watchful waiting or antibiotics, depending on the patient's age and overall clinical picture.

Cholesteatoma: A cyst that is an abnormal accumulation of keratinizing squamous epithelium, which if not surgically excised, expands over time, causing recurrent ear infections, mucopurulent drainage, hearing loss, vertigo, facial nerve palsy, and potentially life-threatening complications (e.g., meningitis, brain abscess).

Ramsay-Hunt syndrome: This is caused by **reactivation of herpes zoster virus (shingles)** in the geniculate ganglion, which affects cranial nerve VII. As a result, facial muscle movement, sensation of part of the ear and ear canal, and taste function of the anterior two thirds of the tongue can be affected. Typically, a patient presents with a **seventh nerve palsy** (Bell's palsy), but on inspection of the tympanic membrane, tongue, and/or hard palate, **eruptive erythematous vesicles** are seen.

Hearing impairment

This can be a concerning symptom for many, but careful examination (Weber and Rinne tests) should be done to differentiate between conductive hearing loss, which is often reversible, from sensorineural hearing loss, which is not. **Conductive hearing** loss is caused by a problem with sound wave conduction, which can occur in the external ear (e.g., cerumen, otitis externa, tympanic membrane perforation) or middle ear (e.g., AOM or otosclerosis). In conductive hearing loss, the **Weber test,** in which the tuning fork is touched to the midline of the forehead, localizes to the affected ear; the **Rinne test,** which tests air conduction (AC) versus bone conduction (BC), is abnormal (i.e., BC > AC; remember in normal hearing, AC > BC). On the other hand, **sensorineural hearing loss** results from dysfunction of the inner ear, cochlea (e.g., noise-induced), or vestibulocochlear nerve (e.g., ototoxic drugs). The Weber test localizes to the normal ear, whereas the Rinne test is normal.

Eye Pathology

External

Hordeolum: Also known as a stye, this **acute painful external** red bump on the eye is an infection of the **sebaceous glands of Zeis** at the base of the eyelashes, or an infection of the **apocrine sweat glands of Moll.** It can also occur internally, infecting the meibomian (sebaceous) gland lining the inside of the eyelids. Treatment generally consists of a combination of warm compresses, incision and drainage, oral antibiotics, and pain control.

Chalazion: Painless internal nodule caused by **chronic** inflammation of a blocked **meibomian gland.** Initially, topical antibiotics can be used in the acute phase, but chalazions generally go away with time. Further treatment options include corticosteroid injections and surgery.

Coloboma: Present from birth, this defect in the eye is caused by the failure of the choroid fissure to close, resulting in a hole in of the eye structures (retina, optic disc, choroid, and iris).

EOM abnormalities: See Fig. 13.43. Remember the mnemonic $LR_6SO_4R_3$.

- CN III damage: Eye looks down and out because of unopposed superior oblique and lateral rectus. Ptosis caused by levator palpebrae superioris muscle disruption. Mydriasis and loss of accommodation because of parasympathetic disruption.
- CN IV: Downward gaze is defective, so the head is tilted toward side of lesion.
- CN VI: Eye looks medially because of unopposed medial rectus.

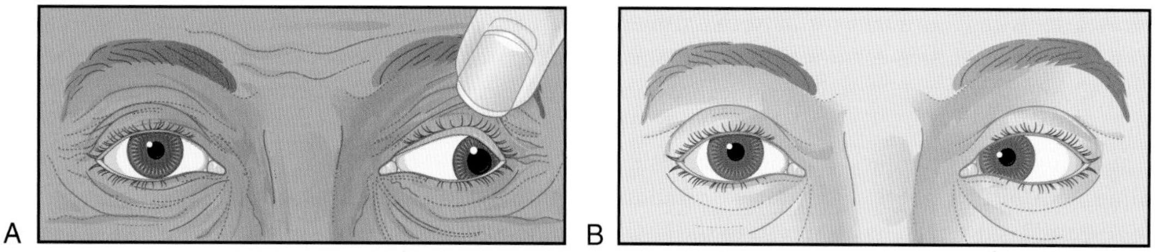

Fig. 13.43 Extraocular movement abnormalities. **A,** Third nerve palsy with a down and out pupil, mydriasis (caused by lack of parasympathetic tone from the third nerve), severe ptosis (caused by denervation of the levator palpebrae muscle). **B,** Sixth nerve palsy with lateral rectus muscle paralysis. The eye looks medially because of the unopposed medial rectus muscle. (*From FitzGerald MJT, Gruener G, Mtui E.* Clinical Neuroanatomy and Neuroscience. *6th ed. Philadelphia: Saunders; 2011.*)

Cataracts: Crystalline clouding of the lens or lens capsule that results in opacification and obstruction of light. The two most common causes include senile cataracts (because of old age) or congenital cataracts. However, some can be acquired (e.g., diabetes, trauma, infection, prolonged steroid use).

Pupils:

- **Marcus Gunn:** Often seen in **optic neuritis,** this **afferent pupillary defect (APD)** is seen during the swinging flashlight test, in which shining light in the affected eye produces less pupillary constriction relative to the unaffected eye.
- **Argyll Robertson:** This highly specific sign of **neurosyphilis,** known as prostitute's pupil, presents as pupils that constrict to accommodation (when the eyes move from looking at a distal object to a near object), but do not react to light.

Glaucoma: An eye disease characterized by damage to the optic nerve because of increased pressure in the eye (intraocular pressure). It is typically divided into two main categories based on the angle between the iris and cornea. The vision loss typically begins in the periphery; this is in contrast to macular degeneration, in which vision loss is central.

- **Open-angle (90%) glaucoma: Insidious** onset of **painless** vision loss associated with increased age, which is not noticed until disease has significantly progressed. The only signs of this disease include visual field loss and optic nerve changes (increased cup-to-disc ratio). Secondary causes result from obstruction of the trabecular network from RBCs (e.g., vitreous hemorrhage), WBCs (e.g., uveitis) or retinal elements (e.g., retinal detachment).
- **Closed-angle (10%) glaucoma:** A **sudden** onset of **pain,** a **midsized, nonreactive pupil** and **injected conjunctiva** (red eye), which requires emergency treatment to lower the high intraocular pressure (usually IOP >30 mm Hg). This is classically precipitated by pupillary dilation (e.g., being in a dark room). Further discussion regarding medical treatment to lower intraocular pressure will be discussed later ("Pharmacology"). If medical management fails, surgical methods, such as iridotomy or iridectomy, canaloplasty, and trabeculectomy or trabeculoplasty are available.

Posterior Eye Pathology

Retinal detachment: An ocular emergency characterized by "peeling" of the retina and described as a **veil or curtain being drawn over the visual field,** which is preceded by **flashes of light, eye heaviness,** and **floaters.** Diagnosis is usually made by funduscopy or ultrasound, and treatment generally consists of sealing retinal breaks via surgery.

Papilledema: Asymptomatic optic disc swelling caused by **increased ICP,** which warrants further workup to discover and treat the underlying cause; otherwise, vision loss can result. On fundoscopic examination, typical findings include venous engorgement (earliest sign), loss of venous pulsations, blurring of optic margins, and elevation of the optic disc.

Optic neuritis: Demyelinating inflammation of the optic nerve usually associated with multiple sclerosis (first manifestation), which can lead to complete or partial painful vision loss. On fundoscopic examination, the optic disc is usually pale, but can be normal. Treatment generally consists of steroids.

Central retinal artery occlusion (CRAO): Acute onset of unilateral **painless** vision loss caused by occlusion (embolic, thrombotic, inflammatory, or traumatic) of the central retinal artery that can be irreversible if not corrected within 90 minutes. On examination, there can be an APD, **Hollenhorst plaque** (cholesterol embolus), pale optic nerve, and a **cherry red spot** (the ischemia causes whitening of the retina, however the macula receives its vascular supply from a different source; note that this can also be seen in carbon monoxide poisoning). Treatment generally includes eye massage, eye paracentesis (lowers IOP to allow embolus to move), oxygen therapy, and consideration of thrombolytics.

Central retinal vein occlusion (CRVO): Acute onset of unilateral **painless** vision loss caused by occlusion of the central retinal vein, leading to macular edema, ischemia, and neovascular glaucoma. Typically on fundoscopic examination, there is extensive hemorrhage, giving a so-called **blood and thunder** appearance. Treatment generally includes intravitreal administration of steroids.

Retinitis: Inflammation of the retina that results in retinal edema and necrosis often leading to scaring and visual changes/loss. Normally it is the result of infectious etiologies, including viral (CMV, HSV, VZV), bacterial, and parasitic causes, especially in immunosuppressed individuals.

Retinitis pigmentosa: Inherited progressive degeneration of retinal rod photoreceptors leading to progressive vision impairment, starting from peripheral vision and dim light compromise to eventual night blindness (nyctalopia). On fundoscopic examination, bone spicules accumulate with time.

Visual Field Defects

Depending on the lesion location in the visual pathway, a characteristic visual field loss is typically seen. Below are common visual field anomalies and their corresponding lesions (Fig. 13.44).

- Unilateral macular degeneration → central scotoma
- Optic nerve → right anopsia
- Optic chiasm → bitemporal hemianopsia
- Optic tract → left homonymous hemianopsia
- Meyer's loop (located in temporal lobe) → left upper quadrantic anopsia
- Dorsal optic radiation (located in parietal lobe) → left lower quadrantic anopsia
- Posterior cerebral lesion → left hemianopsia with macular sparing

Internuclear ophthalmoplegia (INO): Also known as **MLF syndrome.** INO is a disorder in which there is a lesion to the **medial longitudinal fasciculus (MLF),** which essentially connects the abducens nucleus (CN VI) to the contralateral oculomotor nucleus (CN III) in the brainstem. As a result, there is **medial rectus nerve palsy,** with **nystagmus** and **horizontal diplopia** in the abducting eye on attempted lateral gaze, but **convergence remains normal** (Fig. 13.45). In young patients with bilateral INO, multiple sclerosis is often the cause. In older patients with unilateral INO, stroke is usually the cause.

PHARMACOLOGY

Glaucoma

As noted, the goal of glaucoma therapy is to lower IOP to prevent further damage to the optic nerve. Five pharmacologic groups can be used (Table 13.10).

Opioids

Opioids are a large class of drugs that act as agonists by binding to opioid receptors (mu [μ] = morphine, delta [δ] = enkephalin, kappa [κ] = dynorphin), which are found in the central and peripheral nervous system and the GI tract, leading to decreased synaptic transmission of various neurotransmitters (e.g., **acetylcholine [Ach],** serotonin [5-hydroxytryptamine—5-HT], **norepinephrine [NE],** glutamate, substance P). Common opioids that you will encounter in the clinical setting include morphine, fentanyl, codeine, hydromorphone, oxycodone, dextromethorphan, methadone, and meperidine. Clinically, they are used for analgesia, but some are used for cough suppression (dextromethorphan), diarrhea (loperamide, diphenoxylate), maintenance therapy for heroin addicts (methadone), and acute pulmonary edema (morphine). As a result of frequent or excessive dosing, side effects can develop, such as **miosis** (pinpoint pupils), constipation, **respiratory depression,** and CNS depression. Over time, patients can develop opioid tolerance by neuroadaptation through receptor desensitization, which leads to reduced analgesia effect. No tolerance develops to constipation and miosis. In case of opioid overdose, an opioid receptor antagonist can be used. Naloxone is short-acting and is used intravenously. Naltrexone is longer acting and can be used orally.

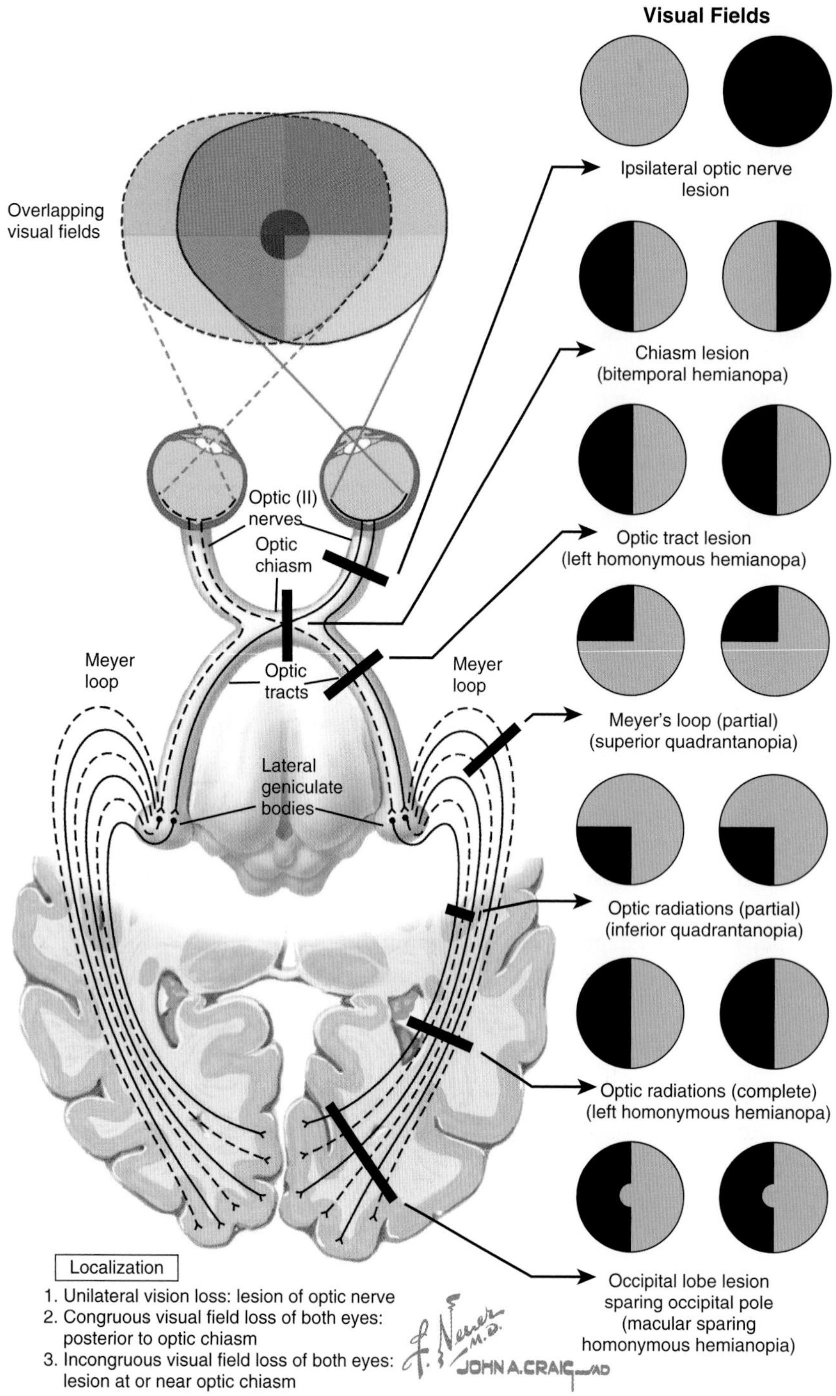

Fig. 13.44 Visual field defects and their corresponding lesions. (*From Felten DL, Shetty AN.* Netter's Atlas of Neuroscience. *Philadelphia: Elsevier; 2009.*)

Newer opioids have been created to reduce side effects. Tramadol, a very weak opioid agonist, is commonly used for chronic pain, but is also known to decrease the seizure threshold. Butorphanol, a kappa agonist and partial mu agonist, is used for migraine headaches and labor and delivery (less respiratory depression).

Epilepsy

Anticonvulsants (also known as antiepileptic drugs [AEDs]) were created with the goal of suppressing rapidly firing neurons that start a seizure. In addition to seizures, anticonvulsants are also used as **mood**

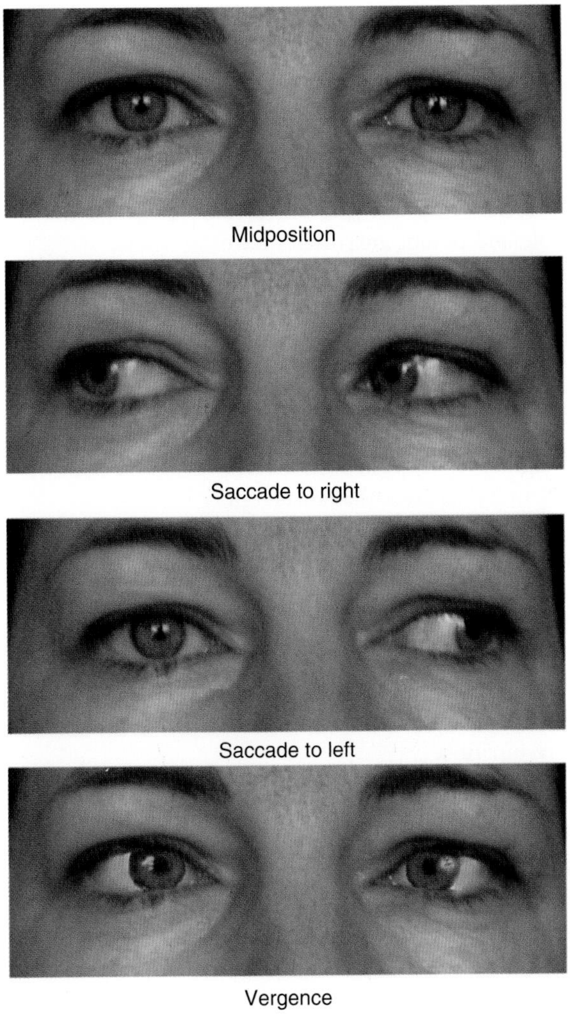

Fig. 13.45 Internuclear ophthalmoplegia. The patient's right eye is unable to perform conjugate left lateral gaze because of destruction of the medial longitudinal fasciculus. Convergence remains normal. *(From FitzGerald MJT, Gruener G, Mtui E. Clinical Neuroanatomy and Neuroscience. 6th ed. Philadelphia: Saunders; 2011.)*

Table 13.10 Pharmacology of Glaucoma

CLASS	DRUG NAMES	MECHANISM OF ACTION	SIDE EFFECTS
Adrenergic agents	Brimonidine, epinephrine	Decrease aqueous humor production	Stinging, mydriasis (contraindicated in closed-angle glaucoma)
Beta blockers	Timolol, betaxolol	Decrease aqueous humor production	Systemic (bradycardia, heart block)
Carbonic anhydrase inhibitors	Acetazolamide, dorzolamide, brinzolamide	Decrease aqueous humor production	Systemic (bitter taste, weight loss, depression, malaise)
Cholinomimetics	Direct—pilocarpine, carbachol Indirect—physostigmine	Increase trabecular outflow via ciliary muscle contraction	Cyclospasm, miosis
Prostaglandin analogs	Latanoprost	Increase uveoscleral outflow	Lengthen eyelashes, hyperemia, iris browning

stabilizers to treat bipolar disorder (see Chapter 14). The **two general mechanisms of action** of AEDs are inactivation of voltage-gated sodium channels or increased GABA signaling ($GABA_A$ receptors, transaminase, or transporter). Table 13.11 lists common AEDs.

Anesthetics

Anesthetics provide a **reversible loss of sensation.** They can be classified as **local** (e.g., injected into a wound) or **general** (e.g., inhaled anesthetics that cause whole-body anesthesia).

General anesthetics are used to cause a reversible loss of consciousness through the inhalation or intravenous administration of the anesthetic to induce and maintain a state of unconsciousness. Inhaled anesthetics, in order from highest to lowest potency, include methoxyflurane, halothane, enflurane, isoflurane, and nitrous oxide. IV anesthetics include barbiturates, benzodiazepines (used in conjunction with opioids), ketamine (phencyclidine [PCP] analog causing dissociative amnesia), etomidate, and propofol. The more lipid-soluble the drug, the more potent it is and the faster the induction and recovery time. This is inversely related to the **MAC (minimal alveolar concentration),** which is used as a marker to compare various anesthetics. Thus the more lipid-soluble and potent anesthetics have a low MAC. Anesthesiologists use the MAC of an anesthetic along with other variables (ventilation rate, tidal volume, atrioventricular [AV] concentration gradient, and blood solubility) to control general anesthesia during surgeries.

Local anesthetics act at a distinct site to prevent transmission of nerve impulses by binding to fast acting sodium channels. The **two general classes** are **esters** (procaine, cocaine, tetracaine) and **amides** (have two Is in the name → lidocaine, bupivacaine, mepivacaine). General side effects include cardiovascular toxicity (arrhythmias seen with cocaine or bupivacaine), methemoglobinemia (seen with benzocaine), seizures, and hypotension or hypertension. It is important to note that if a patient has an allergic reaction to an ester anesthetic, an amide anesthetic should be administered instead.

Malignant hyperthermia (MH) is a rare, life-threatening condition that results from inhaled anesthetics and succinylcholine. It is caused by an **autosomal dominant** inherited mutation in the **ryanodine receptor (RYR1) gene,** which results in uncontrolled increased skeletal muscle metabolism. When MH presents, patients are in a hypercatabolic state, resulting in a high body temperature, tachycardia, tachypnea, rigid muscles, rhabdomyolysis, and increased O_2 consumption and CO_2 production. Treatment consists of stopping the triggering agent, administering **dantrolene,** and providing supportive therapy aimed at correcting the hyperthermia, acidosis, and organ dysfunction.

TABLE 13.11 Common Antiepileptic Drugs

DRUG NAME	GENERAL USES	SIDE EFFECTS	COMMENTS*
Benzodiazepines (lorazepam, diazepam)	First-line acute seizures	Sedation and respiratory depression	Tolerance/dependence may develop
Phenytoin, Fosphenytoin	Partial, first-line tonic-clonic	Pseudolymphoma, megaloblastic anemia, gingival hyperplasia, peripheral neuropathy, hirsutism, nystagmus, ataxia	Can produce SLE-like syndrome. Teratogenic. Class IB antiarrhythmic.
Carbamazepine	Partial, first-line tonic-clonic and trigeminal neuralgia	Agranulocytosis aplastic anemia, liver toxicity; SJS, SIADH, diplopia, ataxia	Need to check CBC & LFTs. Teratogenic.
Gabapentin	Partial and tonic- clonic	Sedation, ataxia and tremor	Used in peripheral neuropathy, bipolar disorder and anxiety disorders.
Topiramate	Partial and tonic- clonic	Mental dulling, sedation, kidney stones, weight loss	Used in migraine HA prophylaxis
Lamotrigine	Partial and tonic- clonic	Dizziness, ataxia, sleepiness, nystagmus, headache, SJS	Contraindicated in myoclonus
Phenobarbital	Partial and tonic- clonic	Respiratory/ cardiovascular/CNS depression in overdose. Dependence.	Exacerbates porphyria, thus contraindicated in those cases. First line in neonates.
Valproic acid	Partial, absence, first-line tonic clonic	Fatal hepatotoxicity, neural tube defects, tremor, weight gain, agranulocytosis	Need to check CBC & LFTs.
Ethosuximide	First-line absence	Fatigue, GI symptoms, headache, rash, SJS	
Vigabatrin	Infantile spasms, complex partial seizures, secondary generalized seizures	Teratogen, retinal toxicity, CNS/GI symptoms	Structural GABA analog acting as suicide GABA transaminase inhibitor
Levetiracetam	Partial onset, myoclonic, or tonic-clonic seizures	CNS (somnolence, HA, etc.), neuropsychiatric, SJS/TEN	Modulates GABA and glutamate release
Lacosamide	Partial-onset seizures, diabetic neuropathic pain	Teratogen, neuropsychiatric, CNS, GI	Functionalized amino acid acting on voltage-gated sodium channels
Tiagabine	Epilespy, anxiety disorder, panic disorder	Dizziness, color perception	Increases GABA levels by blocking GABA reuptake

CBC, Complete blood cell count; LFT, liver function test; SIADH, syndrome of inappropriate antidiuretic hormone secretion; SJS, Stevens-Johnson syndrome; SLE, systemic lupus erythematosus.

*Note: CYP inducers—phenytoin, phenobarbital, and carbamazepine; CYP inhibitors—valproic acid.

Neuromuscular Blockade

Neuromuscular blocking drugs inhibit neuron transmission to muscles by blocking postsynaptic nicotinic acetylcholine (ACh) receptors. Clinically, they are used to produce paralysis, which aids in intubation for mechanical ventilation. They are generally classified as nondepolarizing or depolarizing neuromuscular blocking drugs based on whether or not they depolarize the motor endplate (Table 13.12).

Pharmacologic Treatment of Other Neurologic Disorders

Parkinson Disease

In general, treatment of Parkinson disease involves **increasing** the amount of **dopamine** (DA) in relationship to acetylcholine. Once pharmacotherapy (Table 13.13) has been exhausted, surgical therapies are available, such as deep brain stimulation (DBS).

Table 13.12 Neuromuscular Blocking Drugs

CLASS	COMMENTS
Nondepolarizing (atracurium, pancuronium, rocuronium, cisatracurium)	Drug names generally end in *-curonium* or *-curium*. Competitive antagonists that can be reversed with increase in ACh by acetylcholinesterase inhibitor drugs (AchEIs; e.g., neostigmine) Exhibit tetanic fade (failure of muscles to maintain a fused tetany at high electrical stimulation frequencies)
Depolarizing (succinylcholine)	Resistant to degradation by acetylcholinesterase (fast onset), but short duration because of metabolism by blood cholinesterase (pseudocholinesterase) Noncompetitive antagonist with two phases: • Phase I (depolarizing phase) —sudden muscle fasciculations, twitches followed by flaccidity • Phase II (desensitizing phase)—less responsive to depolarization After phase II, full neuromuscular blockade (paralysis) complete; AChEI potentiates phase I, but can reverse phase II Does not exhibit tetanic fade Complication of hyperkalemia caused by upregulation of receptors as a result of nerve damage or demyelinating disease (e.g., spinal cord injury, MS, chronic burns)

Table 13.13 Pharmacotherapy for Parkinson Disease

DRUG NAME	MECHANISM	SIDE EFFECTS	COMMENTS
L-DOPA (levodopa), carbidopa	L-DOPA crosses BBB to ↑ brain DA; carbidopa prevents peripheral conversion of L-DOPA to DA.	Arrhythmias from peripheral conversion "On effect" = dyskinesia "Off effect" = akinesia Hallucinations and delusions at high dosage	Overdose treatment is pyridoxine (increases peripheral metabolism); high-protein diet competes with L-DOPA.
Amantadine	Increases DA release	Ataxia and livedo reticularis (red-blue fish net mottling)	Good for "on effect" = dyskinesia; also antiviral used for influenza
Bromocriptine, pergolide (ergot), pramipexole, ropinirole (nonergot)	Agonizes DA receptors	Somnolence, hallucinations, compulsive gambling	Good for "on effect"; increased DA activity without increasing concentration so allows ↓ carbidopa-levodopa dose
Selegiline, rasagiline	Selective MAOB inhibitor	HTN crisis at high dosage	Good for "off effect"; rasagiline does not have sympathomimetic action, unlike selegiline.
Tolcapone, entacapone	COMT inhibitor	Central effect and hepatotoxicity	Entacapone does not cross BBB, so less central effect
Benztropine, biperiden, trihexyphenidyl	Antimuscarinic	Anticholinergic toxicity	Used in drug-induced PD; improves tremor and rigidity (not bradykinesia)

BBB, Blood–brain barrier; COMT, catechol-O-methyltransferase; DA, dopamine; HTN, hypertension; MAOB, monoamine oxidase B; PD, Parkinson disease.

Table 13.14 Pharmacotherapy for Alzheimer Disease

NAME	MECHANISM	SIDE EFFECTS
Acetylcholinesterase inhibitors (donepezil, rivastigmine, galantamine, tacrine)	Reduces rate of acetylcholine (ACh) breakdown, thus increasing ACh concentration	Nausea and vomiting because of cholinergic excess
Memantine	Noncompetitive NMDA receptor antagonist	Hallucinations, confusion, dizziness

NMDA, *N*-methyl-D-aspartate.

Table 13.15 Pharmacotherapy for Huntington Disease

DRUG NAME	MECHANISM	SIDE EFFECTS
Tetrabenazine, reserpine	VMAT inhibitor,* so promotes dopamine degradation.	Similar to antipsychotic side effects, such as akathisia, depression, dizziness and parkinsonism, but does not cause tardive dyskinesia

VMAT, Vesicular monoamine transporter.
*By preventing dopamine's repackaging into presynaptic vesicles, it instead will be degraded.

Alzheimer Disease

Current therapy is aimed at counteracting the reduction in cholinergic activity and excitotoxicity of glutamate seen in Alzheimer disease. In addition to pharmacologic therapy (Table 13.14), caregiving and psychosocial intervention needs to be addressed.

Huntington Disease

Symptomatic management of chorea and optimizing quality of life are the main two goals. Chorea is treated in a stepwise system, starting with tetrabenazine (Table 13.15) and then moving to atypical neuroleptics, typical neuroleptics, and eventually a combination of tetrabenazine and a neuroleptic.

Multiple Sclerosis

See Table 13.16.

Headaches

First-line treatment in acute attacks is typically NSAIDs, such as ibuprofen, naproxen, ketorolac, or aspirin. Triptans such as sumatriptan may also be used to treat acute migraines. These are often combined with antiemetics, such as prochlorperazine (Compazine), metoclopramide, or ondansetron. Medications used for migraine prophylaxis include tricyclic antidepressants (TCAs; e.g., amitriptyline or nortriptyline), antiepileptics (valproic acid, divalproex, topiramate), beta blockers (propranolol), and calcium channel blockers (verapamil).

DRUG CLASS	MECHANISM	USE	SIDE EFFECTS/NOTES
Triptans	Serotonin 5-$HT_{1B/1D}$ agonist; causes vasoconstriction and subsequent inhibition of proinflammatory neuropeptides	Acute migraine, cluster headaches (second line)	Risk of coronary vasospasm causing MI in CAD patients; serotonin syndrome; contraindicated in pregnancy
Ergotamines	Similar to triptans, but act at various receptors (5-$HT_{1A/1B}$, D_2, NE), so has more severe side effects than triptans and is rarely used	Acute migraine	Retroperitoneal fibrosis is most serious side effect; can lead to hydronephrosis or varicocele.

CAD, coronary artery disease; D_2, dopamine receptor D_2; MI, myocardial infarction; NE, norepinephrine.

Stroke

Once a thrombus (blood clot) occurs in an ischemic stroke, removing the blockage by mechanically removing it (thrombectomy) or by pharmacologic thrombolysis (clot busting) with tPA are the two definitive therapies available. tPA catalyzes the conversion of plasminogen (inactive enzyme, called a

Table 13.16 Pharmacotherapy for Multiple Sclerosis

DRUG NAME	MECHANISM	SIDE EFFECTS
Interferon-β	Has antiinflammatory properties; improves blood-brain barrier integrity	Flulike symptoms and injection site reactions most common
Glatiramer acetate	By resembling myelin basic protein, it shifts proinflammatory Th1 cells to regulatory Th2 cells to suppress inflammatory response by substituting itself as a target of immune system attack	Injection site and injection reactions; least likely to have flulike symptoms
Mitoxantrone	Topoisomerase inhibitor generally used in cancer chemotherapy	Nausea, vomiting, hair loss, immunosupression, cardiomyopathy
Natalizumab	Monoclonal antibody against cellular adhesion molecules, which reduces influx into the CNS	Fatigue, allergic reaction, hepatotoxicity, PML development
Fingolimod	Sphingosine analog; derived from fungus that modulates sphingosine-1-phosphate receptor to sequester lymphocytes in lymph nodes	Fatal infections, bradycardia, skin cancer, hemorrhagic focal encephalitis.

PML, progressive multifocal leukoencephalopathy; Th cells, T helper cells.

zymogen) to plasmin (active enzyme), which degrades fibrin clots. Therefore tPA activates the body's own clot degradation system. Before giving tPA, a list of inclusion and exclusion criteria is reviewed and risks and benefits discussed with the patient and family. Multiple contraindications exist and include severe hypertension, recent bleeding (GI, intracranial bleeding), and recent surgery. To be most effective, tPA should be given as early as possible. Generally, it is given within 3 hours of the start of neurologic symptoms, but this window can be extended to 4.5 hours depending on certain patient characteristics (age <80 years, no history of stroke or diabetes, not on anticoagulants). Once given, close observation is done to evaluate for hemorrhage, especially intracerebral hemorrhage.

REVIEW QUESTIONS

(1) A 32-year-old woman presents with sudden loss of vision and numbness of her right hand. She has had numbness of her left hand beginning 3 months ago. Her symptoms are worse after she takes a warm bath. An MRI is performed, and she is diagnosed with multiple sclerosis. Which cell type is most commonly damaged in this condition?

(2) A 56-year-old man presents with sudden onset of the worst headache of his life. A CT scan reveals blood in the subarachnoid space. Which artery is most frequently implicated in this condition?

(3) A 36-year-old man presents to the ER with constant seizure activity for 2 hours. Despite rapid control of his seizures, he continues to have neurologic deficits 48 hours after the incident. It is determined that he suffered excitotoxic damage during status epilepticus. Which neurotransmitter is most responsible for excitotoxicty?

(4) Which nerve roots are tested when assessing the patellar reflex?

(5) After suffering an ischemic stroke, a 72-year-old man experiences difficulty speaking. He seems to understand what you are saying, but when he responds he speaks in short broken phrases. What type of aphasia is he suffering, and what area is affected?

(6) A 27-year-old man presents to the ER after being struck in the head with a blunt object. Initially, he appears well, but soon becomes confused and disoriented. A CT scan reveals an epidural hematoma. What bone and artery are usually involved in this condition?

(7) A 67-year-old woman presents with lower extremity weakness, atrophy, spasticity, and hyperreflexia. What condition could explain these findings, and what treatment may delay its course?

(8) A 71-year-old woman presents with a gradual, new-onset headache that is worse whenever she chews. Her vision has started to become blurry. What is the cause of her headache?

(9) In treating Parkinson disease, why is L-DOPA given instead of dopamine? Why are L-DOPA and carbidopa given together?

(10) A male patient with a Glasgow Coma Scale score of 5 is no longer protecting his airway. You determine that he will need endotracheal intubation. You administer succinylcholine, and shortly after the patient begins to twitch. Why do these fasciculations occur? Would they occur if you used rocuronium?

14 PSYCHIATRY

Natalie Villa, Edwin Li, Andrew Yu, and Tiffany Pedigo

PSYCHOLOGY AND DEVELOPMENT

Theories of Learning

The concept of **operant conditioning** says that we may learn a variety of things based on the rewards or negative consequences of our actions. We may learn to acquire a strong drive in education because our loving parents give us hugs and new shiny toys when we bring home *A*s on our report cards; giving rewards is referred to as **positive reinforcement.** Or we can learn to share toys with other kids in school because, if we don't, they call us nasty names. This is called **positive punishment.** This may be confusing at first (after all, what's so positive about calling someone mean names?), so let's break it down.

- **Positive:** *Giving* something ("adding something") to the person as a consequence. You can *give* something good or something bad.
- **Negative:** *Taking away* something ("subtracting something") from the person as a consequence. You *can take away* something good or something bad.
- **Reinforcement:** You like a person's behavior and would like them to continue performing that behavior. You want to reinforce this learning and make it stronger.
  - **Positive reinforcement:** Giving a child candy for cleaning up his toys
  - **Negative reinforcement:** Taking away a teen's chores as a reward for doing well on a math test
- **Punishment:** You do not like a person's behavior and want the person to stop performing that behavior.
  - **Positive punishment:** Punching someone because he insulted your best friend
  - **Negative punishment:** Taking away a child's video game because the child didn't do his or her homework

Negative reinforcement means taking away something bad. Do not confuse this with punishment.

Reinforcement schedules add an additional layer of complexity to operant conditioning. Although it might sound nice and fair to reward children every time they clean up their toys (called **continuous reinforcement**), they'll get too accustomed to this reward system. In the event that parents don't give them candy once or twice, they'll stop cleaning up the toys because they don't think they'll get candy anymore. Thus this learned behavior (cleaning up) is **rapidly extinguished.** In contrast, reinforcement can be applied using a **variable ratio** in which the reward is given only at random intervals. Think of persons who have learned to enjoy gambling because it can be profitable; however, the slot machine they like to play rarely gives them money. The element of surprise and hope that they'll get that big monetary award leads them to continue playing, even if they don't win for a while; this response is **slowly extinguished.**

Another principle of learning is **habituation.** This refers to the observation that in some cases, repeated stimulation can eventually be "ignored." For example, a car alarm outside may at first be overwhelmingly distracting and make it impossible to study. After a while, however, it may be possible to ignore the noise and continue studying. **Sensitization** is the opposite phenomenon, in which repeated stimulation leads to a stronger and stronger response. For example, a woman who has been abused by her husband might startle every time her husband raises his hand, even if it's in a nonthreatening way.

Habituation: Repeated stimulation causes less response.

Sensitization: Repeated stimulation causes more response.

Freudian Theory

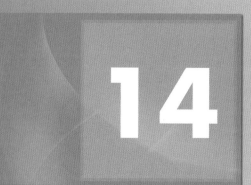

Freud's structural model explains people's impulses and the actions they take. The **id** is the part of a person's personality that drives what you want to do; it consists of hedonistic, impulsive urges such as seeking food and sex. In contrast, the **superego** is like the white angel that sits on your other shoulder, opposite the devilish id; it contains one's **morals** and what you should do. The **ego** is the **mediator** between the two, the source of a person's balance that determines the difference between right and wrong and what you want to do and what you should do.

According to Freud's psychoanalytic theory, the ego has ways to cope with life's stressors unconsciously. Some of these ego defenses are mature and more sophisticated, whereas others are immature and more primitive. For the U.S. Medical Licensing Examination (USMLE), it is important to recognize examples of each of these ego defenses.

Immature Ego Defenses:

- **Acting out:** Feelings of distress are expressed in unacceptable ways, such as **temper tantrums** or taking drugs. Patients who act out aren't able to channel their feelings in productive ways.
- **Denial:** Patients pretend that something isn't real and ignore its existence and significance. They do not want to deal with the consequences of this reality. For example, an alcoholic may deny that she or he has a problem with drinking.
- **Idealization:** Unconsciously inflating the positive qualities of a person relative to his or her negative qualities. A woman may idealize her abusive husband, focusing on how he appears caring, generous, smart, and devoted, while minimizing the harm he causes her to suffer.
- **Passive aggression:** Another unproductive way of dealing with feelings. A patient may express antagonistic feelings in indirect ways, such as **procrastinating** on tasks that he or she has been asked to do. A patient in conflict with the physician may repeatedly arrive late to appointments or perform tasks halfheartedly. This is something that is done consciously (unlike acting out): "I don't like you, so I'm not going to do what you say."
- **Projection:** Patients may have unpleasant feelings or impulses that they don't like and thus cause them anxiety. To relieve this anxiety, they behave as if another person harbors these feelings. For example, a man who has racist feelings may subconsciously projects these feelings onto his neighbor and accuses his neighbor of racist behavior. Another example is someone who is cheating on his or her partner and accuses the partner of being unfaithful.
- **Splitting:** Simply put, this is the idea that everything is black or white, good or bad, or loved or hated, and there are no shades of gray. For example, a patient may absolutely love the nurse taking care of her but may hate the physician she sees or vice versa. This immature ego defense can contribute to chaotic relationships and is commonly seen in people with **borderline personality disorder** (see later).

Splitting is an immature ego defense associated with borderline personality disorder.

Displacement is the shifting of undesirable feelings to a less-threatening person. For example, a boss yells at an employee, so the employee goes home and yells at a child.

Neurotic Ego Defenses:

- **Displacement:** Patients shift their undesirable feelings or impulses to a safer, less threatening person (e.g., Person A → B → C). For example, a husband may yell at his wife, who in turn yells at their son.
- **Dissociation:** May be a reaction to a stressful or traumatic event. Patients try to separate themselves (dissociate) from the trauma and emotion. They may even **change their personalities temporarily** to separate themselves from the reality of the underlying stressor (e.g., being attacked).
- **Identification:** Unconsciously modeling one's behaviors on someone else, although this may be good or bad. A child may grow up to be generous and warm like her mother. A teen who is physically abused by his stepfather may become physically aggressive toward his young brother.
- **Intellectualization:** When faced with a stressful or traumatic event, some patients may focus on the details in an intellectual fashion so that they do not dwell on the difficult emotions. For example, after a man's father passes away, when asked how he is doing, he discusses the medical aspects of how his father passed away instead of discussing his emotions.
- **Isolation of affect:** Like patients who dissociate, patients who use isolation of affect try to separate themselves from a traumatic event. A soldier may describe the death of his friend from a grenade explosion without emotion; he tries to remove his feelings from the situation. He **doesn't change his personality.**
- **Rationalization:** Also known as making excuses, rationalization is done when a person doesn't want to confront his or her true motives or the reason why something occurred. For example, a man who doesn't want to admit he has romantic feelings for a woman may rationalize that he drove an hour out of his way to pick her up from the airport simply because that's what any nice person would do. Or a woman who fails an examination may rationalize that she doesn't even care about the class, so it doesn't matter.

- **Reaction formation:** When a patient has uncomfortable, undesirable feelings or impulses, he or she may deal with them by actually converting them into the ***opposite*** emotion. For example, a woman who falls in love with a close male friend but is afraid to risk initiating a romantic relationship may begin to treat him cruelly. This is done unconsciously.
- **Regression:** These patients deal with stress by reverting back to childlike ways, such as a woman with cancer wanting to cry and be held by her mother.
- **Repression: Unconsciously** pushing a painful or stressful feeling or idea into the subconscious. This is different from denial, in which a patient is purposefully avoiding reality. To an outsider who tries to ask the patient about the feeling or event, it will seem like the patient had a memory lapse.
- **Undoing:** People who feel guilty about something may deal with it by performing actions that partially undo what they did. For example, a man has an affair with another woman and then buys his wife flowers on the way home. He is trying psychologically to cancel out one action with the other.

Repression is unconsciously pushing stressful feelings into the subconscious to avoid reality. Suppression is consciously and temporarily avoiding stressful feelings to deal with more pressing matters.

Mature Ego Defenses:

- **Sublimation:** This is a productive way of channeling an unpleasant or undesirable feeling into an acceptable action. For example, a man who has a bad temper and wants to physically hurt people who wrong him decides to become a judge so that he can punish evildoers via the law.
- **Altruism:** Giving selflessly to others to bring personal satisfaction. A man who feels terrible about hitting his ex-wife volunteers at a women's shelter. Or, a woman whose husband recently died of cancer sets up a charity that benefits cancer research. These people are trying to resolve their own stress or anxiety by helping others.
- **Suppression: Consciously** pushing a painful or stressful thought into the back of one's mind with the intent of addressing it later (which makes it different from repression). For example, a woman whose husband just passed away suddenly puts her grief aside so that she can logically focus on funeral arrangements and making sure the finances are in order. She will deal with the emotions later.
- **Humor:** Another mature defense, humor is just what it sounds like—breaking tension by joking about the stress of a situation. For example, a man who is nervous about his first date with a woman may make jokes to his friends that express his distress but in a comical way.

The USMLE may ask you to recall which ego defenses are mature. They can be remembered by the mnemonic **SASH: mature** women wear a **SASH**.

SASH: **S**ublimation, **A**ltruism, **S**uppression, and **H**umor are the mature ego defenses.

Miscellaneous Concepts in Psychology

Transference is an important concept to recognize for the USMLE and for your career as a physician. It refers to a phenomenon in which a patient redirects feelings about an important person in life onto the clinician. For example, a patient may unconsciously associate his therapist with his neglectful mother. If the therapist then inadvertently glances at the clock on the wall during a session, it might rekindle surprisingly strong feelings of neglect from an otherwise benign action.

Countertransference is the opposite. The patient may remind the physician of someone significant, and this elicits feelings that change how the physician treats the patient. For example, a young patient may remind a physician of her daughter, so she may find herself encouraging the patient to do better in school or saying something critical when the patient mentions her active sex life. Because this can bias how physicians treat their patients, in mental health and other situations, countertransference is quite significant.

PSYCHOPATHOLOGY

The *Diagnostic and Statistical Manual for Mental Disorders,* fifth edition (DSM-5), lays out specific and technical criteria for the diagnosis of mental disorders. In general, however, you will only need to have the general picture of each disorder to answer questions correctly on the USMLE Step 1. A few exceptions are noted.

Psychiatric Disorders of Children

Attention-Deficit/Hyperactivity Disorder

Children with attention-deficit/hyperactivity disorder (ADHD) are commonly described as being unable to sit still in class and often speak out of turn. They have great difficulty focusing on tasks such as homework assignments. Of note, these **traits must be present in more than one setting,** such as at home and at school. These children have **normal intelligence.** Unlike children with conduct disorder, children with ADHD **do not characteristically exhibit criminal behavior.** Unlike children with oppositional defiant disorder, they fail to follow through with instructions for homework assignments or interrupt conversations **not because they are being defiant** but rather because they are forgetful or unable to control their energy.

Tip: These children may stare off into space and appear to ignore others who are speaking to them, so ADHD can be confused with **absence seizures.** A child with ADHD will have additional symptoms, as described, whereas a child with absence seizures may be described as blinking quickly during the staring spells and will not have other symptoms of ADHD.

Treatment: Stimulants, which are thought to help children focus, are the primary treatment. Examples include amphetamines and methylphenidate.

Types of ADHD

Inattention: Makes careless mistakes on schoolwork, has trouble paying attention, doesn't seem to listen when spoken to, fails to follow through with instructions (because of forgetfulness, not because of defiance), avoids activities that require sustained mental effort, easily distracted.

Hyperactivity, impulsivity: Fidgets or squirms in seat, gets out of seat in class, runs or climbs excessively in inappropriate situations, difficulty playing quietly, always "on the go," talks excessively, blurts out answers before questions have been completed, difficulty waiting for one's turn, interrupts others.

Oppositional Defiant Disorder

Children with oppositional defiant disorder are defiant and naughty; they do not like to obey authority figures such as parents or teachers. They may get into arguments with adults and lose their temper, but they **do not exhibit criminal behavior** or overt acts of cruelty, like those with conduct disorder. They may be described as having normal relationships with their peers.

Treatment: Unfortunately, there is no good pharmacologic treatment. Behavior modification is sought through various forms of counseling and psychotherapy.

Conduct Disorder

Children with conduct disorder repeatedly **exhibit cruel or criminal behavior** such as harming animals or people, violating rules, deceitfulness or theft, or destroying property. They are, **by definition, younger than 18 years of age.** (After age 18, they are diagnosed with **antisocial personality disorder.**)

Treatment: Like oppositional defiant disorder, there is no good pharmacologic treatment. Psychotherapy and wraparound services are used to prevent the patient from continuing on to antisocial personality disorder.

Tourette Syndrome

Tourette syndrome is characterized by involuntary tics, usually motor (such as blinking or lip-licking), and including **at least one vocal tic** (such as throat clearing or grunting). Unlike sitcoms would have you believe, patients rarely spew out profanities uncontrollably (called **coprolalia**). Some children exhibit **echolalia** in which they repeat words. These tics may be temporarily suppressible and are often compared with the need to sneeze. Although these children do not necessarily have other symptoms of mental illness, Tourette syndrome is associated with obsessive-compulsive disorder (think: they can't control their grunting, and they also can't control their need to wash their hands).

Treatment: Antipsychotics, which are best known for their use in schizophrenia, are the primary treatment.

Tourette syndrome: Motor tics and at least one vocal tic

Separation Anxiety Disorder

Separation anxiety disorder may manifest in elementary school-age children who are extremely afraid to leave their caregivers. They may pretend to have tummy aches to stay home and avoid leaving their parents.

Pervasive Developmental Disorders

Autism Spectrum Disorders: A new diagnosis in the DSM-5, this is a spectrum of disorders characterized by markedly **impaired social function.** Individuals with autism spectrum disorders have difficulties making friends and relating to others. Their **speech is also abnormal**, ranging from repetition of words and phrases to complete lack of speech. (Don't confuse this with echolalia in Tourette syndrome; children with Tourette syndrome typically have normal friendships and language capabilities, although they may be shy and embarrassed.) Children with autism also have **ritualistic behavior,** such as habitually lining up cars.

Autism: Impaired social function, impaired language, and ritualistic behavior

These disorders have no good medical treatment. However, selective serotonin reuptake inhibitors can help treat certain behaviors, as can atypical antipsychotics such as risperidone; these medications will be discussed later in this chapter.

Asperger Disorder: On the less severe end of the spectrum of autistic disorders is Asperger disorder. In the DSM-5, Asperger disorder is no longer a subdiagnosis of autism spectrum disorders. However, many patients may still use this term, and it is unclear when the USMLE will make this change. These children have **normal intelligence and verbal capabilities** and may be successful academically. However, they have trouble with social skills and tend to fixate on particular interests, such as displaying an obsession with airplanes.

Asperger: Impaired social function and ritualistic behavior; normal language development

Rett Syndrome: The characteristic examination finding in Rett syndrome is a **girl** who **wrings her hands.** These girls initially develop normally but later **lose skills they had acquired**, such as the ability to speak or crawl. (In contrast, children with autism or Asperger disorder never have normal periods of development.) They may also be noted to have decelerating or plateauing head circumference growth. Unlike children with Asperger disorder, children with Rett syndrome become intellectually disabled. Although this disorder is **X-linked,** affected male fetuses die in utero, so the only living patients with this syndrome are female. Rett syndrome is no longer a diagnosis in DSM-5 because it is a genetic disorder that is separate from autism. However, some girls with Rett syndrome may also have autism—the two entities do have an association—so they are not mutually exclusive.

Childhood Disintegrative Disorder: Similar to Rett syndrome in that there is initially a period of normal development, children with childhood disintegrative disorder then lose many of their acquired skills, from language to motor skills to bowel and bladder control. This disorder is more common in **boys** and is not characterized by stereotyped hand wringing, unlike Rett syndrome.

Delirium versus Dementia
Delirium
Acute onset
Waxing and waning
Usually reversible
Dementia
Gradual onset
Steady decline in function
Usually not reversible

Delirium Versus Dementia

Delirium and dementia are often difficult to tell apart in clinical practice, although there are key points that differentiate the two.

Patients who are **delirious** typically have an underlying medical cause for this **acute change in mental status.** They may be hallucinating and are not alert and attentive to the world around them; their level of consciousness **waxes and wanes**—they seem out of it. Older patients are particularly prone to delirium, especially those who have recently undergone surgery, are in a hospital (or other unfamiliar setting), are infected (e.g., urinary tract infection, pneumonia) or are taking **anticholinergic medications.** Think of an old lady who is in a hospital recovering from hip replacement surgery who was previously pleasant and able to carry on conversations normally; one day she becomes febrile and starts to drift in and out of consciousness, speaks somewhat incoherently to her deceased husband, and apparently does not hear hospital staff who attempt to ask her what is wrong. Delirium is **reversible** if the underlying cause is treated.

Patients with **dementia** are also typically older, although they **decline gradually** rather than exhibiting a waxing and waning course as in delirium. In the early stages, they are **alert** and will interact relatively normally with those around them, although they gradually **lose their memory** and may eventually forget certain words (aphasia) and the ability to use certain objects, such as turning on a faucet (apraxia). Eventually, they exhibit personality changes and may become more withdrawn or more aggressive. Think of an older man who started to forget where he put his keys 6 months ago, started to forget to pay his bills 3 months ago, and yesterday took 2 hours to get home from the grocery store because he got lost. Dementia is **not reversible,** with few exceptions—notably normal pressure hydrocephalus and vitamin B_{12} deficiency.

Specific causes of dementia and medications that help slow cognitive decline are discussed in Chapter 13.

Likely cause of hallucinations:
Auditory: schizophrenia
Visual: delirium, LSD, psilocybin
Tactile: cocaine, alcohol withdrawal
Olfactory: temporal lobe epilepsy

Schizophrenia

Schizophrenia can manifest in many different ways and is categorized by five characteristic symptoms, two of which need to be present to diagnose the condition. Only one symptom is necessary if a pathognomonic symptom is present—presence of a bizarre delusion or auditory hallucination consisting of a running commentary, or of two voices conversing. To make the diagnosis, these symptoms have to be present for **more than 6 months**; if not, the appropriate diagnosis may be brief psychotic disorder (<1 month) or schizophreniform disorder (1–6 months).

- **Delusions:** Fixed, false beliefs. Think of a man who believes that the government is spying on him and cannot be convinced otherwise, despite evidence to the contrary.
- **Hallucinations:** Sensing something that is not actually present. **Auditory** hallucinations (e.g., hearing voices) are the most common in schizophrenia. If a patient is having visual hallucinations, consider delirium or other organic causes, such as LSD intoxication. Tactile hallucinations are more common in patients who are withdrawing from alcohol or are abusers of cocaine. **Formications,** the sensation of ants crawling on one's skin, is the most common tactile hallucination. Olfactory hallucinations may be present in temporal lobe epilepsy.
- **Disorganized speech:** Characterized by loose associations (e.g., jumping from one thought to another).
- **Disorganized or catatonic behavior:** A person with disorganized behavior may dress oddly or inappropriately (a purple raincoat with three hats in the summer) or may neglect hygiene (brushing hair or bathing). A person with catatonic behavior is unresponsive and generally unmoving, much like a statue. However, he or she may instead have peculiar movements, such as prolonged grimacing or repeating words that others say (echolalia).
- **Negative symptoms:** Include flat affect, lack of motivation, lack of speech, and social withdrawal. To understand why they are called negative, consider that the previous four symptoms (delusions, hallucinations, disorganized speech, and disorganized behavior) are positive; they involve the **addition** of abnormal characteristics, such as hearing voices that are not truly there. Negative symptoms, in contrast, involve the **absence** of characteristics that normal people have (such as speech and a wide range of emotion). The distinction between positive and negative symptoms of schizophrenia is clinically important because certain medications are more effective against one or the other type of symptoms.
- Interestingly, schizophrenia has a similar prevalence across many socioeconomic, cultural, and ethnic groups (≈1.5%). Unlike most psychological disorders, schizophrenia is evenly divided between men and women, although men tend to present earlier (in their late teens), whereas women tend to present later (in their late 20s).

Positive Symptoms
Hallucinations
Delusions
Disorganized speech and behavior

Negative Symptoms
Flat affect, apathy
Neglect of hygiene
Social withdrawal
Lack of motivation
Lack of speech

Neurobiological Mechanism

Schizophrenia is thought to result primarily from an **excess of dopaminergic signaling in the mesolimbic** (connecting the midbrain to the limbic system) **and mesocortical** (connecting the midbrain to the frontal cortex) **pathways of the brain.**

Treatment

The mainstay of medical treatment is with **antipsychotics.** Their efficacy relates to the degree to which they **block dopamine signaling at D_2 receptors.** Some side effects of antipsychotics can be explained by dopamine blockade in other pathways of the brain.

The **nigrostriatal pathway** connects the substantia nigra to the striatum and is important for control of movement. In fact, patients with Parkinson disease have profound reductions in dopamine signaling in this pathway; thus antipsychotics can actually cause abnormalities of movement. The nigrostriatal pathway is part of the extrapyramidal system, so called because this group of motor regulatory pathways does not pass through the pyramids of the medulla. The symptoms that antipsychotics cause are referred to as **extrapyramidal symptoms (EPS)** and include **acute dystonic reactions** (muscle spasms, especially those of the neck [torticollis] and eyes [oculogyric crisis]), **akathisia** (restless legs), **pseudoparkinsonism** (bradykinesia, resting tremor, and other symptoms commonly seen in Parkinson disease), and **tardive dyskinesia** (involuntary movements such as tongue darting out of the corner of the mouth or lip smacking). Treatment of acute dystonic reactions is with **anticholinergics,** such as diphenhydramine or benztropine. Beta blockers (e.g., propranolol) may be used for akathisia.

The **tuberoinfundibular pathway** connects the hypothalamus and pituitary gland to regulate pituitary hormone secretion. Particularly important is the control of prolactin, a hormone that can cause symptoms such as galactorrhea (milky discharge from the nipples), gynecomastia (breast enlargement), and loss of libido. Normally, dopamine signaling **inhibits** prolactin secretion. When dopamine signaling is blocked, as with antipsychotics, this inhibition is taken away, and hyperprolactinemia results.

Table 14.1 First-Generation (Typical) Antipsychotics (Neuroleptics)

MEDICATION	POTENCY	SPECIAL NOTES
Chlorpromazine	Low	This low-potency drug is usually associated with sleepiness and orthostatic hypotension. With long-term use, patients may note gray-blue skin pigmentation.
Thioridazine	Low	Known for causing prolonged QT, it can accumulate in the eyes and cause retinitis pigmentosa, which may lead to blindness.
Haloperidol	High	Known in hospitals as vitamin H, haloperidol is commonly used intramuscularly when a patient becomes acutely aggressive or delirious. The incidence of EPS is high.
Trifluoperazine, perphenazine, fluphenazine	High	—

Other side effects of antipsychotics relate to other receptor types that are inadvertently **also blocked.**

- **Histamine H_1:** Antihistamine side effects include sleepiness and weight gain.
- **α_1:** Blocking these receptors may result in orthostatic hypotension.
- **Muscarinic:** Anticholinergic effects include dry mouth, urinary retention, constipation, and blurry vision.

NMS: Hyperthermia, rigidity, and elevated CPK.

Finally, there are some side effects of antipsychotics that are not attributable to a single mechanism, as far as we know.

- **QT prolongation:** This dangerous cardiac side effect can lead to torsades de pointes.
- **Seizures:** Many antipsychotics lower the seizure threshold.
- **Neuroleptic malignant syndrome** (NMS): This life-threatening syndrome is characterized by fever **(hyperthermia),** lead pipe muscle **rigidity, autonomic instability** (tachycardia, sweating), tremor, leukocytosis, and **elevated creatine phosphokinase** (CPK) level. It is treated by immediately stopping the offending drug and cooling the patient. As the hyperthermia associated with NMS is related to blockade of the D_2 receptor in the hypothalamus and subsequent increase in the body's temperature set point, **bromocriptine** (a dopamine agonist) may be used in treatment. **Dantrolene** inhibits calcium release through ryanodine receptor channels and can also be useful for relaxing muscles.

First-Generation (Typical) Antipsychotics: This class of medications is relatively successful at **reducing positive symptoms,** but they do not work well in treating negative symptoms (Table 14.1). The information given earlier about mechanism of action and side effects applies to typical antipsychotics.

Of note, the drugs that have **lower potency** (more drug required to achieve therapeutic levels of D_2 receptor blockade) are **less likely to cause EPS** but are **more likely to cause autonomic side effects** such as drowsiness and hypotension because the higher doses cause blocking of the **H_1** (drowsiness) and **α_1** (vasodilation, hypotension) receptors described earlier. Conversely, the drugs that have **higher potency** are **more likely to cause EPS** but are **less likely to cause autonomic side effects.**

Second-Generation (Atypical) Antipsychotics: Atypical antipsychotics actually **block serotonin 2A (5-HT_{2A}) receptors** and α_1, and H_1 receptors in addition to D_2 receptors (Table 14.2). They are somewhat less effective than typical antipsychotics at treating positive symptoms, but they **treat negative symptoms** well. They are **less likely to cause EPS and anticholinergic side effects** than their typical counterparts. However, they do cause **significant H_1 blockade** and are thus associated with **weight gain and the metabolic syndrome,** which is of great concern for many patients.

Unfortunately, despite medical treatment and cognitive-behavioral interventions, most patients with schizophrenia are affected for their lifetime, with many of them experiencing significant impairment; they are often unable to keep jobs or maintain relationships.

Similar Disorders

The following disorders are characterized by symptoms similar to the symptoms of schizophrenia, but there are key differences among these diagnoses. Patients with schizophrenia-like symptoms can all be described as **psychotic** because psychosis is a description of this constellation of symptoms, but it is not a formal diagnosis.

Table 14.2 Second-Generation (Atypical) Antipsychotics (Neuroleptics)

MEDICATION	SPECIAL NOTES
Clozapine	May cause agranulocytosis; this leukopenia can be fatal, so the CBC must be monitored. It also lowers the seizure threshold. Because of these concerns, clozapine is never considered as a first-line medication. Associated with weight gain and insulin resistance.
Olanzapine	Strongly associated with weight gain and insulin resistance. Think of an obese person looking very round, like the letter *O* in *olanzapine.*
Risperidone	Particularly associated with hyperprolactinemia.
Aripiprazole	In addition to the listed mechanisms of action, aripiprazole is also a partial agonist at dopamine and 5-HT_{1A} receptors.
Quetiapine	Makes people very sleepy. It can even be used as a sedative for patients who have trouble sleeping. Think of sleeping during "quiet time," which sounds similar to "quetiapine." It may also be associated with cataracts, so patients need their eyes checked regularly.
Ziprasidone	Known for QT prolongation; causes less weight gain than other atypical antipsychotics.

CBC, Complete blood cell count.

Brief psychotic disorder is similar in the type of symptoms to schizophrenia, but the time course is different. In brief psychotic disorder, the symptoms have been present for **less than 1 month** and are usually precipitated by a major stressor, such as being expelled from college.

Schizophrenia: Bizarre delusions—not plausible

Delusional disorder: Nonbizarre delusions—plausible

Schizophreniform disorder also is like schizophrenia. Its duration is longer than a brief psychotic disorder but shorter than schizophrenia. The symptoms have been present for **1 to 6 months.** Thus it is critical that you note the time course in the question stem, because this will affect the diagnosis of a patient with psychotic symptoms.

Schizoaffective disorder is similar to schizophrenia **plus mood symptoms** such as depressive symptoms or manic symptoms (see later). The mood disorder must be present for a substantial portion of the illness. How do we tell the difference between schizoaffective disorder and a mood disorder with psychotic features if both include psychosis and mood disorders (mania or depression)? In a mood disorder with psychotic features (e.g., MDD with psychotic features), the psychotic episodes will occur during a mood episode. In schizoaffective disorder, the psychotic features must persist for longer than 2 weeks without a mood episode.

Delusional disorder may be difficult to distinguish from schizophrenia. Patients with delusional disorder have delusions, as the name suggests, but they are **not bizarre.** Such delusions are actually plausible but unwavering. For example, nothing you say can make the patient shake his belief that members of the CIA are following him every time he leaves his house. Contrast this with a schizophrenic, who may believe that aliens have implanted a device in his brain that controls his thoughts and actions; this delusion is bizarre and certainly not plausible. Unlike patients with schizophrenia, those with delusional disorder lack disorganized speech and behavior, are **not severely impaired,** and may lead otherwise normal lives, with stable jobs and relationships. You may encounter a question regarding a man with delusional disorder whose wife also begins to develop delusions; this is a **shared psychotic disorder** (or folie à deux). His wife has a reasonable chance of recovery if separated from him because he unwittingly induced the delusions in her.

Women attempt suicide more often than men, but men are more likely to be successful. Men tend to use guns or more lethal means, whereas women more often try a medication overdose or poisoning.

Depression

To meet the criteria of a **major depressive episode,** a person must have at least five of the **SIG E CAPS** criteria for at least 2 weeks. Also, one of the symptoms must be **depressed mood** or **anhedonia** (loss of interest in pleasurable activities):

- **S**leep—insomnia or hypersomnia
- **I**nterest—loss of interest in pleasurable activities (anhedonia)
- **G**uilt—feelings of guilt or worthlessness
- **E**nergy—fatigue or loss of energy
- **C**oncentration—diminished ability to concentrate or focus
- **A**ppetite—increase or decrease in appetite or weight
- **P**sychomotor retardation or agitation
- **S**uicidality or thoughts of self-harm (active or passive)

The proportion of people who experience a major depressive episode at least once in their lifetime is significant, 5% to 12% for men and 10% to 25% for women. These symptoms must interfere with

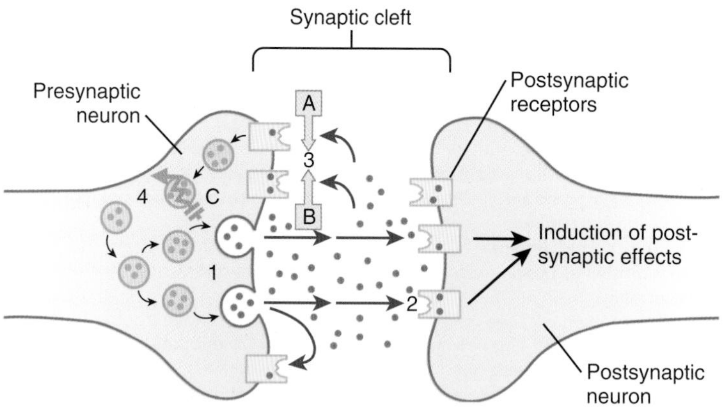

Physiological processes at the synapse:
1. When an electrical signal reaches the presynaptic terminal, presynaptic amine vesicles fuse with the neuronal membrane and release their contents into the synaptic cleft.
2. Amines in the synaptic cleft bind to postsynaptic receptors to produce a post synaptic response.
3. Amines may be removed from the synaptic cleft by reuptake into the presynaptic neuron.
4. The monoamine oxidase enzyme breaks down presynaptic amines.

Effects of antidepressants:
A. Tricyclics prevent presynaptic reuptake of the amines nonadrenaline and serotonin
B. SSRIs predominantly block reuptake of serotonin.
C. MAOIs reduce the activity of monoamine oxidase in breaking down presynaptic amines (leaving more available for release into the presynaptic cleft).

Fig. 14.1 Mechanism of action of the major classes of antidepressants. MAOIs, Monoamine oxidase inhibitors; SSRIs, selective serotonin reuptake inhibitors. (*From Bennett PM, Brown MJ.* Clinical Pharmacology. *10th ed. Philadelphia: Elsevier; 2008.*)

the patient's functioning and must not be attributable to any other medical condition (e.g., increased fatigue in a patient with newly diagnosed hypothyroidism).

It is occasionally difficult to distinguish between major depressive disorder and grief in a patient who just underwent a major stressor such as losing a spouse. The major symptom that will allow you to diagnose a patient with major depressive disorder is excessive guilt to the point of feeling worthless. Patients who state that they feel worthless because they did not spend more time with their loved one are usually clinically depressed. Additionally, major depressive disorder extends far longer than usual feelings of grief (i.e., longer than a few months).

Risk factors for suicide completion:
Previous attempts
Concurrent medical illness
Organized plan (including access to weapons)
Lacking social support
Suicidal ideation

Neurobiological Mechanism

The neurotransmitter abnormalities in depression are less clear than those in schizophrenia. It appears that patients with depression have **decreased levels of serotonin** (5-HT), **norepinephrine, and dopamine**, because drugs that increase signaling in these pathways tend to improve patients' symptoms.

Treatment

See Fig. 14.1 for an explanation of the mechanism of action of the major classes of antidepressants.

Tricyclic antidepressants (TCAs) are an older class of medications that work by **blocking reuptake of norepinephrine and serotonin into the presynaptic neuron,** thereby prolonging their action in the synapse. These medications are rarely used for depression now because they can prolong the QRS, QT, and PR intervals and cause cardiac arrhythmias; they are **lethal in overdose.** TCAs also have anticholinergic side effects, including dry mouth, constipation, and urinary retention. As noted previously in the "Delirium" section, anticholinergic side effects can produce altered mental status, especially in elderly patients. One of these side effects can be exploited for another medical use; **imipramine** is a TCA that is still used in children who suffer from **bedwetting** (enuresis) because it promotes urinary retention. Other TCAs such as **amitriptyline** and **nortriptyline** have found a role in treating neuropathic pain, such as in diabetics. TCAs are used in lower doses in these situations, with a more favorable side effect profile.

SSRIs are an important potential cause of sexual dysfunction, as are other medications, such as beta blockers. Organic diseases such as diabetes (impaired neurovascular functioning) can also be culprits. Psychological causes such as depression and anxiety may also contribute.

Monoamine oxidase inhibitors (MAOIs) **inhibit monoamine oxidase,** an enzyme that breaks down amine neurotransmitters, including serotonin, norepinephrine, and dopamine. Therefore higher levels of these neurotransmitters are available. The MAO enzyme is located within the neuron's cytoplasm, not in the synapse where other medications have their effects. The use of MAOIs for depression is limited by two major side effects. First, patients who consume foods rich in tyramine (such as smoked meats, aged cheeses, and wine) while taking an MAOI are at risk of a hypertensive crisis. Both lead to an increase in the amount of norepinephrine, a potent vasoconstrictor: Tyramine is a precursor in the biosynthesis of norepinephrine, and MAOIs increase the availability of norepinephrine. Second, patients taking multiple medications that increase the availability of serotonin (such as MAOIs and selective serotonin reuptake inhibitors) are at risk for **serotonin syndrome** (see later). Despite these side effects, it is notable that MAOIs are particularly effective for **atypical depression,** which is characterized by hypersomnia, hyperphagia, and leaden paralysis. However, they are almost never used as a first-line medication.

Selective serotonin reuptake inhibitors (SSRIs) are typically first-line treatments for depression because they are effective and have a more favorable side effect profile than other classes of antidepressants. As their name suggests, they **inhibit the reuptake of serotonin** into the presynaptic neuron, allowing for longer duration of serotonin action in the synapse. Common side effects include weight gain, gastrointestinal (GI) upset, and **sexual dysfunction,** which limit their use in many patients. Examples of SSRIs include fluoxetine, sertraline, paroxetine, and citalopram. SSRIs usually must be tapered or else patients can experience SSRI discontinuation syndrome (dizziness, headache, fatigue, agitation). The risk is highest with paroxetine and lowest with fluoxetine.

Serotonin-norepinephrine reuptake inhibitors (SNRIs) are newer medications that **inhibit the reuptake of both serotonin and norepinephrine.** Like SSRIs, they are more widely used today because they are safer than MAOIs and TCAs in overdose. Their side effects are also similar to SSRIs; although some patients do experience decreased sexual drive and anorgasmia, some patients actually have an *increased* sexual drive while taking SNRIs. Interestingly, like TCAs, they can be used for neuropathic pain, possibly because they both increase norepinephrine signaling. The increase in norepinephrine levels can lead to hypertension, tachycardia, and other stimulant effects. Commonly used SNRIs include venlafaxine, duloxetine, milnacipran, and sibutramine.

Bupropion is a newer antidepressant that has stimulant qualities because of its **norepinephrine and dopamine reuptake inhibition.** Bupropion **does not cause weight gain** (it actually can cause weight loss) and it **does not cause sexual dysfunction** (it can actually increase libido). It is important to note that bupropion **decreases the seizure threshold,** so patients who are prone to seizures should not take this medication. These patients include those with epilepsy, brain tumors, anorexia nervosa, and bulimia nervosa (see later), as well as those with the potential for withdrawal from alcohol or benzodiazepines. Bupropion is also used as a smoking cessation aid.

> Bupropion can be used for smoking cessation because it reduces cravings and withdrawal symptoms.

Electroconvulsive therapy (ECT) is a safe and effective therapy used for depression that is refractory to antidepressant medications. It can also be used if a patient is actively suicidal because it works more quickly than medications, which take at least 3 to 6 weeks to have noticeable effect. After the patient is sedated and paralyzed, electricity is passed through the brain to induce a seizure. The main side effect of ECT is retrograde amnesia. It is contraindicated in patients with space-occupying lesions because it causes a temporary increase in intracranial pressure (ICP).

Serotonin Syndrome: Of note, TCAs, MAOIs, SSRIs, and SNRIs all increase synaptic levels of serotonin. When patients take multiple serotonergic medications, they are at risk for serotonin syndrome, a condition marked by sweating, diarrhea, fever, autonomic instability, and seizures. The presentation of serotonin syndrome is similar to neuroleptic malignant syndrome (NMS). On Step 1, a patient with NMS will have lead pipe rigidity and elevated CPK, whereas a patient with serotonin syndrome will not. Additionally, NMS is caused by antipsychotics, so patient history can be highly relevant in distinguishing the two.

> On Step 1, a patient with NMS will have lead pipe rigidity and elevated CPK, whereas a patient with serotonin syndrome will not.

Persistent Depressive Disorder (Dysthymia)

Dysthymia can be thought of as a **milder form of depression that is more chronic (lasting at least 2 years, or 1 year in children and adolescents).** Patients with this disorder have depressed mood for most of the time on most days, and they also may experience sleep disturbances and other depressive symptoms. These patients usually do not require hospitalization because they typically can care for themselves. Think of a patient who has felt "down" for many years, doesn't take joy in anything, and is always tired.

> Unlike depression, which is more common in women, bipolar disorder is equally prevalent in men and women.

Bipolar Disorders

Bipolar I

A woman notices that her husband has been acting strangely for the past 2 weeks. He has barely been sleeping, only an hour a night, because he says he has to get back to his "big research project." He eagerly tells everyone within shouting distance about his exciting plan to achieve world peace and how he is going to meet with one of the President's advisors to tell him all about it; however, it is hard to understand him because he talks so quickly and jumps from one idea to another. He has also drained their savings by buying an expensive new suit and sports car. This is a classic example of a patient with bipolar I disorder.

Patients with bipolar I disorder by definition have had **at least one manic episode** (lasting at least 7 days, or for any length of time if hospitalization is required) that includes at least three of the **DIG FAST** criteria:

- **D**istractibility
- **I**nsomnia (decreased need for sleep)
- **G**randiosity (increased self-esteem)
- **F**light of ideas or racing thoughts
- **A**ctivity or **A**gitation, such as putting in significantly more work into projects or an increase in sexual activity
- **S**peech—pressured, rapid speech
- **T**houghtlessness— engaging in pleasurable activities with negative consequences, such as gambling or shopping sprees

Patients experiencing a manic episode can have an elevated/expansive mood or an irritable mood; if irritability is the predominant feature, then four DIG FAST criteria must be met. Note that a patient only needs to have a manic episode to be diagnosed with bipolar I disorder, although most patients also cycle through periods of major depression.

Bipolar II

Patients with bipolar II disorder have had at least one major depressive episode and at least one **hypomanic episode (both are required for the diagnosis)** and they **have never had a manic episode.** A hypomanic episode still fulfills at least three of the DIG FAST criteria but only needs to last 4 days (unlike 7 days for a manic episode) and is less severe than a manic episode; these patients have DIG FAST symptoms but are not as severely impaired. Any episode with symptoms severe enough to result in hospitalization should be considered to be a manic episode. Similarly, the presence of psychotic features also qualifies as mania.

Cyclothymic Disorder

Cyclothymic patients experience a chronic cycling mood disorder that varies between hypomanic symptoms that don't fulfill criteria for either a manic or hypomanic episode and depressive symptoms that fulfill criteria for a major depressive episode. These symptoms must last at least 2 years with no symptom-free period longer than 2 consecutive months and must impair the functioning of the patient. Approximately 15% to 50% of patients will go on to develop bipolar I or II disorders.

Treatment for Bipolar I and Bipolar II Disorders: Lithium helps stabilize mood and decreases the risk of a manic or depressive episode and is usually the first-line treatment. Important side effects include its antidiuretic hormone (ADH) antagonist effects on the kidney (causing **nephrogenic diabetes insipidus**) and **hypothyroidism.** It is associated with **Ebstein anomaly** in the infant, in which the opening of the tricuspid valve is displaced downward toward the apex of the right ventricle; this makes the right atrium too large and the right ventricle too small. Lithium can be toxic in overdose: Mild lithium toxicity is manifested by tremor and nausea, with higher levels of toxicity progressing to seizures, coma, and death.

Antiepileptic drugs (AEDs), such as valproate, are also used as mood stabilizers. Side effects of valproate include hepatotoxicity and neural tube defects in prenatal exposure. Carbamazepine is another AED that also increases liver function test results and carries a risk of agranulocytosis as well as Stevens-Johnson syndrome. (Do you recall which antipsychotic is also strongly associated with agranulocytosis? Answer: clozapine.)

Electroconvulsive therapy can also be used for patients with bipolar disorder.

Lithium is the first-line drug in the treatment of bipolar disorders, except in pregnancy, when haloperidol is preferred.

Anxiety Disorders

Panic Disorder

Patients with panic disorder have panic attacks and are constantly afraid of having another embarrassing panic attack. Panic attacks are characterized by intense fear, sweating, palpitations, shortness of breath, chest pain, nausea, numbness or tingling, feeling like one is choking, and/or feeling like one is going to die. In order to be diagnosed, patients also must have persistent worry about having another panic attack in the future or have made a significant change in their behavior as a result of the panic attacks (such as avoiding certain places out of fear of having an attack while there, also known as agoraphobia).

Of note, panic attacks can occur out of the blue and **do not have a clear trigger.** Patients can be awoken from sleep by their symptoms.

Neurobiological Mechanism: Panic disorder is associated with **increased norepinephrine** signaling and **decreased serotonin and γ-aminobutyric acid (GABA).** In brief, this makes sense because of the autonomic symptoms that patients have (increased norepinephrine) and inability to relax (decreased GABA).

Treatment

- **Benzodiazepines:** These drugs allosterically alter GABA receptors in the brain and promote GABA binding. Given the known neurotransmitter abnormalities, it should make sense that these GABA-ergic medications should help a patient relax during a panic attack. However, these medications are habit forming and should not be used long term.
- **SSRIs:** Useful for long-term maintenance because of the lower baseline serotonin levels in patients with panic disorder. Recall that SSRIs are also a mainstay of treatment for depression.

Common Phobias
Flying
Heights
Water
Snakes
Spiders
Blood

Specific and Social Phobias

The term *phobia* is used to describe an exaggerated or irrational fear of an object or situation. Those with a phobia are so affected by this fear that it interferes with their social life, job, or other activities of daily living.

Patients with social phobia have similar anxious reactions to social situations. Patients with performance anxiety have a specific fear of public speaking but are otherwise not anxious in public.

Some patients may experience actual panic attacks in reaction to their phobia. Such patients are not considered to have panic disorder. Although the distinction between panic disorder and a specific or social phobia may seem hazy, the key point is that panic disorder is characterized by **unprovoked** panic attacks, whereas patients with a specific or social phobia have symptoms of anxiety or panic specifically when confronted by their fear.

Treatment: Unlike for panic disorder, medications are not particularly effective for specific phobias. This disorder is best treated by **systematic desensitization,** in which the patient is gradually exposed to their fear in a controlled environment.

In contrast, sufferers of social phobia do benefit from paroxetine, an **SSRI. Beta blockers** such as propranolol are also useful for social phobia to blunt the sympathetic response that causes a person's heart to race.

Generalized Anxiety Disorder

Unlike those with panic disorder or specific phobia, patients with generalized anxiety disorder (GAD) are always anxious (as the name of the disorder suggests). They worry about multiple aspects of their daily lives, such as their job, finances, or grades. They can also worry about social situations, but look for anxiety about other aspects of their lives to differentiate from social phobia. These symptoms are chronic and must last for **at least 6 months**; many patients complain of "being anxious my whole life." GAD is common, with a lifetime prevalence of about 4%.

Like major depressive disorder, GAD is more common in women than in men.

Neurobiological mechanism: There is no one neurotransmitter implicated in GAD, although it appears that there is **increased norepinephrine, decreased GABA, and decreased serotonin signaling.** Also, functional MRI studies link GAD to abnormal processing in the amygdala, an area of the brain that has important roles in emotions and memory.

Treatment

- **SSRIs and SNRIs:** Recall that depression and GAD are associated with decreased levels of serotonin.
- **Buspirone:** A unique medication that is a **partial agonist at serotonin 5-HT_{1A} receptors,** it is also a D_2 antagonist; however, it is not clear if this contributes to its anxiolytic effects. Unlike benzodiazepines, buspirone does not have potential for tolerance or dependence. Also, it is not sedating and does not interact with alcohol.
- **Benzodiazepines:** May be used for the treatment of GAD. However, as is the case with panic disorder, they are not ideal for monotherapy or for prolonged periods because of the risk of tolerance and dependence. Furthermore, because benzodiazepines are GABA-ergic depressants, there is a risk of respiratory depression and death when mixed with alcohol.

Because depression, GAD, and OCD are all associated with decreased serotonin signaling, SSRIs are used to treat all three. Think of depression and anxiety as being related illnesses.

The prognosis for GAD is not as poor as for other disorders such as schizophrenia; 50% of patients will fully recover.

Obsessive-Compulsive Disorder

Patients with obsessive-compulsive disorder (OCD) experience both obsessions and compulsions.

Obsessions are recurrent thoughts that cause distress to the patient. Unlike hallucinations (e.g., what a schizophrenic might have), a patient with OCD is **aware that the distressing obsession is "all in the head."** (The fact that patients with OCD are aware of their irrational thoughts and behavior is termed *ego-dystonic;* they are not comfortable with these obsessions.) For example, someone might have recurring thoughts that he or she has forgotten to turn off the stove. Another patient may feel that performing a task, from folding clothes to cutting carrots, has to be done in an exact fashion or else it will not feel "right." Other common obsessions relate to symmetry (of an arrangement of objects) or cleanliness (and the presence of germs).

Compulsions are compensatory **actions** that the patient does to relieve the anxiety caused by the obsessions. Patients who worry about whether the stove is on or off may go to the kitchen to check it repeatedly; this urge may be so strong that it causes them to be late for work or get out of bed when trying to sleep. Patients who have less well-defined obsessions regarding daily tasks may count in their head while chopping carrots to make sure they finish on a "safe" number. Patients may spend significant amounts of time moving and rearranging objects so that their alignment is good or may wash their hands repeatedly to the point that their skin becomes raw. Patients with OCD are very distressed by their obsessions, and the resulting compulsions interfere with the flow of their daily lives.

OCD is associated with tic disorders and Tourette syndrome. However, Tourette syndrome is better treated with antipsychotics.

Neurobiological Mechanism

Although this is not well understood, researchers postulate that **serotonin signaling is decreased** in OCD patients as well. This is based on the finding that SSRIs are an effective treatment.

Treatment: SSRIs are used to treat OCD. **TCAs,** particularly clomipramine, can also be used. Behavioral therapy, such as relaxation techniques, is equally important.

Stress Disorders

Posttraumatic Stress Disorder (PTSD)

PTSD develops in some patients after experiencing or witnessing a traumatic, or potentially life-threatening, event. Such events include rape, war, and motor vehicle accidents. For **at least 1 month,** they experience symptoms such as the following:

Patients with PTSD are also more likely than the general population to have depression and substance abuse.

- Hyperarousal—a state of increased alertness and tension that can lead to trouble sleeping, jumpiness, or angry outbursts.
- Intrusive thoughts—the patient has persistent dreams or flashbacks of the event.
- Numbness—patients may have limited emotions and affect, and they may feel detached from the world around them.

- Avoidance—patients avoid anything that reminds them of the traumatic event, such as a war veteran avoiding fireworks shows, shooting ranges, or other locations that have loud, sudden noises.

Treatment: Antidepressants such as **SSRIs, TCAs, and MAOIs** may be used for PTSD. Counseling and behavioral therapy are of great importance for patients with PTSD. Support groups and relaxation training are especially valuable. Benzodiazepines can be prescribed to help with sleep.

Acute Stress Disorder

Patients with acute stress disorder have similar reactions to a traumatic event as those with PTSD, but symptoms of acute stress disorder last **less than 1 month.** When symptoms last longer than a month, it is considered PTSD. It is treated similarly to PTSD.

Adjustment Disorder

Adjustment disorder involves an excessive, maladaptive reaction to a stressful life event. Symptoms must start within 3 months of the onset of the stressor. Unlike PTSD, the life event need not be life threatening; it may involve starting at a new school or divorcing one's spouse. Although most people do have some sadness or anxiety in response to such situations, those with adjustment disorder have more severe reactions that impair the patient's ability to function. For example, a teenager may develop symptoms of depression after leaving his childhood friends and moving to a new town; he loses his appetite and feels sad all the time. This particular patient developed depressive symptoms, whereas others with adjustment disorder may develop anxiety or aggression. Note that patients who meet criteria for major depressive disorder will be diagnosed with that condition instead, not adjustment disorder, regardless of the presence of a trigger.

Of note, normal grief after the death of a loved one does not constitute an adjustment disorder.

Malingering

A patient who is malingering **fakes a disorder** for **secondary gain** (a goal that would benefit the patient). For example, an inmate may fake psychotic symptoms to be removed from jail. Or the disorder may be physical; a man may fake or greatly exaggerate back pain to receive opiates or time off work from a physician. **Symptoms may resolve once the patient's secondary gain has been achieved.**

Factitious Disorder

Like malingering, patients with factitious disorder **consciously fake symptoms, both physical and psychological.** However, they do not have a secondary goal in mind (e.g., avoiding work); their aim is to **be a sick patient** and thus get attention and sympathy from medical providers (also called primary gain). This can be difficult to diagnose and requires a high degree of suspicion and some detective work on the part of the physician. For example, for a patient who complains of terrible stomach pain, an examiner may stand near the patient and subtly bump into the patient or the bed while talking. This should elicit a grimace in a patient with truly severe abdominal pain, but patients with a factitious disorder may not react because they do not believe they are being examined. Another commonly tested example is a patient who secretly injects insulin to purposely induce hypoglycemia. The treating physician should measure levels of C-peptide to distinguish factitious disorder from organic causes (C-peptide is produced with endogenous insulin and will be low in a factitious disorder [exogenous insulin] but high with an organic cause [endogenous insulin]). Unfortunately, factitious disorder has a poor prognosis, and there is no good treatment.

Munchausen syndrome is the term used to describe a factitious disorder that is chronic (rather than a few isolated episodes). Think of a woman who complains of awful, chronic abdominal pain who has been to numerous doctors. On two occasions, her abdominal pain has even appeared to be acute on examination, and she has actually consented to and undergone two exploratory surgeries. She visits new doctors to continue to receive care. However, imaging, laboratory work, and the history and physical have all failed to reveal an organic reason for her pain. (On the USMLE, the question stem will likely tell you that all testing has been negative, and you should infer that the disorder is being faked. In real life, though, don't be too quick to blame the patient if you are unable to find an answer, because there are certainly actual diseases that elude explanation for quite some time.)

Related Disorders with Important Time Differences
PTSD: > 1 month
Acute stress disorder: < 1 month
Schizophrenia: > 6 months
Schizophreniform disorder: 1 to 6 months
Brief psychotic disorder: < 1 month
Depression: > 2 weeks
Dysthymic disorder: > 2 years

Adjustment disorder has a clear trigger, and the symptoms resolve within 6 months after the trigger has been removed.

Stages of grief:
Denial
Anger
Bargaining
Depression
Acceptance

In both malingering and factitious disorders, the symptoms (physical or psychological) are not real; the patient is actively and willingly making them up. The difference is in the purpose for the fake symptoms.

Malingering: Symptoms are not real, specific secondary gain.

Factitious disorder: Symptoms are not real; goal is to assume sick role.

Somatoform disorders: The patient believes the symptoms are real.

Munchausen syndrome by proxy or factitious disorder by proxy is almost always a case of a parent faking an illness in a child. For example, a mother may take her young son to a number of physicians, saying that he has joint pains, headaches, vomiting, and a rash. She may appear to have a lot of knowledge about medicine and may even work in a health care setting. In the hospital, she is always by her son's side and demands near-constant attention and always wants more tests or procedures. Mysteriously, when she is not present, her son doesn't seem to have any symptoms at all. Testing doesn't support any of her claims or point to a diagnosis. When told that there is nothing more to be done and that it is time for discharge, the patient may suddenly get worse, and the mother may demand transfer to a "better" hospital. This is a very unfortunate situation and is a form of child abuse that must be reported.

Somatoform disorders are much more common in women than men. The exception is hypochondriasis, which affects the two genders equally.

Somatoform Disorders

Patients with somatoform disorders have physical symptoms that have no identifiable explanation, like malingering and factitious disorder. However, the key difference is that patients with somatoform disorders are not consciously creating symptoms for primary or secondary gain. The reason for their symptoms and health care–seeking behavior is **unconscious,** and they are not creating their symptoms willfully.

Somatization Disorder: These patients have multiple complaints that span **several organ systems.** Their symptoms must include pain (e.g., leg or neck pain) and sexual (e.g., discomfort with intercourse), gastrointestinal (e.g., diarrhea or bloating), and neurologic symptoms (e.g., tingling in hands and feet). This tends to be a chronic disorder and, sadly, can be debilitating. The best way for the physician to handle a patient with somatization disorder is **frequently scheduled visits** with the same primary care provider to help the patient feel nurtured and discuss any new concerns. Medication does not help. Excessive diagnostic testing should be avoided.

Mnemonic: **Soma**tization disorder has **so many** symptoms (pain, sexual, gastrointestinal, neurologic).

Conversion Disorder: Characterized by a psychological trigger being converted into a **neurologic symptom** in the absence of an organic cause, conversion disorder's symptoms are often **transient.** Examples include motor deficits, paresthesias, seizures, blindness, and the sensation of a lump in the throat (called "globus hystericus"). These patients tend to be young adults. In older patients, be vigilant for organic causes such as transient ischemic attacks. Patients may display *la belle indifference,* a surprising lack of concern for their severe symptom. Often the symptom will resolve and never return; the prognosis is much better than for other somatoform disorders.

Illness Anxiety Disorder: The distinguishing feature of illness anxiety disorder (previously called hypochondriasis) is that patients are **fearful that they have a disease** and repeatedly seek health care and testing to prove that they have a disease. They may actually have symptoms, but they misinterpret them in a way that produces extreme anxiety; for example, a man who has bloating after meals may fear that he has some type of gastrointestinal cancer and is **not reassured by multiple negative tests.** This can be distinguished from somatization disorder, in which there is a fixation on a **multitude of symptoms** and how they feel (not an underlying disease).

Body Dysmorphic Disorder: These patients are preoccupied with aspects of their appearance that they believe to be flawed, despite all evidence to the contrary. An example is a woman who hates how her nose looks. She refuses to look at herself in the mirror and won't allow her friends to take pictures of her nose. Even after having plastic surgery on her nose twice, she still thinks it is ugly, although her friends see no problem with it. Other examples include muscle dysmorphia (the belief that one is not muscular enough) or skin, hair, or weight concerns. **SSRIs** can reduce symptoms in some of these patients.

Personality Disorders

Personality is something that is **stable** across multiple situations and affects how people react to different events in their life. Patients with personality disorders have atypical or troubling aspects of their personality that **cause significant distress or impair daily functioning.** Personality disorders are difficult to treat and most have a chronic course.

Cluster A: Weird

Cluster A personality disorders include people who are just odd. Some of these disorders have a familial association with schizophrenia (i.e., the patient has a family history of schizophrenia; the patients themselves do not meet criteria for schizophrenia).

- **Paranoid:** These people just **don't trust others.** They always think that others have ulterior motives. In contrast to psychotic patients (who may be paranoid that the CIA has implanted a mind-controlling device in their brain), their mistrust is less bizarre. They bear grudges and are easily offended by perceived slights.
- **Schizoid:** Despite the name, patients with schizoid personality disorder do not share many characteristics with schizophrenics. These people are **cold, withdrawn, and have little interest in friends, romance, or sex.** They have no friends or close contacts, and they prefer it this way. Mnemonic: "Schizoid" rhymes with "android"). They do not have any delusions or hallucinations.
- **Schizotypal:** Again, these patients do not meet criteria for schizophrenia, but their personality is characterized by **odd magical beliefs** (e.g., a belief in telepathy or aliens), ideas of reference, or eccentric clothing. Like those with schizoid personality disorder, these people have difficulty with relationships, but they may have some **anxiety** about it. (Recall that schizoid patients are indifferent to relationships.)

Cluster B: Wild

Patients with wild-type personality disorders are impulsive, emotional, and dramatic. Many of them have a family history of mood disorders.

- **Antisocial:** Patients with antisocial personality disorder demonstrate a persistent disregard for the rights of others and commit serious crimes. Recall the description of **conduct disorder;** when those patients reach the age of 18, they gain the diagnosis of antisocial personality disorder. Similarly, these patients are prone to breaking the law (e.g., **stealing, assault, and even murder**). They are **impulsive** and poor planners; they do not think about consequences of their actions for either themselves or others.
- **Borderline:** These are the "crazy girls." Driven by a fear of abandonment, they frequently dance in and out of friendships and romantic relationships. Relationships are often passionate and intense at first and then end quickly and dramatically. Patients may be **impulsive** sexually as well. These women do not have a stable self-image and do not make good decisions for themselves because of this. A key point for the USMLE (as well as with real patients) is that patients with borderline personality disorder often engage in **self-mutilation** (e.g., cutting wrists) and **threaten suicide** as a result of the **frequent ups and downs** in their lives, particularly when friends or partners threaten to leave the relationship. They classically use **splitting** as an ego defense; they either love people or hate them. In the clinical setting, this may present as a patient effusively praising the physician while deriding the nursing staff (or vice versa). In general, these patients can be thought of as **whirlwinds of emotion and instability.**
- **Histrionic:** These are the "drama queens." Think of a woman who always **dresses provocatively, flirts** to an inappropriate degree, and **hates it when she isn't the center of attention,** which makes it difficult to be her friend. She is known for overdramatizing things. Because of this air of drama and exaggeration she constantly carries, she **inflates the significance of the tenuous relationships she does have,** and she is surprised to find that the "absolutely perfect, divine" man that she went on two dates with is not, in fact, intending to propose to her. (This may sound a bit like borderline personality disorder, but histrionic patients tend to lack the tendency toward self-harm.)
- **Narcissistic:** These are the "guys with an ego bigger than their zip code." They think they're the best and most important thing since sliced bread, and they **believe that everyone envies them.** This may be a business executive who is obsessed with making money, is **arrogant** toward people with less financial success, and only associates with other wealthy businessmen. He has **no problem taking advantage of others** as long as he benefits in the long run. He has a sense of **entitlement** and yells at waitresses who don't treat him like royalty. Surprisingly, his feelings can be easily hurt if people don't shower him with compliments or treat him the way he thinks he deserves.

Gender differences in Cluster B
Antisocial: Men > women
Borderline: Women > men
Histrionic: Women > men
Narcissistic: Men > women

Reasons for Social Isolation
Avoidant: Fear of rejection
Schizoid: No desire to interact
Social phobia: Fear of embarrassment

Cluster C: Worried

Cluster C patients are anxious and fearful. There is often a family history of anxiety disorders.

- **Avoidant:** These patients are so **intensely afraid of being rejected** by others that they **avoid engaging in social contact.** They even avoid jobs that require interpersonal interaction because they are so worried about being criticized. Although they may appear to be loners, like those with schizoid personality disorder, remember that the robotic schizoids have no interest in making friends. In contrast, patients with avoidant personality disorder would very much like to have relationships; they're just too scared to try because of the risk of failure. This dichotomy produces a lot of anxiety. Social phobia may also sound similar, but such patients are afraid of interacting with others primarily because of a deep-seated fear of embarrassment; avoidant patients are primarily driven by a fear of rejection as a consequence of their actions.

- **Dependent:** Although these patients also worry about rejection and failure, their main issue is a **submissive** nature and **extreme lack of self-confidence.** Unlike avoidant patients, dependent patients often do have relationships and cling to them as tightly as they can because they perform any task without reassurance or guidance from their partner. They are **afraid of being alone** and will immediately seek another relationship when one ends. Think of a woman who has to call her boyfriend to **ask for his approval, even for the smallest things,** such as choosing a brand of ketchup at the grocery store. She always lets him have his way because she doesn't want to argue and make him unhappy.
- **Obsessive-compulsive:** Obsessive-compulsive personality disorder (OCPD) is a different and separate entity from the similarly named obsessive-compulsive disorder. Patients with OCPD are often known as **strict and perfectionistic.** They **love to follow rules** and become very distraught if they or other people do not follow the rules. They **obsess over their work** and will spend so much time making every little bit of it perfect that they **fail to turn in projects on time.** This is exacerbated by their inability to trust others to do it perfectly and **failure to delegate** tasks. Note that this is not like OCD, in which patients have obsessive thoughts that cause them to perform compulsive actions to relieve the anxiety caused by those thoughts. Also, recall that OCD is an *ego-dystonic* disorder, in that the patients know that their obsessions and compulsions are unreasonable and they wish they did not have them. In contrast, OCPD is an *ego-syntonic* disorder, in which patients see no wrong in their ways and they think everyone should be as perfectionistic as they are.

Dissociative Disorders

Patients with dissociative disorders somehow dissociate from themselves in that they lose their memory or sense of who they are. These disorders are associated with stressful life events.

In **dissociative amnesia,** a **traumatic event** such as a robbery leaves a patient unable to remember what happened to him. He may even **forget his name** and where he lives. This can be thought of as a psychological defense that prevents a patient from dealing with the difficult situation that occurred. (Note that this is different from repression as a defense mechanism, in which a patient involuntarily pushes the memories out of awareness.) This often resolves spontaneously.

Dissociative fugue is also an amnestic disorder in which patients **forget who they are** and suddenly **travel** someplace new. Think of a man who finds himself in Oklahoma City and calls himself "Charles." He doesn't remember anything about how he got there or what happened in his past. These fugues usually end spontaneously as well; after a couple of weeks, "Charles" remembers that his name is actually Arthur, he goes home to resume his normal life as a stockbroker in San Francisco, and he forgets everything about the fugue episode.

Known colloquially as multiple personality disorder, **dissociative identity disorder** (DID) is an extremely rare disorder in which a patient develops **multiple unique personalities** that are thought to defend the patient and fill important roles for his or her survival and well-being. DID may develop as a **consequence of sexual abuse.** For example, the female victim may develop a strong male personality who emerges when she is feeling threatened; he will act strong for her or will confront people who are threatening her. Strangely, each personality has a unique voice, vocal inflections, and body language. These patients may have gaps in their memory from life events (e.g., getting married) to learned skills (e.g., driving). They can also experience **dissociative fugue.** Unlike the previous two dissociative disorders, patients with DID are unlikely to recover.

Depersonalization disorder does not involve amnesia but rather a **feeling of being separated from one's body.** Patients may describe themselves as "**being outside my body, watching myself** like I'm on TV." During these episodes, reality testing is intact and they are not psychotic. This is an unsettling feeling for many patients and causes anxiety or panic attacks.

Depersonalization is different from **derealization,** which is not a disorder but rather a symptom of anxiety or panic disorders. Derealization is characterized by a patient **feeling that what she is experiencing is not real**; she may feel like she is behind a thick pane of glass watching an unreal world, or perhaps the world looks like it is merely a cartoon.

Eating Disorders

Anorexia Nervosa

Patients with anorexia nervosa have a distorted sense of body image. They **believe themselves to be overweight,** even if they are very thin. They have an **extreme fear of gaining weight,** and they go to **extreme lengths to lose weight or not gain weight.** One criterion for anorexia nervosa is **body weight at least 15% less than normal.** Their personality is often **controlling and type A**; they may actually be successful in other areas of their life (e.g., straight A student, accomplished gymnast), and they transfer this strict attitude toward controlling their weight. There are two main types of anorexia nervosa:

- **Restrictive:** These patients **restrict what they eat**; a **young woman** may put only a few leaves of lettuce and a few small pieces of broccoli on her plate and call that salad her dinner. Even then, she may pick at it and not finish all the food. She also **exercises excessively** to help her get thin.
- **Binge-eating and purging:** As the name suggests, these patients alternate between **binging** (losing control and eating a very large amount of food at once) and **purging** (getting rid of the food to avoid gaining weight). Some patients may induce vomiting, whereas others may abuse laxatives.

Women are more likely than men to suffer from eating disorders.

Patients with eating disorders are also likely to suffer from **mood disorders.** Because patients with poor self-image who harm their bodies in this way are likely to be unhappy or anxious, antidepressants can sometimes be helpful.

In addition to these behaviors, there are several physical changes that are commonly found in those with anorexia nervosa. Patients may have **dry skin** and develop fine body hair called **lanugo.** Their **teeth may erode** and develop cavities as a result of repeated emesis, particularly on the lingual surface of the molars and front teeth. They may have **calluses on their knuckles** (Russell sign) from sticking their fingers into their mouths to induce emesis. Because of their starvation, they may develop **amenorrhea, infertility, anemia, and osteoporosis.** With intense exercise they may develop **stress fractures.** They may develop **hypotension and bradycardia** because their bodies are depleted of volume and their sympathetic drive is low. Another classic finding and test question is that laxative abuse can cause **melanosis coli,** in which the colonic mucosa becomes darkened.

Particularly for those who binge and purge, electrolyte abnormalities are relatively common and can be dangerous. They typically have a **hypochloremic hypokalemic metabolic alkalosis** because emesis contains chloride and potassium ions. From purging volume from their body, they develop a contraction alkalosis; subsequent activation of the renin-angiotensin-aldosterone axis causes more potassium secretion in the distal tubule. These electrolyte abnormalities can be deadly because of the potential for prolonged QT and **arrhythmias.**

These electrolytes abnormalities can worsen when severely malnourished patients resume eating. Eating stimulates insulin release, causing cells to rapidly take up potassium, magnesium (for enzyme cofactors), and phosphate (to make adenosine triphosphate [ATP]). These patients may already have depleted systemic stores of these electrolytes. This can lead to **refeeding syndrome,** which is characterized by hypokalemia, hypomagnesemia, and **hypophosphatemia.** Without phosphate to make ATP, the heart and diaphragm can fail.

In addition, patients may die of **starvation or suicide;** the mortality rate is approximately 10%. Patients whose body weight is 20% or more below normal should be hospitalized for treatment, which includes therapy and possibly **antidepressants,** as well as treatment of the electrolyte and nutrition abnormalities. Only 50% of patients will recover completely.

Bulimia Nervosa

Unlike patients with anorexia nervosa, patients with bulimia nervosa are usually of **normal weight** (or may be overweight) and **do not have amenorrhea** as a result of their disease (Table 14.3). If they ever drop to 15% less than normal body weight, the diagnosis is changed to anorexia. Instead of being control freaks, bulimics can be thought of as **lacking control** (many patients also suffer from impulse control disorders and drug abuse). Patients with bulimia frequently **binge-eat** and then try to **compensate for their overeating** by exercising or purging. This part of the clinical picture sounds similar to the binge-eating and purging type of anorexia nervosa. There are also two types of bulimia nervosa:

- Purging: These patients try to get rid of food and weight by inducing **emesis,** taking **laxatives,** or taking **diuretics.**
- Nonpurging: These patients try to get rid of weight by **exercising excessively** or having periods of **fasting.**

Table 14.3 Anorexia Nervosa and Bulimia Nervosa

DISORDER	GENERAL PATIENT CHARACTERISTICS	EATING HABITS	COMPENSATION FOR FOOD INTAKE
Anorexia Nervosa			
Restrictive type	Controlling	Minimal intake	Excessive exercise
Binge-eating, purging type	High achieving; thin, starving; amenorrheic	Binge-eating episodes (uncontrollably eating large amounts)	Purging—vomiting, laxatives, diuretics
Bulimia Nervosa			
Purging type	Impulsive, normal weight, normal menses	Binge-eating episodes	Purging—vomiting, laxatives, diuretics
Nonpurging type		Binge-eating episodes	Excessive exercise

Because of these purging behaviors, patients with bulimia nervosa can also have **hypochloremic hypokalemic metabolic alkalosis** for the same reasons described earlier. They may also have **knuckle calluses** and **eroded teeth.** However, because they are not starving, they will not develop lanugo, anemia, osteoporosis, and amenorrhea like anorexic patients. Repeated episodes of retching put them at risk for Mallory-Weiss tears and the severe complication of Boerhaave syndrome (rupture of the esophagus, see Chapter 10 for details).

If a bulimic patient drops 15% below normal body weight, the diagnosis is changed to anorexia.

Though patients with bulimia nervosa may binge and purge more frequently in times of stress, they have lower morbidity and mortality rates than patients with anorexia nervosa. A diagnosis requires that binge-purging behavior occur at least weekly (on average) for 3 months. Because their lack of control is closely linked to mood and impulse control disorders, **SSRIs** can be beneficial. Therapy is also important.

Gender Dysphoria

An easy way of remembering the difference between sex and gender is that **sex is between the legs** (men have a penis and testicles; women have a vagina), whereas **gender is between the ears** or in the brain (some people feel that they are a man, want to dress like a man, and want to be treated like a man). For some people, their sex and gender are not the same; for example, someone may be born XY and have male genitalia but feel that he was **born with the wrong body** and in fact should be a female. **Gender dysphoria** refers to **distress** from this difference between expressed and assigned gender. **Transgenderism** broadly refers to individuals who **persistently identify** with a gender different than their sex at birth. They may take hormones or seek sex reassignment surgery to make their body match their gender. People like this are commonly known as **transsexuals.** Although they may dress like the gender that they believe they are, note that this is **not the same as cross dressing;** a man may enjoy wearing dresses and high heels every now and then because it makes him feel sexy, but he still feels fundamentally that he is a man. Unfortunately, patients with gender dysphoria often struggle internally and with their family, friends, and society, and many of them subsequently deal with depression or suicide.

Withdrawal can occur in patients with substance abuse or dependence, although it is only a criterion for the latter. Withdrawal can occur in a person who does not meet either criterion. For example, a medical student drinks two cups of coffee daily. Doing so does not cause distress or legal problems, and he doesn't feel the need to cut down. However, when he doesn't drink caffeine, he feels tired and has headaches. Do not use withdrawal as the sole distinguishing factor between abuse and dependence.

Disorders of Substance Use

Substance abuse is a **psychological** disorder in which patients use a substance such as alcohol, cocaine, or opiates in a **maladaptive pattern that negatively affects their life**. Specifically, a man who abuses alcohol may **neglect to arrive to work on time, not perform his household chores, put himself in dangerous situations** by driving while intoxicated, and **get in trouble with the law.** He **continues to use alcohol despite all these problems.** Note that patients with a substance abuse diagnosis have never met the criteria for substance dependence.

Substance dependence consists of **physical** and **psychological** symptoms. First, these patients may experience **withdrawal** (defined later) when they decrease the amount of drug used or stop using it entirely. Second, they may develop **tolerance;** their body becomes accustomed to the drug and therefore more drug is required to achieve the same effect. They **try to cut back** but are unsuccessful. They **spend a lot of time and effort** getting their drug of choice, resulting in less time spent with friends, family, and their job. Finally, similar to those with substance abuse, patients with substance dependence **continue**

TABLE 14.4 Substance Intoxication and Withdrawal

TYPE	SUBSTANCE	INTOXICATION	WITHDRAWAL
Stimulant	Amphetamines (e.g., methamphetamine, MDMA [ecstasy])	Dilated pupils, agitation, euphoria, heightened attention (recall—used for ADHD), decreased inhibitions, hallucinations, delusions, insomnia, tachycardia, hypertension, cardiac arrhythmias	For both amphetamines and cocaine: depressed and crummy-feeling "crash," fatigue, depression, suicidality, constricted pupils
	Cocaine	Similar to amphetamines; more likely to cause paranoia and myocardial infarction	Same as for amphetamines
	Nicotine	Improved mood and relaxation initially, then anxiety, restlessness, insomnia, increased GI motility, cardiac arrhythmias	Severe craving, irritability, depression, anxiety, increased appetite, weight gain
	Caffeine	Anxiety, fast speech, restlessness, insomnia, increased GI motility, flushed face, tinnitus, cardiac arrhythmias	Headache, nausea, fatigue, hypersomnolence, depression, anxiety
Depressant	Alcohol	Impaired fine motor control and balance, impaired judgment, ataxia, coma, respiratory depression	Mild—tremor, anxiety, palpitations, sweating; moderate—alcoholic hallucinosis; severe—seizures, delirium tremens
	Barbiturates (e.g., amobarbital, pentobarbital)	For both barbiturates and benzodiazepines—decreased anxiety, ataxia, somnolence, respiratory depression, coma	For both barbiturates and benzodiazepines: anxiety, tremors, hallucinations, insomnia, tachycardia, diaphoresis, seizures
	Benzodiazepines (e.g., lorazepam [Ativan], diazepam [Valium])	Benzodiazepines are safer than barbiturates.	
	Opioids (e.g., heroin, oxycodone [Oxycontin])	Slurred speech, constipation, nausea, pinpoint pupils, seizures, respiratory depression, coma	Anxiety, dysphoria, yawning, lacrimation, rhinorrhea, diaphoresis, diarrhea, dilated pupils, piloerection
Hallucinogen	PCP	Aggressiveness, suicidality, increased physical strength, delusions, hallucinations, euphoria, vertical nystagmus, tachycardia, ataxia	Anxiety, depression, irritability, fatigue, restlessness
	LSD	Delusions, hallucinations, depersonalization, tachycardia, diaphoresis, pupillary dilation	None
	Marijuana	Euphoria, paranoid delusions, psychosis, increased appetite, tachycardia, conjunctival injection, dry mouth	Irritability, insomnia, nausea, decreased appetite

LSD, Lysergic acid diethylamide; PCP, phencyclidine.

to use their drug despite the physical or psychological problems it causes; for example, a young man may continue to use cocaine even though he has had a myocardial infarction as a result.

Substance withdrawal (Table 14.4) is characterized by **physical and mental symptoms** that arise as a result of **stopping or reducing substance use.** These symptoms typically do not appear unless a person has been using the substance for a long sustained period. (Thus, if a question presents unusual symptoms after a young woman's first experience with heroin, her symptoms are not caused by withdrawal.) Withdrawal symptoms are typically the opposite of intoxication symptoms. When a patient is in withdrawal, administering that drug will cause withdrawal symptoms to cease, making it difficult for patients to quit.

Commonly Abused Substances

Stimulants: These drugs, known as uppers, tend to make patients excited, agitated, energetic, and restless.

Amphetamines and Cocaine: Amphetamines (such as methamphetamine, MDMA, or ecstasy) cause similar intoxication and withdrawal symptoms to cocaine because both **increase dopamine signaling,** although their mechanisms of action are slightly different. **Amphetamines induce the release of dopamine** from presynaptic vesicles, whereas **cocaine blocks reuptake of dopamine** from the synapse. This contributes to the happy and crazy symptoms of intoxication, which include **euphoria, decreased inhibitions, hallucinations, delusions, and agitation.** (Recall that psychosis is also associated with increased dopamine; you can see some similarities in their symptoms.) Because they both **increase norepinephrine signaling** as well, they cause sympathetic effects such as **pupillary dilation, tachycardia, hypertension,** and **cardiac arrhythmias.** Cocaine is particularly known as a cause of **myocardial infarction.** If a patient has a myocardial infarction suspicious for cocaine use, **do not use beta blockers**—they take away the vasodilatory effects of active β-adrenergic receptors and allow α-adrenergic receptors to worsen coronary arteries spasm. Further details are available in Table 14.4. **Synthetic canthinones (bath salts)** are mixtures of drugs with an amphetamine-like action and physical effects. However, they are not detected on clinically available drug tests. If a patient comes in with symptoms of stimulant use and a negative drug screen, consider bath salt abuse.

Patients report a crash after they cease using amphetamines or cocaine. They feel crummy and unhappy; they may complain of **fatigue and depression.** Examination reveals **constricted pupils.** Fortunately, withdrawal from amphetamines and cocaine is not typically fatal, although on occasion patients may be so depressed that they attempt suicide. Patients who snort stimulants may have mucosal injury including nasal septum perforation. Patient who use amphetamines chronically may have tooth decay from dry mouth ("meth mouth").

Nicotine: Nicotine is another commonly abused stimulant, typically via cigarette smoking (also, chewing tobacco, snuff). Many people say they enjoy smoking because it **relaxes** them. However, nicotine in large quantities is not at all pleasant and can cause **anxiety, restlessness, insomnia,** and **increased GI motility** (diarrhea). It tends to **reduce appetite**. Furthermore, **cardiac arrhythmias** may occur.

With cessation of smoking, patients experience **extreme cravings**. They feel **unhappy** and **anxious.** Many patients have constipation as well as **increased appetite** and **weight gain** after they stop smoking.

Caffeine: Caffeine use is also common. Patients may feel **jittery** and **anxious.** They have **trouble sleeping.** Their **faces become red and flushed,** they **sweat,** and they also have **increased GI motility.** Cardiac arrhythmias can also result as well. The symptoms of nicotine and caffeine intoxication are similar; the USMLE will not ask you to distinguish between the two unless the history makes the answer clear.

Many people are acquainted with the symptoms of caffeine withdrawal. **Headaches** are a key symptom. Patients may also experience **nausea.** They are frequently **tired** and can even feel **anxious** or **depressed.**

Depressants or Sedatives: These drugs, known as downers, tend to make people calm, slow (mentally and physically), and sleepy.

Alcohol: At lower doses, patients experience impaired fine motor control, coordination, and judgment. With more alcohol, vertigo may develop because the alcohol permeates into the inner ear and changes the density of the endolymph. With prolonged use, patients also exhibit emotional lability. More dangerous consequences occur with yet larger quantities of alcohol, such as coma and respiratory depression, which are potentially fatal. There is no specific cure or antidote for this situation, but it is important to provide supportive care, including intubation and intravenous (IV) fluids. The liver will eventually metabolize the alcohol, but large quantities will take quite some time because of alcohol's zero-order kinetics.

Alcohol enhances GABA signaling in the brain, accounting for its relaxing and sedating effects. Because neurons grow accustomed to this exogenous GABA enhancement, they compensate by decreasing GABA receptor responses to bring signaling back to baseline. When alcohol is removed, the patient is left with less GABA signaling than normal, and this global neuronal excitability can cause seizures.

Patients who consume significant amounts of alcohol over a long period are susceptible to **Wernicke encephalopathy,** an acute syndrome characterized by the triad of **ataxia, ophthalmoplegia** (paralysis of extraocular muscles), **and confusion.** Because the syndrome is thought to be precipitated by **thiamine deficiency** (vitamin B_1), patients who present with alcohol intoxication and altered mental status are often given thiamine. Pathologic examination demonstrates neuron death in the **mammillary bodies,** medial thalamus, and cerebellar vermis. If untreated, this may progress to **Korsakoff psychosis;** these patients have **anterograde and retrograde amnesia,** and they are known for **confabulation,** making up stories to fill the gaps in their memory. For example, when asked how his day is going, a man with Korsakoff psychosis may not remember and thus fabricate a story about waking up at 9 AM, making pancakes, and enjoying a TV show. In contrast to someone who is consciously lying, he is not actually aware that these supposed memories are false and may even insist they are real if questioned. Thiamine may help, but unfortunately Korsakoff psychosis is **usually irreversible.**

Disulfiram is a medication that causes unpleasant symptoms such as flushing and vomiting when taken with alcohol and thus is used as an aversive therapy to help patients quit. It inhibits aldehyde dehydrogenase (see Chapter 7). Of note, the antibiotic metronidazole has a disulfiram-like reaction and will cause similar symptoms when mixed with alcohol.

Though withdrawals to most substances are uncomfortable, alcohol withdrawal can be dangerous and presents in myriad ways. Starting **6 to 12 hours** after the last drink, patients may have minor symptoms such as **tremors, anxiety, headache, palpitations, diaphoresis, and insomnia.** Approximately **12 to 48 hours** after the last drink, some patients experience **alcoholic hallucinosis,** which is characterized by visual, auditory, or tactile hallucinations (e.g., formication, the sensation of bugs crawling on the skin). Starting **24 to 48 hours** after the last drink, a minority of patients develop **seizures** because of the loss of GABA-ergic signaling in the brain. Finally, starting **48 to 72 hours** after the patient's last drink, a small percentage of patients develop **delirium tremens,** which includes hallucinations (typically visual, such as seeing rats or snakes), altered mental status, and **autonomic instability** (tachycardia, hypertension, fever, and diaphoresis). Delirium tremens symptoms peak at 5 days after the last drink. Mortality for delirium tremens is 5% to 15%. **Benzodiazepines,** which are also GABA-ergic, are used to treat alcohol withdrawal.

Barbiturates have few clinical uses; these include treatment for epilepsy (phenobarbital), anesthesia for **electroconvulsive therapy (ECT;** methohexital), and lethal injection. They are rarely used because of their significant danger in overdose. They have been largely replaced by drugs such as benzodiazepines (for anxiety and insomnia) and propofol (for induction of anesthesia).

Barbiturates and Benzodiazepines: Barbiturates act as central nervous system (CNS) depressants to varying degrees by binding to the GABA receptor, prolonging the duration of channel opening and chloride flux, and therefore potentiating GABA signaling. Recall that benzodiazepines also increase GABA signaling, although they do so by increasing the frequency of chloride channel opening. Because they bind at different sites and have slightly different mechanisms, barbiturates and benzodiazepines can act synergistically and are much more dangerous when taken together.

The effects of barbiturates and benzodiazepines span a spectrum from decreased anxiety, drowsiness, and ataxia to amnesia, respiratory depression, and coma. (This sounds just like alcohol intoxication, which makes sense because of their similar mechanisms of action.) Barbiturates have a worse safety profile than benzodiazepines and thus are rarely used therapeutically in medicine. Because barbiturates are acidic, alkalinizing the urine with sodium bicarbonate can help speed excretion. Benzodiazepines do have a specific antidote—**flumazenil** is a competitive inhibitor at the benzodiazepine binding site on the GABA receptor. Again, flumazenil does not work for barbiturate overdose because barbiturates bind at a different site.

For alcohol, barbiturates, and benzodiazepines, intoxication and withdrawal can be life threatening.

In withdrawal, as was the case with alcohol, patients may have **seizures** because of decreased GABA tone and increased excitability of the brain. They also may experience **anxiety, tremors, and hallucinations.** Their bodies also respond to withdrawal of these sedatives with **insomnia, tachycardia, and diaphoresis.**

Opiates

Opiates, whose main medical use is control of moderate to severe pain, work primarily by binding to **μ (mu) opioid receptors** in the CNS. The endogenous agonists for these receptors are the endorphins and enkephalins. Synthetic agonists, technically called opioids, include morphine, oxycodone, and hydromorphone (all pain medications), as well as heroin. The term *opiates* is often used as a blanket term to cover endogenous and synthetic opioid receptor agonists.

Naloxone is very effective and can bring a patient back from a stupor in just several minutes. However, its duration of action is briefer than that of most opiates, so the medical team must be watchful for recurrent overdose symptoms.

In intoxication, like the other depressants, **drowsiness, respiratory depression, or coma** can result. Patients may also develop **seizures** (recall that this is a symptom of withdrawal of the depressants discussed earlier). Clearly, overdose can be fatal and is a major public health problem. On examination, **pupils are constricted;** they are so small that they are referred to as pinpoint pupils (recall that pupillary constriction is also seen in amphetamine and cocaine withdrawal). Like benzodiazepines, opiates do have a specific antidote; **naloxone** is a competitive antagonist at the opioid receptor and thus prevents opiates from exerting their effect.

One notable side effect of opiates is **constipation.** This is because there are also μ opioid receptors in the gut, and their function is to decrease gut motility.

Withdrawal from opiates is not deadly, but it is certainly unpleasant. Patients experience **anxiety, dysphoria, and insomnia,** and they frequently **yawn.** Other symptoms collectively can be thought of as secretory—**rhinorrhea, lacrimation, and diarrhea** (because the brakes on gut motility have now been removed). On examination, the patient withdrawing from opioids will have **dilated pupils** and **piloerection.**

Hallucinogens

Hallucinogens can cause hallucinations and delusions and mood changes.

Phencyclidine (PCP, Angel Dust): The most notable aspect of PCP is that it tends to make people very **aggressive.** The combination of the **hallucinations** and **euphoria** they experience gives them a sense of great power and **surprising strength.** Patients have also **committed suicide** as a result of PCP intoxication. PCP is one of the few causes of vertical nystagmus.

In a patient with agitation and vertical nystagmus, think PCP.

Physiologic effects can be remembered using the mnemonic RED DANES:

- **R**age
- **E**rythema of the skin
- **D**ilated pupils (like amphetamine or cocaine intoxication or opiate withdrawal)
- **D**elusions
- **A**mnesia
- **N**ystagmus
- **E**xcitation
- **S**kin dryness

In withdrawal, patients are **anxious, depressed, and irritable;** they have lost the intense euphoria. They may be **fatigued or restless.**

Lysergic Acid Diethylamide (LSD, Acid)

Many symptoms of lysergic acid diethylamide (LSD) intoxication overlap with those of PCP. **Delusions and hallucinations** are common; some people may see **beautiful rippling colors** amid everyday objects. People may feel **depersonalized** from themselves. These feelings are interpreted by some as profound religious or spiritual experiences. Patients can also become paranoid. They experience **tremors, tachycardia, diaphoresis, and pupillary dilation.**

Fortunately, LSD is not addictive and does not cause a withdrawal syndrome. However, patients may have flashbacks—years after their last dose of LSD, they may experience episodes of LSD's perceptual effects.

Marijuana

Marijuana is used relatively commonly because it **improves mood** and induces **euphoria.** With higher doses, it can cause **anxiety and paranoid delusions,** possibly even severe enough to require temporary hospitalization. Physiologically, marijuana causes tachycardia, dry mouth, conjunctival injection, and increased appetite.

Although most people do not experience withdrawal symptoms, some may suffer from **irritability, insomnia, nausea, and decreased appetite.**

Dronabinol (Marinol) is a cannabinoid analog used to suppress vomiting and increase appetite. It is used for chemotherapy-induced nausea and vomiting when conventional medications do not give adequate control.

Medication Summary

Now that the specific characteristics of several classes of medications have been described, it may be helpful to oversimplify for the sake of committing them to memory (Table 14.5). Please note that side effects are not thoroughly covered in this table, but they are commonly tested on the USMLE; refer to the earlier descriptions in this chapter for details.

Table 14.5 Summary of Medications

CLASS AND MECHANISM	PURPOSE	USES	OTHER COMMENTS
SSRIs; block reuptake of serotonin	Increase happiness (extremely gross oversimplification!)	Major depressive disorder; panic disorder; generalized anxiety disorder; anorexia, bulimia; PTSD; OCD; body dysmorphic disorder	Think of people who are depressed, panicked, anxious, obsessive-compulsive, or suffer from eating disorders and posttraumatic stress as unhappy in general.
SNRIs; block reuptake of norepinephrine and serotonin	Increase happiness because of both the serotonin and norepinephrine	Major depressive disorder; neuropathic pain; GAD (duloxetine)	Increased norepinephrine can cause hypertension and other stimulant effects.
Bupropion; blocks reuptake of norepinephrine and dopamine	Increases happiness because of both the norepinephrine and dopamine	Major depressive disorder; smoking cessation	Lowers the seizure threshold; no weight gain or sexual dysfunction.
TCAs; block reuptake of norepinephrine and serotonin	Increase happiness because of both the norepinephrine and serotonin	Formerly, major depressive disorder; now, bedwetting (imipramine), neuropathic pain (amitriptyline, nortriptyline), OCD (clomipramine)	Can cause QT prolongation and arrhythmias.
MAOIs; decrease breakdown of serotonin, norepinephrine, and dopamine	Increase happiness because of all three listed neurotransmitters	Formerly, major depressive disorder; now, atypical depression	Eating tyramine-containing foods leads to hypertensive crisis from norepinephrine overload; risk of serotonin syndrome when taking with SSRIs and other serotonin boosters.
Antipsychotics; block dopamine D_2 receptors	Decrease craziness	Schizophrenia; psychosis; mania; Tourette syndrome	Typical—better for positive symptoms. Atypical—good for positive symptoms, better for negative symptoms, less EPS, more weight gain.
Mood stabilizers (e.g., lithium, valproic acid, carbamazepine)	Stabilize mood	Bipolar disorder	Easy to remember that people with bipolar disorder unstably flip between mania and depression.
Benzodiazepines; bind allosterically to GABA receptor, promoting GABA binding	Promote relaxation, sort of like alcohol	*Short-term use only!* Panic disorder; generalized anxiety disorder; alcohol withdrawal	Risk for tolerance and dependence; think of people who are panicked, anxious, or withdrawing from alcohol as not relaxed.
Buspirone; partial $5\text{-}HT_{1A}$ agonist	Promotes relaxation	GAD	In contrast to benzodiazepines, causes no tolerance or dependence, no interaction with alcohol.

REVIEW QUESTIONS

(1) If your favorite pet dies the week before your USMLE Step 1 and you push the thoughts out of your mind just for that week so you can focus on your test (but then grieve afterward), what ego defense are you using? Is this mature or immature?

(2) If you're frustrated and stressed and studying 16 hours a day and neglecting the rest of your life to study for the USMLE Step 1, but then see someone else in the library studying and berate that person for "studying way too hard" and tell her she really needs to "take a break and see some sunlight," what ego defense is this? Is this mature or immature?

(3) A 2-year-old girl had been meeting most developmental milestones but recently began having difficulty walking. Her fine motor skills have also deteriorated and she often is seen wringing her hands without purpose. What are the genetics of this condition?

(4) A 7-year-old boy is brought to your office because his mother says he is uncontrollable at home. He plays loudly and often loses focus when performing chores. His report cards show that he is getting good marks and gets along well with other students and teachers. Does this patient meet criteria for ADHD?

(5) First-generation antipsychotics are very effective in treating the positive symptoms of schizophrenia. Which would not be effectively treated: (1) delusions; (2) hallucinations; (3) bizarre behavior; (4) flat affect?

(6) You interview a 75-year-old woman in the emergency room. She is oriented to person only and has difficulty focusing on the examination. At times, she stares past you and appears to be reacting to something that is not there. Is she more likely to be suffering from delirium or dementia?

(7) A 30-year-old man recently had an increase in his haloperidol dosing. Shortly after, he presents to your office with his neck twisted to the side in spasm. What is the neurologic reason for this reaction?

(8) If patient A intentionally made himself appear sick and did so to receive opioid pain medication, what is his diagnosis? If patient B intentionally made herself appear sick but did so just to take on the sick role and not for any specific gain, what is her diagnosis?

(9) A previously healthy teenage boy comes into the emergency department unable to move the right half of his body. His mother recently had a stroke and as a result can also not move the right half of her body. Extensive workup of the teenage boy shows that there is no organic cause of his weakness. What is his diagnosis?

(10) Which personality disorder is characterized by the immature ego defense of splitting? What cluster is this?

(11) A patient cleans her apartment daily, including sweeping, mopping, vacuuming, and washing her clothes. She has a strict regimen for doing this. If she knows that this is irrational and just cannot help herself from doing it, what is her likely diagnosis?

(12) A 47-year-old woman has been using alcohol on a regular basis for 15 years. Although she used to get drunk after three beers, she now requires eight beers to get drunk. She lost her job because she arrived to work drunk, so she asks family and friends for money to buy beer, and she has even stolen money from a charity's collection jar for her beer fund. She doesn't like the financial burden or the fact that she spends so much time drinking every day, but every time she tries to quit, she gets terrible anxiety and her hands start to shake. How would you describe this disorder?

(13) A 28-year-old man is screaming about "demons" and "the devil" and is punching an already bleeding and unconscious man outside a bar. When police arrive, they are unable to restrain him initially; it takes eight men to hold him down. On physical examination, you note vertical nystagmus. What drug do you suspect he may have been using?

(14) A 52-year-old man with chronic back pain comes to the doctor complaining of "feeling like I got hit by a truck." He also brusquely demands a medication refill. He seems dysphoric and snaps back at the doctor with sarcastic answers. He is sniffling and has goosebumps on his arms. The doctor also immediately notes dilated pupils. What do you suspect is going on?

(15) A 10-year-old boy is angry at his mother because she punished him for not cleaning his room. Instead of yelling back at his mother, he kicks the family dog out of anger. What ego defense mechanism is he using?

(16) A 40-year-old married man finds himself attracted to another woman. Instead of addressing these feelings directly, he accuses his wife of flirting with a stranger. What ego defense mechanism is he using?

15 NEPHROLOGY

Ryan A. Pedigo

ANATOMY

Kidneys

- Paired bean-shaped retroperitoneal organs, each with an adrenal gland located on the upper pole (kidney's "beanie hat"; Fig. 15.1A).
- The outermost part of the kidney is the cortex, and the inner part is the medulla (Fig. 15.1B).

Blood Supply

Each kidney is perfused by a **renal artery,** which branches off the aorta. Both renal arteries further branch into smaller vessels to perfuse the glomeruli (site of blood filtration in each nephron); each glomerulus has an **afferent and efferent arteriole,** which modulate blood flow and glomerular filtration pressure.

After the glomeruli and efferent arteriole, the blood flows through **peritubular capillaries,** sites in which secretion and reabsorption of various substances occur. These capillaries run down the nephron into the medulla. Because the **medulla** is the last to be perfused, it has the lowest oxygen tension and is **most susceptible to hypoxia and hypoxic injury.** These peritubular capillaries also serve an endocrine role, mediating release of erythropoietin (EPO) when local hypoxia occurs to stimulate red blood cell production.

The kidneys are drained by renal veins that drain into the **inferior vena cava** (IVC). Because the IVC is on the right side, the **left renal vein is longer** and is therefore preferred for transplantation (more plumbing to work with).

Left renal vein: Longer because it is farther away from the inferior vena cava (IVC is on right side of body).

Of note, the left **gonadal vein** drains into the left renal vein (as opposed to the right gonadal vein, which drains directly into the IVC). Because the renal vein is of smaller caliber compared with the IVC (higher resistance; resistance is proportional to $1/r^4$), there is greater potential for venous congestion in the left gonadal vein—hence, greater risk for testicular varicoceles on the left side compared with the right side. For this reason, right-sided varicoceles should always raise suspicion of malignant invasion into the venous system, whereas left-sided varicoceles are usually benign.

Urinary Collecting System

The **renal pelvis** has projections into the kidney to facilitate urine collection; the smallest projections are termed ***minor calices,*** with groups of them joining to become ***major calices.***

- The area where the minor calyx interfaces with the renal medulla is called the **renal papilla.** This becomes important in **renal papillary necrosis** (see later).
- The major calices then unite and become the **renal pelvis,** which drains into the ureter.
- The ureters drain urine from the renal pelvis into the bladder for storage (Fig. 15.1C).

Ureters have three sites of relative constriction in which obstruction of urine flow can easily occur (e.g., limiting kidney stone passage): (1) ureteropelvic junction (UPJ), where the renal pelvis meets the ureter; (2) pelvic inlet, where the ureter crosses over and is mildly compressed by the iliac arteries; and (3) ureterovesical junction (UVJ), where the ureters insert into the bladder. In other words, stones can get stuck where the ureter starts, where it enters the pelvis, or where the ureter ends.

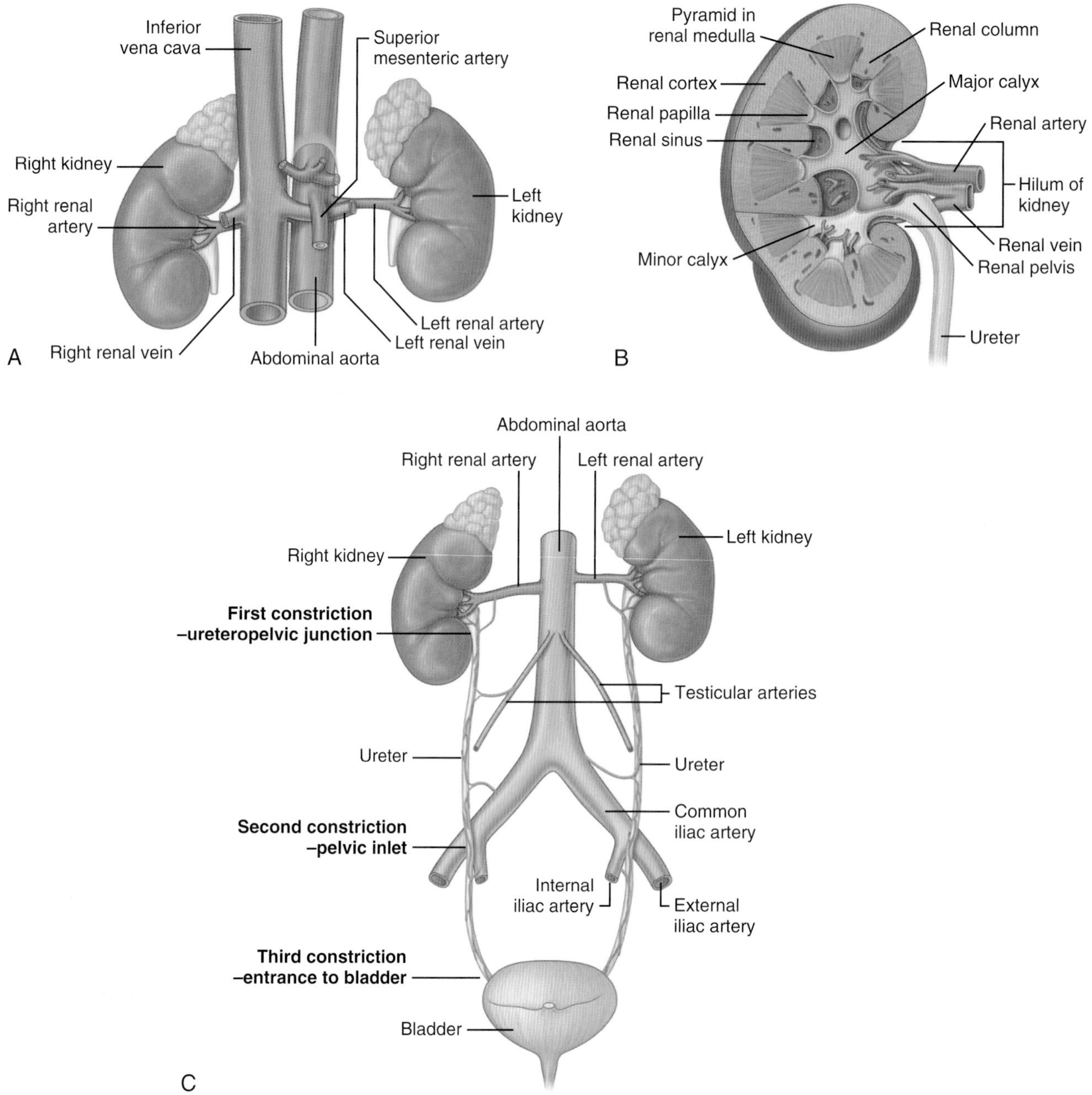

Fig. 15.1 **A,** Kidneys and their relationship to the inferior vena cava and aorta. **B,** Coronal view of a kidney, detailing the interior anatomy. **C,** The urinary tract, including the kidneys, ureters, and bladder. (*From Drake RL, Vogl AW, Mitchell AWM.* Gray's Anatomy for Students. *2nd ed. Philadelphia: Elsevier; 2009.*)

The ureters pass **under** the uterine artery (female) and vas deferens (male). Mnemonic: **Water** (ureters) **under the bridge** (uterine artery, vas deferens). This is important to know during surgery to ensure the ureters are not damaged. It should be intuitive that the ureters are under these structures; the kidneys are retroperitoneal.

PHYSIOLOGY

Overview and Terminology

The **kidneys** have important functions:

1. **Endocrine:** (1) Synthesizes **erythropoietin** to stimulate red blood cell production; (2) **converts 25-OH-vitamin D into its active form**, 1,25-$(OH)_2$-vitamin D, by the **1-α- hydroxylase** enzyme

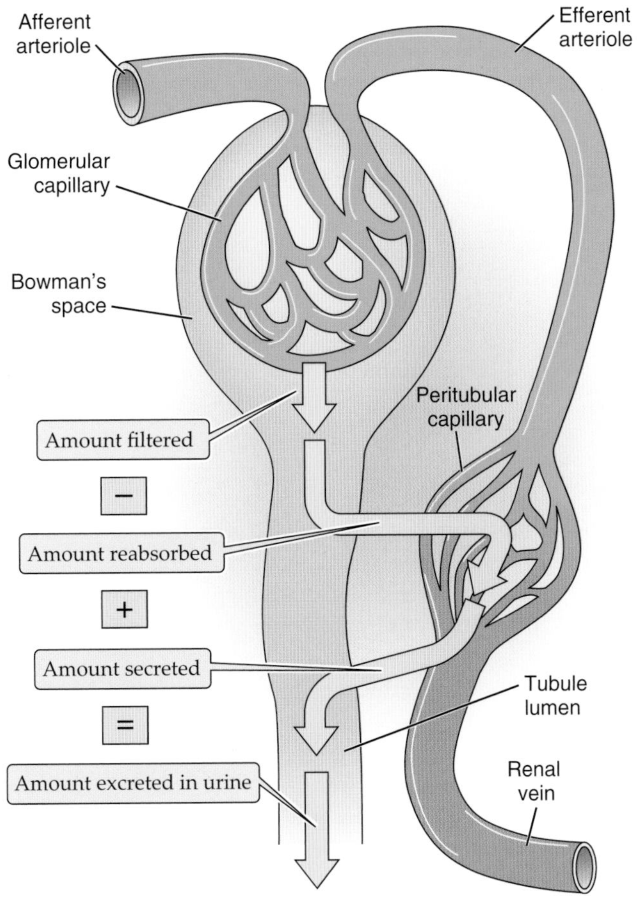

Fig. 15.2 Terminology of the nephron. (1) Filtration, when a substance enters the nephron via the glomerulus through Bowman's space. (2) Secretion, when a substance is pumped into the nephron at a site other than the glomerulus. (3) Reabsorption, when a substance is moved from the nephron back into the peritubular capillaries (and therefore back into the general circulation). (*From Boron WF, Boulpaep EL.* Medical Physiology. *2nd ed. Philadelphia: Elsevier; 2008.*)

Kidneys: Activate vitamin D, produce erythropoietin to stimulate red blood cell production, secrete renin to activate the RAA axis, and filter the blood.

located in the proximal tubule; and (3) secretes the enzyme **renin** into circulation to start the **renin-angiotensin-aldosterone** (RAA) axis to increase blood pressure.

2. **Homeostatic: (1) Eliminates waste products and water as urine;** and (2) controls blood **pH**, **electrolyte** concentrations, and **volume** status.

There are some **terms** that must be covered before an in-depth discussion of renal physiology can occur; familiarize yourself with these before moving forward (Fig. 15.2):

- **Filtration:** When a substance in question passively travels into Bowman's space from the glomerular capillary, which takes place within the glomerulus (the kidney's filter)
- **Secretion:** When a substance is actively delivered into the nephron from the peritubular capillaries (located downstream from the glomerulus)
- **Reabsorption:** When a substance is returned into peritubular capillaries from the nephron
- **Clearance (of a substance X into the urine):** The total plasma volume that is completely cleared of substance X per unit time (i.e., mL/min) where C_X = clearance of substance X, $[P]_X$ = plasma concentration of X, $[U]_X$ = urine concentration of X, and V = urine flow rate. A high amount of X in the urine (high urine concentration of X ($[U]_X$) and/or a high urine flow rate, V; large numerator) in association with a low plasma concentration of X ($[P]_X$,) (not much left to excrete; small denominator) indicates high clearance.

Creatinine is used as a marker for glomerular filtration rate: Higher creatinine means a lower GFR.

Glomerular Filtration Rate

The amount of fluid being **filtered through the glomerulus** per unit time is the glomerular filtration rate (GFR). It is normally 100 to 120 mL/min but is significantly reduced in renal failure. Clearance of **inulin** (not to be confused with in**su**lin) is used to calculate GFR because it is a substance that is only filtered through the glomerulus and not significantly secreted or reabsorbed, thus providing a good estimate of the capacity of the glomerulus for filtration. Because infusing patients with inulin is unwieldy in the real world, **creatinine** (breakdown product of creatine phosphate, used as a phosphate source by muscle to quickly regenerate adenosine triphosphate [ATP] when needed), which is always present in the blood, is used as an endogenous surrogate for GFR. There are formulas that can approximate GFR based on creatinine levels (higher creatinine levels in the blood = lower GFR, because the creatinine is not being removed and is building up).

$$\text{GFR} = \text{C(inulin)} = \frac{[\text{U}]\text{inulin } \dot{\text{V}}}{[\text{P}]\text{inulin}}$$

$$\text{GFR} \approx \text{C(creatinine)} = \frac{[\text{U}]\text{creatinine } \dot{\text{V}}}{[\text{P}]\text{creatinine}}$$

Clearance and GFR

Clearance of substance X = glomerular filration of substance X + renal tubular secretion of substance X into the urinary space - renal tubular reabsorption of substance X back into circulation

When substance X is creatinine, the latter two processes are relatively small and presumed negligible; hence, creatinine clearance is traditionally used as an estimate of so-called pure glomerular filtration.

Hence:

- **C_X > GFR:** Indicates that more of the substance got into the urine than by filtration alone (therefore there was **net tubular secretion** of the substance as well).
- **C_X < GFR:** Indicates that less of the substance got into the urine than expected from filtration (therefore there was **net tubular reabsorption** of the substance as well).
- **C_X = GFR:** Exactly the same amount of substance got into the urine as was expected from filtration. This either means that no secretion or reabsorption occurred or that they occurred to the same extent (i.e., no **net** secretion or reabsorption occurred).

Effective Renal Plasma Flow (ERPF): ERPF estimates total amount of plasma flowing through the kidney based on the **clearance of *para*-aminohippuric acid (PAH).** This substance is used because it has an incredibly high clearance; it is **filtered** (at the glomerulus) **and secreted** (by the proximal tubule of the kidney). Essentially 100% of the PAH is cleared from the bloodstream into the urine by these two processes. Renal plasma flow is important because the glomeruli filter plasma; red blood cells are normally too big to be filtered through the glomerular membrane (unless there is a disease process going on; **nephritic syndromes** can result in passage of blood through the glomeruli).

$$\text{ERPF} = \text{C(PAH)} = \frac{[\text{U}]\text{PAH } \dot{\text{V}}}{[\text{P}]\text{PAH}}$$

Renal Blood Flow (RBF): Related to **renal plasma flow** (RPF), because plasma is a component of blood, RBF also takes into account the red blood cells (RBCs) that are flowing through; knowing the plasma flow makes it an easy conversion based on the hematocrit (HCT; the percentage of the blood that is RBCs).

$$\text{RBF} = \frac{\text{RPF}}{1 - \text{HCT}}$$

Logically, this makes sense, because if there were no RBCs in the blood (HCT = 0), it would all be plasma and the RBF would be the same as the RPF. With a normal hematocrit (e.g., 45%, [0.45]) the RBF would be higher than the RPF because it is taking into account red blood cells and plasma, which has a larger volume than just plasma alone.

Filtration Fraction (FF): Representing the percentage of the plasma going through the glomerulus that actually passes into the nephron, normally FF is approximately 20%. Therefore it is the simple fraction of how much is put into the nephron through the glomerulus (GFR) divided by all the plasma that went through the glomerulus (RPF).

$$FF = \frac{GFR}{RPF}$$

You should know the formulas provided in this section for Step 1 and should know which compounds are used as to calculate which values (i.e., inulin and creatinine are used to calculate clearance, and PAH is used to calculate RBF).

The Glomerulus and Filtration

The **glomerulus** is the **interface between the blood and the nephron.** The goal of the glomerulus is to **prevent cells and proteins** in the blood from entering the nephron while still allowing filtration of plasma to occur, creating a **plasma ultrafiltrate** composed of electrolytes and low-molecular-weight solutes. The glomerulus has a specialized **filtration barrier** that helps ensure minimal loss of larger solutes with filtration (Fig. 15.3). From the blood to Bowman's space, these barriers, in order, are as follows:

1. **Fenestrated capillary endothelium:** Fenestrations (holes) in the capillary endothelium act as a **size barrier,** preventing cells from entering Bowman's space.
2. **Basement membrane:** The basement membrane has **three layers:** the lamina rara interna (*interna,* internal, nearest to the capillary), lamina densa, and lamina rara externa (*externa,* external). The membrane is **heavily negatively charged** because of the presence of **heparan sulfate** (not to be confused with hepar**in**, an anticoagulant). Because **almost all blood proteins** are negatively charged, this acts as a charge barrier to **prevent proteins from being filtered into Bowman's space.**
3. **Podocytes:** On the epithelium of Bowman's space, the podocytes are attached to the basement membrane by means of **foot processes,** which have small **slits** between them that are also coated in heparan sulfate to ensure further that no proteins are filtered.

The charge barrier is lost in **nephrotic syndrome, allowing** large proteins such as albumin and immunoglobulins to be filtered and lost in the urine.

Mnemonic: **Nephrotic** rhymes with **oncotic;** proteins produce oncotic pressure in the glomerular and peritubular capillaries, and severe protein loss in the urine is observed in nephrotic syndromes. Think also of the *O* found in both prOtein and nephrOtic but not in nephritic.

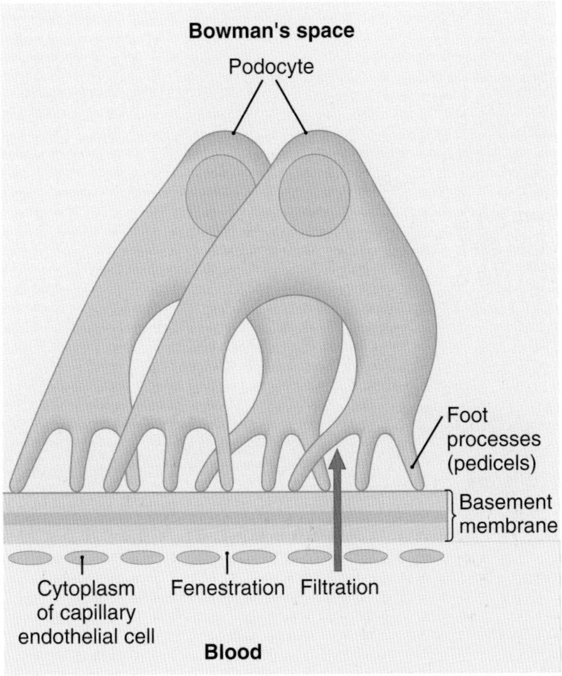

FIG. 15.3 Layers through which a filtered molecule must pass, from the glomerular capillary bed *(bottom)* to Bowman's space inside the nephron *(top)*. (From *Page CP, Hoffman B, Curtis M, Walker M.* Integrated Pharmacology. *3rd ed. Philadelphia: Elsevier; 2006.*)

Nephrotic-oncotic (rhymes). The mnemonic is used to remember that in nephrotic syndrome, proteins (which make up oncotic pressure) are lost in the urine (>3.5 g/day).

If inflammation allows entire cells to pass through, red blood cells can be filtered and lost in the urine, leading to **nephritic** syndrome. These syndromes will be covered later, in the "Pathology" section.

The nephrons can only filter what the glomerulus is able to deliver. The blood that flows through the renal arteries eventually makes it to the glomeruli, first encountering the **afferent arteriole,** then the **glomerular capillaries,** and exiting out the **efferent arteriole** (the afferent arteriole comes before the efferent arteriole, **A before E,** just like the alphabet, or A for "arriving" and E for "exiting") into the peritubular capillaries, which provide oxygen to the nephron and are conduits for reabsorption and secretion (Fig. 15.4). The fluid that passes through the glomerular capillaries goes into **Bowman's space** and subsequently the nephron. Just like all capillary beds, the driving forces for fluid moving out of the capillary are the **Starling forces** of oncotic and hydrostatic pressure from the blood in the capillary bed and the interstitium surrounding the capillary bed.

As the fluid moves from afferent arteriole to efferent arteriole, fluid, not protein, is pushed into Bowman's space, which would normally reduce hydrostatic pressure as fluid leaves the capillaries. However, **glomerular capillary hydrostatic pressure is constant along the entire capillary bed** (unique to glomerular capillaries) because of vasoconstriction of the efferent arteriole acting as a dam that backs up the pressure into the glomerulus. Because fluid is leaving (and not protein), the **glomerular capillary oncotic pressure** will **increase** along the capillary bed until forces reach equilibrium. **Therefore alterations in any of the Starling forces will change the glomerular filtration rate** (Table 15.1):

$$GFR = K_f(\text{forces favoring filtration} - \text{forces preventing filtration} = K_f([P_{gc}] - [\pi_{gc} + P_{bs}]))$$

where K_f = filtration coefficient, P_{gc} = hydrostatic pressure in the glomerular capillaries (pushing fluid into Bowman's space), π_{gc} = oncotic pressure in glomerular capillaries (osmotic gradient pulling fluid back into glomerular capillaries), P_{bs} = hydrostatic pressure in Bowman's space, and π_{bs} = oncotic pressure in Bowman's space (omitted because proteins are not filtered; normally, this is zero).

Note the following:

- P_{gc} **increases with** efferent arteriolar vasoconstriction and afferent arteriolar vasodilation and **decreases with** efferent arteriolar vasodilation and afferent arteriolar vasoconstriction.
- π_{gc} **decreases with** protein wasting (malnutrition, nephrotic syndrome).
- P_{bs} **increases with** urinary obstruction (**back pressure** from obstruction goes to Bowman's space).
- π_{bs} **increases with** nephrotic syndrome, because protein now leaks into Bowman's space.

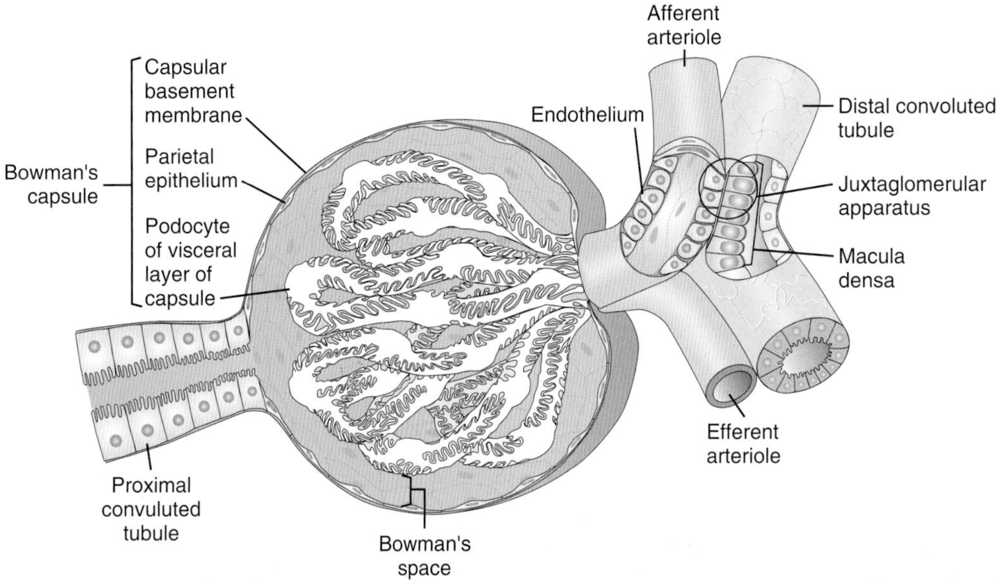

Fig. 15.4 Blood flows into the glomerular capillary bed through the afferent arteriole, into the glomerular capillary bed, and out the efferent arteriole (A before E, just like the alphabet) into the peritubular capillaries. (*From Bargmann W.* Histologie und Mikronscopische Anatomie des Menshen. *Stuttgart, Germany: Georg Thieme; 1977:86.*)

TABLE 15.1 Starling Force Alterations: Effects on Renal Plasma Flow, Glomerular Filtration Rate, and Filtration Fraction

PARAMETER	CHANGE	RPF	GFR	FF
Afferent constriction	$\downarrow P_{gc}$	↓	↓	No change
Efferent constriction	$\uparrow P_{gc}$	↓	↑	↑
Increased plasma oncotic pressure	$\uparrow \pi_{gc}$	No change	↓	↓
Decreased plasma oncotic pressure	$\downarrow \pi_{gc}$	No change	↑	↑
Urinary obstruction	$\uparrow P_{bs}$	No change	↓	↓

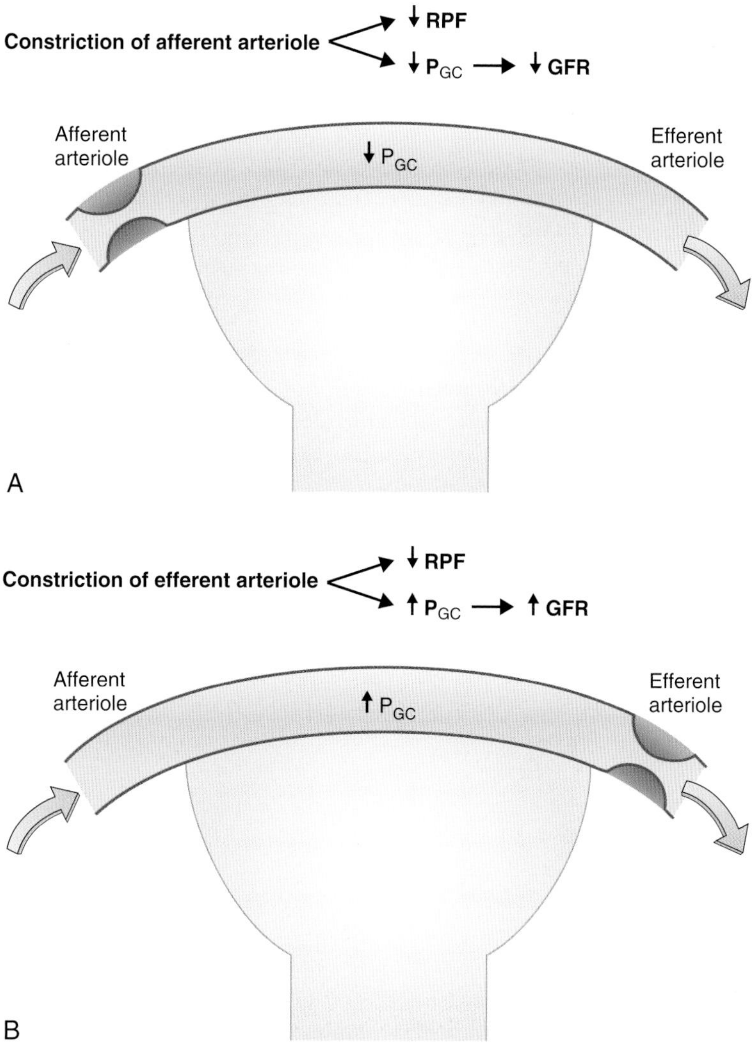

FIG. 15.5 Effects of afferent arteriole constriction **(A)** and efferent arteriole constriction **(B)** on renal plasma flow (RPF), glomerular hydrostatic pressure (P_{GC}), and glomerular filtration rate (GFR). (*From Costanzo LS.* Physiology. *4th ed. New York: Elsevier; 2009.*)

Changes in Starling forces may also alter the **filtration fraction;** higher glomerular capillary hydrostatic pressures (e.g., with efferent arteriole constriction) will "push" more plasma into Bowman's space and a higher filtration fraction will result. Lower glomerular capillary oncotic pressures (e.g., hypoalbuminemia) will cause the capillaries to have less "pull" to keep fluid in and will result in a higher filtration fraction because a larger proportion of plasma is now going into Bowman's space. The opposite conditions (efferent vasodilation, high capillary oncotic pressure) will cause a lower filtration fraction. Changes in the afferent arteriole do not modify filtration fraction because it is before the glomerular capillary bed (Fig. 15.5A); dilation of the afferent arteriole, for example, increases **renal plasma flow**

Filtration fraction: Increases with constriction of the efferent arteriole (higher capillary hydrostatic pressure)

and GFR to the same degree, so the **fraction** of plasma is unchanged (numerator and denominator increase the same).

Angiotensin II (AT II): Part of the RAA axis, AT II is a vasoconstrictor that the body uses to maintain blood pressure when the patient becomes hypotensive. By preferentially constricting the **efferent arteriole,** it **increases glomerular pressure** (acts as a dam, preventing blood exiting the glomerulus) and therefore attempts to **maintain GFR** in spite of hypotension (Fig. 15.5B). With high levels of AT II (e.g., in severe hypotension), the afferent arteriole will constrict as well, which lowers the GFR because the blood is needed elsewhere (e.g., the brain).

Angiotensin II (AT II) preferentially constricts the efferent arteriole, increasing glomerular pressure and attempts to maintain GFR even in the presence of hypotension.

Prostaglandins: Prostaglandins vasodilate the afferent arteriole, increasing renal plasma flow. **Nonsteroidal antiinflammatory drugs** (NSAIDs) prevent prostaglandin synthesis and in turn cause decreased renal plasma flow. In hypotensive or hypovolemic patients who already have low blood flow to the kidneys, taking NSAIDs can further cut off blood supply to the kidney, leading to ischemic damage.

Remember that when a substance is filtered, it does not necessarily end up in the urine; it can be **reabsorbed** into the bloodstream during passage through the nephron. Similarly, when a substance is not filtered, it can still end up in the urine; it can be **secreted** into the nephron from the bloodstream. Next, the nephron and its segments and pumps will be discussed.

THE NEPHRON AND ITS SEGMENTS

See Fig. 15.6 for an overview of the nephron.

Proximal Tubule

The proximal tubule is the only site of the nephron that has **isosmotic** reabsorption; there are small gaps between cells that allow water to move back into the peritubular capillaries along with solutes, so the osmolality does not change from the urinary to blood space.

Proximal tubule: **Isosmotic** reabsorption because of "leaky" tight junctions.

Proximal tubule: Na^+/H^+ exchanger is efficient because of H^+ molecules are recycled with the aid of the carbonic anhydrase enzyme, which is upregulated by AT II.

Functions of the Proximal Tubule:

- **Reabsorbs all glucose and amino acids** if present at normal levels. However, high levels overwhelm the resorptive capacity of these transporters, leading to the presence of glucose in the urine (glucosuria) at blood glucose levels greater than 200 mg/dL (all transporters are fully saturated at 350 mg/dL), or protein in the urine (proteinuria), with large amounts of filtered protein as in nephrotic syndrome.

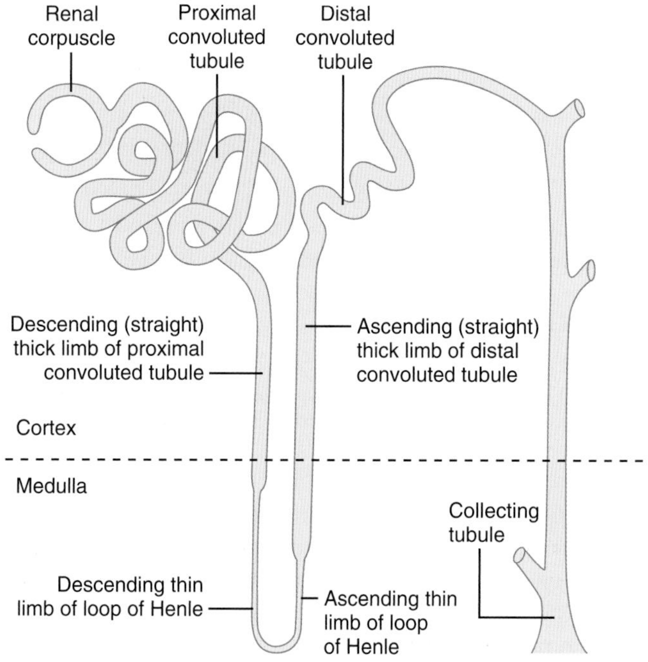

Fig. 15.6 Overview of the nephron. (*From Telser AG, Young JK, Kate M, Baldwin KM.* Elsevier's Integrated Histology. *Philadelphia: Elsevier; 2007.*)

- **Reabsorbs Na^+** into the blood via the Na^+/H^+ exchanger, with H^+ being secreted into the lumen of the tubule in exchange. This H^+ will eventually be recycled (put back into the proximal tubule cell and secreted again into the lumen (Fig. 15.7) in the following fashion: (1) the Na^+/H^+ exchanger secretes H^+ into the lumen of the proximal tubule to reabsorb Na^+, (2) this H^+ combines with bicarbonate to make H_2CO_3; (3) H_2CO_3 becomes H_2O and CO_2, catalyzed by carbonic anhydrase (carbonic anhydrase inhibitors such as **acetazolamide** block this step, shutting down this recycling); (4) CO_2, a freely diffusible gas, diffuses back into the cell; and (5) again with carbonic anhydrase, the CO_2 and H_2O become H_2CO_3, breaking down into H^+ and HCO_3^-. The $[HCO_3^-]$ is pumped into the peritubular capillaries and the H^+ is put back into the tubular lumen to restart the process. This Na^+/H^+ exchanger is upregulated by AT II (see earlier). The mechanism of the Na^+/H^+ exchanger functions well because the H^+ secreted into the lumen is buffered (mostly by phosphate) and therefore the H^+ gradient continues to be favorable by ensuring that the concentration of free H^+ in the urine remains low. This provides one method of **buffering excess acid** (e.g., during respiratory acidosis).

1-α-Hydroxylase enzyme: Activates vitamin D, found in proximal tubule, upregulated by PTH.

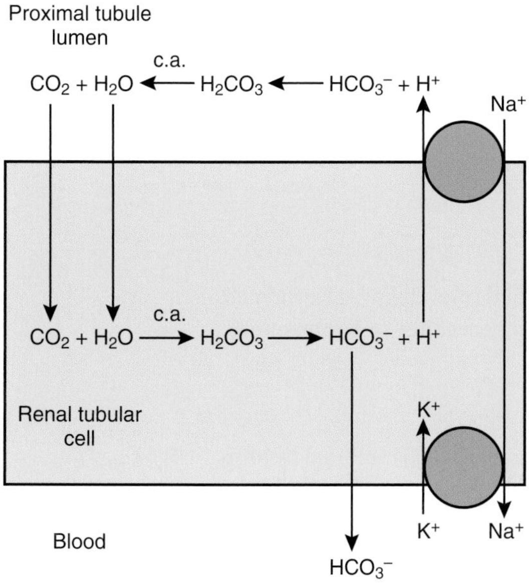

FIG. 15.7 The proximal tubule. Shown is the H^+ recycling system mediated by the Na^+/H^+ exchanger and carbonic anhydrase enzyme to help reabsorb bicarbonate. This process is inhibited by carbonic anhydrase (c.a.) inhibitors such as acetazolamide. (*From Goljan EF, Sloka KI.* Rapid Review Laboratory Testing in Clinical Medicine. *St. Louis: Mosby Elsevier; 2008:32.*)

- Also gets rid of additional H^+ and **generates additional** HCO_3^- by metabolizing **glutamine.** One molecule of **ammonia** (NH_3) is removed from glutamine, leaving **α-ketoglutarate** behind, which can enter into the Krebs cycle and be metabolized to CO_2 and water. The CO_2 and H_2O can be changed into HCO_3^- and H^+ by carbonic anhydrase activity. This H^+ can be secreted into the lumen with NH_3, creating NH_4^+; the bicarbonate left over is reabsorbed into the bloodstream, and in effect, a new HCO_3^- is generated and the ammonium will be excreted (Fig. 15.8).
- **Reabsorbs phosphate. Parathyroid hormone (PTH)** inhibits this process, hence PTH promotes phosphaturia (see Chapter 9).
- Absorbs and secretes **organic cations and anions,** such as uric acid and lactic acid.
- Converts vitamin D into its active form, calcitriol (1,25-dihydroxycholecalciferol). The enzyme **1-α-hydroxylase** adds a hydroxyl group to position 1 of 25-(OH)-vitamin D, producing 1,25-$(OH)_2$-vitamin D; this activity is upregulated by PTH. Calcium homeostasis is covered in detail in Chapter 9.

Thin Loop of Henle

The **descending** thin limb of the loop of Henle is highly permeable to **water,** whereas the **ascending** limb is permeable to **solutes.** There is an **osmotic gradient** (corticopapillary gradient) where the medulla has a much higher osmolarity of the interstitial fluid than the cortical area; the thin loop of Henle takes advantage of this because water and solutes are permeable in this part of the nephron (the part of the nephron furthest toward the medulla). It uses a **countercurrent multiplication** system to generate and maintain this gradient.

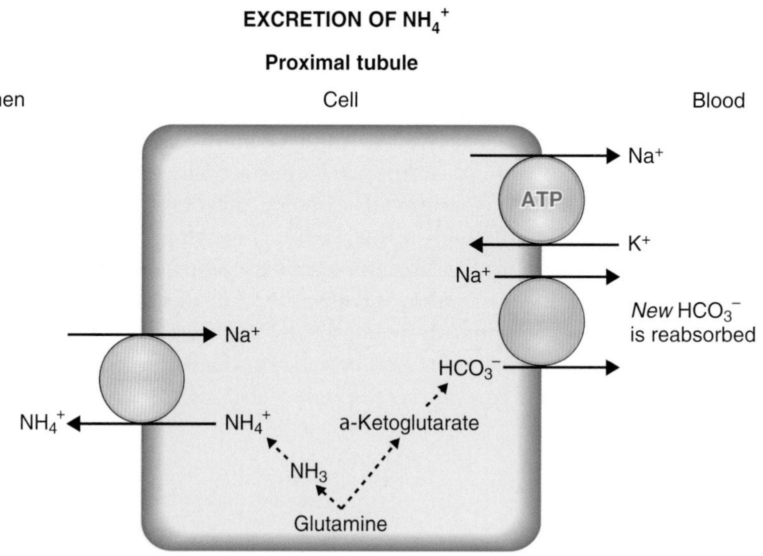

FIG. 15.8 The proximal tubule. Shown is the method for generating new bicarbonate to be excreted into the bloodstream via the breakdown of glutamine and secretion of ammonium into the urine. (*From Costanzo LS.* Physiology. *4th ed. New York: Elsevier; 2009.*)

Function of the Thin Loop of Henle:

- The net effect of the thin loop of Henle is that **more solutes are reabsorbed** (moved out of the tubular lumen) **than water** (because the ascending limb is permeable to solutes), leading to **hypoosmotic fluid** generation.

Thick Ascending Loop of Henle

The thick ascending loop of Henle uses the NKCC2 (Na^+-K^+-Cl^--Cl^-) cotransporter (inhibited by **loop diuretics**; Fig. 15.9). This ATP-driven pump pumps two cations (Na^+ and K^+) and two anions (Cl^- and Cl^-) into the thick ascending limb cell, but **the potassium can leak back into the lumen** via a potassium channel (see Fig. 15.9). Therefore although the pump itself does not directly generate an electric gradient, it does do so indirectly by allowing a cation back into the tubular lumen. The sodium and chloride are reabsorbed into the peritubular capillaries. Because the cation leaked back into the lumen, there is a more net positive voltage in the tubular lumen, aiding in the reabsorption of other cations, especially **calcium and magnesium,** via a paracellular (between cells) route. Shutting this pump off with a loop diuretic then causes decreased magnesium and calcium reabsorption as well ("loops loose calcium").

Thick ascending limb: Generates positive electrical gradient for reabsorption of Ca^{2+} and Mg^{2+} via the NKCC2 transporter (blocked by loop diuretics).

Functions of the Thick Ascending Limb:

- Na^+ and K^+ are reabsorbed.
- K^+ leaks back into the filtrate, which produces an electrical gradient.
- This electrical gradient drives reabsorption of Ca^{2+} and Mg^{2+}.
- Cl^- is secreted into the filtrate.
- Tight junctions prevent reabsorption of water; **only the concentrations of solutes** are modified here.

Distal Convoluted Tubule

Distal convoluted tubule: Reabsorbs sodium using a NaCl cotransporter; site of action of thiazide diuretics.

Functions of the Distal Convoluted Tubule:

- Sodium and chloride are reabsorbed in equal amounts by an **NaCl cotransporter,** which can be inhibited by **thiazide diuretics** (Fig. 15.10).
- Calcium is reabsorbed from the urine. Because the voltage gradient for reabsorption is only so large, whenever sodium is reabsorbed into this cell, fewer calcium molecules can be reabsorbed (both cations are "fighting" for the same electrochemical gradient). Therefore blockage of the NaCl cotransporter with a thiazide diuretic will allow increased calcium reabsorption (opposite of loop diuretics).

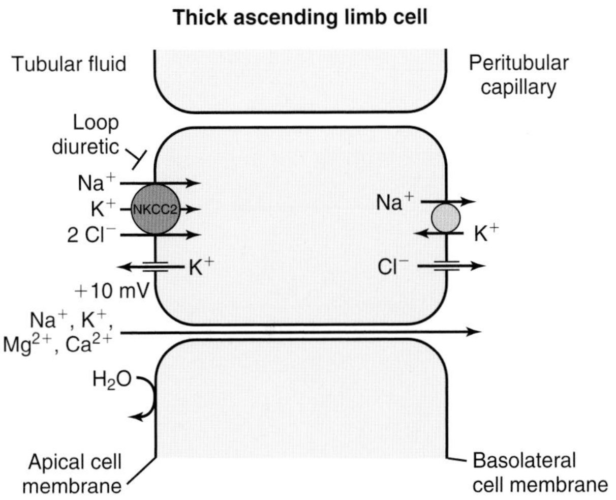

FIG. 15.9 The thick ascending limb of loop of Henle, showing the NKCC2 cotransporter blocked by loop diuretics, such as furosemide. (*From Wecker L, Crespo L, Dunaway G, et al.* Brody's Human Pharmacology. *5th ed. Philadelphia: Elsevier; 2009.*)

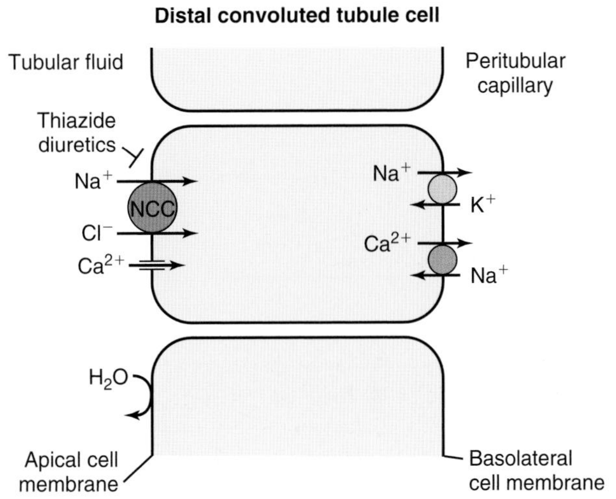

FIG. 15.10 The distal convoluted tubule, showing the NaCl cotransporter blocked by thiazide diuretics such as hydrochlorothiazide. NCC, NaCl cotransporter. (*From Wecker L, Crespo L, Dunaway G, et al.* Brody's Human Pharmacology. *5th ed. Philadelphia: Elsevier; 2009.*)

Collecting Duct

Collecting duct: Site of action of aldosterone (sodium reabsorption, potassium and acid excretion) and antidiuretic hormone (water reabsorption).

The collecting duct consists of several different cell types, which each have their own functions.

- **α-Intercalated cells** (Fig. 15.11A) **secrete acid** (remember: **a**lpha, **a**cid) into the lumen using an ATP-dependent pump. Their activity is upregulated by aldosterone.
- **β-Intercalated cells** exchange bicarbonate for chloride and **reabsorb acid** using a pump.
- **Principal cells** (Fig. 15.11B) are responsible for the **reabsorption of sodium** at the expense of secreting potassium. Their activity is upregulated by aldosterone. The principal cells are the final place in the nephron at which sodium and potassium balance can be adjusted before excretion. Any increased sodium delivery to the principal cells (i.e., by a high-salt diet) causes this excess sodium to be reabsorbed from the lumen of the nephron into the principal cell through the epithelial Na^+ channel (ENaC) because of an increased electrochemical gradient (increased difference in sodium concentration from tubular lumen to distal convoluted tubule cell). This Na^+ is subsequently pumped into the blood by the Na^+/K^+ ATPase, but recall that this pumps sodium out and potassium **in.** Therefore the more sodium is pumped out, the more potassium is moved into the principal cell. This potassium then flows through a potassium channel into the tubular lumen, with eventual excretion in the urine. Aldosterone upregulates this (see discussion of the RAA axis) in an effort to increase intravascular volume by reabsorbing more sodium, but in the process it causes K^+ secretion and also stimulates H^+ secretion in the α-intercalated cells.

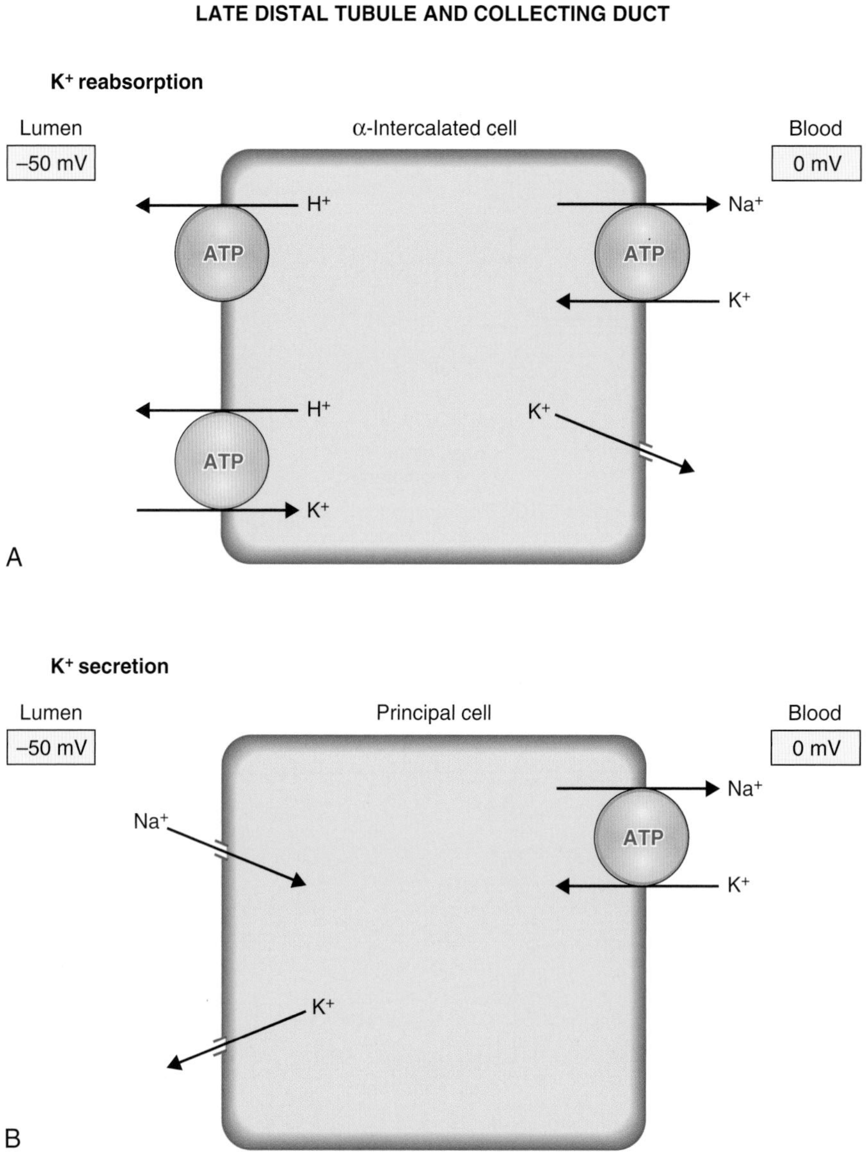

Fig. 15.11 The late distal tubule and collecting duct. **A,** α-Intercalated cells, which secrete acid into the urine. **B,** Principal cells that reabsorb sodium at the expense of excreting potassium. Both these cells increase their activity in response to aldosterone by synthesizing new proteins, such as increasing the number of epithelial sodium channels (ENaCs) in the principal cells. (*From Costanzo LS.* Physiology. *4th ed. New York: Elsevier; 2009.*)

The collecting duct also has an important effect on **water balance** through the effect of antidiuretic hormone (ADH), which promotes increased water reabsorption (diuretics increase urine output, **anti**diuretic hormone decreases it by reabsorbing water). Increased water reabsorption leads to concentrated urine. The function of ADH and its mechanism of action are covered later (see "Antidiuretic Hormone and Free Water Clearance").

Antidiuretic hormone increases water reabsorption, concentrating urine.

Body Fluid Compartments and Maintenance

The human body, by weight, is **mostly water.** This water is present inside the cells (intracellular) and outside the cells (extracellular). The **60-40-20 rule** is that **60% of an average person's body weight is water,** with two-thirds **(40% of body weight)** of that water in the intracellular fluid and one-third **(20% of body weight)** in the extracellular fluid. The extracellular compartment is divided into **plasma** (or **intravascular**; i.e., in the bloodstream) and **interstitial fluid,** the area between the cells and capillary beds. Of the extracellular fluid, 25% is plasma volume and 75% is interstitial volume (Fig. 15.12).

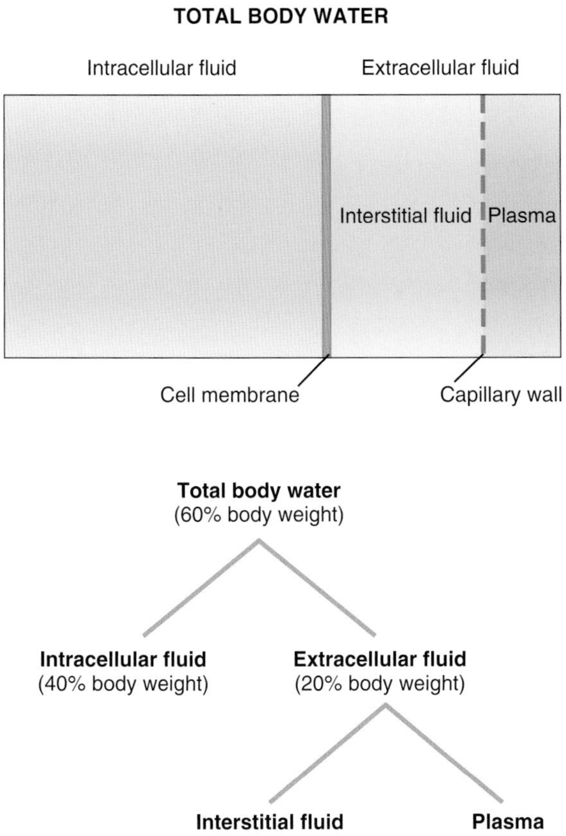

Fig. 15.12 Distribution of fluid in the body. Note the 60-40-20 rule—60% of a person's body weight is water (more if lean, less if fat), 40% of the body weight (two-thirds of the water) is intracellular fluid, and 20% of the body weight (one-third of the water) is extracellular fluid. Of the extracellular fluid, 75% is interstitial fluid and 25% is plasma. (*From Costanzo LS.* Physiology. *4th ed. New York: Elsevier; 2009.*)

- **Total body water** (60% total body weight): Represents all fluid compartments (intracellular plus extracellular compartments); can be measured by using deuterated water, D_2O (water with deuterium, hydrogen with an extra neutron, taking place of the hydrogen atoms), because water will come to equilibrium with the rest of the body.
- **Intracellular fluid** (ICF; two-thirds of total body water): Impossible to measure directly because you cannot measure the amount of water inside each cell. Therefore measurement of this is **indirect** by taking the total body water and subtracting the extracellular water, leaving you with only intracellular water. The major cation here is **potassium** and the major anion is **phosphate.**
- **Extracellular fluid** (ECF; one-third of total body water): Represents **plasma volume and interstitial volume together** (because both of these compartments are outside the cells). **ECF** can be measured by using sugars that cannot be metabolized by the body, such as **mannitol or inulin.** These sugars cannot get into the cells but can go into plasma and the interstitial compartment. The major cation in the extracellular compartment is **sodium** because cells have Na^+/K^+ ATPases that continually pump sodium out of the cells in exchange for pumping potassium into the cells.

The 60-40-20 rule: Of a person's total body weight, 60% is water (intracellular + extracellular), 40% is intracellular water, and 20% is extracellular water.

- **Plasma volume** (25% of the ECF): Contains **albumin,** the major anion of plasma, which also provides **oncotic pressure** to keep fluid inside the vessels. Therefore **radioactive albumin** can measure the plasma volume (or Evans blue, a blue dye that attaches strongly to albumin).
- **Interstitial fluid** (75% of the ECF): Just like plasma, except no plasma proteins or cells, because the capillaries do not normally permit their passage. Cannot be directly measured, but if the ECF and plasma volume are known, then the ECF minus the plasma volume must be the interstitial volume.

Measurement of Compartments
Total body water: Deuterated water
Extracellular fluid (plasma + interstitial): Mannitol, inulin
Plasma volume: Radioactive albumin, Evans blue

The normal osmolarity of these compartments is 290 mOsm/L. The osmolarity of the intracellular and extracellular compartments should be identical because any changes will lead to **osmotic water shifts** to balance the osmolarities. For example, if someone urinates extremely hypotonic fluid (almost urinating water, as in diabetes insipidus), the ECF will increase in osmolarity because water, but not solute, is being lost, in effect concentrating the blood. The ICF, now relatively lower in osmolarity, will have water move from the ICF (lower osmolarity) to the ECF (higher osmolarity) to balance the osmolarity; this is termed

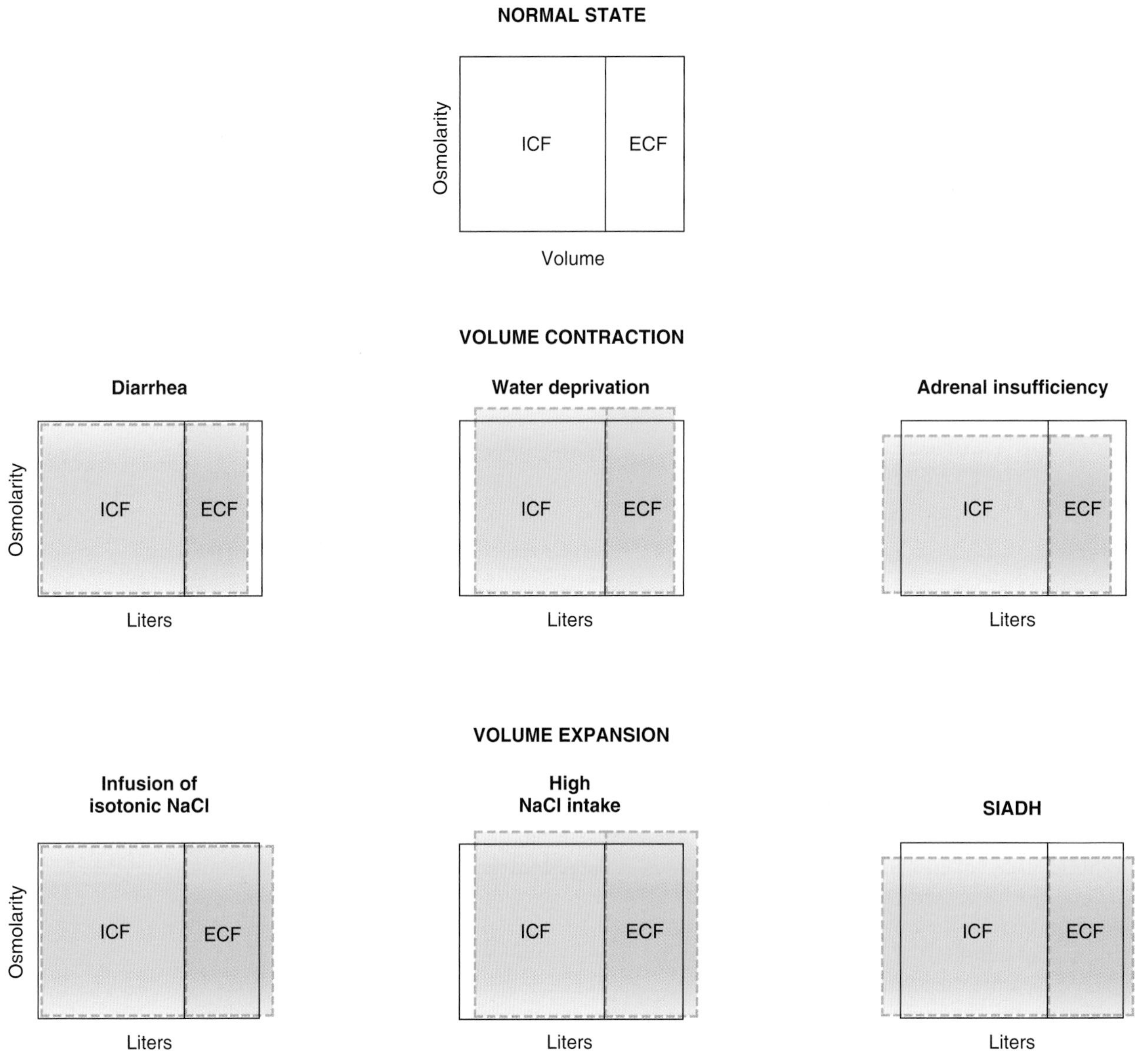

FIG. 15.13 Changes to ICF and ECF volumes after various disturbances (*middle row,* volume contraction; *bottom row,* volume expansion). ECF, Extracellular fluid; ICF, intracellular fluid. (*From Costanzo LS.* Physiology. *4th ed. New York: Elsevier; 2009.*)

osmosis. On the other hand, if a patient has diarrhea, which is isosmotic to the body's fluids (because the colon does not have pumps to generate a gradient and therefore reaches equilibrium with the cells), fluid would be lost but no changes in osmolarity would occur and therefore no fluid shifts.

It is important to remember that **all changes begin in the ECF** because the cells themselves cannot generate water or solute (therefore, changes do not begin in the ICF), but urinary or gastrointestinal (GI) losses can take fluid and electrolytes out of the interstitial and plasma volumes, just as drinking or eating sodium will put fluid or sodium into your interstitial or plasma volumes. Because with loss of fluid **(volume contraction)** or gain of fluid **(volume expansion)** there can also be changes in **solute,** the concentration of the fluid lost or gained is important. It is important to understand that osmolarity and volume do not necessarily move together; it is possible to lose volume and have higher or lower osmolarity, just as it is possible to gain volume and have higher or lower osmolarity. It just depends on the concentration of the fluid lost or gained.

Refer to Fig. 15.13 when analyzing the following:

- Loss of isosmotic fluid (e.g., diarrhea) will take fluid just from the ECF (with no osmotic gradient generated because the ECF osmolarity will be unchanged).

- Loss of more water than solute (e.g., diabetes insipidus or insensible fluid loss, as in sweating or breathing) will lead to the ECF becoming hyperosmotic, with an osmotic gradient now favoring water moving from the ICF (osmolarity = 290 mEq/L) to the ECF (osmolarity > 290 mEq/L) until equilibrium is reached.
- Loss of more solute than water (e.g., adrenal insufficiency, leading to decreased ability to reabsorb sodium in the kidney because of lack of aldosterone) will cause the ECF to become hypoosmotic, favoring water movement from ECF (osmolarity < 290 mEq/L) to ICF (osmolarity = 290 mEq/L) until equilibrium is reached.
- Gain of isosmotic fluid (e.g., 0.9% normal saline intravenous [IV] infusion) will lead to ECF expansion with no osmotic gradient because the ECF will still be 290 mEq/L.
- Gain of more solute than water (e.g., 3% normal saline IV infusion) will cause the ECF to be hyperosmotic, leading to water moving from ICF to ECF until equilibrium is reached.
- Gain of less solute than water (e.g., syndrome of inappropriate antidiuretic hormone secretion [SIADH] or increased ADH secretion, leading to abnormally high amounts of water reabsorption from the kidney), will cause the ECF to become hypoosmotic, leading to water moving into the ICF until equilibrium is reached.

Renin-Angiotensin-Aldosterone Axis

The **RAA axis** plays a critical role in the following: (1) maintenance of blood pressure; (2) altering urinary sodium excretion; and (3) altering renal blood flow parameters. The RAA axis is initially triggered when **the juxtaglomerular apparatus (JG cells) in the afferent arteriole of the kidney sense a decrease in perfusion** (hypovolemia, hypotension). See Fig. 15.14 when referring to the following explanation of the axis pathway.

1. The **JG cells,** in response to decreased blood flow (decreased stretch of the afferent arteriole), secrete the proteolytic enzyme **renin** into the bloodstream. Another important stimulus for renin release includes sympathetic outflow via stimulation of the β_1-adrenergic receptors on the JG cells.
2. **Renin** cleaves angiotensinogen in the bloodstream (produced by the liver) into angiotensin I.
3. Angiotensin I is converted to **angiotensin II** by **angiotensin-converting enzyme (ACE),** found mostly in the pulmonary endothelium.

RAA axis: Renin released by JG cells when they sense decreased perfusion → renin cleaves angiotensinogen to angiotensin I → ACE converts angiotensin I to angiotensin II → AT II stimulates the zona glomerulosa of the adrenal cortex to release aldosterone.

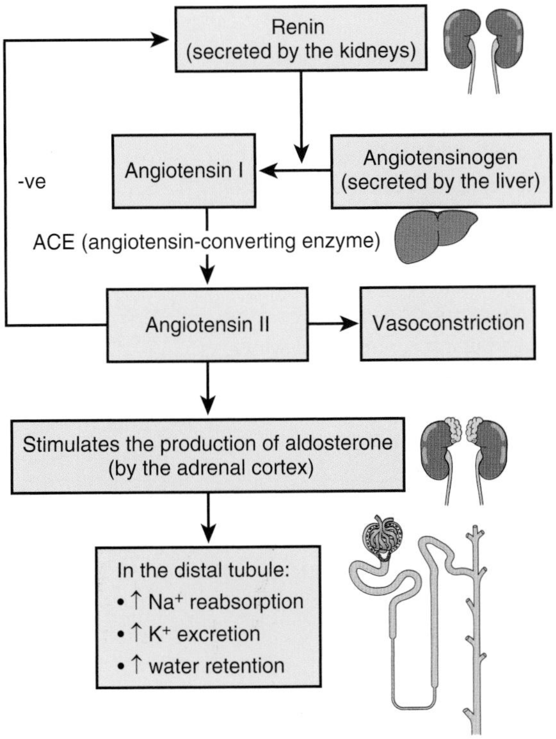

Fig. 15.14 The renin-angiotensin-aldosterone axis. (*From Jones TC.* Crash Course: Renal and Urinary Systems. *3rd ed. Philadelphia: Elsevier; 2007.*)

4. **Angiotensin II** is a potent vasoconstrictor, increasing blood pressure by increasing systemic vascular resistance. It also preferentially constricts the **efferent** arteriole in the kidney to maintain GFR in low blood pressure states by increasing glomerular capillary hydrostatic pressure. In addition, it **increases the activity of the Na^+/H^+ exchanger** in the proximal tubule of the nephron to increase sodium and water reabsorption, leading to increased blood pressure. Finally, it is a potent **dipsogen,** meaning that it stimulates thirst to aid in replenishing intravascular volume.
5. Angiotensin II stimulates release of the hormone **aldosterone** from the zona glomerulosa of the adrenal gland cortex.
6. **Aldosterone** acts on the distal tubules to increase sodium reabsorption (at the expense of potassium excretion). When more sodium is reabsorbed, water is also reabsorbed to maintain chemical gradients; the end result is expanded blood volume and increased blood pressure. Because aldosterone is a steroid hormone, it works by entering the nucleus and **increasing transcription** of new sodium channels (luminal side) and the Na^+/K^+ ATPase pumps (basolateral side) to assist in reclaiming sodium. This means that there is a lag on the order of hours before aldosterone can have an effect because it takes time to make the new proteins.

Aldosterone increases sodium reabsorption at the expense of potassium secretion; it also increases acid secretion.

Antidiuretic Hormone and Free Water Clearance

ADH: Causes aquaporin-2 (AQP2) channel fusion into cell membrane in collecting duct (increased water reabsorption) and increased thick ascending limb function.

Antidiuretic hormone (the "no pee" hormone; just as the diuretic medication class causes urination, *anti*diuretic hormone stops it) is released by the posterior pituitary gland. ADH increases water reabsorption, leading to decreased urine volume and concentrated urine (decreased free water clearance). ADH **increases water permeability at the late distal tubule and collecting duct;** these cells have V_2 receptors that are coupled to the G_s signaling pathway, leading to protein kinase A–mediated phosphorylation of proteins, with various effects:

- **Primary effect: Fusion of preformed aquaporin 2 (AQP2) channels into the cell membrane,** leading to increased water permeability but with no effect on solutes and therefore leading to concentrated urine.
- **Additional effects:** Increased water reabsorption would destroy the osmotic gradient in the loop of Henle because it would get overly diluted with all the water moving into the interstitial space. Therefore ADH also **increases the activity of the NKCC2 cotransporter in the thick ascending limb** to ensure that more solutes are available to maintain the gradient and **increase urea permeability** to maintain the gradient further.

The two primary stimuli for ADH release are **increased plasma osmolarity** and **low intravascular volume (the volume that effectively circulates in the blood vessels),** such as what might happen when someone stops drinking water (while insensible hypotonic fluid loss from sweating and respiration are ongoing). **SIADH** when ADH is secreted abnormally, as well as **diabetes insipidus** (DI), in which the ability to make ADH is impaired (central DI) or the receptor on the kidney does not function correctly (nephrogenic DI), are discussed later ("Pathology" section).

ADH is the primary determinant of **free water clearance** (C_{H2O}). Free water clearance is simply a way to express if the urine is hypotonic (dilute urine) with respect to the plasma, or hypertonic (concentrated urine). Plasma osmolarity is about 290 mOsm/L and the urine concentration can range from 50 mOsm/L (very hypotonic, very positive free water clearance, because the urine is almost all water) to 1200 mOsm/L (very hypertonic, very negative free water clearance).

Positive free water clearance: Loss of free water in the urine, low ADH levels.

Negative free water clearance: Water retention, high ADH levels.

$$C_{H2O} = \dot{V} - C_{osm} = \dot{V} - \frac{[U]osm\ \dot{V}}{[P]osm}$$

- C_{H2O} is **positive:** This means that **free water is being removed in the urine** and therefore the urine must be **more dilute than plasma.** Imagine the most extreme case, in which the urine is almost all water (50 mOsm/L). The kidney must have **essentially no ADH activity** and therefore no water in the distal nephron and collecting duct is reabsorbed. Therefore because the urine is essentially all water, free water is being removed from the body.
- C_{H2O} is **negative:** This means that **free water is not being removed;** the urine must be **more concentrated than plasma.** The term *negative free water clearance* may be confusing; just remember this is essentially free water "kept" by the body as opposed to free water "cleared" by the body.

○ C_{H2O} is **zero:** This means that the urine has the exact same osmolarity as plasma, isosmotic. This can occur in **renal failure** when the kidney loses the ability to concentrate or dilute urine because of extensive damage or with **loop diuretic** usage because the thick ascending limb with the NaKCC channels is the site of dilution of the filtrate (remember that the proximal tubule has isosmotic reabsorption). Because loop diuretics inhibit this channel, it will lead to zero free water generation.

Other Endocrine Functions of the Kidneys

The kidney also functions as an endocrine organ in addition to the RAA axis described earlier. It plays a role in (1) red blood cell synthesis via **erythropoietin** production and (2) **activation of vitamin D via 1-α-hydroxylase** enzyme in the proximal tubule of the kidney.

Erythropoietin stimulates the hematopoietic stem cells in the bone marrow to increase red blood cell synthesis. The stimulus for this release is **hypoxia** in the **peritubular capillary endothelium.** A small amount of erythropoietin can also be created in the liver, a remnant from when it was mostly generated there in utero. Of interest, hepatocellular carcinoma (liver cancer) is associated with erythrocytosis, or excess red blood cell production, for this reason.

Vitamin D metabolism and effects are discussed in depth in Chapter 9. The kidney is responsible for the final step of turning vitamin D into its active form, calcitriol (1,25-dihydroxycholecalciferol), by adding a hydroxyl group to position 1 of 25-hydroxyvitamin D by **1-α-hydroxylase** enzyme in the proximal tubule of the kidney. Active vitamin D increases intestinal absorption of both calcium and phosphate. The activity of 1-α-hydroxylase is primarily dependent on PTH.

pH Homeostasis and Acid–Base Disturbances

The body is normally kept at a pH of 7.40 ± 0.05 (**7.35–7.45**). Whenever the pH is **lower** than this, it is termed ***acidemia;*** if the pH is **higher** than this, it is termed ***alkalemia.*** Two types of acids are continually being created in the body, **fixed acids** (e.g., sulfuric and phosphoric acid, acids that cannot be breathed out and must be excreted by the kidney) and **CO_2 (carbon dioxide),** which is a **volatile acid** because it can be breathed out. The reason that our pH does not vary wildly over the course of the day is due to **buffers,** which resist changes in pH (remember your chemistry courses), with **bicarbonate** being the most important buffer. It is especially important because of **carbonic anhydrase,** which catalyzes the italicized part of the following reaction: H^+ and HCO_3^- to H_2O and CO_2 ($H^+ + HCO_3^- \leftrightarrow H_2CO_3 \leftrightarrow H_2O + CO_2$). Because CO_2 is highly diffusible, it can move from the blood to the alveoli of the lungs with ease; this CO_2, a volatile acid, can then be removed from the body simply by exhaling. When we talk about the various acid–base disturbances, this reaction is why hyperventilation is a compensation for metabolic acidosis; the body is attempting to expel CO_2 to get rid of acid as a compensatory mechanism. The **kidneys** play a role in **fixed acid** balance, because they **reabsorb bicarbonate** and **excrete H^+**, and can even **generate ammonia** as a third method to help buffer H^+. This is why individuals with **renal failure** develop a **metabolic acidosis;** they have lost this important regulatory mechanism. Therefore it should be apparent that there are two main organs responsible for acid–base balance, the lungs (managing the volatile acid CO_2) and the kidneys (managing the fixed acids).

There are four basic processes that account for all acid–base disturbances (although more than one may be present at any time)—**metabolic acidosis or alkalosis**, and **respiratory acidosis or alkalosis.** See Fig. 15.15 and follow the explanations.

Metabolic Acidosis: Caused by a **decrease in bicarbonate** because of **increased fixed acids** (e.g., lactate) that have been buffered by free bicarbonate molecules or direct **loss of bicarbonate** (e.g., through the stool in diarrhea), metabolic acidosis is further divided into an **anion gap** metabolic acidosis (when the calculated anion gap is **≥ 12**) or a **nongap** metabolic acidosis (when the calculated anion gap is normal, or < 12). The **anion gap** is the difference between unmeasured anions and cations. It is derived from the fact that the total number of cations must always be equal to the total number of anions in the plasma (for electroneutrality, total cations = total anions). That is,

> Metabolic acidosis: Calculate the anion gap to see if it is an anion gap acidosis or a nongap acidosis.

$$Na^+ + \text{unmeasured cations} = Cl^- + HCO_3^- + \text{unmeasured anions}$$

Rearranging the equation,

$$Na^+ - (Cl^- + HCO_3^-) = \text{unmeasured anions} - \text{unmeasured cations}$$

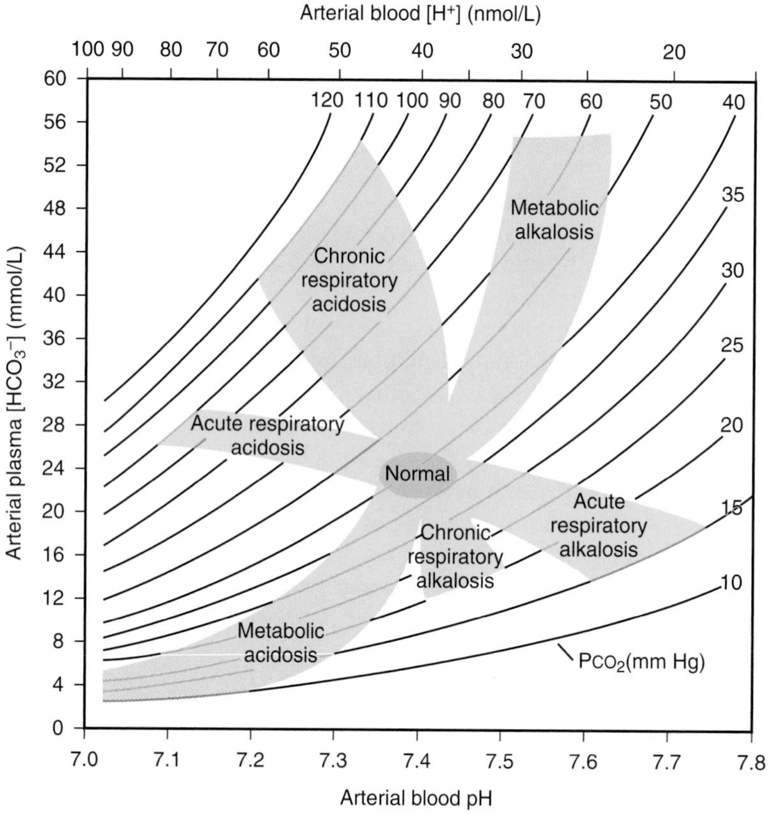

Fig. 15.15 Acid–base nomogram showing the normal pH range and various acid–base disturbances that can occur. (*From Taussig LM, Landau LI.* Pediatric Respiratory Medicine. *2nd ed. Philadelphia: Elsevier; 2008.*)

The quantity (unmeasured anions – unmeasured cations) is defined as the **anion gap.** In anion gap metabolic acidosis, the acid HA enters circulation as an acid H^+ and an anion A^- (e.g., lactic acid = H^+ + lactate$^-$). The acid H^+ molecules are buffered by an equivalent number of basic HCO_3^- molecules, which leaves behind the same number of anion A^- molecules in the plasma that are not measured in the formula just provided. These excess unmeasured A^- molecules cause the anion gap to increase, resulting in an anion gap metabolic acidosis. A **nongap** metabolic acidosis can be caused by diarrhea (colonic secretion of bicarbonate in exchange for chloride; hence no change in anion gap, because for every bicarbonate lost, there will be a chloride gained, and the measured anions [chloride + bicarbonate] will therefore not change) or by renal tubular acidosis (equivalent loss of urinary bicarbonate and sodium in proximal renal tubular acidosis; increased urinary sodium loss with reduced acid H^+ secretion in distal renal tubular acidosis. In both types of renal tubular acidosis, there is no change in anion gap, defined by the equation provided above).

Metabolic Alkalosis: Metabolic alkalosis is caused by **loss of acids** or **retention/gain of bicarbonate.** Kidney loss of acids is predominantly regulated by aldosterone. Any condition with increased aldosterone production can induce metabolic alkalosis because of increased acid H^+ secretion at the collecting tubule. Hyperaldosteronism can be primary (a tumor or hyperplasia of the adrenal glands causing increased aldosterone release) or secondary (secondary to renal artery stenosis, making the JG cells secrete more renin and increase activation of the RAA axis). Kidney retention of bicarbonate predominantly occurs when there is no chloride delivery distally to the collecting tubules. Bicarbonate secretion at this nephron segment requires an exchange for a urine chloride. In volume-depleted states, most of the filtered sodium chloride is reabsorbed in the proximal tubules, which severely limits chloride delivery to the collecting tubules to exchange for a bicarbonate secretion. Finally, there's one cause of metabolic alkalosis that results from the **gain of bicarbonate:** excessive ingestion of the antacid calcium carbonate. The body will respond by attempting to retain CO_2 (volatile acid) and so the respiratory rate will be slow.

Breathing more rapidly removes CO_2, a volatile acid, from the body.

Respiratory Acidosis: Respiratory acidosis is caused by **hypoventilation** because CO_2 (volatile acid) is not being adequately expelled by the lungs. There can be many reasons for this, from the blood–alveolar interface (fibrosis, edema), to the muscles of inspiration (diaphragmatic paralysis from phrenic nerve damage), to obstruction of the airway, to loss of inspiratory drive from a central nervous system (CNS) insult (especially in the medulla, where the respiratory center is located) or medications (especially opiates). Any cause of hypoventilation will result in respiratory acidosis. In all cases, the kidneys will respond by attempting to excrete more acid and generate more bicarbonate.

Respiratory Alkalosis: Respiratory alkalosis is caused by (you guessed it) **hyperventilation,** blowing off too much of the volatile acid CO_2, leading to alkalosis. Any stimulus to breathe above normal will cause this, from a panic attack to hypoxemia (the normal drive to breathe is usually CO_2 but can be O_2 if severe hypoxemia exists). The kidneys will attempt to compensate by **retaining fixed acids** and getting rid of bicarbonate by decreasing reabsorption.

In all acid–base disturbances, the body will attempt to compensate to adjust the pH back to normal, because all enzymes and physiologic processes were intended to function at a normal pH (Table 15.2). Changes in this pH can cause abnormal organ function. However, **compensation** takes time; the lungs are more easily able to respond to a metabolic acidosis or alkalosis because changes in respiratory rate occur quickly. The kidneys, on the other hand, have to adjust the reabsorption and secretion of acids and bases, which takes longer. It is also important to remember that **compensation is never complete.** This is helpful because even if a metabolic acidosis is well compensated, the pH will never return to 7.40; it will be slightly less, allowing you to determine that the initial disturbance was an acidosis.

Winter's formula: Used in metabolic acidosis to calculate the appropriate respiratory response (CO_2).

Understanding whether an acidosis or alkalosis is properly compensated is difficult to remember because each has specific criteria. In general, **if the pH is close to normal, it is compensating appropriately,** whereas if the pH is significantly abnormal, it is uncompensated. It is important to remember that the **normal P_{CO_2} is 40 mm Hg** and the **normal bicarbonate concentration is 24 mEq/L.** There are also two formulas to remember as well that will be important on Step 1:

Winter's Formula for Metabolic Acidosis:

$$\text{Expected } PCO_2 = 1.5\,[HCO_3^-] + 8 \pm 2$$

Table 15.2 Acid–Base Disturbances: Their Effects on pH, P_{CO_2}, and HCO_3^-

DISTURBANCE	PH	P_{CO_2}	HCO_3^-	COMPENSATION
Metabolic acidosis	↓	↓*	↓	Hyperventilation (lung)
Metabolic alkalosis	↑	↑*	↑	Hypoventilation (lung)
Respiratory acidosis	↓	↑	↑*	↑ HCO_3^- (renal)
Respiratory alkalosis	↑	↓	↓*	↓ HCO_3^- (renal)

* Denotes a compensatory response to attempt to keep pH as close to normal as possible, but compensation is never complete.

Because the expected compensation for metabolic acidosis is hyperventilation to get rid of CO_2, if the bicarbonate level goes from 24 (normal) to 16 mEq/L (low), then the P_{CO_2} should be = 1.5 (16) + 8 ± 2 = 32 ± 2 (30 – 34) mm Hg, which is less than the normal value of 40 mm Hg, indicating that CO_2 has been blown off to compensate for the metabolic acidosis. If the patient's actual P_{CO_2} is within this range, then he or she is adequately compensated. If the P_{CO_2} is greater than expected, then there is also a respiratory acidosis occurring. If the P_{CO_2} is lower than expected, then there is a concurrent respiratory alkalosis.

Metabolic Alkalosis: P_{CO_2} should increase by 0.7 mm Hg for every 1-mEq/L increase in $[HCO_3^-]$. This is because the increased bicarbonate will cause alkalosis, leading the lungs to compensate by retaining CO_2; if it has retained 0.7 mm Hg for every 1-mEq/L increase in $[HCO_3^-]$, there has been adequate compensation.

This is a lot of information. Therefore a systematic approach can help narrow down the possibilities; ask yourself these questions in order when you are faced with an acid–base problem. Refer to Table 15.3 for causes of various acid–base disturbances once you have learned to identify them.

1. Is the pH less than or greater than 7.40?

Table 15.3 Common Causes of Acid–Base Disturbances

DISTURBANCE	CAUSES AND COMMENTS
Anion gap metabolic acidosis • Methanol: Found in ink toner and homemade alcohol, metabolized to formic acid and formaldehyde; causes organ damage, including optic nerve injury and blindness • Uremia: Found in renal failure because of severely reduced excretion of organic anions (e.g., sulfates, phosphates, urates) • Diabetic ketoacidosis (DKA): Ketoacids formation from increased fatty acid oxidation caused by lack of insulin • Propylene glycol • Isoniazid: Antituberculosis agent (also iron and isopropyl alcohol) • Lactic acidosis: Seen with hypoxemia, hypoperfusion and anaerobic metabolism • Ethylene glycol: Found in antifreeze; metabolized into oxalic acid (oxalate), causing renal crystallizations and stones and kidney injury • Salicylates: Metabolic acidosis seen later (>6 hr) in course of overdose; initially causes primary respiratory alkalosis by directly stimulating medullary respiratory centers in the brain	**Anion gap: MUDPILES mnemonic** On Step 1, any person presenting an intermediate amount of time after a salicylate ingestion (ie, between 1 and 6 hours), might have a normal pH secondary to a combination of these two processes. Within one hour, expect them to have a predominantly respiratory alkalosis, and after 6 hours, expect them to have a predominantly metabolic acidosis. However, this is only a rule of thumb; you should still run through the below questions to determine what process is going on.
Non–anion gap metabolic acidosis: Hyperchloremic acidosis caused by increased Cl^- anions replacing bicarbonate anions • Diarrhea: GI loss of bicarbonate • Renal tubular acidosis: Renal loss of bicarbonate or retention of acid (H^+) • Carbonic anhydrase inhibitors: Lead to inability of kidney to reabsorb bicarbonate	
Metabolic alkalosis • Vomiting: Loss of acid leading to alkalosis, contraction alkalosis from volume loss, and RAA stimulation • Diuretic use: RAA stimulation leading to alkalosis • Hyperaldosteronism: Overactive aldosterone causing increased H^+ secretion into nephron, alkalosis • Antacid use: Contains bicarbonate, leading to increased bicarbonate levels and alkalosis	
Respiratory acidosis • Respiratory muscle paralysis: Phrenic nerve damage, autoimmune diseases (e.g., Guillain-Barré) • Lung disease: Inability for CO_2 to diffuse out of bloodstream into alveoli effectively • Loss of respiratory drive: Brain damage, sedatives, intoxication, opioid use	Caused by hypoventilation from any cause:
Respiratory alkalosis • Anxiety: Leading to hyperventilation • Salicylate (aspirin) toxicity: Direct stimulation of medullary respiratory centers causing hyperventilation	Caused by hyperventilation from any cause:

Because compensation is never complete, even if the acid–base disturbance is fully compensated, the pH will never return completely to normal. The direction of the deviation from normal will allow you to determine the primary disturbance (acidosis or alkalosis). If it is **less than 7.40,** the initial process was an **acidosis** (metabolic or respiratory). If it is **greater than 7.40,** the initial process was an **alkalosis** (metabolic or respiratory).

2. What is the P_{CO_2}?

The P_{CO_2} will determine whether the problem is respiratory or metabolic. If the primary process is an acidosis and the P_{CO_2} (an acid) is **high,** the acidosis is caused by the increased P_{CO_2} and therefore it is a **respiratory acidosis.** If the P_{CO_2} is **normal or low,** it indicates that the problem cannot be with

CO_2 and therefore it is a **metabolic acidosis** (and the bicarbonate will be low); in the latter case, in which the Pco_2 is low, it indicates that the lungs are compensating.

If an **alkalosis** and the **Pco_2 is low,** it indicates that the acid CO_2 is being removed from the body excessively to cause the alkalosis, and the issue is a **respiratory alkalosis**. On the other hand, if the Pco_2 is normal or high, it indicates that the CO_2 is not the primary problem (and in the case where the Pco_2 is high, the lungs are compensating), and the problem must be a **metabolic alkalosis** (and the bicarbonate level will be high).

3. Bonus step—if it is a metabolic acidosis, calculate the anion gap to assess if the anion gap is elevated:

$$\text{Anion gap (normal} \leq 12) = Na^+ - (Cl^- + HCO_3^-)$$

The cation potassium is not included in the calculation.

Another important item to remember is that **cells have K^+/H^+ exchangers,** meaning that they can swap K^+ for H^+ and vice versa. This is important in acidosis because the excess H^+ in the bloodstream gets taken into the cells to help buffer, but in turn the cells release K^+ into the bloodstream, leading to **hyperkalemia.** The opposite effect can occur with alkalosis.

PATHOLOGY

Hyponatremia and Hypernatremia

A normal sodium concentration is from 135 to 145 mEq/L. A sodium concentration less than 135 mEq/L is **hyponatremia** and greater than 145 mEq/L is **hypernatremia.** It is important to consider the overall volume status of the patient as well as whether or not this is an acute or chronic process. Sodium concentration is based not only on gain or loss of sodium but also on gain or loss of free water; disturbances in either of these can lead to sodium concentration abnormalities, but **changes in total body water** are more common. Important regulatory hormones implicated include **antidiuretic hormone** and **aldosterone.**

Hyponatremia

Hyponatremia can be caused by the following: (1) net sodium loss in excess of net free water loss; (2) net free water gain in excess of net sodium gain; or (3) free water shift. Severe, symptomatic hyponatremia ($[Na^+] < 120$ mEq/L) is almost always caused by **SIADH.** The third cause of hyponatremia is observed in a hyperosmotic hyperglycemic state in which intracellular free water shifts extracellularly to maintain osmotic balance. The extracellular free water shift induces a dilutional state for sodium—hence, hyponatremia. The total body sodium, however, is not reduced in this case. Hyponatremia associated with hyperglycemia can be corrected by the control of hyperglycemia alone. Pseudohyponatremia is due to conditions that interfere with laboratory tests such as hyperlipidemia or hyperparaproteinemia; the actual level of sodium in the body is normal, but the laboratory test will indicate hyponatremia as a result of this interference. The hyponatremia associated with hyperglycemia may be corrected as follows. **For each 100 mg/dL of glucose over normal (e.g., normal is ≈ 100 mg/dL), add 2.4 mEq/L of sodium as a correction.** Hyponatremia can be further classified into hypovolemic, euvolemic, or hypervolemic.

Hypovolemic Hyponatremia: This is caused by hypotonic to hypertonic fluid loss plus concomitant pure free water or relatively hypotonic fluid replacement. Stated another way, hypovolemic hyponatremia occurs when the patient has lost volume and sodium but has lost more sodium. Examples include hypotonic fluid loss (diarrhea, sweating, respiration), in which the urine sodium would be low (kidney trying to actively reabsorb sodium and water), as well as hypertonic fluid loss (diuretics, aldosterone insufficiency), in which the urine sodium would be high (kidney cannot reabsorb the sodium or water).

Euvolemic Hyponatremia: This is usually caused by excess free water reabsorption with SIADH. Causes of SIADH are many, including malignancy; pulmonary or CNS lesions; antipsychotic, antidepressant, or antiepileptic drugs; pain medications; acute nausea and vomiting; and pain. A classic example is a smoker with **small cell carcinoma of the lung** (also known as oat cell carcinoma, a nickname given to it because of the histologic appearance of the cells), which can secrete ADH (among other hormones; see Chapter 9). Hyponatremia caused by SIADH is considered euvolemic, even though the body is reabsorbing large amounts of water because the accumulation of volume can stimulate the intravascular pressure-sensing receptors (baroreceptors) to induce a natriuretic effect to enhance sodium and water excretion. Other causes of euvolemic hyponatremia include excessive ingestion of free water and poor oral intake. The former overwhelms the maximal ability of the kidneys to excrete water and the latter is caused by the need of the kidneys to pull out solutes with free water excretion. Limited solute intake (poor oral intake as in alcoholics ["beer potomania"] or "tea and toast diet") limits the ability of the kidneys to excrete free water. The difference between SIADH and the others is that with SIADH, the urine will be concentrated (reabsorbed all the water), but the urine will be dilute in the other conditions. Other causes of euvolemic hyponatremia are hypothyroidism, hypocortisolism, and nephrogenic syndrome of inappropriate diuresis.

Hypervolemic Hyponatremia: In hypervolemic hyponatremia, the hypervolemia is caused by volume overload from heart, liver, or kidney failure or hypoalbuminemia (nephrotic syndrome), leading to significant interstitial fluid overload.

Acute hyponatremia results in decreased osmoles in the intravascular space, leading to water rushing into the cells (down the osmotic gradient). This precipitates cellular swelling and **cerebral edema,** leading to altered mental status, headache, vomiting, and seizures. The treatment of hyponatremia can involve the following: (1) restrict water and allow the kidneys to fix the problem by urinating out the excess water; (2) give salt-containing fluids IV or sodium tablets to correct the sodium; or (3) give medications (e.g., ADH receptor antagonists, vaptans, demeclocycline [ADH antagonist]) to increase free water excretion. **Care must be taken not to correct hyponatremia too quickly.** This is because with chronic hyponatremia (with decreased intravascular osmoles), the body has made intracellular adjustments to the fewer osmoles; increasing the osmoles in the bloodstream rapidly by introducing a large sodium load from IV fluids will pull water out of the cells because of the osmotic gradient. This pull of water out of the cells is particularly destructive to myelin, potentially causing a syndrome called osmotic demyelinating syndrome (ODS), previously called **central pontine myelinolysis (CPM),** which is a condition that may cause permanent neurologic damage or death.

> Fixing hyponatremia too quickly: Osmotic demyelination syndrome (formerly known as central pontine myelinolysis; "from low to high your pons will die").
>
> Fixing hypernatremia too quickly: Cerebral edema ("From high to low your brain will blow").

Hypernatremia

Hypernatremia can occur from the following: (1) gain of sodium; (2) loss of free water (more common); or less commonly (3) intracellular free water shift. It may not be intuitive that loss of water could cause hypernatremia. Wouldn't people just drink water? That's true and is why hypernatremia is often seen in those with altered mental status (e.g., nursing home patients) or intubated patients, people who cannot get access to free water. Another way to lose water is to have **diabetes insipidus,** which causes polyuria (increased urine production) of very dilute urine. Symptoms of hypernatremia include altered mental status and coma.

- In **central DI**, the problem is centrally located in the posterior pituitary gland. If it fails to secrete ADH, hypernatremia will result via lack of water reabsorption in the distal nephron, producing a large loss of free water in the urine. This is sometimes seen after head trauma if the posterior pituitary is damaged. This condition will respond to desmopressin (DDAVP; synthetic ADH) administration.
- **Nephrogenic diabetes insipidus** occurs when there is a problem with the V_2 ADH receptors in the kidney: There is ADH but the kidney can't respond to it. This can be caused by chronic **lithium use, hypokalemia, or hypercalcemia** or by mutations of the ADH receptors (rare). This condition does not respond to desmopressin administration.

> Diabetes insipidus: Differentiate central (problem of ADH production) from nephrogenic (problem of ADH receptor function).

Differentiation of the two types of DI can be done by administration of desmopressin, a synthetic ADH analog. In **central DI,** the body will respond to desmopressin because the problem is a lack of ADH and not a problem with the receptor pathway; the urine osmolarity should increase (become more concentrated as fluid is reabsorbed from the collecting duct) by at least 50%. If the urine remains dilute, it indicates that the problem may be with the kidney's ability to use ADH and therefore suggests **nephrogenic DI.** Interestingly, the treatment of nephrogenic DI is a thiazide diuretic; this is counterintuitive, but as salt and water is lost (instead of just water) with diuretic use, the increased RAA axis activation will cause increased sodium (and water) reabsorption in earlier parts of the nephron (e.g., upregulation of the Na^+/H^+ exchanger in the proximal tubule by angiotensin II), leading to a net decrease in water loss.

If **primary polydipsia** is thought to be in the differential diagnosis of dilute polyuria (although this causes hyponatremia, it would also lead to dilute urine), then **fluid restriction** can lead to a diagnosis. If the patient does not take in fluids with primary polydipsia, the urine will concentrate normally (which is not the case with diabetes insipidus).

Hypokalemia and Hyperkalemia

Changes in potassium levels alter the resting membrane potential, leading to abnormal cellular activity. Potassium homeostasis is controlled by the kidneys, with **aldosterone** being the key regulatory hormone, leading to excretion of potassium in the urine. As mentioned in the acid–base section, cells also have a H^+/K^+ exchanger, leading to changes in potassium levels with changes in pH (acidosis causing cells to take in H^+ in exchange for putting K^+ into the bloodstream, alkalosis causing cells to give H^+ to the bloodstream in exchange for taking in K^+).

Hyperkalemia

Hyperkalemia is defined as potassium level greater than 5.0 mEq/L.

Causes: Hyperkalemia can be caused by many factors, with the main causes involving the following: (1) decreased renal excretion; (2) cell lysis; and (3) transcellular movement. Causes of decreased renal excretion include **renal failure** (inability to excrete potassium), **hypoaldosteronism** (because aldosterone causes potassium loss in urine), and **potassium-sparing diuretic use** (prevents elimination of potassium). Cell lysis as occurs with **rhabdomyolysis** (skeletal muscle breakdown) or high cell turnover, such as in some **leukemias and lymphomas,** can cause hyperkalemia because it is spilling the intracellular potassium into the bloodstream. **Lysis of cells during blood draws** (hemolysis) can lead to **elevated potassium of the blood sample** as well, so it is important to keep in mind. If hemolysis is suspected, the sample should be redrawn. Transcellular movement, as noted earlier, can occur in **acidosis** as the excess H^+ in the bloodstream moves into the cells in exchange for K^+. Insulin and activation of the sympathetic nervous system both activate the Na^+/K^+ ATPases in cells (promoting K^+ uptake in cells); loss of either of these can cause hyperkalemia.

Findings: Electrocardiographic findings include **peaked T waves** (from vigorous accelerated repolarization), PR interval prolongation, QRS widening, and eventually a sinusoidal tracing, which is a sign of life-threatening hyperkalemia. **Ventricular arrhythmias** can also occur from abnormal excitability of the heart. **Muscle weakness** can occur as well because of higher resting membrane potential, leading to sodium channels not being able to reset fully (repolarization not complete).

Hyperkalemia ECG findings: (1) peaked T waves, (2) PR prolongation, (3) QRS widening.

Treatment: Treatment is threefold: (1) Reduce myocardial irritability to prevent arrhythmia and death; (2) move potassium intracellularly to temporarily reduce potassium; and (3) promote potassium loss through the urine and stool. Reduction of myocardial irritability is via immediate **calcium** gluconate administration, which helps stabilize the cell membranes. This should always be the first step when faced with an unstable hyperkalemic patient. Next, potassium can be moved intracellularly by increasing Na^+/K^+ ATPase activity via **insulin** (administered with glucose to prevent hypoglycemia) and **sympathetic stimulation** (albuterol) or by causing an alkalosis and promoting H^+/K^+ exchange across the cell via **bicarbonate** administration. However, these actions only shift potassium into cells, which is a temporary measure. The excess potassium must eventually be removed from the body, usually via **potassium-wasting diuretics** (e.g., furosemide), **potassium-binding resins** that bind potassium in the intestines (sodium polystyrene sulfonate [Kayexalate]), or **dialysis.**

Hypokalemia

Hypokalemia is defined as potassium level less than 3.5 mEq/L.

Causes: The causes of hypokalemia, in general, are the opposite of the causes of hyperkalemia and involve the following: (1) increased renal excretion; (2) transcellular movement; and (3) gastrointestinal loss. Increased renal excretion occurs with **hyperaldosteronism** from any cause, **hypercortisolism** because high levels of cortisol can bind the aldosterone receptor, and **potassium-wasting diuretic use.** Hypokalemia can also be seen in states of increased diuresis, such as in diabetes from glucosuria leading to polyuria. Hypokalemia can be seen with **alkalosis** because the cells give up some H^+ to help replenish the lost serum H^+ and exchange it by taking in potassium through the H^+/K^+ exchangers we have already mentioned. Finally, the gastrointestinal fluids are generally potassium rich (stomach acid and stool), so vomiting and diarrhea can lead to potassium loss, further exacerbated by volume loss, leading to RAA axis stimulation and increased potassium loss via aldosterone action.

Findings: Electrocardiographic findings include the presence of a U wave (a small hump after the T wave), and altered membrane potentials can also lead to arrhythmias with hypokalemia. There is muscle weakness caused by a more negative membrane resting potential (hypokalemia or hyperkalemia causes muscle weakness).

Treatment: Potassium repletion and correction of the underlying cause. Avoid alkalinization and use of glucose or insulin in patients with severe hypokalemia because both of these can increase intracellular potassium uptake and exacerbate the existing hypokalemia.

Urinalysis and Urine Microscopy

Understanding basic urinalysis (UA) and urine microscopy will help you understand the pathology of the kidney. A typical urinalysis has many findings, which give clues to the function or dysfunction of the kidney.

Color

Gross appearance of the urine can be yellow (concentrated urine), clear (dilute urine), tea-colored, or red (blood or myoglobin in the urine). Ingestion of certain red foods, such as beets, can also cause a reddish coloration to the urine (known as beeturia).

Specific Gravity

The specific gravity of plasma is 1.010; any higher and the urine is more concentrated than plasma, any less and the urine is more dilute than plasma. In renal failure, the kidney loses the ability to concentrate or dilute urine and the specific gravity can be stuck at 1.010.

pH

The pH can have a wide range, depending on the acid–base status of the patient. In a urinary tract infection or with urolithiasis (kidney stones), a high pH can signify the presence of ammonia from urease-splitting bacteria, such as *Proteus.*

Protein

Normally, the urine should be relatively free of protein. Proteinuria can occur when the glomerulus does not adequately prevent large proteins such as albumin from being filtered **(nephrotic syndrome)** or the proximal tubules fail to absorb normally filtered low-molecular-weight proteins. Routine urinalysis is not sensitive enough to detect small amounts of albumin. In addition, it does not detect Bence-Jones proteins, seen in multiple myeloma. Detection for the latter may be done with prior addition of sulfosalicylic acid to the urine. More sensitive testing for a low degree of albuminuria (microalbuminuria) may be done separately to detect early glomerular injury in diabetic patients.

Glucose

Normally, glucose is filtered and then reabsorbed in the proximal tubule. With hyperglycemia, the excess glucose can overwhelm the transporters and lead to glucose in the urine, called glucosuria.

Ketones

Present when the body is using fatty acids for energy, ketones can be a clue to **diabetic ketoacidosis (DKA)** or **starvation,** with subsequent fat catabolism for nutrition. In DKA, there are two main ketones produced—acetoacetate and β-hydroxybutyrate—but UA cannot detect the latter.

Urinary ketones: Only detects acetoacetate, not β-hydroxybutyrate.

Bilirubin

Can be seen with increased levels of conjugated (water-soluble) bilirubin, such as in liver or gallbladder disease.

Urobilinogen

Formed by bacterial modification of bilirubin in the gut, if urobilinogen is present, it means that **bilirubin is making it to the intestines;** therefore it is less likely that an obstructive jaundice is present because if there is no bile getting to the gut, there can be no urobilinogen produced to be excreted in the urine.

Blood

The blood dipstick will turn positive with the presence of either **blood** or **myoglobin** in the urine. Blood in the urine can be from broken down red blood cells being excreted in the urine from hemolysis, red blood cell casts from nephritic syndrome, or red blood cells from a lower urinary tract bleed. Myoglobin can be from rhabdomyolysis (skeletal muscle breakdown, where myoglobin is stored). Differentiation of these entities can only be done by microscopy; with myoglobinuria, there will be **no red blood cells on microscopy.**

Nitrites

Many gram-negative bacteria reduce nitrates to nitrites, which can be seen on UA. The most common urinary tract infection (UTI) pathogen, *Escherichia coli,* is a nitrate reducer. However, this reduction reaction takes time to occur and may be negative, even in the setting of a UTI, if the patient is urinating frequently or has an infection by an organism that is not a nitrate reducer. Therefore it is specific **(positive result almost guarantees UTI)** but not sensitive (negative result does not rule out UTI).

Nitrites: Most specific UA finding for UTI (positive result almost guarantees UTI).

Leukocyte Esterase

Leukocyte esterase is an enzyme released by white blood cells. The presence of leukocyte esterase indicates the presence of white blood cells and suggests a UTI or other inflammatory condition of the urinary tract (e.g., renal tuberculosis, *Chlamydia* urethritis), stones, or stents that irritate the ureters.

Microscopy allows the analysis of any cells, casts, or crystals in the urine. This is important because it can give insight into some of the urinalysis abnormalities described.

Cells

Red blood cells (RBCs) may indicate glomerular bleeding, lower urinary tract bleeding, or contamination from menstruation in women. **White blood cells** (WBCs) indicate the presence of an infection or inflammation. **Bacteria** can indicate a urinary tract infection but can also be a contaminant if the specimen was not collected in a clean fashion.

Casts

Red blood cell casts indicate glomerular bleeding or acute glomerulonephritis. **White blood cell casts** indicate an ongoing intrinsic kidney infection (pyelonephritis) or allergic reaction (interstitial nephritis). **Granular casts** indicate varying degrees of degenerated cellular casts (e.g., degenerated RBC or WBC casts) and are thus nonspecific. **Muddy brown casts** indicate the presence of dead necrotic renal tubular cells seen with acute tubular necrosis. **Waxy casts** are acellular and indicate advanced kidney disease. Finally, **fatty casts** are seen in nephrotic syndrome (see explanation of nephrotic syndrome).

Crystals, Stones

Precipitation may reflect dietary intake (calcium oxalate stones with high oxalate-containing food) or drugs (e.g., acyclovir) in association with low urine flow. Excessive precipitation of specific crystals may indicate increased stone risks.

Kidney Stones (Urolithiasis)

Kidney stones come in many types and sizes (Table 15.4). Clinically, symptomatic stones cause **hematuria** and **sudden-onset flank pain,** in which patients continue to move because they are trying to find

TABLE 15.4 Types of Stones and Their Characteristics

STONE	RISK FACTORS	RADIOGRAPH	SHAPE ON MICROSCOPY	TREATMENT
Calcium oxalate	Hypercalcemia Hyperoxaluria	Radiopaque	Envelope	Hydration Thiazide diuretic Stop loop diuretics
Magnesium ammonium phosphate	Urinary tract infection with urease-producing bacteria	Radiopaque	Coffin lid*	Antibiotics to eradicate infection
Uric acid	Hyperuricemia Gout	**Radiolucent**	Diamond	Allopurinol Alkalinization of urine
Cystine	Cystinuria	Faintly radiopaque	Hexagon	Alkalinization of urine

*Mnemonic: magnesium ammonium phosphate crystals can cause the entire renal pelvis to fill with stones and destroy the kidney, killing it and putting a **coffin lid** on it!

a less painful position (but cannot). The pain is often so severe as to cause **nausea and vomiting.** Stones can cause **obstruction** and **hydronephrosis** from the increased back pressure, potentially leading to kidney damage. **Inadequate fluid intake** is a predisposing factor for all stones because the concentration of the compounds making up the stones is higher, promoting precipitation and stone formation. Most stones (except uric acid) can be seen by radiography and are termed ***radiopaque,*** although cystine stones are only faintly radiopaque; ultrasound can show obstruction (hydronephrosis) but not the stone itself.

Calcium Stones

The most common (80%) stones are composed of calcium oxalate (adults) or calcium phosphate (children). Predisposing factors include anything that causes hypercalcemia or increases oxalate concentration. One classic scenario is the presence of stones after ethylene glycol (antifreeze) ingestion because its final metabolite is oxalate (oxalic acid). Other predisposing factors include vegan diets (some vegetables, such as spinach, are high in oxalates) and inflammatory bowel disease (poor fat absorption causes calcium to bind to fat instead of oxalate in the gut, leading to oxalate absorption). These stones appear as envelopes or dumbbells on microscopy. Treatment for recurrent stones is hydrochlorothiazide because it increases calcium reabsorption in the distal nephron, thereby decreasing its concentration in the urine. Avoid loop diuretics in these patients because they increase calcium excretion in the urine.

Calcium stones: Most common; associated with dehydration, hypercalcemia, or diets high in oxalates.

Magnesium Ammonium Phosphate (Struvite)

Ammonium can be produced by organisms that split urea with their **urease** enzyme, typically *Proteus* spp. The ammonium is a **base** and therefore the urine will become **alkaline** (high urine pH), which is a key finding. Unfortunately, these stones can get so large that they fill the entire renal pelvis, termed ***staghorn calculus*** because it looks like antlers. Treatment involves **antibiotics** to kill the urease-producing organism and potentially **surgery** for removal of very large stones.

Uric Acid Stones

The only truly **radiolucent** (not seen on x-ray examination) stone, uric acid stones often occur in those with high uric acid levels (hyperuricemia), such as patients with **gout** or those with high cell turnover rates (because uric acid is a purine nucleotide breakdown byproduct) in conditions such as **leukemia.** Treatment is **allopurinol,** which inhibits xanthine oxidase and prevents uric acid production in the purine breakdown pathway. These stones appear kite shaped on microscopy. Initial treatment can also include high fluid intake and **alkalinization** of the urine to shift the uric acid molecules into their ionized (soluble) form. These stones are radiolucent; remember, **U**ric acid stones are radiol**U**cent and therefore **U**nseen on radiographs. They can be diagnosed with a computed tomography (CT) scan.

Cystine Stones

Cystine stones are rare, essentially only found in those with **cystinuria,** an autosomal recessive disease. Consider this condition in patients who have a family history of renal stones. They appear hexagonal on microscopy. Treatment is with high fluid intake and **alkalinization** of the urine to keep the cystine in its ionized (soluble) form.

Glomerular Diseases

The **glomerulus** is implicated in a wide variety of pathologic conditions. Generally, glomerular diseases will allow large amounts of **protein** (**nephrotic** syndromes) or **red blood cells** and some protein (**nephritic** syndromes) to pass through the glomerulus, leading to hematuria and/or proteinuria. Excretion of more than 3.5g of protein over 24 hours or a result of more than 3+ proteinuria on urine dipstick are considered nephrotic-range proteinuria, with lesser amounts more typically seen in nephritic syndromes. There are many nephrotic syndromes and many nephritic syndromes. The terminology describing the syndromes (e.g., *focal segmental glomerulosclerosis,* a nephrotic syndrome) can be confusing but is explained here; all these are histologic determinations after a **percutaneous kidney biopsy** has been obtained.

- **Focal versus diffuse:** Defines the **number of glomeruli on the biopsy affected.** If less than half the glomeruli on the biopsy are affected, it is **focal.** If more than half are affected, it is **diffuse.**

- **Segmental versus global:** Defines **how much of each individual glomerulus is affected.** For each affected glomerulus, if only part is affected, then it is **segmental.** If the entire glomerulus is affected, it is **global.** (Therefore, **focal segmental glomerulosclerosis** means that less than half of the glomeruli are affected [**focal**] and, of those affected, only part of each glomerulus is affected [**segmental**].)
- **Membranous versus proliferative versus membranoproliferative:** In **membranous,** the glomerular basement **membrane** becomes thickened in parts; those thickenings appear as **spikes and domes** on microscopy because of the bulging membrane. **Proliferative** indicates that the **cells are proliferating** and numerous nuclei will be seen on microscopy from the added cell count. **Membranoproliferative** just indicates that there is membranous thickening **and** proliferation. This leads to a so-called **tram track** appearance because the basement membrane is rebuilt on top of the damaged deposits.

Glomerulosclerosis versus glomerulonephritis: Sclerosis means hardening; in glomerulosclerosis, there are sclerotic, scarred areas that lose the ability to filter, secondary to capillary collapse. In **glomerulonephritis** (*-itis* means inflammation), there is ongoing glomerular inflammation.

Crescentic: Used to describe the appearance when inflammatory cells and fibrin fill Bowman's space, leading to a crescent appearance, which is always indicative of a **rapidly progressive glomerulonephritis** (bad).

The best way to remember **nephrotic** syndrome is the mnemonic **nephrotic-oncotic** (rhymes) because the oncotic pressure is based on protein, which is what is lost in nephrotic syndromes (to a much greater degree than in nephritic syndromes), leading to decreased oncotic pressure and subsequent edema.

- **Criteria:** More than 3.5 g/24 hr of protein lost in the urine.

Nephrotic syndromes are usually caused by destructive cytokines produced by immune cells that cause loss of the negative charge barrier (loss of heparan sulfate leading to loss of negative repelling forces between podocytes, with subsequent **fusion of the podocytes**) or by an intrinsic abnormality in various podocyte proteins. This leads to the passage of negatively charged proteins into the urine, especially albumin, leading to **hypoalbuminemia, low intravascular oncotic pressure, and edema.** The **edema** is further exacerbated by the decreased effective arterial volume (from the hypoalbuminemia), leading to RAA axis activation, sodium retention, and worsening edema. There is also evidence that there is an intrinsic increase in sodium reabsorption independent of the RAA axis in nephrotic syndrome.

The liver reacts to hypoalbuminemia and loss of other large proteins by increasing its synthetic function, but unfortunately it also increases the synthesis of apolipoproteins, leading to **hypercholesterolemia.** Loss of cholesterol in the urine leads to **fatty casts** with a so-called **Maltese cross** appearance under polarized light.

Loss of other proteins is significant as well. The loss of **antithrombin III** (ATIII), an anticoagulant molecule (among other anticoagulants), leads to **hypercoagulability** and increased risk for **renal vein thrombosis, lower extremity deep venous thrombosis, and pulmonary embolism.** The loss of immunoglobulins makes patients more susceptible to infections.

In **nephritic** syndromes, red blood cells can pass through the glomerulus (and also usually proteins, because if large red blood cells can pass through, so can smaller proteins).

- **Criteria:** Red blood cell **casts** in the urine on microscopy.

Nephrotic syndrome: Loss of protein in urine (>3.5 g/day).

Nephritic syndrome: Loss of blood through the glomerulus (red blood cell casts) and smaller amounts of protein in urine.

It is important to remember that **when red blood cells pass through the glomerulus, they become red blood cell casts** (protein coated) and can be seen as such in the urine on microscopy. Imagine that the red blood cell gets banged up when it passes through the nephron and needs a cast. This can differentiate blood that has passed through the kidney (glomerulonephritis) from bleeding at a site after the kidney, such as a lower urinary tract bleed (bleeding from the ureter, bladder, urethra).

The larger permeability of the glomerulus in this case is attributed to **inflammation** and **damage by neutrophils,** usually a response to **complement deposition in the glomerulus** (type III hypersensitivity) or **antibodies directed at the basement membrane of the glomerulus itself** (type II hypersensitivity). See Chapter 6 for an explanation of the various hypersensitivities.

The severe glomerular inflammation decreases glomerular performance and leads to a decreased glomerular filtration rate with oliguria (decreased urinary output). Remember that this is a problem with the glomerulus; the tubules in the nephron work just fine, but because the glomerulus is not functioning properly, the performance of the whole kidney suffers.

As a result of the decreased GFR, the functioning tubules attempt to increase sodium reabsorption to try to correct the decreased GFR, potentially leading to **hypertension and edema.**

Nephrotic and Nephritic Syndromes

Table 15.5 details common glomerular diseases and their characteristics.

Table 15.5 Common Types of Glomerular Diseases and Their Characteristics

SYNDROME	IMPORTANT INFORMATION	BIOPSY FINDINGS	CAUSES
Nephrotic Syndromes			
Minimal change disease (Nil disease, lipoid nephrosis; Fig. 15.16) 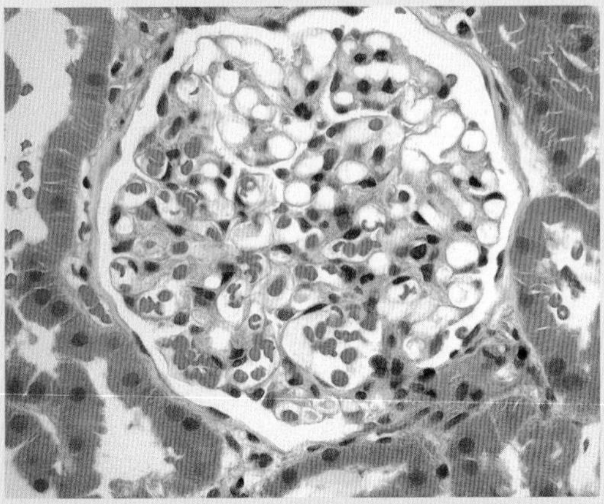 **Fig. 15.16** Normal-appearing glomerulus. (*From Kumar P, Clark M. Clinical Medicine. 6th ed. Philadelphia: Elsevier; 2005.*)	Most common cause of nephrotic syndrome in children Selective albuminuria (essentially only albumin is lost in urine) Responds to corticosteroids; only rarely causes permanent renal dysfunction but recurrence common	Nothing on light microscopy (LM); hence, the name Fusion and loss of podocytes on electron microscopy (EM)	Cytokines from T cells reduce heparan sulfate production from basement membrane, leading to anion charge barrier loss. Recent infections can trigger this because increased cytokines are implicated in the disease. Hodgkin lymphoma is a secondary cause, most likely because of increased cytokine production from the abnormal T cells.
Focal segmental glomerulosclerosis (FSGS) (Fig. 15.17) 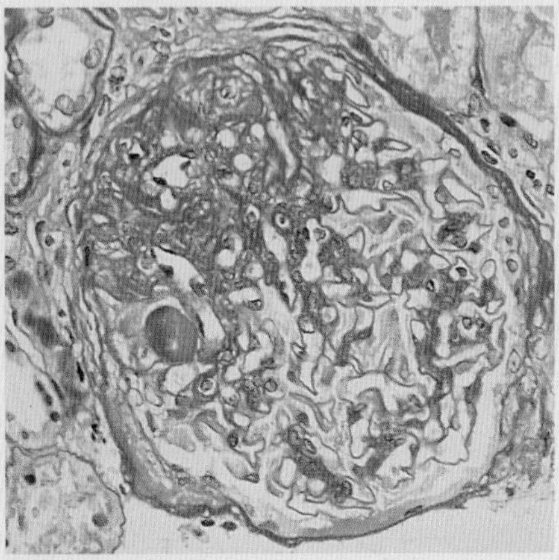 **Fig. 15.17** Focal segmental glomerulosclerosis (FSGS). (*From Kumar V, Fausto N, Abbas AK. Robbins Basic Pathology. 7th ed. Philadelphia: Elsevier; 2002.*)	Most common cause of nephrotic syndrome in adults Can be primary (no underlying cause) or secondary Treatment—corticosteroids, but response typically poor, often leading to progressive renal failure	LM—as the disease name implies, there is scarring (sclerosis) of parts (segmental) of some (focal) of the glomeruli	Secondary causes include obesity, HIV, sickle cell disease, and heroin usage. The most severe subtype, the collapsing variant, is more often seen in African Americans.
Membranous glomerulopathy (MGN)	Second most common cause of nephrotic syndrome in adults Most is primary (idiopathic) but many secondary causes Caused by circulating immune complexes depositing in the subepithelial space of the glomerulus (type III hypersensitivity)	LM: Diffuse GBM thickening EM: Membranous, so focal thickening of the basement membrane, spike and dome pattern in the subepithelial space	Secondary causes include any disorder that can create antigen–antibody complexes, such as autoimmune disease (especially SLE), infections (especially hepatitis B), drugs such as NSAIDs and gold salts, and some solid organ malignancies.

TABLE 15.5 Common Types of Glomerular Diseases and Their Characteristics—cont'd

SYNDROME	IMPORTANT INFORMATION	BIOPSY FINDINGS	CAUSES
Membranoproliferative Glomerulonephritis (MPGN)			
Type I	More common than MPGN II; associated with hepatitis B or C Subendothelial immunocomplex deposition (under the capillaries) Poor prognosis; treatment aimed at treating underlying disease causing MPGN I	EM: Membranoproliferative diseases have tram track appearance from basement membrane rebuilding on top of immunocomplex deposits	Hepatitis B or C (or cryoglobulinemia, which is also associated with hepatitis C), can cause MPGN I.
Type II	Associated with autoantibody against C3 convertase, which normally helps clear complement; disabling this with an antibody leads to overactive complement activity, subsequent deposition in the glomerulus, and depleted C3 levels	EM: Membranoproliferative diseases have tram track appearance from basement membrane rebuilding on top of immunocomplex deposits EM also shows dense deposits	Caused by defective complement regulation from autoantibodies.
Nephritic Syndromes			
IgA glomerulopathy (Berger disease) (Fig. 15.18) 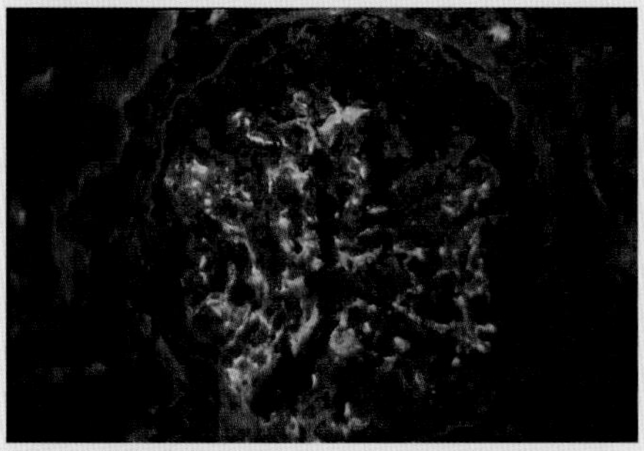 **FIG. 15.18** Granular immunofluorescence. (*From Damjanov I, Linder J. Pathology: A Color Atlas. St. Louis; Mosby; 2000: 224.*)	Most common glomerulonephritis. Termed *synpharyngitic* because it occurs after a viral pharyngitis or upper respiratory infection; glomerulonephritis starts during illness *(syn)*, often within 24–48 hr Associated with Henoch-Schonlein purpura. Can have recurrences	LM shows mesangial IgA immunocomplex deposition, granular immunofluorescence staining (from haphazard deposition of immunocomplexes)	Can occur or recur after viral upper respiratory infection or gastroenteritis (usually within 1 wk).
Poststreptococcal glomerulonephritis (PSGN) (Fig. 15.19) 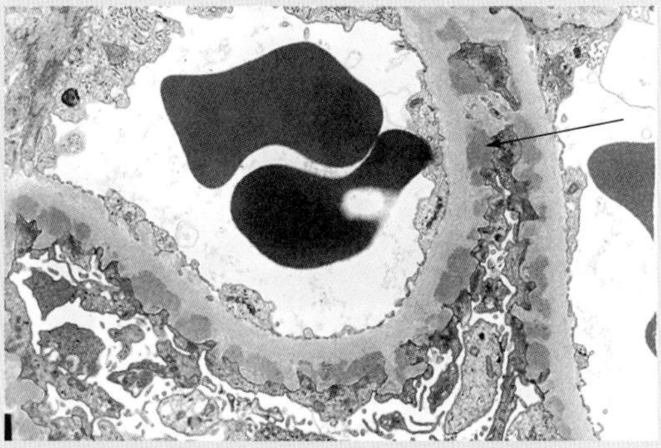 **FIG. 15.19** Subepithelial deposits (arrow). (*From Damjanov I. Pathology for the Health-Related Professions. 2nd ed. Philadelphia: WB Saunders; 2000: 341.*)	Delayed immunocomplex deposition after streptococcal infection Occurs regardless of antibiotic treatment for initial infection Resolves spontaneously; often seen in children	LM: Neutrophil infiltration and hypercellular glomeruli EM: Subepithelial granular deposits IF: Granular immunofluorescence (IF)	Occurs after streptococcal infection: • 1–3 wk after strep throat (strep pharyngitis) • 2–6 wk (twice as long) after strep skin infection

Continued

Table 15.5 Common Types of Glomerular Diseases and Their Characteristics—cont'd

SYNDROME	IMPORTANT INFORMATION	BIOPSY FINDINGS	CAUSES
Rapidly progressive (crescentic) glomerulonephritis (RPGN; Fig. 15.20)	Very serious; can quickly lead to renal failure or death. This is a syndrome and can be caused by a few diseases: • Goodpasture disease: Type II hypersensitivity affecting mostly men; antibodies against basement membrane leading to linear immunofluorescence (every spot on basement membrane covered, making linear pattern; remember that linear is associated with Goodpasture); can also attack lung basement membrane, leading to hemoptysis and pulmonary edema. Treatment is plasmapheresis to remove antibodies, steroids to prevent new ones from being made, and potential renal transplantation. • Granulomatous polyangiitis (formerly known as Wegener granulomatosis) (predominantly c-ANCA): See Chapter 8 for details on this vasculitis; can affect the kidneys and lead to renal failure. • Microscopic polyarteritis (predominantly p-ANCA): See Chapter 8 for details on this vasculitis; can affect the kidneys and lead to renal failure.		

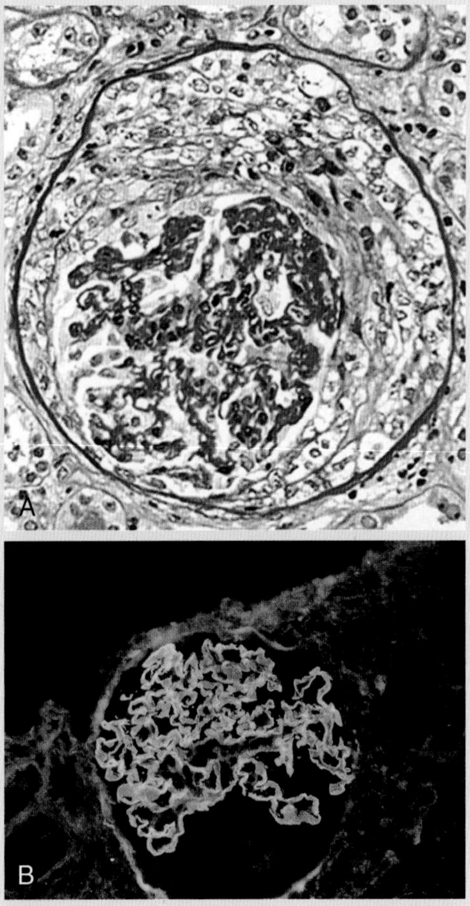

Fig. 15.20 Rapidly progressive (crescentic glomerulonephritis (RPGN). **A,** Crescentic glomerulonephritis demonstrating crescent formation around the glomerulus. **B,** Linear immunofluorescence, associated with Goodpasture disease. (**A** *from Kumar V, Abbas AK, Fausto N, Aster J.* Robbins & Cotran Pathologic Basis of Disease. *8th ed. New York: Elsevier; 2009;* **B** *from Kumar V, Fausto N, Abbas AK.* Robbins & Cotran Pathologic Basis of Disease. *7th ed. Philadelphia: Saunders; 2004: 969.*)

Table 15.5 Common Types of Glomerular Diseases and Their Characteristics—cont'd

SYNDROME	IMPORTANT INFORMATION	BIOPSY FINDINGS	CAUSES
Diffuse proliferative glomerulonephritis (lupus nephritis; Fig. 15.21) 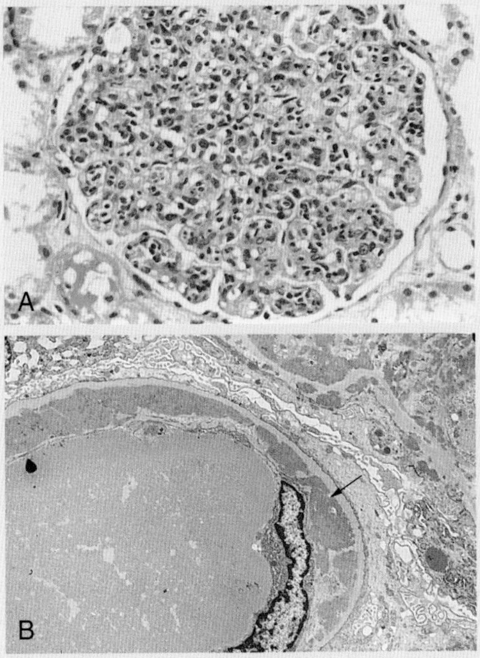 **Fig. 15.21** Subendothelial deposits *(arrow)* **(A)** as seen under a light microscope and **(B)** as seen under an electron microscope. (**A** *from Kumar V, Fausto N, Abbas AK.* Robbins Basic Pathology. *7th ed. Philadelphia: Elsevier; 2002;* **B** *from Damjanov I, Linder J.* Pathology: A Color Atlas. *St. Louis: Mosby; 2000: 224.*)	Most common glomerular disease in SLE patients, although SLE patients can also have other types of glomerulopathies Poor prognosis	Subendothelial immunocomplexes (under endothelium of capillary) leads to wire loop appearance of capillaries (a way to remember lupus nephritis as subendothelial is that DNA–anti-DNA complexes are big because DNA strands are big and can only fit under capillary endothelium; PSGN has subepithelial deposits that are smaller and can travel to subepithelial area) IF: Granular	Patients with SLE, an autoimmune disease, can have DNA–anti-DNA immunocomplex deposition in the glomeruli.

GBM, glomerular basement membrane; IgA, immunoglobulin A; SLE, systemic lupus erythematosus.

Other Systemic Diseases Causing Glomerular Damage

Diabetes is a very common cause of renal damage (diabetes causes the triad of retinopathy, neuropathy, and nephropathy as part of its microvascular disease) and is the **most common cause of chronic renal failure** in the United States. Disease severity is based on glycemic control; good glycemic control will prevent or slow the progression of the **diabetic glomerulopathy.** The pathogenesis is **nonenzymatic glycosylation (NEG) of the basement membrane,** which is a fancy term for molecules of glucose attaching themselves to the proteins of the basement membrane (without the aid of enzymes; hence, nonenzymatic). This modification prevents the negative charge barrier from functioning properly, leading to **proteinuria.**

Diabetes: Nonenzymatic glycosylation of basement membrane leads to **diabetic glomerulopathy** characterized by proteinuria and Kimmelstiel-Wilson nodules.

- NEG of basement membrane: Thickening, loss of charge barrier, proteinuria.
- NEG of arterioles: **Efferent** arterioles are affected first, before afferent arterioles, leading to **hyaline arteriolosclerosis** (narrowing and hardening). This causes increased hydrostatic pressure on the glomerulus, with subsequent glomerular hyperfiltration (initial increased GFR) and damage. This is why **ACE inhibitors** are nephroprotective in diabetics.
- Early kidney damage can be detected by checking for **microalbuminuria,** a sensitive test for small amounts of albumin leaking in the urine. Diabetics should be regularly screened for microalbuminuria.
- On biopsy, **Kimmelstiel-Wilson nodules** can be present (Fig. 15.22). These are focal nodules of pink hyaline material that forms in the glomerulus from NEG.

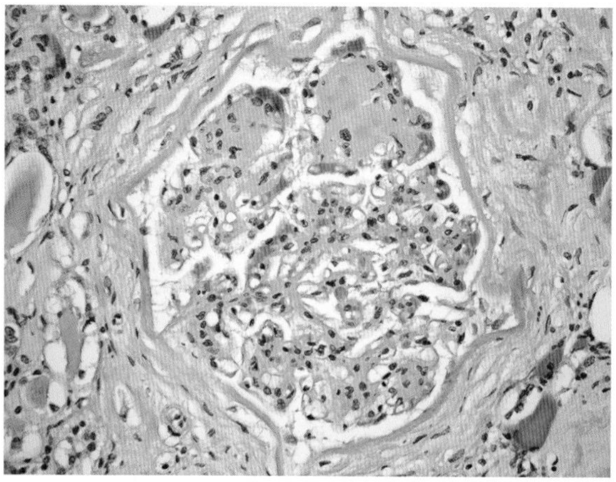

Fig. 15.22 Kimmelstiel-Wilson nodules in a patient with diabetic glomerulopathy. Focal nodules of pink hyaline material can be seen, most notably at the top of the glomerulus shown. (*From King T. Elsevier's* Integrated Pathology. *Philadelphia: Elsevier; 2006.*)

Amyloidosis describes any disease in which abnormal proteins deposit in tissues, leading to organ damage. These amyloid plaques are improperly folded proteins in a beta-pleated sheet configuration. Several types of proteins can form deposits:

- AL amyloidosis (**A**myloid **L**ight chains): Seen in **multiple myeloma,** in which **Bence-Jones proteins** are present (immunoglobulin **light** chains, hence AL).
- AA amyloidosis (**A**myloid-**A**ssociated): Caused by any disorder that has long-standing cell breakdown with **chronic inflammation,** including autoimmune diseases such as **rheumatoid arthritis** and ankylosing spondylitis, but also chronic infections such as **tuberculosis.**

There are other miscellaneous diseases that require brief mention:

- **Alport syndrome** (mostly X-linked recessive): Hereditary mutation of type IV collagen, preventing proper basement membrane (BM) formation in many areas, leading to splitting of the BM in the glomerulus and nephritic syndrome. Also implicated in **eye problems (lenticonus), deafness,** and **nerve disorders** for the same reason.
- **Thin basement membrane disease** (autosomal dominant): Characterized by thin basement membranes, leading to proteinuria and microscopic hematuria. Also known as benign familial hematuria because the disease itself does not lead to serious renal problems.

Tubular and Interstitial Disorders

This section will discuss acute tubular necrosis, drug-induced interstitial nephritis, renal papillary necrosis, and diffuse cortical necrosis.

Acute tubular necrosis (ATN) occurs when tubules of nephrons die of lack of blood flow (**ischemic** ATN), the most common type, or from drugs that cause kidney damage to the point of necrosis (**nephrotoxic** ATN). In both cases, the nephrons that are shed will be lost in the urine, leading to microscopic findings of **muddy brown casts.**

Acute tubular necrosis (ATN) is usually caused by ischemic injury or by the use of nephrotoxic agents.

- **Ischemic ATN:** The kidney requires a constant supply of blood; any condition that significantly diminishes blood flow, and therefore oxygen, to the kidney can result in ischemic ATN. Usually, **hypovolemia** will be the precipitating factor, such as in hypovolemic shock from hemorrhage. Treatment is aimed at correcting the underlying cause of the low renal perfusion.
- **Nephrotoxic ATN:** There are many nephrotoxic agents. The most common two are **aminoglycoside antibiotics** (e.g., gentamicin), and **iodinated radiocontrast agents,** such as those used in contrast-enhanced CT scans. Treatment is aimed at adjusting or discontinuing the responsible medication(s) and providing supportive care.

Drug-induced interstitial nephritis is triggered by a drug (as the name implies) and causes inflammation in the interstitium of the kidney, often starting 1 to 2 weeks after beginning a drug. The mnemonic **FARE** can be used as a memory aid to remember the symptoms: **F**ever, **A**rthralgias, **R**ash, and **E**osinophilia. Common offenders include penicillins and sulfa drugs. Treatment is simply stopping the inducing drug.

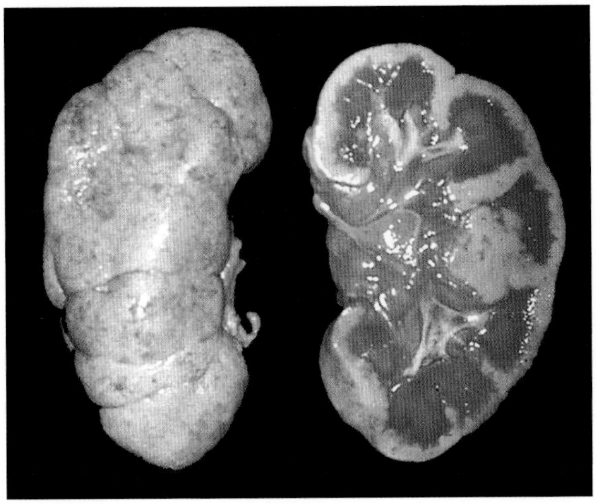

FIG. 15.23 Diffuse cortical necrosis, displaying coagulation necrosis in the outer part (cortex) of the kidney. (*From Kumar V, Abbas AK, Fausto N, Aster J. Robbins & Cotran Pathologic Basis of Disease. 8th ed. New York: Elsevier; 2009.*)

Renal papillary necrosis is characterized by necrosis of the renal papilla, which is the innermost tip of the medulla and therefore the last section of the kidney to receive oxygen and nutrients (recall that the peritubular capillaries run downward after the glomerulus). Renal papillary necrosis occurs most often after chronic acetaminophen, aspirin, or NSAID use, called **analgesic nephropathy.** In those with **sickle cell disease,** sickle formation in the ischemic medullary papilla leads to occlusion and infarction. Infections such as **acute pyelonephritis** and systemic diseases such as **diabetes mellitus** can also cause this.

Diffuse cortical necrosis (Fig. 15.23) is a rare occurrence that causes necrosis of the outer parts of the kidneys (the cortex). This occurs almost exclusively during **obstetric emergencies** such as abruptio placentae but can also be seen in sepsis. It is thought that disseminated intravascular coagulation (DIC) is implicated in this disease, but the mechanism of cortical death is unknown. In Fig. 15.23, **coagulation necrosis** has occurred on the cortical area of the kidney only.

Renal Tubular Acidosis

Renal tubular acidosis causes a nongap metabolic acidosis.

Renal tubular acidosis (RTA) refers to metabolic acidosis caused by the inability of the kidneys to secrete acid or reabsorb bicarbonate adequately to regulate body pH. The diagnosis of RTA implies that the degree of tubular dysfunction in acid–base regulation is out of proportion to the degree of renal failure.

Type 1 RTA: In type 1 RTA (distal RTA), the **collecting tubules** (specifically the α-intercalated cells) in the distal nephron are unable to secrete H^+ and reclaim K^+. This leads to a **normal anion gap hypokalemic metabolic acidosis** and also a risk of developing **calcium oxalate** kidney stones because of the alkalotic urine (remember that the kidneys are **unable to acidify the urine,** so the urine is alkalotic and the body is acidotic from the retained acids). The pH of the urine is alkaline (>5.5).

Type 2 RTA: In type 2 RTA (proximal RTA), the **proximal tubules** are **unable to reabsorb** HCO_3^- (bicarbonate) from the urine, leading to **bicarbonate wasting in the urine** and therefore metabolic acidosis from loss of base. This can be a standalone disease but more often occurs in **Fanconi syndrome,** in which the **entire proximal tubule** is dysfunctional. Recalling the normal functions of the proximal tubule makes the symptoms logical—rickets from hypovitaminosis D and inability to reabsorb phosphate, acidosis from bicarbonate wasting, and decreased sodium reabsorption, leading to RAA axis activation and hypokalemia from increased distal nephron sodium reuptake. Type 2 RTA will have an acidic urine (pH <5.5) because, although the proximal tubule cannot reabsorb bicarbonate, the downstream α-intercalated cells are still intact and can secrete H^+ to try and compensate for the acidosis.

Whereas the previous types of RTA were characterized by tubular dysfunction, **type 4 RTA** (aldosterone failure) is not a problem with the tubules at all. It is a consequence of **hypoaldosteronism** (low aldosterone) or **aldosterone resistance,** such as in those taking spironolactone. Recall that aldosterone allows the distal nephron to reabsorb sodium at the expense of secreting potassium and hydrogen ions. Lack of aldosterone therefore would cause sodium not to be reabsorbed (hypotension), and also results in the inability to excrete potassium (hyperkalemia) and hydrogen ions (acidosis). Interestingly, the acidosis may be exacerbated in patients with concurrent hyperkalemia caused by reduced **ammonia secretion**. Cells have a H^+/K^+ exchanger; the hyperkalemia causes excess K^+ to move into the cell, with H^+ exiting; this intracellular alkalosis inhibits ammoniagenesis. The reduced urinary level of ammonia associated with hypoaldosterone-induced hyperkalemia leads to reduced H^+ buffering in the urine—hence, acidic **urine and low urine pH (typically < 5.5).**

You may wonder about type 3 RTA. It's simply a combination of types 1 and 2 RTA.

Azotemia and Renal Failure

The term ***azotemia*** implies that there are high serum levels of nitrogen-containing waste products, especially **urea** (measured as blood urea nitrogen [**BUN**]). Azotemia in general is caused by a **lack of filtration by the kidney,** but that can be caused by a lack of blood flow to the kidney **(prerenal azotemia);** the kidney itself is damaged and unable to filter properly **(renal azotemia),** or urine produced by the kidney is unable to leave the body and backs up into the ureters and kidney, preventing proper function (**postrenal azotemia;** Fig. 15.24). Differentiating among these three disorders is important because it gives a clue about the underlying cause of the decreased renal function and how best to manage it.

Azotemia: Must establish if it is prerenal, renal, or postrenal (Table 15.6).

The determination of **prerenal** azotemia (problem is **before** the kidney) versus **renal** azotemia (problem is **in** the kidney) versus **postrenal** azotemia (problem is **after** the kidney) is often elucidated by the **BUN-to-creatinine** (Cr) ratio, urine sodium level, and fractional excretion of sodium, Fe_{Na}. Remember before reading the explanations that **urea can be** reabsorbed **by the kidney**, but **creatinine cannot;** this will become important in understanding BUN/Cr ratios.

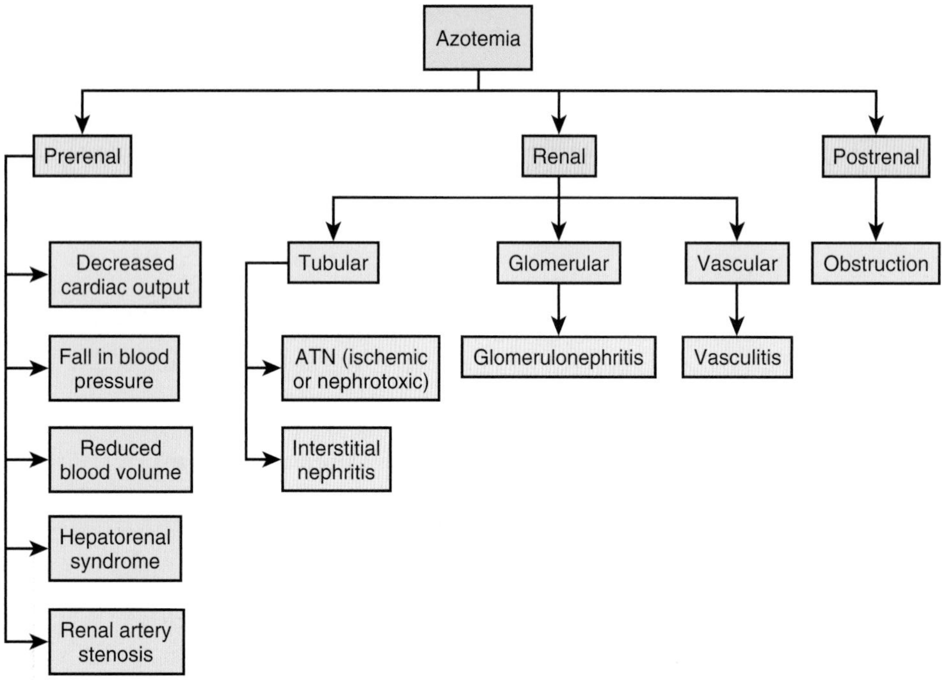

Fig. 15.24 Diagrammatic representation of the prerenal, renal, and postrenal causes of azotemia.

Table 15.6 Characteristics of Prerenal, Renal, and Postrenal Azotemia

PARAMETER	PRERENAL AZOTEMIA	RENAL AZOTEMIA	POSTRENAL AZOTEMIA
Serum BUN/Cr ratio	>15:1	<15:1	>15:1
Urine (Na^+) (mEq/L)	<20 (low)	>20	Varies
Fe_{Na}	<1% (low)	>2%	Varies
Urine osmolality (mOsm/L)	>500 (concentrated)	300–350	Varies

$$Fe_{Na} = \frac{[Na]\ urine/[Na]\ plasma}{[Cr]\ urine/[Cr]\ plasma} = \frac{[Na]\ urine \times [Cr]\ plasma}{[Na]\ plasma \times [Cr]\ urine}$$

Fe_{Na} is simply a measure of the percentage of sodium filtered by the nephron that is excreted in the urine. In azotemia, if the Fe_{Na} is low (<1%), the nephron is actively trying to reclaim all the sodium possible and is able to do so; if it is higher, it is possible that the nephrons are dysfunctional and unable to reclaim sodium properly.

Prerenal Azotemia

In prerenal azotemia, there is **not enough blood going to the normally functioning kidney** to allow for an adequate GFR, leading to buildup of waste products. The **reduced renal perfusion** may be caused by hypovolemia, poor cardiac output (e.g., cardiomyopathy, congestive heart failure, severe aortic valvular dysfunction, pericardial effusions), renal artery stenosis, or medications that cause afferent arteriolar vasoconstriction or efferent arteriolar vasodilation. Other causes can include hepatorenal syndrome, a serious disorder caused by cirrhosis, and subsequent hemodynamic changes that can lead to poor renal perfusion. **The serum creatinine level** will increase because of the decreased overall GFR, but all the creatinine that is filtered is excreted because creatinine is not reabsorbed. However, **urea** can go back into the bloodstream because it is freely diffusible and can be reabsorbed. The low flow through the nephron caused by low perfusion allows more time for **urea to move back into the bloodstream,** leading to significantly **increased BUN** with a smaller increase in creatinine, which results in a **BUN/Cr ratio greater than 15:1**. Next, because of the low-volume state, the RAA axis is fully active, leading to **low urine sodium** from increased sodium reabsorption to promote volume expansion. The urine will be **concentrated** because ADH is also present to reabsorb the water.

Renal Azotemia

In renal azotemia, there is **intrinsic renal parenchymal dysfunction,** which can be **tubular** (**ATN** [most common] or interstitial nephritis), **glomerular** (glomerulonephritis), or **vascular** (vasculitis). Although the BUN and Cr levels are both elevated, the **BUN/Cr ratio** is similar to what is seen in a **normal** patient (<15:1) because **both BUN and Cr are elevated to the same degree.** This is because the functioning nephrons are not in a low-flow state, as in prerenal azotemia, with not as much time to reabsorb BUN. Damage to the tubules also prevents reabsorption of BUN. Additionally, the damaged kidney does not reabsorb sodium as efficiently; the Fe_{Na} and urine sodium levels will be elevated as sodium remains in the urine.

Prerenal azotemia: Not enough blood delivered to the kidney.

Renal azotemia: Kidney damage.

Postrenal azotemia: Blockage after the kidney.

Postrenal Azotemia

In postrenal azotemia, there is enough blood flow to the kidney, and the kidney is (at least initially) functioning normally, but there is a **urinary tract obstruction** preventing formed urine from leaving the body. This can be anywhere in the lower urinary tract (ureteral obstruction if **bilateral,** bladder outlet obstruction, urethral obstruction) and is usually caused by benign prostatic hyperplasia (BPH) in older men. Treatment is aimed at the underlying cause, draining the urine (e.g., Foley catheterization in those with BPH). The **BUN/Cr ratio is more than 15:1**, similar to prerenal azotemia, but for a different reason. The urinary blockage increases back pressure in the kidney, decreasing GFR, but there is a low-flow state because the urine cannot exit out of the kidney, leading to urea reabsorption and increase in BUN. Prolonged blockage, however, leads to intrinsic renal damage and renal failure, with laboratory values similar to those of renal azotemia.

Urinary Tract Infections

Almost all **UTIs** are **ascending infections;** that is, the normally present bacteria in the perineal area (mostly *E. coli* from fecal material) start around the urethra and climb up the urethra into the bladder (causing **cystitis**), eventually trying to climb further up into the ureters and kidneys (**pyelonephritis;** Fig. 15.25). Because the urethra is significantly shorter in women, **women are at higher risk for UTIs.** Both cystitis and pyelonephritis are characterized by painful urination **(dysuria),** frequency, and urgency, as well as **bacteriuria** (bacteria in the urine). Because the kidneys are highly vascular, when bacteria reach them in pyelonephritis, the bacteria have the opportunity to enter the bloodstream, leading to **fever, chills, nausea, and vomiting** and the possibility for sepsis (termed ***urosepsis*** because the sepsis is of urinary origin). In addition, with pyelonephritis, the inflamed kidneys will be tender, leading

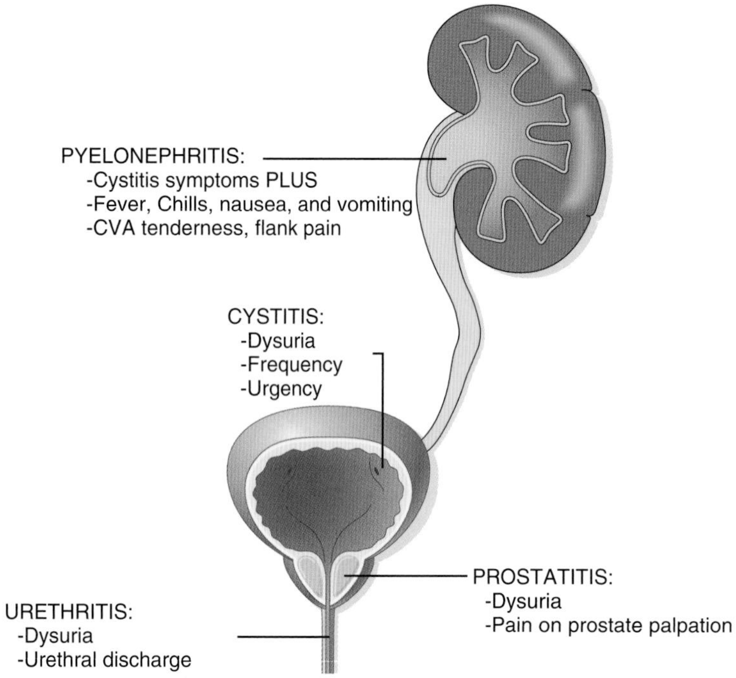

FIG. 15.25 The urinary tract, showing what occurs when each part becomes infected. *CVA*, Costovertebral. (*Modified from Kumar V, Abbas AK, Fausto N, Aster J.* Robbins & Cotran Pathologic Basis of Disease. *8th ed. New York: Elsevier; 2009.*)

to costovertebral (CVA) angle tenderness and flank pain. With cystitis, on the other hand, there is generally no fever because the bacteria are confined to the bladder.

Because the **urethra** is part of the urinary tract, inflammation can occur here too, termed ***urethritis.*** However, this is usually caused by a sexually transmitted infection, characterized by **dysuria** and **urethral discharge.** Usually, this is caused by chlamydia or gonorrhea. Gonorrhea will display gram-negative diplococci on staining of the discharge, whereas chlamydia, because it is intracellular, will not stain (stain will not reach the bacteria).

Finally, the prostate can become inflamed, termed ***prostatitis.*** The main clinical clue here is an exquisitely tender prostate on digital rectal examination.

Although *E. coli* is the most common pathogen in UTIs (>80%), other bacteria can be implicated:

- *Escherichia coli* (>80%): Have pili that allow adhesion to the epithelial cells of the urethra
- *Staphylococcus saprophyticus* (5% to 10%): Implicated in sexually active young women
- *Klebsiella, Proteus, Pseudomonas, Enterobacter* spp.: Implicated in those with urinary catheters in place

UTIs: Cystitis (infection confined to bladder) does not have a fever or systemic symptoms because the bacteria do not have access to the bloodstream.

E. coli is the most common cause, by far, of UTIs.

There are many **risk factors** for UTIs. The most common is **female gender,** because of a short urethra providing an easy path for bacteria to ascend into the bladder. Second, **older men** are at risk as a result of BPH. Urination flushes out the bacteria climbing up the urethra; with BPH, the urinary stasis and decreased ability to void urine lead to increased risk for UTIs. Also, **catheterization** is a risk factor because there is an instrument placed into the bladder that can serve as a nidus for infection.

Malignancies and Benign Tumors of the Urinary Tract

There are a few important malignancies of the urinary tract: (1) **renal cell carcinoma**; (2) **transitional cell carcinoma**; and (3) **nephroblastoma.**

Renal Cell Carcinoma

Renal cell carcinoma (RCC) is the most common malignancy affecting the kidney, with **smoking** being the most common risk factor because the kidney filters the carcinogenic substances. Another rare but important risk factor is **von Hippel–Lindau** disease. Patients with this disease can develop bilateral RCC. Histologically, the most common appearance of RCC is that of clear cell carcinoma caused by the

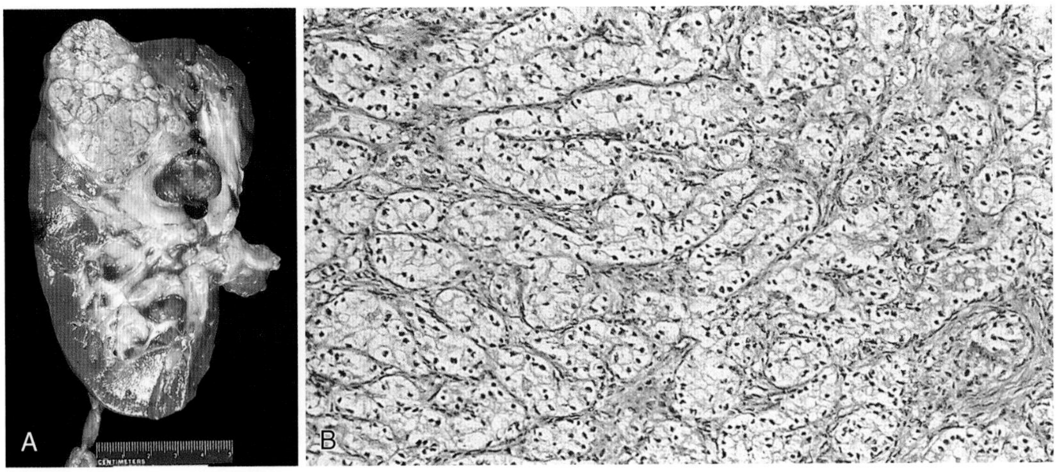

Fig. 15.26 Renal cell carcinoma (RCC). **A,** Histologic appearance, showing the vacuolated appearance of clear cell carcinoma. **B,** Gross image of RCC. (**A** *from Stevens A, Lowe J, Scott I.* Core Pathology. *3rd ed. Philadelphia: Elsevier; 2008;* **B** *from Kumar V, Abbas AK, Fausto N, Aster J.* Robbins & Cotran Pathologic Basis of Disease. *8th ed. New York: Elsevier; 2009.*)

histologic appearance of the vacuolated cells (Fig. 15.26A). The tumor spreads **hematogenously** (unlike most carcinomas, which spread via lymphatics) by traveling through the renal vein to the IVC. It often metastasizes to lung and bone as well. In the gross section of the RCC shown in Fig. 15.26B, a tumor in the renal vein can be seen causing thrombosis. Hemorrhagic areas of the tumor lead to **hematuria and flank pain;** the size often allows for a **palpable mass** to be felt; this triad should raise immediate suspicion for RCC. Because the kidney is involved in the endocrine system, **paraneoplastic syndromes** can occur from ectopic hormone production, especially **erythropoietin,** causing secondary polycythemia.

Renal cell carcinoma: Most common malignancy affecting the kidney; spreads via the renal vein.

Transitional Cell Carcinoma

The area from the renal calices to the renal pelvis, ureters, and bladder is lined with transitional epithelium (to allow stretch), and therefore malignancies in this area are termed *transitional cell carcinoma.* The unique feature of this type of malignancy is the **field effect,** in which multiple primary tumors can arise simultaneously. This is because the carcinogens responsible are in the urine and bathe the entire urinary tract in carcinogens, leading to the development of multiple foci of malignancy in the urinary tract. Those carcinogens include **smoking** (just like RCC), but also **aniline dyes** used in the manufacture of some plastics and medications such as **cyclophosphamide** (a chemotherapeutic agent and immunosuppressant).

Nephroblastoma (Wilms Tumor)

Nephroblastoma is a rare malignancy occurring in children (although rare, it is the most common primary renal tumor in children) between the ages of 2 to 4 years (Fig. 15.27). Although mostly sporadic, it can be associated with the **WAGR** syndrome, an acronym standing for **W**ilms tumor, **A**niridia (absent iris), **G**enitourinary abnormalities, and mental **R**etardation. Nephroblastoma is also associated with **Beckwith-Wiedemann syndrome,** which is characterized by hemihypertrophy of the extremities (e.g., one but not both arms with hypertrophy) and organomegaly. This tumor is derived from **mesonephric mesoderm** and has numerous histologic characteristics: (1) primitive blastema cells (undifferentiated cells); (2) primitive glomeruli and tubules; and (3) rhabdomyoblasts (creating muscle and connective tissue strands). Grossly, the tumor appears as a large, tan-colored mass. Like RCC, there is often a palpable abdominal mass. Unique to nephroblastoma is that some of the cells can secrete **renin,** leading to **hypertension** (see Fig. 15.27).

Nephroblastoma: Can secrete renin, causing hypertension. Remember the association with WAGR syndrome and Beckwith-Wiedemann syndrome.

Angiomyolipomas

Angiomyolipomas are **benign** tumors of the kidney and, as the name implies, are composed of **blood vessels** (*angio*), **smooth muscle** (*myo*), and **fat** (*lipo*). A commonly tested association is with **tuberous sclerosis,** a rare genetic disease that causes benign tumor formation in multiple organs, developmental delay, and characteristic skin findings—**adenoma sebaceum,** a facial rash of reddish bumps that are

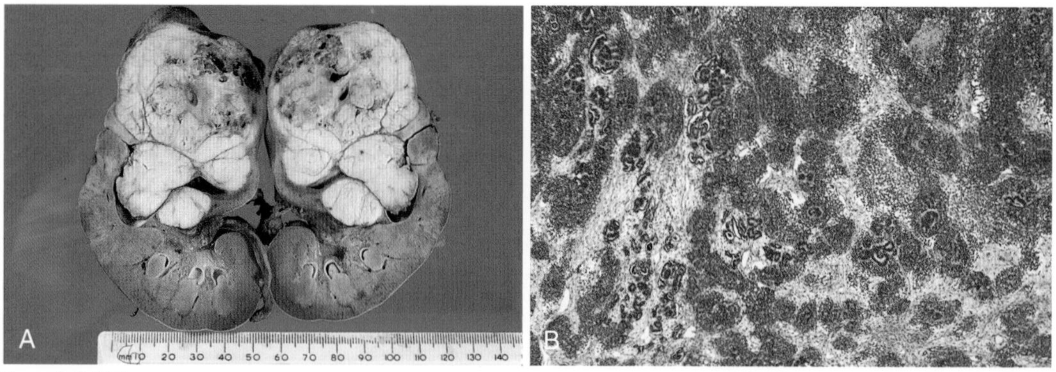

FIG. 15.27 Nephroblastoma (Wilms tumor). **A,** Gross image of bilateral nephroblastoma. **B,** Histologic appearance, showing primitive glomeruli as a prominent feature interspersed with connective tissue strands. (**A** *from Stevens A, Lowe J, Scott I. Core Pathology. 3rd ed. Philadelphia: Elsevier; 2008;* **B** *courtesy Nephron, Wikimedia Commons/ CC-BY-SA-3.0/GFDL;* http://en.wikipedia.org/wiki/File:Wilms_tumor_-_low_mag.jpg.)

angiofibromas, and areas of hypomelanosis called **ash leaf spots,** because the lack of melanin causes an ashen appearance.

Congenital and Inherited Renal Disorders

There are a few congenital and inherited renal disorders that are important to know, especially **polycystic kidney disease (PKD)** and **horseshoe kidney.**

Polycystic Kidney Disease

Autosomal Dominant PKD: This disease is characterized by a **generalized abnormality of collagen,** leading to numerous problems, especially **multiple bilateral renal cysts** that develop during adolescence and adulthood, with the eventual development of renal failure later in life (Fig. 15.28A). These cysts can **rupture,** leading to a localized peritonitis and flank pain if on the outside of the kidney, or **hematuria,** if rupturing into the renal pelvis. Because it is a generalized collagen defect, other organs are affected—**berry aneurysms** in the circle of Willis from arterial wall weakening, resulting in **subarachnoid hemorrhage** if ruptured; weakening of the colonic wall, leading to **diverticulosis**; and **mitral valve prolapse** from valvular collagen abnormalities.

Autosomal recessive PKD: Oligohydramnios (no baby urine), Potter's sequence, congenital hepatic fibrosis.

Autosomal Recessive PKD: PKD causes bilateral cystic disease that occurs **during development in utero.** Unfortunately, this severe disease is usually fatal. Normally, the kidneys of the fetus generate urine, which the fetus expels, becoming amniotic fluid. This fluid protects the fetus and also helps the

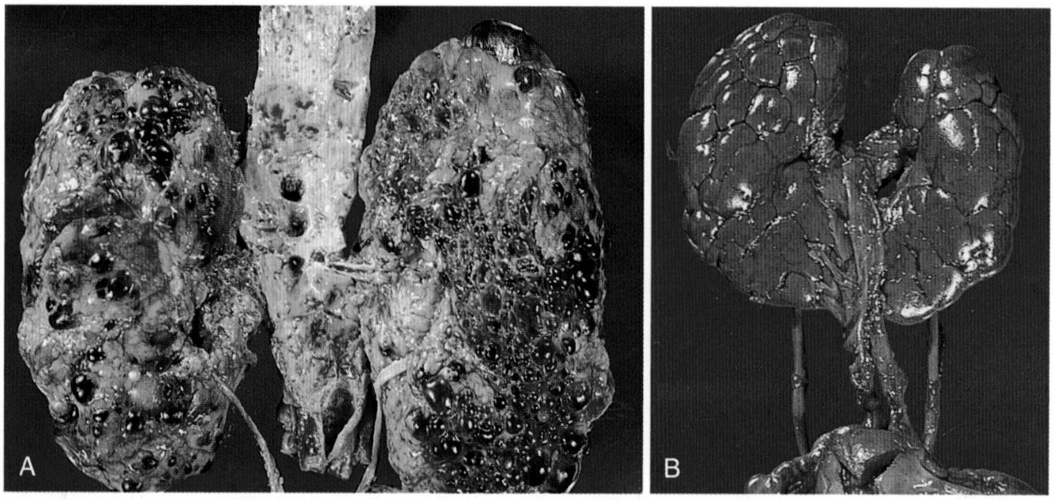

FIG. 15.28 A, Polycystic kidney disease, depicting multiple hemorrhagic cysts. **B,** Horseshoe kidney with kidneys typically fused on the lower pole, stuck at the inferior mesenteric artery during migration. (*From Damjanov I, Linder J.* Pathology: A Color Atlas. *St. Louis: Mosby; 2000.*)

lung develop when the fluid and accompanying growth factors fill the lungs. Without functioning kidneys, **oligohydramnios** (decreased amniotic fluid) occurs, leading to **Potter's sequence**—loss of the protective cushion with subsequent trauma leading to facial abnormalities, pulmonary hypoplasia because of decreased growth factors, and renal insufficiency. Autosomal recessive PKD is also associated with **congenital hepatic fibrosis.**

Horseshoe Kidney

Horseshoe kidney may be associated with **Turner syndrome** (genotype 45,X), characterized by **fusion of the kidneys at the lower pole,** forming a U shape. As the kidneys ascend to their normal place in the retroperitoneum, the horseshoe kidney will get stuck on the **inferior mesenteric artery** (Fig. 15.28B). Mnemonic: I'm a horseshoe ("IMA" for inferior mesenteric artery).

Chronic Kidney Disease

Chronic kidney disease (CKD) is becoming more and more common, with most causes linked to **diabetes, hypertension,** and **glomerular diseases.** CKD implies any chronic impairment in kidney function, but chronic renal failure (CRF) implies severe dysfunction. A normal GFR is 100 to 120 mL/min, but patients with CRF will have a GFR less than 10 mL/min, with some producing no urine at all. The hallmark of irreversible renal damage on imaging is small, shrunken kidneys. Remembering the vital functions of the kidneys already described, the changes in CRF can be understood:

- **Fluid retention:** Without the kidney's ability to regulate sodium and water balance, fluid overload and edema develop.
- **Electrolyte disturbances: Hyperkalemia** is particularly common, because the kidney normally is responsible for the excretion of potassium. Also, because the kidney normally excretes fixed acids to maintain pH, a **metabolic acidosis** can occur. Phosphoric acid is one of those fixed acids, so **hyperphosphatemia** develops.
- **Uremia:** This is a consequence of nitrogenous waste products building up, leading to **altered mental status, uremic pericarditis,** and **platelet dysfunction,** because the byproducts prevent normal platelet aggregation. The patient will still have a normal platelet count. With severe uremia, it is possible for urea to be secreted in sweat in such high amounts that urea crystals develop on the skin, termed ***uremic frost*** for the white color.
- **Anemia:** The kidneys use the hypoxic stimulus of the peritubular capillaries to release **erythropoietin,** which stimulates **red blood cell production.** Loss of this hormone leads to anemia.

Renal Osteodystrophy

Renal osteodystrophy encompasses a triad of (1) osteomalacia, (2) osteitis fibrosa cystica, and (3) osteoporosis. Recall that the kidneys are responsible for the hydroxylation of vitamin D into its active form, 1,25-$(OH)_2$-vitamin D, by 1-α-hydroxylase in the proximal tubule. In renal failure, vitamin D cannot be activated because of decreased GFR (vitamin D doesn't make it to the proximal tubule), and therefore **osteomalacia** occurs from hypovitaminosis D. This leads to **decreased mineralization of bone.** Because vitamin D also acts to raise the calcium level by promoting GI absorption, hypocalcemia causes **sustained PTH release** to attempt to correct it. This is termed ***secondary hyperparathyroidism*** (see Chapter 9). The resultant hyperparathyroidism induces a high-turnover bone disease (associated with increased bone reabsorption, lytic lesions, and hemorrhage into bones) known as **osteitis fibrosa cystica.** Overly aggressive suppression of secondary hyperparathyroidism may lead to the opposite of high-turnover bone disease, termed ***adynamic bone disease***. Finally, the impaired mineralization and increased demineralization lead to **osteoporosis** and predisposes patients to pathologic fractures. Osteoporosis is further exacerbated by metabolic acidosis because H^+ ions are not effectively excreted by the kidneys. More often, renal patients suffer from mixed bone lesions.

Renal osteodystrophy: Osteomalacia, osteitis fibrosa cystica, osteoporosis.

Treatment

Treatment is multimodal. **Dialysis** targets many of the problems with volume and electrolyte disturbances, but pharmacologic therapy is important as well. **Phosphate-binding agents** (e.g., sevelamer) prevent phosphate absorption from the gut, **erythropoietin** supplementation can correct low erythropoietin levels, **activated vitamin D** supplementation can correct low levels of active 1,25-$(OH)_2$ vitamin D, and low-sodium diets can help slow volume overload.

PHARMACOLOGY

The main diuretic classes, from most proximally acting to most distally acting, are **carbonic anhydrase inhibitors, osmotic agents, loop diuretics, thiazide diuretics, and potassium-sparing diuretics** (Fig. 15.29). Each class will be individually covered in detail. All diuretics increase the rate of urination, but each works in a different manner. Any diuretic that provides increased delivery of Na^+ to the collecting tubule's principal cells will cause potassium wasting because some of that sodium will be absorbed at the expense of K^+ caused by the Na^+/K^+ ATPase activity there.

Carbonic Anhydrase Inhibitors (Acetazolamide)

Carbonic anhydrase catalyzes this reaction:

$$H^+ + HCO_3^- \leftrightarrow H_2CO_3 \leftrightarrow H_2O + CO_2$$

This reaction is why there is a continuous gradient for H^+ secretion and bicarbonate reabsorption into the proximal nephron by the Na^+/H^+ exchanger. The gradient is normally maintained by the action of carbonic anhydrase because once the H^+ is secreted into the lumen, it binds with HCO_3^- in the lumen; with the aid of carbonic anhydrase, it can become CO_2 and H_2O. The CO_2 can then diffuse back into the proximal tubular cells, dissociating again to H^+ and HCO_3^-, with the H^+ recycled into the lumen and the HCO_3^- (bicarbonate) reabsorbed into the bloodstream.

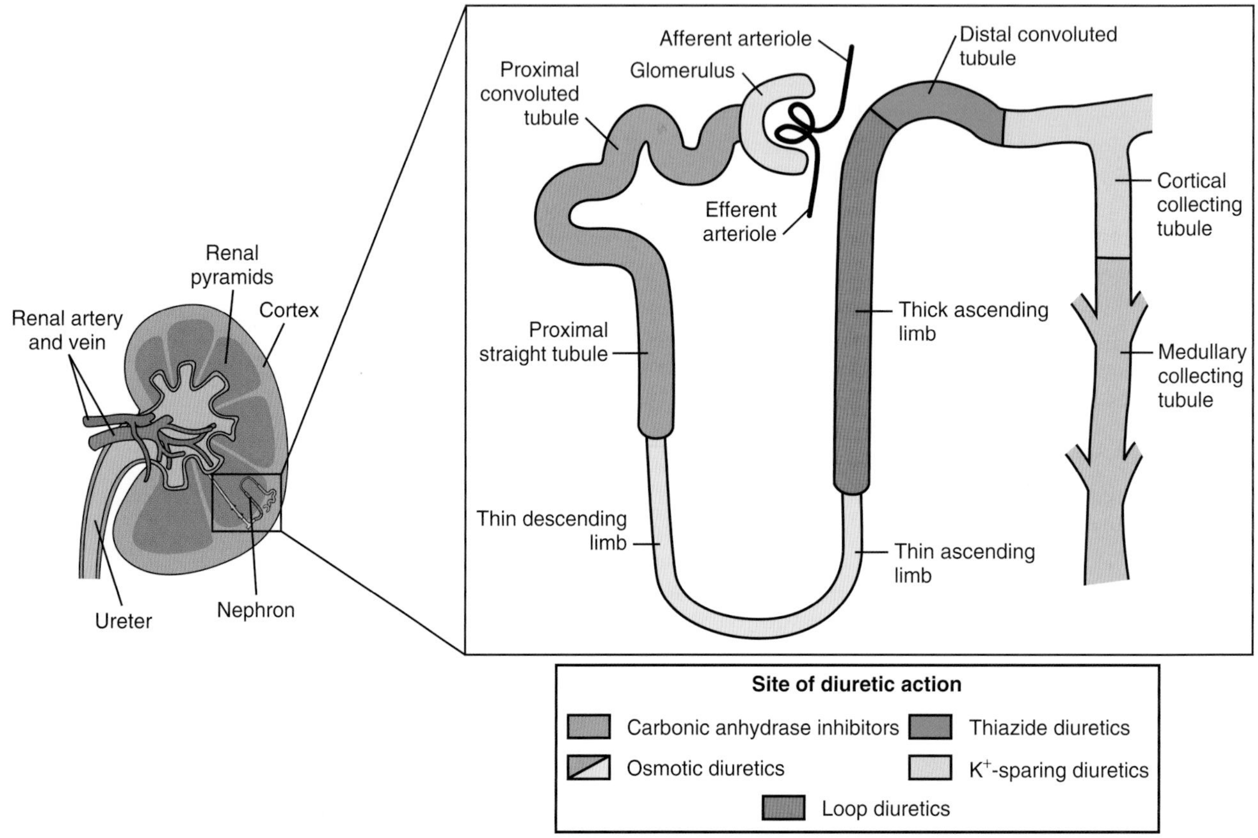

FIG. 15.29 Overview of the pharmacologic agents that act on the kidney and their primary location of action. (*From Wecker L, Crespo L, Dunaway G, et al.* Brody's Human Pharmacology. *5th ed. Philadelphia: Elsevier; 2009.*)

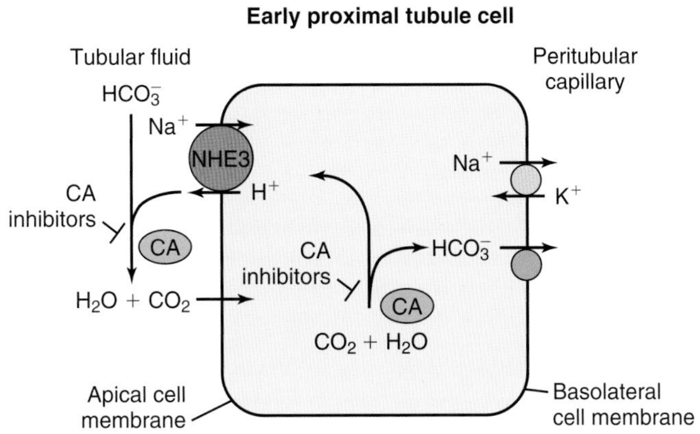

FIG. 15.30 Proximal tubule of the nephron and the action of carbonic anhydrase (CA) inhibitors. (*From Wecker L, Crespo L, Dunaway G, et al.* Brody's Human Pharmacology. *5th ed. Philadelphia: Elsevier; 2009.*)

Carbonic anhydrase inhibitors: Block carbonic anhydrase, leading to increased bicarbonate excretion in the urine.

Blocking carbonic anhydrase, therefore, prevents this recycling and leads to **bicarbonate wasting in the urine** (Fig. 15.30), causing a metabolic acidosis. Blockage of this pathway, because it ultimately impedes the Na^+/H^+ exchanger, also prevents Na^+ reabsorption.

- **Uses:** For glaucoma (decreases aqueous humor secretion, because the aqueous humor is bicarbonate-rich); for altitude sickness (high altitudes), because the resultant metabolic acidosis causes compensatory hyperventilation by the lungs (respiratory alkalosis) and improved oxygenation; and for alkalization of the urine, as with toxic ingestions of acids (to keep the acid in the conjugate base; charged form to promote excretion).
- **Side effects:** Causes a hyperchloremic (non–anion gap) metabolic acidosis. It is a sulfa drug (contraindicated in those with sulfa allergies).

Osmotic Agents

Mannitol: Used to treat cerebral edema to increase serum osmolarity, promoting fluid to return to the bloodstream.

Mannitol is a nonabsorbable sugar that when given intravenously, will be filtered through the glomeruli and act as an osmotic agent to keep water in the lumen of the nephron. This leads to **increased urination** (polyuria). This is similar to the mechanism of polyuria in diabetes, except endogenous glucose acts as the osmotic agent. While in the bloodstream, the mannitol acts as an osmotic agent there too, causing fluid to move into the extracellular fluid from the intracellular tissue (increased osmolarity of the ECF); for this reason it is used in the treatment of **cerebral edema** to draw out the excess water.

- **Uses:** Decreasing **cerebral edema,** promoting diuresis and therefore renal clearance of certain **drug overdoses.**
- **Side effects:** Giving mannitol leads to a large expansion of extracellular fluid because it draws water out of the cells via osmosis, potentially leading to or exacerbating existing **congestive heart failure** and **pulmonary edema** in those with poor cardiac and/or renal function. With the increased diuresis, eventual **dehydration** is also a concern.

Loop Diuretics

Loop diuretics (e.g., furosemide, torsemide, bumetanide, ethacrynic acid) are potent, **high-volume** diuretics that block the NKCC2 cotransporter in the thick ascending limb of the loop of Henle, with far-reaching implications (see Fig. 15.9). First, it causes increased delivery of sodium, potassium, and chloride to the distal nephron. The distal nephron can absorb sodium at the expense of potassium (enhanced by aldosterone), leading to further potassium loss in the urine. Therefore loop diuretics are **potassium-wasting diuretics.** Normally some of the potassium that is pumped into the thick ascending limb cells leaks back into the lumen of the nephron via a K^+ channel, leading to a more positive charge in the lumen. This positive charge enhances the paracellular reabsorption of calcium and magnesium (also positively charged). Therefore blocking the NKCC2 pump prevents this, leading to a decreased ability to reabsorb calcium and magnesium and potentially leading to hypocalcemia and hypomagnesemia.

Loop diuretics: High-volume diuretics, potassium-wasting, work on thick ascending loop of Henle.

- **Uses:** Hypertension, any edematous state in which unloading volume is advantageous (e.g., congestive heart failure [CHF], hypoalbuminemia from any cause [hepatic failure or loss in urine, as in nephrotic syndrome]), hypercalcemia because loop diuretics have calciuretic effects.

- **Side effects:** A common mnemonic is **OH DANG—o**totoxicity, **h**ypo (-kalemia, -calcemia, -magnesemia), **d**ehydration, **a**llergy (sulfa drug, except for ethacrynic acid), **n**ephritis (drug-induced interstitial), **g**out. The reason for ototoxicity is that the ear uses the NKCC2 transporter to maintain proper endolymph and perilymph electrolyte concentrations; blockage can lead to damage.

Thiazide Diuretics

Thiazide diuretics (e.g., hydrochlorothiazide [HCTZ], chlorthalidone, metolazone) work in the distal convoluted tubule of the nephron on the NaCl cotransporter (see Fig. 15.10). Blockage of this transporter leads to increased sodium loss but also to increased potassium loss because of increased sodium delivery to the collecting tubule (where again, sodium is reclaimed at the expense of potassium caused by Na^+/K^+ ATPase activity). Therefore it is a **potassium-wasting diuretic.** As shown in Fig. 15.10, sodium and calcium are both cations and are therefore competing for uptake in the distal convoluted tubule cell (both can't be reabsorbed because cell voltage would become too positive; there is not enough of a gradient). Blockage of sodium uptake here by thiazide diuretics leads to **increased calcium** reabsorption.

Loop diuretics can cause hypocalcemia. Thiazide diuretics can cause hypercalcemia.

- **Uses:** Hypertension, hypercalciuria (thiazides will help reclaim calcium from the urine, the opposite effect as a loop diuretic), nephrogenic diabetes insipidus. It is ironic that a thiazide diuretic (which produces more urine) would be used to treat nephrogenic diabetes insipidus because lack of ADH responsiveness already leads to increased urination of pure water. With thiazide diuretics, there is now water **and sodium** loss, leading the body to activate the RAA axis and increase proximal tubule sodium and water reabsorption (via an AT II stimulatory effect on Na^+/H^+ exchange), which limits water delivery distally to the collecting tubules for potential loss in the urine.
- **Side effects:** Hypokalemia, hypercalcemia, hyperglycemia, hyperlipidemia, hyperuricemia.

Potassium-Sparing Diuretics

Potassium-sparing diuretics (e.g., spironolactone, eplerenone, amiloride, triamterene; Fig. 15.31) all work on the principal cells because these cells have the final input on potassium excretion. Whenever there is excess sodium delivered here, it will move through the epithelial (luminal side) sodium channel (ENaC) into the cell and be pumped out into the peritubular capillaries via the Na^+/K^+ ATPase in exchange for potassium. That potassium will then leak into the lumen of the nephron and be excreted. Aldosterone increases activity of the Na^+/K^+ ATPase pump and ENaC channel synthesis to facilitate volume repletion by reabsorbing more sodium, at the expense of more potassium. This cell's activity can be impeded by two main mechanisms: (1) blocking the ENaC (amiloride, triamterene) or (2) blocking aldosterone's upregulation of these cells (spironolactone, eplerenone).

Potassium-sparing diuretics: Either block the ENaC or block aldosterone.

- **Uses:** Spironolactone and eplerenone are used in hyperaldosteronism to prevent the effects of the abnormally elevated aldosterone on the kidney, as well as finding use as a general diuretic. Amiloride and triamterene are also used as diuretics if hypokalemia is a concern.
- **Side effects:** Too much of a good thing—preventing potassium excretion by shutting down the principal cell can lead to hyperkalemia. Also, spironolactone is nonspecific and can also block the testosterone receptor, leading to gynecomastia in men; eplerenone is aldosterone-specific and does not have this side effect.

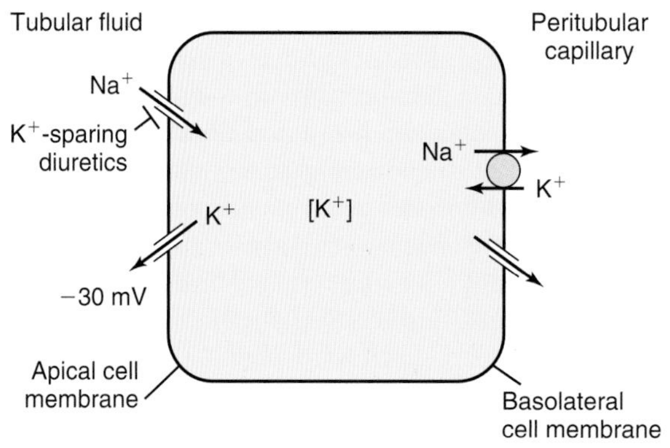

FIG. 15.31 Collecting duct and the site of action of potassium-sparing diuretics. (*From Wecker L, Crespo L, Dunaway G, et al. Brody's Human Pharmacology. 5th ed. Philadelphia: Elsevier; 2009.*)

REVIEW QUESTIONS

(1) Which part of the kidney has the least oxygen tension? Why is this important?
(2) Glucose can move through the glomerulus and into Bowman's space. It can also be put back into the bloodstream after it has been in the nephron. It cannot be pumped into the nephron. What are each of these three processes called?
(3) If the clearance of a molecule is greater than the glomerular filtration rate, what does that suggest?
(4) Which portion of the nephron acts to turn vitamin D into its active form? What enzyme does it use, and how is it regulated?
(5) How are calcium and magnesium reabsorbed in the thick ascending loop of Henle? How do loop diuretics alter this?
(6) How much total body water (a), intracellular fluid (b), and extracellular fluid (c) will a 70-kg man have?
(7) A patient comes from a nursing home with low blood pressure, fever, tachypnea, and tachycardia and is found to have lactic acidosis. The patient is diagnosed with sepsis. What would the patient's pH, anion gap, bicarbonate, and Pco_2 likely be?
(8) A patient is diagnosed with primary hyperaldosteronism (Conn syndrome), a tumor in the zona glomerulosa of the adrenal cortex that secretes high levels of aldosterone. What acid–base disturbance does this patient have, and why? What is the potassium level?
(9) A patient recently had a flulike illness and then developed ascending weakness. She was diagnosed with Guillain-Barré syndrome. Unfortunately, on the second day of her hospitalization, the paralysis ascended to her diaphragm, causing her to have difficulty breathing. What acid–base disturbance does she have?
(10) What are the three main components in treating hyperkalemia? Before treating hyperkalemia, what must be checked to ensure that it is true hyperkalemia?
(11) What are the classic findings on urinalysis in rhabdomyolysis?
(12) What is the most common composition of kidney stones? Can these stones typically be seen on radiographs? What do they look like on microscopy?
(13) What stone is associated with a urinary tract infection from urease-producing bacteria? Why?
(14) Why do diabetic patients sometimes initially have increased glomerular filtration rates?
(15. In a severely dehydrated patient, if the creatinine level were found to be 2, what would the most likely BUN be: (a) 2, (b) 10, (c) 20, or (d) 40?
(16) In a patient with an aldosterone-secreting tumor, which of these pharmacologic agents would work best to counteract the problem before surgery could definitively remove the tumor?
(17) A patient with congestive heart failure is started on diuretics. A chemistry panel the following month shows that he is hypocalcemic, hypokalemic, and hypomagnesemic. Which diuretic is he likely on, and what is the basis for his laboratory findings?

16 REPRODUCTIVE SYSTEM

Theodore X. O'Connell and Tina Roosta Storage

ANATOMY

Female Reproductive Anatomy

See Fig. 16.1 for an overview of the female reproductive anatomy.

- **Infundibulopelvic ligament:** Also known as the suspensory ligament of ovaries. Connects the ovaries to the pelvic wall and contains the **ovarian blood vessels.**
- **Ovarian ligament:** Connects the ovaries to the lateral surface of the uterus. It does not contain any vessels.
- **Round ligament:** Connects the uterine fundus to the labia majora by passing through the deep inguinal ring. The round ligament is a derivative of the embryologic gubernaculum.
- **Cardinal ligament:** Connects the cervix to the pelvic side wall. It contains the **uterine blood vessels.**
- **Broad ligament:** Connects the ovaries, fallopian tubes, and uterus to the pelvic floor and side wall (Fig. 16.2). Made up of three parts: mesosalpinx, mesoovarium, and mesometrium.
- **Pouch of Douglas:** The anatomic space between the rectum and uterus. It can be palpated via a digital rectal examination. It is an important anatomic area because it can be a collecting site of blood (from ruptured ectopic pregnancy), pus (from pelvic inflammatory disease), malignant cells (from ovarian cancer), or endometrial implants (from endometriosis). Also called the rectouterine pouch for the two surrounding organs.
- **Course of the female ureters:** Cross over the bifurcation of the common iliac arteries, then lateral to the internal iliac arteries. They enter the retroperitoneal space in the uterosacral ligaments, then the cardinal ligaments, and **dive under** the uterine artery. Mnemonic: Water (urine) under the bridge (artery). The ureters are sometimes injured in surgeries involving ligation of the uterine artery because of their anatomic proximity. Surgeons must be wary!

DON'T cut the Infundibulopelvic ligament, Cardinal ligament, or Ureter OR your patient will end up in the **ICU**!

The pouch of Douglas can be a collecting site for blood, pus, malignant cells, or endometrial implants.

Male Reproductive Anatomy

- **Pathway of sperm:** Remembered by the mnemonic **SEVEN UP**—Seminiferous tubules (sperm created) → Epididymis (sperm stored) → Vas deferens → Ejaculatory ducts →"Nothing"→ Urethra → Penile urethra (Fig. 16.3).

Composition of Semen

- Sperm (10%)
- Prostatic fluid (20%): **zinc,** citric acid, and enzymes that help sustain sperm
- Seminal vesicle fluid (70%): **fructose**, ascorbic acid

Male Sexual Response

In order for an **erection** to occur, the parasympathetic fibers in the pelvic plexus release nitric oxide (NO), which increases cyclic guanosine monophosphate (cGMP), resulting in smooth muscle relaxation of the helicine artery, which results in increased blood flow into the paired corpus cavernosa and corpus spongiosum (Fig. 16.4).

During **emission,** smooth muscle contractions by the vas deferens and ejaculatory ducts push sperm into the prostatic urethra. This is a sympathetic response from the hypogastric nerve.

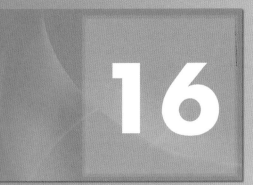

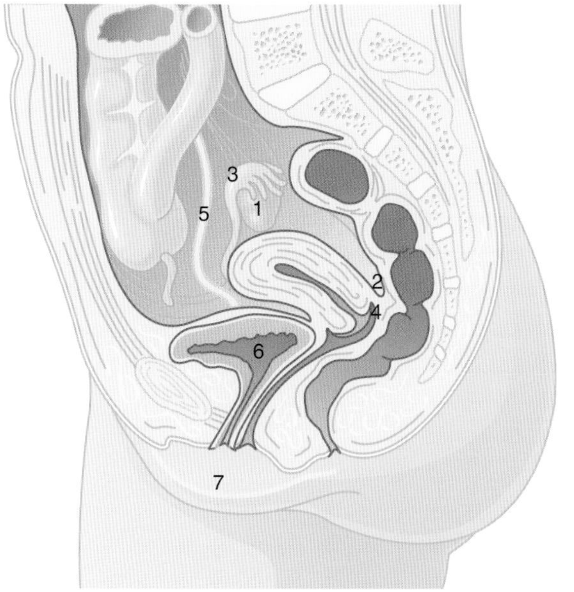

FIG. 16.1 Sagittal view of female reproductive anatomy. 1, Ovary; 2, pouch of Douglas; 3, fallopian tubes; 4, vagina; 5, ureter; 6, urinary bladder; 7, vulva. *(From Hacker NF, Gambone JC, Hobel CJ.* Hacker & Moore's Essentials of Obstetrics and Gynecology, *5th ed. Philadelphia: Elsevier; 2009.)*

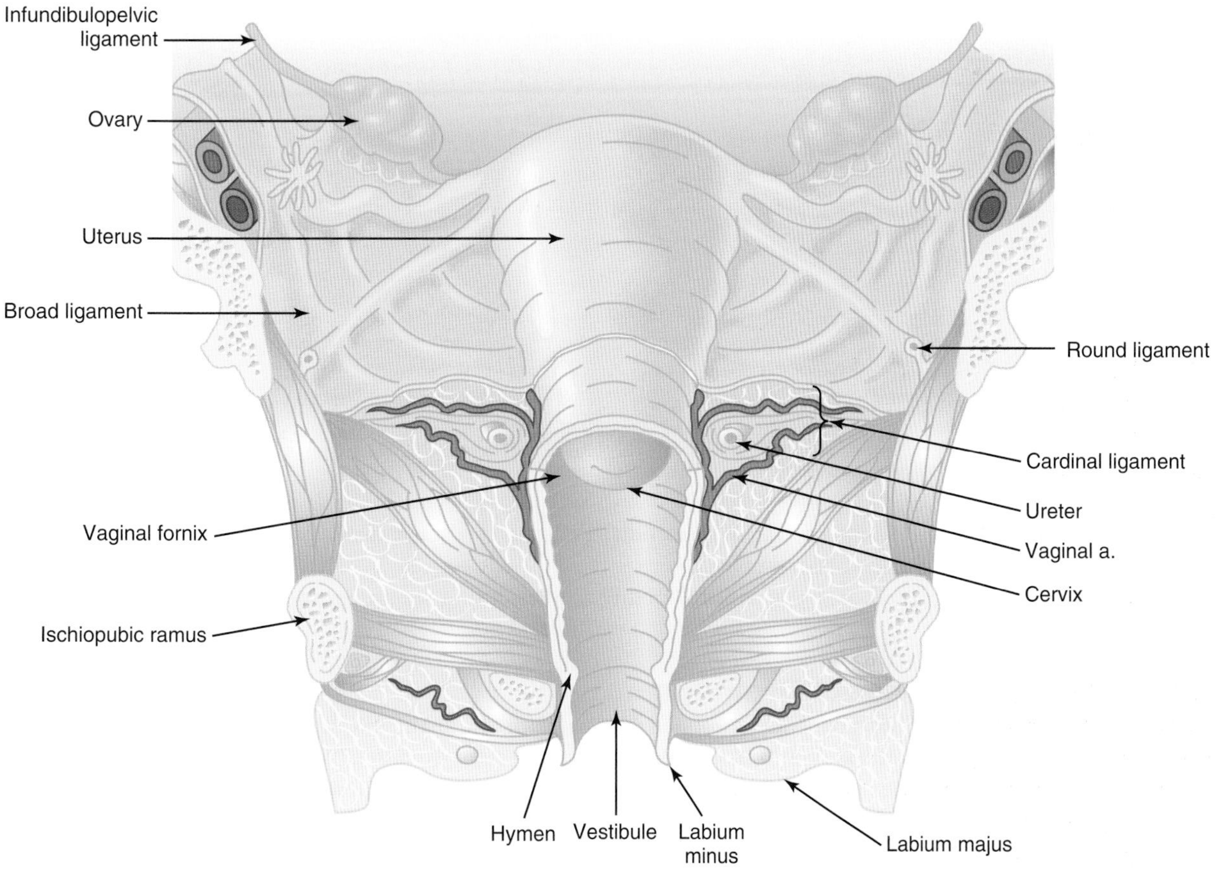

FIG. 16.2 Coronal section of pelvis demonstrating the ligaments of the female reproductive tract.

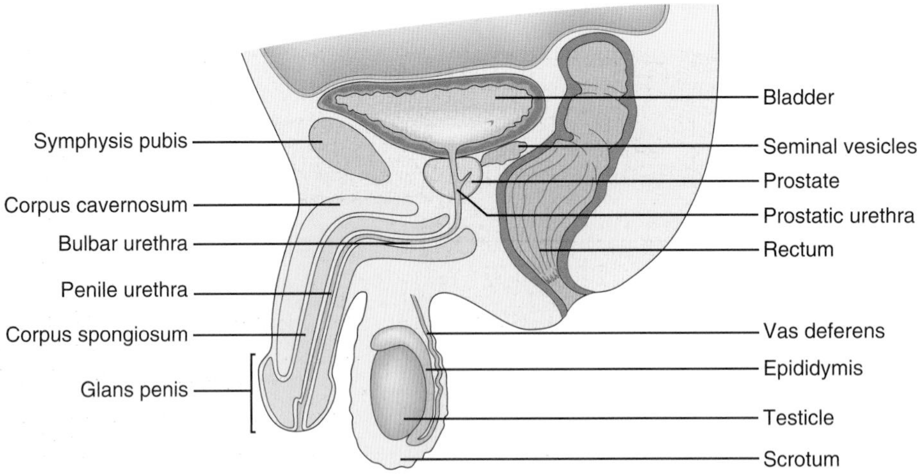

FIG. 16.3 Pathway of sperm and anatomy of the male reproductive tract. *(From Garden OJ, Bradbury AW, Forsythe JLR, Parks RW.* Principles and Practice of Surgery. *5th ed. Philadelphia: Elsevier; 2007.)*

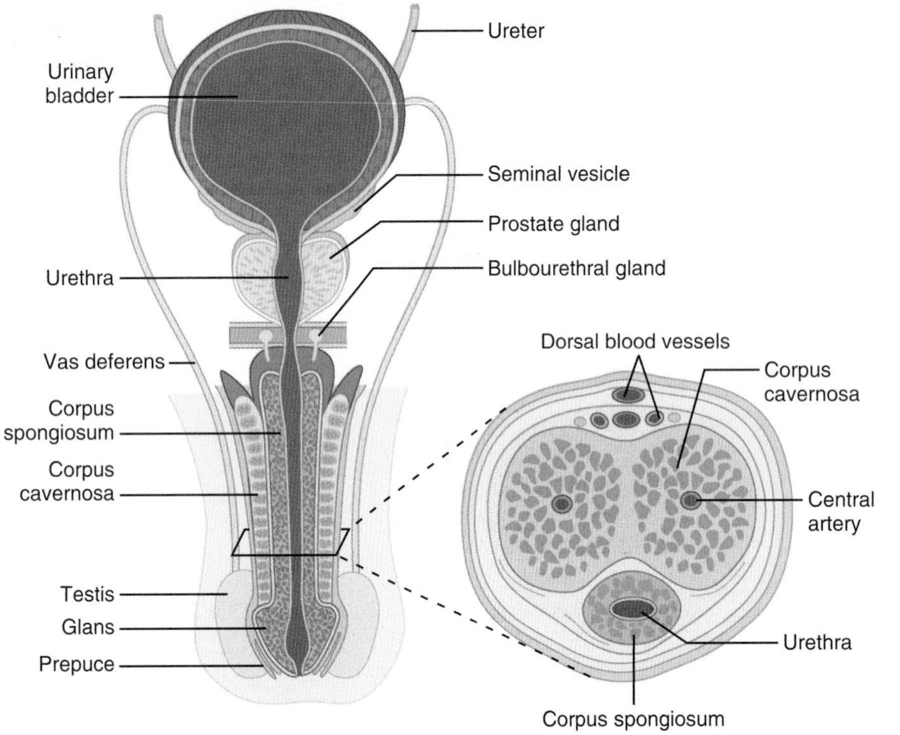

FIG. 16.4 Cross-sectional anatomy of the penis. *(From Carroll RG.* Elsevier's Integrated Physiology. *Philadelphia: Elsevier; 2006.)*

Remember the mnemonic "**P**oint and **S**hoot." Erection (**P**oint) is a **P**arasympathetic response, whereas emission (**S**hoot) is a **S**ympathetic response.

During **ejaculation,** sperm is released through the urethra as a result of a **somatic response** from the pudendal nerve.

Erection is a **P**arasympathetic response, whereas emission is a **S**ympathetic response. "**P**oint and **S**hoot."

Male and Female Gonadal Drainage

It is important to understand the venous and lymphatic drainage of the male and female gonads (Fig. 16.5). The venous drainage of the right ovary or testis is into the right ovarian or testicular vein and then into the inferior vena cava. The venous drainage of the left ovary or testis is into the left ovarian or testicular vein, then into the left renal vein, and then into the inferior vena cava. The extra step in left testicular venous drainage causes increased hydrostatic pressure. That is why **varicoceles are more common on the left side.**

Varicoceles are more common on the left side because the left testicular vein drains into the left renal vein before the inferior vena cava (IVC).

The lymphatic drainage from the ovaries or testes is into the paraaortic nodes (this drainage pattern occurs because the ovaries and testes descended from the abdomen with their blood source from the aorta). The lymphatic drainage of the scrotum and distal third of the vagina is into the superficial inguinal nodes. The uterus and proximal two-thirds of the vagina drain into the external iliac, obturator, and hypogastric nodes.

Testicular lymphatic drainage is to paraaortic lymph nodes. Scrotal drainage is to superficial inguinal nodes.

PHYSIOLOGY

Hypothalamic-Pituitary-Gonadal Axis

The hypothalamus secretes gonadotropin-releasing hormone (GnRH) in a pulsatile fashion to stimulate the anterior pituitary to produce luteinizing hormone (LH) and follicle-stimulating hormone (FSH). If GnRH were secreted continuously, it would paradoxically suppress the production of LH and FSH.

In males (Fig. 16.6A), LH stimulates Leydig cells to secrete testosterone. FSH stimulates Sertoli cells (Support cells) to maintain spermatogenesis. Some testosterone is further converted by 5-α-reductase into the more potent dihydrotestosterone (DHT). As in most of the endocrine system, a negative feedback loop maintains homeostasis. For example, administration of exogenous testosterone decreases LH, FSH, and testicular synthesis of testosterone. Interestingly, because spermatogenesis requires high local concentrations of testosterone in the seminiferous tubules, administering

Exogenous testosterone decreases LH, FSH, and endogenous testosterone production by negative feedback. Spermatogenesis will decrease because testosterone will not be concentrated in the testicles.

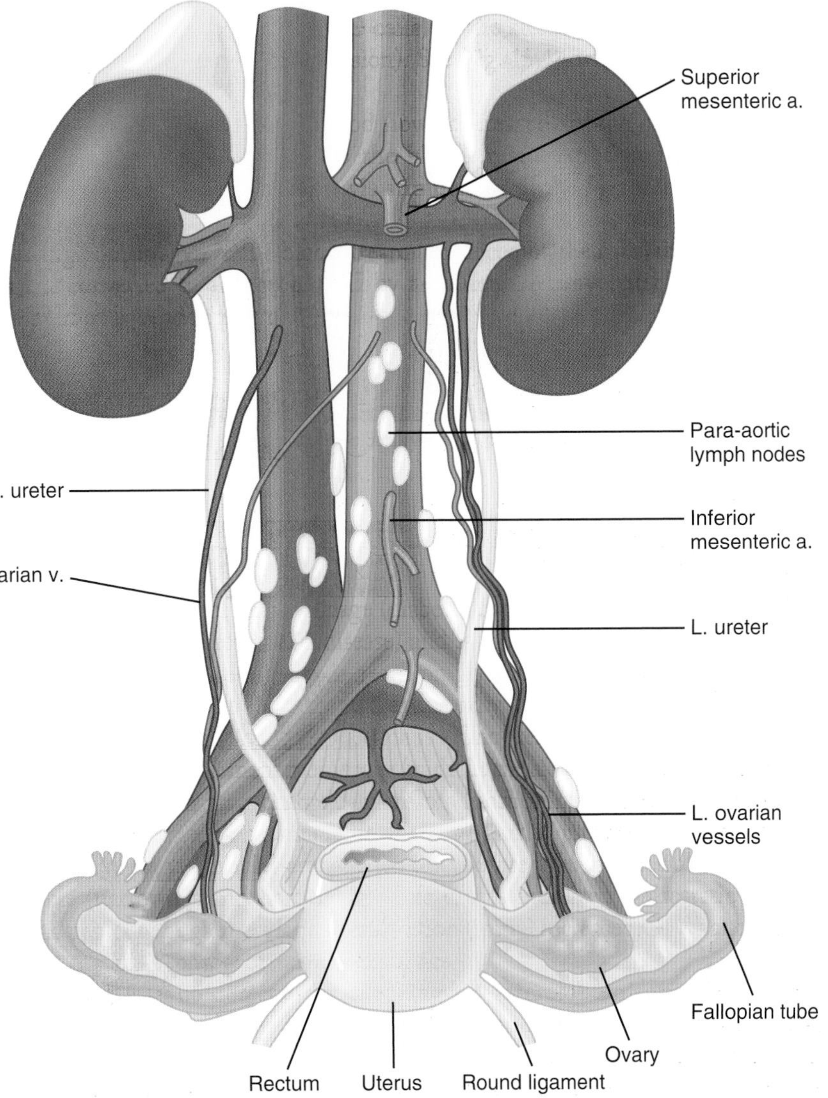

FIG. 16.5 Vascular and lymphatic system of the female reproductive tract. IVC, Inferior vena cava.

exogenous testosterone actually inhibits spermatogenesis because it will not be sufficiently concentrated in the testicles.

- Dihydrotestosterone is the most potent androgen, followed by testosterone, and finally by androstenedione.

In females (Fig. 16.6B), LH stimulates theca cells to secrete androgens. FSH stimulates granulosa cells to convert those androgens into estradiol by aromatization. FSH, as the name implies, helps stimulate and mature the ovarian follicles.

Of note, *estrogen* refers to a group of hormones (unlike testosterone, which is a single molecule). In humans, estradiol is the most potent estrogen. It is produced by the ovary and is the most abundant estrogen in premenopausal women. Estrone is less potent. Adipose tissue produces estrone by aromatization of androstenedione (released from the adrenal cortex and gonads) through the enzyme aromatase. Because estrone production does not require ovaries, it is the most abundant estrogen in postmenopausal women and men. Estriol is the least potent estrogen and is only present

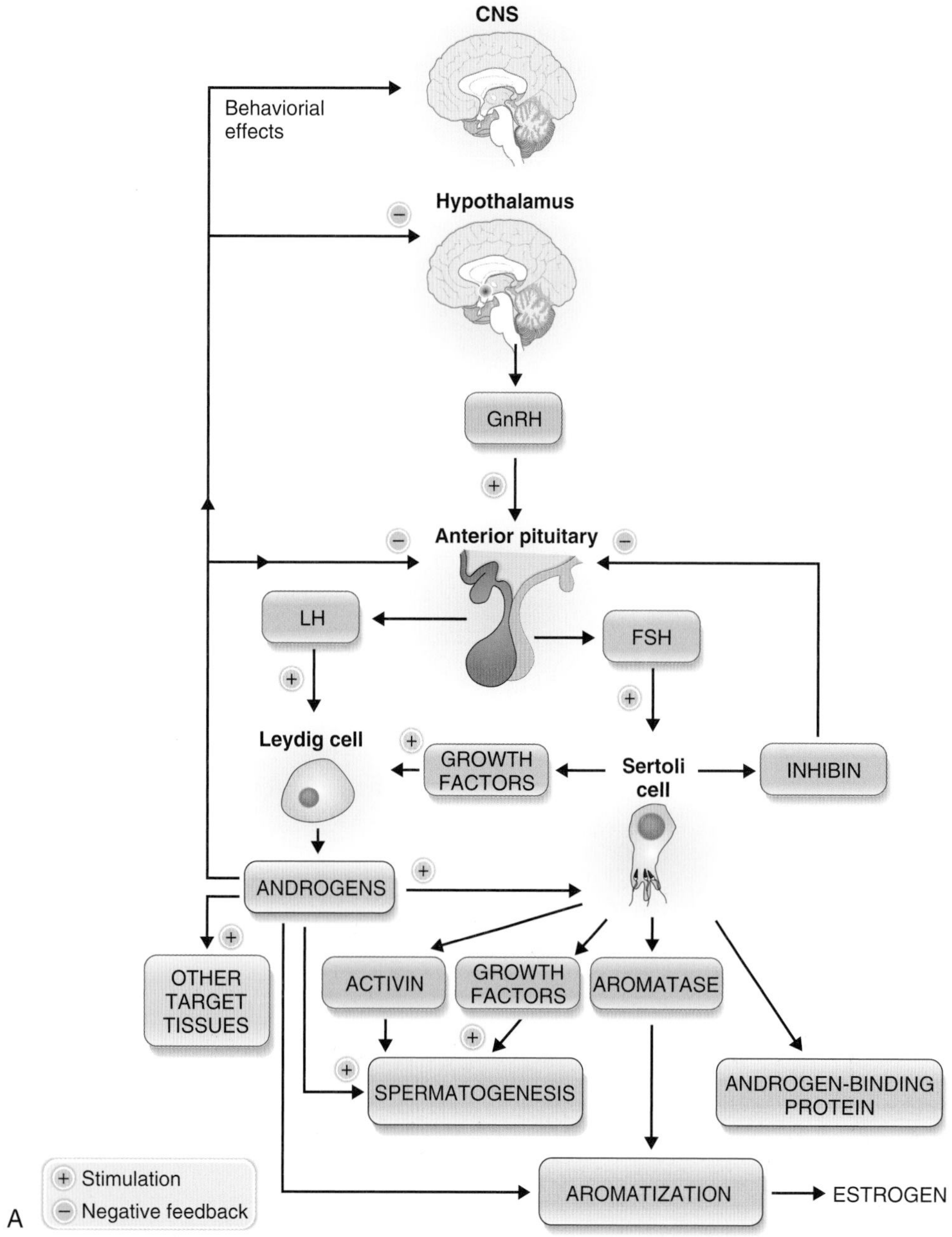

in significant levels during pregnancy. The placenta produces estriol by aromatization of fetal androgens. It can be used as a marker of fetal well-being.

Mnemonic: During reproductive years, there are two (husband and wife) in the house— estra**DI**ol. During pregnancy there are three (husband, wife, and baby)—es**TRI**ol. During menopause, sadly you might be a widow: estr**ONE.**

Spermatogenesis

Sertoli cells are tall columnar Support cells that nurture spermatogenesis. They are located in the parenchyma of the seminiferous tubules and are stimulated by **FSH.** At puberty, Sertoli cells form tight junctions with each other, creating the basal and adluminal compartment and the **blood–testis barrier.** This barrier protects the maturing sperm in the adluminal compartment from autoimmune attack because they otherwise would be seen as foreign cells. Sertoli cells secrete three products: (1) **inhibin,** which provides negative feedback and inhibits FSH secretion that normally would stimulate the Sertoli cells; (2) **androgen-binding protein** (ABP), which maintains a high testosterone level in the seminiferous

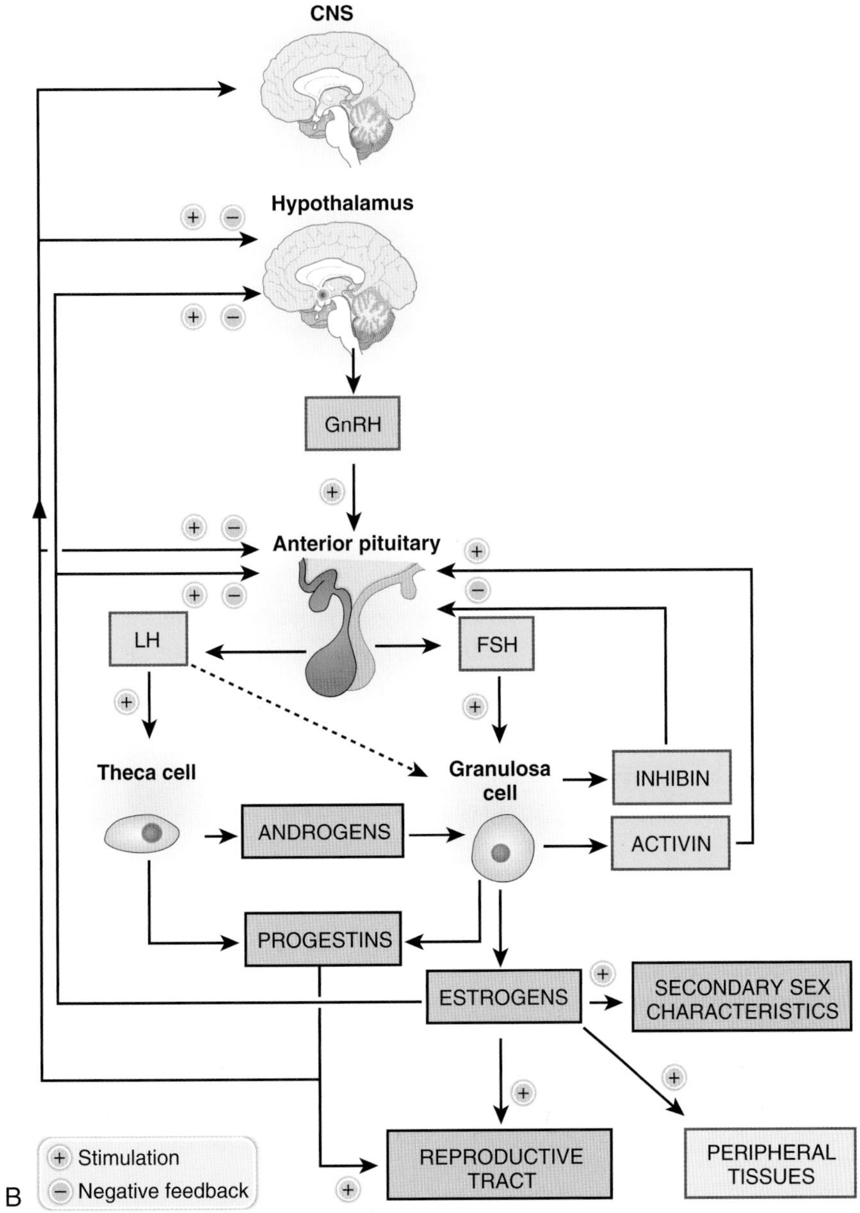

FIG. 16.6, cont'd Hormonal control of the hypothalamic-pituitary-testicular axis **(A)** and hypothalamic-pituitary-ovarian axis **(B)**. CNS, Central nervous system. *(From Damjanov I. Pathophysiology. Philadelphia: Elsevier; 2008.)*

tubules; and (3) **Müllerian inhibiting hormone,** which during fetal development inhibits the default female Müllerian system from developing.

Leydig cells are endocrine cells in the interstitium or stroma that secrete testosterone. They are stimulated by LH. Testosterone helps increase sperm production and libido. (Remember, however, because spermatogenesis requires a high concentration of testosterone within the seminiferous tubules, exogenous administration of testosterone will decrease spermatogenesis.)

Spermatogonia are the most immature spermatogenic cells, located close to the basement membrane of the seminiferous tubules, and divide by **mitosis** to regenerate. Spermatogenesis begins at puberty and takes about 64 days for completion (Fig. 16.7).

1. **Spermatogonia:** Diploid, 2 N. The most immature spermatogenic cells, located close to the basement membrane of the seminiferous tubules. They divide by mitosis. One of the daughter cells serves

Sertoli cells **s**upport spermatogenesis. They secrete ABP, inhibin, and Müllerian inhibiting hormone. They also form the blood–testis barrier. Leydig cells secrete testosterone.

The sperm's flagellum is derived from the centriole. The acrosome is derived from the Golgi apparatus.

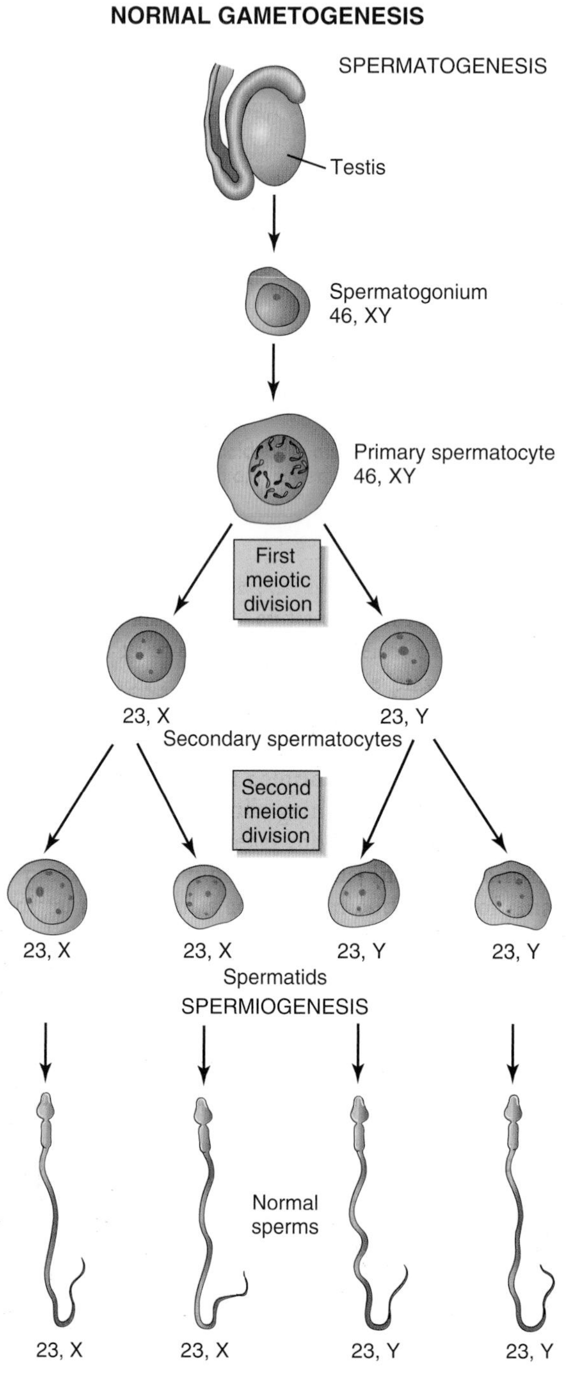

FIG. 16.7 Spermatogenesis. Primordial germ cells mature into spermatogonia during puberty. Spermatogonia will undergo mitosis to become primary spermatocytes, which then undergo meiosis I to become secondary spermatocytes. Secondary spermatocytes undergo meiosis II to divide into spermatids. *(From Moore KL, Persaud TVN, Torchia MG.* Before We Are Born. *8th ed. Philadelphia: Elsevier; 2011.)*

as a stem cell and remains near the basement membrane. The other daughter cell starts the differentiation process and becomes a primary spermatocyte.

2. **Primary spermatocyte:** Diploid, 4 N. Migrates toward the adluminal compartment and undergo meiosis I to become a secondary spermatocyte. **Failure of meiosis I** results in primary spermatocyte accumulation.
3. **Secondary spermatocyte:** Haploid, 2 N. Undergoes meiosis II very quickly and becomes a spermatid. **Failure of meiosis II** results in accumulation of secondary spermatocytes.
4. **Spermatids:** Haploid, N. Undergo **spermiogenesis,** the process whereby spermatids transform into mature **spermatozoa** (haploid, N). Spermiogenesis results in a decreased amount of cytoplasm, formation of a flagellum (derived from a centriole), and an acrosome (derived from the Golgi apparatus). The head of a mature sperm contains chromatin and acrosomal enzymes needed for penetration of the ovum's outer zona pellucida. The midpiece contains abundant mitochondria for adenosine triphosphate (ATP) production. The tail contains specialized cilia for efficient transport.

Male and Female Hormones

See Table 16.1 for a summary of steroid hormones and their functions.

TABLE 16.1 Summary of Steroid Hormones and Their Functions

PARAMETER	ESTROGENS	TESTOSTERONE	DHT	PROGESTERONE
Synthesis	Estradiol: Ovarian granulosa cell conversion of theca cell androgen Estrone: Adipose tissue conversion of adrenocortical androgen Estriol: Placental conversion of fetal androgen	Leydig cells in the testes under stimulation of LH	Synthesized from conversion of testosterone to DHT via the enzyme 5-α-reductase	Corpus luteum, placenta, adrenal cortex
Functions	Development of female secondary sex characteristics (breast and genitalia) Increase HDL Decrease LDL Follicular growth, endometrial proliferation, and hyperplasia Increase myometrial contractions	In utero: Maturation of internal genitalia except prostate (epididymis, vas deferens, seminal vesicles) Puberty: Growth spurt, deepening of voice, increased libido, epiphyseal plate closure	In utero: Virilization of external genitalia During the postpubertal period, contributes to BPH and balding (androgenetic alopecia)	Everything is PRO-GESTATION: Goal is to maintain pregnancy Increase in secretory endometrium Decrease in myometrial contractions (through smooth muscle relaxation) and decreased estrogen receptors (not progestation) Thickened cervical mucus
Effect on sex hormone-binding globulin (SHBG)	Increase synthesis of SHBG in the liver Also increase synthesis of other transport proteins (transcortin, TBG) SHBG has higher affinity for testosterone than estrogen When there is high SHBG, testosterone binds first, thus decreasing free testosterone	Decreases synthesis of SHBG, so increases free testosterone (FT) levels Obesity and hypothyroidism also decrease SHBG levels, thus increasing FT → hirsutism	None	None

BPH, Benign prostatic hypertrophy; HDL, high-density lipoprotein cholesterol; LDL, low-density lipoprotein cholesterol; TBG, thyroxine-binding globulin.

Female Physiology

Menstrual Cycle

Day 1 of the menstrual cycle is defined as the day menstruation begins.

The menstrual cycle (Fig. 16.8) normally lasts 28 days (±7 days), with day 1 defined as the day menstruation begins. The cycle is divided into a follicular phase (before ovulation) and a luteal phase (after ovulation; Fig. 16.9).

Follicular (Proliferative) Phase: Ovarian follicles are spherical ovarian structures that contain oocytes, theca cells, and granulosa cells. They are the basic unit of female reproductive physiology. The *follicular phase* of the menstrual cycle refers to the growth of the follicles through various stages.

The LH surge occurs at the end of the follicular phase when estrogen switches from a negative to a positive feedback loop.

In the early follicular stage (during menstruation), estrogen levels are low, which means the anterior pituitary can produce abundant LH and FSH without much negative feedback. FSH stimulates several ovarian follicles to grow and will eventually create a dominant follicle. As the ovarian follicles grow, they will produce more and more estrogen. Although increasing estrogen will inhibit FSH production, the dominant follicle will upregulate FSH receptors, which will increase their sensitivity to FSH, so estrogen levels can continue to rise.

At the end of the follicular phase, estrogen switches from a negative feedback loop with the pituitary to a positive feedback loop. This creates a surge of LH, which causes rupture of the dominant follicle and release of its oocyte into the fallopian tube. There is also a smaller surge of FSH at this time, the significance of which is unknown.

The follicular phase is also known as the proliferative phase because, during this time, the endometrium (uterine lining) sees mostly estrogen, so the glands are "proliferating." Histologically, the glands appear **short, narrow, and slightly wavy.**

If it is not rescued by hCG, the corpus luteum degenerates in 2 weeks.

Of note, in the preovulatory phase, the LH surge causes the granulosa cells to make progesterone (released 24 hours before ovulation, causing the increase in basal body temperature) and prostaglandins.

Luteal (Secretory) Phase: The *luteal phase* refers to the **corpus luteum** (yellow body), which forms from the follicle once the oocyte has been expelled. The theca cells in the corpus luteum produce estrogen and progesterone. These hormones again provide negative feedback on LH and FSH, resulting in their declining levels. The luteal phase is also known as the secretory phase because the elevated progesterone causes the endometrium to become secretory as it prepares for implantation.

The corpus luteum degenerates in a fixed 2 weeks if it is not stimulated by human chorionic gonadotropin (hCG). The degenerated corpus luteum is now called the **corpus albicans** (white body). The loss of the corpus luteum causes a decline in estrogen and, more significantly, progesterone. Without progesterone to support it, the endometrial lining is sloughed off and menstruation occurs.

If the corpus luteum is rescued by pregnancy and hCG produced by the conceptus, it will linger for 8 to 10 weeks until the placenta takes over producing progesterone, which is required for the maintenance of the pregnancy.

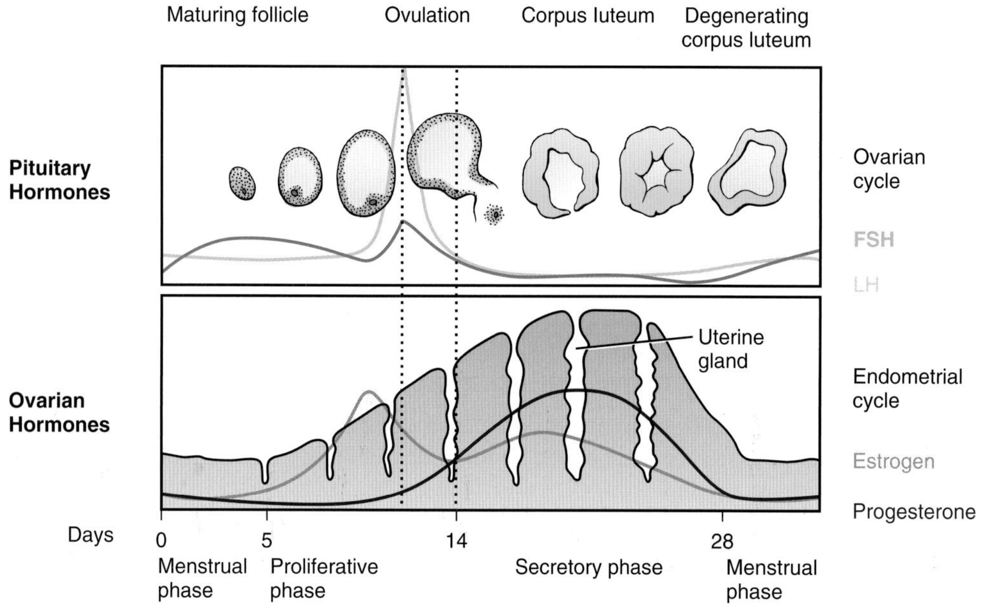

FIG. 16.8 The menstrual cycle. *(From Brauer PR, Francis-West PH, Schoenwolf GC, Bleyl SB.* Larsen's Human Embryology. *4th ed. Philadelphia: Elsevier; 2008.)*

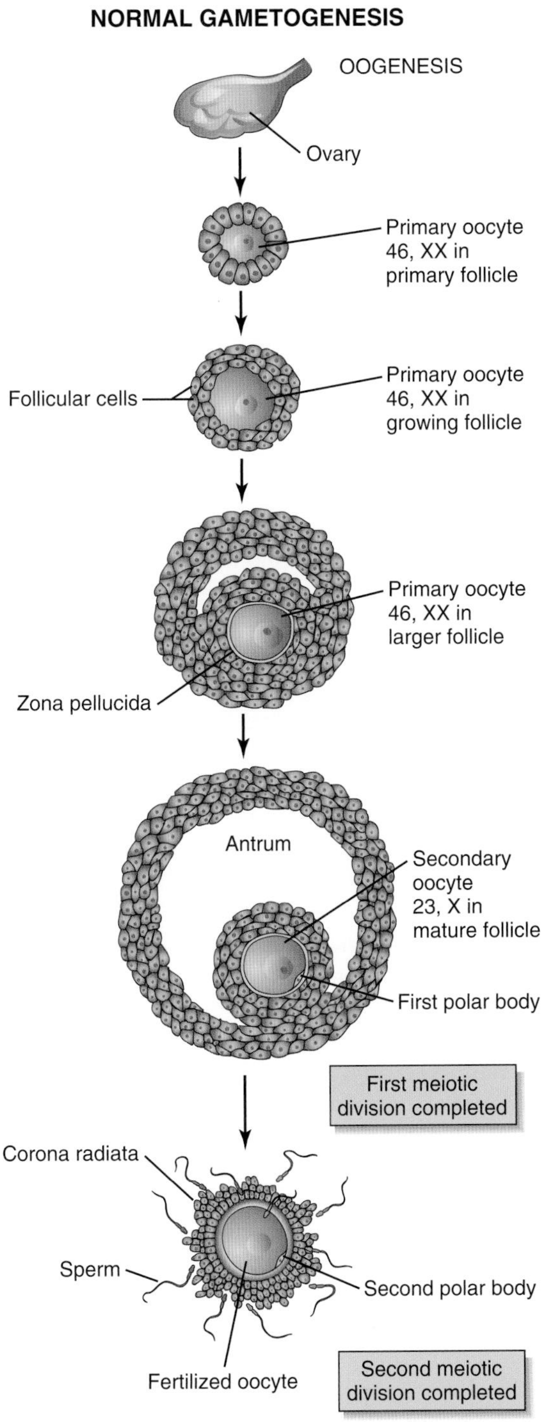

FIG. 16.9 During the first month of fetal life, germ cells of a female embryo undergo extensive mitosis to become oogonia (diploid, 2 N). By the third month of gestation, these oogonia enter meiosis I and pass through the different phases of **prophase I.** They are now called **primary oocytes** (diploid, 4 N), and these primary oocytes are arrested in prophase I until **puberty.** Hours before **ovulation,** these primary oocytes complete meiosis I and become **secondary oocytes** (haploid, 2 N). Immediately, these secondary oocytes enter **meiosis II** and are arrested in **metaphase II** until **fertilization.** Once fertilization occurs, meiosis II is complete and becomes a mature **ovum** (haploid, N). *(From Moore KL, Persaud TVN, Torchia MG.* Before We Are Born. *8th ed. Philadelphia: Elsevier; 2011.)*

Of note, the luteal phase is fixed at 14 days long (the amount of time the corpus luteum can survive without hCG), whereas the length of the follicular phase may vary. It is therefore the follicular phase that is responsible for the variability in the length of a woman's menstrual cycle.

Definitions of Abnormal Menses: See Table 16.2 for descriptions of disorders of menstruation.

Oogenesis

See Fig. 16.9 for a detailed description of oogenesis.

Table 16.2 Disorders of Menstruation

NAME	CYCLE FREQUENCY	CYCLE LENGTH	BLEEDING FREQUENCY	BLEEDING VOLUME	BLEEDING DURATION
Menorrhagia	Normal	21–35 days	Regular	Increased	Increased
Polymenorrhea	Short	<21 days	Regular	Normal	Normal
Oligomenorrhea	Long	>35 days	Regular		
Metrorrhagia	Irregular frequency of breakthrough bleeding between normal menstrual cycles				
Menometrorrhagia	Varies	Varies	Irregular	Increased	Increased

Pregnancy and hCG

Fertilization: Once ovulation has occurred, the secondary oocyte can typically survive for 24 hours before it degenerates. The ampullary portion of the fallopian tube is the most common location of fertilization. From there, the fertilized egg typically spends an average of 3 days in the fallopian tube and then 2 days in the uterine cavity, where it will implant on day 6.

Hormones of Pregnancy

Human growth hormone, human placental lactogen, prolactin, progesterone, and estriol are all increased during pregnancy.

Human chorionic gonadotropin is produced by the syncytiotrophoblast of the placenta, peaks at about 9 to 10 weeks gestation, and then falls. In the first trimester, hCG functions by binding to the LH receptor on the corpus luteum and stimulates it to produce progesterone. The beta subunit of hCG is used clinically as the first indicator of pregnancy. It is detectable in the blood by 1 week of gestation and in the urine by 2 weeks' gestation. The peak level of β-hCG in a normal pregnancy is 90,000 to 100,000 mIU/mL. Anything significantly higher than this usually signifies a pathologic state, such as a molar pregnancy or gestational trophoblastic disease (see later). The alpha subunit of hCG is identical to the alpha subunit of LH, FSH, and TSH.

hCG's beta subunit is unique and can therefore be used to detect pregnancy. The alpha subunit is shared with LH, FSH, and TSH.

Progesterone is initially produced by the corpus luteum, but by gestational week 12 the placenta produces enough progesterone to maintain pregnancy. Everything it does is **progestation.** It increases secretory endometrium in preparation for implantation, it decreases myometrium contractility, and it thickens cervical mucus. Progesterone is a marker of fetal viability in early pregnancy. The smooth muscle relaxation that progesterone causes is responsible for some of the physiologic changes seen in pregnancy, such as decreased peripheral vascular resistance.

Estriol, as discussed earlier, is produced by the placenta by aromatization of fetal androgens. It can be used as a marker of fetal well-being later in pregnancy.

Human placental lactogen is produced by the synctiotrophoblasts of the placenta. It decreases maternal insulin sensitivity and thus raises maternal serum glucose levels. Maintaining adequate glucose is crucial to fetal development.

Human placental lactogen decreases maternal insulin sensitivity and can contribute to gestational diabetes.

Prolactin is involved in milk production and simultaneously inhibits GnRH, serving as a natural form of contraception for the first 6 weeks postdelivery.

Oxytocin is produced by the posterior pituitary. During pregnancy, the uterus upregulates oxytocin receptors so that an oxytocin surge at the onset of labor facilitates uterine contractions. It is also involved in the letdown of milk that was already produced through the actions of prolactin.

Corticotropin-releasing hormone is a hypothalamic hormone involved in the cortisol pathway thought to induce the beginning phases of labor.

Menopause

Physiologic menopause occurs after 40 years of age, with the average age being **51** years. Most women experience perimenopausal symptoms for 3 to 5 years preceding menopause, after which time anovulation, amenorrhea, and menopausal symptoms occur (see later). The physiology behind menopause is the gradual loss of ovarian follicles, leading to decreased estradiol production, and thus increases in LH and FSH. The rise

Menopause: ↓ Follicles → ↓ estrogen → ↓ LH and FSH.

in LH and FSH can be used to diagnose menopause when the cause of amenorrhea is uncertain. **Estrone** becomes the principal estrogen that continues to circulate through peripheral conversion of androgens.

Symptoms of menopause include hot flashes, night sweats, amenorrhea, and mood swings. Conditions associated with menopause include atrophic vaginitis, urinary incontinence, cardiovascular disease (↓ high-density lipoprotein [HDL], ↑ low-density lipoprotein [LDL]), and **osteoporosis.** Risk factors for osteoporosis include fair skin, thin body habitus, smoking, alcohol and caffeine intake, and positive family history. The most common osteoporotic fracture site is the **vertebral bodies.**

Menopause before 40 years of age can indicate **premature ovarian failure,** which can be caused by oophorectomy, radiation, chemotherapy, infection, autoimmune conditions, or mosaic karyotype.

FEMALE PATHOLOGY

Pathology in Pregnancy

Ectopic pregnancy is a condition in which the embryo implants outside the uterus. The most common site of ectopic pregnancy is the ampulla of the fallopian tube. Ectopic pregnancy often results in the triad of **vaginal bleeding, pelvic pain, and adnexal mass.** The patient with an ectopic pregnancy has elevated hCG levels signifying the presence of a pregnancy; however, the hCG level does not double in 48 hours as in most normal early uterine pregnancies. Risk factors include **pelvic inflammatory disease** causing scarring of the tubes, prior ectopic pregnancy, tubal ligation, and adhesions from previous abdominal surgeries. Confirmation can be made with ultrasound, which may show an adnexal mass. Decidualized endometrium without chorionic villi may also be present because the pregnancy is not in the uterine cavity. Treatment is often necessary before ultrasonographic findings are present. Methotrexate may be used to terminate the pregnancy or surgery can be used to remove the embryo.

> Ectopic pregnancy:
> Vaginal bleeding (minimal to moderate)
> Pelvic pain
> Adnexal mass

Molar pregnancy is a benign proliferative abnormality of the placenta or chorionic epithelium that has malignant potential if it transforms to gestational trophoblastic tumor or choriocarcinoma. The most common form is **complete mole,** which is dispermic fertilization of an anuclear ovum, resulting in 46,XX or 46,XY. There are no fetal parts because it is a complete mole. There is a 20% chance of progressing to malignancy. On ultrasound, there are grapelike vesicles and a "snowstorm" appearance. **Incomplete mole** is dispermic fertilization of a normal ovum resulting in 69,XXY. An incomplete mole contains fetal parts and no vesicles. There is a 5% chance of progressing to malignancy. Presenting signs and symptoms include abnormal vaginal bleeding, nausea and vomiting (from extremely elevated hCG levels), theca lutein cysts, and hyperthyroidism (as a result of alpha subunit recognition of the TSH receptor because hCG and TSH share a nearly identical alpha subunit). Treatment is dilation and curettage and follow-up of hCG levels until they reach zero. This ensures that no tissue is retained that will progress to malignancy.

Miscarriages are extremely common, and one or two miscarriages do not imply maternal pathology. First-trimester losses are usually caused by aneuploidy, more specifically an autosomal trisomy. Second-trimester losses usually have maternal causes, such as uterine anomaly (bicornuate uterus), cervical insufficiency, maternal infection, or maternal hypercoagulable state.

Third-trimester bleeding is commonly secondary to placenta previa or placenta abruption.

- **Placenta previa** is when the placenta attaches to the lower uterine segment and partially covers the cervix ("prev"ents exit of the fetus). This commonly causes **painless vaginal bleeding.** Risk factors include prior cesarean section and multiparity. Patients with placenta previa are at higher risk for **placenta accreta,** in which the placenta attaches to the myometrium.
- **Placental abruption** is premature separation of the placenta, causing **painful vaginal bleeding,** fetal distress, and tetanic (constant maximal) contractions. Risk factors include cocaine use, smoking, hypertension, and trauma. The mother is at risk for disseminated intravascular coagulation (DIC) and shock.

> On Step 1:
> Painless third trimester bleeding is placenta previa.
> Painful third trimester bleeding is placental abruption.

Preeclampsia is a triad of pregnancy-induced hypertension, proteinuria, and edema of the face and hands, all of which result from placental artery vasoconstriction. The hypertension is defined as more than 140/90 mm Hg and usually occurs after 20 weeks' gestation and subsides by 6 weeks postpartum. Other symptoms include oliguria, headache, vision changes, and right upper quadrant (RUQ) abdominal pain. Newer guidelines do not require proteinuria for diagnosis because many women don't meet the proteinuria cutoff, which could delay diagnosis and treatment. Risk factors include previous hypertension, diabetes, or kidney disease. Severe preeclampsia can be manifested as blood pressure >140/90 with massive proteinuria (>3+ on dipstick) or as HELLP syndrome (**H**emolysis, **E**levated **L**FTs [liver function tests], **L**ow **P**latelets). **Eclampsia** is preeclampsia with the addition of seizures. Preeclampsia is treated with delivery whenever possible (usually after 34 weeks), and magnesium sulfate is given to prevent progression to eclampsia. Magnesium levels must be monitored during treatment with magnesium to prevent toxicity. An early sign of magnesium toxicity is loss of deep tendon reflexes. Later signs are respiratory depression and cardiac arrest. Treatment of eclampsia involves immediate delivery regardless of gestational age.

An early sign of magnesium toxicity is loss of deep tendon reflexes. Later signs are respiratory depression and cardiac arrest.

Amniotic Fluid Disorders

Polyhydramnios is an excess of amniotic fluid. Duodenal atresia and tracheoesophageal fistula lead to polyhydramnios because the fluid cannot go through the fetal gastrointestinal tract. Anencephaly causes polyhydramnios as the central nervous system leaks excess fluid into the amniotic sac. Maternal diabetes is also associated with polyhydramnios.

Oligohydramnios is a deficit of amniotic fluid related to urogenital abnormalities (e.g., renal agenesis, posterior urethral valves), premature rupture of membranes, or placental insufficiency (preeclampsia or postterm pregnancy).

Benign Gynecologic Conditions

Mittelschmerz is abdominal pain secondary to ovulation. When ovulation occurs, blood from the ruptured follicle may cause peritoneal irritation.

Endometriosis is a condition in which endometrial glands and stroma are located outside the uterus, resulting in cyclic bleeding and dysmenorrhea. The most common sites are the ovaries, pouch of Douglas, fallopian tubes, and intestines. These growths can coalesce into small masses of ectopic endometrial tissue called endometriomas (or "chocolate cysts" because of their color and consistency). The pathogenesis is thought to be as follows: (1) retrograde menstrual flow through the fallopian tubes; (2) coelomic metaplasia into endometrial cells; or (3) vascular or lymphatic spread. Patients may experience dyspareunia (pain with intercourse) and are at increased risk for infertility. Definitive diagnosis is by laparoscopy, and treatment begins with oral contraceptive pills (OCPs; birth control pills). **Adenomyosis** is endometrial glands and stroma within the myometrium, resulting in an enlarged uterus on bimanual examination.

A **leiomyoma (fibroid)** is a common benign smooth muscle tumor that is more common in African American women. These tumors are responsive to estrogen and commonly become larger during pregnancy and shrink in size after menopause. They are generally asymptomatic, but clinical findings include heavy menstrual bleeding, constipation, and urinary frequency or urgency. Complications include obstructing delivery or iron deficiency anemia from bleeding of submucosal fibroids. This tumor is commonly stained with smooth muscle actin. **Leiomyosarcoma** occurs de novo and not as malignant transformation of an existing leiomyoma. Leiomyosarcomas are aggressive, irregularly shaped tumors with atypical mitotic changes and necrotic areas. This tumor is commonly stained with desmin.

Anovulation occurs as a result of an increase in the estrogen-to-progesterone ratio, resulting in unopposed estrogen that puts the patient at increased risk of endometrial hyperplasia and thus cancer. Because there is not enough progesterone, there is no LH surge and ovulation does not occur. Regular menses also does not occur because of the absence of progesterone withdrawal. Therefore anovulatory bleeding occurs when the proliferative endometrium outgrows its blood supply, resulting in irregular bleeding. Common causes of anovulation include obesity, hypothalamic-pituitary abnormalities, polycystic ovarian syndrome (PCOS), thyroid disorders, and Cushing syndrome.

Polycystic ovarian syndrome is a disorder in which there is increased LH and decreased FSH released from the pituitary. The ratio is usually >2:1. Because of the increased LH, there is increased testosterone, which is converted into estrogen in adipose tissue (this is why patients with PCOS are at increased risk of endometrial cancer). This estrogen has negative feedback on the production of FSH, thus decreasing FSH levels, which results in follicular degeneration and bilateral cystic ovaries. Clinical findings associated with PCOS include obesity, insulin resistance, hirsutism as a result of elevated testosterone, amenorrhea, and infertility. Treatment includes OCPs, leuprolide, and metformin.

Ovarian cysts are follicular cysts, the most common ovarian mass; they result from fluid buildup in a follicle, usually right before ovulation. They are unilateral and regress spontaneously. Corpus luteum cysts are similarly unilateral and regress spontaneously. Corpus luteum cysts are most common during pregnancy. Theca lutein cysts are usually bilateral and usually associated with molar pregnancies.

Gynecologic Malignancies

Vaginal cancer is the fourth most common gynecologic malignancy. Risk factors include human papillomavirus (HPV) 16 and 18 infection, obesity, and chronic hypertension. **Squamous cell carcinoma** is also associated with HPV infection. **Clear cell adenocarcinoma** is associated with diethylstilbestrol exposure in utero. **Sarcoma botryoides** is a rhabdomyosarcoma that typically occurs in very young females (<8 years) and stains desmin-positive. The name *botryoides* comes from the Greek word for "grape bunches" because of the gross appearance of the tumor, resembling a bunch of grapes.

Incidence and average age of gynecologic cancer (CA; years): endometrial (55) > ovarian (65) > cervical (45) > vaginal

Best prognosis of gynecologic CA: ovarian > cervical > endometrial

Cervical dysplasia—cervical intraepithelial neoplasia (CIN) refers to the potentially premalignant transformation of the normal columnar epithelium to squamous epithelium at the transformation zone of the cervix. These dysplastic changes are mostly caused by HPV 16 and 18 (the most high risk of the HPV types), which inactivate p53 and Rb tumor suppressor genes. Risk factors include **multiple sexual partners,** early age of sexual intercourse, smoking, immunosuppression, and OCP use. Low-grade dysplasia normally regresses on its own. High-grade dysplasia has a greater chance of progressing to invasive cancer; however, this process usually takes about 10 years. Vaccines are now available that protect against HPV types 16 and 18 (as well as other types).

Cervical cancer is the least common gynecologic malignancy. The most common tumor type is squamous cell carcinoma; less common is adenocarcinoma. Patients typically present with postcoital bleeding. The most common cause of death is renal failure from lateral invasion of the ureters.

Endometrial hyperplasia is abnormal proliferative endometrium related to prolonged estrogen exposure. Therefore risk factors include nulliparity, late menopause, early menarche, anovulatory cycles, PCOS, and hormone replacement therapy, along with systemic diseases such as diabetes mellitus, chronic hypertension, and obesity. The most common presenting sign is **postmenopausal bleeding.** Because endometrial hyperplasia progresses to endometrial carcinoma, any woman older than 35 years with abnormal vaginal bleeding requires an endometrial biopsy to rule out endometrial hyperplasia or cancer.

Endometrial carcinoma is the most common gynecologic malignancy, with adenocarcinoma being the most common tumor type. Risk factors are similar to endometrial hyperplasia, with the greatest risk factor being a history of endometrial hyperplasia. OCPs are protective.

Ovarian tumors (Table 16.3) are the second most common gynecologic malignancy. Risk factors include the *BRCA1* gene mutation, **positive family history,** higher lifetime ovulation (early menarche, late menopause, nulliparity), and white ethnicity. OCPs are protective (fewer lifetime ovulations). Early disease is asymptomatic, which is why most patients present in later stages of the disease. Later disease has nonspecific symptoms and signs such as bloating, constipation, nausea, and vomiting. The most common tumor type is epithelial (65%–70%), followed by germ cell (15%–20%), gonadal-stromal (3%–5%), and metastatic (5%).

Breast Disorders and Malignancy

Common Breast Conditions

Acute mastitis is an infection around the areola that can lead to a breast abscess and usually results from breastfeeding. Common organisms included *Staphylococcus aureus* and *Streptococcus pyogenes.* Purulent nipple discharge may be present. Treatment is dicloxacillin and continued breastfeeding. **Fat necrosis** is a painless lump secondary to breast trauma. **Mammary duct ectasia** occurs when the main ducts are filled with debris, causing inflammation and greenish nipple discharge. **Gynecomastia** is a glandular proliferation in the male breast caused by increased estrogen. Causes include puberty, old age, cirrhosis, Klinefelter syndrome, estrogen, marijuana use, spironolactone, digitalis, cimetidine, and ketoconazole (displaces estrogen from sex hormone–binding globulin). The classic presentation of gynecomastia is a pubertal boy presenting with a lump in his breast; the high levels of testosterone during puberty lead to high levels of estrogen when the aromatase enzyme converts the androgens into estrogens, causing gynecomastia. This usually self-resolves and is of no serious consequence.

Benign Breast Disorders

Fibroadenoma is the most common benign tumor in young women. It is a small, well-circumscribed, mobile mass in the breast stroma. It is often tender during periods of increased estrogen, such as pregnancy and menstruation. Fibroadenoma does not commonly progress to breast cancer. Intraductal papilloma is a papillary growth within the lactiferous ducts of the breast, usually presenting with unilateral bloody discharge. It does not pose an increased risk for cancer. Phyllodes tumor is a large bulky tumor

Table 16.3 Summary of Ovarian Tumors

NAME	TUMOR TYPE	DESCRIPTION	TUMOR MARKER
Serous cystadenoma	Epithelial	Most common benign ovarian tumor; bilateral; Lined by ciliated cells	CA-125, CEA
Serous cystadenocarcinoma	Epithelial	Most common malignant ovarian tumor; bilateral Psammoma bodies on histology	CA-125, CEA
Mucinous cystadenoma	Epithelial	Large, benign, ovarian mass lined by mucous-secreting cells (endocervix-like)	CA-125, CEA
Mucinous cystadenocarcinoma	Epithelial	Large malignant mass that can cause pseudomyxoma peritonei (mucinous material in the peritoneal space from seeding)	CA-125, CEA
Brenner tumor	Epithelial	Benign tumor that has transitional-like epithelium (bladder-like) Mnemonic: B = bladder = Brenner	CA-125, CEA
Dysgerminoma	Germ cell	Most common malignant germ cell tumor Undifferentiated germ cells with stroma infiltrated by lymphocytes on histology Can be seen in Turner syndrome	hCG, LDH
Endodermal sinus tumor or yolk sac	Germ cell	Second most common germ cell tumor Yolk sac cells with Schiller-Duvall bodies (structures that look like glomeruli on histology)	AFP
Choriocarcinoma	Germ cell	Rare, malignant tumor that can progress from molar pregnancy or arise sporadically Trophoblastic differentiation on histologic examination Associated with bilateral theca lutein cysts	hCG
Teratoma	Germ cell	Mature teratoma (dermoid cyst) is benign and contains cells from two or three germ layers, especially ectoderm (hair, teeth) Immature: Malignant, contains neural element Struma ovarii: Contains thyroid tissue, potentially leading to hyperthyroidism	
Fibroma	Gonadal-stromal	Benign tumor Spindle-shaped fibroblasts on histologic examination Leads to Meig syndrome: ascites and pleural effusion from fibroma	
Granulosa cell tumor	Gonadal-stromal	Low-grade, estrogen-producing tumor that can cause endometrial hyperplasia and carcinoma Call-Exner bodies on histologic examination	Estrogen
Sertoli-Leydig	Gonadal-stromal	Benign androgen-producing tumor that causes masculinization	Testosterone
Krukenberg tumor	Metastatic	Gastrointestinal malignancy that metastasizes to ovaries, producing a signet cell adenocarcinoma on histologic examination	CEA, CA-125

AFP, alpha-fetoprotein; CA-125, cancer antigen 125; CEA, carcinoembryonic antigen; hCG, human chorionic gonadotropin; LDH, lactate dehydrogenase.

derived from the stroma that has malignant potential. Although a fibroadenoma is the most common benign tumor in young women, the most common cause of a breast lump in a young woman is **fibrocystic change,** which occurs in more than half of women at some point during their reproductive years. This causes multiple lumps in the breast, which are usually painful and vary in size and tenderness with the reproductive cycle. This is often concerning and bothersome for the patient but is benign.

Breast Cancer

Breast cancer (Fig. 16.10) is the most common cancer in postmenopausal women and the second most common cancer resulting in death in women. The mean age at diagnosis is 64 years. Risk factors include increased estrogen exposure (nulliparity, early menarche, late menopause), *BRCA1* and *BRCA2* gene mutations, positive family history in first-generation relatives, obesity, and hormone replacement therapy. Malignancy is most commonly found in the upper outer quadrant, which drains into the axillary lymph nodes (important prognostic indicator). The inner quadrant drains to the internal mammillary lymph nodes and is a less common site for breast cancer. Breast cancer commonly metastasizes to lungs, bone, liver, brain, and ovaries. Breast cancers can also be classified by the presence or absence of hormone receptors—estrogen receptor (ER), progesterone receptor (PR), and human epidermal growth factor receptor 2 (HER2/neu). ER-positive cancers carry a better prognosis and can be treated with selective estrogen receptor modulators (SERMs) such as tamoxifen. HER2/neu-positive cancers carry a worse prognosis but can be treated with the monoclonal antibody trastuzumab, which binds the receptor.

See Table 16.4 for a summary of breast tumors.

BRCA1 mutation results in an 80% lifetime risk of breast cancer and 40% lifetime risk of ovarian cancer. *BRCA1* breast cancer has a higher grade and typically is HER2/neu positive. Survival rates have improved because of the drug trastuzumab.

BRCA2 mutation results in a 40% lifetime risk of breast cancer and a 20% lifetime risk of ovarian cancer. *BRCA2* breast cancer is better differentiated and is ER-PR positive.

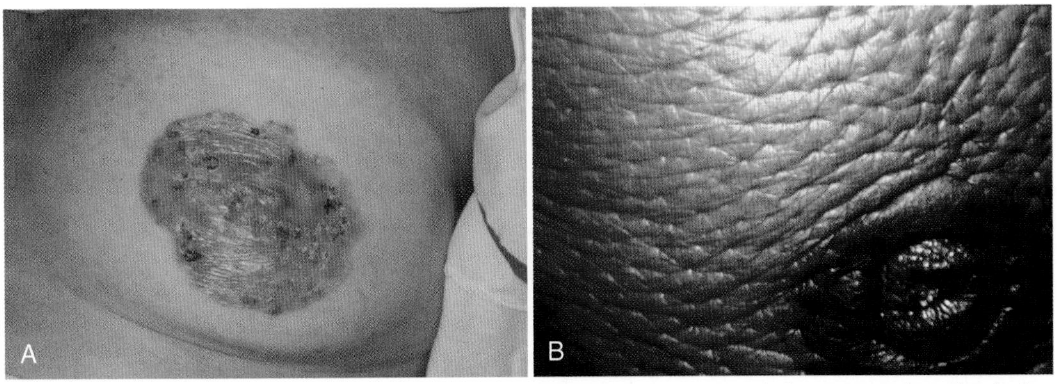

Fig. 16.10 Breast cancer. **A,** Paget disease of nipple. **B,** Peau d'orange. French for "orange skin," this finding is caused by lymphedema and dimpling secondary to lymphatic plugging. *(From Swartz MH.* Textbook of Physical Diagnosis. *6th ed. Philadelphia: Elsevier; 2009.)*

Table 16.4 Summary of Breast Tumors

TYPE	DESCRIPTION
Ductal carcinoma in situ (DCIS)	Ductal hyperplasia that can invade past basement membrane in one-third of cases Not palpable, detected via mammography because of microcalcifications
Paget disease of nipple	Dermal invasion of DCIS resulting in rash and possible nipple retraction (see Fig. 16.10A) Paget cells are **large** cells in the epidermis with halos
Invasive ductal carcinoma	Most common type of breast cancer Firm, hard, sharply demarcated, invasive mass with stellate morphology One-third have HER2/neu amplification and can be treated with trastuzumab
Lobular carcinoma in situ (LCIS)	Nonpalpable, often found incidentally on breast biopsy—not identified via mammography because there are no calcifications One-third invade ER and PR positive
Invasive lobular carcinoma	Row of cells or concentric circles that have a bull's-eye appearance on histologic examination Often bilateral, although the other breast does not have to have lobular cancer
Medullary carcinoma	Related to *BRCA1* mutation Typically HER2/neu positive and ER, PR negative
Inflammatory	Poor prognosis Tumor plugs up dermal lymphatic lumens, resulting in lymphedema and dimpling (peau d'orange; see Fig. 16.10B)

Sex Chromosome and Hormone Disorders

Turner syndrome (45,XO) is a disorder that results in follicle deterioration and ovarian dysgenesis (streak ovary) by 2 years of age. This puts those with this disorder at risk for dysgerminoma. Because of the nonfunctioning ovaries, there is decreased estrogen and increased FSH and LH. Clinical signs and symptoms include short stature, shield chest, preductal coarctation of aorta, bicuspid aortic valve, horseshoe kidney, cystic hygroma (from dilated lymphatics), amenorrhea, and a shortened fourth metacarpal.

Female pseudohermaphrodites (XX) have normal internal genitalia and virilized external genitalia from excessive exposure to androgens. Common causes include congenital adrenal hyperplasia and androgen exposure during pregnancy.

MALE PATHOLOGY

Benign Prostatic Hyperplasia

Benign prostatic hyperplasia (BPH) of the prostate gland is age related. It is thought that in later adult male life, there is an increase in estrogen levels, along with an increased synthesis of androgen receptors that respond to DHT. Enlargement of the transitional and periurethral lobes (Fig. 16.11) results in increased urinary frequency, urgency, hesitancy, and nocturia from anatomic compression of the urethra. Complications include obstructive uropathy leading to bilateral hydronephrosis, bladder infections, and prostatic infarcts. Prostate-specific antigen (PSA) level is normal (0–4 ng/mL) or mildly elevated (4–10 ng/mL). Medical treatment includes α-adrenergic antagonists (e.g., terazosin, tamsulosin), which relax the smooth muscle around the urethral sphincter, or 5-α-reductase inhibitors (e.g., finasteride) that block the conversion of testosterone to DHT. Surgical treatment is most commonly transurethral resection of the prostate (TURP).

Mnemonic: TerazoSIN and TamsuloSIN are sinners because they ANTAGONIZE the α-adrenergic receptor.

Prostatic Adenocarcinoma

Prostate cancer is the most common cancer in men, usually affecting the peripheral or posterior lobe of the prostate (see Fig. 16.11). For this reason, it is often diagnosed via digital rectal examination, in which a hard mass is palpated. Risk factors include increasing age, family history, and African American ethnicity. Clinically, prostate cancer is silent until advanced stages, at which time patients may report

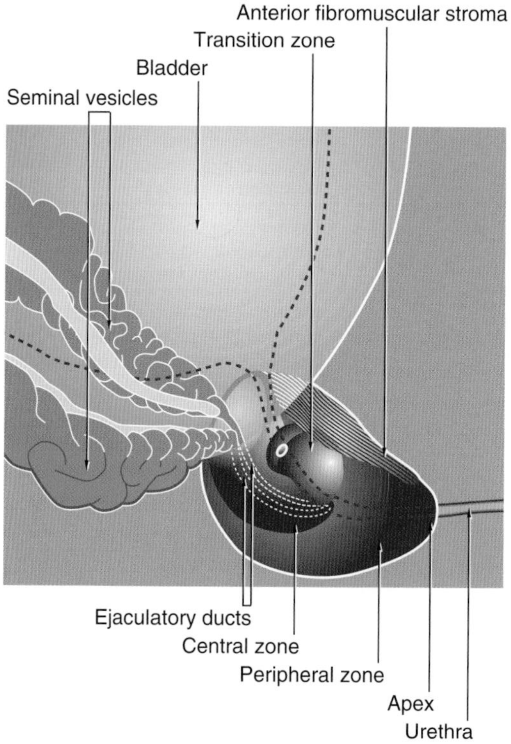

FIG. 16.11 The prostate. Note the lobes of the prostate and their relation to pathology. Because prostate cancer affects the peripheral zone on the posterior of the prostate, it can be detected on digital rectal examination. Because BPH affects the transition zone, it is more likely to obstruct the urethra. *(From Young B, Lowe JS, Stevens A, Heath JW. Wheater's Functional Histology. 5th ed. Philadelphia: Elsevier; 2006.)*

back pain from **osteoblastic** metastasis to the bone (spread via the Batson venous plexus), resulting in high alkaline phosphatase levels. PSA levels are elevated (usually >10 ng/mL). Diagnosis is made by needle biopsy. Radiation, chemotherapy, and surgery may all be used in treatment. Side effects of surgery are common, including erectile dysfunction and urinary incontinence.

Although serum PSA testing can be useful in detecting recurrences of prostate adenocarcinoma or in monitoring response to therapy, its use as a general screening tool in asymptomatic men has not been found to be helpful. You may use PSA to screen patients who request it after a conversation about the risks and benefits of screening, but in general its use is not recommended.

Cryptorchidism is undescended testicle(s), most often found in the inguinal canal. Patients are at risk for infertility (increased body temperature), germ cell tumors, and testicular torsion (twisting of spermatic cord).

Testicular Tumors

Testicular cancer is the most common malignancy between ages 15 and 35 years in males (Table 16.5). The most common types of testicular tumors are germ cell in origin (95%), followed by gonadal-stromal (5%), which are mostly benign. Risk factors include cryptorchidism, Klinefelter syndrome, and inguinal hernias.

Penile Disorders and Pathology

- **Peyronie disease:** Bending of the penis caused by fibrous tissue deposition secondary to previous trauma.
- **Priapism:** Persistent penile erection secondary to sickle cell disease, spinal cord trauma, or medications (e.g., trazodone, sildenafil). Failure of detumescence leads to impaired venous drainage and causes compartment syndrome, which can eventually lead to ischemia and necrosis of penile tissue.
- **Carcinoma in situ (CIS; Bowen disease):** Leukoplakia (white plaques) of the penis and/or scrotum associated with HPV 16 that progresses to squamous cell carcinoma in 10% of cases.
- **Erythroplasia of Queyrat:** Erythroplakia (red plaques) on the glans penis, also associated with HPV 16.
- **Bowenoid papulosis:** Red papular lesions on the external genitalia associated with HPV 16 that does not have the potential to become invasive squamous cell carcinoma (SCC).
- **Squamous cell carcinoma:** Associated with HPV 16 and 18. Other risk factors include uncircumcised status and smoking.

Table 16.5 Summary of Testicular Tumors

NAME	DESCRIPTION	TUMOR MARKER
Seminoma	Most common germ cell tumor Malignant Affects men 30–35 years old Large cells with *fried-egg* appearance on histologic examination Good prognosis, radiosensitive	Can have increase in hCG
Embryonal carcinoma	Big, painful tumor with bloody necrotic areas Mixed with other tumor types Worse prognosis	AFP, hCG
Endodermal sinus tumor (yolk sac)	Most common testicular tumor in young children (<5 years old) Schiller-Duvall bodies on histologic examination	AFP
Choriocarcinoma	Aggressive tumor of trophoblastic tissue that spreads hematogenously	hCG
Teratoma	Benign in children, malignant in adult	AFP, hCG
Leydig cell	Androgen-producing tumor that causes precocious puberty in boys Reinke crystals on histologic examination	Testosterone
Testicular lymphoma	Most common testicular tumor in men >60 years old Bilateral testicle involvement Poor prognosis	LDH (lymphoma marker)

AFP, alpha-fetoprotein; hCG, human chorionic gonadotropin; LDH, Lactate dehydrogenase.

Scrotal Sac Disorders

A **varicocele** is dilation of the spermatic pampiniform venous plexus from increased pressure. It is most common on the left side because the left testicular vein drains into the left renal vein (not directly to the inferior vena cava), resulting in increased pressure. Varicocele on the right side should raise suspicion for cancer. A varicocele feels like a "bag of worms." Patients are asymptomatic or may complain of pain and a pulling sensation in the scrotum. If large, a varicocele can lead to infertility (theoretically because of elevated scrotal temperature from local pooling of blood that inhibits spermatogenesis).

A **hydrocele** is an incomplete fusion of the tunica vaginalis causing serous fluid accumulation around the testicle, resulting in scrotal swelling. Hydroceles are asymptomatic but are associated with inguinal hernias if there is total failure of fusion and therefore communication with the peritoneal cavity. Hydroceles will **transilluminate,** meaning that a bright light will pass through the fluid-filled sac (as opposed to testicular tumors, which will block light).

A **spermatocele** is a cystic mass derived from a tubule of the rete testis or the head of the epididymis. It can be palpated superior to the testicle. It contains spermatozoa and is generally asymptomatic.

Sex Chromosome and Hormone Disorders

Klinefelter syndrome (47,XXY) is a disorder in which hyalinization and dysgenesis of the seminiferous tubules lead to decreased inhibin. Because inhibin normally has a negative feedback on FSH, its absence causes an increase in FSH. There are also decreased testosterone levels from excess aromatization of testosterone to estrogen, leading to an increase in LH. Clinical symptoms include testicular atrophy, tall and long extremities (lack of testosterone to close epiphyseal plates), gynecomastia, female hair distribution, and infertility. Klinefelter syndrome is an example of primary hypogonadism (a defect of the gonad itself).

XYY syndrome occurs as a result of paternal nondisjunction. Patients are phenotypically tall and affected by acne. There are some reports of increased antisocial behavior. Fertility is unaffected.

Androgen insensitivity syndrome (46,XY) results in a nonfunctional androgen receptor, so there is no functional exposure to androgens. Testosterone levels are elevated but cannot bind the androgen receptor. This allows for the development of a phenotypically female-appearing individual with female external genitalia (because of peripheral conversion of testosterone to estrogen). The upper vagina, cervix, uterus, and fallopian tubes are absent because Müllerian inhibiting hormone is still produced by the testes. Testicles are normally found in the labia majora and are removed surgically to prevent malignancy. There are **high** levels of LH and testosterone because testosterone cannot feed back negatively on the anterior pituitary to regulate LH levels because the testosterone receptors on the anterior pituitary are similarly defective. High LH levels thus stimulate even more testosterone production. This is an example of male pseudohermaphroditism because the individual has testes (male) but female-appearing external genitalia. High testosterone levels in utero can cross the placenta and result in virilization of the mother during pregnancy, which resolves after delivery.

In **5-α-reductase deficiency,** there are normal male internal genitalia because of normal testosterone levels. However, they are phenotypically female-appearing males until puberty. This is because early in life, as a result of the defective enzyme, males cannot convert testosterone to DHT, which is important in developing male external genitalia and masculinization. When puberty occurs, the patient will become virilized as a result of high levels of testosterone that are produced at that time. This is because although testosterone has a weaker affinity for the androgen receptor than does DHT, the level of testosterone increases to such an extent that it is able to stimulate the androgen receptor and cause these changes to occur, regardless of DHT levels.

PHARMACOLOGY

See Table 16.6 for a summary of reproductive pharmacology.

Table 16.6 Summary of Reproductive Pharmacology

NAME	MECHANISM	CLINICAL USE	SIDE EFFECTS
Leuprolide	GnRH analog Increases FSH, LH when used in pulsatile fashion Inhibits FSH, LH when used in continuous fashion	Pulsatile: Infertility Continuous: Prostate cancer, fibroids, precocious puberty	Nausea, vomiting
Finasteride	5-α-reductase inhibitor	Treatment of BPH and male pattern baldness	Gynecomastia
Flutamide	Competitive inhibitor at testosterone receptor	Used with leuprolide to treat prostate cancer	
Spironolactone	Blocks testosterone receptor and is a potassium-sparing diuretic	Used to treat hirsutism in PCOS. Spironolactone also has uses in the treatment of hypertension and congestive heart failure (CHF)	Gynecomastia, amenorrhea, hyperkalemia
Clomiphene	Partial agonist at estrogen receptor; prevents negative feedback → increased LH, FSH, which induces ovulation	Promotes ovulation in PCOS and infertility	Hot flashes, multiple pregnancies
Tamoxifen	Estrogen antagonist at breast; agonist on endometrial tissue	Treatment of ER-positive breast cancer	Increased risk of endometrial cancer
Raloxifene	Estrogen agonist at bone; antagonist at breast and endometrium	Treatment of osteoporosis	Leg cramps, deep venous thrombosis, pulmonary embolism
Anastrozole	Aromatase inhibitor	Treatment of breast cancer in postmenopausal women	
Mifepristone RU-486	Competitive progesterone receptor antagonist	Elective abortion	Heavy bleeding, abdominal pain
Oral contraceptives	Prevent estrogen surge and thus the LH surge by keeping estrogen and progesterone at baseline levels	Contraception Do not protect against STDs Regulate irregular or painful menses Protective against ovarian and endometrial cancer	Depression, weight gain, hypertension, deep venous thrombosis, pulmonary embolism Contraindicated in women >35 years who smoke or have history of thromboembolic disease Also contraindicated in women with history of estrogen-sensitive tumors (e.g., breast or endometrial cancer)
Dinoprostone	Prostaglandin E_2 (PGE_2) analog	Makes the cervix favorable and induces labor (dilates cervix and promotes uterine contractions) Can also be used as an abortive therapy	Nausea, abdominal pain
Ritodrine/terbutaline	β_2 agonists at uterine smooth muscle	Reduce uterine contractions	Tachycardia
Terazosin/tamsulosin	$\alpha_{1A,D}$-adrenergic antagonist (selective for prostate)	Treatment of BPH if urinary symptoms are present	Hypotension because they can bind other alpha receptors on the vasculature
Sildenafil, vardenafil, tadalafil	Increases cGMP by inhibiting its breakdown by phosphodiesterase-5 (PDE5); this causes smooth muscle relaxation in the vasculature. Increased blood flow leads to erection.	Treatment of erectile dysfunction (ED) Can also be used to treat Raynaud syndrome or pulmonary hypertension	Headache and flushing; life-threatening hypotension in patients also taking nitroglycerin

STD, Sexually transmitted disease.

REVIEW QUESTIONS

(1) A woman has undergone a total abdominal hysterectomy. Postoperatively, she has a fever and is having trouble urinating. What happened?
(2) True or false: The ovarian artery is contained in the ovarian ligament.
(3) True or false: Erection is a parasympathetic response, and ejaculation is a sympathetic response.
(4) A woman at 38 weeks' gestation comes in with a blood pressure of 156/100 mm Hg, hemolytic anemia, and elevated liver enzymes. She states that she is having vision changes and RUQ pain. What is your next step?
(5) A 19-year-old woman presents with LLQ abdominal pain, vaginal spotting, and hypotension. On physical examination, she appears pale and diaphoretic. What diagnostic test would you order, and what treatment options are available?
(6) True or false: BPH is hypertrophy of the prostatic tissue.
(7) A mother refuses treatment for her son, who has one undescended testicle. What risk factors do you counsel her on if she refuses treatment for him?
(8) What is a pseudohermaphrodite? Give an example.
(9) Oral contraceptive pills (OCPs) are protective for which gynecologic cancers?
(10) A woman comes in with a diffuse rash on her nipple that has not responded to steroids or antibiotics. Breast examination shows no palpable masses. What is on the differential diagnosis and what is your next step?

17 PULMONOLOGY

Theodore X. O'Connell and Masood Memarzadeh

ANATOMY OF THE RESPIRATORY SYSTEM

The Lungs

The **right lung has three lobes,** whereas the **left has two lobes and a lingula** (Fig. 17.1). The left lung has one fewer lobe to accommodate space occupied by the heart. Each lung is located in its respective pleural cavity enclosed by parietal pleura. The parietal pleura are innervated by somatic sensory nerves, which allow the sensation of sharp and localized pain. Inflammation of the pleura causes pain that **worsens** on inspiration and is referred to as pleuritic chest pain. This characteristic pain can help distinguish pulmonary pathologic conditions (e.g., pneumonia, pneumothorax, pulmonary embolism) from cardiac pathologic conditions (e.g., myocardial infarction).

One can remember the position of a pulmonary artery relative to its main bronchus at each lung hilum by **RALS**—**R**ight **A**nterior **L**eft **S**uperior.

The trachea bifurcates into the left and right main bronchi at the carina. For the U.S. Medical Licensing Examination (USMLE) Step 1, it is important to know that the **right main bronchus is wider, shorter, and more vertical** than the left main bronchus. Consequently, **aspirated foreign bodies are far more likely to enter and obstruct the bronchi of the right side of the lung.** An object aspirated while standing or sitting upright will usually be found in the inferior portion of the right lower lobe, whereas an object aspirated while supine will most often end up in the superior portion of the right lower lobe (Fig. 17.2).

Bronchopulmonary Segments

Each **bronchopulmonary segment** of the lung has its own neurovascular supply that is not shared with surrounding bronchopulmonary segments (see Fig. 17.2). This is important because each bronchopulmonary segment can function independently; a single segment can be removed surgically (e.g., to remove a tumor) without affecting the other segments. The trachea bifurcates into the right and left main bronchi at the carina. These main bronchi divide further into lobar bronchi, which subsequently divide into segmental bronchi, totaling 10 in each lung. A single segmental bronchus is the core of each bronchopulmonary segment. In addition to a segmental bronchus, each bronchopulmonary segment is also composed of two arteries, located centrally within each segment, and veins and lymphatics, located peripherally. Specifically, these include the following:

- One branch of the **pulmonary artery.** These branches carry **deoxygenated** blood from the right side of the heart and are centrally located within the bronchopulmonary segment.
- **Pulmonary veins** that return **oxygenated** blood to the left atrium. These are located peripherally within each segment.
- One branch of the **bronchial artery.** These branches originate from the thoracic aorta and carry highly oxygenated blood to supply the lung parenchyma and stroma. Like the pulmonary artery branch, the bronchial artery is also centrally located within each segment.
- **Bronchial veins,** located peripherally along each segment. These return deoxygenated blood that has circulated through the lung parenchyma and stroma to the azygous venous system.
- **Lymphatics,** located peripherally along each segment.
- **Autonomic fibers**, located around the segmental bronchi and blood vessels. These are composed of parasympathetic branches from the vagus nerve, which innervate smooth muscle in the walls of terminal bronchioles, and sympathetic fibers, which innervate vascular smooth muscle.

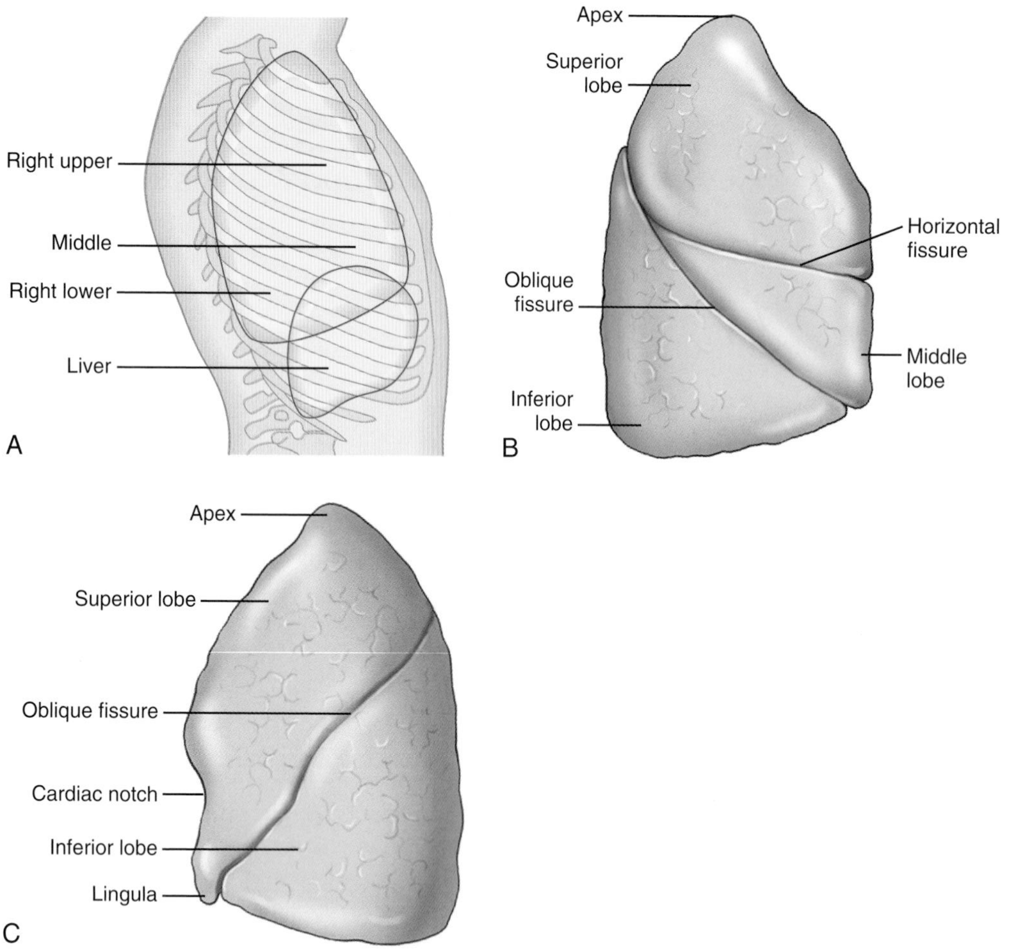

Fig. 17.1 **A,** Lobes of the lung. **B,** Detailed anatomy of the right lung, demonstrating the horizontal fissure (separating the superior from middle lobe) and the oblique fissure (separating the middle from inferior lobe). **C,** More detailed anatomy of the left lung, demonstrating the lingula at the base of the superior lobe. *(**A** from Douglas G, Nicol F, Robertson C.* Macleod's Clinical Examination. *11th ed. Philadelphia: Elsevier; 2005;* ***B, C*** *from Morton DA, Albertine KH, Peterson KD.* Gray's Dissection Guide for Human Anatomy. *2nd ed. Philadelphia: Elsevier; 2006.)*

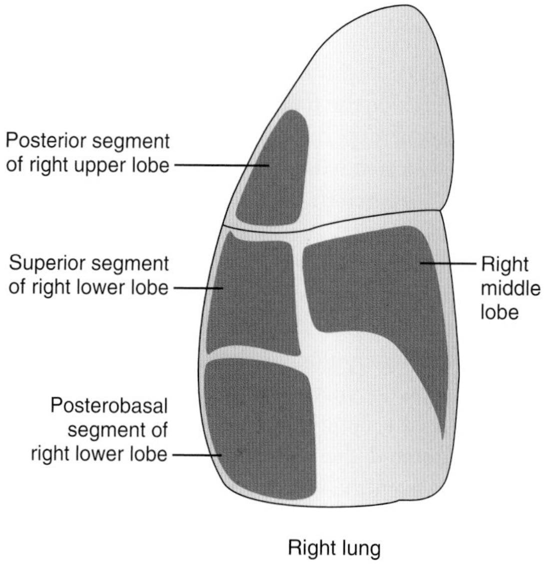

Fig. 17.2 Bronchopulmonary segments, each of which has its own neurovascular supply. An object aspirated while standing or sitting will usually be found in the inferior (posterobasal) segment of the right lower lobe; an object aspirated while supine will usually be found in the superior segment of the lower lobe. *(From Goljan EF.* Rapid Review Pathology. *3rd ed. Philadelphia: Mosby Elsevier; 2010.)*

Pulmonary Airways

The pulmonary airways can be divided into a **conducting zone** and an **alveolar-respiratory zone.** This division is based on a fundamental distinction in the function of these two zones.

Conducting Zone: The function of this zone is to **conduct air** from outside into the alveolar-respiratory zone, where gas exchange occurs. **No actual gas exchange occurs** in the conducting zone; thus **it comprises the anatomic dead space.** The conducting zone is composed of the first 16 generations (branches) of the respiratory tree (Fig. 17.3) and consists of the nose, pharynx, trachea, bronchi, and terminal bronchioles. As the generation number increases (and the airways decrease in size), there is a decrease in the amount of mucus-secreting cells, cilia, submucosal glands, and cartilage in the airway walls. At the level of the terminal bronchioles, the airway resistance is also the lowest; although the area of an individual bronchiole is small, the total cross-sectional area of all the bronchioles is high, which results in an overall low resistance.

Respiratory Zone: This zone participates in **gas exchange.** It begins with the respiratory bronchioles and alveolar ducts, terminating blindly as alveolar sacs or acini. **The alveolus (singular form of alveoli) is the fundamental unit of gas exchange.**

> The *terminal* bronchioles are the *terminal* part of the conducting zone.
>
> The *respiratory* bronchioles are the first part of the *respiratory* zone.

Cells of the Respiratory System

There are many specialized cells of the respiratory system; the important types are covered here.

The mucosa of the conducting zone of the respiratory system is composed primarily of **ciliated pseudostratified columnar cells.** These **ciliated** cells play a critical role in sweeping mucus secretions and debris out of the lungs and toward the mouth. The density of these cells gradually decreases as the airway progresses distally from the conducting to respiratory zones, and the respiratory bronchioles are the last segment of the airway in which these ciliated cells can be found. At the level of the bronchioles,

> Patients with **primary ciliary dyskinesia (Kartagener syndrome** when accompanied by situs invertus) do not have functioning cilia. These patients are predisposed to recurrent respiratory infections.

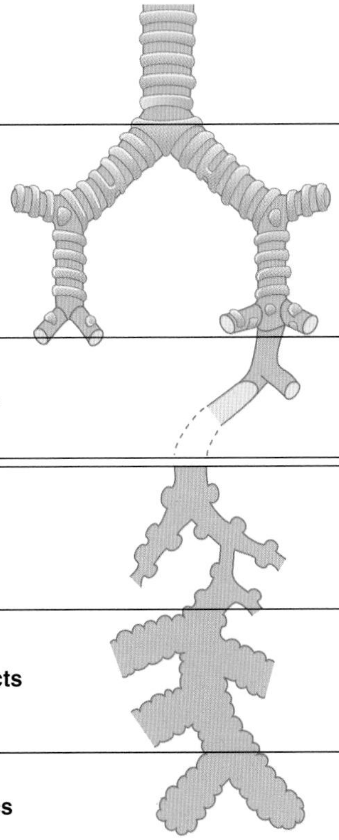

		Number	Epithelium	Smooth Muscle	Cartilage
CONDUCTING ZONE	Trachea	1	Pseudostratified columnar ciliated	Yes	Yes
	Bronchi	2 4 8	Pseudostratified columnar ciliated	Yes	Patchy
	Bronchioles	–	Simple cuboidal	Yes	No
RESPIRATORY ZONE	Respiratory bronchioles	–	Simple cuboidal	Some	No
	Alveolar ducts	–	Simple squamous	Some	No
	Alveolar sacs	6×10^8	Simple squamous	No	No

FIG. 17.3 Schematic of the airway, including the conducting zones (trachea, bronchi, bronchioles) and respiratory zones (respiratory bronchioles, alveolar ducts, alveolar sacs). *(From Costanzo LS.* Physiology. *4th ed. New York: Elsevier; 2009.)*

the epithelium transitions to a **simple cuboidal epithelium.** At the transition to the alveoli, the epithelium becomes a **simple squamous epithelium** that helps to facilitate gas exchange (with the exception of the type II pneumocytes).

Goblet cells are also abundant within the conducting zone epithelium and **produce mucus secretions** that trap particulate matter and help moisten the air. These cells (like the ciliated pseudostratified columnar epithelial cells) also progressively decrease in number as the airway progresses distally. They are no longer found beyond the terminal bronchioles. Thus they are **exclusive to the conducting zone** and are not found in the respiratory zone. This **is logical,** because if goblet cells were present distal to the ciliated pseudostratified columnar cells, mucus would be produced that could not be cleared.

Kulchitsky cells (enterochromaffin cells) are neuroendocrine cells found throughout the conducting zone. Because they are neuroendocrine cells, they stain positive for chromogranin A. These cells secrete peptide hormones that regulate airway and vascular tone. They are important for the USMLE because they are the cells of origin for **small cell carcinoma** of the lung, a particularly aggressive form of lung cancer that will be discussed later in more detail.

Clara cells are nonciliated, dome-shaped cells found within the airways of the conducting zone and respiratory bronchioles. These cells secrete a surfactant-like material. These secretions coat the luminal surface of the bronchioles to prevent luminal adhesion so that should they collapse (as they often do), these bronchioles are able to reexpand.

Type I alveolar cells (pneumocytes) are membranous pneumocytes that comprise 95% of the single-layered alveolar wall. These cells are extremely thin, **simple, squamous epithelial cells** that can no longer divide. Their luminal surfaces face the air space; their function is to **participate in gas exchange across the alveolar-capillary membrane** (Fig. 17.4A).

Type II alveolar cells (pneumocytes) are cuboidal cells that comprise the remaining 5% of the single-layered alveolar wall. These cells have two critical functions:

- They are the **regenerative cells of the lung.** When lung damage occurs, these cells proliferate and have the ability to **regenerate type I cells.**
- Type II alveolar cells also contain foamy vesicles called **lamellar bodies, which continuously produce pulmonary surfactant** that covers the luminal surface of the alveoli (Fig. 17.4B).

Surfactant is a protein-lipid material that reduces surface tension on the surface of the alveoli so they can expand more easily during inspiration. The main lipid component of surfactant is **dipalmitoylphosphatidylcholine.** It is important to know that corticosteroids help to increase surfactant production, whereas high levels of insulin (as seen in infants of diabetic mothers) inhibit surfactant production. Mature levels of surfactant are not reached until 34 to 35 weeks of gestation. Thus premature neonates may experience respiratory distress if the mother is not given corticosteroids before delivery to help increase surfactant production.

Diaphragm and Accessory Respiratory Muscles

The diaphragm is the primary respiratory muscle and is essentially the only muscle used during quiet inspiration at rest in healthy individuals. **Active downward movement or contraction of the diaphragm generates an increase in negative pleural pressure that causes the lungs to expand and fill with air during inspiration.** Similarly, passive upward movement or relaxation of this crucial muscle causes an increase in pleural pressure and results in an increased pressure in the airways, facilitating expiration. The diaphragm is innervated by the **phrenic nerve,** which originates from the **C3, C4, and C5** spinal nerves. In addition to the motor fibers to the diaphragm, the phrenic nerve also contains pain fibers, which is why pain originating from the diaphragm can be referred to the shoulders.

> Mnemonic: C3, C4, and C5 keep the diaphragm alive.

The diaphragm also forms the boundary between the thoracic and abdominal cavities, so a number of important structures found in both these compartments must traverse the diaphragm:

- The inferior vena cava traverses the diaphragm at the T8 level.
- The esophagus and two trunks of the vagus nerve traverse the diaphragm at the T10 level.
- The aorta (red), thoracic duct (white), and azygous vein (blue) traverse the diaphragm at T12 level.

Mnemonic: I ate 10 eggs at 12 (**I**VC, T**8** ["ate"], T**10, e**sophagus, **a**orta, T**12**).

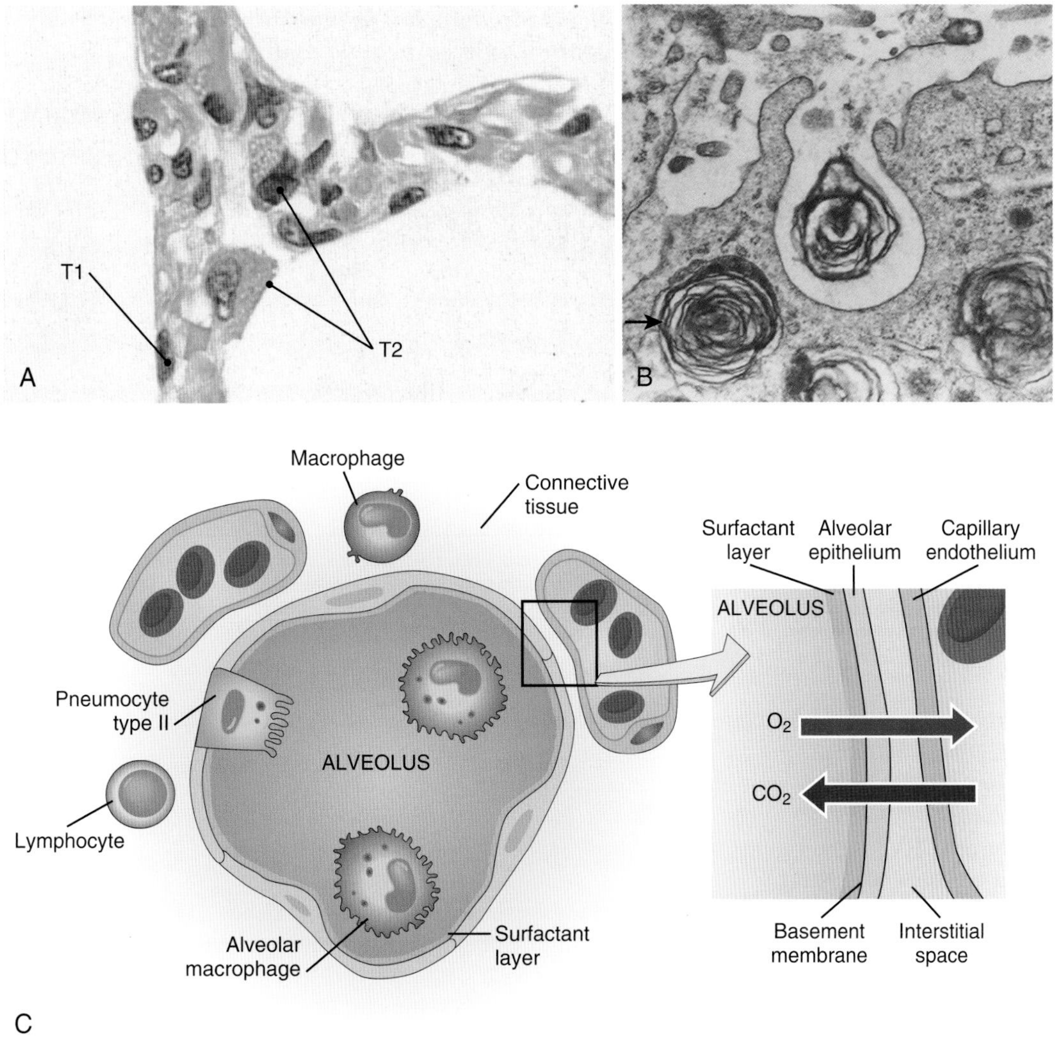

FIG. 17.4 A, Alveolar cells, demonstrating the simple squamous epithelial nature of type I pneumocytes (T1) as well as type II pneumocytes (T2). **B,** Electron microscopy of a type II pneumocyte, demonstrating lamellar bodies that produce surfactant. **C,** Illustration of an alveolus showing a type II pneumocyte, alveolar macrophages inside the alveolus, and the area in which type I pneumocytes interface with the pulmonary capillary beds to exchange oxygen and carbon dioxide. *(**A** from Stevens A, Lowe JS.* Human Histology. *3rd ed. Philadelphia: Elsevier; 2004;* ***B*** *from Goljan EF.* Rapid Review Pathology. *3rd ed. Philadelphia: Mosby Elsevier; 2010;* ***C*** *from Corrin B:* Pathology of the Lungs. *London: Churchill Livingstone; 1999.)*

Although the diaphragm is the predominant muscle of respiration used by healthy individuals during quiet inspiration and expiration, several other muscles assist in respiration during exercise and in certain diseases in which airway resistance is increased (e.g., asthma). During vigorous inspiration, the **external intercostal, scalene, and sternocleidomastoid** muscles may be used. During exercise and conditions of increased airway resistance, expiration is aided by the **abdominal muscles** and **internal intercostal muscles,** which pull the ribs inward and downward.

RESPIRATORY PHYSIOLOGY

Spirometry

Spirometry is an important clinical tool used to measure a variety of lung volumes. When at least two lung volume measurements are added together, it is termed *lung capacity,* and alterations in these lung capacities are important in diagnosing several diseases (see later). For now, let us briefly review the different lung volume measurements and capacities (Fig. 17.5).

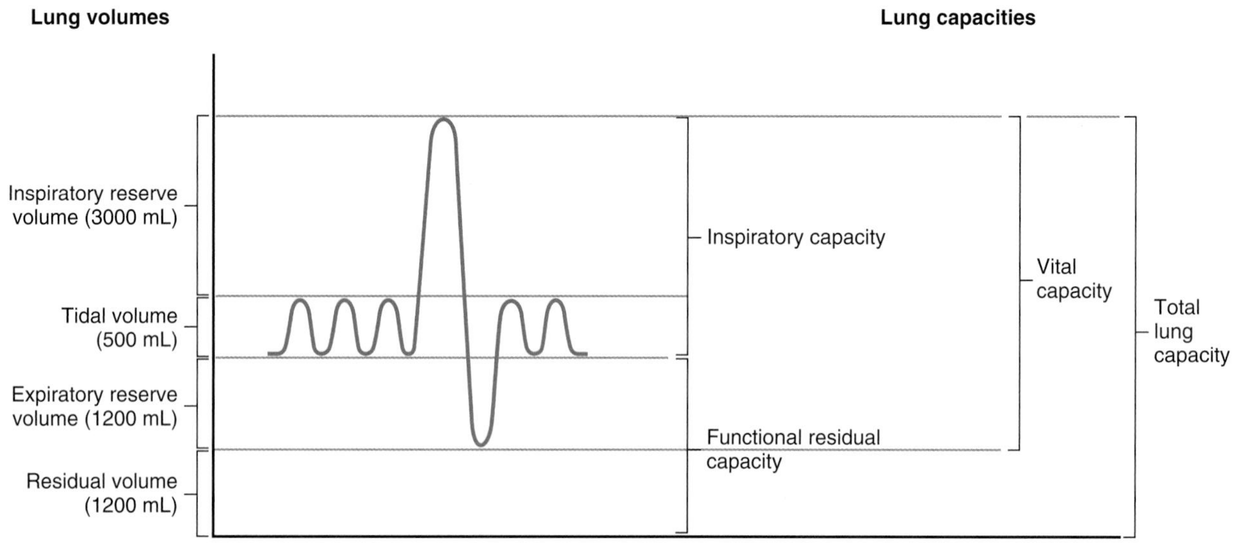

FIG. 17.5 Diagram of the various volumes and capacities in the lung. The first three breaths recorded are tidal volume breaths (500 mL each). At the end of a normal exhalation, the subject is at his or her functional residual capacity (residual volume and expiratory reserve volume). The subject then takes in a deep breath and forcibly exhales as much as possible; that volume is the vital capacity. Note that the lungs are not completely deflated because there is a residual volume (1200 mL) that cannot be exhaled. *(From Costanzo LS.* Physiology. *4th ed. New York: Elsevier; 2009.)*

Tidal volume (TV) is the amount of air drawn into the lungs during normal respiration. In a 70-kg adult, it normally measures around 500 mL.

Inspiratory reserve volume (IRV) is the volume of air that can be inhaled during a maximal inspiration, beyond the tidal volume.

Expiratory reserve volume (ERV) is the volume of air that can be exhaled in a forced expiration, beyond the tidal volume. It is normally 1200 mL.

Residual volume (RV) is the amount of air that remains in the lungs at the end of a maximal exhalation. It actually cannot be measured by simple spirometry and requires use of either helium dilution or body plethysmography to characterize. It is normally about 1200 mL as well.

Total lung capacity (TLC) is derived from combining all of the lung volumes:

$$TLC = RV + ERV + TV + IRV$$

Vital capacity (VC) is the volume that can be exhaled after maximal inspiration. It includes everything except the RV. VC increases with male gender, physical conditioning, and body size and decreases with age:

$$VC = ERV + TV + IRV$$

Functional residual capacity (FRC) is the volume remaining in the lungs after a normal expiration. It is the resting or equilibrium volume of the lungs. The pulmonary vascular resistance is lowest at the FRC. Because it includes the RV, it cannot be calculated with normal spirometry:

$$FRC = ERV + RV$$

Inspiratory capacity is the maximum volume that can be inspired after a normal expiration:

$$IC = IRV + TV$$

Now it's time to practice using this information:

If a patient's total lung capacity is 6000 mL, functional residual capacity is 2400 mL, and inspiratory reserve volume is 3000 mL, what is the tidal volume?

Answer: 6000 – 2400 = inspiratory capacity = 3700 mL. Because IC = TV + IRV, 3700 – 3000 = 700 mL = TV.

This is a classic type of USMLE Step 1 question that doesn't require tertiary thinking but does require mastery of the equations and their relationships to one another in order to solve the problem quickly.

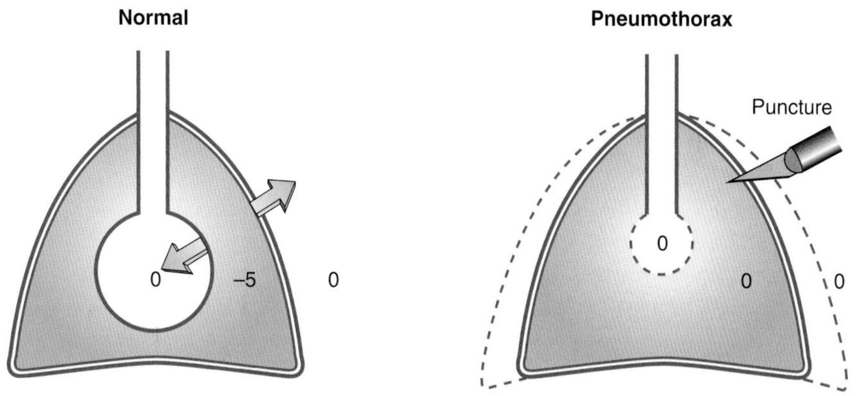

Fig. 17.6 In the resting state, the alveoli are attempting to collapse and the chest wall is attempting to expand, forming an equilibrium with negative intrapleural pressure. In a pneumothorax, the negative intrapleural pressure becomes atmospheric (or elevated, as in the case of a tension pneumothorax), and the alveoli collapse as the chest wall expands. *(From Costanzo LS.* Physiology. *4th ed. New York: Elsevier; 2009.)*

In addition to the previously stated lung volumes and capacities, there are three important spirometric measurements you should know:

- **Forced expiratory volume in 1 second (FEV_1)** is the volume of air that can be forcibly expired in 1 second after a full inspiration.
- **Forced vital capacity (FVC)** is the volume of air that can be **forcibly** expired after a full inspiration.
- The **FEV_1/FVC ratio** is normally about 0.8, meaning that about 80% of the VC can be forcibly expired in the first second. Obstructive lung disease generally produces a reduced FEV_1/FVC ratio (<0.8), whereas restrictive disease often produces a preserved or elevated FEV_1/FVC ratio (≥0.8). This will be discussed in greater detail later.

There are also two definitions of ventilation one should know: minute ventilation and alveolar ventilation. *Ventilation* refers to how much volume is being exchanged given a certain amount of time.

- Minute ventilation (V_E) = V_T × respiratory rate. This is the total volume moving in or out of the lungs per minute.
- Alveolar ventilation (V_A) = ($V_T - V_D$) × respiratory rate. This is the total volume of air that actually participates in gas exchange per minute. (V_D = volume of dead space).

Compliance and Elastance

Compliance refers to the **distensibility** of a system and is a measure of how volume changes in response to changes in pressure:

$$\text{Compliance} = \frac{\text{volume}}{\text{pressure}}$$

Compliance is inversely proportional to **elastance** because something that is very elastic requires a lot of pressure to change the volume a small amount (resists expansion, does not comply with expansion). At rest, the lung volume equals the FRC and the pressure in the lungs and airways is equal to atmospheric pressure. In this state of equilibrium, the lungs have a natural tendency to collapse, whereas the chest wall has an equal and opposite tendency to expand. These opposing forces create a negative intrapleural pressure. Thus, if air is introduced into the intrapleural space, as occurs in **pneumothorax,** the chest wall will follow its natural tendency to expand outward while the lungs collapse (Fig. 17.6).

Lung compliance varies in different disease states. Patients with **emphysema** have an increase in lung compliance because of destruction of elastic fibers in the terminal bronchioles and alveolar walls. At FRC, these patients' lungs have a decreased tendency to collapse relative to the tendency of the chest wall to expand. Their lung–chest wall system will therefore be in equilibrium at a higher FRC, and these patients will **often** have higher total lung capacities and **barrel-shaped** chests.

In **pulmonary fibrosis,** on the other hand, lung compliance is decreased because of the fibrotic tissue in the lung parenchyma. At FRC, these patients' lungs have an increased tendency to collapse relative to the tendency of the chest wall to expand. Their lung–chest wall system will be in equilibrium at lower FRCs, and these patients tend to have lower total lung capacities.

Gas Exchange

Gas exchange is the process whereby O_2 and CO_2 diffuse between the lungs and blood in the pulmonary capillaries and between the peripheral tissues and systemic capillaries. The rates of diffusion of O_2 and CO_2 are directly proportional to the partial pressure difference of the gas and surface area along which diffusion will take place, and inversely proportional to the thickness of the membrane barrier. This is given by the following equation, known as Fick's law (please note that the equations in this chapter should be understood, but not memorized, for Step 1):

$$\dot{V}x = DA\left(\frac{\Delta P}{\Delta X}\right)$$

where $\dot{V}\mathbf{x}$ is the volume of gas transferred per unit time, **D** is the diffusion coefficient of the gas, **A** is the surface area, **ΔP** is the difference in partial pressures of the gas between the membrane barrier, and **ΔX** is the thickness of the membrane. This is mostly intuitive; for a high volume of gas transferred per unit time (high $\dot{V}\mathbf{x}$), you must have a high diffusion coefficient (the gas must "like" crossing the membrane), a high surface area (as created collectively by the millions of alveoli), a high difference in partial pressure (if this is zero, it is at equilibrium and no gas exchange occurs), and a thin membrane (like the simple squamous epithelium of the type I pneumocyte).

Diffusion is decreased in certain lung diseases because of alterations in these variables. For example, diffusion impairment in emphysema results from destruction of the alveolar-capillary membranes, reducing the surface area (A) along which diffusion can occur. In pulmonary fibrosis and pulmonary edema, diffusion is impaired because of increases in the membrane thickness and interstitial volume (ΔX), respectively.

Gas exchange across the alveolar/capillary membrane can be classified as being **diffusion or perfusion limited** (Fig. 17.7).

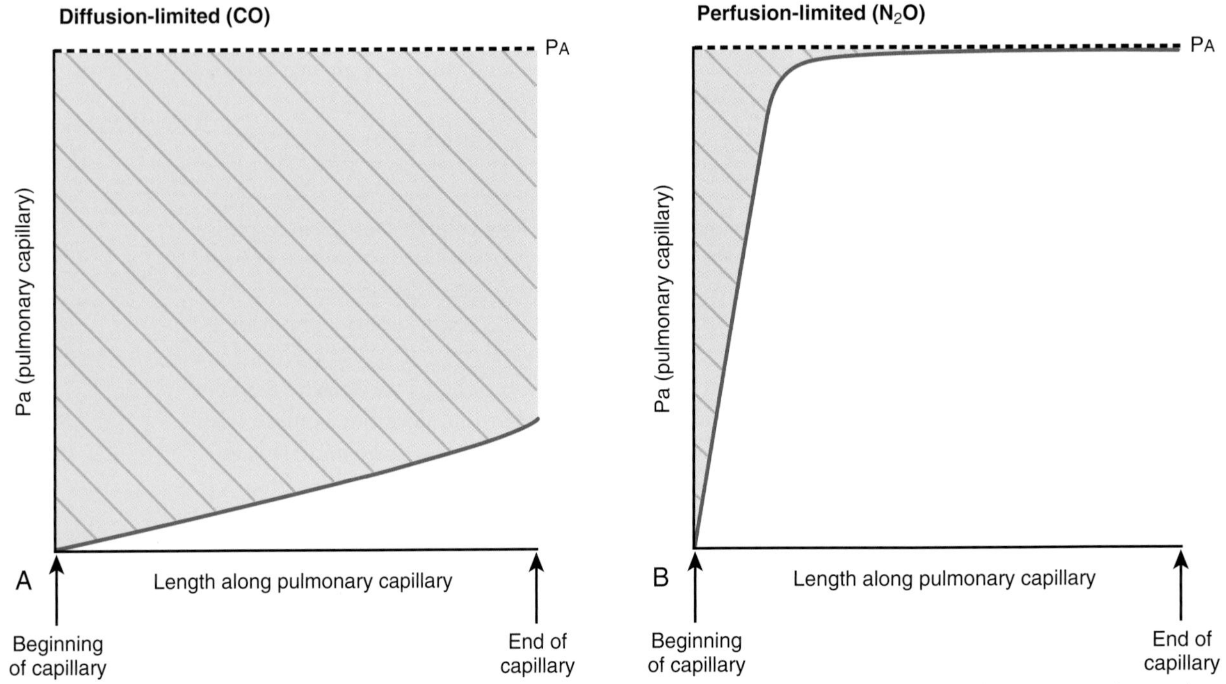

FIG. 17.7 A, Diffusion-limited exchange (e.g., carbon monoxide, CO) is characterized by relatively slow diffusion across the membrane, meaning that equilibrium is not reached by the time the blood reaches the end of the pulmonary capillary bed. **B,** Perfusion-limited exchange (e.g., oxygen in healthy individuals at rest) is characterized by complete equilibrium (ΔP is zero) by the end of the capillary bed. P_a, Arterial partial pressure; P_A, alveolar partial pressure. *(From Costanzo LS. Physiology. 4th ed. New York: Elsevier; 2009.)*

Diffusion-Limited Exchange

In diffusion-limited exchange, gas in the **alveoli does not equilibrate with blood by the time it reaches the end of the pulmonary capillary.** Thus the partial pressure gradient for the gas is maintained through the length of the capillary, and diffusion will continue to occur until the blood has left the alveolar-capillary membrane. In diffusion-limited exchange, the partial pressure of the gas in the alveoli and blood will not equilibrate (i.e., **ΔP** is never zero). Carbon monoxide (CO) is the classic example of a gas that undergoes diffusion-limited exchange. O_2 exchange can be diffusion-limited in disease states such as pulmonary fibrosis and emphysema, as well as in healthy individuals during strenuous exercise. Diffusion-limited exchange is largely why patients with severe pulmonary fibrosis and emphysema are hypoxemic and are unable to saturate their circulating hemoglobin at near 100%, like healthy individuals.

Perfusion-Limited Exchange

Under normal circumstances, in healthy individuals, O_2 exchange is perfusion limited. This means that in healthy individuals, O_2 normally equilibrates at some point earlier along the length of the pulmonary capillary, such that the partial pressure of oxygen in the alveoli (P_{AO_2}) and blood will equalize before the blood leaves the alveolar-capillary membrane. Thus in perfusion-limited exchange, the only way to increase the diffusion of a gas is to increase the blood flow through the pulmonary capillaries along the alveolar-capillary membrane. Nitrous oxide (N_2O), an inhaled anesthetic, is a classic example of another gas that undergoes perfusion-limited exchange.

Dead Space

The dead space is the volume of the lungs and airways that **does not take part in gas exchange.** It is a general term that includes both the actual anatomic dead space of the conducting airways and the physiologic dead space in the alveoli.

Anatomic dead space is the volume of the conducting airways (the conducting zone, discussed earlier), from the nose all the way down to the terminal bronchioles. Because there are no alveoli in the conducting airways, no gas exchange can occur and the conducting airways are dead space. The volume of the conducting airways is approximately 150 mL, approximately one-third of each 500-mL tidal volume. This means that only about 350 mL of air actually fills the alveoli and participates in gas exchange during a tidal volume breath.

Physiologic dead space (functional dead space) is a more abstract concept. Recall first that by definition, dead space is any part of the lungs or airways that does not participate in gas exchange. Gas exchange not only requires airflow into the alveoli but also requires perfusion (blood flow). If a portion of the lung is not adequately perfused for any reason, the alveoli in that portion will be unable to participate in gas exchange because there will not be any blood flow to those alveoli. This situation is called a ventilation-perfusion (V/Q) defect or mismatch, and the ventilation to the nonperfused alveoli is wasted. V/Q mismatch occurs in pathologic conditions, reducing perfusion to the lungs (e.g., an occlusive pulmonary embolus), but also occurs to a minor degree in normal healthy individuals at baseline. When upright, the apical portions of the lung are better ventilated than they are perfused; thus, some of this ventilation is wasted and contributes to the physiologic dead space in normal individuals. The volume of physiologic dead space is about equal to the anatomic dead space in normal lungs but can be significantly greater in conditions causing V/Q mismatch. The concept of V/Q mismatch will be discussed in greater detail later.

The volume of dead space can be calculated as follows:

$$V_D = V_T \times [(Pa_{CO_2} - Pe_{CO_2})/Pa_{CO_2}]$$

where V_D = dead space, V_T = tidal volume, Pa_{CO_2} = arterial P_{CO_2}, and Pe_{CO_2} = expired air P_{CO_2}.

Although this equation appears complex, it is relatively intuitive. The dead space is equal to the fraction of the tidal volume that does not participate in gas exchange. For example, if the entire tidal volume breath participated in gas exchange, the Pa_{CO_2} (arterial CO_2) and the expired air P_{CO_2} would be identical because everything has come to equilibrium. Therefore the dead space would be zero. In actuality, the arterial CO_2 will be higher than the expired CO_2 because the expired CO_2 (that was received by gas exchange) will mix with the air that did not participate in gas exchange (e.g., **the dead space**).

Oxygen Transport

Hemoglobin

Oxygen is transported in the blood in two forms, dissolved oxygen and oxygen bound to hemoglobin (Fig. 17.8), the latter of which is the most important. Hemoglobin A (comprising 97% of adult hemoglobin) is a globular protein composed of four polypeptide (two alpha [α] and two beta [β]) subunits and an iron-containing (Fe^{2+}) heme moiety. O_2 is poorly soluble in blood, so at a normal Pao_2 of 100 mm Hg, the amount of oxygen dissolved in blood is negligible and insufficient to meet the body's metabolic requirements. Hemoglobin solves this problem by reversibly binding O_2 and **carrying 98% of the total oxygen content of blood within erythrocytes.** Hemoglobin can bind four O_2 molecules when the iron is in the ferrous form (Fe^{2+}).

Adult hemoglobin (HbA) is composed of two alpha and two beta subunits and accounts for 97% of the total hemoglobin in children older than 6 months. During embryonic development, however, another type of hemoglobin, known as **fetal hemoglobin (HbF),** predominates. HbF is made from two alpha and two gamma (γ) subunits and has a **much higher affinity for O_2** than HbA because HbF binds more poorly with 2,3-bisphosphoglycerate (2,3-BPG), a potent modulator of the affinity of hemoglobin for O_2. HbF is physiologically critical to the growing fetus because it facilitates the transport of O_2 across the placenta by ensuring that the Hb circulating in the fetal circulation will be oxygenated by drawing O_2 from oxygenated maternal HbA.

Oxygen Content of Blood (Cao_2)

The O_2 content of arterial blood can be calculated using the following equation, in which Cao_2 is the O_2 content of blood; Hb is the concentration of hemoglobin in blood (in g/dL); Sao_2 is the percentage saturation of hemoglobin, with O_2 expressed as a fraction (e.g., 100% saturation corresponds to a Sao_2 of 1.00); and Pao_2 is the partial pressure of O_2 in the arterial blood:

$$Cao_2 = (\text{amount of oxygen bound to hemoglobin, major}) + (\text{amount of oxygen dissolved in plasma, minor})$$

$$Cao_2 = (1.34 \times Hb \times Sao_2) + \left(\underline{0.003} \times Pao_2\right)$$

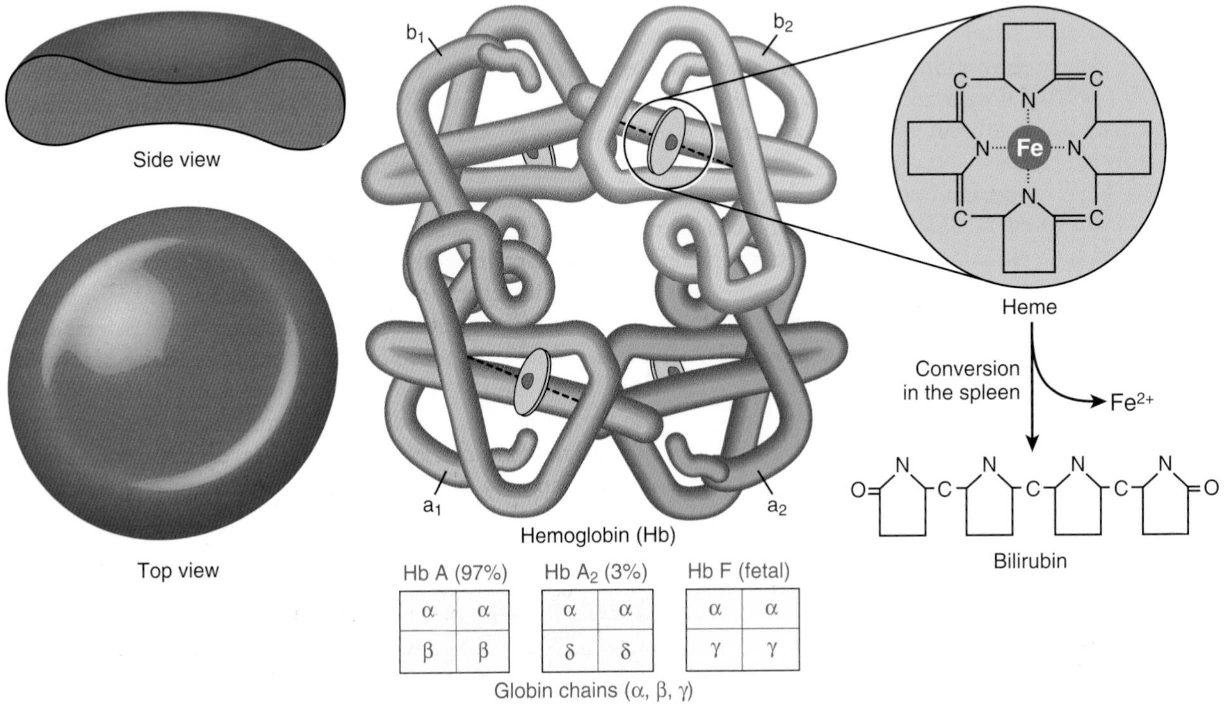

FIG. 17.8 Hemoglobin in red blood cells, showing the biconcave disc of the red blood cell *(left)*, hemoglobin A, composed of four subunits *(middle)*, and the structure of an individual heme group, with its Fe^{2+} group in the center *(right)*. *(From Damjanov I. Pathophysiology. Philadelphia: Elsevier; 2008.)*

This equation is not important to memorize, but its value is to demonstrate that the **vast majority of the O_2 content carried by blood is bound to hemoglobin,** with O_2 dissolved in blood (**0.003** × PaO_2) contributing only negligibly. We also see from this equation that each gram of hemoglobin binds approximately 1.34 mL of O_2, so assuming a normal Hb concentration of 15 g/dL at 100% saturation, the O_2 binding capacity of all the Hb in a healthy individual is about 20.1 mL/dL of blood.

Oxygen Delivery to Tissues

The O_2 that enters the bloodstream via the lungs is carried to the tissues by the cardiac output (Q). Oxygen delivery to the tissues (DO_2) can be calculated using the Q and CaO_2 as follows:

$$DO_2 = (\text{rate of pumping the oxygenated blood through the body}) \times (\text{oxygen content of that blood})$$

$$DO_2 = Q \times CaO_2$$

We can see from this equation that the two ways to increase O_2 delivery to the tissues in a clinical context are to increase the Q or CaO_2. Q can be increased by ensuring adequate preload (e.g., giving intravenous [IV] fluids), increasing contractility (e.g., using β_1-adrenergic agonists such as dobutamine), or decreasing the afterload (e.g., using an arteriolar vasodilator such as nitroprusside). Because Hb contains almost all the oxygen content of blood, CaO_2 is best increased by ensuring maximum oxygen saturation (SaO_2; such as through supplemental oxygen to maximize oxygenated Hb) and increasing the blood Hb concentration (e.g., through a red blood cell transfusion). Note that increasing the oxygen further after 100% saturation will not significantly change the CaO_2 because once the Hb molecules are saturated with oxygen, the dissolved fraction in plasma (the PaO_2) is negligible because it is being multiplied by 0.003.

Hemoglobin-O_2 Dissociation Curve

The Hb-O_2 dissociation curve (Fig. 17.9) plots the percentage saturation of Hb as a function of partial pressure of O_2 (PO_2). The curve is **sigmoidal in shape** because of a fascinating property of hemoglobin known as **positive cooperativity.** Hemoglobin exits in two forms, a **tensed (T) state** and a **relaxed (R) state.** It is in a tensed state when no O_2 is bound to the heme moiety, and this tensed conformation sterically inhibits the approach of O_2. When enough O_2 molecules bind to Hb, it snaps into the relaxed state, in which it has 150 times more affinity for O_2 than the tensed state. Thus, when one molecule of O_2 binds to Hb, Hb relaxes and increases its affinity for a second molecule of O_2. Once the second molecule of O_2 has bound, its affinity for a third molecule of O_2 is still greater, and so on, until it is fully saturated, with a maximum of four O_2 molecules. This property is that of positive cooperativity.

Because of the sigmoidal shape of the Hb-O_2 dissociation curve, a PO_2 of 100 mm Hg results in 100% hemoglobin saturation, whereas a PO_2 of only 25 mm Hg still yields 50% saturation ($P_{50} = PO_2$,

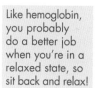

Like hemoglobin, you probably do a better job when you're in a relaxed state, so sit back and relax!

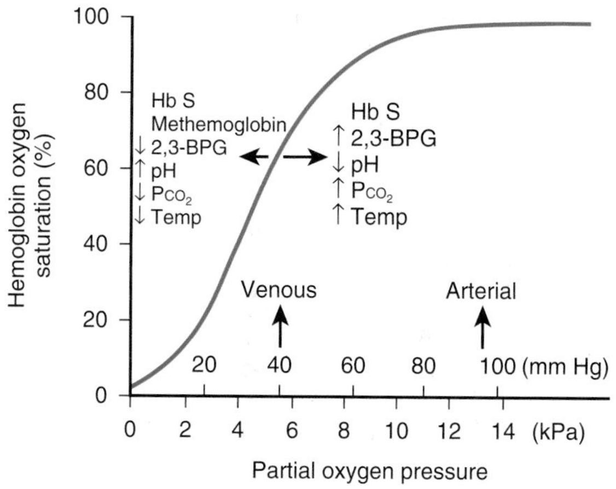

FIG. 17.9 Hemoglobin-oxygen dissociation curve. A rightward shift will cause a decreased affinity for oxygen because a higher partial pressure of oxygen will be required for the same oxygen saturation; examples include increased 2,3-DPG, decreased pH (acidemia), increased PCO_2, and increased temperature. A leftward shift will cause an increased affinity for oxygen, meaning that hemoglobin wants to hold onto the oxygen as much as possible; most of the examples are the opposite of the causes of a rightward shift, but also includes fetal hemoglobin (HbF) because it cannot bind 2,3-DPG as effectively. *(From Damjanov I.* Pathophysiology. *Philadelphia: Elsevier; 2008.)*

at which hemoglobin is 50% saturated). The curve is flattest between 60 and 100 mm Hg, indicating that humans can tolerate a fair degree of reduction in Po_2 without dramatically reducing the oxygen content of hemoglobin.

Shifts in the Hemoglobin-O_2 Dissociation Curve: Changes in the local environment through which hemoglobin circulates also change the affinity of hemoglobin for O_2, causing the Hb-O_2 dissociation curve to shift to the right or shift to the left. The definition of Hb affinity for O_2 is defined as the P_{50}. The P_{50} is the partial pressure of O_2 at which the hemoglobin saturation is 50% (see Fig. 17.9). In other words, for high affinity, there is a low partial pressure of O_2 that will result in 50% saturation of hemoglobin, and vice versa.

Shifts to the Right: The Hb-O_2 dissociation curve will shift rightward (increased P_{50}) when there is a **decreased affinity** for O_2. This decreased affinity facilitates unloading of O_2 for use by the tissues. Increases in Pco_2, temperature, and 2,3-BPG and decreases in pH cause a rightward shift of the curve. If one thinks about each of the factors that causes a rightward shift, it becomes readily apparent that improved unloading of O_2 is physiologically advantageous in these situations. For example, an increase in peripheral tissue metabolic activity, such as that which occurs with vigorous exercise, will result in increased production of CO_2 by active skeletal muscle, an increase in H^+ production, and a decrease in pH. Metabolically active tissue, such as the exercising skeletal muscle in this scenario, has a higher O_2 demand. Thus the resultant rightward shift facilitates the unloading of O_2 from Hb to these tissues, which need it most. The effect of decreased pH and increased Pco_2 on the Hb-O_2 dissociation curve is known as the **Bohr effect.** Hypoxemia at high altitudes facilitates production of 2,3-BPG, which causes a rightward shift and helps facilitate delivery of O_2 to the tissues.

Shifts to the Left: The curve will shift leftward (decreased P_{50}) when there is an **increased affinity** of Hb for O_2. This increased affinity makes the unloading of O_2 more difficult. Decreases in Pco_2, temperature, and 2,3-BPG and increases in pH cause a leftward shift of the curve. Leftward shifts of the curve are also physiologically advantageous because when demand for O_2 is lower, O_2 is more strongly bound to hemoglobin and less of it is unloaded to the tissues. As noted, HbF has a left-shifted Hb-O_2 dissociation curve because of its much higher affinity for O_2, which is beneficial to the fetus.

Carboxyhemoglobin

Carboxyhemoglobin is a form of Hb created when carbon monoxide is bound to Hb instead of O_2. **CO binds to Hb with a 250-fold greater affinity than O_2 and reduces the O_2-carrying capacity of Hb** by binding where O_2 normally would. CO also causes a leftward shift of the Hb-O_2 dissociation curve, making it even harder for carboxyhemoglobin to unload the reduced amount of O_2 it can carry to the tissues. The excessive amount of carboxyhemoglobin that is seen in CO poisoning is highly lethal and must be immediately treated with 100% O_2 at very high flow rates to displace the CO bound to Hb with O_2. For some patients who are extremely hypoxemic, O_2 may be administered inside a hyperbaric chamber because O_2 delivered at elevated pressures helps displace CO from the Hb. Of importance, a patient with carbon monoxide poisoning may actually have a pulse oximetry reading that is falsely normal. The best test for oxygen saturation in carbon monoxide poisoning would be an arterial blood gas.

Patients with CO poisoning are often described as having cherry red skin.

Methemoglobin

Hemoglobin normally contains iron in the reduced ferrous state (Fe^{2+}) because this is the only form of iron that can bind O_2. When the Fe^{2+} in Hb is oxidized to ferric iron (Fe^{3+}), it is called methemoglobin and is unable to bind O_2. Methemoglobinemia is caused by drug exposures (e.g., nitrates, dapsone), hemoglobinopathies, and enzyme deficiencies. It is treated by administering methylene blue intravenously.

Interestingly, methemoglobin has an affinity for cyanide (CN^-) that is cleverly used in the treatment of CN^- poisoning. CN^- antidote kits contain nitrites and sodium thiosulfate. Nitrites are administered to oxidize hemoglobin and cause an intentional increase in methemoglobin levels. Because of its natural affinity for CN^-, the methemoglobin quickly binds CN^-, keeping CN^- from exerting its lethal inhibition of the cytochrome oxidase system. Then, thiosulfate is administered to bind the CN^- and form thiocyanate, which can be excreted renally.

Patients with methemoglobinemia poisoning may have "chocolate brown" blood and cyanosis.

Oxygen Disorders

Hypoxemia (Low Pa_{O_2}): Hypoxemia is defined as a **low arterial P_{O_2} (Pa_{O_2}).** The **A-a gradient** (alveolar-arterial P_{O_2} gradient) is an indirect measure of ventilation-perfusion abnormalities (discussed in greater detail later) and is essential to differentiating causes of hypoxemia. The A-a gradient is calculated as follows:

$$A - a \text{ gradient} = (\text{alveolar } P_{O_2}\text{, calculated by alveolar air equation}) - (\text{arterial } P_{O_2}\text{, measured by arterial blood gas})$$

$$A - a \text{ gradient} = P_{AO_2} - Pa_{O_2}$$

Pa_{O_2} is measured directly by performing arterial blood gas analysis in the laboratory. P_{AO_2}, on the other hand, is calculated using the **alveolar gas equation,** as follows:

$$P_{AO_2} = (\text{pressure of inspired oxygen}) - \left(\begin{array}{l}\text{pressure of } CO_2\text{, modified by amount of} \\ CO_2 \text{ produced per oxygen consumed}\end{array}\right)$$

$$P_{AO_2} = P_{IO_2} - \frac{Pa_{CO_2}}{R}$$

P_{IO_2} in turn is calculated as follows:

$$P_{IO_2} = \text{fraction of inspired air that is oxygen (barometric pressure} - \text{water vapor pressure)}$$

$$P_{IO_2} = F_{IO_2}\,(P_B - P_{H_2O})$$

Because F_{IO_2} = 0.21 (at all altitudes, unless using supplemental oxygen), P_B = 760 mm Hg and P_{H_2O} = 47 mm Hg at sea level while breathing room air, and P_{IO_2} = 150 mm Hg, P_{AO_2} can be approximated under these conditions as follows:

$$P_{AO_2} = 150 - \frac{Pa_{CO_2}}{R}$$

where R is usually 0.8.

The A-a gradient in healthy individuals is normally less than 10 mm Hg because O_2 normally equilibrates between the alveolar gas and arterial blood. However, O_2 is unable to equilibrate fully in certain conditions such as diffusion impairments (e.g., pulmonary fibrosis), V/Q mismatch, or right-to-left cardiac or pulmonary shunts, resulting in an elevated A-a gradient. On the other hand, high altitudes and conditions resulting in hypoventilation (e.g., obstructive sleep apnea, obesity, depressed respiratory drive, opiate overdose) do not interfere with the ability of alveolar gas and arterial blood to equilibrate and therefore do not result in an elevated A-a gradient. Some common causes of hypoxemia and their effect on the A-a gradient are summarized in Table 17.1.

Hypoxia (Low DO_2): Hypoxia is defined as reduced O_2 delivery to the tissues. If we recall the equation for O_2 delivery (D_{O_2} = Q × Ca_{O_2}), we see that the two factors that can reduce D_{O_2} are a reduced cardiac output (Q) or reduced blood O_2 content (Ca_{O_2}). Because the two most important components of Ca_{O_2}— Ca_{O_2} = (1.34 × **Hb** × **Sa_{O_2}**) + (0.003 × Pa_{O_2})—are the concentration of Hb in blood and the percentage saturation of Hb with O_2 (Sa_{O_2}), we can reason that hypoxemia (↓ Pa_{O_2} → ↓ Sa_{O_2}) and anemia (↓ hemoglobin concentration) are causes of hypoxia, in addition to a reduced Q. Moreover, because CO poisoning and methemoglobinemia dramatically impede hemoglobin's ability to bind O_2 and therefore reduce the Ca_{O_2}, CO poisoning and methemoglobinemia are other

P_{AO_2} = alveolar P_{O_2}

Pa_{O_2} = arterial P_{O_2}

P_{IO_2} = inspired air P_{O_2}

Pa_{CO_2} = arterial P_{CO_2}

R = respiratory quotient = CO_2 produced/O_2 consumed ≅ 0.8

F_{IO_2} = fractional concentration of inspired O_2 ≅ 0.21 in room air

P_B = barometric pressure = 760 mm Hg at sea level

P_{H_2O} = partial pressure of H_2O in humidified gas = 47 mm Hg

TABLE 17.1 Common Causes of Hypoxemia and Their Effect on the A-a Gradient

CAUSES OF HYPOXEMIA	A-a GRADIENT
High altitude (because of low P_B)	Normal
Hypoventilation (because of increased Pa_{CO_2} resulting in low P_{AO_2})	Normal
Diffusion impairment (e.g., pulmonary fibrosis, edema)	Elevated
V/Q defects	Elevated
Right-to-left cardiac or pulmonary shunt	Elevated

important causes of hypoxia that must be considered. Several causes of hypoxia and their mechanisms are summarized in Table 17.2.

CO_2 Transport

CO_2 is a major product of oxidative metabolism in the tissues and is transported to the lungs by venous blood in three forms:

Bicarbonate: This is the predominant form of CO_2 transport in the blood, comprising about **90% of CO_2 transported in blood** (Fig. 17.10). CO_2 produced by the peripheral tissues enters the erythrocytes through diffusion, where it combines with H_2O to produce H_2CO_3 in a reaction catalyzed by **carbonic anhydrase**. H_2CO_3 instantaneously dissociates into H^+ and HCO_3^-. The H^+ generated is buffered by deoxyhemoglobin; this buffering is important in maintaining the pH in the venous blood and within the erythrocytes in physiologic range. Finally, a large portion of the HCO_3^- that is generated is pumped into the plasma in exchange for chloride. When the erythrocytes enter the pulmonary circulation, all these reactions reverse, and the generated CO_2 is expired through the lungs.

Bound Directly to Hemoglobin: A small fraction of CO_2 that enters the erythrocytes binds directly to the N terminus of Hb, forming carbaminohemoglobin. This accounts for about 5% of the CO_2 content of blood.

Dissolved CO_2: Like O_2, CO_2 is poorly soluble in blood. Dissolved CO_2 accounts for approximately 5% of the CO_2 content of blood.

Haldane effect: Desaturated Hb has a greater buffering capacity than saturated Hb, allowing deoxyhemoglobin in the tissues to bind more CO_2. Saturation of Hb with O_2 upon entering the lungs promotes the release of buffered H^+, thus promoting the formation of CO_2, which can then be expired.

Pulmonary Circulation

The pulmonary circulation is a lower pressure and lower resistance system than the systemic circulation. Because the circulatory system is a closed circuit, the cardiac output of the right ventricle equals the pulmonary blood flow, which in turn equals the left ventricular output.

TABLE 17.2 Causes of Hypoxia and Their Mechanisms

CAUSE OF HYPOXIA	MECHANISM
↓ Cardiac output (Q)	↓ Blood flow to tissues
Hypoxemia	↓ Pao_2 → ↓ Sao_2 → ↓ Cao_2
Anemia	↓ Hemoglobin → ↓ Cao_2
Carbon monoxide poisoning	↓ Sao_2 → ↓ Cao_2
Methemoglobinemia	↓ Sao_2 → ↓ Cao_2
Cyanide poisoning (technically causes intracellular hypoxia)	Prevents O_2 uptake by tissues through inhibition of cytochrome oxidase in mitochondria

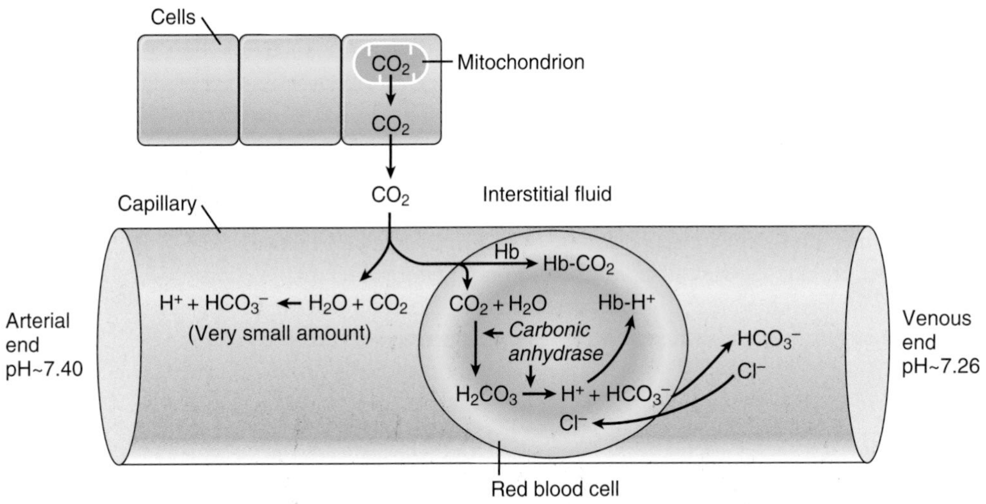

FIG. 17.10 Carbon dioxide transport. The CO_2 diffuses into the red blood cell (RBC), combines with water, and is catalyzed by carbonic anhydrase to make carbonic acid (H_2CO_3). This breaks down into H^+ (buffered by deoxyhemoglobin) and HCO_3^- (bicarbonate), the latter of which is exchanged for chloride. *(From Brown T. Rapid Review Physiology. 2nd ed. Philadelphia: Elsevier; 2011.)*

Regulation of Pulmonary Perfusion

Oxygen exerts an elegant regulatory effect on the flow of blood through the pulmonary circulation that is crucial to maximizing gas exchange in the lungs. When the partial pressure of O_2 within alveoli (PAO_2) decreases, the pulmonary vasculature around alveoli with a low PAO_2 will constrict to shift blood flow away from these alveoli toward alveoli with a higher PAO_2. This **hypoxic vasoconstriction** ensures that blood flows preferentially to regions of lung that are better ventilated so that ventilation and perfusion are matched as well as possible. Understanding the concept of hypoxic vasoconstriction is essential to understanding the mechanism whereby certain lung diseases and chronic hypoxemia can result in pulmonary hypertension, discussed later in greater detail.

Ventilation-to-Perfusion Ratio

The ratio of alveolar ventilation (V) to pulmonary perfusion (Q) is the **ventilation-to-perfusion** or **V/Q** ratio. Although having an equal amount of V and Q (V/Q = 1) is ideal in maximizing gas exchange, the normal value of V/Q ratio across the entire lung in a person who is standing happens to be about 0.8. This means that the amount of alveolar ventilation (measured in L/min) is about 80% of the amount of the perfusion (L/min) in the lungs. The unevenness of V/Q across the entire lung is the result of perfusion being uneven across the three lung zones (Fig. 17.11) when a person is standing. Because of the effect of gravity in the upright lung, the more dependent portions of the lung receive more blood flow and are better perfused than the less dependent portions of the lung (i.e., blood flow is greatest in zone 3 and least in zone 1). Although there is some regional variation in ventilation as well, it is not nearly as dramatic as the regional variation in perfusion, so **the V/Q ratio is greatest in zone 1** (where V/Q = 3) and **lowest in zone 3** (where V/Q = 0.6). Thus one could say that when standing upright, the apical portions of the lung are better ventilated than they are perfused (V/Q >1), resulting in so-called wasted ventilation, whereas the lung bases are better perfused than they are ventilated (V/Q <1), resulting in wasted perfusion. When a person is supine, however, the effect of gravity is removed and blood flow is almost uniform throughout the lung, resulting in an average V/Q closer to 1 across the lungs.

The regional variations in V/Q lead to corresponding variation in the efficiency of gas exchange in the different lung zones. Because of these differences, the apical portions of the lungs (where V/Q is higher) have a relatively higher Po_2 and lower Pco_2 because gas exchange is greatest here. Similarly, the lung bases (where V/Q is lower) have a relatively lower Po_2 and higher Pco_2 because less gas exchange occurs at the bases, given the low V/Q ratio there.

V/Q Mismatch: There are two extremes of V/Q mismatch that are important to understanding the pathophysiology of certain lung conditions (Fig. 17.12). A **shunt** describes a situation in which blood flow is normal but zero ventilation takes place (i.e., V/Q = 0). A shunt can occur in a small segment of the lungs (e.g., lobar pneumonia with alveolar infiltrates), an entire lung (e.g., endobronchial tumor occluding a mainstem bronchus), or even in both lungs (e.g., piece of food occluding the trachea). In this situation, no gas exchange can take place in the portion of lung that is perfused but not ventilated. In this shunt physiology, the portion of blood entering the region of lung with airway obstruction (the shunt fraction) has the same Po_2 and Pco_2 as mixed venous blood. When this blood mixes with systemic arterial blood, it lowers the overall Pao_2 and can cause **significant** hypoxemia, depending on the amount of lung affected by the shunt physiology and whether or not the affected individual has underlying pulmonary disease, such as emphysema. The reduction in Pao_2 caused by

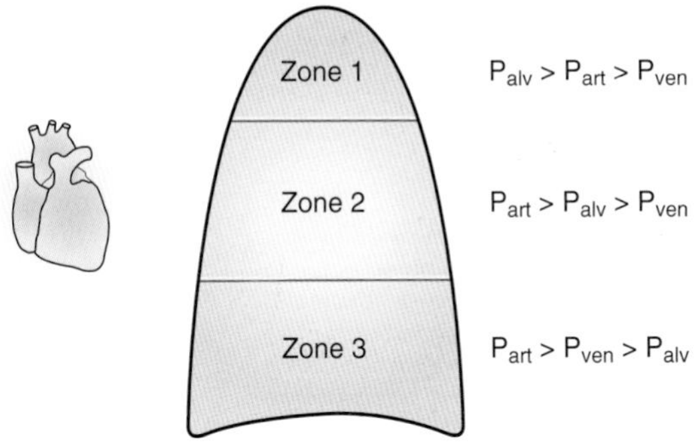

FIG. 17.11 Zones of the lung. *Zone 1,* Alveolar pressure is higher than arterial or venous pressure. *Zone 2,* Alveolar pressure is lower than arterial but higher than venous pressure. *Zone 3,* Alveolar pressure is lower than arterial or venous pressure. P_{alv}, ***; P_{art}, ***; P_{ven}, ***. *(From Brown T. Rapid Review Physiology. 2nd ed. Philadelphia: Elsevier; 2011.)*

shunting causes a **widening of the A-a gradient.** Shunting as a result of the extreme V/Q mismatch described is identical to the effect from right-to-left cardiac shunts that occur with abnormalities of cardiac anatomy.

The other extreme of V/Q mismatch occurs when areas of lung that are well ventilated are not perfused (V/Q = ∞), resulting in additional **dead space.** Recall that dead space is the volume of the lungs and airways that does not take part in gas exchange. Because no gas exchange can occur in the absence of perfusion, the ventilation of nonperfused alveoli is wasted ventilation, and the Po_2 and Pco_2 of the alveolar gas will be similar to that of inspired air in the trachea or other airways of the conducting zone that do not participate in gas exchange. Dead space physiology is best illustrated by a pulmonary embolus occluding blood flow to a portion of lung or even an entire lung in the case of an embolus in one of the main pulmonary arteries.

Both extremes of V/Q mismatch result in elevations of the A-a gradient but **can be differentiated by the administration of 100% O_2.** In a significant shunt, administering 100% O_2 cannot overcome the hypoxemia caused by the shunt. On the other spectrum of V/Q mismatch, in which dead space is created because of occlusion of blood flow to well-ventilated lung, 100% O_2 should result in some improvement in Pao_2. This method of using 100% O_2 delivery to differentiate shunt from other causes of V/Q mismatch is often referred to as a shunt study in the clinical setting.

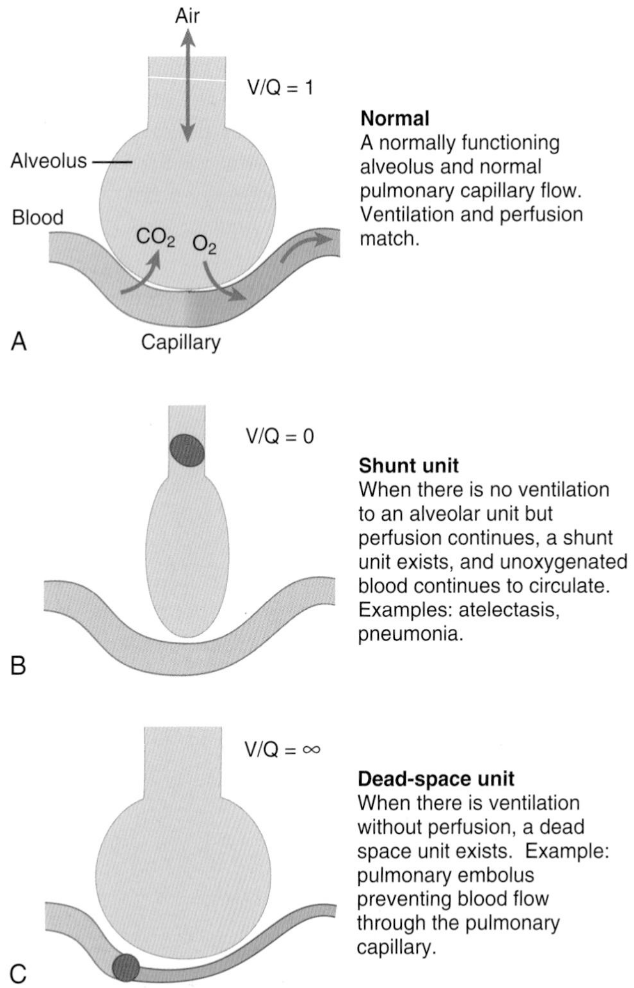

Air
V/Q = 1
Normal
A normally functioning alveolus and normal pulmonary capillary flow. Ventilation and perfusion match.
Alveolus
Blood
CO2 O2
A
Capillary
V/Q = 0
Shunt unit
When there is no ventilation to an alveolar unit but perfusion continues, a shunt unit exists, and unoxygenated blood continues to circulate. Examples: atelectasis, pneumonia.
B
V/Q = ∞
Dead-space unit
When there is ventilation without perfusion, a dead space unit exists. Example: pulmonary embolus preventing blood flow through the pulmonary capillary.
C

FIG. 17.12 Examples of V/Q mismatch. **A,** Normal, in which the ventilation and perfusion match each other for optimal gas exchange. **B,** Shunt, in which there is perfusion without ventilation. This leads to deoxygenated blood going to the systemic circulation, because the blood passing through the shunt does not participate in gas exchange. Examples include atelectasis, pneumonia, and foreign bodies. **C,** Dead space, in which there is ventilation without perfusion. This is normally present as anatomic dead space in the conducting zones of the respiratory system (e.g., the trachea) but is abnormal in the alveoli. In this example, the patient has a pulmonary embolus blocking blood flow to a portion of the lung. *(From Carroll RG.* Elsevier's Integrated Physiology. *Philadelphia: Elsevier; 2006.)*

RESPIRATORY PATHOLOGY

Pneumonia

Infections of the pulmonary parenchyma are referred to as pneumonia. Pneumonia can be classified based on anatomic distribution, causative organism, or whether it is community or hospital acquired.

Typical (lobar) pneumonia is usually caused by ***Streptococcus pneumoniae.*** Occasionally, *Klebsiella pneumoniae, Staphylococcus aureus, Haemophilus influenzae,* or other gram-negative rods may be the causative organism. Lobar pneumonias are characterized by intraalveolar exudates that create areas of **dense consolidation.** Consolidations may be lobar or multilobar or even involve the entire lung and are often readily visible on chest x-ray examination (Fig. 17.13A).

Atypical pneumonia is so-named because it presents **without prominent consolidation** and has a less aggressive course than lobar or bronchopneumonia. This type of pneumonia results in patchy and diffuse inflammation in the **alveolar interstitium.** It is caused by **viral infections** (adenoviruses, respiratory syncytial virus [RSV]) and bacterial infections not seen in lobar pneumonias: ***Mycoplasma*** (most common cause), ***Legionella,*** and ***Chlamydia.*** Atypical pneumonia can be treated with **macrolide antibiotics** (erythromycin, azithromycin, clarithromycin), fluoroquinolones (ciprofloxacin, levofloxacin), or doxycycline.

Bronchopneumonia begins initially as an acute bronchitis that extends into adjacent lung parenchyma. Bronchopneumonias are most often caused by *S. aureus, Streptococcus pyogenes,* or *H. influenzae.* Unlike lobar pneumonia, bronchopneumonia is **multifocal, heterogeneous, and patchy** on chest x-ray examination, with no clear lobar distribution.

Hospital-acquired pneumonia is most often caused by gram-negative rods such as *Pseudomonas aeruginosa* (especially in patients on ventilators), *Klebsiella,* and *Escherichia coli. P. aeruginosa* is also a common cause of pneumonia and chronic infection in patients with cystic fibrosis (CF).

***Pneumocystis* pneumonia (PCP)** is caused by *Pneumocystis jirovecii,* which before highly active antiretroviral therapy was the most common pneumonia-causing pathogen in patients with AIDS (CD4 count <200/μL; Fig. 17.13B). PCP is often suspected by the presence of its characteristic appearance on chest radiographs and hypoxemia in an immunocompromised patient. It is also often **associated with an elevated level of lactate dehydrogenase (LDH).** First-line treatment is TMP-SMX; second choice is dapsone.

Lung Abscess

Lung abscesses are confined collections of pus within the lung parenchyma and are **usually caused by aspiration of oropharyngeal secretions.** Risk factors for aspiration include any condition that causes

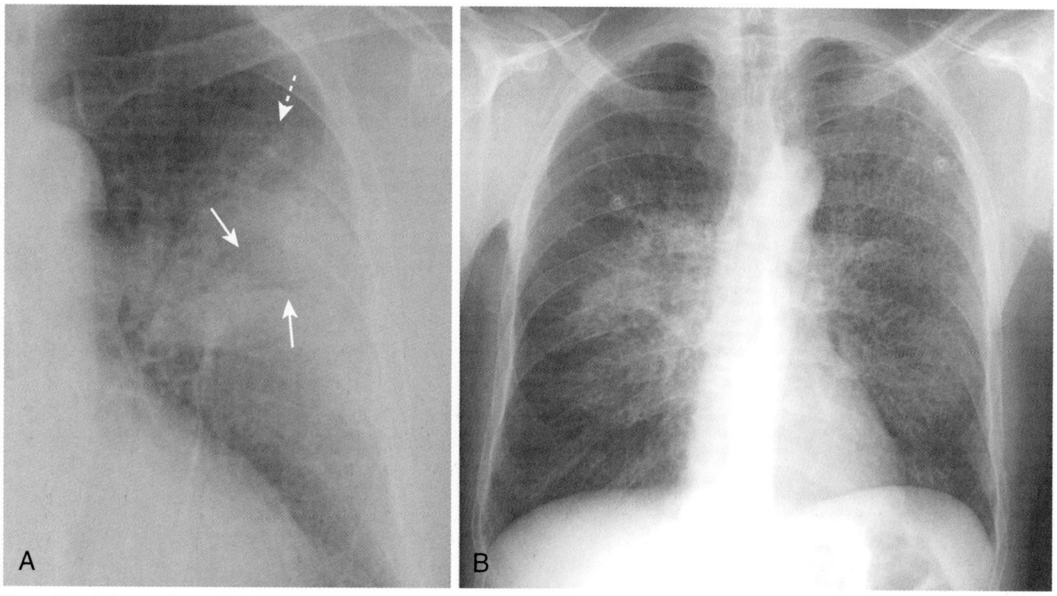

Fig. 17.13 A, Left upper lobe pneumonia. **B,** *Pneumocystis* pneumonia with diffuse interstitial lung disease (reticular) shown. *(From Herring W. Learning Radiology. 2nd ed. Philadelphia: Elsevier; 2011.)*

altered mental status and impairs one's ability to protect the airway, such as alcoholism, dementia, or epilepsy. The pathogens found in lung abscesses are usually a mix of aerobes and anaerobes, such as *S. aureus, Peptostreptococcus,* and *Fusobacterium.* Clinical findings include spiking fevers and **cough productive of foul-smelling sputum.** Chest radiography and chest computed tomography (CT) demonstrate cavitation with an air-fluid level. The initial antibiotic of choice is often **clindamycin,** which provides gram-positive, methicillin-resistant *S. aureus* (MRSA), and anaerobic coverage.

Lung Cancer

Despite advances in cancer therapy, primary lung cancer (bronchogenic carcinoma) unfortunately is still the **leading cause of cancer death in men and women** in the United States (Table 17.3).

TABLE 17.3 Lung Cancer

CANCER TYPE AND LOCATION IN LUNGS	COMMENTS
Adenocarcinoma, bronchial; location, peripheral	Often develops at sites of previous lung injury or inflammation (e.g., healed tuberculous granuloma) **Most common type in women and nonsmokers** Can have well-differentiated glandular elements (stains positive for mucin) or papillary lesions on histopathologic examination
Adenocarcinoma, bronchoalveolar; location, peripheral	**Unrelated to smoking** Can coalesce to give appearance of pneumonia-like consolidation on chest radiograph Possible paraneoplastic syndrome is hypertrophic osteoarthropathy, a syndrome of digital clubbing, periostitis of long bones, and arthritis (may present as pain along ulna or fibula) Originates from **Clara cells** Malignant cells grow along existing alveolar structures without destroying them
Squamous cell carcinoma (SCC); location, central	**Strongly linked to smoking** Hilar masses often seen on imaging Tendency toward cavitation Possible paraneoplastic syndrome is **PTHrP** overproduction, which can cause **hypercalcemia** On histopathologic examination, keratin pearls and intercellular bridges often visible
Small cell (oat cell) carcinoma; location, central	Strongly linked to smoking Highly malignant with early metastases Common paraneoplastic syndromes are **ectopic ACTH** production (Cushing syndrome), **ectopic ADH** production (SIADH), **Lambert-Eaton syndrome** (weakness from antibodies against presynaptic calcium channels) Originates from the neuroendocrine Kulchitsky cells On histopathologic examination, small highly basophilic cells that are poorly differentiated Generally inoperable because of frequent metastases, but **highly responsive to initial chemotherapy**
Large cell carcinoma; location, peripheral	Unrelated to smoking Highly malignant with early metastases Undifferentiated and anaplastic on histopathologic examination, with large nuclei May secrete β-hCG Poorly responsive to chemotherapy; often treated surgically Prognosis very poor
Bronchial carcinoid; location, random	Low-grade malignant neuroendocrine tumor that rarely metastasizes **Serotonin-secreting tumor** Sometimes presents with wheezing in addition to more typical symptoms of lung cancer Carcinoid syndrome rarely occurs but may present with flushing, diarrhea, wheezing, and hypotension Most resistant to radiation and chemotherapy; surgical excision necessary
Mesothelioma; location, adjacent to pleura	Rapidly progressive malignancy arising from pleural serosa Strongly associated with asbestos exposure, although adenocarcinoma still more common in those exposed to asbestos Unrelated to smoking Causes pleural effusions that are often hemorrhagic Surgery, chemotherapy, and radiation often unsuccessful **Psammoma bodies** visible on histopathologic examination
Pancoast (superior sulcus) tumor; location, lung apex	Not a histopathologically distinct type of lung cancer because most are actually SCCs Anatomically distinct given apical location, which may affect cervical sympathetic plexus, causing **Horner syndrome** (ptosis, miosis, anhydrosis) May cause shoulder weakness if affecting the brachial plexus
Metastasis to the lungs; location, random	**More common than primary lung cancers** Breast, colon, prostate, and renal cell carcinomas most common primary cancers to metastasize to lungs Often present with **multiple lung nodules** on chest imaging

ACTH, Adrenocorticotropic hormone; ADH, antidiuretic hormone; PTHrP, parathyroid hormone–related protein; SIADH, syndrome of inappropriate antidiuretic hormone.

Smoking is the greatest risk factor for developing lung cancer and is believed to cause more than 90% of cases. Patients with lung cancer may present with a **new cough, change in a chronic cough, dyspnea, hemoptysis, anorexia, or unintentional weight loss.** Patients with primary lung cancers present more often with cough, whereas those with metastases to the lung from a different primary cancer more commonly present with dyspnea. Patients may also present with symptoms or signs related to paraneoplastic syndromes associated with certain types of lung cancer (see Table 17.3). Almost all patients with lung cancer have abnormal findings on chest radiographs or chest CT, such as lung nodules, hilar lymphadenopathy, or infiltrates (Fig. 17.14). A tissue or cytology specimen is needed to make the diagnosis.

Superior vena cava (SVC) syndrome is an infrequent complication of lung cancer that you should know about in addition to the paraneoplastic syndromes. SVC syndrome occurs when a primary lung cancer compresses the SVC, **resulting in swelling of the face, neck, and bilateral upper extremities,** as well as **visibly dilated veins on the anterior chest wall** (Fig. 17.15). The SVC is located in the mediastinum, so the presence of SVC syndrome suggests that cancer has spread to the mediastinum, a poor prognostic indicator.

Pulmonary Embolism

Pulmonary embolism is a potentially lethal condition that occurs when a pulmonary artery or one of its branches is occluded by something that has traveled (embolized) from elsewhere in the body. The vast majority of pulmonary emboli originate from a thrombus formed in the femoral veins and other deep veins of the leg, known as a **deep venous thrombosis.** When a thrombus is the source, this condition is called **pulmonary thromboembolism.** The three categories of risk factors for deep venous thrombosis and pulmonary embolism are collectively known as **Virchow's triad—stasis** (e.g., long airplane flights, immobility after hip surgery), **hypercoagulability** (e.g., factor V Leiden, oral contraceptives, malignancy), and **endothelial damage.** The basic pathophysiology of this condition relates to the severe V/Q mismatch that takes place, as well as the impediment to forward flow and resultant pulmonary hypertension. Patients who suffer an acute pulmonary embolism often experience dyspnea, tachypnea, tachycardia, hypoxemia, and pleuritic chest pain.

Patients suspected of having a pulmonary embolism should undergo **CT angiography** (Fig. 17.16), which allows visualization of the emboli, or less commonly a **V/Q scan,** which looks for areas of lung that are well ventilated but not perfused. Pulmonary thromboembolism is generally treated with **anticoagulation** using unfractionated or low-molecular-weight (LMW) heparin initially and switching to warfarin or a factor Xa direct inhibitor (e.g., rivaroxaban) for long-term therapy. Occasionally a massive pulmonary thromboembolism, or **saddle embolus,** may cause hemodynamic instability and precipitate acute right-sided heart failure because of the increased afterload. Saddle emboli can result in sudden death, and in these cases the use of **thrombolytics** or **surgical thrombectomy** is warranted. Most deep

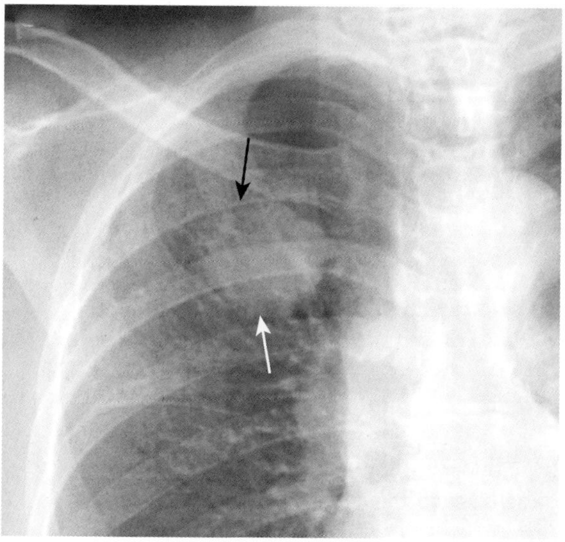

FIG. 17.14 Adenocarcinoma in the right upper lobe (outlined in *arrows*). *(From Herring W. Learning Radiology. 2nd ed. Philadelphia: Elsevier; 2011.)*

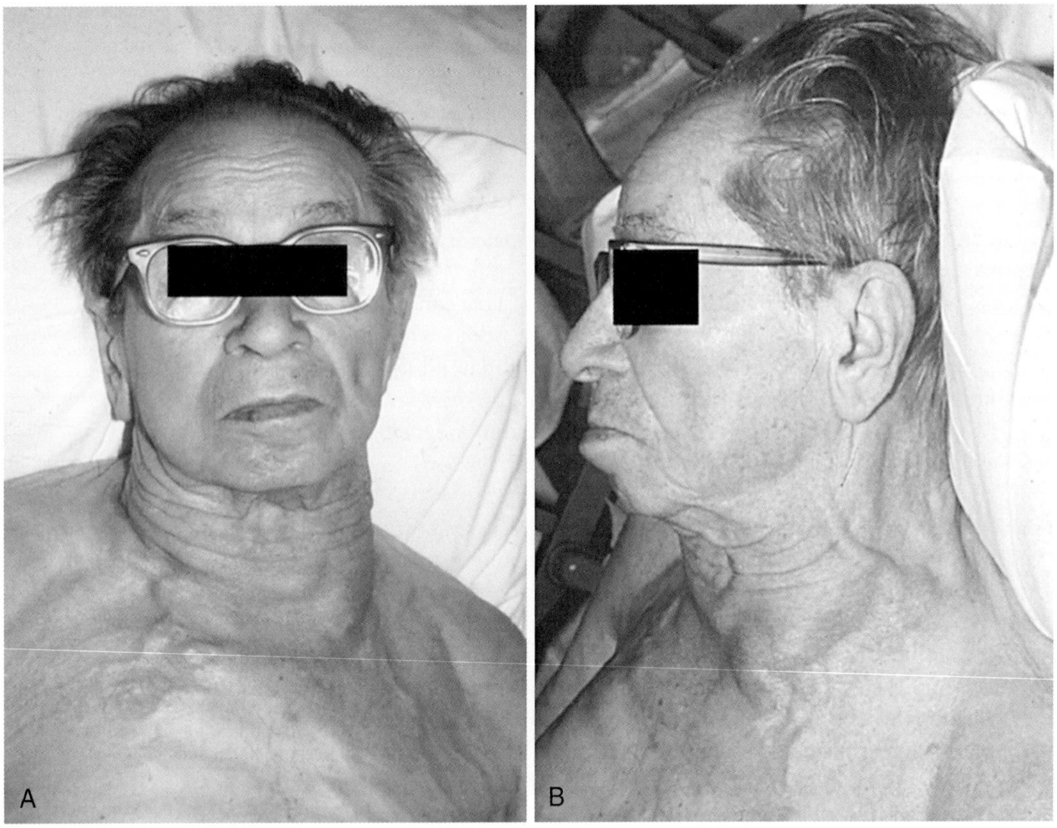

FIG. 17.15 A and **B,** Superior vena cava syndrome demonstrating swelling of the face and dilated veins on the anterior chest wall and neck. *(From Mangione S.* Physical Diagnosis Secrets, *2nd ed. Philadelphia: Elsevier; 2007.)*

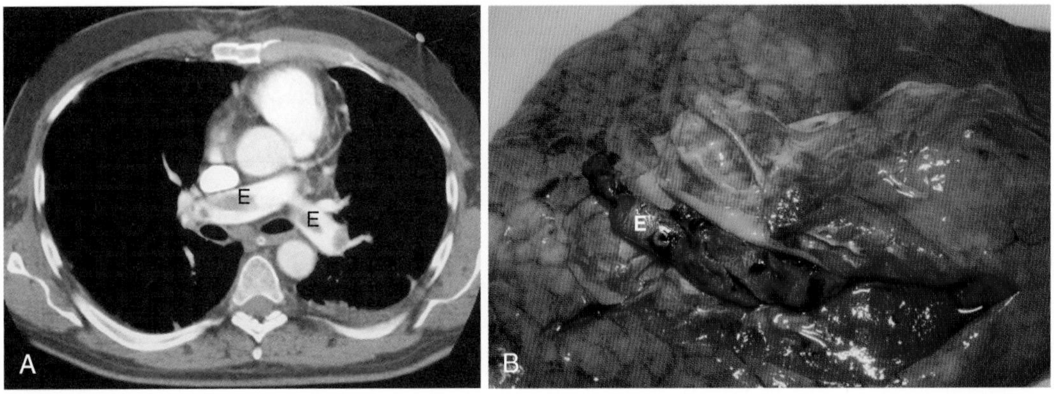

FIG. 17.16 A, CT angiography of the pulmonary artery, displaying emboli (E) in the right and left main pulmonary arteries. **B,** Gross dissection of one of the pulmonary arteries shows a large clot. *(From Burkitt HG.* Essential Surgery. *4th ed. Philadelphia: Elsevier; 2007.)*

venous thromboses and pulmonary emboli occur in hospitalized patients, so many hospitalized patients are provided with prophylactic dosing of unfractionated or LMW heparin to prevent development of this potentially devastating condition.

In addition to a thromboembolism originating from the lower extremity veins, other causes of pulmonary embolism include fat, air, septic, and amniotic fluid emboli:

- **Fat emboli** are typically associated with **fractures of long bones** (e.g., midshaft femoral fractures) and often present with **petechiae** over the chest and upper extremities. Less commonly, they can be associated with neurologic deficits (upper motor neuron signs, seizure).

- **Air emboli** are fairly rare but may occur if large amounts of air are infused into the bloodstream, as may occur if air is not properly expelled from a syringe before administering IV medication, or when divers rise to the surface too quickly, resulting in precipitation of nitrogen bubbles (decompression sickness, aka "the bends").
- **Septic pulmonary emboli** are typically associated with **right-sided bacterial endocarditis** (e.g., tricuspid valve endocarditis in an IV drug abuser) because right-sided valvular vegetations can break off and lodge in the pulmonary circulation.
- **Amniotic fluid emboli** may occur in pregnant women during delivery or immediately postpartum. They are often very abrupt in onset and may present with profound hypotension and **disseminated intravascular coagulation (DIC).**

Pulmonary Hypertension

Pulmonary hypertension (PH) is defined as a sustained elevation in pulmonary artery pressure (normally 10–14 mm Hg) to more than 25 mm Hg at rest or more than 30 mm Hg with exercise. PH has recently undergone a change in how it is classified, and there are now five different groupings that will be reviewed. PH increases the afterload of the right ventricle and can lead to right-sided heart failure. PH causing right ventricular strain or failure is called **cor pulmonale** only if the reason for the pulmonary hypertension **began in the pulmonary circulation** itself (e.g., pulmonary embolism, chronic obstructive pulmonary disease [COPD], familial [previously called primary] PH) and not from another cause, such as left-sided heart failure.

Pulmonary Arterial Hypertension

Pulmonary arterial hypertension (PAH) includes all conditions in which the primary abnormality is confined to the small pulmonary arterioles. There is a familial form of PAH associated with a mutation in the gene that encodes for **bone morphogenetic protein receptor type 2 (BMPR2), a receptor of the transforming growth factor β (TGF-β)** family that plays a role in the regulation of apoptosis and growth. It is thought that this mutation prevents normal apoptosis, resulting in the overgrowth of smooth muscle cells and consequent PAH. Certain diseases are also associated with PAH, such as **connective tissue disease (most often systemic sclerosis, scleroderma) and HIV infection. Schistosomiasis** is a parasitic disease caused by several species of *Schistosoma* that is uncommon in the United States but is the **most common cause of PH worldwide.**

Pulmonary Hypertension Caused by Left-Sided Heart Disease

Functional abnormalities in the left side of the heart can result in increased resistance to the drainage of the pulmonary veins that can subsequently cause PH. The pulmonary veins and venules are affected by pulmonary venous hypertension and can undergo hypertrophy and fibrosis, resulting in PH. Thus any condition associated with left ventricular systolic dysfunction (e.g., congestive heart failure [CHF] secondary to myocardial infarction) or diastolic dysfunction (long-standing hypertension [HTN] causing left ventricular hypertrophy [LVH]) can cause PH. Valvular disease, such as mitral stenosis, can also cause increased back pressure in the pulmonary venous circulation and lead to PH.

Pulmonary Hypertension Associated with Lung Disease and/or Hypoxemia

Patients with restrictive or obstructive pulmonary disease often have PH. Recall that the pulmonary vasculature around alveoli with a low PAO_2 will constrict to shift blood flow away from these alveoli toward those alveoli with a higher PAO_2. This process of **hypoxic vasoconstriction** is critical to ensuring a good match between ventilation and perfusion (V/Q) but can also result in PH if chronic hypoxemia persists. Patients with **COPD** and **obstructive sleep apnea,** as well as healthy individuals living at a very high altitude, are often chronically hypoxemic and can develop PH when permanent remodeling of the pulmonary vasculature occurs over time in response to their hypoxemia. Destruction of the pulmonary vascular bed, as seen in **interstitial lung disease,** is also associated with PH.

Chronic Thromboembolic Pulmonary Hypertension

As discussed earlier in the section on pulmonary embolism, emboli to the pulmonary vascular bed create resistance to forward flow and can thus cause PH. Some patients chronically suffer small pulmonary thromboemboli that may not even cause symptoms, and these patients are at particularly high risk of developing permanent PH.

Pulmonary Hypertension with Unclear Multifactorial Mechanisms

This grouping includes a number of miscellaneous causes. The most important of these is **sarcoidosis.** Sickle cell anemia can also cause PH through unclear mechanisms thought to be related to hemolysis.

Sleep Apnea

Apnea is defined as cessation of breathing. Sleep apnea can be obstructive or central. **Obstructive sleep apnea (OSA)** is the most common form of sleep apnea. The biggest risk factor for OSA is **obesity** (present in 70%), although male gender and age are also risk factors.

Cause: Obese individuals with OSA have redundant soft tissue in their pharynx. When they fall asleep, the redundant soft tissue causes pharyngeal collapse and blocks airflow for periods of more than 10 seconds at a time.

Findings: Although they often do not notice it themselves, these patients frequently wake up for very brief periods after these apneic episodes and often suffer from **daytime sleepiness and chronic tiredness.** Partners of patients with OSA often notice that they **snore loudly** and may even be able to observe apneic periods.

Because OSA patients become hypoxemic during their frequent nighttime apneic episodes, **their pulmonary vasculature undergoes hypoxic vasoconstriction.** When left untreated, this chronic pulmonary vasoconstriction results in permanent pulmonary hypertension and can lead to cor pulmonale (right-sided heart failure secondary to pulmonary hypertension).

Diagnosis and Treatment: OSA is **diagnosed by polysomnography,** a sleep study in which the patient is monitored while sleeping. Treatment for OSA includes **weight loss** and use of **continuous positive airway pressure (CPAP),** which helps prevent pharyngeal collapse. Some patients may require surgical removal of excess pharyngeal soft tissue.

Central sleep apnea (CSA) is far less common than OSA and is caused by a **neurologic impairment to respiration** and **lack of respiratory effort,** rather than a physical obstruction to airflow. Risk factors for CSA include congestive heart failure, cerebrovascular accident, advancing age, and male gender. CSA is also diagnosed by polysomnography.

Obstructive Versus Restrictive Lung Disease

A number of lung diseases can be classified as having an underlying pathophysiologic component that is obstructive (e.g., COPD, asthma) or restrictive (e.g., pulmonary fibrosis, acute respiratory distress syndrome) based on pulmonary function tests (PFTs). Before discussing several of these diseases in detail, certain PFT findings are helpful in diagnosing and differentiating obstructive versus restrictive disease and will be reviewed here (Fig. 17.17).

Obstructive Disease PFTs

In general, lung volumes in patients with obstructive disease are greater than normal because of air trapping and hyperinflation that result from difficulty exhaling fully. On spirometry, this is reflected as an **increased TLC and increased RV**, and it often correlates with hyperinflated lung fields on chest x-ray examination. **FEV_1 and FVC are reduced in obstructive lung disease,** although **FEV_1 is more dramatically reduced than FVC**; this results in a **reduced FEV_1/FVC ratio of less than 0.8.** Two classic obstructive lung diseases are COPD and asthma.

Restrictive Disease PFTs

Restrictive lung diseases are characterized by **reduced TLC and reduced RV.** Like obstructive diseases, the **FEV_1 and FVC are also reduced** in restrictive lung disease, but importantly, **FEV_1 is less dramatically reduced than the FVC,** resulting in an **FEV_1/FVC ratio that is normal or increased beyond 0.8.** Thus restrictive lung disease is suspected when PFTs show reduced TLC in the setting of a normal or

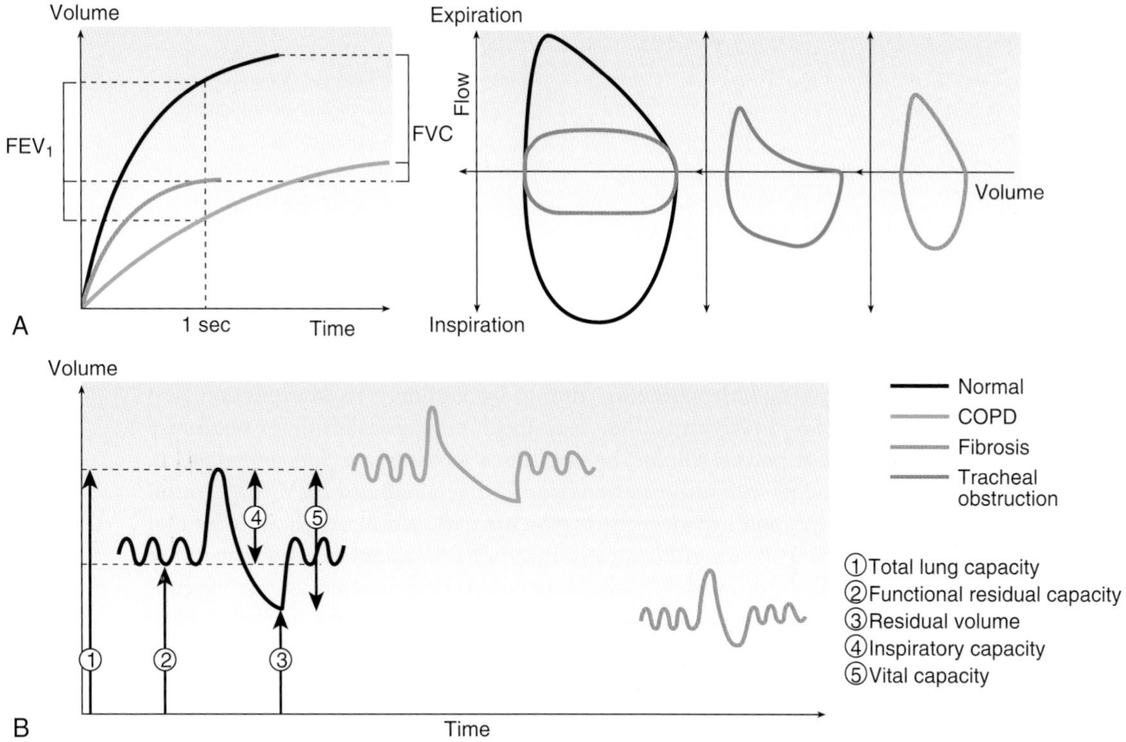

FIG. 17.17 ***A, left,*** Forced expiration curves showing a normal expiration (black) compared with fibrosis (red) and COPD (green). ***A, right,*** Flow-volume loops that compare the flow and volume of the lungs during expiration and inspiration in a normal lung (black) with COPD (green, higher volumes) and fibrosis (red, lower volumes). **B,** Spirometry showing normal tidal volumes followed by a vital capacity breath in a normal subject (black) compared with those with COPD (green) with chronic hyperinflation from decreased elasticity and increased compliance, compared with a patient with fibrosis (red) with lower lung volumes because of increased elasticity and decreased compliance. *(From Colledge NR, Walker BR, Ralston SH.* Davidson's Principles and Practice of Medicine. *21st ed. Philadelphia: Elsevier; 2010.)*

increased FEV_1/FVC ratio. Pulmonary fibrosis, sarcoidosis, acute respiratory distress syndrome, pneumoconiosis, Goodpasture syndrome, Wegener granulomatosis, and certain drug toxicities leading to pulmonary fibrosis (e.g., bleomycin, amiodarone, busulfan) are examples of restrictive lung diseases. However, extrapulmonary processes that negatively affect breathing mechanics can also cause a restrictive physiology. Such extrapulmonary processes include those with poor diaphragmatic or muscular effort, such as **myasthenia gravis** or **polio,** as well as those in which there is structural restriction on the lungs, such as **severe obesity, severe scoliosis, or severe ankylosing spondylitis.**

Pathology of Obstructive Lung Diseases

Asthma

Affecting millions of people worldwide, asthma is a chronic inflammatory disorder of the airways characterized by airway hyperresponsiveness and reversible, bronchoconstriction- induced airway obstruction (Fig. 17.18) that is episodic.

Pathogenesis: Asthma can result from intrinsic or extrinsic causes. Intrinsic asthma does not involve an immune reaction or elevations of immunoglobulin (IgE) levels. An example of intrinsic asthma is the so-called asthma triad related to aspirin sensitivity, in which patients have symptoms consistent with **asthma, nasal polyps, and sensitivity to aspirin** or nonsteroidal antiinflammatory drugs (NSAIDs).

Extrinsic asthma is far more common and is strongly related to atopy and type I hypersensitivity reactions. Environmental allergens stimulate IgE production by plasma cells (B cells) as well as eosinophil recruitment into the mucosal lining of the airways.

Findings: Patients with asthma suffer from **wheezing, cough, dyspnea, and a sensation of chest tightness,** and their symptoms are often worse at night. A variety of triggers can induce an asthma attack, including respiratory irritants (e.g., smoke), allergens (e.g., pet dander, pollen, dust), infections (upper respiratory infection, bronchitis), medications (aspirin, NSAIDs), cold air, and exercise. On physical

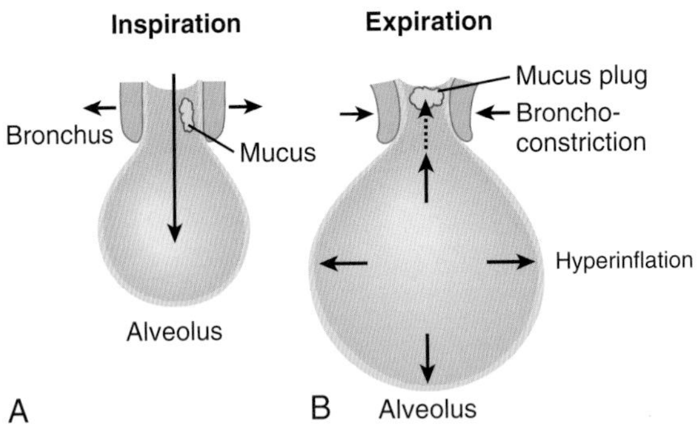

Fig. 17.18 Pathophysiology of asthma, demonstrating air trapping during expiration because of bronchoconstriction and mucus plugging. *(From Damjanov I. Pathophysiology. Philadelphia: Elsevier; 2008.)*

examination, these patients often have **audible wheezing** (during inspiration [I] and expiration [E]) and a **prolonged expiratory phase (i.e., ↓ I/E ratio).** They may also have physical findings suggestive of an atopic component, such as nasal polyps, rhinitis, or rash. Because asthma is fundamentally an obstructive lung disease, PFTs in patients with asthma often demonstrate a **reduced FEV_1/FVC ratio.** The reversibility of the bronchoconstriction experienced by patients with asthma is characteristic of the disease, and this is reflected on PFTs by **a significant increase in FEV_1 after bronchodilators are administered.** The role of eosinophils in the pathogenesis of asthma is corroborated by the presence in sputum samples from patients with asthma of **Charcot-Leyden crystals,** which are breakdown products of eosinophils. Sputum samples from patients with asthma typically contain **Curschmann spirals,** which reflect desquamated epithelium from the airways.

Treatment: The aggressiveness of treatment depends on the frequency of asthma symptoms. Generally, an inhaled β_2-adrenergic agonist such as albuterol is used alone to treat mild disease and acute asthma attacks. Other medications are used to control symptoms and prevent acute attacks. These include inhaled corticosteroids, long-acting inhaled β_2-adrenergic agonists (e.g., salmeterol), leukotriene modifiers (e.g., montelukast), and, less commonly, theophylline or cromolyn. Oral corticosteroids are sometimes used for short periods to treat more severe asthma exacerbations.

Chronic Obstructive Pulmonary Disease

COPD is divided into two subtypes, **chronic bronchitis** and **emphysema,** that will be reviewed here. It is worth noting, however, that **patients with COPD often exhibit characteristics of both chronic bronchitis and emphysema** subtypes, which is why many pulmonologists consider these designations to be increasingly irrelevant. Nevertheless, you should learn them for the USMLE Step 1 and know that regardless of the subtype, COPD is fundamentally characterized by **chronic airflow limitation and obstruction that is not fully reversible** and that its **biggest risk factor is cigarette smoking.** This obstruction and **premature airway closure** results in **air trapping** and **hyperinflation.** Consequently, PFTs of COPD patients typically demonstrate an obstructive pattern—**increased RV** (caused by air trapping), **increased TLC** (caused by air trapping), and a **decreased FEV_1/FVC ratio** (Fig. 17.17).

Chronic Bronchitis: This condition is defined as a productive cough lasting at least 3 months per year for 2 consecutive years. Its pathophysiology relates to hypertrophy and hypersecretion of mucus-secreting glands in the terminal bronchioles. This mucous gland hypertrophy can be characterized histologically by measuring the **Reid index,** which is the ratio of mucous gland depth to the thickness of the bronchial wall. COPD patients with chronic bronchitis often have a **Reid index** of more than **50%.** Clinically, in addition to frequent productive cough, chronic bronchitis patients tend to be **CO_2 retainers** (have high $Paco_2$), tend to become **hypoxemic and cyanotic earlier in their disease course,** and tend to have an **obese body habitus,** which is why they are sometimes referred to as **blue bloaters.**

Emphysema: The underlying pathophysiology of this COPD subtype is characterized by abnormal permanent alveolar airspace distention distal to the terminal bronchioles (the area affected in chronic bronchitis) resulting from destruction of the alveolar walls and surrounding elastic tissue. Because of the destruction of elastic tissue in and around the respiratory bronchioles and alveolar walls, these patients have increased lung compliance and decreased lung elastance. Moreover, the destruction of elastic tissue in the most distal portions of the terminal bronchioles results in a loss of radial traction that normally keeps these tiny airways open during expiration, predisposing them to collapse and air trapping behind

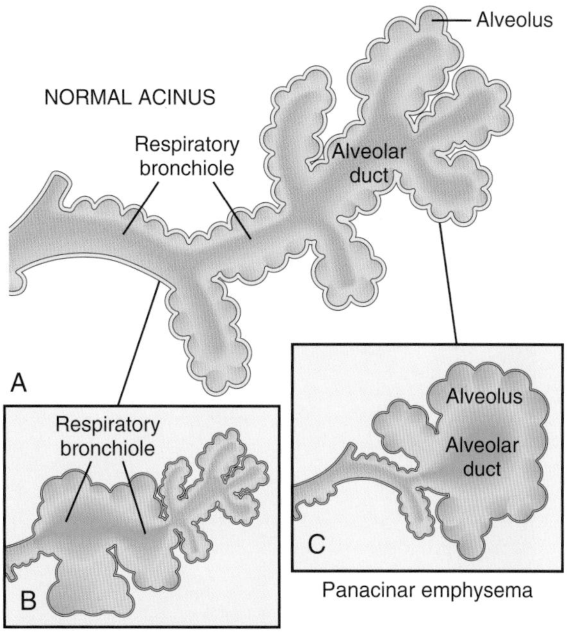

Fig. 17.19 A, Normal acinus. Comparison between centriacinar emphysema (common in COPD and in smokers) in which the respiratory bronchioles are dilated and the distal alveoli are spared (**B**), and panacinar emphysema (**C**), in which the entire acinus is dilated. *(From Kumar V, Abbas AK, Aster J.* Robbins Basic Pathology. *9th ed. St. Louis: Elsevier; 2012.)*

these collapsed airways. All these factors result in hyperinflation with **increased TLC** that can present as a barrel-chested habitus (increased anterior-posterior chest diameter), reduced breath sounds, and wheezes on physical examination. Chest radiographs will reveal hyperexpanded-hyperlucent lung fields, with flattening of the hemidiaphragms. As you might expect, these patients often experience shortness of breath that slowly progresses.

There are a few different types of emphysema classified according to its anatomic distribution within the lobule. The three major types are centriacinar, panacinar, and paraseptal (Fig. 17.19).

- **Centriacinar emphysema** involves the **central parts of the acini formed by the distal terminal bronchioles** but spares the distal alveoli. This type of emphysema is **associated with heavy smokers** and is often accompanied by chronic bronchitis. Centriacinar emphysema more commonly **affects the upper lobes and apical segments** (to remember this, recall that **"smoke rises."**)
- **Panacinar emphysema** involves the **entire acinus,** including the distal terminal bronchioles and terminal alveoli. Unlike centriacinar emphysema, the panacinar type predominantly affects the lower lung lobes. It is associated with **α-1 antitrypsin deficiency,** a condition that also commonly results in liver cirrhosis.
- **Paraseptal emphysema** predominantly involves only the **distal parts of the acinus,** leaving the more proximal areas unaffected. This type of emphysema notably **affects areas of lung adjacent to pleura** and is associated with bullae that can rupture and result in a **spontaneous pneumothorax.** Paraseptal emphysema is thought to be the underlying mechanism of spontaneous pneumothoraces that occur in otherwise healthy young men.

Bronchiectasis

Bronchiectasis is a condition characterized by destruction of elastic tissue and muscle, resulting in a permanent dilation of the bronchioles and bronchi (Fig. 17.20). It is highly associated with **chronic necrotizing infections.** Patients with bronchiectasis may present with a **cough productive of copious amounts of sputum,** recurrent pulmonary infections, and hemoptysis. Primary ciliary dyskinesia, allergic bronchopulmonary aspergillosis, chronic bronchial obstruction (e.g., by tumor, foreign body), and certain inflammatory disorders can cause bronchiectasis, but the most common and important cause for the USMLE Step 1 is **cystic fibrosis.**

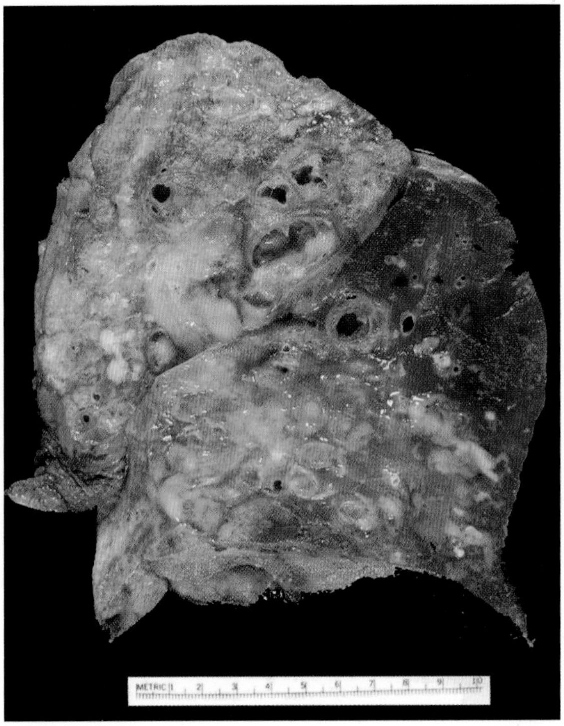

Fig. 17.20 Bronchiectasis showing dilated bronchioles filled with purulent material. This patient had cystic fibrosis. *(From Kumar V, Abbas AK, Aster J. Robbins Basic Pathology. 9th ed. St. Louis: Elsevier; 2012.)*

Cystic Fibrosis

Cystic fibrosis (CF) is a life-shortening autosomal recessive disease most commonly caused by a 3-nucleotide deletion on chromosome 7 coding for a phenylalanine residue (**ΔF508,** shorthand referring to the deletion [Δ] of a sequence coding for phenylalanine [F] at position 508), resulting in abnormal function of special chloride channels known as cystic fibrosis transmembrane conductance regulators (CFTRs). The mutation affects the CFTR channels by causing them to be prematurely degraded in the cell's Golgi apparatus, preventing CFTRs from reaching the epithelial cell membrane, where they are needed. Lack of these functional chloride channels in sweat glands of the skin inhibits absorption of chloride and sodium by the epithelial cells lining the glands. The consequent increase in NaCl in the sweat is the basis for the **sweat test** that can be used to diagnose CF (Fig. 17.21, *top*). In epithelial cell membranes, the lack of CFTR prevents secretion of chloride into the luminal space and promotes increased resorption of sodium and H_2O from the luminal space into the epithelial cells. In the lung, this results in dehydrated airway mucus and secretions that are difficult for ciliated cells in the airway to sweep toward the mouth as intended (Fig. 17.21, *bottom*). Because mucociliary clearance is impaired, the thick dehydrated mucus that remains in the airways becomes a nidus for bacterial growth (most commonly with ***Pseudomonas aeruginosa***), predisposing CF patients to chronic necrotizing respiratory infections and **bronchiectasis.** Clinically, CF presents with chronic productive cough, airway obstruction, and nasal polyps. Respiratory infection is the most common cause of death in CF.

Because CFTR channels are found in the exocrine glands and epithelial linings of the gastrointestinal and reproductive systems as well, patients with CF suffer from widespread problems in all these organs, in addition to the respiratory difficulties mentioned. In the gastrointestinal system, CF often initially presents as **meconium ileus** in the young infant, where the infant is unable to produce his or her first stool after birth because of intestinal obstruction caused by dehydrated stool. In the exocrine system, **chronic pancreatitis resulting in malabsorption** and **diabetes mellitus secondary to pancreatic dysfunction** are common complications. Infertility affects men and women with CF, although it is more severe in men. In men with CF, infertility is caused by an **absent vas deferens,** whereas thickened cervical mucus secretions and malnutrition are often why women with CF have fertility problems.

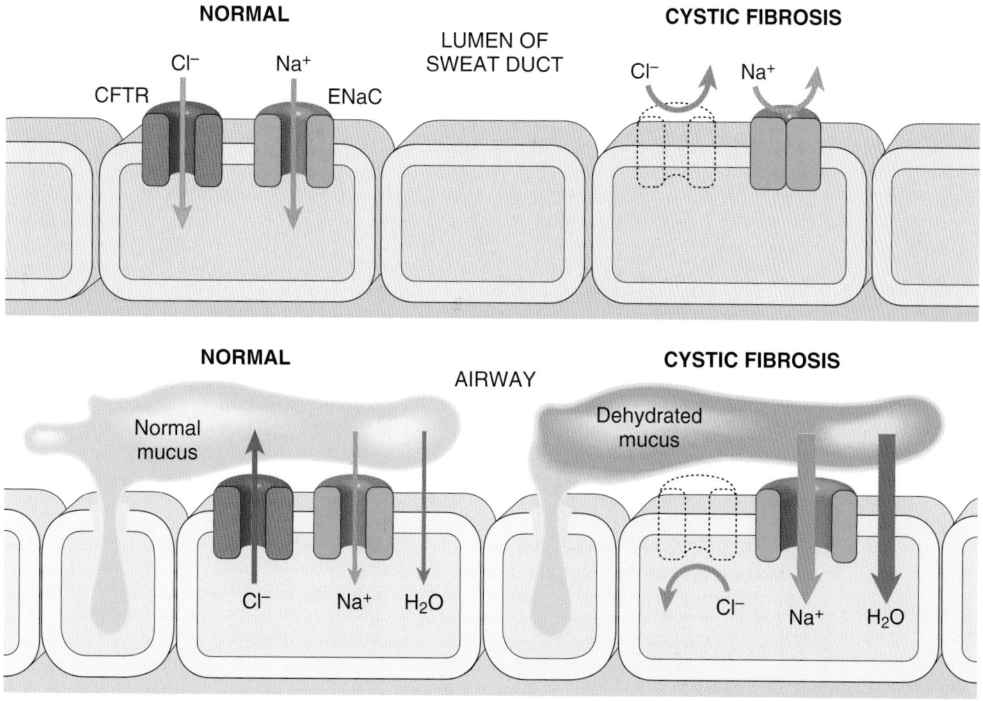

FIG. 17.21 ***Top,*** Inability of cystic fibrosis (CF) patients to resorb sodium chloride from sweat before being excreted. ***Bottom,*** Inability of CF patients to hydrate mucus properly. Both these effects are caused by lack of functional chloride channels. Note that the orientation of the CFTR is reversed in sweat ducts compared with respiratory epithelium (i.e., chloride is not properly absorbed in sweat glands, whereas it is not properly secreted in respiratory epithelium). *(From Kumar V, Abbas AK, Aster J.* Robbins Basic Pathology. *9th ed. St. Louis: Elsevier; 2012.)*

Pathology of Restrictive Lung Diseases

Acute Respiratory Distress Syndrome

Acute respiratory distress syndrome (ARDS) is the leading cause of acute respiratory failure in the United States. Its underlying pathogenesis relates to a **diffuse inflammatory process involving both lungs,** resulting in a **noncardiogenic pulmonary edema** and **bilateral lung consolidations.** It is the final common pathway of lung injury, and a number of conditions predispose patients to developing ARDS, including sepsis, pneumonia, pulmonary contusions, intracranial hypertension, blood product transfusions, cardiopulmonary bypass, pancreatitis, amniotic fluid embolism, and long bone fractures.

When critical damage to the alveolar-capillary membranes occurs, the permeability of these membranes increases and **a massive influx of inflammatory cells such as neutrophils and macrophages enter the alveoli** (Fig. 17.22). This constitutes the exudative inflammatory phase of ARDS. In the fibroproliferative phase of the disease, chronic inflammatory cells release cytokines, chemokines, growth factors, and angiogenic mediators, eventually **resulting in fibrosis and stiff noncompliant lungs that are edematous and atelectatic.** The marked infiltration of inflammatory cells in the alveolar spaces **increases V/Q mismatch and results in significant shunting,** which presents **as profound hypoxemia** and respiratory distress.

ARDS is diagnosed by observing profound hypoxemia unresponsive to 100% O_2, an elevated A-a gradient, and bilateral fluffy infiltrates on chest x-ray examination, all in the presence of a pulmonary capillary wedge pressure less than 18 mm Hg (wedge pressures >18 mm Hg suggest a likely cardiogenic component). The poor oxygenation and shunting in ARDS patients is treated with careful fluid management, endotracheal intubation, and mechanical ventilation, using positive end-expiratory pressure (PEEP). **PEEP is used to recruit alveoli** that are collapsed or otherwise filled with fluid and an inflammatory infiltrate, improving their ability to participate in gas exchange, thus reducing shunting and alleviating the patient's hypoxemia. An important adverse effect of **PEEP** is that it **can reduce cardiac output** (except in heart failure patients, in whom PEEP may increase CO by decreasing afterload). Cardiac output is reduced because the positive intrathoracic pressure that PEEP creates can reduce venous return to the heart. The positive pressure used in PEEP can also cause alveoli to rupture, resulting in a spontaneous pneumothorax.

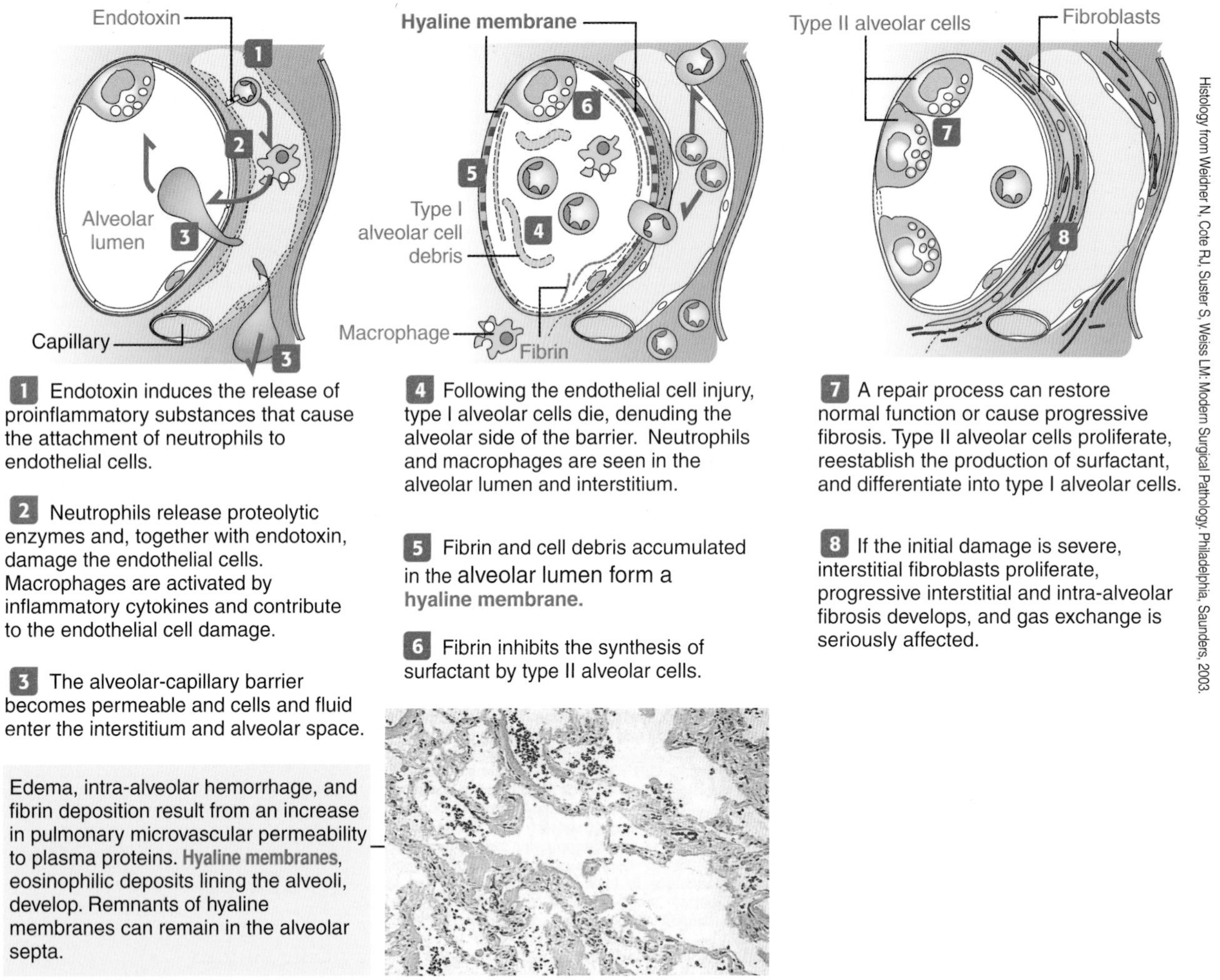
Endotoxin
1
2
Alveolar lumen
3
Capillary
3
Hyaline membrane
6
5
Type I alveolar cell debris
4
Macrophage
Fibrin
Type II alveolar cells
Fibroblasts
7
8
1 Endotoxin induces the release of proinflammatory substances that cause the attachment of neutrophils to endothelial cells.
2 Neutrophils release proteolytic enzymes and, together with endotoxin, damage the endothelial cells. Macrophages are activated by inflammatory cytokines and contribute to the endothelial cell damage.
3 The alveolar-capillary barrier becomes permeable and cells and fluid enter the interstitium and alveolar space.
4 Following the endothelial cell injury, type I alveolar cells die, denuding the alveolar side of the barrier. Neutrophils and macrophages are seen in the alveolar lumen and interstitium.
5 Fibrin and cell debris accumulated in the alveolar lumen form a hyaline membrane.
6 Fibrin inhibits the synthesis of surfactant by type II alveolar cells.
7 A repair process can restore normal function or cause progressive fibrosis. Type II alveolar cells proliferate, reestablish the production of surfactant, and differentiate into type I alveolar cells.
8 If the initial damage is severe, interstitial fibroblasts proliferate, progressive interstitial and intra-alveolar fibrosis develops, and gas exchange is seriously affected.
Edema, intra-alveolar hemorrhage, and fibrin deposition result from an increase in pulmonary microvascular permeability to plasma proteins. Hyaline membranes, eosinophilic deposits lining the alveoli, develop. Remnants of hyaline membranes can remain in the alveolar septa.
Histology from Weidner N, Cote RJ, Suster S, Weiss LM: Modern Surgical Pathology. Philadelphia, Saunders, 2003.

Fig. 17.22 Histology and pathophysiology of ARDS. *(From Kierszenbaum A, Tres L.* Histology and Cell Biology: An Introduction to Pathology. *3rd ed. Philadelphia: Elsevier; 2011.)*

Neonatal Respiratory Distress Syndrome

Neonatal respiratory distress syndrome (NRDS) is a feared complication in newborns caused by a **deficiency of surfactant.** Recall that surfactant is made by type II alveolar cells and reduces surface tension on the surface of the alveoli so they can expand more easily during inspiration. Therefore, when an insufficient amount of surfactant is present, widespread alveolar collapse ensues. This leads to intrapulmonary shunting because of massive atelectasis, resulting in hypoxemia and respiratory distress. Neonates with NRDS present with grunting, intercostal retractions, and tachypnea. It is worth recalling that neonates depend on increased oxygen tension after birth to close the ductus arteriosus, so neonates who are hypoxemic because of NRDS often have patent ductus arteriosus.

> Although it is often used to treat hypoxemia, **supplemental O_2 has toxic potential.** Too much O_2 can cause cell injury and death from superoxide generation. One consequence of this in neonates is retinopathy.

Prematurity is the greatest risk factor for NRDS because the lamellar bodies in type II alveolar cells that produce surfactant first appear late in gestation. Recall that surfactant production is not mature until approximately 34 to 35 weeks gestation. Fetal exposure to corticosteroids is important in inducing surfactant production, and the stress of vaginal delivery on the fetus often increases fetal corticosteroid production. Neonates who undergo cesarean delivery are at increased risk for NRDS because they are not exposed to the stress of vaginal delivery and may not experience the stress-induced increase in corticosteroids that stimulates surfactant production. Finally, elevated insulin levels in the fetus also reduce surfactant production, making maternal diabetes another risk factor for NRDS.

> Fetal lung maturity is assessed by the lecithin-to-sphingomyelin ratio of amniotic fluid. A ratio >2.0 indicates sufficient lung maturity.

NRDS can be prevented by assessing fetal lung maturity when risk factors for NRDS are present or anticipated. Fetal lung maturity is assessed by checking the lecithin-to-sphingomyelin ratio of amniotic

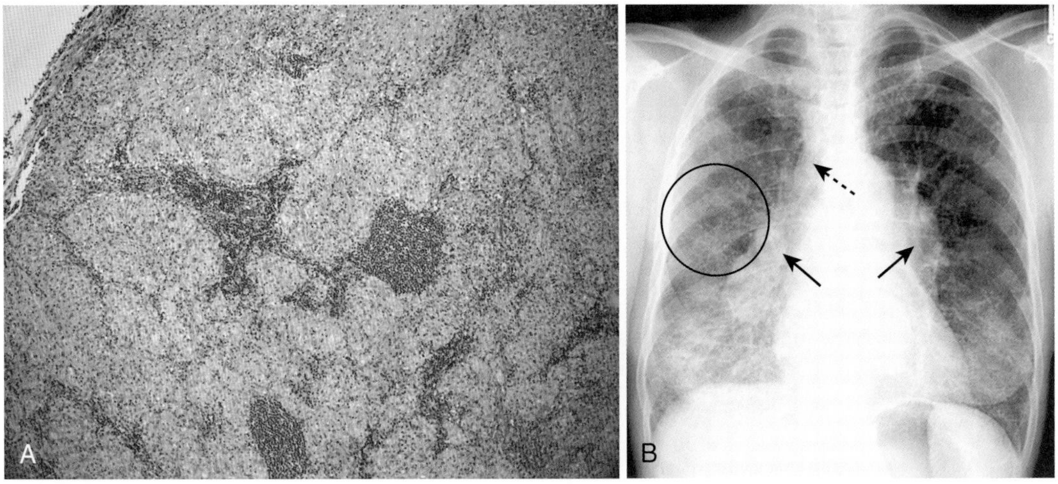

Fig. 17.23 A, Noncaseating granulomas of sarcoidosis. **B,** Chest radiograph of a patient with sarcoidosis, showing adenopathy, especially in the hilar (*black solid arrows*) and paratracheal (*dashed arrow*) areas, as well as interstitial lung disease (*black circle*). (**A** *from King T.* Elsevier's Integrated Pathology. *Philadelphia: Elsevier; 2006;* **B** *from Herring W.* Learning Radiology. *2nd ed. Philadelphia: Elsevier; 2011.)*

fluid. A ratio more than 2.0 indicates sufficient lung maturity, and a ratio less than 1.5 is concerning for the development of NRDS after birth. If a low lecithin-to-sphingomyelin ratio is detected, surfactant production can be increased by giving the mother a course of **corticosteroids.** Thyroxine can also be given to the mother to increase lung maturity, although this is not commonly done. The actual treatment of neonates suffering from NRDS involves the administration of exogenous surfactant and provision of oxygen-assisted ventilation.

Sarcoidosis

Sarcoidosis is a multisystem, immune-mediated granulomatous disease of unknown cause that accounts for approximately 25% of interstitial lung diseases. It is more common in women and in African Americans, and many examination questions involving sarcoidosis feature female African American patients. The pathogenesis of sarcoidosis involves the CD4 helper T (Th) cells interacting with unknown antigens, releasing inflammatory cytokines and causing the formation of noncaseating granulomas (Fig. 17.23A).

Sarcoidosis is a diagnosis of exclusion but has certain patterns and findings that assist in diagnosis. The disease affects multiple organs, but the lung is most commonly involved. In the lungs, **granuloma formation in the parenchyma and hilar lymph nodes** is characteristic of sarcoidosis, and dyspnea is a common symptom. **Chest x-ray examination often shows enlarged mediastinal and hilar lymph nodes** and often **demonstrates** interstitial lung disease (Fig. 17.23B). **Angiotensin-converting enzyme (ACE) levels** are sometimes elevated in sarcoidosis, although this is a nonspecific finding. **Hypercalcemia** may also occur **because of hypervitaminosis D** caused by increased synthesis of 1-α-hydroxylase within the granulomas. Because it is a primarily CD4 Th cell–mediated disease, the ratio of **CD4 to CD8 cells is high** when measured in bronchoalveolar lavage fluid. Lung biopsy showing noncaseating granulomas not caused by a detectable infectious **organism** is also highly suggestive of sarcoidosis.

Nonpulmonary manifestations of sarcoidosis are also often seen and can assist in diagnosis. Nodular skin lesions containing noncaseating granulomas may occur. As in other granulomatous diseases, such as Crohn disease, **erythema nodosum** (painful erythematous nodules caused by subcutaneous fat inflammation) may be seen on the shins of patients with sarcoidosis. **Uveitis** is a painful inflammation of the middle layer of the eye that may also be seen in sarcoidosis. The disease often goes into remission spontaneously but may require treatment with corticosteroids.

Hypersensitivity Pneumonitis

Hypersensitivity pneumonitis (HSP) is an **extrinsic allergic alveolitis caused by a known inhaled antigen.** It is not a type I hypersensitivity reaction (does not involve IgE antibody production) and does not cause eosinophilia. The diagnosis is difficult to make but can be reached by obtaining a thorough exposure history and confirming the relationship of a known antigen with a patient's symptoms. In some cases, bronchoalveolar lavage can be helpful because in HSP it may show dramatic lymphocytosis and a **low ratio of CD4 to CD8 cells** (the opposite of sarcoidosis). The best treatment for HSP is avoidance of the precipitating antigen and proper occupational measures, such as wearing a face mask.

There are a few specific varieties of HSP of which you should be aware:

- **Farmer's lung** is most often caused by **exposure to thermophilic actinomycetes in moldy hay or grain** that results in type III (immune complex–mediated) and type IV (delayed type T cell–mediated) hypersensitivity reactions.
- **Byssinosis** is often seen **in textile workers who are exposed to linen, cotton, and hemp products.**
- **Silo filler's disease** is associated with the inhalation of **gases containing oxides of nitrogen.**
- **Bird fancier's lung** is caused by exposure to an antigen found in bird droppings (pigeons, parrots, etc.).

Pneumoconioses

Pneumoconioses are lung diseases that result from the inhalation of mineral dust and other small microparticles. With time, inhalation of these microparticles can cause significant lung and pleural damage, leading to interstitial fibrosis, and can also increase the risk of developing certain lung cancers. There are several pneumoconioses with which you should be familiar that will be reviewed here. Pay close attention to the exposures associated with each disease, because they are likely to be helpful in differentiating them on the USMLE Step 1.

Silicosis: This is the most common occupational pneumoconiosis and is most often **associated with work in foundries, mines, and sandblasting.** Quartz is a highly fibrogenic material that deposits in the upper lung lobes, activates macrophages there, and causes them to release cytokines that promote collagen deposition and fibrogenesis. The quartz is actually believed to destroy macrophages as well, which may be why patients with silicosis are at **increased risk for tuberculosis.** Patients with silicosis also have an **increased risk of developing primary lung cancer.** The classic finding of silicosis on chest x-ray is eggshell calcification of the hilar lymph nodes.

Coal Worker's Pneumoconiosis (CWP): This occurs with the chronic inhalation of anthracotic pigments (coal dust) and is **associated with coal mining.** The disease predominantly affects the upper lobes and upper portions of the lower lobes. Simple CWP is characterized by fibrotic opacities smaller than 1 cm. Complicated CWP results in progressive massive fibrosis and is characterized by fibrotic opacities larger than 1 to 2 cm, possibly with necrotic centers. The complicated form of CWP can be debilitating and is often called black lung disease because of the black coloration caused by anthracotic pigment deposition in the lung tissue. On histologic examination, blackened masses of coal dust particles gathered by macrophages, called dust cells, may be seen along the alveolar walls. CWP is **not** associated with an increased risk of tuberculosis or primary lung cancer, but patients with CWP **may develop cor pulmonale** and are at increased risk for developing **Caplan syndrome.** Caplan syndrome can be diagnosed in the **presence of *any* pneumoconiosis** presenting **with intrapulmonary nodules** and **rheumatoid arthritis.** The feared complication of CWP is **progressive massive fibrosis** in which, as the name implies, severe pulmonary fibrosis occurs and progresses.

Asbestosis: This is associated with asbestos inhalation from exposure to **shipbuilding, insulation around plumbing, roofing material, floor tile, and ceiling tile.** Asbestos fibers deposit inside the alveoli when inhaled. Alveolar macrophages phagocytose the asbestos fibers and coat them with iron, creating golden brown, fusiform, dumbbell-shaped rods within the macrophages called **asbestos bodies** or **ferruginous bodies.** Unlike CWP and silicosis, asbestosis predominantly affects the lower lobes. Asbestosis **usually causes benign calcified pleural plaques,** which are not malignant precursors. Asbestosis is associated with an **increased risk of mesothelioma,** a malignancy with a poor prognosis that arises from the pleural serosa and eventually encases and traps the lung. Despite the strong association with mesothelioma, the **most common malignancy associated with asbestosis is bronchogenic carcinoma.** Asbestosis can cause **interstitial fibrosis** and may also present with Caplan syndrome. There is no increased risk of tuberculosis with asbestosis.

Berylliosis: This is strongly **associated with exposure in the aerospace and nuclear industries.** Berylliosis causes diffuse interstitial pulmonary fibrosis. Noncaseating granulomas, similar to those seen in sarcoidosis, are often seen on histopathologic examination. Patients with berylliosis have a higher risk of developing **primary lung cancer** and can also develop cor pulmonale.

Pleural Disorders

Each lung is located in its respective pleural cavity enclosed by parietal pleura. A number of disorders involve the pleural cavity.

Pleural effusions are collections of fluid that develop in the pleural cavity. Normally, a small amount of pleural fluid moves from the parietal pleura into the pleural space, is absorbed by the visceral pleura on the lungs, and ultimately drains into the lymphatic system. This fluid movement depends on a parietal capillary hydrostatic pressure greater than the visceral capillary hydrostatic pressure and a parietal capillary oncotic pressure equal to the visceral oncotic pressure. Pleural effusions develop when these pressures are altered by disease processes.

- Elevated hydrostatic pressure within the visceral pleura is the mechanism whereby **CHF** and **pulmonary embolism** cause pleural effusions. **CHF is the most common cause of pleural effusions.**
- Reduced oncotic pressure within the visceral pleura is the mechanism whereby **cirrhosis, nephrotic syndrome,** and other conditions resulting in low albumin levels cause pleural effusions.
- Elevated permeability of the visceral pleural capillaries caused by inflammatory conditions such as **systemic lupus erythematosus (SLE)** and **pneumonia** can cause pleural effusions. This is also the mechanism whereby malignancies affecting the pleura (**mesothelioma** or cancer metastatic to the pleura) cause pleural effusions.
- Lymphatic obstruction that interferes with drainage from the visceral pleura can result in pleural effusions. This may occur in **primary lung cancer.**

The cause of the pleural effusion can be determined by performing thoracentesis to sample and analyze the pleural fluid. Pleural effusions are classified as being **transudative** or **exudative** based on fulfilling one of the three **Light's** criteria shown in Table 17.4.

Transudates are caused by conditions that disturb capillary hydrostatic or oncotic pressure (e.g., CHF, cirrhosis). Exudates are protein rich, have a cloudy appearance, and are caused by increased vessel permeability secondary to inflammation (e.g., pneumonia, SLE, cancer). If an effusion is due to lymphatic obstruction (also called a "chylothorax"), the fluid appears milky and has elevated triglycerides; suspect this in malignancies, such as lymphomas. Physical examination of patients with pleural effusions may reveal dullness to percussion, decreased tactile fremitus, and reduced breath sounds in the areas of effusion. On chest x-ray examination, pleural effusions will often cause blunting of the **costophrenic angles** and **conceal the border of the diaphragm** (Fig. 17.24). Treatment of pleural effusions generally involves treatment of the underlying cause and possibly drainage, which removes risk of infection and may provide symptomatic improvement.

Spontaneous Pneumothorax

Spontaneous pneumothorax occurs when an intrapleural or subpleural bleb ruptures, creating a **hole in the pleura.**

Pathogenesis: Recall that the intrapleural pressure is normally negative at rest and that at equilibrium the lungs have a natural tendency to collapse, whereas the chest wall has an equal and opposite tendency to expand (see Fig. 17.6). Thus a hole in the pleura causes an equalization of the intrapleural and atmospheric pressures, causing the lung to collapse and the chest wall to expand. Primary spontaneous pneumothoraces occur in the absence of underlying lung disease, are caused by blebs, and **occur most commonly in thin and tall young men.** Secondary pneumothoraces occur in the presence of underlying lung disease, with **COPD being the most common secondary cause.**

Table 17.4 Classification of Pleural Effusions by Light's Criteria

	EFFUSION	
COMPONENT	**TRANSUDATIVE**	**EXUDATIVE**
Total $protein_{Effusion}$/total $protein_{Serum}$	<0.5	>0.5
$LDH_{Effusion}/LDH_{Serum}$	<0.6	>0.6
$LDH_{Effusion}$	<Two-thirds of the upper limit of normal	>Two-thirds of the upper limit of normal

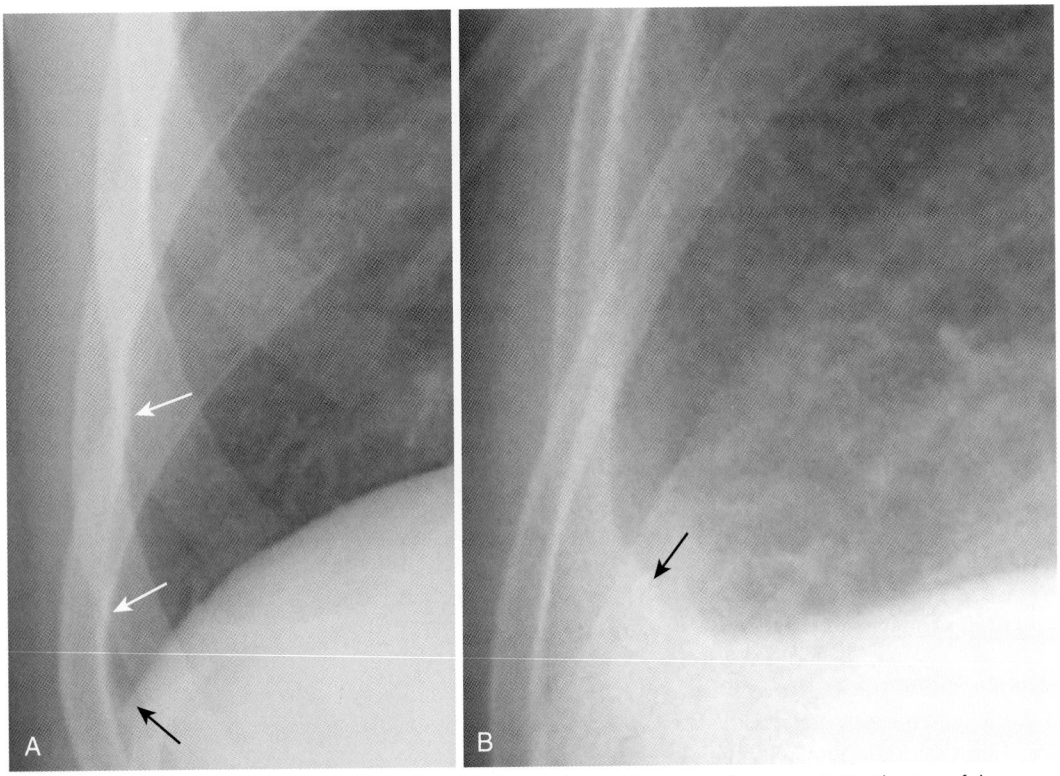

Fig. 17.24 **A,** Normal chest x-ray (CXR) showing a normal costophrenic angle *(arrows)*. **B,** Blunting of the costophrenic angle *(arrow)*, suggesting a pleural effusion. *(From Herring W. Learning Radiology. 2nd ed. Philadelphia: Elsevier; 2011.)*

Findings: Patients often report **sudden-onset pleuritic chest pain** and **dyspnea.** On physical examination, there may be reduced breath sounds and tympany to percussion on the affected side, with **tracheal deviation *toward* the affected side.** Chest radiographs may show loss of lung markings, a clear pleural reflection, and tracheal deviation **toward** the side of collapse (Fig. 17.25).

Treatment: The vasculature beneath the visceral pleura gradually resorbs air, so small pneumothoraces may be treated with observation alone if the patient is asymptomatic. However, administration of 100% oxygen dramatically increases the rate of resorption. In patients in whom the pneumothorax is large and symptomatic, a chest tube may be inserted to evacuate the pleural air and reexpand the lung.

Tension Pneumothorax

Tension pneumothorax is a **life-threatening emergency** that must be diagnosed and treated rapidly.

Pathogenesis: Penetrating trauma to the lung or chest wall **can create** a **one-way valve, flaplike tear in the lung parenchyma, which causes air leakage** from the lung into the pleural space but prevents air escape. As air continues to enter the pleural space without exiting, it accumulates, increases the pleural pressure, causes the lung to collapse, and compresses nearby structures such as the vena cava by placing them under tension. When the vena cava is compressed, **preload to the heart is dramatically reduced,** impairing cardiac output and resulting in **hypotension** and eventual death if not treated emergently.

Findings: As with spontaneous pneumothorax, these patients present with a history **of sudden onset pleuritic chest pain** and **dyspnea.** Physical examination may reveal **jugular venous distention, hypotension,** evidence of hypoperfusion, reduced or absent breath sounds on the affected side, tympany to percussion on the affected side, and **tracheal deviation *away* from the affected side.** Because of the urgency and seriousness of this condition, diagnosis is best made clinically because taking time to confirm with imaging may result in prolonged hypotension and death. Nevertheless, when chest radiography is performed, common findings include hyperlucent lung fields on the affected side with absent markings, diaphragm flattening on the affected side, and tracheal-mediastinal deviation away from the affected side (Fig. 17.26).

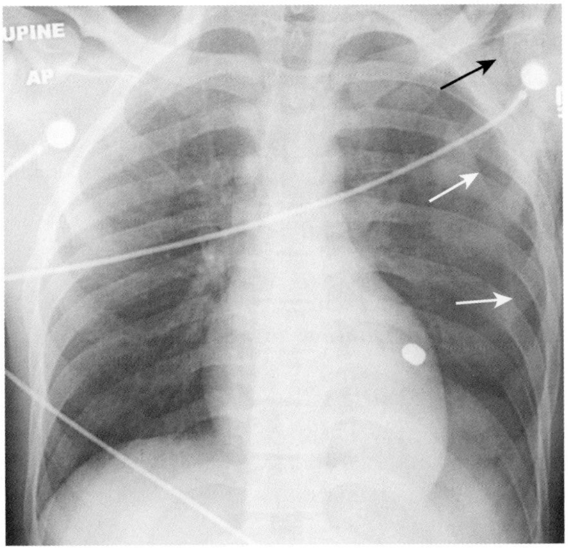

FIG. 17.25 Pneumothorax of the left lung, outlined in *white arrows*. Also present is subcutaneous emphysema *(black arrow)* and a bullet (superimposed over the heart). *(From Herring W.* Learning Radiology. *2nd ed. Philadelphia: Elsevier; 2011.)*

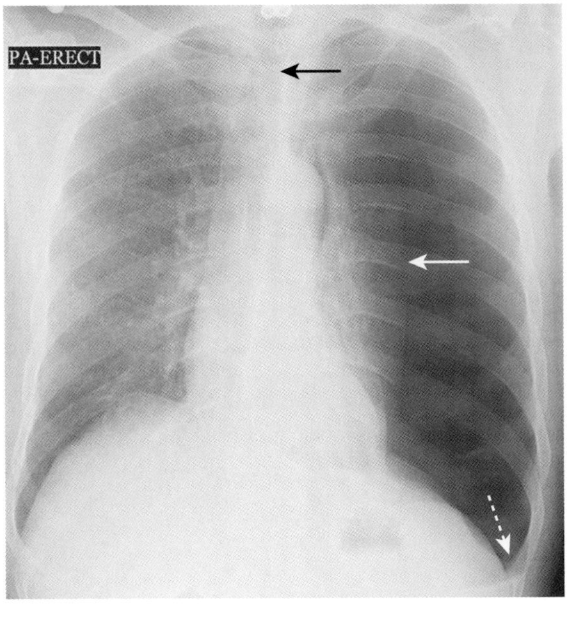

FIG. 17.26 Large left-sided tension pneumothorax (*white arrows*). Note that this is a tension pneumothorax because the trachea is displaced away from the side of the pneumothorax *(black arrow)*. *(From Herring W.* Learning Radiology. *2nd ed. Philadelphia: Elsevier; 2011.)*

Treatment: Pressure is first relieved via needle thoracotomy, which involves inserting a large-bore IV needle into the second intercostal space along the midclavicular line. This relieves the tension on the vena cava and resolves the hypotension, providing enough time for a chest tube to be placed.

PHARMACOLOGY

Inhaled β_2-Adrenergic Selective Agonists

Inhaled β_2-adrenergic selective agonists can be short acting, such as albuterol or levalbuterol, or long acting, such as salmeterol or formoterol.

Mechanism of Action: They act on β_2 receptors of intracellular adenyl cyclase, the enzyme that catalyzes the conversion of adenosine triphosphate (ATP) to cyclic adenosine monophosphate (AMP). This action results in **increased cyclic AMP levels in bronchial smooth muscle, causing bronchial smooth muscle relaxation.** They are also thought to inhibit mast cell release of immediate hypersensitivity mediators.

Clinical Uses: These agents are used to alleviate acute bronchospasm in acute asthma exacerbations (most common); as prophylaxis against exercise-induced asthma; to alleviate bronchospasm in COPD; during general anesthesia; in NRDS or RSV infection; and as rapid treatment of critical hyperkalemia (drive K^+ into cells).

Side Effects: These include tachycardia and palpitations (caused by some β_1 effects, although levalbuterol is more β_2 selective than albuterol and causes less tachycardia), tremors, anxiety, and hypokalemia.

Muscarinic Antagonists

Examples of muscarinic antagonists are ipratropium (short acting) and tiotropium (long acting).

Mechanism of Action: Muscarinic antagonists **antagonize acetylcholine at muscarinic receptors,** prevent bronchoconstriction by preventing increase in cyclic guanosine monophosphate (cGMP) caused by interaction of acetylcholine with muscarinic receptors on bronchial smooth muscles, and reduce secretions from mucous glands.

Clinical Uses: Uses include COPD maintenance therapy and, off-label, asthma exacerbations.

Side Effects: Side effects include nasal mucosa dryness, xerostomia, bronchitis, and sinusitis.

Phosphodiesterase-4 Inhibitors

An example of a phosphodiesterase-4 (PDE4) inhibitor is roflumilast.

Mechanism of Action: These agents selectively inhibit PDE4 leading to accumulation of cyclic AMP (cAMP) within inflammatory and structural cells important in the pathogenesis of COPD.

Clinical Uses: They are used in the treatment of COPD.

Side Effects: Side effects include headache, diarrhea, and weight loss.

Methylxanthines

An example a methylxanthine is theophylline.

Mechanism of Action: Methylxanthines are believed to cause **bronchodilation through inhibition of phosphodiesterase,** the enzyme that breaks down cyclic AMP, thus increasing cyclic AMP levels, which causes bronchial smooth muscle relaxation. Also thought to increase contraction force of diaphragm by increasing Ca^{2+} uptake into the muscle.

Clinical Uses: Uses include as an asthma controller medication and treatment for COPD.

Side Effects: Side effects include tremor, irritability, nausea, vomiting, and tachyarrhythmia. These agents have a narrow therapeutic index and so are used as a last-line controller medication in patients with poorly controlled asthma.

Cromolyn

Mechanism of Action: Cromolyn is a **mast cell stabilizer** (blocks histamine release) and **antiinflammatory** agent. It prevents bronchoconstriction in response to inhaled antigens.

Clinical Uses: It is used as an asthma controller medication and to treat allergic rhinitis.

Side Effects: Cromolyn has minimal toxicity.

Omalizumab

Mechanism of Action: Omalizumab is an anti-IgE monoclonal antibody.

Clinical Uses: Uses include treatment of asthma that is poorly controlled with steroids or beta agonists.

Side Effects: Omalizumab has minimal toxicity.

Leukotriene Inhibitors

Leukotrienes are mediators synthesized by leukocytes that promote bronchoconstriction and neutrophil chemotaxis. Inhibition of leukotriene production and activity is therefore an important target for asthma therapy.

Montelukast, Zafirlukast

Mechanism of Action: These agents selectively antagonize leukotriene receptors.

Clinical Uses: They are used as asthma controller medication and are especially useful in triad asthma (asthma induced by aspirin, NSAID use). Montelukast is also indicated for acute prevention of exercise-induced bronchoconstriction and for allergic rhinitis.

Side Effects: Leukotriene inhibitors have minimal toxicity. Headache can be a side effect.

Zileuton

Mechanism of Action: Zileuton selectively inhibits 5-lipoxygenase, the enzyme that catalyzes the formation of leukotrienes from arachidonic acid.

Clinical Uses: Zileuton is used as an asthma controller medication.

Side Effects: This agent has minimal toxicity.

Corticosteroids

- Inhaled: Beclomethasone, budesonide, fluticasone, mometasone
- Oral: Prednisone and dexamethasone

Mechanism of Action: Corticosteroids exert **antiinflammatory** effects by inhibiting inflammatory cells and production of inflammatory mediators.

Clinical Uses: Inhaled corticosteroids are first-line asthma controller medications; oral corticosteroids are used to treat asthma exacerbations unresponsive to other measures, **as well as other** inflammatory conditions.

Side Effects

- Inhaled: Minimal systemic absorption and therefore minimal toxicity.
- Oral: Osteoporosis, immunosuppression, hypertension, Cushing syndrome, hyperglycemia, cataracts, glaucoma, fluid retention, avascular necrosis of femoral head, depression, mania, adrenal insufficiency (on cessation).

Expectorants

Guaifenesin

Mechanism of Action: Guaifenesin has an expectorant effect by reducing the viscosity of tracheal and bronchial secretions.

Clinical Uses: It is used as an expectorant in over-the-counter medications (e.g., Robitussin, Mucinex) and in intensive care units to help patients on mechanical ventilation clear secretions.

Side Effects: Guaifenesin has minimal toxicity.

N-Acetylcysteine

Mechanism of Action: *N*-Acetylcysteine cleaves disulfide bonds in mucous glycoproteins, thus loosening thick sputum. It functions as a glutathione donor in acetaminophen overdose.

Clinical Uses: It is a mucolytic used for cystic fibrosis, tracheostomy care, or any respiratory condition with abnormal or inspissated mucous secretions and in acetaminophen overdose.

Side Effects: *N*-Acetylcysteine has minimal toxicity.

Pulmonary Arterial Hypertension Medications

Oral Phosphodiesterase Inhibitors

Examples of oral phosphodiesterase inhibitors are sildenafil and tadalafil.

Mechanism of Action: Oral phosphodiesterase inhibitors inhibit phosphodiesterase type 5 (PDE-5) in smooth muscle in the pulmonary vasculature, resulting in increased cGMP, which relaxes the pulmonary vasculature.

Clinical Uses: These agents are used to treat pulmonary arterial hypertension and also erectile dysfunction.

Side Effects: Side effects include flushing, headache, visual disturbance, dyspepsia, and epistaxis.

Prostacyclin Pathway Agonists

Examples of prostacyclin pathway agonists are epoprostenol, trepostinil, iloprost, and selexipag.

Mechanism of Action: These agents have vasodilatory effects on pulmonary arterial vascular beds through the prostacyclin pathway.

Clinical Uses: They are used to treat pulmonary arterial hypertension.

Side Effects: Side effects include flushing and jaw pain.

Endothelin Receptor Antagonists

Examples of endothelin receptor antagonists include bosentan, ambrisentan, and macitentan.

Mechanism of Action: These agents function by antagonizing the endothelin-1 receptor. Endothelin-1 is a potent vasoconstrictor that can promote cell proliferation, fibrosis, and tissue remodeling and is thought to play a role in pulmonary arterial hypertension.

Clinical Uses: They are used to treat pulmonary arterial hypertension.

Side Effects: Side effects include headache, aspartate transaminase (AST)–alanine aminotransferase (ALT) elevation, lower extremity edema, and hypotension.

REVIEW QUESTIONS

(1) A 5-year-old boy is eating peanuts while lying in bed and accidentally aspirates one. A pulmonologist evaluates him and performs a bronchoscopy. In which bronchopulmonary segment is the pulmonologist most likely to find the peanut?

(2) A 64-year-old man is having a severe congestive heart failure exacerbation. On physical examination, you notice he is having increased work of breathing. Which accessory muscles of inspiration is he likely using? Your next patient is having a severe asthma attack and has difficulty exhaling. Which accessory muscles is he using to aid in exhalation?

(3) A 69-year-old woman with a 55-pack/yr smoking history presents to your office with proximal muscle weakness. Physical examination confirms the weakness, but you notice strength increases with repeated testing. A chest radiograph reveals a centrally located pulmonary mass. What may be responsible for this patient's symptoms?

(4) A premature infant develops tachypnea, grunting, and retractions shortly after birth. Symptoms improve with oxygen, assisted ventilation, and administration of exogenous surfactant. Why did the neonate have a deficiency of endogenous surfactant, and from where does endogenous surfactant arise?

(5) A 62-year-old smoker with COPD presents to your office with the results of his pulmonary function tests. What are they likely to reveal? How will they compare with the PFTs of your patient with pulmonary fibrosis?

(6) A 7-year old boy with mild intermittent asthma has an episode of wheezing and shortness of breath relieved with his albuterol inhaler. What is the mechanism of action of this medication?

ANSWERS

CHAPTER 1

1. Answer:

2.5%. 1 SD contains 68% of values, 2 SDs contain 95% of values, and 3 SDs contain 98% of values. Therefore 5% of his values will be >2 SDs away; 2.5% will be >145; and 2.5% will be <135.

2. Answer:

This test appears to be very good at identifying sick people but not good at identifying healthy people. It is therefore sensitive but not specific.

		DISEASE	
		YES	**NO**
Test	**Yes**	Tp = 195	Fp = 35
	No	Fn = 5	Tn = 115

$$\text{Sensitivity} = \frac{\text{Tp}}{(\text{Tp}+\text{Fn})} = \frac{195}{(195+5)} = 97.5\,\%.$$

$$\text{Specificity} = \frac{\text{Tn}}{(\text{Tn}+\text{Fp})} = \frac{115}{(115+35)} = 77\,\%.$$

$$\text{PPV} = \frac{\text{Tp}}{(\text{Tp}+\text{Fp})} = \frac{195}{(195+35)} = 85\,\%$$

$$\text{NPV} = \frac{\text{Tn}}{(\text{Tn}+\text{Fn})} = \frac{115}{(115+5)} = 96\,\%$$

3. Answer:

		OUTCOME	
		YES	**NO**
Exposure	**Yes**	**A** = 9	**B** = 2
	No	**C** = 1	**D** = 8

$$\text{Risk in exposed} = \frac{\text{a}}{(\text{a}+\text{b})} = \frac{10}{(10+190)} = 0.05 = 5\,\%.$$

$$\text{Risk in unexposed} = \frac{\text{c}}{(\text{c}+\text{d})} = \frac{30}{(30+170)} = 0.15 = 15\,\%.$$

$$\text{ARR} = 15\,\% - 5\,\% = 10\,\%.$$

$$\text{NNT} = \frac{1}{\text{ARR}} = \frac{1}{0.1} = 10.$$

$$\text{RR} = \frac{\text{risk in exposed}}{\text{risk in unexposed}} = \frac{5\,\%}{15\,\%} = 33\,\%$$

$$\text{RRR} = \frac{(\text{risk in exposed} - \text{risk in unexposed})}{\text{risk in unexposed}} = \frac{(15\,\% - 5\,\%)}{15\,\%} = 67\,\%.$$

4. Answer:

		OUTCOME	
		YES	**NO**
Exposure	Yes	**A** = 10	**B** = 190
	No	**C** = 30	**D** = 170

OR = (a/b)/(c/d) = ad/cb = 36. The odds of having Buerger's disease in smokers are 36 times those of non-smokers. We cannot calculate prevalence using these data because we intentionally selected 10 patients with the disease and 10 without. Because this is a case-control study, we calculate odds ratio, not relative risk.

5. Answer:

A chi-square test is the appropriate choice to determine whether there is a difference in proportions of categorical data. Note that even though age is continuous, you chose the nominal variable >65 and <65.

6. Answer:

ANOVA is the appropriate test to compare continuous data between more than two groups.

7. Answer:

The patient's reproductive health concerns can be addressed without parental consent. After counseling the patient, it would be appropriate to begin treatment for chlamydia and gonorrhea and consider starting an oral contraceptive. Suturing her laceration will require the consent of her mother.

8. Answer:

The physician must inform the patient unless it will be so distressing as to cause the patient to become suicidal (therapeutic privilege). A family member's request is not enough to prevent disclosure of a diagnosis (unless it is the guardian of a minor).

9. Answer:

The patient's autonomy to refuse care must be respected. Every effort should be made, however, to ensure she understands the acuity of the situation.

10. Answer:

Yes, a patient is considered competent unless legally declared incompetent. He is considered to have decision-making capacity unless the physician notes overwhelming evidence to the contrary.

CHAPTER 2

1. Answer:

ALA dehydratase and ferrochelatase are inhibited by lead, causing reduction in heme synthesis.

2. Answer:

PKU is diagnosed by finding elevated phenylalanine caused by an autosomal recessive deficiency of phenylalanine hydroxylase. This prevents conversion of phenylalanine to tyrosine. Treatment consists of a low-phenylalanine diet.

3. Answer:

The branched-chain amino acids leucine, isoleucine, and valine will be found in the patient's urine in increased levels as a result of an autosomal recessive enzyme deficiency known as maple syrup urine disease.

4. Answer:

Vitamin C deficiency can result in scurvy. Vitamin C is an important cofactor that allows the cross-linkage of collagen. Without vitamin C, connective tissue becomes fragile.

5. Answer:

For competitive inhibitors, K_m is increased but V_{max} is unchanged. For noncompetitive inhibitors, K_m is unchanged but V_{max} is decreased.

6. Answer:

This patient has orotic aciduria and should be fed synthetic uridine to supply needed pyrimidines.

7. Answer:

Allopurinol is a xanthine oxidase inhibitor. Xanthine oxidase converts hypoxanthine to xanthine, and then converts xanthine to uric acid. Hypoxanthine and xanthine are more soluble than uric acid and do not form crystal deposits, thereby decreasing uric acid crystal formation.

8. Answer:

Xeroderma pigmentosum. Patients with this disorder have a mutant ultraviolet (UV) radiation–specific endonuclease and are unable to repair thymine dimers created by DNA damage by UV radiation.

9. Answer:

This infant has a deficiency in galactose metabolism causing severe galactosemia, which if untreated could lead to death. The treatment should include eliminating all galactose and lactose from the diet.

10. Answer:

This patient likely has G6PD deficiency, and the oxidant drug sulfamethoxazole was enough oxidative stress to cause red blood cell lysis and thus hemolytic anemia. The red blood cells of patients with G6PD deficiency have characteristic Heinz bodies, which are clumps of denatured hemoglobin that form from the oxidative damage.

11. Answer:

As levels in insulin increase and levels of glucagon decrease after a meal, there is an increase in fructose 2,6-bisphosphate. This causes activation of PFK-1 and an increase in the rate of glycolysis when glucose is plentiful.

12. Answer:

Mitochondrial diseases such as Leber hereditary optic neuropathy, mitochondrial encephalomyopathy with lactic acidosis and strokelike episodes (MELAS), and myoclonic epilepsy and ragged red fibers (MERRF) are transmitted only from affected women to their offspring. This is because the egg has the mitochondria that are passed on, not the sperm. His chance of passing on his condition to his offspring is 0%.

13. Answer:

This one is more difficult. The man's father has cystic fibrosis ("aa") and the man's mother presumably is not a carrier (and is therefore "AA"). Therefore all the offspring are carriers ("Aa"). The man must be a carrier, and the man's wife must also be a carrier. Therefore the four options for their offspring are AA, Aa, Aa, and aa. There is a 25% chance their children will have cystic fibrosis, and there is a 50% chance their children will be carriers.

14. Answer:

The answer to both questions is 0%. The son must get the Y chromosome and not the X chromosome from the father; therefore, the son could not have hemophilia A. The daughter would get the affected X chromosome from the father but the normal X chromosome from the mother. Therefore all the daughters would be carriers, but none of them would have hemophilia A.

CHAPTER 3

1. Answer:

In Addison disease, adrenal insufficiency causes elevated levels of ACTH. ACTH cleavage produces melanocyte-stimulating hormone, which stimulates melanocytes to produce more melanin (and darker skin). Of note, adrenal insufficiency also leads to decreased production of aldosterone and thus the given electrolyte imbalances.

2. Answer:

The presence of joint pain, nail pitting, and a rash that improves with sunlight is suspicious for psoriatic arthritis. Psoriatic arthritis is associated with HLA-B27, as are the other seronegative spondyloarthropathies: inflammatory bowel disease, ankylosing spondylitis, and reactive arthritis.

3. Answer:

The presence of tense bullae that spare mucous membranes is suggestive of bullous pemphigoid. Linear deposits of IgG and C3 along the basement membrane confirm that hemidesmosomes have been targeted, leading to subepidermal blisters.

4. Answer:

Tinea versicolor from infection with *Malassezia globosa* or *Malassezia furfur.* These lesions should be differentiated from vitiligo, which will present as asymptomatic depigmented patches without scaling.

5. Answer:

The patient's rash was initially thought to be tinea corporis; however, it was actually the herald patch of pityriasis rosea. When the patient returned, he had the full presentation of the rash in a "Christmas tree" distribution. This self-limited condition will likely improve on its own. Topical antifungals will be of no use.

6. Answer:

The severity, rapid onset, high fever, and presence of skip lesions all are concerning for necrotizing fasciitis as opposed to a simple diabetic foot infection. This patient should be admitted to the hospital for intravenous antibiotics and debridement of necrotic tissue.

7. Answer:

This patient likely has postinfectious glomerulonephritis from a previous episode of streptococcal impetigo. The diagnosis can be confirmed if studies show high titers of antistreptolysin O (ASO) antibodies, low complement, and the presence of RBC casts in the urine. Management is supportive, and children tend to have complete recovery. Any ongoing infection should be treated.

8. Answer:

This patient has evidence of sarcoidosis. Among other findings, she may have tender nodules of the skin representing the panniculitis of erythema nodosum.

9. Answer:

No. Acanthosis nigricans is a result of elevated insulin, usually as a result of type 2 diabetes. Given this patient's early age of onset, history of DKA, and early requirement of insulin, it is likely that her diagnosis is type 1 diabetes and that native insulin levels will be negligible.

10. Answer:

As in the treatment of dermatologic conditions, retinoids bind retinoic acid receptors and induce transcription. In APL, this vitamin A analog induces differentiation of leukemic promyelocytes into mature granulocytes.

CHAPTER 4

1. Answer:

The T3 vertebral body is caudal, medial, and dorsal to the left clavicle.

2. Answer:

During ovulation, eggs are arrested in metaphase II and will not complete the cell cycle unless fertilization occurs.

3. Answer:

This is a monochorionic, monoamniotic set of twins. Because they share so many structures, the split must have occurred later, after day 8, because the cells by then were too differentiated to make their own placenta and amniotic sac.

4. Answer:

The epidermis of the skin (a) originates from ectoderm. The GI tract (b) originates from endoderm. The muscles (c) originate from myotome, which is from the mesoderm.

5. Answer:

The neural tube closes at 4 weeks' gestation. Recall ovulation occurs 14 days before the onset of menses, so the fetus will be at least 2 weeks old before a woman's menstrual cycle is "late." Therefore, it is possible that a woman may not know she is pregnant until the fetus is at least 3 weeks old. Folate supplementation must occur before the neural tube closes to help prevent spina bifida, so supplementation before pregnancy is known is important.

6. Answer:

Spina bifida with myelomeningocele (see Fig. 4.7C) is the term for spina bifida when the defect is large enough for both the spinal cord and meninges to protrude. This can lead to spinal cord damage at this level and therefore cause paralysis and sensory loss below this level.

7. Answer:

Levothyroxine is not teratogenic; in fact, not taking it can be harmful to the fetus if there is not enough thyroid hormone available to it before its own thyroid is developed. Lisinopril, an ACE inhibitor, is teratogenic and can cause renal agenesis and should be stopped. Lithium is also teratogenic and associated with Ebstein anomaly.

8. Answer:

She is at increased risk for clear cell carcinoma of the vagina.

9. Answer:

The three main shunts are (1) the ductus venosus, which shunts blood away from the liver to the heart, closing and becoming the ligamentum venosum after birth; (2) the foramen ovale, shunting blood from right to left atrium to bypass the lungs, closing and becoming the fossa ovalis after birth; and (3) the ductus arteriosus, shunting blood from the pulmonary artery to aorta to bypass the lungs, closing and becoming the ligamentum arteriosum after birth.

10. Answer:

It can be kept open by prostaglandin E_1 (alprostadil) and closed by indomethacin.

11. Answer:

Omphalocele. An umbilical hernia is also midline but will be covered by skin. Gastroschisis will be lateral, and viscera will not be covered by a peritoneal sac.

12. Answer:

Thyroglossal duct cyst.

13. Answer:

This chromosomal anomaly is a variant of Klinefelter syndrome (most commonly XXY). By the genotype alone, however, one could deduce that the patient would have testicles because the Y chromosome contains the testis-determining factor, *SRY.*

14. Answer:

A branchial cleft cyst has likely been growing as a result of failure of obliteration of the second branchial cleft.

15. Answer:

These milestones are consistent with a 2 year old.

CHAPTER 5

1. Answer:

Gram-positive bacteria have a thick peptidoglycan cell wall and Gram stain blue; gram-negative bacteria have a thin peptidoglycan cell wall and an additional outer LPS membrane and Gram stain red.

2. Answer:

(a) Requires oxygen for ATP synthesis; (b) requires fermentation for ATP synthesis and cannot survive in the presence of oxygen; (c) prefers oxygen but can ferment; (d) prefers fermentation but can survive in low oxygen; (e) cannot make ATP and therefore requires host ATP; (f) can survive if phagocytosed because enzymes protect it against digestion by superoxide radicals.

3. Answer:

Asplenic patients cannot destroy encapsulated organisms because the spleen is where phagocytosis of opsonized bacteria takes place; encapsulated organisms are detected either by India ink stain or the Quellung reaction.

4. Answer:

S. aureus causes disease through direct invasion or toxin release; *S. pyogenes* causes disease by direct invasion, toxin release, and postinfectious autoimmunity. See the tables in this section for examples.

5. Answer:

All three are cause by both *S. aureus* and *S. pyogenes* and can present with erythema, pain over the affected area, and fever. However, erysipelas generally has a well-demarcated erythematous border, cellulitis has no well-demarcated border, and necrotizing fasciitis may have a blue-purple discoloration with blisters and is generally much more painful.

6. Answer:

(a) Scarlet fever; (b) group A strep; (c) throat swab showing gram-positive cocci in chains that are β-hemolytic and bacitracin sensitive, or presence of anti–streptolysin O antibodies; (d) penicillin G; (e) the child may experience desquamation of palms and soles after the rash subsides.

7. Answer:

Streptococcus pneumoniae; gram-positive diplococci.

8. Answer:

N. meningitidis causes meningitis, sepsis, and Waterhouse-Friderichsen syndrome. *N. gonococcus* causes gonorrhea (urethritis, epididymitis, prostatitis in men, urethritis, endometritis, pelvic inflammatory disease in women), Fitz-Hugh-Curtis syndrome, septic arthritis, and ophthalmia neonatorum.

9. Answer:

Both *N. meningitidis* and *N. gonococcus* appear as gram-negative diplococci and selectively grow on Thayer-Martin media; in the laboratory they can be distinguished because *N.* **m***eningitidis* metabolizes **m**altose and glucose, whereas *N.* **g***onococcus* only metabolizes **g**lucose.

10. Answer:

The HACEK organisms cause "culture-negative endocarditis" and are ***H****aemophilus*, ***A****ctinobacter*, ***C****ardiobacter*, ***E****ikinella*, and ***K****ingella.*

11. Answer:

B. anthracis causes anthrax, including woolsorter's disease (inhalation anthrax); *B. cereus* causes gastroenteritis. *B. anthracis* is the only encapsulated bacteria with a protein rather than polysaccharide capsule.

12. Answer:

C. botulinum releases a toxin that blocks acetylcholine release at nerve synapses of the autonomic system and motor endplates, causing paralysis; *C. tetani* releases a toxin that blocks GABA/glycine release from Renshaw interneurons, causing spasm; *C. perfringens* and *C. tetani* release toxins that cause local tissue damage.

13. Answer:

At risk are those with compromised cell-mediated immunity (immunocompromised patients, older adults), pregnant women (third trimester), and neonates. *L. monocytogenes* is the only gram-positive bacterium that produces endotoxin.

14. Answer:

Diagnose with culture on potassium tellurite and Loeffler coagulated blood serum; treat with antitoxin immunoglobulin, antibiotics (penicillin or erythromycin), and TDaP vaccine.

15. Answer:

(a) ETEC, *V. cholera;* (b) EHEC; (c) EIEC, Shigella, C. jejuni, *S. typhi, Y. enterolitica;* (d) K. *pneumoniae;* (e) *K. pneumoniae, P. mirabilis*; (f) *H. pylori;* (g) *P. aeruginosa;* (h) *P. aeruginosa;* (i) EHEC strain O157:H7.

16. Answer:

Pneumonia (especially with intubation or sedation), sepsis, and urinary tract infections (especially with indwelling catheter).

17. Answer:

Bacteroides and *Fusobacterium* species, which generally cause disease after tissue damage, especially in the GI tract, mouth, and vagina. In addition, *B. melaninogenicus* can cause aspiration pneumonia, and *F. necrophorum* is implicated in Lemierre disease.

18. Answer:

Immunized individuals are still susceptible to *H. influenzae* otitis media (kids) and upper respiratory infections (adults with COPD); unimmunized individuals are susceptible to *H. influenzae* meningitis, acute epiglottitis, and septic arthritis (mainly children aged 6 months to 3 years).

19. Answer:

(a) Bacterial vaginosis: dysuria, labial itching, and foul-smelling discharge, demonstrates "clue cells" on wet mount; (b) pertussis: fever, nasal discharge, sneezing, and later a paroxysmal "whooping" cough, diagnosed by culture on Bordet-Gengou medium; (c) atypical pneumonia: lobar pneumonia with bradycardia, elevated LFTs, hyponatremia, and hypophosphatemia.

20. Answer:

(a) *Y. pestis,* (b) *F. tularensis.*

21. Answer:

They grow like mycelia, live in water and soil, and are saprophytes, all of which are characteristics of fungi.

22. Answer:

Nocardia is diagnosed by acid-fast stain and treated with TMP-SMX; *Actinomyces* is diagnosed by observation of yellow granules in pus from an abscess and treated with drainage and penicillin G.

23. Answer:

Starts as a metabolically inactive but infectious *elementary body,* then switches to *reticulate body* inside the host cell, which can form proteins but not ATP. Serotypes A to C cause trachoma; serotypes D to K cause inclusion conjunctivitis, pneumonia, and sexually transmitted infections; serotypes L1 to L3 cause lymphogranuloma venereum.

24. Answer:

Both are extremely small and require host ATP and hence are obligate intracellular organisms; whereas chlamydial species prefer to infect columnar epithelium and can be spread host to host, rickettsial species prefer to infect endothelial cells lining blood vessels and require an arthropod vector.

25. Answer:

Rickettsia rickettsii, or Rocky Mountain spotted fever. Patients will often not be aware they have been bitten by a tic, especially if in a nonvisible area such as the back of the leg or in an area covered by hair.

26. Answer:

(a) Herpes simplex, chancroid caused by *H. ducreyi,* and syphilis; (b) FTA-ABS (antitreponemal antibodies); (c) desensitization to penicillin; (d) primary; (e) primary and secondary; (f) all trimesters; (g) no, the baby will require further treatment after birth because the patient is already in her third trimester.

27. Answer:

(a) *Borrelia burgdorferi;* (b) annular, expanding rash with central blue discoloration; (c) early disseminated phase; (d) skin, nervous system, heart, joints.

28. Answer:

Treat immediately with penicillin to cover empirically for leptospira.

29. Answer:

Mycobacterium and *Nocardia;* the high lipid content of their cell walls causes them to resist decolorization by acid after staining with carbolfuchsin.

30. Answer:

(a) Active tuberculosis infection; (b) sputum culture and stain for acid-fast bacteria; (c) secondary/reactivation TB; (d) rifampin, isoniazid, pyrazidamole with vitamin B_6, and ethambutol.

31. Answer:

Because *Mycobacterium* spp. are intracellular organisms, the host response is purely cell mediated, and therefore the skin tests rely on a type IV hypersensitivity reaction to take place, which takes 48 to 72 hours.

32. Answer:

The cooler areas of the body are most affected: skin (lumps, leonine facies), peripheral nerves (glove-and-stocking paresthesias), nasal cartilage (saddlenose deformity), testes (infertility), and eyes (blindness).

33. Answer:

Cold agglutinin test, PCR for DNA or DNA probe, sputum cultures.

34. Answer:

Urease in urine.

35. Answer:

Both single-stranded and double-stranded DNA viruses require the host cell's DNA and RNA polymerases located in the nucleus in order to create viral progeny and mRNA for translation into viral proteins, respectively. Members of the family Poxviridae have a viral DNA-dependent RNA polymerase contained within the virus particle to create the transcriptional machinery necessary to replicate in the host cell's cytoplasm.

36. Answer:

Enveloped viruses usually require their lipid bilayer membrane for transmission—often direct contact of mucous membranes, eyes, or bloodstream with virus-containing body fluids. Anything that destabilizes that membrane (heat, detergents, desiccation) will interfere with their ability to infect. Naked viruses do not have a membrane and thus are often stable in the environment for longer periods. They are transmitted by direct transfer as described, and also by indirect transmission through fomites or aerosols.

37. Answer:

Patient is in the equivalence zone or "window period" of hepatitis B infection. Test for anti-HBc antibody to prove infection with HBV.

38. Answer:

DNA viruses (adenovirus, EBV, CMV); RNA viruses (coxsackievirus, orthomyxoviruses, primary HIV); bacteria (group A strep, *Mycoplasma pneumoniae, Corynebacterium diphtheriae*).

39. Answer:

Parvovirus B19 infection. Pregnant women in the first trimester, because of the risk for hydrops fetalis; and patients with hemoglobinopathies including sickle cell disease or hereditary spherocytosis, because of the risk for precipitating an aplastic crisis.

40. Answer:

Positive-sense single-stranded RNA viruses, because their genome represents mRNA that can readily undergo translation. Linear, double-stranded DNA viruses, because their genome can be incorporated into the host cell's DNA by double-stranded break repair mechanisms. All other viruses require a viral polymerase, or reverse transcriptase, in order to be used by the host cell's transcription/translation machinery.

41. Answer:

Rubella is a much milder illness; onset begins with truncal maculopapular erythematous rash with rapid distal spread. Rubeola or "measles" begins with 3 days of fever and the 3 *C*s (cough, coryza, and conjunctivitis); on the third day, maculopapular erythematous rash begins on the head and spreads caudally, eventually darkens, and coalesces. Rubella can cause congenital syndrome if the mother is infected in the first or second trimester, including cataracts, sensorineural hearing loss, and cardiac defects (patent ductus arteriosus, pulmonary artery stenosis). Rubeola can cause a persistent infection in the CNS that manifests 6 to 15 years later as subacute sclerosing panencephalitis (SSPE), a progressive neurodegenerative disease that is often fatal.

42. Answer:

Selected influenza strains from previous years contained within the vaccine may be sufficiently different from the current year's circulating strains to cause poor antibody recognition and insufficient immunity (genetic drift); circulating influenza strains may have undergone cross-species recombination in animal reservoirs, creating serotypes unrelated to any recently circulating strains, rendering vaccine-derived antibodies useless (genetic shift).

43. Answer:

A, contaminated water or food source; B, needle stick injuries, sexually transmitted, blood contact with ocular or mucocutaneous surface; C, IV drug use, multiple transfusions; D, *only* in HBV chronic carriers, similar risk factors as HBV, transplant or immunosuppression; E, contaminated water or food source, pregnancy increases risk for fulminant hepatitis.

44. Answer:

CNS toxoplasmosis, primary CNS B-cell lymphoma. Progressive multifocal leukoencephalopathy or PML, caused by infection with JC virus in AIDS patients.

45. Answer:

Fungal cell membranes are composed of ergosterol, a sterol unique to fungi. Ergosterol is a target in multiple antifungal drugs, including ketoconazole, nystatin, and amphotericin B.

46. Answer:

Hyphae are the branching filaments of a budding fungus. True hyphae consist of connected cells with dividing septa; pseudohyphae lack septa. This distinction is important for the identification of a fungus. For example, *Candida* spp. may form pseudohyphae, whereas *Aspergillus* spp. form true septated hyphae.

47. Answer:

He likely has a superficial *Tinea versicolor* infection. *Tinea versicolor* damages melanocytes, so affected skin does not tan. Diagnosis is confirmed by microscopic evaluation of a skin scraping for fungal elements ("spaghetti and meatballs").

48. Answer:

Because the patient is immunocompromised, he is at risk for developing opportunistic infections. This patient has oral thrush, caused by *Candida* infection of the mucous membranes. Diagnosis is confirmed by examining the white exudate under the microscope for *Candida* fungal elements, such as pseudohyphae.

49. Answer:

In an immunocompromised patient with oral thrush and pain with swallowing, *Candida* esophagitis should be considered in the differential diagnosis. CMV and HSV esophagitis should also be considered in the differential.

50. Answer:

This landscraper has sporotrichosis, caused by cutaneous inoculation with *Sporothrix schenckii.* She likely has developed ascending lymphangitis. Treat with potassium iodide or itraconazole.

51. Answer:

Dimorphic fungi are found as mold forms in the environment and morph to yeast forms at higher temperatures.

52. Answer:

Coccidiomycosis, endemic to southern California ("San Joaquin Valley fever") and the U.S. Southwest; histoplasmosis, endemic to the Ohio River Valley; blastomycosis, endemic mostly to the Mississippi River Valley and the Great Lakes region. Paracoccidiomycosis is endemic mostly to Central and South America.

53. Answer:

(a) Coccidiomycosis; (b) blastomycosis; (c) histoplasmosis.

54. Answer:

In immunocompetent individuals, *Aspergillus* may cause allergic bronchopulmonary aspergillosis (ABPA). ABPA is characterized by bronchospasm and, left untreated, with bronchiectasis, pulmonary fibrosis, and irreversible pulmonary changes. ABPA is caused by an IgE-mediated hypersensitivity reaction to pulmonary *aspergillosis,* rather than primary infection with the fungus.

55. Answer:

Immunocompromised state, particularly in those with immunodeficiency (CGD) or those taking immunosuppressive medications (transplant recipients, patients taking high-dose steroids).

56. Answer:

Immunocompromised states, diabetes mellitus, trauma/burns, iron overload, and deferoxamine therapy.

57. Answer:

For HIV-positive individuals with a CD4 count <100 and meningitic symptoms, suspect *Cryptococcus* meningitis. Treat with amphotericin B and suppressive doses of fluconazole thereafter.

58. Answer:

(a) Although this man has HIV and a depressed CD4 count, community-acquired pneumonia (i.e., *Streptococcus pneumoniae*) is still the most likely diagnosis. (b) *Pneumocystis* pneumonia is likely in this patient with low CD4 count, diffuse interstitial infiltrates on chest radiograph, and low O_2 saturation. Other expected findings may include high LDH, ground-glass opacities on CT scan, and yeast forms (flying-saucer shaped) in induced sputum. Treat with high-dose TMP-SMX, pentamidine, or dapsone with trimethoprim.

59. Answer:

Suspect *Toxoplasma gondii* infection in an HIV-infected individual with progressive mental status changes and ring-enhancing lesions of the brain on CT imaging. CNS lymphoma should also be considered in the differential diagnosis.

60. Answer:

The triad of chorioretinitis, hydrocephalus, and intracranial calcifications in a newborn is considered diagnostic for congenital *Toxoplasma gondii.* Other congenital infections that should be considered in the differential include rubella, CMV, and syphilis.

61. Answer:

(a) Cryptosporidium; (b) *Entamoeba histolytica;* (c) *Giardia lamblia.*

62. Answer:

Suspect IgA deficiency in an individual with recurrent *G. lamblia* infection, recurrent otitis, sinusitis, bronchitis, and/or pneumonia. Family history of recurrent infection and/or known IgA deficiency may also be elicited.

63. Answer:

(a) *Babesia microti,* Ixodes tick; (b) *Plasmodium* sp., *Anopheles* mosquito; (c) *Leishmaniasis* sp., sandfly; (d) *Trypanosoma cruzi,* reduviid bug; (e) *Trypanosoma brucei* sp., tsetse fly.

64. Answer:

Acute manifestations of Chagas disease include Romaña sign at the site of the bite, fever, lymphadenopathy, hepatosplenomegaly, and myositis. Chronic manifestations include organomegaly: dilated cardiomyopathy, megaesophagus, and megacolon.

65. Answer:

Thick smears screen for the presence of *Plasmodium* sp. in the blood. Thin smears are used to identify specific *Plasmodium* sp.

66. Answer:

(a) 48 hours; (b) 72 hours; (c) irregular intervals.

67. Answer:

P. falciparum infects both young and old red blood cells. Infected RBCs can adhere to capillary walls, causing congestion and infarct of the brain, lung, and kidney.

68. Answer:

The most likely diagnosis is the sexually transmitted disease trichomoniasis, caused by the flagellate *Trichomonas vaginalis.* She should be treated with metronidazole. Her partner should also be treated to prevent reinfection.

69. Answer:

This patient likely has cutaneous larva migrans from hookworm infection. Cutaneous larvae migrans ("creeping eruption") is caused by cutaneous penetration and migration of hookworm. It can be accompanied by elevated IgE and peripheral eosinophilia (Loeffler syndrome).

70. Answer:

This boy likely has enterobiasis ("pinworm"), caused by infection with *Enterobius vermicularis.* Diagnosis can be made at home—adult worms moving near the anus can be visualized with a flashlight at night.

Eggs deposited near the anus can be picked up with a piece of transparent tape ("the Scotch tape test") and evaluated under a light microscope. Treat with a benzimidazole and preventive hygienic measures.

71. Answer:

Trichinosis, caused by infection with the parasite *Trichinella spiralis,* is acquired by the consumption of raw or undercooked meat (usually pork) infected with *Trichinella* cysts. Cysts exist in the stomach and migrate into skeletal muscle.

72. Answer:

A-j; B-f; C-d; D-h; E-e; F-i; G-c; H-g; I-a; J-b.

73. Answer:

No, it is a Jarisch-Herxheimer reaction likely caused by the simultaneous accelerated rupture of many treponemal organisms within the bloodstream causing an inflammatory cytokine buildup.

74. Answer:

Pseudomembranous colitis, trichomoniasis. Both are treated with metronidazole.

75. Answer:

Gram-negative enteric and anaerobic bacteria *(Escherichia coli, Klebsiella, Enterococcus, Streptococcus, Bacteroides)*; third-generation cephalosporin, fluoroquinolone, β-lactamase inhibitor combinations with aminopenicillins or antipseudomonal penicillins).

76. Answer:

Ganciclovir [first line] or foscarnet [second line] for CMV esophagitis; acyclovir and famciclovir would be ineffective because CMV cannot perform the initial phosphorylation step to create the nucleotide analog.

77. Answer:

In the first scenario, *Histoplasma* or *Blastomyces* can be treated with itraconazole, or amphotericin B if the presentation is severe or systemic; *Coccidioides* can be treated with fluconazole, IV before PO if the presentation is acute or severe or systemic; *Aspergillus* can be treated with voriconazole, or amphotericin B if the presentation is severe or there is hematogenous spread.

CHAPTER 6

1. Answer:

This patient has a T-cell deficiency as a result of thymic aplasia. The features of DiGeorge syndrome are remembered by the mnemonic **CATCH-22**—**C**ardiac anomalies, **A**bnormal facies, **T**hymic aplasia, **C**left palate, **H**ypoparathyroidism/**H**ypocalcemia caused by a deletion on chromosome **22.**

2. Answer:

These findings of thrombocytosis and Howell-Jolly bodies on the peripheral smear suggest that this sickle cell disease patient has suffered from autosplenectomy as a result of chronic splenic infarctions.

3. Answer:

The patient in this scenario is in septic shock as a result of a gram-negative rod infection. Most likely, lipopolysaccharide (LPS) from the cell wall of the bacteria triggered the innate immune system by binding to Toll-like receptors and other pattern recognition receptors, resulting in a massive cytokine cascade and shock.

4. Answer:

This patient is suffering from an allergic reaction to a bee sting resulting in anaphylaxis causing urticaria (hives) and wheezing (secondary to bronchoconstriction). This is most likely a result of a type I hypersensitivity reaction involving mast cell degranulation and massive histamine release.

5. Answer:

MHC class I is expressed on all nucleated cells; hence, mature red blood cells that have lost their nucleus no longer express MHC class I on their cell membrane. The exception to this is platelets, which lack a nucleus but do express MHC class I.

6. Answer:

False. $CD8^+$ T cells bind to MHC class I to trigger cell destruction. $CD4^+$ T cells bind MHC class II.

7. Answer:

This patient most likely has hyper-IgM syndrome, with the most common type (type 1) resulting from an inability to undergo isotype class switching. Often there is a deficiency of CD40 ligand on Th2 cells.

8. Answer:

False. IgM does not cross the fetoplacental barrier. Rather, IgG is the isotype implicated in erythroblastosis fetalis and is the reason why Rh-negative mothers are administered RhoGAM during each pregnancy.

9. Answer:

IL-8.

10. Answer:

This situation leads to anergy in which the T cell is inactivated to prevent autoimmune disease from developing.

11. Answer:

This patient is at risk for *Neisseria* infections and therefore is at high risk for disseminated meningococcal infection. Thus the patient should receive the meningococcal (MCV-4) vaccine.

12. Answer:

This patient is most likely suffering from a contact dermatitis secondary to exposure to nickel in the backing of the earring. This is an example of a type IV hypersensitivity reaction in which sensitized T cells from prior exposure interact with the substance (nickel) and release various lymphokines, stimulating an inflammatory response.

CHAPTER 7

1. Answer:

Incomplete tablet breakdown, enzymatic or gastric acid destruction, first-pass metabolism, barriers to absorption across the gut mucosa.

2. Answer:

A very high volume of distribution because it is not staying in the bloodstream in the free unbound form.

3. Answer:

St. John's wort induced CYP3A4, increasing metabolism of her birth control pills—rendering them less effective.

4. Answer:

Because it is a weak acid, alkalization of the urine would facilitate excretion by making more of the drug into the A^- form rather than the uncharged HA form.

5. Answer:

Phenytoin, ethanol, aspirin, the PEA mnemonic—they have a constant amount removed per unit time.

6. Answer:

About 4 to 5.

7. Answer:

Loading dose.

8. Answer:

(a) When a competitive antagonist is added, the potency is decreased because more agonist will be required to reach the EC50 of the drug, whereas the efficacy will be unchanged because adding a lot of agonist will drown out and displace the competitive antagonist. (b) Adding a competitive antagonist will decrease the potency and efficacy of the agonist.

9. Answer:

Irreversible mechanism of action.

10. Answer:

α_1-Receptor activation constricts smooth muscle, using the G_q pathway, which causes increased calcium release and muscle contraction.

11. Answer:

The G_s pathway works by activating adenylyl cyclase and activating protein kinase A, phosphorylating downstream targets to have their effects. The β_1 and β_2 receptors use this pathway.

12. Answer:

(a) The hypotension produced by vasodilation will respond to an α_1 agonist, which causes vasoconstriction through the G_q pathway. (b) The bronchospasm will be relieved by the smooth muscle relaxing receptor β_2, which works through the G_s pathway. Epinephrine is used instead of norepinephrine because norepinephrine would not fix the bronchospasm because of its lack of β_2 activity.

13. Answer:

Cocaine is a reuptake inhibitor, and the patient would have increased sympathetic outflow, causing dilated pupils from activation of the α_1 receptor. **D**ilation of the pupil is called my**D**riasis.

14. Answer:

NAPQI formation, a toxic metabolite of acetaminophen, can overwhelm glutathione stores in large quantities. The treatment is *N*-acetylcysteine, which replenishes those stores to allow for detoxification.

15. Answer:

Iron overdose is potentially lethal because of free radical formation, leading to damage to the intestinal wall and increased iron absorption, which subsequently damages mitochondria and leads to lactic acidosis. The treatment is deferoxamine, which chelates the iron.

16. Answer:

Methanol is metabolized into formaldehyde and formic acid, which is **damaging to the optic nerve** and organs, whereas ethylene glycol is metabolized into oxalic acid, which binds calcium and precipitates in the urine, causing kidney stones and **renal failure.** The treatment is blocking this metabolism by using fomepizole, an alcohol dehydrogenase inhibitor.

CHAPTER 8

1. Answer:

Right atrium → tricuspid valve → right ventricle → pulmonary valve → pulmonary artery → pulmonary capillary → pulmonary vein → left atrium → mitral valve → left ventricle → aortic valve → aorta → renal artery → (renal capillary beds, including glomerular capillaries) → renal vein → inferior vena cava → right atrium.

2. Answer:

Decreased capillary oncotic pressure leads to decreased ability to retain fluid in the capillary bed.

3. Answer:

MAP is two-thirds of the diastolic pressure plus one-third of the systolic pressure. Therefore the MAP is 60 + 50 = 110.

4. Answer:

Stroke volume is the absolute amount ejected by the heart, end-diastolic volume minus end-systolic volume, and is therefore 60 mL. The patient's ejection fraction is the stroke volume (total ejected) divided by the end-diastolic volume (how much the heart had to possibly eject to begin with) and is therefore 50%. The patient's cardiac output is the product of the stroke volume (how much volume the heart pumps each beat) and heart rate (how fast it repeats the stroke volume) and is therefore 4800 mL.

5. Answer:

By Poiseuille's equation, it can be seen that the resistance is proportional to radius to the 4th power. Plugging in ½ as *r* in the equation yields resistance = 2^4 = 16. Therefore the resistance has increased by 16-fold.

6. Answer:

Phase 0: the threshold potential for depolarization has been reached, sodium channels open, rapidly depolarizing the cell. Phase 1: sodium channels close, some potassium leaves (effluxes from) the cell, leading to a transient drop in voltage. Phase 2: L-type calcium channels open, leading to the plateau in the action potential as well as providing calcium for calcium-induced calcium release and myocyte contraction. Phase 3: calcium channels close, potassium efflux predominates and repolarizes the cell. Phase 4: resting state, awaiting another depolarizing stimulus.

7. Answer:

With an increase in calcium availability to bind to troponin C and allow for increased actin–myosin interaction, an increased strength of contraction would occur at a given preload (increased contractility)—conditions that lead to this include β_1 stimulation and digoxin administration. Increased preload leads to a stronger contraction of the heart, but not an increased contractility, because that is defined as the strength of contraction **for a fixed preload.**

8. Answer:

In aortic stenosis, there is increased resistance to movement of blood out of the ventricle into the aorta as a result of narrowing of the outlet through the aortic valve. Therefore it would be expected that the left ventricle would have to generate much higher pressures to get the same pressure in the aorta (in Fig. 8.7, the blue line would rise much higher than the green line). Because the aortic valve is stenotic, there is increased afterload, and changes similar to that in Fig. 8.8B would occur.

9. Answer:

Randomly dropped beats without progressive PR prolongation indicates that the patient has a second-degree Mobitz type II AV block. This is dangerous because it can progress to a complete third-degree AV block.

10. Answer:

During hypotension, there is less pressure on the baroreceptors and therefore they fire less frequently. This causes decreased parasympathetic tone and increased sympathetic tone in an effort to increase the blood pressure.

11. Answer:

The most common cause of right-sided heart failure is left-sided heart failure. Left-sided heart failure leads to blood "backing up" into the pulmonary circulation, causing pulmonary hypertension. Pulmonary hypertension is increased afterload for the right side of the heart; with chronic elevations in afterload, the right side of the heart will fail as well.

12. Answer:

Hypertrophic cardiomyopathy is classically inherited in an autosomal dominant fashion. The physical finding on auscultation is a crescendo–decrescendo murmur similar to that of aortic stenosis. However, in aortic stenosis, increased preload is increased blood that gets ejected through the stenotic valve and therefore the murmur intensity would increase. In hypertrophic cardiomyopathy, increased preload allows for the outflow tract to be wider, lessening the obstruction and decreasing the intensity of the murmur.

13. Answer:

The classic presentation is chest pain that is better when leaning forward, worse when supine. The ECG demonstrates diffuse ST-segment elevation from the inflammation around the heart. The most common infectious cause is viral, specifically Coxsackie B.

14. Answer:

In a pediatric patient with fever lasting longer than 5 days, Kawasaki disease must be considered. The diagnostic criteria can be remembered by the "CRASH and burn" mnemonic: **C**onjunctivitis; **R**ash; **A**denopathy; **S**trawberry tongue or other oral findings; **H**and or foot changes such as desquamation, which is a late finding; and fever (burn). Treatment is aspirin and intravenous immune globulin, and the feared complication is a coronary artery aneurysm.

15. Answer:

The diagnosis is likely Henoch-Schönlein purpura, which is a small vessel vasculitis. Other symptoms may include arthritis and abdominal pain and potentially bloody stool. It is also possible to have intussusception.

16. Answer:

At high doses, epinephrine has significant α-agonist activity and at all doses has significant β-agonist activity. Therefore at high doses there would be significant α- and β-agonist effect, but the beta blocker would prevent epinephrine from attaching to the β receptor, and only α activity would occur. Therefore the patient would have an increase in blood pressure as a result of an increase in systemic vascular resistance. This would trigger the baroreceptor reflex and decrease the heart rate to attempt to counteract this change, and a decrease in heart rate would occur.

17. Answer:

All class I antiarrhythmics are sodium channel blockers. Class Ia: disopyramide, quinidine, procainamide (prolongs AP duration); class Ib: lidocaine, mexiletine, tocainide (does not change AP duration); encainide, moracizine, flecainide, propafenone (shortens AP duration). Class II antiarrhythmics are beta blockers and includes all -lol drugs except for sotalol. Class III antiarrhythmics are potassium channel blockers; sotalol and amiodarone are class III antiarrhythmics, but amiodarone has class I, II, III, and IV activity. Class IV antiarrhythmics are calcium channel blockers, such as verapamil and diltiazem.

CHAPTER 9

1. Answer:

The patient likely has MEN I, characterized by the three *P*s of **p**ituitary, **p**ancreas, and **p**arathyroid endocrine tumors.

2. Answer:

Patients with either MEN IIa or MEN IIb are both at risk for pheochromocytoma and medullary carcinoma of the thyroid. However, only patients with MEN IIa are at increased risk for primary hyperparathyroidism; patients with MEN IIb are instead at risk for developing oral or intestinal ganglioneuromatosis.

3. Answer:

Steroid hormones typically have nuclear receptors to alter gene expression. Therefore the receptor is more likely to be found on the nucleus, rather than on the cell surface.

4. Answer:

(a) Hypothyroidism causes increased TRH and therefore increased stimulation for prolactin release. (b) Dopamine is the negative feedback mechanism for prolactin; dopamine antagonists such as antipsychotic medications increase prolactin by removing the negative feedback inhibition. (c) A prolactinoma will directly cause increased prolactin production.

5. Answer:

FLAT PeG. FSH and LH are involved in reproduction and sex hormone production. ACTH is involved in release of cortisol from the zona fasciculata of the adrenal cortex and androgens from the zona reticularis of the adrenal cortex. TSH is involved in stimulating thyroid hormone production. Prolactin is involved in breast milk production. Growth hormone is involved in linear growth and organ growth.

6. Answer:

The thyroid migrates downward from the base of the tongue to its normal position in the neck. The entire migration is midline, via the thyroglossal duct. If a remnant of the thyroglossal duct remains, a cyst can form; therefore, these cysts are midline as well. This is in contrast to branchial cleft cysts, which are classically lateral.

7. Answer:

False. Thyroglobulin is a protein found normally only in the colloid inside of thyroid follicles. Thyroid-binding globulin is found in the bloodstream. Because thyroglobulin is not normally found in the bloodstream, in inflammatory conditions where thyroglobulin may leak into the bloodstream, antithyroglobulin antibodies can form (and are found in conditions such as Hashimoto thyroiditis).

8. Answer:

The patient has Graves disease. This is characterized by antibodies that stimulate the thyroid's TSH receptor, consistently giving the thyroid the false signal to make more hormone. These antibodies also stimulate fibroblasts behind the eye, leading to increased collagen deposition and proptosis. Proptosis is also due to lymphocytic infiltrate behind the eye in this autoimmune condition.

9. Answer:

The most common form of thyroid cancer is papillary thyroid cancer. Histologic findings include Orphan Annie nuclei and psammoma bodies.

10. Answer:

Remember the mnemonic GFR: zona glomerulosa, zona fasciculata, zona reticularis. They make mineralocorticoids (aldosterone), glucocorticoids (cortisol), and androgens (DHEA), respectively.

11. Answer:

Patients with Addison disease have hyperpigmentation because the decreased level of hormones such as cortisol increase the level of ACTH as a result of loss of negative feedback. The ACTH breaks down into multiple fragments, one of which is α-melanocyte–stimulating hormone (α-MSH). α-MSH stimulates melanocytes, causing hyperpigmentation. The loss of aldosterone causes hyperkalemia because aldosterone activity causes the principal cells of the kidney to increase sodium reabsorption at the expense of potassium excretion. Therefore less aldosterone activity means less potassium excretion, resulting in hyperkalemia.

12. Answer:

The high levels of catecholamines in pheochromocytoma necessitate the use of an irreversible α antagonist to ensure that it is not outcompeted by the catecholamines. Phenoxybenzamine, an irreversible α antagonist, is therefore a good choice. Phentolamine is also an α antagonist, but it is reversible and therefore could be outcompeted.

13. Answer:

High blood glucose levels cause increased glucose to move into the β cell of the islets of Langerhans in increased quantity via the GLUT-2 channel. This glucose is then metabolized; the ATP closes the cell's potassium channel, removing the hyperpolarization of the cell. This relative depolarization causes a voltage-gated calcium channel to open. This calcium influx causes release of preformed insulin. Bonus: The incretin pathway only works when nutrition is orally ingested. GLP-1 and other mediators are released, causing insulin release even before the glucose enters the blood.

14. Answer:

Absolute insulin deficiency leads to hyperglycemia in the blood, but no sugar inside the cells (no insulin to import sugar into the cells via GLUT-4). Insulin inhibits lipolysis; lack of insulin and lack of glucose inside cells leads to widespread lipolysis. Fat breakdown has ketoacids as a byproduct, and this leads to the acidosis in diabetic ketoacidosis.

15. Answer:

The first reason is that in any state of acidosis (including diabetic ketoacidosis), cells will take up some of that H^+ in exchange for putting K^+ into the blood via an H^+/K^+ exchanger (the opposite occurs in alkalosis). The second reason is that insulin promotes cellular uptake of potassium. Absolute insulin deficiency therefore causes a lack of cellular uptake and hyperkalemia in the blood.

16. Answer:

(a) If the calcium and PTH are both high, this must be primary hyperparathyroidism because the PTH is still high even in the face of a high calcium level (the gland is not responding properly). (b) If the calcium is high and the PTHrP is high, this indicates that there must be a malignancy. PTHrP is secreted by some tumors, especially squamous cell carcinoma of the lung, and has a PTH-like action. The parathyroid gland is responding normally by shutting off its own PTH secretion given the hypercalcemia. (c) If the calcium and PTH are low, then the parathyroid gland is not appropriately secreting PTH in response to hypocalcemia. Therefore the diagnosis is hypoparathyroidism.

17. Answer:

Hypoalbuminemia will decrease the total calcium but not the ionized calcium. That is because a certain percentage of calcium is bound to albumin in the normal state. A loss of albumin therefore will create a new equilibrium where there is less calcium overall but the same amount of ionized calcium. Acid–base disturbances, on the other hand, do not change the total calcium. However, because H^+ can displace Ca^{2+} on the negatively charged albumin sites, acidosis causes an increase in ionized calcium as the calcium is "bumped off" the albumin by the H^+. In alkalosis, there is less H^+ and therefore more open sites for Ca^{2+} to bind. This causes a decrease in the free, ionized calcium level.

CHAPTER 10

1. Answer:

Skin, Camper fascia, Scarpa fascia, linea alba, transversalis fascia, extraperitoneal fascia, parietal peritoneum.

2. Answer:

The myenteric plexus innervates the inner and outer circular muscles of the muscularis propria. These layers contract around the products of digestion (chyme) to propel it through the GI tract.

3. Answer:

Intrinsic factor is secreted by gastric parietal cells, which facilitates absorption of B_{12} in the ileum. As an infectious disease bonus correlate, remember that the tapeworm *Diphyllobothrium latum* is the parasitic intestinal fluke that absorbs its host's B_{12}.

4. Answer:

CCK stimulates the gallbladder to releases bile salts. They enter the duodenum via the ampulla of Vater, emulsify dietary fats, and eventually create micelles. Although the lipid portions of micelles are absorbed in the jejunum, the bile salts remain in the intestinal lumen until they are absorbed in the ileum. The portal vein then takes the bile acids back to the liver, where hepatocytes efficiently extract and recycle them.

5. Answer:

Lingual lipase in the mouth and gastric lipase in the stomach contributes slightly to fat digestion. Most fat digestion, however, occurs after bile salts have emulsified the fats, thereby increasing their surface area. This process allows pancreatic lipase to digest most of the lipids.

6. Answer:

Destruction of the esophageal myenteric plexus leads to achalasia. Similarly, destruction of the colonic myenteric plexus leads to megacolon.

7. Answer:

The patient has physical findings of calloused knuckles, damage to dental enamel, and parotid enlargement. These signs are associated with repeated vomiting from bulimia nervosa; her hypochloremia is also the result of vomiting. Retching may have led to Boerhaave syndrome. A chest radiograph may be suggestive and CT scan can be confirmatory. A water-soluble contrast esophagram would also be diagnostic.

8. Answer:

This patient may have an untreated peptic ulcer and may be suffering acute perforation. If so, air under the diaphragm will be seen on chest x-ray examination. The patient should be immediately evaluated for surgical intervention.

9. Answer:

This patient likely has dermatitis herpetiformis as a result of untreated celiac disease. The presence of anti–tissue transglutaminase antibody would support the diagnosis. The GI and dermatologic symptoms will improve with a gluten-free diet.

10. Answer:

This patient may have IBS because she meets all three of the Rome criteria and all other studies are negative. It is important to rule out other pathologic conditions, however, before giving a diagnosis of IBS. Giardiasis, for example, can also present with long-standing abdominal cramping and diarrhea, but an ova and parasite stool study would be positive.

11. Answer:

Cholangitis and hepatitis may both present in this manner. Note that this patient has cholestatic laboratory findings and fulfills all three criteria of Charcot triad. The elevation in AP and bilirubin levels implies something more complicated than simple cholecystitis. Hepatitis A IgM antibodies will be diagnostic for viral infection. The presence of gallstones on ultrasound would be suggestive of cholangitis, whereas ERCP would be definitive and allow for intervention.

12. Answer:

Gallstone disease from pigment stones, which may accumulate in conditions with high RBC turnover, such as sickle cell anemia or spherocytosis.

13. Answer:

Acute pancreatitis secondary to familial hypertriglyceridemia. Lipase is more specific than amylase for the diagnosis of pancreatitis. Extremely elevated triglyceride levels will confirm the cause. Simply examining the patient's blood may reveal a milky discoloration caused by high levels of chylomicrons.

14. Answer:

The chronic consumption of alcohol has likely led to cirrhosis and subsequent portal hypertension. Furthermore, the impaired synthetic function of the liver has impaired the production of albumin. These factors combine to produce an increased transudative leak of fluid across the interstitium. The ascites may also communicate with the scrotum, causing local swelling.

15. Answer:

The differential diagnosis includes the following: (1) congenital megacolon (passage of copious stool after rectal examination); (2) meconium ileus (pathognomonic for cystic fibrosis); and (3) anal atresia (should be immediately apparent on physical examination; association with VACTERL anomalies).

16. Answer:

The differential diagnosis includes the following: (1) duodenal atresia (bilious vomiting, association with Down syndrome); (2) pyloric stenosis (projectile, nonbilious vomiting, voracious appetite, palpable abdominal mass); and (3) annular pancreas (bifid ventral pancreatic bud).

17. Answer:

Painless hematochezia in an otherwise healthy infant should be immediately concerning for Meckel diverticulum; painful hematochezia should be considered intussusceptions or volvulus in this age group. Ectopic gastric and pancreatic tissue from a remnant of the vitelline duct is the underlying mechanism of this disease process.

18. Answer:

Ranitidine antagonizes the H2 receptors on parietal cells, thereby inhibiting cAMP activation of the H^+,K^+-ATPase and subsequently raising the gastric pH. A more direct way to accomplish this would be with a PPI.

19. Answer:

To reach sufficient concentrations for the antiinflammatory properties to improve the patient's Crohn disease, the patient would likely suffer significant GI side effects. Sulfasalazine is able to reach high concentrations in the intestines without excessive systemic absorption.

20. Answer:

The patient likely began taking an opioid analgesic for his pain, which resulted in opioid-induced cholinergic inhibition of the enteric nervous system. The result was constipation. Patients on opioids should also be given a stool softener to prevent constipation. Loperamide acts as an antidiarrheal via the same mechanism but does not affect the central nervous system. It therefore slows GI motility but lacks analgesic properties.

CHAPTER 11

1. Answer:

CMP cells produce RBCs, platelets, and all WBCs except lymphocytes. Therefore you would expect an elevation in any one or all of these cell types.

2. Answer:

CLP cells produce lymphocytes, so you would expect a proliferation of T and/or B cells.

3. Answer:

Neoplasms, ***a***sthma, ***a***llergic processes, ***c***ollagen vascular diseases, and ***p***arasites (NAACP).

4. Answer:

Neutrophils are usually the first responders of the innate immune system to fight off infection, so patients with neutropenia will have an increased risk of infection. The patient will have increased susceptibility to infection with endogenous organisms in the skin, oropharynx, and intestine.

5. Answer:

Administer RhoGAM to prevent sensitization. The patient is Rh negative and is in the postpartum period.

6. Answer:

Proteins C and S help decrease the production of thrombin; a deficiency leads to increased clotting or thrombosis. Clinically these conditions may present as unprovoked deep vein thromboses or pulmonary emboli.

7. Answer:

Bernard-Soulier syndrome, an autosomal recessive disorder leading to deficiency of GP Ib receptors on platelets. There is a functional absence of vWF despite normal vWF because it can no longer bind platelets.

8. Answer:

The patient developed sideroblastic anemia from his INH therapy. Vitamin B_6 should be started in patients taking INH to prevent development of sideroblastic anemia. An increase in ALA, protoporphyrin, and serum iron levels is expected.

9. Answer:

The older patient's anemia and positive heme occult stool represent adenocarcinoma of the colon until proven otherwise. His symptoms are nonspecific but consistent with anemia. His peripheral smear would show a microcytic and hypochromic anemia, with increased RDW.

10. Answer:

IDA (most common), thalassemia, lead poisoning, and sideroblastic anemia.

11. Answer:

This patient has a hemoglobinopathy, specifically sickle cell disease, given his frequent pain crises and typical physical examination and family history.

12. Answer:

This patient most likely has G6PD deficiency, which is often asymptomatic until faced with an oxidative challenge. Heinz bodies and bite cells will be seen on peripheral smear.

13. Answer:

(1) G6PD deficiency, (2) hereditary elliptocytosis, (3) DIC or TTP-HUS, or traumatic hemolysis, (4) hereditary spherocytosis or IHA, (5) α-thalassemia or G6PD deficiency, (6) asplenic patients or sickle cell disease, (7) liver disease or thalassemia, (8) liver disease, and (9) myelofibrosis.

14. Answer:

Folate and vitamin B_{12} are required for DNA synthesis; a deficiency in either leads to a cessation in DNA synthesis. This halts the maturation process of the nucleus so the red blood cells remain in hypersegmented or immature form. The cytoplasm matures normally, resulting in a dissociation of maturity levels between the nucleus and cytoplasm.

15. Answer:

The patient likely has vitamin B_{12} deficiency and was treated inappropriately with folate alone.

16. Answer:

CONDITION	BT	PT	PTT	PLATELET COUNT
vWD disease	High	Normal	High	Normal
ITP, TTP, HUS	High	Normal	Normal	Low
DIC	High	High	High	Low
Hemophilia A	Normal	Normal	High	Normal
NSAIDs	High	Normal	Normal	Normal
Warfarin or heparin	Normal	High	High	Normal
Vitamin K deficiency	Normal	High	High	Normal
Bernard-Soulier syndrome	High	Normal	Normal	Low
Glanzmann disease	High	Normal	Normal	Normal

BT, Bleeding time; DIC, disseminated intravascular coagulation; HUS, hemolytic-uremic syndrome; ITP, idiopathic thrombocytopenia purpura; NSAIDs, nonsteroidal antiinflammatory drugs; PT, prothrombin time; PTT, partial thromboplastin time; TTP, thrombotic thrombocytopenic purpura; vWD, von Willebrand disease.

17. Answer:

Both disorders present with thrombocytopenia, renal failure, and microangiopathic hemolytic anemia. The main differentiating feature is the development of neurologic deficits in TTP, which do not develop in HUS. Additionally, HUS usually occurs in children because of an infection, whereas TTP occurs in adults and results from a defect in the ADAMTS-13 enzyme.

18. Answer:

Sepsis, trauma, obstetric problems, pancreatitis, malignancy, nephrotic syndrome, transfusion.

19. Answer:

On the test, you can often answer a leukemia question by looking only at the age. It is important to memorize these age ranges: (1) ALL = newborn to 14 years; (2) AML = 15 to 39 years; (3) CML = 40 to 60 years; (4) CLL ≥60 years.

20. Answer:

The patient is 3 years old, so he most likely has ALL. Think of ALL when you see a child with fever, HSM, and lymphadenopathy with increased blasts on peripheral smear.

21. Answer:

The patient is 60 years old, so he most likely has CLL. Smudge cells in an older patient are characteristic of CLL. In CLL, warm antibody type HA can develop—hence, the positive direct Coombs test and the anemia.

22. Answer:

The patient most likely has the sporadic variant type of Burkitt lymphoma. This type of lymphoma presents with abdominal lymphadenopathy and biopsy with a starry sky appearance. It is associated with EBV.

23. Answer:

The patient likely has follicular lymphoma, given the biopsy results. It is associated with the t(14;18) translocation, which results in bcl-2 activation.

24. Answer:

Based on these findings, the patient most likely has nodular sclerosing Hodgkin lymphoma.

25. Answer:

The patient in this case presents with symptoms of hypercalcemia secondary to MM. In addition to the bone lesions, you will see BJ proteins in the urine, an M spike on serum proteins, anemia, and rouleaux formation of RBCs.

26. Answer:

The patient likely has MGUS. She will require frequent follow-up to quantify the monoclonal protein because she is at increased risk of developing MM later in life.

27. Answer:

Leukocyte alkaline phosphatase will be decreased in CML and increased in PV.

28. Answer:

This patient likely has PV; the RBC mass and count will be elevated and the EPO level will be low.

29. Answer:

This patient likely has acute intermittent porphyria. Psychiatric disturbances include delirium, depression, emotional lability, schizophreniform psychoses, and hysteria. Her AIP episode was likely precipitated by antipsychotic medications she received during the admission.

CHAPTER 12

1. Answer:

PTH will activate osteoclasts and increase resorption of bone. The result will be an increased serum calcium level and decrease in bone matrix. In cases of severe resorption, osteitis fibrosa cystica will occur (woven bone without matrix).

2. Answer:

Without ATP generation, the Ca^{2+} ATPase cannot sequester Ca^{2+} in the SR. The presence of Ca^{2+} permits actin-myosin cross-bridge formation, but without ATP there is a consistently high affinity of myosin for actin, which results in rigor.

3. Answer:

An ice pack test might further suggest the diagnosis of myasthenia gravis and anti–acetylcholine receptor antibodies would confirm it. Pyridostigmine, an acetylcholine esterase inhibitor, would improve her symptoms. She should also be evaluated for thymoma.

4. Answer:

Yes. Spiral fractures are often suspicious for child abuse; however, toddler's fractures are the exception in the right age group. At 3 months old, however, this child should not be able to roll over. This makes his parents history suspicious for nonaccidental trauma. Child services should be notified and a skeletal survey should be performed.

5. Answer:

Polymyalgia rheumatica (PMR) is highly associated with temporal arteritis. Untreated temporal arteritis may result in vision loss secondary to involvement of the ophthalmic artery. PMR characteristically presents as muscle pain and elevated ESR. Polymyositis, on the other hand, presents with weakness and elevated creatine kinase (CK).

6. Answer:

A, SCFE. B, Legg-Calvé-Perthes disease. C, Congenital hip dysplasia.

7. Answer:

This woman has classic sarcoidosis, with pulmonary involvement and erythema nodosum. Lymph node biopsy will reveal noncaseating granulomas.

8. Answer:

A, Giant cell. B, Osteosarcoma. C, Osteochondroma. D, Ewing sarcoma. E, Osteoid osteoma.

9. Answer:

This patient likely has septic arthritis. A joint aspirate will be needed. If it reveals more than 50,000 neutrophils, he will need surgical washout of the joint and IV antibiotics.

10. Answer:

Paget disease of bone could be suggested by an elevated alkaline phosphatase level, but radiography would be diagnostic. Bisphosphonates such as alendronate are beneficial in preventing pathologic remodeling.

11. Answer:

Glucocorticoids have side effects, including weight gain, purple striae, and an elevated blood sugar level. These steroids function by inhibiting the production of inflammatory cytokines by phospholipase A_2.

12. Answer:

Patients with OA often self-medicate with over-the-counter NSAIDs. Although NSAIDs inhibit the pain and inflammation of OA, they also vasoconstrict the glomerular afferent arteriole. This may lead to a temporary bump in the creatinine level or permanent renal damage.

CHAPTER 13

1. Answer:

MS is a demyelinating autoimmune phenomenon that causes destruction of oligodendrocytes in the CNS. This patient has optic neuritis and neurologic weakness consistent with MS. Worsening of symptoms with heat is also characteristic.

2. Answer:

The anterior communicating artery is the most common site of aneurysms. Ruptured aneurysms cause subarachnoid hemorrhage.

3. Answer:

Glutamate is the major excitatory NT. In conditions such as seizure and stroke, excessive excitatory transmission can cause neuronal damage and death.

4. Answer:

The patellar reflex assesses the reflex arc at L3–L4 level.

5. Answer:

He is experiencing Broca aphasia. This is an expressive aphasia in which comprehension remains intact. The lesion is located on the inferior frontal gyrus of the frontal lobe.

6. Answer:

Epidural hematomas are frequently the result of a temporal bone fracture from trauma to the pterion. This causes rupture of the middle meningeal artery (not to be confused with middle cerebral artery).

7. Answer:

The combination of upper and lower motor neuron findings is consistent with ALS. Riluzole may improve survival by indirectly preventing glutamate excitotoxicity.

8. Answer:

Temporal arteritis should be considered in any older individual with a headache, especially with jaw claudication or tenderness over the temporal artery. Diagnosis is confirmed with temporal artery biopsy, and treatment is with steroids.

9. Answer:

L-Dopa is the precursor of dopamine. L-Dopa, unlike dopamine, is able to cross the blood–brain barrier. Carbidopa prevents the peripheral conversion of L-dopa into dopamine. This allows for greater CNS concentration of the drug and limits side effects.

10. Answer:

Succinylcholine is a depolarizing neuromuscular blocker. It activates nicotinic acetylcholine receptors, which cause fasciculations followed by persistent depolarization at the motor endplate (resulting in paralysis). Rocuronium is simply a nicotinic acetylcholine receptor antagonist, so it does not cause fasciculations.

CHAPTER 14

1. Answer:

This is suppression because you are consciously choosing to push a painful thought out of your mind to address it later. This is a mature ego defense.

2. Answer:

This is projection because you are taking your own frustrations of studying too hard and projecting them onto someone else, accusing them of neglecting their life from studying too hard. This is an immature ego defense.

3. Answer:

This child is likely suffering from Rett syndrome. It has an X-linked dominant pattern of inheritance; affected male fetuses die in utero.

4. Answer:

With the information given, this child does not currently meet criteria for ADHD because the inattentive or hyperactive traits must be present in more than one setting. More information should be gathered about the structure of the home environment.

5. Answer:

Positive symptoms are those that are added to a person with schizophrenia; these include adding delusions, hallucinations, or bizarre behaviors. These are in addition to what a normal person would do. Negative symptoms are things that are removed from what an unaffected person would be expected to do. For example, a flat affect is removal of the normal range of affect that someone has and is therefore a negative symptom.

6. Answer:

Delirium. Disorientation is a common feature of both conditions; however, inattention and hallucinations are more likely to be signs of delirium.

7. Answer:

Torticollis is a known side effect of antipsychotics. It is caused by dopamine antagonism in the nigrostriatal pathway. Treatment is with anticholinergics.

8. Answer:

Although in both malingering and factitious disorders, the decision to make themselves appear sick is conscious, the difference lies in the motive. Patient A wants to gain something specific, narcotic pain medication, and is therefore malingering. Patient B wants to assume the sick role and does not want to gain something specific; therefore she has a factitious disorder.

9. Answer:

Conversion disorder is one in which a psychological trigger, such as his mother's stroke, causes a physical manifestation in the patient—namely, the teenage boy having the same "symptoms" as his mother.

10. Answer:

Borderline personality disorder is characterized by splitting. This is a cluster B personality disorder ("wild").

11. Answer:

Obsessive-compulsive disorder is ego dystonic, meaning that the patient understands that this is unreasonable and wishes she or he could stop. Therefore in this patient's case, her symptoms are more consistent with OCD than the personality disorder OCPD.

12. Answer:

Alcohol dependence. The diagnosis of substance dependence supersedes that of substance abuse. Look at the whole clinical picture. Although it might seem like she could meet the criteria for abuse, she suffers from withdrawal and tolerance in addition to the psychological aspects of dependence, so this is the best answer.

13. Answer:

PCP. Although hallucinations can occur with multiple substances, including LSD intoxication and alcohol withdrawal, the intense aggression and strength point to PCP.

14. Answer:

Opiate withdrawal. This man was likely overusing opiates for quite some time, and now that he has run out of pills, he is experiencing withdrawal symptoms. The scenario of a chronic pain patient running out of pills makes other answers such as LSD intoxication (which also causes dilated pupils) or cocaine withdrawal (which also causes significant dysphoria, along with constricted pupils) unlikely.

15. Answer:

He is using the immature ego defense mechanism of displacement. His impulses toward his mother are shifted to a less threatening being.

16. Answer:

He is using the immature ego defense mechanism of projection. He projects his anxiety-provoking feelings on his wife in order to relieve his own guilt and discomfort.

CHAPTER 15

1. Answer:

The medulla of the kidney has the lowest oxygen tension, which becomes important in hypoxia. It is important because the nephrons can be damaged in ischemic acute tubular necrosis, but also because the peritubular capillaries can detect hypoxia and release erythropoietin in response.

2. Answer:

Filtration, resorption, secretion.

3. Answer:

Because the molecule is being cleared faster than filtration alone, it suggests that the molecule is also being secreted into the nephron.

4. Answer:

The proximal tubule has 1-α-hydroxylase activity, which converts 25-vitamin D into 1,25-vitamin D, the active form. PTH upregulates 1-α-hydroxylase activity.

5. Answer:

Calcium and magnesium are absorbed via the paracellular route when the charge of the lumen increases (becomes more positive), pushing the magnesium and calcium cations out of the lumen into the paracellular space for resorption back into circulation. The favorable positive electrical gradient is created by the recycling of K^+ back into the tubular lumen after its coresorption with Na^+ and $2Cl^-$ via the NKCC2 cotransporter.

6. Answer:

The 60-40-20 rule says that he will have 60% total body water by weight, so (a) is 70 kg × 0.60 = 42 L total body water; 40% of the weight will be ICF (two-thirds of the water), so (b) is 70 kg × 0.40 = 28 L ICF volume; and 20% of the weight will be ECF (one-third of the water), so (c) is 70 kg × 0.20 = 14 L ECF volume.

7. Answer:

The patient has an anion gap metabolic acidosis (recall that lactic acidosis from anaerobic metabolism is a cause of an anion gap metabolic acidosis). Therefore the pH will be low (<7.4), the bicarbonate will be low (<24 mEq/L), and the Pco_2 will also be low (<40 mm Hg) because the patient is mounting a respiratory compensation (hyperventilation to blow off CO_2) to the metabolic acidosis with the tachypnea.

8. Answer:

Aldosterone upregulates the α-intercalated cells in the collecting duct, causing them to excrete more acid. Therefore the patient will have a metabolic alkalosis and also have hypokalemia because the principal cells are also upregulated by aldosterone. The principal cells resorb sodium into the bloodstream at the expense of secreting potassium into the lumen of the nephron to be excreted in the urine.

9. Answer:

She would have a respiratory acidosis from retaining the volatile acid CO_2 because she is not ventilating adequately.

10. Answer:

The three main components of treating hyperkalemia are (1) reduce myocardial irritability (calcium), (2) temporarily drive potassium into cells (insulin, sympathomimetics, bicarbonate), and (3) eliminate potassium from the body (with potassium-wasting diuretics, potassium binders, dialysis). Ensure that it is true hyperkalemia by making sure that the blood sample was not hemolyzed. Hemolysis of red blood cells releases intracellular potassium into the blood sample, falsely elevating readings.

11. Answer:

Rhabdomyolysis typically has positive blood on the dipstick, but on microscopy, no red blood cells are seen. This is because in rhabdomyolysis, the muscle cell breakdown releases myoglobin. Myoglobin turns the dipstick test positive for blood, but because there is no actual blood in the urine, red blood cells will not be seen.

12. Answer:

The most common type of kidney stone is a calcium oxalate stone. It is radiopaque (can be seen by radiograph if large enough) and has an envelope shape on microscopy.

13. Answer:

Urease-producing bacteria such as *Proteus* are associated with magnesium ammonium phosphate crystals; the splitting of urea allows free ammonium to form the stones.

14. Answer:

Nonenzymatic glycosylation occurs preferentially at the efferent arteriole first, increasing the filtration fraction by increasing glomerular pressure and therefore increasing GFR.

15. Answer:

The correct answer is d. In a severely dehydrated patient, it would be expected that the patient would have a prerenal azotemia, characterized by a BUN/Cr ratio of at least 15:1. The other answer choices have a BUN/Cr ratio less than 15:1.

16. Answer:

Spironolactone or eplerenone would work best because they have aldosterone antagonist activity and would attempt to counteract the increased aldosterone secreted by the tumor.

17. Answer:

He is likely on a loop diuretic, which blocks the NKCC2 channel in the thick ascending loop of Henle. Because potassium leaks back into the lumen of the nephron, there is a net positive charge in the lumen, which promotes calcium and magnesium resorption. Blocking this pump causes increased excretion and loss of potassium, magnesium, and calcium.

CHAPTER 16

1. Answer:

In a hysterectomy or any procedure that essentially requires ligation of the uterine artery, it is possible to damage the ureter because of its anatomic course deep to the uterine artery. Most patients with damage to the ureter have a fever and decreased urine output.

2. Answer:

False. The ovarian artery is contained in the infundibulopelvic ligament (suspensory ligament) of the ovary. There are no vessels in the ovarian ligament; its function is simply attachment to the uterus.

3. Answer:

False. Yes, erection is a parasympathetic response; however, the act of ejaculation is a somatic response carried out by the pudendal nerve. It is emission that is a sympathetic response.

4. Answer:

Delivery. Because this woman is full term (>37 weeks), it is necessary and prudent to induce delivery, and the preeclampsia will thus resolve.

5. Answer:

Ectopic pregnancy should be at the top of your differential for any hypotensive female patient of reproductive age. Pregnancy can be confirmed with a urine β-hCG and quantified with a serum β-hCG. A stable patient can be evaluated with ultrasound, and methotrexate may be sufficient to treat the condition. An unstable patient will need surgery without delay.

6. Answer:

False. BPH is hyper**plasia** of the prostatic tissue.

7. Answer:

Patients with cryptorchidism are at increased risk for malignancy, infertility, and testicular torsion.

8. Answer:

In a pseudohermaphrodite, phenotypic sex and gonadal sex are opposite. An example is androgen insensitivity syndrome, in which the individual has testicles but female-appearing external genitalia. Another example is congenital adrenal hyperplasia, in which the individual appears to have male external genitalia but has ovaries.

9. Answer:

It is thought that OCPs are protective for endometrial and ovarian cancers because they prevent high levels of estrogen exposure and prevent ovulation, respectively. OCPs are not protective for cervical cancer.

10. Answer:

The differential includes Paget disease of the breast, which is invasion of ductal carcinoma in situ to the skin. Your next step should be biopsy to look for Paget cells. There is no palpable mass because DCIS is nonpalpable. A mammogram might show microcalcifications.

CHAPTER 17

1. Answer:

An aspirated foreign body while supine will often be found in the superior segment of the right lower lobe. If aspirated while standing or sitting, it will usually be found in the inferior (posterobasal) segment of the right lower lobe.

2. Answer:

Accessory muscles of inspiration include external intercostal, scalene, and sternocleidomastoid. Abdominal muscles and internal intercostals muscles aid in forced expiration.

3. Answer:

This patient's smoking history and radiograph are concerning for lung cancer. The location is consistent with small cell cancer, so her weakness may be the paraneoplastic Lambert-Eaton syndrome, in which antibodies against presynaptic calcium channels cause weakness.

4. Answer:

Surfactant is found in lamellar bodies in type II alveolar cells. These lamellar bodies first appear late in gestation.

5. Answer:

Patients with obstructive lung disease often have increased TLC and RV because of air trapping and hyperinflation. FEV_1 and FVC are often reduced, with an FEV_1/FVC ratio <0.8. Patients with restrictive lung disease, on the other hand, have decreased TLC and RV. FEV_1 and FVC are also reduced, but with a ratio >0.8.

6. Answer:

Albuterol is an inhaled, short-acting β_2-selective agonist. This leads to increased cAMP levels within bronchial smooth muscle, causing bronchial smooth muscle relaxation and relief of bronchospasm.

INDEX

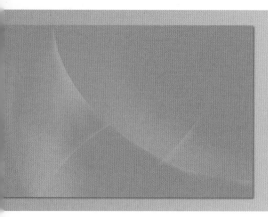

Note: Pages followed by *b*, *t*, or *f* refer to boxes, tables, or figures, respectively.

F

G

I

M

N

O

Q

R

S